Fourth Edition

Current
C A N C E R
Therapeutics

John M. Kirkwood, MD

Professor and Chief, Division of Medical Oncology, University of Pittsburgh School of Medicine;
Chief, Melanoma Center, University of Pittsburgh Cancer Institute, Pittsburgh, Pennsylvania

Michael T. Lotze, MD

Vice President and Director, Departments of Inflammation, Tissue Repair, and Oncology,
SmithKline Beecham Pharmaceuticals, King of Prussia, Pennsylvania

Joyce M. Yasko, PhD

Professor, School of Nursing, University of Pittsburgh;
Associate Director, Clinical and Network Programs, University of Pittsburgh Cancer Institute, Pittsburgh, Pennsylvania

With 69 contributors

CM
CURRENT
MEDICINE

Developed by Current Medicine, Inc., Philadelphia

CURRENT MEDICINE, INC.

400 Market Street
Suite 700
Philadelphia, PA 19106

DEVELOPMENTAL EDITOR: *Elise M. Paxson*
DESIGNER: *Christine Keller-Quirk*
ASSISTANT PRODUCTION MANAGER: *Simon Dickey*
EDITORIAL ASSISTANT: *Janet Gilmore*
ILLUSTRATOR: *Wiesia Langenfeld*

The Editors thank Rowena Schwartz, Pharm. D., for pharmaceutical review of the manuscripts.

Current Medicine Inc. grants authorization to photocopy items for educational, class-room, or internal use, and to republish in print, Internet, CD-ROM, slide, or other media, provided that the appropriate fee is paid directly to Copyright Clearance Center Inc. (CCC), 222 Rosewood Drive, Danvers, MA 01923, USA (Tel: (978) 750-8400; Fax: (978) 750-4470; E-mail: info@copyright.com; Website: http://www.copyright.com). For permission for other uses, please contact the Permissions Department, Current Medicine Inc., 400 Market Street, Suite 700, Philadelphia, PA 19106-2514, USA.

Although every effort has been made to ensure that drug doses and other information are presented accurately in this publication, the ultimate responsibility rests with the prescribing physician. Neither the publishers nor the authors can be held responsible for errors or for any consequences arising from the use of information contained herein. Products mentioned in this publication should be used in accordance with the prescribing information prepared by the manufacturers. No claims or endorsements are made for any drug or compound at present under clinical investigation.

For more information please call 1-800-427-1796 or e-mail us at inquiry@phl.cursci.com
www.current-science-group.com

ISBN: 1-57340-176-5
ISSN: 1074-2816

Printed in the United States of America by Port City Press.
5 4 3 2 1

CONTRIBUTORS

JAMES L. ABBRUZZESE, MD
Professor
Department of GI Medical Oncology
University of Texas;
Chairman
University of Texas M.D. Anderson
  Cancer Center
Houston, Texas

EDWIN ALYEA, MD
Instructor in Medicine
Department of Adult Oncology
Harvard Medical School
Boston, Massachusetts

JANET A. AMICO, MD, FACP
Professor of Medicine and
  Pharmaceutical Sciences
Department of Medicine
University of Pittsburgh School of Pharmacy
Pittsburgh, Pennsylvania

CARLOS WILLIAM DE ARAUJO, MD
Department of Medicine
University of Colorado Medical School;
Hematology/Oncology Fellow
University of Colorado Cancer Center
Denver, Colorado

ROBERT M. ARNOLD, MD
Associate Professor
Department of Medicine;
Physician
University of Pittsburgh Health System
Divison of General Internal Medicine
Pittsburgh, Pennsylvania

EDWARD D. BALL, MD
Professor of Medicine
Department of Medicine;
Director and Chief
Blood & Marrow Transplantation Division
University of California San Diego
La Jolla, California

DAVID L. BARTLETT, MD
Assistant Professor
Department of Surgery
University of the Health Sciences;
Senior Investigator
Surgery Branch
National Cancer Institute, National
  Institutes of Health
Bethesda, Maryland

MICHAEL J. BECICH, MD, PHD
Associate Professor of Pathology and
  Information Sciences and
  Telecommunications
Director, Center for Pathology Informatics
University of Pittsburgh School of Medicine;
Chairman of Pathology
UPMC Shadyside
Pittsburgh, Pennsylvania

JULIE BEITZ, MD
Director
Division of Drug Risk Evaluation I
Food and Drug Administration
Rockville, Maryland

JAMES R. BERENSON, MD
Professor of Medicine
Department of Hematology/Oncology
UCLA School of Medicine;
Director
Multiple Myeloma and Bone Metastasis
  Programs
Division of Hematology/Oncology
Cedars-Sinai Medical Center
Los Angeles, California

JOHANN SEBASTIAN DE BONO, MD
Clinical Research Fellow
Department of Medicine
University of Texas Health Science
  Center at San Antonio;
Clinical Research Fellow
Institute for Drug Development
Cancer Therapy and Research Center
San Antonio, Texas

RONALD H. BLUM, MD
Director
Cancer Center
Phillips Ambulatory Care Center
Beth Israel Medical Center
New York, New York

PAUL A. BUNN JR., MD
Grohne/Stapp Professor and Director
University of Colorado Cancer Center
Professor
Department of Medicine
University of Colorado Medical School;
Denver, Colorado

PAUL P. CARBONE, MD, MACP, D.SC. (HON.)
Professor of Medicine Emeritus
Director Emeritus, University of
  Wisconsin
Comprehensive Cancer Center
Madison, Wisconsin

JUDY H. CHAIO, MD
Division of Oncology Drug Products
Food and Drug Adminstration
Rockville, Maryland

JONATHAN CEBON, MD
Ludwig Institute Oncology Unit
Austin & Repatriation Medical Centre
Heidelberg, Victoria, Australia

BERNARD F. COLE, PHD
Assistant Professor
Department of Community and Family
  Medicine
Dartmouth University Medical School
Lebanon, New Hampshire

ROBERT J. DELAP, MD, PHD
Food and Drug Administration
Rockville, Maryland

JAYESH DESAI
Ludwig Institute Oncology Unit
Austin & Repatriation Medical Centre
Heidelberg, Victoria, Australia

GERARD M. DOHERTY, MD
Associate Professor
Department of Surgery
Washington University School of Medicine;
Attending Surgeon
Barnes-Jewish Hospital
St. Louis, Missouri

AFSHIN DOWLATI, MD
Assistant Professor of Medicine
Department of Medicine
Division of Hematology/Oncology
Case Western Reserve University;
University Hospitals of Cleveland
Cleveland, Ohio

MARC S. ERNSTOFF, MD
Professor of Medicine
Department of Medicine
Dartmouth Medical School;
Section Chief
Hematology/Oncology Section
Hitchcock Clinic;
Deputy Director
Norris Cotton Cancer Center
Lebanon, New Hampshire

YUMAN FONG, MD
Professor of Surgery
Cornell University Medical College;
Attending Surgeon
Memorial Sloan-Kettering Cancer Center
New York, New York

CONTRIBUTORS

SONIA FULLERTON, MD
Ludwig Institute Oncology Unit
Austin & Repatriation Medical Centre
Heidelberg, Victoria, Australia

RICHARD D. GELBER, PHD
Professor
Department of Pediatrics
Harvard Medical School;
Senior Biostatistician
Dana-Farber Cancer Institute
Boston, Massachusetts

SHARI GELBER, MS, MSW
Biostatistician
Frontier Science
Chestnut Hill, Massachusetts

STANTON L. GERSON, MD
Professor of Medicine
Department of Hematology Oncology
Case Western Reserve University;
Asa and Patricia Schiverick Professor of
    Hematological Oncology
Chief, Division of Hematology Oncology
Associate Director, Cancer Center
University Hospitals of Cleveland
Cleveland, Ohio

MICHELLE GOLD, MD
Ludwig Institute Oncology Unit
Austin & Repatriation Medical Centre
Heidelberg, Victoria, Australia

MICHAEL S. GORDON, MD
Associate Professor
Department of Medicine;
Associate Dean for Research
University of Arizona College of
    Medicine (Phoenix Campus)
Phoenix, Arizona

JEAN L. GREM, MD
Chief
Cellular and Clinical Pharmacology
    Section
Medicine Branch-Department of
    Developmental Therapeutics
National Cancer Institute/National
    Institutes of Health
Bethesda, Maryland

JOHN A. HEANEY, MD, BCH
Professor
Department of Surgery
Dartmouth University Medical School;
Chief
Section of Urology
Dartmouth-Hitchcock Medical Center
Lebanon, New Hampshire

HOWARD HOCHSTER, MD
Associate Professor of Medicine
Department of Internal Medicine
Division of Medical Oncology
New York University School of Medicine;
Attending Physician
Department of Internal Medicine
New York Tisch Hospital
New York, New York

JOHN HOHNEKER, MD
Clinical Assistant Professor
Department of Medical Oncology
University of North Carolina–Chapel Hill
Chapel Hill, North Carolina
Vice President, Medical Affairs–Oncology
Novartis Pharmaceuticals Corporation
East Hanover, New Jersey

JEAN L. HOLLEY, MD
Professor of Medicine
Department of Medicine
Nephrology Unit
University of Rochester Medical Center
Rochester, New York

SANDRA J. HORNING, MD
Associate Professor
Department of Medicine
Division of Oncology
Stanford University;
Stanford University Medical Center
Stanford, California

DAVID M. JABLONS, MD
Assistant Professor of Surgery in Residence
Department of Surgery
UCSF School of Medicine;
Chief
Department of General Thoracic Surgery
Mount Zion Medical Center
San Francisco, California

ULRICH KEILHOLZ, MD
Department of Medicine III
UKBF, Frewe University Berlin
Berlin, Germany

DAVID T. KIANG, MD
Professor Emeritus
Department of Medicine
University of Minnesota
Minneapolis, Minnesota

LINDA A. KING, MD
Assistant Professor of Medicine
Division of General Internal Medicine
Section of Palliative Care and Medical Ethics
University of Pittsburgh Medical Center
Pittsburgh, Pennsylvania

JOHN M. KIRKWOOD, MD
Professor and Chief, Division of Medical
    Oncology, University of Pittsburgh
    School of Medicine;
Chief, Melanoma Center, University of
    Pittsburgh Cancer Institute,
    Pittsburgh, Pennsylvania

THOMAS A. LAMPKIN, PHARM D
Clinical Research Program Head
GlaxoSmithKline
Research Triangle Park, North Carolina

MARC E. LIPPMAN, MD
John G. Searle Professor
Department of Internal Medicine
University of Michigan School of Medicine;
Chair
Department of Internal Medicine
University of Michigan Health System
Ann Arbor, Michigan

MINETTA C. LIU, MD
Chief Fellow
Division of Hematology/Oncology
Lombardi Cancer Center
Georgetown University Hospital
Washington, District of Columbia

MICHAEL T. LOTZE, MD
Vice President and Director
Departments of Inflammation, Tissue
    Repair, and Oncology
SmithKline Beecham Pharmaceuticals
King of Prussia, Pennsylvania

JENNIFER LOWNEY, MD
Senior Resident
Department of Surgery
Washington University School of Medicine;
Senior Resident
Surgery Housestaff Officer
Barnes-Jewish Hospital
St. Louis, Missouri

STEPHEN F. LOWRY, MD
Professor and Chairman
Department of Surgery
Robert Wood Johnson Medical School
University of Medicine and Dentistry of
    New Jersey
New Brunswick, New Jersey

DOROTHY PAN, MD
Department of Medicine
Weill Medical College of Cornell
    University;
Fellow in Medical Oncology
Memorial Sloan-Kettering Cancer Center
New York, New York

CONTRIBUTORS

CAROL S. PORTLOCK, MD
Professor
Department of Medicine
Weill Medical College of Cornell
  University;
Attending Physician
Memorial Sloan-Kettering Cancer Center
New York, New York

TJEERD J. POSTMA, MD
Department of Neurology
University Hospital/Vrije Universiteit
Amsterdam, The Netherlands

MICHAEL D. PRADOS, MD
Professor
Department of Neurological Surgery;
Director
Clinical Neuro-Oncology Program;
Principal Investigator
Brain Tumor Research Center
UCSF School of Medicine
San Francisco, California

SAI SUBHODHINI REDDY, MD
Senior Instructor of Medicine
Department of Medicine
Nephrology Unit
University of Rochester Medical Center
Rochester, New York

SCOT C. REMICK, MD
Associate Professor
Department of Medicine
Division of Hematology/Oncology
Case Western Reserve University;
Program Leader
Developmental Therapeutics
University Hospitals of Cleveland
Cleveland, Ohio

JEROME RITZ, MD
Professor of Medicine
Department of Adult Oncology
Harvard Medical School;
Dana-Farber Cancer Institute
Boston, Massachusetts

LINDA BARRY ROBERTSON, RN, MSN, CCRC
Adjunct
School of Health Sciences
University of Pittsburgh;
Director
Clinical Research Services
University of Pittsburgh Cancer Institute
University of Pittsburgh Medical Center
  Health System
Pittsburgh, Pennsylvania

ERIC K. ROWINSKY, MD
Clinical Professor of Medicine
University of Texas Health Science
  Center at San Antonio;
Director
Department of Clinical Research
Institute for Drug Development
Cancer Therapy and Research Center
San Antonio, Texas

JOHN C. RUCKDESCHEL, MD
Professor of Medicine and Director
H. Lee Moffitt Cancer Center and
  Research Institute
University of South Florida
Tampa, Florida

KEVIN F. STAVELEY-O'CARROLL, MD
Assistant Professor of Surgery
Section of Surgical Oncology
Pennsylvania State University
Milton S. Hershey Medical Center
Hershey, Pennsylvania

ROGER STUPP, MD
Attending Physician
Multidisciplinary Oncology Center
University Hospital CHUV
Lausanne, Switzerland

MARGARET A. TEMPERO, MD
Chief, Medical Oncology
Department of Hematology/Oncology
University of California, San Francisco,
  School of Medicine;
Deputy Director
University of California at San Francisco
  Comprehensive Cancer Center
San Francisco, California

MELANIE B. THOMAS, MD
Senior Fellow
Division of Cancer Medicine
M.D. Anderson Cancer Center
University of Texas
Houston, Texas

ANTHONY W. TOLCHER, MD
Clinical Assistant Professor of Medicine
University of Texas Health Science
  Center at San Antonio;
Associate Director
Department of Clinical Research
Institute for Drug Development
Cancer Therapy and Research Center
San Antonio, Texas

CHRISTOPHER TRETTER, MD, CM
Instructor
Department of Medicine
Dartmouth University Medical School;
Clinical Fellow
Department of Hematology/Oncology
Dartmouth-Hitchcock Medical Center
Lebanon, New Hampshire

EVERETT E. VOKES, MD
Duchssois Professor of Medicine and
  Radiation Oncology;
Director
Section of Hematology/Oncology
University of Chicago School of Medicine
Chicago, Illinois

MATTHEW VOLM, MD
Clinical Instructor
Department of Medicine
New York University School of Medicine;
Bellevue Hospital Center
New York, New York

SCOTT WADLER, MD
Professor
Departments of Medicine,
  Obstetrics/Gynecology, and Women's
  Health
Albert Einstein College of Medicine;
Associate Director
Albert Einstein Comprehensive Cancer
  Center
Bronx, New York

PAUL S. WISSEL, MD
Clinical Associate Professor
Department of Medicine
University of North Carolina;
Head Clinical Development, Oncology
GlaxoWellcome
Research Triangle Park, North Carolina

DOUGLAS YEE, MD
Professor of Medicine
Department of Medicine
Division of Hematology, Oncology, and
  Transplantation
University of Minnesota Cancer Center
Minneapolis, Minnesota

ALAN YUEN, MD
Assistant Professor
Department of Medicine
Stanford University School of Medicine
Stanford, California

HERBERT J. ZEH, MD
Johns Hopkins School of Medicine
Baltimore, Maryland

FOREWORD

Cancer management has become increasingly complex with the enormous influx of information from cancer molecular biology and genetics. In addition there has been a rapid introduction of new agents, biologicals, and combinations. The information base has expanded exponentially, making therapy decisions difficult to manage the more than 100 human malignancies. Unlike the large cancer centers, where sub-specialists in oncology manage specific diseases, the practicing oncologist must be aware of and be ready to manage the broad spectrum of cancers. Likewise the pharmacists and nurses who work with oncologists must always deal with a wide variety of agents and protocols.

The fourth edition of *Current Cancer Therapeutics*, edited by three international experts, provides a useful tool to keep the oncology team up to date. This edition, with more than 60 authors, provides accurate information on the many biologic and chemotherapy agents, protocols on managing specific diseases, as well as supportive care.

The drug section provides a stylized set of drug pages on pharmacokinetics, indications, and toxicities as well as nursing and patient information. The information is presented in uniform panels on a gray background, making searching for specific information easy.

The disease sections are comprehensive, but include concise summaries of epidemiology, risk factors, screening, staging, and therapy. Tabular information is presented on specific treatment protocol results and combinations. A flow decision diagram is also provided, defining pathways for specific stage subsets.

The supportive care section contains concise information on management of complications such as hematologic, allergic and immunologic, nausea and vomiting, mucositis, neurologic, and cardiopulmonary toxicities.

The editors are to be commended on putting together this comprehensive survey of a large field of medicine. The book will be useful to the library of the oncologist, nurse, or pharmacist. It will serve as an up-to-date resource on management issues not usually available in standard texts.

Paul P. Carbone, MD, MACP, D.Sc. (hon.)
Professor of Medicine Emeritus
Director Emeritus, University of Wisconsin
Comprehensive Cancer Center
Madison, Wisconsin

INTRODUCTION

This fourth edition of *Current Cancer Therapeutics* comes to print at a particularly important time in clinical oncology. Not only are the molecular bases of cancer increasingly understood, but these findings are finally being brought to the clinic with apparent efficacy and enhancement of survival and decreased toxicity. In this edition we have substantially revised every chapter with the addition of an entire section on clinical trials management with appropriate synoptic reporting forms, revised the organization of the first section on therapeutic agents and their overviews, and extended the number and apparent reach of world class oncologists providing their unique vantage on current therapies. Fully one third of the chapters have new authors, all of them leaders in their field. This edition should provide the busy clinician, informed patients, and clinicians in training with the most up to date information about the current status of cancer therapies.

We have every reason to believe that this edition reflects those therapies currently approved and applied. Novel therapies will be the province of the future and, it is hoped, future editions of this text. It is probably worthwhile here to signal some of these future agents. The development of kinase inhibitors, long thought to be difficult because of targeting of a common ATP binding site, are falling to a set of kinase inhibitors with great specificity. Apparent success in the clinic, targeting the activated kinase product of the Philadelphia chromosome, in patients with chronic myelogous leukemia, has led to increased enthusiasm for their application to other kinases. In the near future, agents targeting the VEGFR and Tie2 kinase receptors of the angiopoietins, at various stages of investigation, appear promising for inhibiting tumor-related angiogenesis. Similarly, targeting the cell-cycle kinases Polo kinase, checkpoint kinase 1 and 2, and myt1 kinase allow some enthusiasm for new classes of agents to focus on the mitotic checkpoints important in cancer progression. The application of novel tubulin-targeting agents is well demonstrated with the vinca alkaloids and the paclitaxel-associated agents. A new class of mitotic cytokinesins which traffic on the tubulin bundles are currently in evaluation for their ability to function to disrupt migration of the chromosomal material along tubulin bundles without the associated neurotoxicity.

Development of sponsored clinical trials proceeds apace with the perceived problems of a dearth of patients with early disease amenable to testing with experimental agents. The death of a patient on an academic/biotech sponsored gene therapy trial has led to widespread consternation related to the safeguards within such "boutique" trials and led to the more rigorous oversight and review of clinical trials. With many of the riches of cancer investigation now being ushered into the clinic, we can be optimistic about the novel therapies destined to find their way into current cancer therapies.

CONTENTS

CHAPTER 1: ALKYLATING AND PLATINATING AGENTS
Stanton L. Gerson

Alkylating agents form the backbone of many anticancer regimens and are used in both conventional and high-dose therapy settings. The biologic and chemical activities of the nitrogen mustards were studied extensively between the World Wars. Because of their vesicant activity on the skin, eyes, and respiratory tract, the mustards also were studied for their effects on lymphosarcomas in mice during World War II. This led to the start of clinical studies, in 1942, and kicked off the era of modern cancer chemotherapy [1].

Alkylating agents are polyfunctional compounds that have the ability to substitute alkyl groups for hydrogen ions. These compounds react with phosphate, amino, hydroxyl, sulfhydryl, carboxyl, and imidazole groups, which are part of the molecular make-up of the body. In neutral or alkaline solution, these drugs ionize and produce positively charged ions that attach to susceptible nuclear proteins, with the most likely site of alkylation being the N-7 position of guanine. This alkylation reaction leads to abnormal base pairing, cleaving of the imidazole ring of guanine, cross-linking of DNA, depurination of DNA, and interference with DNA replication, transcription of RNA, and the disruption of nucleic acid function. These actions lead to an interruption in the normal cell functions of both cancerous and normal tissues [1,2]. Cytotoxicity, in large part, is due to DNA alkylation at N or O. Disruption of DNA synthesis by the DNA adducts formed (particularly crosslinks or induction of apoptosis during the process of DNA repair) represents predominant mechanisms of cytotoxicity.

The alkylating agents are cell cycle phase–nonspecific agents because they exert their activity independently of the specific phase of the cell cycle. The nitrogen mustards and alkyl alkone sulfonates are most effective against cells in the G_1 or M phase. Nitrosoureas, nitrogen mustards, and aziridines impair progression from the G_1 and S phases to the M phase.

CLASSES

The alkylating agents traditionally are divided into five classes; however, the platinum-containing compounds have been added as a sixth class owing to their ability to bind to DNA and produce crosslinks in the DNA helix. The traditional classes of alkylators include the bischloroethylamines (nitrogen mustards), the aziridines (ethylenimines), the alkyl alkone sulfonates, the nitrosoureas, and the nonclassical alkylating agents [1–4].

The bischloroethylamines, commonly referred to as the nitrogen mustards, include mechlorethamine, melphalan, chlorambucil, cyclophosphamide, ifosfamide, and uracil mustard. Thiotepa is a member of the aziridine class. Busulfan belongs to the alkyl alkone sulfonate class. Carmustine, lomustine, and streptozocin are members of the nitrosourea family. The nonclassical alkylating agents include procarbazine, and altretamine (formerly called hexamethylmelamine) and the triazenes, dacarbazine and temozolamide. Carboplatin and cisplatin are the platinum compounds that exhibit alkylating activity.

Table 1-1 lists the mechanisms of action for each class of alkylating agents as well as the trade name, manufacturer, and dosage forms for each member of the class.

PHARMACOKINETICS

As shown in Table 1-2, most of the alkylating agents are hepatically metabolized prior to renal excretion. Active metabolites are formed in the liver from cyclophosphamide, ifosfamide, chlorambucil, and carboplatin [3,5–7]. Melphalan is uniquely cleared by hydrolysis to monohydroxy- and dihydroxymelphalan. Cisplatin and mechlorethamine are not metabolized prior to renal elimination. Carmustine primarily is cleared by the kidneys but a small portion is eliminated from the lungs [8,9].

The half-lives of the alkylators range from 10 minutes for procarbazine up to 290 hours for cisplatin. No half-life is given for mechlorethamine because it undergoes rapid chemical transformation in body fluids until the drug is no longer present in active form within a few minutes after administration. Dacarbazine, temozolamide, lomustine, streptozocin, and thiotepa have both initial and terminal phase half-lives [10].

APPROVED INDICATIONS

The alkylating agents are active against a wide variety of neoplastic diseases, with significant activity in the treatment of leukemias and lymphomas as well as many solid tumors. This group of drugs is routinely used in the treatment of acute and chronic leukemias; Hodgkin's disease; non-Hodgkin's lymphoma; multiple myeloma; primary brain tumors; carcinomas of the breast, ovaries, testes, lungs, bladder, cervix, head, and neck, and malignant melanoma [4,5,11–14].

A list of the indications for the alkylating agents is included in Table 1-3.

Table 1-1. Classes of Alkylating Agents and Mechanisms of Action

Alkylating Agent	Trade Name	Manufacturer	Dosage Forms
Bischloroethylamines (nitrogen mustards)*†			
Chlorambucil	Leukeran	Glaxo-Wellcome	PO
Cyclophosphamide	Cytoxan	Mead Johnson Oncology	PO, IV
	Neosar	Adria	IV
Ifosfamide	Ifex	Mead Johnson Oncology	IV
Mechlorethamine	Mustargen	Merck, Sharpe, & Dohme	IV
Melphalan	Alkeran	Glaxo-Wellcome	PO, IV
Uracil mustard	Uracil Mustard	Upjohn	PO
Aziridines*			
Thiotepa	Thioplex	Immunex	IV
Alkyl alkone sulfonates*			
Busulfan	Myleran	Glaxo-Wellcome	PO
Nitrosoureas†			
Carmustine	BiCNU	Bristol-Myers Oncology	IV
Lomustine	CeeNU	Bristol-Myers Oncology	PO
Streptozocin	Zanosar	Upjohn	IV
Nonclassic Alkylating Agents‡			
Altretamine	Hexalen	US Bioscience	PO
Dacarbazine	DTIC	Dome	IV
Procarbazine	Matulane	Roche	PO
Temozolamide	Temodal	Schering-Plough	PO
Platinum Compounds§			
Carboplatin	Paraplatin	Bristol-Myers Oncology	IV
Cisplatin	Platinol	Bristol-Myers Oncology	IV

*Interfere with DNA replication and transcription and DNA crosslinks.
†Alkylation of DNA, RNA, DNA crosslinks, and methylate DNA.
‡Alkylation; inhibition of DNA, RNA, and protein synthesis.
§Formation of interstrand and intrastrand DNA cross-links.

DOSAGES

Dosages of the alkylating agents are varied. Many of the drugs are used not only as single-agent therapy but as a part of combination regimens that include other antineoplastic agents. Clinicians should refer to the individual drug monographs for a more complete list of dosing regimens and for adjustments to dosing based on other factors.

Table 1-2. Pharmacokinetics of the Alkylating Agents

Agent	Half-life	Metabolism	Elimination
Bischloroethylamines			
Chlorambucil	90 min (parent drug)	Liver to active metabolites	Renal
Cyclophosphamide	145 min (metabolite)	Liver to active metabolites	Renal
Ifosfamide	4–6.5 h (parent drug)	Liver to active metabolites	Renal
Mechlorethamine	7–14 h (parent drug)	—	Renal
Melphalan	—	Hydrolysis	Chemical hydrolysis to monohydroxy- and dihydroxymel- phalan; low renal clearance
	Oral—90 min		
	IV—6–10 min (initial)		
	40–75 min (terminal)		
Aziridines			
Thiotepa	10 min (initial)	Liver to active metabolites	Renal (60%)
	125 min (terminal)		
Alkyl alkone sulfonates			
Busulfan	1.5–2.6 h	Liver	Renal
Nitrosoureas			
Carmustine	α—6.1 min	Liver	Renal (60%–70%)
	β—21.5 min		Lungs (6%–7%)
Lomustine	6 h (initial plasma)	Liver to active metabolites	Renal
	1–2 d (second plasma)		
Streptozocin	5 min (initial)	Liver and kidneys	Renal (60%–70%)
	35–40 min (terminal)		
Nonclassic alkylating agents			
Altretamine	3–10 h	Liver to active metabolites	Renal
Dacarbazine	19–55 min (initial phase)	Liver	Renal
	5–7.2 h (terminal phase)	Liver	Renal
Procarbazine	10 min	Liver and kidneys	Renal (70%)
Temozolamide	90 min	Spontaneous, liver	Renal
Platinum Compounds			
Carboplatin	α (free drug)— 90 min	Liver to active metabolites	Renal
	β (free drug)— 180 min		
	β (free platinum)— 90 min		
Cisplatin	α—20 min	—	Renal (unchanged)
	β—48–70 min		
	γ—24 h		

TOXICITIES

The major toxicity common to all of the alkylating agents is myelosuppression. Gastrointestinal adverse effects of variable severity occur commonly and various organ toxicities are associated with specific compounds [3,4].

Leukopenia, thrombocytopenia, and anemia are all commonly occurring hematologic toxicities due to the effect of these drugs on the hematopoietic system. Hematologic toxicity is dose-related, cumulative, and can lead to treatment cycle delay or dosage reductions. Although the problem is usually reversible following discontinuation of the alkylator, long-term administration of the alkylating agents can lead to severe and prolonged duration of suppression of the bone marrow. The oral agents, chlorambucil, melphalan, busulfan, lomustine, altretamine, and procarbazine, have slower onset of hematologic toxicity, taking anywhere from 3 to 6 weeks for decreases in blood counts to appear. Nadirs for the IV administered alkylators appear within 1 or 2 weeks and persist for 1 or 2 weeks after discontinuing drug therapy. Prophylactic colony-stimulating factor use may be indicated.

A CBC including hematocrit, hemoglobin, platelets, and total and differential leukocyte counts should be obtained weekly throughout the treatment course to allow the physician to monitor for significant hematologic changes. Other serum chemistries, such as BUN, creatinine, SGPT, SGOT, lactate dehydrogenase, and bilirubin should be obtained at periodic intervals to monitor for adverse effects on liver and kidney function.

Patients being treated for lymphomas and leukemias who have high tumor burdens are especially subject to hyperuricemia. Hyperuricemia is caused by extensive purine catabolism that accompanies rapid cellular destruction and is not a specific toxicity of the drug. Because hyperuricemia is associated with rapid tumor lysis, patients being treated with chlorambucil, cyclophosphamide, mechlorethamine, uracil mustard, busulfan, carboplatin, and cisplatin should have serum uric acid levels monitored throughout the course of therapy.

Treatment of severe hematologic toxicity includes supportive therapy with platelet and erythrocyte transfusions and appropriate antibiotics for febrile neutropenia. Patients who have elevated serum uric acid levels should be treated with allopurinol and advised to increase their oral fluid intake.

Antineoplastic agents, including the alkylators, are toxic to rapidly proliferating cells. Because the gastrointestinal mucosa turns over rapidly, it is susceptible to these agents. Nausea and vomiting are the most common adverse gastrointestinal effects seen with this group of drugs. Stomatitis and anorexia also occur. These adverse effects can lead to decreased nutritional intake.

The gastrointestinal effects can be minimized by prescribing appropriate antiemetic agents as a part of the chemotherapy regimen and providing patients with orally or rectally administered antiemetics to use at home to combat delayed-onset emesis. Adequate fluid is essential to prevent complications associated with dehydration due to loss of excessive fluid volume. Electrolyte replacement may be necessary for patients with severe emesis or diarrhea.

Hemorrhagic cystitis is a major toxicity of ifosfamide as well as high-dose cyclophosphamide therapy and is caused by concentration of the metabolite acrolein in the bladder [3,4,11,15–18]. A urinalysis should be obtained and examined for microscopic hematuria prior to each course of treatment, especially with ifosfamide. To help prevent this complication, patients should be adequately hydrated prior to the start of the ifosfamide or cyclophosphamide infusion. Mesna, a uroprotective agent, should be administered in an intravenous dosage equal to 20% of the ifosfamide dosage (weight/weight) at the time of ifosfamide administration and repeated 4 and 8 hours after each dose of ifosfamide. Other mesna dosing schedules also may be used in patients receiving either ifosfamide or high-dose cyclophosphamide. Patients receiving ifosfamide or high-dose cyclophosphamide therapy on an outpatient basis should be advised to increase their oral fluid intake and to void every 2 hours during the day and once at night on the days they receive their chemotherapy treatments to decrease the risk of hemorrhagic cystitis.

Table 1-4 lists the hematologic, gastrointestinal, and other major toxicities associated with the alkylating agents [2,11,15–21,34].

INVESTIGATIONAL AGENTS

Fotemustine, an amino acid–linked chloroethyl nitrosourea, has activity against disseminated malignant melanoma. It also has been studied in colorectal cancer, non–small cell lung cancer, and high-grade gliomas. Doses of 100 to 500 mg/m² in a variety of treatment regimens have been investigated. Leukopenia, thrombocytopenia, anemia, central nervous system toxicity, and transient liver chemistry abnormalities are the major reported toxicities of fotemustine [22–27].

COST ANALYSIS

The cost of treating cancer patients with the alkylating agents varies based on the treatment course selected, doses of the alkylating agents, and number of cycles of therapy.

MECHANISMS OF RESISTANCE

Resistance to antineoplastic agents is the major cause of treatment failure for many cancer patients. Increasing dosages of drugs may be required to levels where toxicities are prohibitive. Alternatively, changing the treatment to a non–cross-resistant drug or combination of drugs that will be effective against the particular neoplasm is required. Resistance is either primary (natural) or acquired. Primary resistance results when innate resistance is selected out from natural cell lines. Acquired resistance results from drug-induced adaptation or mutation of neoplastic cells. Acquired resistance may be due to decreased intracellular concentrations of the drug, increased degradation of the active compound, decreased conversion of the drug to the active form, changes in cellular metabolism and utilization of separate metabolic pathways, and increased activity or concentration of target enzymes within the cell. Among the alkylating agents, cross-resistance has been reported with carmustine and lomustine.

Two key mechanisms are 1) high levels of O6-alkylguanine-DNA alkyltransferase for resistance to nitrosoureas [28], and 2) glutathione and glutathione-s transformed for alkylating agents [29]. DNA repair processes explain most of the resistance. Recently, tumor defects in mismatch repair have been associated with platinum- and methylating-agent resistance [30,31].

Table 1-3. Approved Indications for Alkylating Agents

Alkylating Agent	Approved Indications
Bischloroethylamines	
Chlorambucil	Chronic lymphocytic leukemia, malignant lymphomas, lymphosarcoma, giant follicular lymphoma, Hodgkin's disease
Cyclophosphamide	Acute lymphocytic leukemia, acute myelocytic leukemia, chronic myelocytic leukemia, chronic lymphoncytic leukemia, acute monocytic leukemia, Hodgkin's and non-Hodgkin's lymphoma, carcinoma of the breast and ovary, multiple myeloma, mycosis fungoides, Burkitt's lymphoma, neuroblastoma, retinoblastoma
Ifosfamide	Third-line therapy for germ cell testicular tumors
Mechlorethamine	Palliative treatment of stage III and IV Hodgkin's disease, lymphosarcoma, chronic myelocytic leukemia, chronic lymphocytic leukemia, polycythemia vera, mycosis fungoides, bronchogenic carcinoma, palliative intraperitoneal treatment of metastatic carcinoma
Melphalan	Palliative treatment of multiple myeloma and nonresectable epithelial ovarian carcinoma
Uracil mustard	Palliative treatment of chonic lymphocytic leukemia, chronic myelocytic leukemia, non-Hodgkin's lymphomas, mycosis fungoides, early polycythemia vera
Aziridines	
Thiotepa	Intravesical treatment of tumors of the bladder, palliative treatment of adenocarcinoma of the breast or ovary, intrathecal treatment of meningeal neoplasms
Alkyl alkone sulfonates	
Busulfan	Chronic myelogenous leukemia, severe thrombocytosis, polycythemia vera
Nitrosoureas	
Carmustine	Palliative treatment of primary and metastatic brain tumors, multiple myeloma, disseminated Hodgkin's disease, non-Hodgkin's lymphomas
Lomustine	Palliative treatment of primary and metastatic brain tumors, disseminated Hodgkin's disease
Streptozocin	Metastatic islet cell carcinoma of the pancreas
Nonclassic alkylating agents	
Altretamine	Palliative treatment of persistent or recurrent ovarian cancer
Dacarbazine	Malignant melanoma, Hodgkin's disease
Temozolamide	Anaplastic astrocytoma
Procarbazine	Advanced Hodgkin's disease
Platinum compounds	
Carboplatin	Advanced ovarian carcinoma
Cisplatin	Metastatic testicular tumors, metastatic ovarian tumors, advanced bladder carcinoma

AREAS OF RESEARCH ACTIVITY

As oncologists strive to improve the treatment of cancer, research studies continue with many drugs being studied for possible new indications [6,32,33]. The alkylating agents, although among the oldest antineoplastic agents, continue to be studied for possible new indications, both alone and in combination with other antineoplastics.

Among the alkylators, ifosfamide and dacarbazine are being examined in the treatment of soft tissue sarcomas. Mechlorethamine and carmustine have been studied for topical application in the treatment of mycosis fungoides [7]. Cyclophosphamide is being studied in small cell lung carcinoma and in carcinomas of the gastrointestinal tract, endometrium, testes, prostate, and bladder and in renal cell carcinoma. Streptozocin has shown activity in metastatic carcinoid tumors and in metastatic colorectal cancer. Cisplatin has shown activity in metastatic squamous cell carcinomas of the head and neck and cervix, and in non–small cell lung carci-

noma. Temozolomide shows promising activity in anaplastic astrocytomas and melanoma.

High-dose chemotherapy is being increasingly utilized with hematopoietic cellular support (*eg*, bone marrow or peripheral blood progenitor cell transfusion and colony-stimulating factor use). Cyclophosphamide, carmustine, carboplatin, cisplatin, melphalan, and thiotepa are among the alkylators that have been used in this approach to cancer chemotherapy [8,32–38]. Recently, a potent inhibitor of O6-alkylguanine-DNA alkyltransferase, O6-benzylguanine, has been identified that potentiates the anti-tumor efficacy of nitrosoureas and methylating agents such as temozolomide [39]. It has now entered phase 1 and 2 clinical trials [40,41]. In addition, d,l-Buthionine-S,R-sulfoximine (L-BSO) has been identified as an inhibitor of the synthesis if glutathione resulting in increased cytotoxicity of many alkylating agents [29,42]. It also has entered phase 1 and 2 clinical trials [43]. Both represent a new class of mechanism-based agents designed to overcome tumor drug resistance.

Table 1-4. Major Toxicities of the Alkylating Agents

Alkylating Agent	Hematologic	Gastrointestinal	Other
Bischloroethylamines			
Chlorambucil	Leukopenia, thrombocytopenia	Nausea, vomiting, diarrhea, gastric discomfort (doses>20 mg)	Hyperuricemia*
Cyclophosphamide	Leukopenia, anemia, thrombocytopenia	Nausea, vomiting, anorexia	Hemorrhagic cystitis, alopecia, hyperuricemia*
Ifosfamide	Leukopenia, thrombocytopenia	Nausea, vomiting	Hemorrhagic cystitis, alopecia
Mechlorethamine	Leukopenia, anemia, thrombocytopenia, hemorrhagic diathesis	Nausea, vomiting	Thrombophlebitis, headache, weakness, hyperuricemia*
Melphalan	Leukopenia, thrombocytopenia	Nausea, vomiting (infrequently PO, more IV), mucositis	
Uracil mustard	Leukopenia, thrombocytopenia	Nausea, vomiting, anorexia, diarrhea, epigastric distress	Hyperuricemia*
Aziridines			
Thiotepa	Leukopenia, anemia, thrombocytopenia, pancytopenia	Nausea, vomiting, anorexia (infrequently), diarrhea	Pain at injection site, headache, dizziness
Alkyl alkone sulfonates			
Busulfan	Leukopenia, anemia, thrombocytopenia	Nausea, vomiting, diarrhea (infrequently)	Hyperuricemia*
Nitrosoureas			
Carmustine	Leukopenia, anemia, thrombocytopenia	Nausea, vomiting	Hepatotoxicity, pulmonary infiltrates
Lomustine	Leukopenia, anemia, thrombocytopenia with prolonged therapy	Nausea, vomiting	
Streptozocin	Mild to moderate leukopenia, anemia, thrombocytopenia	Nausea, vomiting	Nephrotoxicity, pain at injection site
Nonclassic Alkylating Agents			
Altretamine	Leukopenia, anemia, thrombocytopenia	Nausea, vomiting	Peripheral neuropathy
Dacarbazine	Leukopenia, thrombocytopenia	Nausea, vomiting, anorexia	Pain at injection site, fever, myalgia, malaise, hypocalcemia, hypotension (high doses)
Temozolamide	Leukopenia, thrombocytopenia	None	
Procarbazine	Leukopenia, anemia, thrombocytopenia	Nausea, vomiting, anorexia, stomatitis	
Platinum Compounds			
Carboplatin	Leukopenia, anemia, thrombocytopenia	Nausea, vomiting	Peripheral neuropathies, ototoxicity
Cisplatin	Leukopenia, anemia, thrombocytopenia	Nausea, vomiting	Nephrotoxicity, hypomagnesemia, hypocalcemia, hypokalemia, ototoxicity, peripheral neuropathy, hyperuricemia*

*Hyperuricemia is most often associated with leukemia and lymphoma in patients who have a high tumor burden and is not necessarily an adverse effect of the drug.

REFERENCES

1. Calabresi P, Rall T, Nies A, Palmer T. In *Goodman and Gilman's The Pharmacological Basis of Therapeutics*, edn 8. Edited by Gilman A, Rall T, Nies A, Palmer T. New York: Pergamon Press, 1990:1202–1276.

2. Chabner BA, Collins JM, eds: *Cancer Chemotherapy: Principles and Practice*. Philadelphia: JB Lippincott, 1990.

3. Black DJ, Livingston RB: Antineoplastic drugs in 1990: a review (Part I). *Drugs* 1990, 39:489–501.

4. Black DJ, Livingston RB: Antineoplastic drugs in 1990: a review (Part II). *Drugs* 1990, 39:652–673.

5. Alberts DS: Clinical pharmacology of carboplatin. *Semin Oncol* 1990, 7(Suppl):6–9.

6. Whitmore WF, Yagoda Y: Chemotherapy in the management of bladder tumors. *Drugs* 1989, 38:301–312.

7. Zackheim HS, Epstein EH, Carin WR: Topical carmustine (BCNU) for cutaneous T-cell lymphoma: a 15-year experience in 143 patients.
   J Am Acad Dermatol 1990, 22(Part 1):802–810.

8. Henner WD, Peters WP, Eden JP: Pharmacokinetics and immediate effects of high-dose carmustine in man. *Cancer Treat Rep* 1986, 70:877–880.

9. Jones RB, Matthes S, Dufton C, *et al.*: Pharmacokinetic/pharmacodynamic interactions of intensive cyclophosphamide, cisplatin, and BCNU in patients with breast cancer. *Breast Cancer Res Treat* 1993, 26:S11–17.

10. Cohen BG, Egorin MJ, Kohlhepp EA, *et al.*: Human plasma pharmacokinetics and urinary excretion of thiotepa and its metabolites. *Cancer Treat Rep* 1986, 70:859–864.

11. Dechant KL, Brogden RN, Pillington T, Faulds D: Ifosphamide/mesna: a review of antineoplastic activity, pharmacokinetic properties, and therapeutic efficacy in cancer. *Drugs* 1991, 42:428–467.

12. Gad E, Mawla N, *et al.*: Ifosphamide, methotrexate, and 5-fluorouracil: effective combination in resistant breast cancer. *Cancer Chemother Pharmacol* 1990, 26(Suppl):S85–S86.

13. Hansen LA, Hughes TE: Altretamine. DICP, *Ann Pharmacother* 1991, 25:146–152.

14. Loehrer PJ, Einhorn LH: Cisplatin. *Ann Intern Med* 1984, 100:704–713.

15. Dorr RT: Ifosphamide and cyclophosphamide: review and appraisal. 1992.

16. Frasier LH, Kanekal S, Kehrer JP: Cyclophosphamide toxicity: characterizing and avoiding the problem. *Drugs* 1991, 42:781–795.

17. Sanchiz F, Milla A: High-dose ifosphamide and mesna in advanced breast cancer. *Cancer Chemother Pharmacol* 1990, 26(Suppl):S91–S92.

18. Thigpen T, Lambath BW, Vance RB: Ifosphamide in the management of gynecologic cancers. *Semin Oncol* 1990, 17(Suppl 4): 11–18.

19. Finley RS, Fortner CL, Grove WR: Cisplatin nephrotoxicity: a summary of preventative interventions. *Drug Intelligence Clin Pharma* 1985, 19:362–367.

20. Kris MG, Gralla RJ, Clark RA, *et al.*: Incidence, course, and severity of delayed nausea and vomiting following the administration of high-dose cisplatin. *J Clin Oncol* 1985, 3:1379–1384.

21. Smith AC: The pulmonary toxicity of nitrosoureas. *Pharmacol Therapeutics* 1989, 41:443–460.

22. Antico J, Pascon G, Turjansky L, *et al.*: Phase II study of fotemustine in gliomas: preliminary report. *Proc Am Soc Oncol* 1995, 14:151. Abstract.

23. Fishchel JL: Tamoxifen enhances the cytotoxic effects of the nitrosourea fotemustine: results of human melanoma cell lines. *Eur J Cancer* 1993, 29A:2269–2273.

24. Khayat D, Berille J, Gerard B, *et al.*: Fotemustine in the treatment of brain primary tumors and metastases. *Cancer Invest* 1994, 12:414–420.

25. Riviere A, LeCesne A, Berille J, *et al.*: Cisplatin-fotemustine combination in inoperable non-small lung cancer: preliminary report of a French multicenter phase II trial. *Eur J Cancer* 1994, 30A:587–590.

26. Rougier P, Chabot GG, Bonneterre J, *et al.*: Phase II and pharmacokinetics study of fotemustine in inoperable colorectal cancer. *Eur J Cancer* 1993, 29A:288–289.

27. Trachand B, Lucas C, Biron F, *et al.*: Phase I pharmacokinetics study of high dose fotemustine and its metabolite 2-chloroethanol in patients with high-grade gliomas. *Cancer Chemother Pharmacol* 1993, 32:46–52.

28. Pegg AE, Dolan ME, Moschel RC: Structure, function, and inhibition of O6-alkylguanine-DNA alkyltransferase. *Prog Nucleic Acid Res Mol Biol* 1995, 51:167–223.

29. Skapek SX, Colvin OM, Griffith OW, *et al.*: Enhanced melphalan cytotoxicity following buthionine sulfoximine-mediated glutathione depletion in a human medulloblastoma xenograft in athymic mice. *Cancer Res* 1988, 48:2764–2767.

30. Liu L, Markowitz S, Gerson SL: Mismatch repair mutations override alkyltransferase in conferring resistance to temozolomide but not to 1,3-bis (2-chloroethyl) nitrosourea. *Cancer Res* 1996, 56:5375–5379.

31. Fink D, Zheng H, Nebel S, *et al.*: In vitro and in vivo resistance to cisplatin in cells that have lost DNA mismatch repair. *Cancer Res* 1997, 57:1841–1845.

32. Calvert AH, Newell DR, Gore HE: Future directions with carboplatin: can therapeutic monitoring, high dose administration, and hematologic support with growth factors expand the spectrum compared with cisplatin? *Semin Oncol* 1992, 19(Suppl 2):155–163.

33. Batts CN: Adjuvant intravesical therapy for superficial bladder cancer. *Ann Pharmacother* 1992, 26:1270–1276.

34. Corden BJ, Fine RL, Ozols RF, Collins JM: Clinical pharmacology of high-dose cisplatin. *Cancer Chemother Pharmacol* 1985, 14:38–41.

35. Ackland SP, Choi K, Ratain MJ: Human plasma pharmacokinetics following administration of high-dose thiotepa and cyclophosphamide. *J Clin Oncol* 1988, 6:1192–1196.

36. Bishop JF: Current experience with high-dose carboplatin therapy. *Semin Oncol* 1992, 19(Suppl):150–154.

37. Rohaly J: The use of busulfan therapy in bone marrow transplantation. *Cancer Nursing* 1989, 12:144–152.

38. Antman, K, Eder JP, Elias A, *et al.*: High-dose thiotepa alone and in combination regimens with bone marrow support. *Semin Oncol* 1990, 17:33-38.

39. Dolan, ME, Stine L, Mitchell RB, *et al.*: Modulation of mammalian O6-alkylguanine-DNA alkyltransferase in vivo by O6 benzylguanine and its effect on the sensitivity of a human glioma tumor to 1-(2-chloroethyl)-3-(4-methylcyclohexyl)-1-nitrosourea. *Cancer Commun* 1990, 2:371-377.

40. Gerson SL, Willson JK: O6-alkylguanine-DNA alkyltransferase. A target for the modulation of drug resistance. *Hematol Oncol Clin North Am* 1995, 9:431-450.

41. Spiro TP, Gerson SL, Liu L, *et al.*: O2-benzylguanine: a clinical trial establishing the biochemical modulatory dose in tumor tissue for aklytransferase directed DNA repair. *Cancer Res* 1999, 59:2402–2410.

42. Du DL, Volpe DA, Grieshaber CK, Murphy M Jr: Effects of L-phenylalanine mustard and L-buthionine sulfoximine on murine and human hematopoietic progenitor cells in vitro. *Cancer Res* 1990, 50:4038-4043.

43. Lacreta FP, Brennan JM, Hamilton TC, *et al.*: Stereoselective pharmacokinetics of L-buthionine SR-sulfoximine in patients with cancer. *Drug Metab Dispos* 1994, 22:835-842.

44. Lazarus HM, Crilley P, Ciobanu N, *et al.*: High-dose carmustine, etoposide, and cisplatin and autologous bone marrow transplantation for relapsed and refractory lymphoma. *J Clin Oncol* 1992, 10:1682-1689.

45. Jones RB, Matthes S, Shpall EJ, *et al.*: Acute lung injury following treatment with high-dose cyclophosphamide, cisplatin, and carmustine: pharmacodynamic evaluation of carmustine. *J Natl Cancer Inst* 1993, 85:640-647.

ALTRETAMINE

Altretamine (also known as hexamethylmelamine) is an antineoplastic agent structurally similar to triethylenemelamine, a known alkylating agent. The mechanism of action is unknown. It has been postulated that altretamine may act as an alkylator or as an antimetabolite. Altretamine is activated via hepatic microsomal enzymes to cytotoxic intermediates, which may bind to microsomal proteins and DNA. The National Cancer Institute developed altretamine ~18 y ago. The United States Food and Drug Administration approved the drug for market in 1991.

DOSAGE AND ADMINISTRATION

Usual dose is 4–12 mg/kg PO in divided daily doses for 21–90 d, or 240–320 mg/m^2 PO in divided daily doses for 14–21 d; doses are repeated every 6 wk

SPECIAL PRECAUTIONS

All cytotoxic drugs may be embryotoxic or teratogenic; use with caution in pregnant or nursing patients

TOXICITIES

GI: nausea and vomiting occur in approximately 50%–70% of patients and are usually considered dose-limiting; anorexia, abdominal cramps, and diarrhea also have been reported; **CNS:** neurologic side effects are reported in 20% of patients, including paresthesias, numbness, sleep disturbances, confusion, hallucinations, seizures, and Parkinsonian-like syndrome with ataxia; **Hematologic:** mild leukopenia and thrombocytopenia; **Miscellaneous:** alopecia, rash, and pruritus

INDICATIONS

FDA-approved: Treatment of advanced ovarian cancer; Clinical studies show activity in metastatic breast cancer, refractory lymphoma, pancreatic adenocarcinoma, and colorectal, cervical, and endometrial cancers; **investigational uses:** treatment of small cell and non–small cell lung cancer

PHARMACOKINETICS

Absorption—the micronized capsule form exhibits enhanced gastrointestinal absorption; however, oral absorption is extremely variable; peak plasma concentrations can occur from 0.5–3 h after administration; **Distribution**—altretamine is minimally protein bound and highly lipid-soluble; it tends to distribute in tissues with a high lipid content, such as the omentum and subcutaneous tissues; the parent drug does not cross the blood—brain barrier to a significant extent; altretamine metabolites may be more protein bound and also cross the blood–brain barrier more readily. Therefore, the CNS side effects may be due to the metabolites, not the parent drug; **Metabolism**—altretamine is extensively metabolized in the liver; extrahepatic metabolism also may occur; **Elimination**—the elimination half-life varies from 3–10 h, primarily eliminated in the urine as metabolites; a small amount may be excreted through the lungs as expired air and in the feces

DRUG INTERACTIONS

Cimetidine increases the toxicity of altretamine by prolonging its half-life by 29%–80%; phenobarbital may induce the metabolism of altretamine and reduce its antitumor activity; monoamine oxidase inhibitors may result in severe orthostatic hypotension

RESPONSE RATES

When altretamine is used as single-agent treatment for ovarian cancer, response rates of 20%–30% have been reported; in combination with cyclophosphamide, doxorubicin and melphalan response rates increased, ranging from 20%–80% (including complete and partial responses); single-agent therapy for small cell and non–small cell lung cancer ranges from 4%–42%; adding altretamine to cytotoxic agents known to be active against small cell lung cancer produced widely variable results, 7%–94%

PATIENT MONITORING

CBC, including differential leukocyte count and platelet count, should be performed during therapy to monitor for leukopenia and thrombocytopenia; complete neurologic exam should be performed on a routine basis; health care professionals responsible for monitoring patients on altretamine therapy should be familiar with the broad spectrum of other adverse effects that can occur, albeit less commonly, with this treatment

NURSING INTERVENTIONS

Monitor treatment tolerance, weight, and nutritional status; nausea and vomiting are common especially with high doses; appropriate antiemetics should be administered and daily doses should be divided into a four times a day schedule (after meals and at bedtime); neurotoxicity may be decreased by concomitant administration of 100 mg of pyridoxine

PATIENT INFORMATION

Call the doctor immediately if intractable nausea and vomiting occur, unusual bruising or bleeding occurs, fevers above 101°F occur; it is important to continue medication despite nausea and vomiting; GI effects can be controlled so the medication will be better tolerated—please report vomiting episodes that occur soon after the oral dose is taken; take after meals; report signs and symptoms of neurotoxicity

FORMULATION

Available as Hexalen (Applied Analytical Industries, Wilmington, NC, distributed by US Bioscience, West Conshohocken, PA) 50-mg hard gelatin capsules; stored at room temperature

BUSULFAN

Busulfan is an oral alkylating agent that is cell cycle nonspecific and forms interstrand DNA crosslinks. It interferes with DNA replication and transcription of RNA and ultimately results in the disruption of nucleic acid function. Busulfan is primarily used to control chronic myelogenous leukemia because of its selective depression of granulocytopoiesis at low doses. At higher doses the effect on all three hematopoietic cell lines is increased.

DOSAGE AND ADMINISTRATION

Chronic myelogenous leukemia: 0.06 mg/kg or 1.8 mg/m^2 is recommended for both children and adults; therapy varies among clinicians and can be intermittent or continuous (most clinicians discontinue therapy when leukocyte counts decrease to ≤ 10,000/mm^3 and resume therapy when leukocyte counts reach 50,000/mm^3); **Bone marrow transplant preparatory regimens:** high-dose busulfan, 16 mg/kg total dose (4 mg/kg/d for 4 d) (also used in a variety of refractory cancers experimentally)

SPECIAL PRECAUTIONS

Life-threatening pancytopenia can occur with busulfan therapy (extensive monitoring of hematologic parameters is warranted); a rare but life-threatening hepatic venoocclusive disease has been reported with very high dose busulfan; contraindicated in patients with known hypersensitivity to the drug; contraindicated in patients whose chronic myelogenous leukemia has demonstrated resistance to this therapy; all cytotoxic drugs may be embryotoxic or teratogenic; busulfan therapy can cause widespread epithelial dysplasia, chromosomal aberrations, and germ cell aplasia; should be avoided in pregnant and nursing patients

(Continued on next page)

INDICATIONS

FDA-approved: Palliative treatment of chronic myelogenous leukemias; **Clinical studies show activity in** other myeloproliferative disorders including severe thrombocytosis and polycythemia vera; myelofibrosis; and, in high doses, as a component of marrow-ablative conditioning regimens prior to bone marrow transplant for the treatment of malignant and nonmalignant conditions; now used as third-line treatment of chronic myelogenous leukemias after interferon-α and hydroxyurea and in combination with cyclophosphamide in preparative regimens for myeloablative therapy prior to autologous and allogeneic transplantation of bone marrow, peripheral blood, progenitor cell and cord blood

PHARMACOKINETICS

Absorption: rapidly and completely absorbed from the GI tract with measurable blood concentrations obtained within 0.5–2 h after oral administration; **Distribution:** cleared rapidly from the plasma; it is not known whether the drug is distributed into cerebrospinal fluid or into breast milk; **Metabolism:** extensively metabolized by the liver, with 12 metabolites being isolated to date; most of the metabolites have not been identified and it is not known if they possess cytotoxic activity; **Elimination:** ~10%–50% of the dose is excreted in the urine as metabolites within 24 h; monitoring peak blood levels during high-dose therapy is advised to decrease the incidence of venoocclusive disease

DRUG INTERACTIONS

Additive myelosuppression can occur when busulfan is combined with other cytotoxic drugs; hepatoxicity has been reported with the concomitant use of busulfan and thioguanine (more studies are needed to validate this interaction); phenytoin may significantly decrease the clearance of busulfan

RESPONSE RATES

Response rates of 90% have been reported in patients with previously untreated chronic myelogenous leukemia while taking busulfan; although not curative, hematologic remission with regression or stabilization of organomegaly has been noted with relief of symptoms; busulfan is less effective in patients with chronic myelogenous leukemia who lack the Philadelphia chromosome

(Continued on next page)

BUSULFAN (Continued)

TOXICITIES

Hematologic: major dose-related adverse effect is bone marrow suppression (usually reversible but some patients can be very sensitive to the drug and experience an abrupt onset of possibly irreversible toxicity); severe leukopenia, anemia, and thrombocytopenia usually occur approximately 10 d after therapy and can continue 1–2 wk; severe toxicity due to overdose may be prolonged with complete recovery taking 1 mo–2 y; bone marrow fibrosis and chronic aplasia have been reported with busulfan administration; secondary neoplasia is possible

Pulmonary: a syndrome called *busulfan lung* is rare and can occur after long-term therapy; this syndrome is manifested by bronchopulmonary dysplasia with a diffuse interstitial pulmonary fibrosis and is characterized by persistent cough, fever, rales, and dyspnea; discontinuance of busulfan and administration of corticosteroids may improve symptoms and minimize permanent lung damage; in some patients the syndrome progresses to respiratory insufficiency despite intervention, and deaths usually occur within 6 mo

Metabolic: hyperuricemia may occur when the leukemia cell count is rapidly reduced; an Addison-like adrenal insufficiency syndrome is apparent in a small number of patients after long-term therapy

CNS: dizziness, blurred vision, loss of consciousness, and intermittent muscle twitching; myoclonic and generalized tonic-clonic seizures have occurred especially with high-dose therapy; prophylactic anticonvulsant administration has been employed during high-dose therapy for marrow-ablative conditioning regimens prior to bone marrow transplant

Infertility: germinal aplasia and sterility have been reported in rats but not humans; ovarian suppression and amenorrhea with menopausal symptoms commonly occur during busulfan therapy in premenopausal women; ovarian fibrosis and atrophy also have occurred; interferes with spermatogenesis and causes impotence, sterility, azoospermia, and testicular atrophy in male humans

Miscellaneous: mild gynecomastia, cheilosis, glossitis, hepatic dysfunction and cholestatic jaundice, porphyria cutanea tarda, melanoderma, urticaria, rashes, dryness of skin and mucous membranes, anhidrosis, alopecia, cataracts, hemorrhagic cystitis, and fatigue are rare; nausea, vomiting, diarrhea, anorexia, and weight loss are infrequent; venooclusive disease has been seen in high-dose therapy accompanied by hyperbilirubinemia, weight gain, ascites, and hepatic injury

PATIENT MONITORING

A CBC, including differential leukocyte count and platelet count, is generally obtained weekly; leukocyte count generally will not decrease for 10–15 d—this delay should not be interpreted as resistance to the drug nor should the dose be increased; because the effects of busulfan will continue to decrease leukocyte count after discontinuance, the drug should be withheld when leukocyte counts have fallen between 10,000–15,000/mm^3; treatment should be resumed once leukocyte count increases again to ≥ 50,000/mm^3; signs of persistent cough and progressive dyspnea should be carefully monitored; monitor for symptoms of adrenal insufficiency, such as abrupt weakness, unusual fatigue, anorexia, weight loss, nausea and vomiting, and melanoderma; monitoring busulfan serum concentrations and subsequently adjusting the dose may lessen the toxicities observed with high-dose therapy used in bone marrow transplant; health care professionals responsible for monitoring patients on busulfan therapy should be familiar with the broad spectrum of other adverse effects that can occur, albeit less commonly, with this treatment

NURSING INTERVENTIONS

Monitor treatment tolerance, weight, and nutritional status; assure that appropriate lab tests are conducted to monitor for hematologic effects as well as for hyperuricemia and renal function; explain to the patient the importance of weekly blood count monitoring

PATIENT INFORMATION

Call the doctor immediately if the following occurs: unusual bruising or bleeding, temperature over 101°F, sore throat, or other signs of infection; let the doctor or nurse know if you are experiencing a persistent cough or having difficulty breathing; continue to take medication despite the nausea and vomiting; continued monitoring of blood counts is very important and should not be missed; do not take aspirin-containing products they may increase the chance of bleeding; if you forget your because medication, take it as soon as you remember within 24 h of the missed dose (if it has been more than 24 h since the dose was missed, do not take an extra dose but continue with the next regularly scheduled dose)

FORMULATION

Available as Myleran (Glaxo Wellcome Co., Research Triangle Park, NC) 2-mg scored tablets each containing the inactive ingredients magnesium stearate and sodium chloride; now available as IV preparation

CARBOPLATIN

Carboplatin is a second-generation platinum compound that may be classified as a nonclassical alkylating agent and is cell cycle nonspecific. Carboplatin and cisplatin have similar spectrums of activity. This second-generation platinum is used primarily for the treatment of ovarian cancer but also has shown promise in the treatment of seminomas, squamous cell carcinomas of the head and neck, and small cell lung cancer. Carboplatin, "the kinder platinum," is similar to cisplatin but was developed in an attempt to decrease the severe side effects of cisplatin. Nephrotoxicity, ototoxicity, neurotoxicity, and dose-limiting nausea and vomiting are lessened with carboplatin therapy. The major dose-limiting toxicity of carboplatin is myelosuppression. Like cisplatin, carboplatin is a cytotoxic platinum complex that reacts with nucleophilic sites on DNA. This causes interstrand and intrastrand cross-links and DNA-protein cross-links, which inhibits DNA, RNA, and protein synthesis.

DOSAGE AND ADMINISTRATION

Many clinicians routinely use the Calvert formula to dose carboplatin instead of the standard dosing schema mentioned above. This formula is based on a target area under the curve (AUC), the average being 7 mg/mL/min (4–11 mg/mL/min) and the patient's glomerular filtration rate (GFR, mL/min), because the original Calvert formula measured GFR with ^{51}Cr-labeled EDTA. Modifications using estimated creatinine clearance have been used but are less accurate at predicting the actual AUC. Target AUC depends on the patient's previous treatment history, concomitant chemotherapy, and disease state. The Calvert formula is: Total Dose (mg) = target AUC times (GFR + 25). Intraperitoneal doses of 200–650 mg/m^2 have been used. High-dose carboplatin (800–2000 mg/m^2) has been used investigationally with and without bone marrow support. Doses higher than 2000 mg/m^2 have been associated with hepatic toxicity. There is no therapeutic difference between 24-h continuous infusion and bolus dosing. Bolus dosing may be more convenient and does not require hospital admittance

SPECIAL PRECAUTIONS

Myelosuppression is the major dose-limiting toxicity of carboplatin; monitoring for leukopenia, anemia, and thrombocytopenia should be continued throughout therapy; thrombocytopenia can be more severe than leukopenia and anemia; all cytotoxic drugs may be embryotoxic or teratogenic; use with caution in pregnant or nursing patients; contraindicated in patients with a history of severe allergic reactions to cisplatin or other platinum-containing compounds, or mannitol

(Continued on next page)

INDICATIONS

FDA-approved: Initial and secondary treatment of advanced ovarian cancer; clinical studies show activity in lung cancers, squamous cell cancers of the head and neck, gastrointestinal cancer, and testicular cancer

PHARMACOKINETICS

Absorption: AUC increases proportionally with the dose of carboplatin; when administered intraperitoneally, plasma concentrations are approximately one fifth of the peritoneal dose; **Distribution:** 24 h after administration, tissue concentrations of carboplatin can be detected in the kidneys, liver, skin, and ileum; very low concentrations can be found in the spleen, lung, muscle, heart, testes, brain, fat, and bone marrow; 10%–18% of plasma carboplatin is protein bound shortly after bolus administration (some studies have shown protein binding as high as 40%–87% 24 h after carboplatin administration); the volume of distribution has been measured as 16–20 L; **Metabolism:** limited information available; it has been reported that carboplatin is metabolized into highly reactive diamine metabolites that may be similar to cisplatin metabolites; **Elimination:** renal clearance is the main route of excretion of carboplatin and its metabolites; within the first 24 h, 58%–77% of the administered dose is excreted as free platinum and approximately 32% is excreted as unchanged carboplatin; the plasma elimination half lives of carboplatin and free platinum are approximately 3 and 6 h, respectively; renal and total body clearance can be compromised in older or renally impaired patients

DRUG INTERACTIONS

If carboplatin is given concurrently with **nephrotoxic drugs**, myelosuppression and renal toxicity can be enhanced

RESPONSE RATES

Response rates of 25%–28% have been reported in the treatment of ovarian cancer with carboplatin alone in patients previously treated with cisplatin: this may indicate that the two platinum agents are not completely cross-resistant; patients not previously treated with cisplatin achieved responses of 85% with carboplatin; when carboplatin is used in combination with other cytotoxic drugs (*ie*, cyclophosphamide, doxorubicin, 5-fluorouracil, and cisplatin), complete and partial response rates are seen in 30%–83% of patients; intraperitoneal carboplatin has produced 53% response rates in patients previously treated with cisplatin

Varied response rates to carboplatin have been reported in small cell lung cancer and non–small cell lung cancer; responses are usually much higher in patients who have not been previously treated; responses of 0%–60% have been reported in patients with small cell lung cancer treated with carboplatin alone; the combinations of carboplatin with other cytotoxic drugs exhibits slightly improved responses of 50%–77%; in non–small cell lung cancer, combination therapy has produced response rates of 40%–56%

(Continued on next page)

CARBOPLATIN (Continued)

TOXICITIES

Hematologic: dose-limiting thrombocytopenia can occur in 37%–80% of patients receiving carboplatin; contributing factors include increased age, renal impairment, and concurrent and previous chemotherapy; the extent of myelosuppression appears to be proportional to area under the curve (AUC) of ultrafilterable platinum; leukopenia and anemia have been reported in 27%–38% of patients who receive carboplatin alone; myelosuppression is reversible but severity may be cumulative with repeated doses

GI: mild and manageable nausea and vomiting (dose-dependent but rarely dose-limiting); delayed GI toxicity can occur 6–12 h after carboplatin is administered

Renal: although less common than cisplatin, nephrotoxicity can occur with carboplatin therapy, usually caused by chronic tubular damage

Miscellaneous: alopecia is mild but can increase in severity with cumulative therapy; usually mild and infrequent: abnormal liver function tests, mild neurotoxicity, hypersensitivity, stomatitis, mucositis, and flu-like syndrome; with high-dose regimens used in autologous bone marrow transplant, hepatotoxicity, severe renal dysfunction, and severe nausea, vomiting, and electrolyte wasting have been reported

DOSAGE AND ADMINISTRATION*

Treatment Schedule	Dosage, mg/m²		
	Adults		Children
	Previous Therapy	No Previous Therapy	
Bolus every 4 wk	240–270	350–450	560
24 h continuous infusion every 4–5 wk	240	320	
Weekly bolus for 4 consecutive wk with 2 wk of rest	100	125	175
Bolus for 5 consecutive days every 4–6 wk	77	100	

It is preferred to use the Calvert dosing formula to individualize dosing based on patient GFR.

RENAL DOSAGE ADJUSTMENT

Baseline Creatinine Clearance, mL/min	Recommended Dose on Day 1, mg/m²
41–59	250
16–40	200

Dosage adjustment in older or renally impaired patients is recommended. Renal dosage adjustment should only be used for initial therapy. Doses for subsequent courses should be based on hematologic parameters.

HEMATOLOGIC DOSE ADJUSTMENT

Platelets	Neurtrophils	Adjusted Dose (From Prior Course)
>100,000	>2000	125%
50–100,000	500–2000	No adjustment
<50,000	<500	75%

RESPONSE RATES (Continued)

Low response rates averaging 25% are reported when carboplatin is used alone in the treatment of squamous cell carcinoma of the head and neck; when combined with 5-fluorouracil, response rates increase to 62%–92%

Carboplatin alone has demonstrated poor results in the treatment of gastrointestinal cancers; in combination with 5-fluorouracil response rates increase

Promising responses of 84%–86% in patients with seminomatous testicular cancer have been reported; these responses include both previously treated and untreated patients; however, very poor results are reported in the treatment of nonseminomatous testicular cancer

PATIENT MONITORING

CBC, including differential leukocyte count, platelet count, and hemoglobin and hematocrit should be obtained during therapy to monitor for leukopenia, thrombocytopenia, and anemia; routine serum chemistries, especially serum creatinine, should be obtained regularly to monitor electrolyte status and renal function; although the occurrence is infrequent, neurotoxicity is reported—a complete neurologic examination should be performed at the beginning of and then intermittently through therapy; health care professionals responsible for monitoring patients on carboplatin therapy should be familiar with the less common adverse effects that can occur with therapy

NURSING INTERVENTIONS

Monitor treatment tolerance, weight, nutritional status; ensure that appropriate lab tests are conducted to monitor for leukopenia, thrombocytopenia, anemia, and renal function; nausea and vomiting are usually mild to moderate—appropriate antiemetics should be given for management; fluid hydration should be given concurrently; notify physician of uncommon adverse events such as hypersensitivity reactions and skin rashes

PATIENT INFORMATION

Call the doctor immediately if intractable nausea and vomiting occur, unusual bruising and bleeding occur, temperature over 101°F; avoid exposure to people with infections; continue hydration by drinking several glasses of water for 1 or 2 d after therapy

FORMULATION

Available as Paraplatin (Bristol-Myers Oncology Division, Princeton, NJ) in 50-, 150-, and 450-mg vials

Carboplatin is available as a sterile, lyophilized white powder for injection containing equal parts of carboplatin and mannitol; unopened vials should be stored at room temperature and protected from light; the drug must be reconstituted with either sterile water for injection, 0.9% sodium chloride, or dextrose 5% and water yielding a concentration of 10 mg/mL; the reconstituted solution is stable for 8 h and should be discarded because the drug contains no antibacterial preservative; after reconstitution, carboplatin may be further diluted in 0.9% sodium chloride or dextrose 5% water and should be given a 24-h expiration; carboplatin can be infused over 30 or 60 min or 24 h; during preparation and administration, aluminum needles and administration sets should not be used (when carboplatin comes in contact with aluminum the interaction will form a precipitate and result in loss of potency of the drug)

CARMUSTINE

Carmustine (also known a BiCNU or BCNU) is a nitrosourea derivative that has demonstrated cytotoxic activity against a wide variety of malignancies. As with other alkylating agents, carmustine is considered to be cell cycle nonspecific. Active metabolites are responsible for the alkylation, DNA crosslink formation, and carbamoylation activity that interferes with DNA, RNA, and protein synthesis. Cross-resistance between carmustine and lomustine has occurred. Tumors expressing high O6-alkylguanine-DNA alkyltransferase are resistant. Carmustine and its metabolites are distributed rapidly into the cerebrospinal fluid. Nitrosoureas as a class tend to be highly lipophilic, thus enhancing their ability to cross the blood–brain barrier and to be used in the treatment of meningeal leukemias and brain tumors. The long-term use of nitrosoureas has been associated with profound cumulative myelosuppression and renal failure (especially with methyl-CCNU, used investigationally only) with lesions similar to radiation-induced nephritis.

Topical preparations of carmustine have been used to treat mycosis fungoides (cutaneous T-cell lymphoma, or CTCL). Historically topical nitrogen mustard (mechlorethamine) has been used for mycosis fungoides. The mechanism of action is unknown because the alkylating action of mechlorethamine is dissipated shortly after it is dissolved in water but the anti-CTCL activity still remains. The mechanism of action of topical carmustine is similarly unknown.

DOSAGE AND ADMINISTRATION

Adult doses ranging from 30–200 mg/m^2 have been used; may be given as a single slow infusion or divided into multiple infusions over 2–5 d every 6 wk; repeat doses should not be given until leukocyte count is > 4000/mm^3, absolute neutrophil count is < 1500/mm^3, and platelet count is > 100,000/mm^3; doses up to 600 mg/m^2 (as a single dose or divided over 3 d) are used in single-agent or combination therapy in autologous bone marrow transplant protocols for breast cancer or advanced neoplasms [43]

The manufacturer suggests adjusting subsequent doses according to previous treatment nadirs

NADIR AFTER PRIOR DOSAGE (CELLS/MM^3)

Leukocytes	Platelets	Amount of Prior Dose to be Given, %
> 4000	< 100,000	100
3000–3999	75,000–99,999	100
2000–2999	25,000–74,999	70
< 2000	<25,000	50

Some clinicians use absolute neutrophil count (ANC) as the basis of dose adjustment; in which case, reduce the dose by 2.5% for an ANC at nadir of < 1000/mm^3 and by 50% for an ANC < 500/mm^3.

Carmustine is applied topically for mycosis fungoides in a hydroalcoholic solution or ointment in concentrations of 0.05%–0.4%. Topical carmustine is applied once or twice a day. Carmustine can also be given intralesionally at concentrations of 0.1%–0.2% for the management of persistent papules or small nodules associated with mycosis fungoides

INDICATIONS

FDA-approved: Palliative treatment of primary and metastatic brain tumors; used in combination with prednisone and other cytotoxic agents in the treatment of multiple myeloma; used in combination with other chemotherapeutic agents for the treatment of disseminated Hodgkin's disease and non-Hodgkin's lymphoma; clinical studies show activity in carcinoma of the lung, carcinoma of the GI tract, breast carcinoma, Ewing's sarcoma, malignant melanoma, Burkitt's lymphoma; as a topical formulation, carmustine has been shown to have activity in mycosis fungoides

PHARMACOKINETICS

Absorption: not absorbed across the GI tract; absorption from topical application is apparent; **Distribution:** cleared rapidly from the plasma; carmustine and its metabolites rapidly cross the blood–brain barrier; cerebrospinal fluid concentrations of metabolites have been reported to be 15%–70% of the concurrent plasma concentrations; plasma carmustine is ~77% protein bound; is also distributed in breast milk; **Metabolism/Elimination**— rapidly metabolized by the liver; approximately 60%–70% of carmustine and its metabolites are excreted in the urine within 96 h, 6%–7% are excreted as carbon dioxide by the lungs, and 1% is excreted in the feces; average plasma half-life is 22 min; volume of distribution reported in some studies has been as high as 5.1 L/kg; researchers have discovered great patient-to-patient variation in plasma clearance of carmustine—factors causing such variation may include the percent of body fat, serum lipid concentration, and sample collection; some enterohepatic circulation is believed to occur

DRUG INTERACTIONS

Concomitant use of cimetidine and carmustine can result in increased bone marrow toxicity

RESPONSE RATES

When used as a single agent for brain tumors, objective response rates occur in ~50% of patients; similar response rates are reported with carmustine-containing chemotherapy combinations

The use of carmustine and prednisone in multiple myeloma has produced response rates of 39%, as opposed to a response rate of 11% when carmustine is used alone

Response rates of 50% have been demonstrated in patients with advanced Hodgkin's disease refractory to other established treatments; carmustine has been used as a substitute for mechlorethamine in MOPP therapy

For patients with non-Hodgkin's lymphoma, a 28% response rate has been reported using carmustine alone

Carmustine is considered inferior to dacarbazine in the treatment of malignant melanoma; although response rates of 30% have been reported in the treatment of malignant melanoma, carmustine-containing combinations have failed to produce adequate CNS response

A 21% response rate has been reported with carmustine in the treatment of solid tumors: lung, breast, and GI tract

(Continued on next page)

The information here is provided as guidance only. Prescribers should always consult the manufacturer's current prescribing information

12

CARMUSTINE (Continued)

SPECIAL PRECAUTIONS

Because of the prolonged myelosuppression, treatment should not be given more often than every 6 wk; blood counts should be performed weekly for 6–8 wk after administration of carmustine; pulmonary toxicity appears to be related to cumulative dose; pulmonary function tests should be performed prior to therapy, and follow-up tests should be performed if patient becomes symptomatic and particularly after cumulative doses of 400 mg/m^2 or more; drug accumulation may occur in patients with hepatic or renal dysfunction; therefore, routine monitoring of liver and renal function should be performed; carmustine is contraindicated in patients who have demonstrated previous hypersensitivity to the drug; safety and efficacy in children has not been established; all cytotoxic drugs may be embryotoxic or teratogenic; use with caution in pregnant and nursing patients; carmustine has been shown to affect the fertility of male rats receiving higher than usual human doses

TOXICITIES

Hematologic: delayed cumulative hematologic toxicity is the major dose limiting adverse effect; leukocyte nadir occurs first at approximately 15 d after therapy, then a second, lower nadir occurs at approximately 4–6 wk and persists for 1–2 wk after carmustine administration; the degree of leukopenia depends on previous exposure to chemotherapy and can vary among patients; thrombocytopenia is usually the most severe hematologic effect, occurring about 4 wk after therapy and persisting 1–2 wk; anemia can occur but generally is less frequent and less severe than the other hematologic toxicities; bone marrow aplasia occurs at doses of ≥ 600 mg/m^2; rarely, acute leukemias and bone marrow dysplasias have been reported with long-term therapy; **GI:** moderate to severe nausea and vomiting beginning minutes to 2 h after IV administration and lasting 4–6 h after is common; diarrhea, esophagitis, anorexia, and dysphagia occur less frequently; **Pulmonary:** pulmonary infiltrates or fibrosis can be common in patients who have received cumulative doses > 400 mg/m^2; pulmonary toxicity can be progressive and fatal, and its onset may be delayed; oxygen exposure increases the risk of pulmonary fibrosis and should be limited; early use of corticosteroids may prevent fibrosis; **Hepatic:** generally mild and reversible hepatotoxicity has been reported in up to 26% of patients; incidence of hepatic dysfunction may increase with high-dose therapy; **Miscellaneous:** renal toxicity is rare but can occur in patients who have received cumulative doses > 600 mg/m^2; significant hypotension can occur, especially with high-dose therapy; tachycardia and hypotension are associated with intense flushing of the skin of the face and upper chest (this reaction can persist for several hours after the infusion is completed and is believed to be due to the combination of carmustine itself and the alcohol used to reconstitute the drug); dementia has been reported with high-dose regimens; burning at the site of injection; after topical application, dermatologic effects have occurred such as severe dermatitis, petechiae, hyperpigmentation, telangiectasia, and hypersensitivity reactions (occur rarely); mild bone marrow depression incidence is < 10%

RESPONSE RATES (Continued)

Good results have been described in the treatment of mycosis fungoides with topical carmustine; in studies comparing the use of carmustine versus nitrogen mustard, efficacy of the two agents appeared to be equal, with carmustine causing less hypersensitivity reactions and topical side effects; 5-y survival rates are approximately 30% with carmustine depending on the stage of the disease at the time of treatment; in high doses (400–600 mg/m^2), carmustine is effective in combination therapy for refractory breast cancer, non-Hodgkin's lymphoma, Hodgkin's disease, and glioma [51,52]

PATIENT MONITORING

CBC, including differential leukocyte count and platelet count, is generally obtained weekly for 6–8 wk after administration of carmustine to monitor for leukopenia, thrombocytopenia, and anemia—some clinicians suggest waiting 2–3 wk after therapy before obtaining the first CBC and then following up with weekly labs until blood counts are normal or appropriate for subsequent treatment, usually within 6–8 wk; monitor renal, hepatic, and pulmonary status; health care professionals responsible for monitoring patients receiving carmustine therapy should be familiar with the broad spectrum of other adverse effects that can occur, albeit less commonly, with this treatment; pulmonary toxicity may be increased by long radiation

NURSING INTERVENTIONS

Monitor treatment tolerance, weight, and nutritional status; educate patients about neutropenic precautions and self-care at home; wear gloves while administering carmustine and avoid contact with the skin (hyperpigmentation of the skin is common after accidental contact); do not mix with other drugs during IV administration; if pain occurs at the infusion site, dilute solution further or slow the infusion rate; carmustine is considered an irritant—if extravasation occurs, stop infusion immediately and infiltrate the area with injections of 0.5 mEq/mL sodium bicarbonate solution; nausea and vomiting are common (give appropriate antiemetics); intense facial and upper chest flushing may occur due to the alcohol used during reconstitution—this will resolve within 2–4 h and can usually be minimized by slowing the infusion; along with the flushing, significant hypotension (particularly with high-dose therapy) can occur; therefore, blood pressure should be monitored during and after the infusion

PATIENT INFORMATION

Call the doctor immediately if the following occurs: unusual bruising or bleeding, temperature over 101°F, sore throat, or other signs of infection; avoid aspirin and nonsteroidal antiinflammatory agents; avoid exposure to people with infections; follow-up blood counts are essential when receiving carmustine therapy

FORMULATION

Available as BiCNU (Bristol-Myers Oncology Division, Princeton, NJ) 100-mg vial; the drug should appear as dry flakes or as a dry, congealed mass; the drug should be stored at 2–8°C; if an oily film has formed in the vial, the drug has decomposed due to warm temperatures and should be discarded; carmustine powder should be reconstituted with 3 mL dehydrated alcohol provided by the manufacturer followed by 27 mL sterile water for injection; the reconstituted solution must be further diluted in either normal saline or 5% dextrose and water before administration; solutions of 0.2 mg/mL in glass containers are stable for 4–8 h when refrigerated and protected from light; plastic IV bags should not be used due to instability; patients with central IV catheters can tolerate carmustine solutions in a total volume of 250 mL; patients with peripheral IV lines should have the solutions further diluted with a total volume of 500 mL; for preparation of the topical solution, reconstitute a 100-mg vial as per the manufacturer, add the reconstituted drug to a 60-mL light-resistant bottle, and fill it to a total volume of 50 mL with 95% alcohol (concentration = 2 mg/mL); the prepared solution has a shelf-life of 2–3 mo when kept at 4°C

CHLORAMBUCIL

Chlorambucil is a bifunctional alkylating agent of the nitrogen mustard type. It is a cell cycle nonspecific antineoplastic agent that is cytotoxic to nonproliferating cells. Its antineoplastic activity occurs from the formation of an unstable ethyleneimmonium ion, which then alkylates or binds with intracellular structures. The cytotoxicity of chlorambucil is due to cross-linking of strands of DNA and RNA and to inhibition of protein synthesis. Additionally, chlorambucil is metabolized to phenylacetic acid mustard, which is also a bifunctional alkylating agent. Phenylacetic acid mustard has shown antineoplastic activity in some human cell lines approximately equal to that of chlorambucil. Chlorambucil also has immunosuppressant activity. It has the slowest onset of activity and the least toxicity of the classic nitrogen mustard type agents.

DOSAGE AND ADMINISTRATION

Chlorambucil is used alone or in combination with other agents such as prednisone. The incidence and severity of side effects may be altered in combination regimens. Most patients require dose reductions sometime during therapy.
Chronic lymphocytic leukemia: *Remission induction*—0.1–0.2 mg/kg (4–10 mg total) daily for 3–6 wk (given as single or divided doses); *Maintenance*—2–4 mg daily; *Intermittent or pulse therapy*—1.5–2 mg/kg every month; 0.4 mg/kg every 2 wk, increasing by 0.1-mg/kg increments to toxicity or remission; **Hodgkin's and non-Hodgkin's lymphoma:** 0.1–0.2 mg/kg/d or 0.4 mg/kg every 2 wk, increased by 0.1-mg/kg increments to toxicity or remission (duration of therapy is usually 6–12 mo); **immunosuppressant for nephrotic syndrome:** 0.1–0.2 mg/kg/d in a single dose for 8–12 wk
If lymphocytic infiltration of the bone marrow is present or the bone marrow is hypoplastic, do not exceed a dose of 0.1 mg/kg/d; chlorambucil dose should be adjusted to patient response and the dose reduced if there is an abrupt decrease in leukocyte count; short courses of treatment are safer than continuous maintenance therapy although both methods of treatment are effective
Dose adjustments for organ dysfunction: no information

SPECIAL PRECAUTIONS

Do not give at full dosage prior to 4 wk after a full course of radiation therapy or chemotherapy because of the vulnerability of the bone marrow to damage; may treat with a reduced dose if pretherapy leukocyte or platelet counts are depressed from bone marrow disease process prior to institution of therapy; follow patients carefully to avoid life-threatening damage to the bone marrow—decrease dosage if leukocyte or platelet counts fall below normal values; use with caution in patients with a history of seizures or a history of hypersensitivity to the drug; safe and effective use in pediatric patients has not been fully established—it has been used if the potential benefits outweigh the risks

(Continued on next page)

INDICATIONS

FDA-approved: Palliation for chronic lymphocytic leukemia (CLL), malignant lymphomas, lymphosarcoma, giant follicular lymphoma, and Hodgkin's disease; clinical trials show activity in hairy cell leukemia, acute histiocytosis X, autoimmune hepatic anemias, advanced breast cancer, nonseminomatous testicular carcinoma, multiple myeloma, mycosis fungoides, Wegener's granulomatosis, sarcoidosis, macroglobulinemia, polycythemia vera, ovarian cancer, nephrotic syndrome, and thrombocythemia

PHARMACOKINETICS

Absorption: rapidly absorbed from the GI tract with peak plasma levels reached in 1 h; oral bioavailability is estimated to be 50%; **Distribution:** chlorambucil and its metabolites are extensively protein bound (99%) to plasma proteins (primarily albumin); it is not known if chlorambucil crosses the blood–brain barrier, although some adverse CNS effects have been reported; chlorambucil apparently crosses the placenta; it is unknown if the drug or its metabolites are distributed into breast milk; **Metabolism:** extensively metabolized in the liver and its primary metabolite, phenylacetic acid mustard, is pharmacologically active; **Elimination:** reported plasma half-lives of the parent drug and phenylacetic acid are 90 and 145 min, respectively; chlorambucil is excreted via the kidneys almost completely as its metabolites; < 1% is excreted as unchanged chlorambucil or phenylacetic acid mustard; most of the drug is excreted as the monohydroxy and dihydroxy derivatives

DRUG INTERACTIONS

Chlorambucil toxicity is potentiated by barbiturates, possibly by inducing hepatic activation of chlorambucil (discontinue barbiturate if possible); probenecid, sulfinpyrazone, bone marrow depressants, and immunosuppressants also have clinically significant interactions with chlorambucil

RESPONSE RATES

CLL: a decrease in lymphocyte count and lymphadenopathy generally are seen over a minimum of 3–12 mo of therapy; response rates to chlorambucil as a single agent range from 64%–75%; in combination with prednisone, response rates of 38%–87% are reported; recent studies indicate similar responses with fludarabine, and combination therapy has been proposed.
Hodgkin's disease: chlorambucil in combination with vinblastine, procarbazine, and prednisone (Ch1VPP) has been used as a substitute for MOPP therapy, yielding response rates of 70%–89%
Malignant lymphomas: chlorambucil used alone in the treatment of non-Hodgkin's lymphoma has produced complete response rates of 10%–15% and partial response of 40%–70%; intermittent regimens of chlorambucil to treat nodular lymphocytic lymphomas have produced complete responses of 60%–70%

(Continued on next page)

CHLORAMBUCIL (Continued)

TOXICITIES

Hematologic: hematologic effects are the major dose-limiting side effects of chlorambucil; for continuous treatment courses, leukopenia usually appears after the third week of therapy and generally will last between 2–4 wk after discontinuation of therapy; after administration of a single high-dose treatment, leukocyte and platelet nadirs will occur between 7–14 d and will recover in approximately 2–3 wk; thrombocytopenia may continue longer than leukopenia; bone marrow suppression usually is reversible up to a cumulative dose of 6.5 mg/kg in a single-treatment course; acute leukemias and bone marrow dysplasias have been reported with long-term therapy; **GI:** nausea and vomiting (mild), diarrhea, oral ulceration, anorexia, and abdominal pain; **Hepatic:** hepatotoxicity including jaundice, hepatic necrosis, and cirrhosis have rarely been reported; **Pulmonary:** bronchopulmonary dysplasia, pulmonary fibrosis, and interstitial pneumonia (pulmonary effects are rare and occur usually with prolonged therapy); **Reproductive:** sterility (high incidence) in prepubertal and pubertal males, azoospermia, and amenorrhea; **CNS:** tremors, muscular twitching, confusion, agitation, ataxia, flaccid paresis, hallucinations (rare), and seizures; **Miscellaneous:** drug fever, skin hypersensitivity, peripheral neuropathy, sterile cystitis, keratitis, hyperuricemia, and uric acid nephropathy

PATIENT MONITORING

CBC, including hematocrit, hemoglobin, platelet count, and total leukocyte counts should be obtained at periodic intervals (every 2 wk) throughout therapy; other lab tests such as SGPT, SGOT, lactate dehydrogenase and serum uric acid levels are recommended prior to therapy and at periodic intervals; monitor for incidence of leukopenia and thrombocytopenia as these parameters are used to individualize dosage

NURSING INTERVENTIONS

Monitor treatment tolerance, weight, nutritional status; administer antiemetics as necessary; educate patient about most common side effects of chlorambucil, neutropenic precautions, and self-care at home; hyperuricemia can be prevented by adequate hydration and the administration of allopurinol; if patient is unable to swallow tablets, an aqueous suspension can be made from the tablets at a concentration of 2 mg/mL

PATIENT INFORMATION

Call the doctor immediately if vomiting occurs shortly after the dose is taken or a sore throat, fever, or any unusual bruising or bleeding develops; take tablets on an empty stomach; the total daily dose can be taken at one time; chlorambucil may cause permanent or temporary sterility; avoid aspirin and nonsteroidal antiinflammatory agents; avoid exposure to people with infections; follow-up blood counts are essential when receiving chlorambucil therapy

FORMULATION

Available as Leukeran (Glaxo-Wellcome, Research Triangle Park, NC) 2-mg sugar-coated tablets in bottles of 50 tablets; should be stored in a well-closed, light-resistant container at 15–30°C; an oral solution containing 2 mg/mL can be extemporaneously prepared from the tablets using a suspending agent and a syrup; the suspension is stable for 7 d at 5°C

CISPLATIN

Discovered accidentally in 1965 during experiments examining the effects of electricity on the growth of *Escherichia coli*, cisplatin was the first heavy metal compound shown to have antineoplastic activity. During phase I trials cisplatin was nearly discarded due to its extreme gastrointestinal and renal toxicities. However, responses reported with testicular cancer showed promise and researchers developed mechanisms to decrease toxicity.

The mechanism of action of cisplatin is similar to alkylating agents and it is therefore considered a nonclassical alkylator. The *cis*, not the *trans*, isomer of cisplatin is the active moiety. In the relatively high chloride concentrations of plasma, the cisplatin complex is un-ionized and able to pass through cell membranes. In the presence of low chloride concentrations, intracellularly, the chloride ligands of the complex are displaced by water and produce the positively charged platinum compound, which is toxic and probably the active form of the drug. The *cis* isomer forms intrastrand and interstrand cross-links between guanine-guanine pairs of DNA and inhibits synthesis. Cisplatin, to a lesser extent, binds to RNA and protein, ultimately inhibiting synthesis. Other cytotoxic activity may include tumor immunogenicity, and the drug has immunosuppressive, radiosensitizing, and antimicrobial properties.

DOSAGE AND ADMINISTRATION

Testicular cancer: usually used in combination with other cytotoxic drugs such as bleomycin and vinblastine; 20–40 mg/m^2 of cisplatin daily for 5 d *or* 120 mg/m^2 as a single dose every 3–4 wk

Ovarian cancer: usually used in combination with doxorubicin; 30–120 mg/m^2 as a single dose every 3–4 wk

Bladder cancer: 50–70 mg/m^2 as a single dose every 3–4 wk *or* 1 mg/kg once a week for 6 wk then every 3 wk thereafter

Head and neck cancer, cervical cancer, non–small cell lung cancer: treatment varies in dosing schedule and whether single-agent or combination therapy is used; doses range from 50–120 mg/m^2 every 3–6 wk

Bladder cancer, malignant melanoma, osteogenic sarcoma: intraarterial dosing is usually reserved for treatment of regionally confined malignancies such as advanced bladder cancer, malignant melanoma, and osteogenic sarcoma, in doses ranging from 75–150 mg/m^2 as a single dose every 2–5 wk for 1–4 courses

Advanced ovarian carcinoma, carcinoid tumors, and mesotheliomas: intraperitoneal dosing of cisplatin is used primarily in the treatment of advanced ovarian carcinoma, carcinoid tumors, and mesotheliomas, which may or may not be associated with malignant ascites, in doses ranging from 60–270 mg/m^2

Pediatric osteogenic sarcoma or neuroblastoma: reported doses are 90 mg/m^2 once every 3 wk or 30 mg/m^2 once a week

Recurrent pediatric brain tumors: 60 mg/m^2 daily for 2 d every 3–4 wk

High-dose therapy: doses up to 40 mg/m^2 daily × 5 are used in patients receiving combination high-dose therapy for lymphoma

Dose adjustments for renal impairment: clinicians recommend avoiding treatment in patients with a serum creatinine ≥ 1.5 or a creatinine clearance (CLcr) of < 50 mL/min; other guidelines suggest reducing dose to 75% of the usual in patients with CLcr of 10–50 mL/min and 50% of usual in patients with CLcr < 10 mL/min

(Continued on next page)

INDICATIONS

FDA-approved: Treatment of metastatic testicular and ovarian tumors and advanced bladder cancer; clinical studies show activity in head and neck cancer, cervical carcinoma, lung cancer, osteogenic sarcoma, neuroblastoma, recurrent brain tumors, advanced esophageal carcinoma, advanced prostatic carcinoma, malignant melanoma, endometrial cancer, penile carcinoma, breast carcinoma, advanced Hodgkin's disease, malignant lymphomas, advanced soft tissue and bone sarcomas, refractory choriocarcinoma, metastatic adrenal carcinoma, malignant thymoma, medullary carcinoma of the thyroid, and gastric carcinoma

PHARMACOKINETICS

Absorption: cisplatin is not administered orally or intramuscularly; when given by the intraperitoneal route, 50% to 100% of the drug is absorbed systemically

Distribution: after administration of cisplatin, the platinum compound is widely distributed into the tissues exhibiting high concentrations in the kidneys, liver, and prostate; platinum concentrations also can be found in the bladder, muscle, testes, pancreas, spleen, the small and large intestines, adrenals, heart, lungs, lymph nodes, thyroid, gallbladder, thymus, cerebrum, cerebellum, ovaries, and uterus; platinum can accumulate in the tissues and be detected for up to 6 mo after the last dose of cisplatin; the volume of distribution is estimated between 20–80 L; cisplatin is rapidly distributed into pleural effusions and ascitic fluid; it is not known if platinum distributes into breast milk or crosses the placenta; platinum-containing products generally do not penetrate the CNS; low platinum concentrations have been found in tumors of the brain but seldom in healthy brain tissue; cisplatin is extensively and irreversibly protein bound to plasma and tissue proteins—protein binding measures ≥90%

Metabolism: unclear; the drug may undergo some enterohepatic circulation

Elimination: cisplatin is primarily excreted unchanged in the urine; total elimination tends to decrease with time; initial phase half-life is ~25–79 min, whereas a terminal phase half-life of 73–290 h has been reported; hemodialysis minimally removes cisplatin and its platinum-containing products

DRUG INTERACTIONS

The administration of other nephrotoxic drugs, such as aminoglycosides and amphotericin should be avoided (unless clearly indicated) for at least 2 wk after treatment with cisplatin, although evidence of synergistic toxicity is lacking; however, concurrent administration increases the risk of nephrotoxicity and acute renal failure significantly; ototoxicity may be exacerbated by the concomitant administration of the other ototoxic drugs, such as aminoglycosides and diuretics; a synergistic antineoplastic effect has been reported with cisplatin and etoposide; other possibly synergistic agents include bleomycin, doxorubicin, 5-fluorouracil, methotrexate, vinblastine, and vincristine; cisplatin may alter the renal clearance of some drugs as a result of drug-induced nephrotoxicity, thus possibly causing increased systemic toxicity of the renally cleared drug; there may be a possible drug interaction with cisplatin and anticonvulsant drugs—anticonvulsant plasma levels have been reported to be subtherapeutic during cisplatin therapy

RESPONSE RATES

Testicular neoplasms: cisplatin is one of the most active agents used in the treatment of nonseminomatous testicular carcinoma; although cisplatin can be used as a single agent, combination therapy including cisplatin, bleomycin, and vinblastine

(Continued on next page)

CISPLATIN (Continued)

SPECIAL PRECAUTIONS

Safety and efficacy of cisplatin in children has not been established—however, cisplatin therapy has shown encouraging results in the treatment of pediatric osteogenic sarcoma, neuroblastoma, and recurrent brain tumors; cisplatin may be mutagenic and carcinogenic but a direct causal relationship has not been fully elucidated; all cytotoxic drugs may be embryotoxic or teratogenic; use with caution in pregnant or nursing patients; contraindicated in patients who have experienced hypersensitivity reactions to platinum-containing compounds

TOXICITIES

Renal: nephrotoxicity is dose-related and can be severe without appropriate hydration, renal toxicity is associated with increased serum creatinine, BUN, serum uric acid, or decrease in creatinine clearance and glomerular filtration rate; cisplatin-induced renal toxicity is directly associated with renal tubular damage; nephrotoxicity typically appears during the second week after administration of the drug, or within several days after high-dose therapy; renal impairment is usually reversible when associated with low- to moderate-dose regimens but high-dose and repeated therapy may cause irreversible renal insufficiency; recovery generally occurs within 2–4 wk

Electrolyte: due to cisplatin-induced renal tubular dysfunction, electrolyte disturbances are common; hypomagnesemia, hypokalemia, hypocalcemia, hypophosphatemia, and hyponatremia can occur and may persist for several weeks; hypomagnesemia and hypocalcemia can be delayed in onset up to 3–4 wk after therapy

GI: moderate to severe nausea and vomiting are dose-related and may be intractable, especially with rapid infusion of high doses; GI disturbances begin within 1 h of starting cisplatin and can last 8–12 h after administration; delayed nausea and vomiting can occur for up to 5 d and are difficult to manage; anorexia often occurs due to the delayed nausea and vomiting; diarrhea occurs rarely but may increase in frequency when cisplatin is combined with other cytotoxic agents or when high-dose therapy is used

Otic: ototoxicity is usually manifested by tinnitus or high-frequency hearing loss (ototoxicity is reported in up to 31% of patients receiving usual doses); it also may be related to administration time, rapid infusions causing more hearing loss than slow infusions over 1–3 h or 24 h; audiogram abnormalities can be both unilateral and bilateral and may be more severe in children than in adults

Nervous system: neurotoxicity is usually characterized by peripheral neuropathies, including sensory (paresthesias) and motor (gait); neuronal impairment typically is associated with prolonged therapy (4–7 mo) but can occur after single doses; peripheral neuropathy can be irreversible but in most patients it can be partially or completely reversible after discontinuation of the cisplatin; tonic-clonic seizures, slurred speech, loss of taste, memory loss, and intention tremor have also been reported; recovery may take 4–12 mo

Hematologic: leukopenia, thrombocytopenia, and anemia are usually mild to moderate and occur in approximately 25%–30% of patients; an increased incidence of myelosuppression can occur in patients who have been heavily pretreated with cisplatin or other antineoplastic agents; leukocyte and platelet nadirs usually appear 18–23 d after cisplatin therapy with levels returning to baseline by day 39; anemia is suspected to be caused by myelosuppression, decreased erythropoiesis, and hemolysis; acute leukemia has been reported but is rare

(Continued on next page)

RESPONSE RATES *(Continued)*

provides improved responses; patients with stage III disseminated disease receiving combination therapy usually achieve complete remissions ranging from 60%–70%; response rates are higher in patients with minimal stage III disease; disease-free remissions for > 2 y are considered cure; combination of cisplatin and etoposide also has been used in disseminated disease, producing complete remissions of 50%; in seminoma testis and extragonadal germ cell tumors, cisplatin alone or in combination therapy can produce response rates similar to those reported in the treatment of nonseminomatous testicular carcinoma

Cisplatin alone can produce objective responses of 25%–33% in the treatment of advanced ovarian carcinoma refractory to prior chemotherapy or radiation therapy; complete responses are rare; patients who were previously untreated usually achieve increased response rates; combination therapy with doxorubicin can produce overall response rates of 35%–80%; other combinations with cisplatin, cyclophosphamide, and doxorubicin yield improved response rates of 50%–85%—using this three-drug combination and adding altretamine produces response rates of 50%–95%

Intraperitoneal administration of cisplatin for the treatment of advanced ovarian cancers produces varied response rates

Partial response rates lasting 5–7 mo are produced in about one third of bladder cancer patients when treated with cisplatin alone; the superiority of combination cisplatin-based therapy is not established; slightly higher response rates have been reported when cisplatin is combined with cyclophosphamide or with methotrexate and vinblastine

Cisplatin has been reported to produce 30% response rates in patients with metastatic squamous cell carcinoma of the head and neck; several cisplatin-based treatment combinations have been used but most studies are uncontrolled and results are varied

Response rates of 25%–50% have been reported in the treatment of recurrent or advanced squamous cell carcinoma of the cervix. The role of combination therapy has not been established

Lung cancer: cisplatin is one of the more active chemotherapy agents in the treatment of non–small cell carcinoma; objective responses of 15%–20% have been reported with cisplatin therapy; cisplatin-based combinations with cyclophosphamide and doxorubicin or etoposide and vinblastine or vinorelbine have produced slightly increased response rates of 25%–50%; cisplatin alone produces very poor responses in patients with small cell lung carcinoma; when cisplatin is combined with etoposide-containing regimens, high but varied response rates have been produced; median survival after treatment usually averages 12–16 mo

Lymphoma: the combination of cisplatin, carmustine, and etoposide in high doses with autologous progenitor cell infusion has shown a 4% long-term remission in patients with recurrent or refractory disease

PATIENT MONITORING

Renal function should be monitored frequently—the manufacturer recommends avoiding subsequent treatment until renal function has returned to normal; complete serum chemistries should be obtained to monitor electrolyte status, paying particular attention to serum magnesium, potassium, sodium, and calcium concentrations—electrolytes should be supplemented as needed; because cisplatin-induced ototoxicity is cumulative, audiometry should be performed prior to initial and repeated therapies—many clinicians suggest withholding cisplatin until audiometric determinations are within normal limits; neurologic exams should be performed routinely; CBC, including leukocyte count differential and platelet count, should be obtained every week or every other week to monitor for leukopenia, anemia, and thrombocytopenia

TOXICITIES (Continued)

Sensitivity reactions: anaphylactoid reactions usually occur after at least five doses of cisplatin; the mechanism of the hypersensitivity is not known but may be immune mediated; these reactions manifest as facial edema, flushing, wheezing, and respiratory difficulty, tachycardia, and hypotension and will appear within minutes after IV administration; mild hypersensitivity reactions such as urticarial or nonspecific maculopapular rashes, recurrent dermatitis, and erythema

Ocular: optic neuritis, papilledema, and cerebral blindness have been reported

Cardiovascular: bradycardia, left bundle branch block, ST-T wave changes with congestive heart failure, postural hypotension, and hypertension have all been reported but are considered rare; these effects may be due to cisplatin directly or due to electrolyte changes during cisplatin therapy

Miscellaneous: hepatic effects of mild and transient elevations of serum AST (SGOT) and ALT (SGPT) concentrations occur rarely; local effects such as phlebitis and, rarely, severe cellulitis with fibrosis or skin necrosis after extravasation have been reported; the incidence of the following is infrequent: hyperuricemia (due to drug-induced nephrotoxicity), mild alopecia, myalgia, pyrexia, gingival platinum line, aspermia, and syndrome of inappropriate antidiuretic hormone secretion

NURSING INTERVENTIONS

Anaphylactic-like reactions have been reported to occur within minutes of cisplatin administration; these reactions usually occur in patients who have been previously exposed to platinum-containing compounds; antihistamines, epinephrine, oxygen, and corticosteroids should be readily available in case of anaphylaxis

Monitor treatment tolerance, weight, and nutritional status; nausea and vomiting occur in ≥ 90% of patients receiving cisplatin; appropriate antiemetics such as metoclopramide (2 or 3 mg/kg) or serotonin antagonists in combination with dexamethasone or lorazepam or diphenhydramine should be used; phenothiazine antiemetics (ie, prochlorperazine) usually are not effective

Extensive hydration is successful in preventing or decreasing the occurrence and severity of renal toxicity—there are several effective methods of hydration, all routinely include the following: before administering cisplatin, maintain urine output at 100–150 mL/h using 1–2 L of D5W 1/2 NS or 0.9% sodium chloride supplemented with potassium or magnesium; use IV furosemide if urine output is not satisfactory; 12.5 g mannitol can be added to the cisplatin IV bag or given IV push before the cisplatin is administered to maintain appropriate urine output during the infusion; and post-hydration equaling 1–2 L of fluid should be used; hydration should be modified in patients with cardiovascular compromise

Ensure that appropriate labs are drawn to monitor electrolyte status, renal function, and hematologic parameters

Do not use aluminum-containing IV administration sets with cisplatin (aluminum will interact with cisplatin causing a precipitate to form with loss of potency)

Cisplatin is not a vesicant but can cause tissue irritation if extravasated; extent of tissue damage is concentration dependent; fibrosis and necrosis have been reported

When cisplatin is administered intraperitoneally, remember that much of the drug is systemically absorbed and can cause the same side effects; appropriate antiemetics and monitoring of electrolyte, renal, and hematologic status are still warranted

Monitor for ototoxicity and neurotoxicity at each visit

PATIENT INFORMATION

Call the doctor immediately if unusual bruising or bleeding occurs; temperature of ≥ 101°F; intractable nausea and vomiting occur; hearing loss occurs; or numbness or tingling in hands or feet occur; avoid exposure to people with infections; maintain adequate fluid intake for several days after receiving cisplatin, especially if nausea and vomiting are persistent—this will decrease the incidence of kidney damage and dehydration

FORMULATION

Available as an aqueous solution of 1 mg/mL in 50- and 100-mg vials (Platinol-AQ, Bristol-Myers Squibb Oncology Division, Princeton, NJ)

Cisplatin solution for injection should be protected from light and stored at 15–25°C; cisplatin in multiple vials is stable up to 28 d in the dark; refrigeration of the powder and the reconstituted solution should be avoided due to precipitate formation; if cisplatin is accidentally stored in the refrigerator, the precipitate will dissolve at room temperature and no loss of potency is apparent; cisplatin can be further diluted in sodium chloride–containing IV solutions and are stable from 24–72 h; commonly used IV solutions are dextrose 5% and water (D5W) with 0.9% or 0.45% sodium chloride (NS or 1/2 NS) or varied concentrations of sodium chloride solutions; cisplatin is not compatible with sodium bicarbonate; the use of aluminum needles should be avoided in the preparation of cisplatin.

CYCLOPHOSPHAMIDE

Cyclophosphamide is a cell cycle nonspecific alkylating agent of the nitrogen mustard type. It is a prodrug, metabolized in the liver to active metabolites that alkylate nucleic acids. Cyclophosphamide prevents cell division by cross-linking DNA and RNA strands, resulting in an imbalance of growth within the cell, leading to cell death. Cyclophosphamide also has phosphorylating properties that enhance its cytotoxicity and it possesses significant immunosuppressive activity.

DOSAGE AND ADMINISTRATION

Cyclophosphamide is administered over a wide dosing range depending on the disease process being treated. It may be administered orally or parenterally, alone or in combination with other agents, as a part of a chemotherapy regimen. It can be given to both adults and children.

Adults: 50–100 mg/m^2 PO × 10–14 d; 50–1000 mg/m^2 as a single IV dose on d 1 and 8 (or every 14–21 d); *High-dose therapy*—2000–7000 mg/m^2 over 1–4 d; 1875 mg/m^2/d × 3 d × 1 course; 50 mg/kg/d × 4 d; *Maintenance dose*—1–5 mg/kg PO daily; 10–15 mg/kg IV q 7–10 d; 3–5 mg/kg IV twice weekly; **Children:** 2–8 mg/kg or 60–250 mg/m^2 PO or IV qd × 6 d (divide PO dosages; IV doses are given once a week); *Maintenance dose*—2–5 mg/kg or 50–150 mg/m^2 PO twice weekly; **Dosage adjustment in organ dysfunction:** patients with compromised renal function may show significantly prolonged retention of active alkylating metabolites, but no dosage adjustment is necessary; *High-dose therapy*—addition of bladder irrigation will reduce the complication of hemorrhagic cystitis; administer mesna at 20% dose equivalence of cyclophosphamide concurrently and repeat 4, 8, and 12 h later; alternatively, give 100% dose equivalency as a 24-h infusion at the start of the cyclophosphamide infusion

(Continued on next page)

INDICATIONS

FDA-approved: Cyclophosphamide is used alone or in combination with other drugs in the treatment of the following malignancies: ALL, AML, CML, CLL, acute monocytic leukemia, Hodgkin's or non-Hodgkin's lymphoma, carcinoma of the ovary or breast, multiple myeloma, Burkitt's lymphoma, neuroblastoma, retinoblastoma; cyclophosphamide is also used as an immunosuppressant in the following conditions: polymyositis, rheumatoid arthritis, Wegener's agranulomatosis, and nephrotic syndrome in children; clinical studies show activity in bronchogenic carcinoma, small cell lung carcinoma, rhabdomyosarcoma, Ewing's sarcoma, carcinomas of the GI tract, endometrium, testes, prostate, bladder, and renal cell, Wilm's tumor, squamous cell tumors of the cervix, head, and neck; it also has been used as an immunosuppressant to control rejection following kidney, heart, liver, and bone marrow transplants

PHARMACOKINETICS

Absorption: almost completely absorbed from the GI tract in doses < 100 mg; higher doses are 75% absorbed; cyclophosphamide is administered both orally and parenterally; **Distribution:** throughout the body, with minimal amounts found in saliva, sweat, and synovial fluid; crosses the blood–brain barrier to a limited extent but not enough to treat meningeal leukemia; active metabolites are approximately 50% bound to plasma proteins; **Metabolism:** metabolized to 4-hydroxycyclophosphamide, by hepatic microsomal enzymes, which is then able to cross cellular membranes and subsequently is metabolized to the active alkylating species; this metabolite is further metabolized to activate the alkylating moieties phosphoramide mustard and nornitrogen mustard and inactive metabolites; **Excretion:** primarily in the urine with 15%–30% as unchanged drug; acrolein is thought to be the metabolite that is most responsible for causing hemorrhagic cystitis; plasma half-life of the parent compound is 4–6.5 h; however, drug can be detected in the plasma for up to 72 h after administration

DRUG INTERACTIONS

Barbiturates, phenytoin, and chloral hydrate alter the metabolism of cyclophosphamide, leading to an increase in toxic metabolites; ondansetron may increase clearance of cyclophosphamide and increase formation of active metabolites; effects of other antiemetics have not been studied; corticosteroids initially inhibit cyclophosphamide activation, leading to a decreased antineoplastic effect; cyclophosphamide can potentiate the cardiotoxic effects of doxorubicin; interactions with probenecid, chloramphenicol, sulfinpyrazone, bone marrow depressants, radiation therapy, cocaine, and cytarabine all have some clinical significance; the interaction with allopurinol is controversial; allopurinol can increase the cyclophosphamide level and prolong the half-life of cyclophosphamide, leading to an increase in the side effects; the use of these two drugs in combination should be followed closely

RESPONSE RATES

Hodgkin's disease: 60% objective response rate when treated with cyclophosphamide alone
Lymphoma: 10%–20% complete response and 40%–70% objective response rate with cyclophosphamide alone; when used as part of a combination regimen, the complete response rate rose to 50%
Burkitt's lymphoma: 90% complete response rate with cyclophosphamide alone
Multiple myeloma: 30% objective response rate
ALL: 20%–40% objective response rate
AML: 10% objective response rate
Neuroblastoma: 65% objective response rate
Ovarian cancer: 60% objective response rate
Breast cancer: 35% objective response rate with cyclophosphamide alone; up to 90% objective response in combination therapy
High-dose therapy: 30%–50% response rates in patients with active disease when used in combination therapy for lymphoma, myeloma, breast cancer, and chronic myelogenous leukemias
Progenitor cell transplantations: used with busulfan and other agents as preparation prior to cell reinfusion for autologous and allogenic progenitor cell transplants for leukemias (acute and chronic) and lymphomas

(Continued on next page)

CYCLOPHOSPHAMIDE (Continued)

SPECIAL PRECAUTIONS

As with all cytotoxic drugs, use with caution in myelosuppressed patients or patients with infection due to the potential for severe immunosuppression; use with caution in patients with renal impairment; hemorrhagic myocarditis may occur within 1 wk after therapy in patients receiving high-dose cyclophosphamide; all cytotoxic drugs may be embryotoxic or teratogenic; use with caution in pregnant or nursing patients; cyclophosphamide is excreted in breast milk

TOXICITIES

Hematologic: leukopenia, bone marrow depression, thrombocytopenia, anemia; **GI:** nausea (increased incidence in high-dose regimens), vomiting, diarrhea, anorexia; **Dermatologic:** skin rash, hives, itching, increased sweating, redness, swelling, and pain at the injection site; **Renal and genitourinary:** uric acid nephropathy, hemorrhagic cystitis, nephrotoxicity, hyperuricemia (especially when used as therapy for leukemias and lymphomas); **Cardiac:** acute myopericarditis (with doses > 5 g/m^2, but rarely at lower doses); **Pulmonary:** pneumonitis, interstitial pulmonary fibrosis; **Miscellaneous:** hyperglycemia, alopecia, hepatitis, syndrome of inappropriate diuretic hormone secretion, azoospermia

PATIENT MONITORING

CBC, including hematocrit, hemoglobin, platelet count, and total and differential leukocyte counts should be obtained weekly; other serum chemistries such as BUN, serum creatinine, SGPT, SGOT, lactate dehydrogenase, and serum bilirubin should be obtained at periodic intervals throughout treatment; urinary output and specific gravity determinations are recommended following high-dose IV administration; urine should be examined for microscopic hematuria prior to and during therapy

NURSING INTERVENTIONS

Monitor treatment tolerance, weight, nutritional status; encourage good oral hygiene; administer antiemetics as necessary; encourage the patient to increase fluid intake and to void every 2 h to avoid development of hemorrhagic cystitis; educate patient regarding side effects of cyclophosphamide, and when to notify the physician; educate patient regarding care of central venous access devices; educate patient regarding self-care at home

PATIENT INFORMATION

Advise patient to avoid use of aspirin and nonsteroidal antiinflammatory agents; neutropenic precautions should be observed following treatment to reduce the risk of infection; explain side effects of cyclophosphamide (alopecia is a common side effect); stress ample fluid intake (up to 3 L/d) and to void every 2 h to reduce the risk of hemorrhagic cystitis; oral doses may be divided and given with or after a meal to lessen nausea; cyclophosphamide may be given with cold foods to improve tolerance; notify physician if blood is present in the urine

FORMULATION

Oral tablets available as Cytoxan (Bristol-Myers Oncology Division, Princeton, NJ); injection form available as Cytoxan (Bristol-Myers Oncology Division), as Neosar (Elkins-Sinn, Adria Laboratories, Dublin, OH), and as Endoxan (Asta-Werke) Available as oral tablets containing 25 or 50 mg of cyclophosphamide per tablet and as an injection in vials of 100 mg, 200 mg, 500 mg, 1 g, and 2 g of powder for reconstitution; the tablets and injection should be stored at temperatures not to exceed 25°C; the injection may be reconstituted with sterile water for injection with the resulting concentration equal to 20 mg/mL for all vial sizes; the reconstituted solution is stable for 24 h at room temperature and for 6 d under refrigeration; it is compatible with 5% dextrose in water, 5% dextrose and 0.9% sodium chloride injection, 5% dextrose and Ringer's injection, lactated Ringer's injection, 0.45% sodium chloride injection, and sodium lactate injection; an oral solution may be extemporaneously prepared from the injection using aromatic elixir, NF as a diluent and vehicle; the concentration range is 1–5 mg/mL; it should be stored tightly sealed in the refrigerator and is stable for up to 14 d

The information here is provided as guidance only. Prescribers should always consult the manufacturer's current prescribing information

20

DACARBAZINE

Dacarbazine (also known as DTIC) is a cell cycle nonspecific alkylating agent that is a synthetic analogue of the naturally occurring purine precursor, 5-amino-1H-imidazole-4-carboxamide. It is believed to exert its cytotoxic activity by three mechanisms: 1) formation of methylating carbonium ions leading to DNA alkylation at O6 of guanine; 2) antimetabolite activity as a false precursor for purine synthesis; and 3) binding with sulfhydryl groups in proteins. Cytotoxicity appears predominantly due to recognition of a methyl guanine by the mismatch repair system, resulting in apoptotic cell death. Dacarbazine is metabolized in the liver to an active hydroxylated and *N*-dimethylated species. Exposure to light also can lead to formation of an active moiety, which can contribute to cytotoxicity.

DOSAGE AND ADMINISTRATION

Dacarbazine is administered parenterally alone or in combination with other agents as part of a chemotherapy regimen. **Malignant melanoma:** 2–4.5 mg/kg/d x 10 d, every 28 d; up to 250 mg/m^2/d x 5 days, every 21 d; dosage regimens of 400–500 mg/m^2 on d 1 and 2 every 3–4 wk also have been used **Hodgkin's disease (in combination with doxorubicin, bleomycin, and vinblastine):** 150 mg/m^2 x 5 d, every 4 wk; 375 mg/m^2 on d 1, repeated every 15 d, in combination with other agents
Dosage adjustment for organ dysfunction: may be needed in patients with renal or hepatic impairment receiving repeated courses; dacarbazine therapy should be temporarily suspended if leukocyte counts fall below 3000/mm^3, absolute neutrophil count < 1000 mm^3, and platelet counts fall below 100,000/mm^3; given the frequency of nausea and vomiting, adequate antiemetics should be coadministered

(Continued on next page)

INDICATIONS

FDA-approved: Used in the treatment of malignant melanoma and Hodgkin's lymphoma; dacarbazine is rarely used as a single agent in the treatment of Hodgkin's lymphoma; combination therapy with doxorubicin, bleomycin, vinblastine, and dacarbazine (ABVD) is clearly superior to single-agent therapy; clinical studies show activity in treatment of soft-tissue sarcomas (leiomyosarcoma, fibrosarcoma, rhabdomyosarcoma), neuroblastoma, and malignant glucagonoma

PHARMACOKINETICS

Absorption: not absorbed across the GI tract; **Distribution:** localizes in body tissues, especially the liver; crosses the blood–brain barrier to a limited extent; low plasma-protein binding, approximately 20%; exhibits poor cerebrospinal fluid penetration; **Metabolism:** rapid oxidative metabolism by the liver to several compounds, some of which are active; **Elimination:** biphasic elimination with initial phase half-life of 19 min and terminal phase half life of 5 h in patients with normal renal and hepatic function; in patients with renal or hepatic impairment, the initial phase half-life is 55 min and the terminal phase half-life is 7.2 h; 30%–45% of a dose is excreted in the urine within 6 h, about half as unchanged dacarbazine and half as metabolites

DRUG INTERACTIONS

Barbiturates and phenytoin increase the metabolism of dacarbazine leading to a decrease in activity; reports of enhanced efficacy of dacarbazine in combination with bacillus Calmette-Guérin (BCG) immunotherapy in advanced malignant melanoma are controversial; dacarbazine is physically incompatible with solutions containing hydrocortisone sodium succinate

RESPONSE RATES

About 20% of metastatic malignant melanoma patients obtain an objective response of > 50% reduction in measurable tumor mass; dacarbazine in the combination regimen (ABVD) is used as a second-line therapy in advanced Hodgkin's disease after relapse with MOPP (mechlorethamine, vincristine, procarbazine, and prednisone) therapy—3-y survival rates of approximately 60% have been reported with ABVD alone; regimens alternating MOPP and ABVD have not significantly improved survival rates compared with using ABVD alone

PATIENT MONITORING

CBC, including hematocrit, hemoglobin, platelets, and total and differential leukocyte counts, should be obtained weekly to monitor for hematologic changes; hematologic toxicity (leukocyte count < 3000/mm^3 and a platelet count < 100,000 mm^2) may require delaying treatment; other serum chemistries such as BUN, creatinine, SGPT, SGOT, lactate dehydrogenase, bilirubin, and uric acid should be obtained at periodic intervals throughout treatment; monitor temperature daily

(Continued on next page)

DACARBAZINE (Continued)

SPECIAL PRECAUTIONS

Because of its severe hematologic effects, leukocyte, erythrocyte, and platelet counts should be performed prior to and at regular intervals; dacarbazine has been reported to cause anaphylactic reactions and should not be administered to patients who have demonstrated hypersensitivity to the drug; all cytotoxic drugs may be embryotoxic or teratogenic; use with caution in pregnant or nursing patients

TOXICITIES

Hematologic: dose-limiting bone marrow depression, leukopenia, thrombocytopenia, and anemia occur with nadirs between 2–4 wk; the occurrence of acute leukemias has been reported but is considered rare; **GI:** severe nausea and vomiting occur within 1–3 h after therapy in 90% of patients; usually subsiding approximately 12 h after completion of therapy; anorexia, stomatitis, and diarrhea have been reported rarely; **Dermatologic:** phototoxicity, urticaria, and alopecia; **CNS:** confusion, lethargy, blurred vision, seizures, and headache; **Local:** pain, burning, and irritation at the injection site; extravasation can cause tissue damage and severe pain; **Miscellaneous:** flu-like syndrome (fever, myalgia, malaise), numbness and flushing of the face; hypotension can be a dose-limiting toxicity; the citrate salt drug formulation can cause hypocalcemia

NURSING INTERVENTIONS

Monitor treatment tolerance, weight, nutritional status; encourage good oral hygiene; educate patients about neutropenic precautions and self-care at home; care should be taken to avoid extravasation—dacarbazine can be given IV push over 1–2 min or further diluted in D5W or normal saline to a total volume of 100, 250, or 500 mL; further dilution and a slower infusion rate can decrease the pain at the injection site; dacarbazine is considered an irritant and rarely causes extravasation necrosis—if extravasation occurs, treat by applying ice to relieve burning sensation, local pain, and irritation; nausea and vomiting are common—appropriate antiemetics should be given; the oral intake of food and fluids should be avoided 4–6 h before treatment due to the high incidence of nausea and vomiting; some clinicians suggest hydrating the patient 1 h before treatment to avoid dehydration from vomiting

PATIENT INFORMATION

Avoid the use of aspirin and nonsteroidal antiinflammatory agents; call if any moderate or severe adverse effects develop such as sore throat, fever ≥ 101°F, or unusual bruising or bleeding; avoid sun exposure and exposure to sunlamps for at least 2 d posttreatment; avoid exposure to people with infections; treat flu-like symptoms with acetaminophen; maintain good nutrition—modify eating patterns, use dietary supplements as needed to maintain adequate caloric intake

FORMULATION

Available as DTIC-Dome (Bayer Pharmaceutical Division, West Haven, CT).

The information here is provided as guidance only. Prescribers should always consult the manufacturer's current prescribing information.

22

FOTEMUSTINE

Fotemustine, a chloroethylnitrosourea compound, was synthesized and developed by the Servier Research Institute. Fotemustine is a lipophilic chemical structure with a phosphonoalanine group grafted onto a nitrosourea radical. Chloroethylnitrosoureas are the most active agents in brain tumors and may be used with radiotherapy for added efficacy.

DOSAGE AND ADMINISTRATION

In phase II clinical trials the dosage recommendation is 100 mg/m^2 IV over 1 h, weekly for 3 consecutive wk followed by a 5 wk rest period. If response or stabilization of disease occurs after the initial dose a maintenance dose of 100 mg/m^2 every 3 wk is suggested; high-dose regimens with autologous bone marrow transplant consist of total doses of 500–1000 mg/m^2; intraarterial infusions are given through the carotid or vertebrobasilar artery (the artery supplying the tumor), at 100–200 mg every 6 wk

SPECIAL PRECAUTIONS

Myelosuppression is the major toxicity of fotemustine; monitoring for leukopenia, thrombocytopenia, and anemia should be continued throughout therapy; all cytotoxic drugs may be embryotoxic or teratogenic; investigational agents should not be used in pregnant or nursing patients

TOXICITIES

Hematologic: grade III and IV reversible leukopenia, thrombocytopenia, and anemia have been observed at several doses; no aplasia-related deaths have been reported; **GI:** mild nausea, vomiting, and epigastric pain; abnormal liver function tests have been noted in 22% of treated patients but no hepatotoxicity has been observed; **CNS:** CNS toxicity has been reported with intraarterial administration; mild to severe ocular pain during the infusion, depending on the dose; severe loss of vision, blindness, and encephalopathy-related neurotoxicity have been observed with intraarterial administration; **Miscellaneous:** rare allergic reaction (fever and rash) during the infusion; rare supravenous hyperpigmentation

INDICATIONS

FDA-approved: none—fotemustine is an investigational agent in phase II clinical trials.
Clinical studies have shown activity in recurrent malignant glioma, brain metastases of non–small cell lung cancer and malignant melanoma, and colon cancer

PHARMACOKINETICS

Absorption: not given by the oral or intramuscular route at this time; **Distribution:** rapid distribution into the brain tissue occurs, representing approximately 17%–30% of the concomitant plasma concentration; volume of distribution is estimated at 33 L/m^2; **Metabolism:** limited information available; chemical degradation of fotemustine to an active metabolite, 2-chloroethanol; **Elimination:** short elimination half-life of $\leq$ 20 min; total body clearance ranges from 8.96–83.49 L/h; parent drug and metabolite are renally eliminated with urinary metabolite measuring 50%–60% of the delivered dose

DRUG INTERACTIONS

Fotemustine toxicity may be enhanced if given with other myelosuppressive drugs and therapies; fotemustine given in combination with tamoxifen may have synergistic cytotoxicity

RESPONSE RATES

Objective response rates of 24% are reported in patients with melanoma; these studies also revealed a 25% (8.3% 60%) median response rate of brain metastases in these patients; studies are ongoing using fotemustine in combination with dacarbazine, cisplatin, and tamoxifen to increase response rates; in patients with recurrent malignant gliomas, a 26.3% objective response is reported; fotemustine combined with radiotherapy may increase response rates to 29%; a 16.7% response rate has been shown in brain metastases of non–small cell lung cancer; studies are ongoing in this patient population combining cisplatin and fotemustine; only 7% partial response has been reported with colorectal cancer

PATIENT MONITORING

CBC, including differential leukocyte count, platelet count, and hemoglobin and hematocrit should be obtained to monitor for leukopenia, thrombocytopenia, and anemia; if an intraarterial infusion is used, monitor for sudden change or loss in vision and headache; monitor liver chemistries intermittently; health care professionals responsible for monitoring patients on fotemustine therapy should be familiar with the less common adverse effects that can occur with therapy

NURSING INTERVENTIONS

Monitor treatment tolerance, weight, nutritional status; ensure that appropriate lab tests are conducted to monitor for leukopenia, thrombocytopenia, and anemia; ensure appropriate documentation and notify physician of all adverse effects and patient complaints in patients receiving investigational drugs; ensure that a consent form is signed by the patient to receive investigational drugs; nausea and vomiting are mild to moderate—appropriate antiemetics should be given

PATIENT INFORMATION

Call the doctor immediately if intractable nausea and vomiting, unusual bruising and bleeding, temperature over 101°F, change or loss in vision, or severe headache occurs; avoid exposure to people with infections

FORMULATION

Fotemustine for injection is mixed in 50–250 mL of 5% dextrose in water (D5W) and protected from light. IV infusion is over 1 h. Intraarterial and intrahepatic infusions are also mixed in D5W and given over 4 h

IFOSFAMIDE

Ifosfamide is a cell cycle nonspecific alkylating agent of the nitrogen mustard type. It is a synthetic analogue of cyclophosphamide that must be activated by hepatic microsomal enzymes to exert its antineoplastic effect. It is hydroxylated to 4-hydroxyifosfamide (an active metabolite) and then metabolized to 4-ketoifosfamide and to 4-carboxyifosfamide (neither of which is cytotoxic). The active metabolites interact with DNA, forming cross-linking strands of both DNA and RNA as well as inhibiting protein synthesis.

DOSAGE AND ADMINISTRATION

Many dosage schedules and regimens exist for ifosfamide. It may be used alone or in combination with other agents. Dose fractionation, vigorous hydration, and the administration of the uroprotector mesna should be part of the therapeutic regimen to decrease the risk of hemorrhagic cystitis.

Non-Hodgkin's lymphoma: 700–1000 mg/m^2/d x 5 d, repeated q 3 wk;
Nonseminomatous germ cell tumors: 1.2 g/m^2/d x 3 d, repeated q 3 wk;
Non–small cell lung cancer: 2400 mg/m^2/d x 3d, repeated q 3 wk; **Advanced lung cancer:** up to 5000 mg/m^2 as a single dose **Non–small cell cancer:** 2400 mg/m^2/d x 3d; repeat q 3 wk

Ifosfamide should be given with the uroprotective agent, mesna, for the prophylaxis of ifosfamide-induced hemorrhagic cystitis. Mesna is given as an IV bolus in a dosage equal to 20% of the ifosfamide dosage (weight/weight) at the time of ifosfamide administration and 4 and 8 h after each dose of ifosfamide. Alternatively, mesna may begin at 100% of the ifosfamide dose as a 24-h continuous infusion. Mesna can be given orally by doubling the IV dose and mixing in juice, soda, or milk immediately prior to administration of the mesna dose

(Continued on next page)

INDICATIONS

FDA-approved: Third-line therapy for germ-cell testicular tumors; clinical studies show activity in treatment of soft tissue sarcomas, Ewing's sarcoma, Hodgkin's and non-Hodgkin's lymphoma, carcinoma of the breast, lung, pancreas, and ovaries, ALL, and CLL

PHARMACOKINETICS

Absorption: not administered orally; **Distribution:** crosses the blood–brain barrier but its metabolites do not; **Metabolism:** 50% of a dose is metabolized in the liver; doses of 3.8–5 g/m^2 have a biphasic decay and a half-life of 15 h; doses of 1.6–2.4 g/m^2 have a monophasic decay and a half-life of 7 h; **Elimination:** 70%–86% of a dose is renally excreted, with 61% excreted unchanged at single doses of 5 g/m^2 and 12%–18% excreted unchanged at doses of 1.2–2.4 g/m^2; plasma elimination half-life is approximately 14 h

DRUG INTERACTIONS

Phenobarbital, phenytoin, and chloral hydrate may increase ifosfamide activity due to induction of microsomal enzymes; corticosteroids inhibit these enzymes, leading to decreased ifosfamide activity; allopurinol increases the activity and bone marrow toxicity of ifosfamide; bone marrow depressants, radiation therapy, and live virus vaccines also have the potential for clinically significant interactions with ifosfamide; in the kidney, mesna interacts with the urotoxic ifosfamide metabolites, acrolein and 4-hydroxyifosfamide, resulting in the detoxification of these metabolites

(Continued on next page)

IFOSFAMIDE (Continued)

SPECIAL PRECAUTIONS

Use with caution in elderly patients due to age-related renal function impairment; contraindicated in patients who have demonstrated a previous hypersensitivity to ifosfamide; do not administer to patients with leukocyte count < 2000 μL or platelet counts below 50,000 μL; all cytotoxic drugs may be embryotoxic or teratogenic; use with caution in pregnant and nursing patients; breast-feeding is not recommended because ifosfamide is excreted in breast milk

TOXICITIES

Hematologic: severe myelosuppression that is dose-related and dose-limiting is frequently observed, especially when given in combination with other antineoplastic agents; leukopenia and thrombocytopenia are the most common; **GI:** nausea and vomiting are most common; anorexia, diarrhea, and in some cases constipation may occur; **CNS:** lethargy, confusion, hallucinations, encephalopathy; **Renal:** hemorrhagic cystitis is the most frequent; others are dysuria, urinary frequency and renal insufficiency; **Pulmonary:** cough, shortness of breath; **Miscellaneous:** phlebitis, infection, hepatotoxicity, alopecia

RESPONSE RATES

Nonseminomatous germ cell tumors (in combination with cisplatin and etoposide or vinblastine): 21% complete response rate

Nonseminomatous germ cell tumors (in combination with etoposide, cisplatin, and mesna): 26% complete response rate

Bulky seminoma (in combination with cisplatin and vinblastine): 87% complete response rate

Small cell lung cancer (in combination with etoposide and radiation therapy): 76% complete response and 14% partial response

Recurrent or disseminated lung cancer treated with high-dose ifosfamide: 33% response rate

Non–small cell lung cancer treated with ifosfamide alone: 24% response rate

Non–oat cell lung cancer treated with ifosfamide alone: 30% response rate

Advanced non–small cell lung cancer (in combination with cisplatin and etoposide): 26% response rate

Advanced non–small lung cancer (in combination regimen with cyclophosphamide): 38% response rate (7% complete response rate)

PATIENT MONITORING

CBC should be obtained weekly and should include hematocrit, hemoglobin, platelet count, and total and differential leukocyte counts; other serum chemistries such as BUN, serum creatinine, SGPT, SGOT, lactate dehydrogenase, and serum bilirubin should be obtained at periodic intervals; the urine should be examined for microscopic hematuria prior to each course of treatment

NURSING INTERVENTIONS

Monitor treatment tolerance, weight, nutritional status; encourage good oral hygiene; administer antiemetics as necessary; encourage patient to increase fluid intake to prevent hemorrhagic cystitis; encourage patient to void every 2 h during the day and once at night to decrease the risk of hemorrhagic cystitis; educate patient regarding care of central venous access devices and self-care at home

PATIENT INFORMATION

Avoid the use of aspirin and nonsteroidal antiinflammatory agents; ensure adequate fluid intake and frequent voiding; continue therapy in spite of nausea and vomiting; notify doctor if you see blood in the urine or have clinical signs of infection; maintain good nutrition—modify eating patterns and use dietary supplements as needed to maintain adequate caloric intake

FORMULATION

Available as Ifex (Bristol-Myers Oncology Division, Princeton, NJ) in a combination package with mesna

LOMUSTINE

Lomustine (also known as CeeNU and CCNU) is a nitrosourea derivative that has demonstrated cytotoxic activity against a wide variation of malignancies. As with other alkylating agents, lomustine is considered to be cell cycle nonspecific. Within 1 to 6 hours after oral administration of lomustine, peak metabolite concentrations occur. These metabolites are responsible for the alkylation and carbamoylation activity, which interfere with DNA, RNA, and protein synthesis. Cross-resistance between lomustine and carmustine has occurred. Lomustine and its metabolites are widely distributed in the body. Nitrosoureas as a class tend to be highly lipophilic, thus enhancing their ability to cross the blood-brain barrier and to be used in the treatment of meningeal leukemias and brain tumors. The long-term use of nitrosoureas has been associated with profound cumulative myelosuppression and renal failure (especially with methyl-CCNU) with lesions similar to radiation-induced nephritis.

DOSAGE AND ADMINISTRATION

For adults and children 75–130 mg/m^2 by mouth once every 6–8 wk. Repeated doses should not be given until leukocyte count is > 4000/mm^3 and platelet count is > 100,000/mm^3

The manufacturer suggests adjusting subsequent doses according to previous treatment nadirs

NADIR AFTER PRIOR DOSE (CELLS/MM^3)

Leukocytes	Platelets	Amount of Prior Dose to be Given (%)
> 4000	< 100,000	100
3000–3999	75,000–99,999	100
2000–2999	25,000–74,999	70
< 2000	<25,000	50

Some clinicians use absolute neutrophil count (ANC) as the basis of dose adjustment; in which case, reduce the dose by 2.5% for an ANC at nadir of < 1000/mm^3 and by 50% for an ANC < 500/mm^3

(Continued on next page)

INDICATIONS

FDA-approved: Palliative treatment of primary and metastatic brain tumors; used in combination regimens for the treatment of disseminated Hodgkin's disease in disease refractory to other established treatment regimens; clinical studies show activity in bronchiogenic carcinoma, non-Hodgkin's lymphoma, malignant melanoma, breast carcinoma, renal cell carcinoma, and carcinoma of the GI tract

PHARMACOKINETICS

Absorption: rapidly absorbed from the GI tract; oral bioavailability is considered high (60%–90%); **Distribution:** widely distributed; lomustine and its metabolites rapidly cross the blood–brain barrier; cerebrospinal fluid concentrations of metabolites have been reported to be 15%–50% or greater than concurrent plasma concentrations; **Metabolism and elimination:** oral dose is completely metabolized within 1 h after administration; half-life of the metabolites is biphasic; initial plasma half-life is 6 h; second plasma half-life is 1–2 d; 15%–20% of the metabolites may remain in the body for 5 d after oral administration; lomustine is excreted completely in the urine as metabolites within 4–5 d

DRUG INTERACTIONS

Interactions with phenobarbital and cimetidine have been described, although the significance is controversial; cimetidine has been reported to potentiate the neutropenic side effects of lomustine; phenobarbital is a hepatic microsomal enzyme inducer and may decrease the effects of nitrosoureas

RESPONSE RATES

Precise response rates for patients with refractory Hodgkin's disease have not been established; some studies in a limited number of patients with brain tumors have demonstrated a partial response rate of 40%

PATIENT MONITORING

CBC, including differential leukocyte count and platelet count, is generally obtained weekly for 6–8 wk after the oral administration of lomustine to monitor for leukopenia, thrombocytopenia, and anemia; some clinicians suggest waiting 2–3 wk after therapy before obtaining the first CBC and then following up with weekly labs until blood counts are normal or appropriate for subsequent treatment, usually within 6–8 wk; monitor renal and hepatic status; health care professionals responsible for monitoring patients on lomustine therapy should be familiar with the broad spectrum of other adverse effects that can occur, albeit less commonly, with this treatment

(Continued on next page)

LOMUSTINE (Continued)

SPECIAL PRECAUTIONS

Because of the prolonged myelosuppression, treatment should not be given more often than every 6 wk; blood counts should be performed weekly and for 6–8 wk after administration; contraindicated in patients who have demonstrated previous hypersensitivity to the drug; all cytotoxic drugs may be embryotoxic or teratogenic; use with caution in pregnant and nursing patients

TOXICITIES

Hematologic: delayed hematologic toxicity is the major dose-limiting adverse effect; leukocyte nadirs occur first at approximately 15 d after therapy, then a second, lower nadir occurs at approximately 6 wk and persists for 1–2 wk after an oral dose; the degree of leukopenia depends on previous exposure to chemotherapy and can vary among patients; thrombocytopenia generally occurs about 4 wk after therapy and persists approximately 1–2 wk; refractory anemia, acute leukemias, and bone marrow dysplasias have been reported with long-term therapy; **GI:** mild to moderate nausea and vomiting occur beginning 4–5 h after administration of oral lomustine and can last up to 24 h; anorexia often occurs 2–3 d following therapy; stomatitis has occurred infrequently; **CNS:** lethargy, ataxia, and dysarthria occur rarely; **Miscellaneous:** mild hepatotoxicity evidenced by transient elevation in liver enzymes; nephrotoxicity and progressive azotemia are uncommon at total doses < 1000 mg/m^2; pulmonary fibrosis is uncommon at total doses of < 1000 mg/m^2; alopecia

NURSING INTERVENTIONS

Monitor treatment tolerance, weight, and nutritional status; administer antiemetics if necessary; educate patient about neutropenic precautions and self-care at home

PATIENT INFORMATION

Call the doctor immediately if vomiting occurs shortly after the dose is taken, or a sore throat or fever or any unusual bruising or bleeding develops; the medication should be taken on an empty stomach, 2–4 h after meals; anorexia may persist for 2–3 d after the dose is given; avoid aspirin and nonsteroidal antiinflammatory agents; avoid exposure to people with infections

FORMULATION

Available as CeeNU (Bristol-Myers Oncology Division, Princeton, NJ); available as 10-, 40-, and 100-mg capsules; also available as a dose kit containing a total of 300 mg (two 10-mg capsules, two 40-mg capsules, and two 100-mg capsules)
Store in tightly closed containers at a temperature < 40°C

MECHLORETHAMINE

Mechlorethamine hydrochloride, also known as nitrogen mustard, is a nitrogen analogue of sulfur mustard. It is a bifunctional alkylating agent that interferes with DNA replication and transcription of RNA in rapidly proliferating cells, eventually resulting in disruption of nucleic acid function. Mechlorethamine also possesses weak immunosuppressive activity. The drug is cell cycle nonspecific. Its cytotoxic activity is most pronounced on rapidly proliferating cells. The activity of mechlorethamine is due to the transfer of an alkyl group to cellular constituents such as phosphate, amino, hydroxyl, sulfhydryl, carboxyl, and imidazole groups. In neutral or alkaline solution, the drug is ionized to produce a positively charged carbonium ion, which then attaches to susceptible nuclear proteins at the N-7 position of guanine, a nucleoside found in DNA. This leads to abnormal base pairing of guanine with thymine, cleaving of the imidazole ring of guanine, cross-linking of DNA, and depurination of DNA. Mechlorethamine also inhibits glycolysis, respiration, and RNA-directed protein synthesis.

DOSAGE AND ADMINISTRATION

Mechlorethamine is used in combination with other agents. The drug may be given as follows: 0.4 mg/kg for each course either as a single dose or in 2–4 divided doses of 0.1–0.2 mg/kg/d; *or* 6 mg/m^2 on d 1 and 8, repeated every 28 d, for 6 cycles as part of a combination regimen; *or* 6 mg/m^2 on d 1 and 8, repeated every other month as part of a combination regimen.
Dose adjustment for myelosuppression: delay treatment 1 wk for absolute neutrophil count (ANC) < 1500/mm^3 or platelet count < 100,000/mm^3 at time of treatment; after the 1-wk delay, reduce subsequent dose 25% for ANC of 1000–1500/mm^3 or platelets of 75,000–100,000/mm^3; hold treatment an additional week for patients with values below these.

(Continued on next page)

INDICATIONS

FDA-approved: Palliative treatment of Hodgkin's disease (stage III and IV), lymphosarcoma, chronic myelocytic leukemia, chronic lymphocytic leukemia, polycythemia vera, mycosis fungoides, bronchogenic carcinoma, palliative intraperitoneal treatment of metastatic carcinoma; clinical studies show activity in topical application on cutaneous lymphoma, mycosis fungoides, and psoriasis

PHARMACOKINETICS

Absorption: incompletely absorbed following intracavitary administration due to rapid chemical transformation in water or body fluids, so that the drug is no longer present in the active form a few minutes after administration; **Metabolism:** 0.01% of an IV dose is excreted unchanged in the urine; **Elimination:** apparently renal

DRUG INTERACTIONS

Adjust the doses of uricosuric agents because mechlorethamine raises the blood uric acid concentration; patients on blood dyscrasia–causing medications should have their mechlorethamine dosage adjusted based on their blood counts; use mechlorethamine with extreme caution, if at all, in any patient who is receiving radiation therapy; mechlorethamine may increase the likelihood of infections following the use of live virus vaccines (avoid these in patients receiving immunosuppressive therapy)

RESPONSE RATES

70%–80% of previously untreated patients with advanced Hodgkin's disease showed a complete response while receiving MOPP therapy; of this group, 60%–70% will remain disease-free at 10 y, and cures in these patients are likely; the use of mechloroethamine in other clinical settings has been supplanted by other agents

PATIENT MONITORING

Patients should be monitored throughout their course of treatment; hematocrit and hemoglobin status should be followed as well as platelet counts and total (or differential) leukocyte counts; audiometric testing is warranted at periodic intervals in patients receiving high doses of mechlorethamine; other lab tests that should be followed include SGPT, SGOT, serum bilirubin, lactate dehydrogenase, and uric acid concentrations; radiographic examination is recommended to detect reaccumulation of fluid after intracavitary administration

(Continued on next page)

MECHLORETHAMINE (Continued)

SPECIAL PRECAUTIONS

Mechlorethamine is highly toxic and has a low therapeutic index; avoid inhalation of dust and vapors and contact of the drug with skin or mucous membranes; can predispose the patient to bacterial, viral, or fungal infection due to its immunosuppressive activity; use with extreme caution in patients with leukopenia, thrombocytopenia, or anemia caused by infiltration of the bone marrow with malignant cells; chronic lymphocytic leukemia patients appear to be especially sensitive to the hematopoietic effects of mechlorethamine and should receive the drug with caution if at all; can lead to hematologic complications if combined with irradiation; in the event of extravasation, aspirate as much as possible and neutralize the area with 1/6-molar sterile, isotonic sodium thiosulfate and apply cold compresses for 6–12 h; breast-feeding is not recommended because of the risks to the infant (it is not known whether the drug is excreted in breast milk); if skin contact occurs, irrigate the affected area immediately with large amounts of water for 15 min, then irrigate with a 2% sodium thiosulfate solution

TOXICITIES

Hematologic: lymphocytopenia, granulocytopenia (occurs 6–8 d after treatment and lasts for 10 d–3 wk), agranulocytosis, thrombocytopenia, severe leukopenia, anemia, hemorrhagic diathesis; depression of the hematopoietic system may be found up to 50 d or more after starting therapy; **GI:** nausea, vomiting (onset 1–3 h after use), diarrhea, jaundice, anorexia; **Dermatologic:** maculopapular skin eruptions, alopecia, erythema multiforme; **Reproductive:** delayed menses, oligomenorrhea, temporary or permanent amenorrhea, impaired spermatogenesis, azoospermia, total germinal aplasia; **Local toxicity:** thrombosis, thrombophlebitis, extravasation; **Miscellaneous:** weakness, vertigo, tinnitus, diminished hearing, chromosomal abnormalities

NURSING INTERVENTIONS

Monitor treatment tolerance, weight, nutritional status; administer antiemetics as necessary to control delayed-onset nausea and vomiting; educate patient regarding care of central venous access devices and self-care at home

PATIENT INFORMATION

Avoid use of aspirin and nonsteroidal antiinflammatory agents; call if any moderate or severe adverse effects develop, particularly nausea or fever, or other signs of serious infection; maintain good nutrition and adequate fluid intake—modify eating patterns, use dietary supplements as needed to maintain adequate caloric intake; if the drug is to be applied topically (either ointment or topical solution), shower and rinse carefully just before application unless otherwise directed; wear rubber or plastic gloves when applying; mechlorethamine should be applied more lightly to the groin, inside the elbow, and behind the knees; avoid contact with the eyes, nose, and mouth

FORMULATION

Available as Mustargen (Merck, West Point, PA)
Available in vials containing 10 mg of mechlorethamine triturated with 100 mg of sodium chloride; unopened vials are stored at room temperature and protected from light; mechlorethamine is reconstituted with 10 mL of sterile water for injection or 0.9% sodium chloride for injection; the resultant solution contains 1 mg/mL of mechlorethamine; a topical solution can be made by diluting mechlorethamine 10 mg in 60 mL of sterile water; to prepare the topical ointment, dissolve 10 mg of mechlorethamine in 1 mL of sterile water for injection and blend into 100 g of soft white paraffin

MELPHALAN

Melphalan, also known as L-phenylalanine mustard, L-PAM, or L-sarcolysin, is a bifunctional alkylating agent that is a phenylalanine derivative of nitrogen mustard. It is a cell cycle nonspecific agent. Because it is an alkylator of the bischlorethamine type, its antineoplastic activity occurs due to the formation of an unstable ethyleneimmonium ion. This unstable ion alkylates with many intracellular molecular components including nucleic acids. The result is cross-linking of strands of DNA (at the N-7 position of guanine) and RNA and disruption of cellular division leading to cellular death. Melphalan also inhibits protein synthesis and exhibits immunosuppressant activity. It is active against both resting and rapidly dividing tumor cells.

DOSAGE AND ADMINISTRATION

Melphalan is used either alone or in combination with other drugs in various chemotherapy regimens. The following regimens have been used in specific carcinomas.

Multiple myeloma: usual oral dose is 6 mg qd adjusted on the basis of weekly blood counts; 10 mg/d x 7–10 d with maintenance dose of 2 mg/d when leukocytes > 4000 and platelets > 100,000; 0.15 mg/kg/d for 7 d, off for 3 wk, then maintenance dose of 0.05 mg/kg/d; 7 mg/m^2 or 0.25 mg/kg/d x 5 d every 5–6 wk; 16 mg/m^2 IV q 2 wk x 4 doses, then, after recovery from toxicity, at 4-wk intervals; **ovarian carcinoma:** 0.2 mg/kg/d x 5 d every 4–5 wk; **high-dose regimens:** 30–40 mg/m^2 IV q 21 d; 120–200 mg/m^2 IV x 1 dose with hematopoietic cellular support

Dosage adjustment in organ dysfunction: patients with BUN ≥ 30 mg/dL should be monitored closely and IV dosage reductions of 50% should be made; in patients with moderate to severe renal impairment, current data do not support an absolute recommendation on oral dosage reduction, but it may be prudent to initially decrease the dose

SPECIAL PRECAUTIONS

Use with caution in patients who have had prior radiation or chemotherapy; use with caution in elderly patients due to age-related renal impairment; all cytotoxic drugs may be embryotoxic or teratogenic; use with caution in pregnant or nursing patients

TOXICITIES

Hematologic: bone marrow suppression, leukopenia, thrombocytopenia, and hemolytic anemia are most common; leukocyte and platelet nadirs usually occur 2–3 wk posttreatment with recovery in 4–5 wk; irreversible bone marrow failure has been reported; **GI:** nausea, vomiting, diarrhea, oral ulceration (dose-dependent, common with high-dose regimens), esophagitis; **Dermatologic:** skin hypersensitivity, allergic reaction hyperpigmentation; **Pulmonary:** pulmonary fibrosis, interstitial pneumonitis; **Renal:** proteinuria, elevated SGT and BUN; **Miscellaneous:** vasculitis, fever, chill, cough, hoarseness, alopecia, hematuria

INDICATIONS

FDA-approved: Palliative treatment of multiple myeloma and nonresectable epithelial ovarian carcinoma; clinical studies show activity in carcinoma of the breast and testes

PHARMACOKINETICS

Absorption: oral doses variably and incompletely absorbed in the GI tract; **Distribution:** rapidly and widely distributed in total body water; initial plasma protein binding is 50%–60% and increases to 80%–90% over time; ~30% is irreversibly bound; penetration across the blood–brain barrier is low; **Metabolism:** deactivated in body fluids and tissues by the process of hydrolysis; plasma half-life is 90 min for oral dosing and biphasic for IV dosing with an initial half-life of 6–10 min and a terminal half-life of 40–75 min; **Elimination:** eliminated from the plasma primarily by chemical hydrolysis to monohydroxy- and dihydroxymelphalan; renal clearance is apparently low

DRUG INTERACTIONS

Concomitant administration with cimetidine, famotidine, nizatidine, and ranitidine has reduced the bioavailability of oral melphalan because these drugs increase gastric pH; severe renal failure has occurred in patients receiving high-dose melphalan and cyclosporine; use with caution with other bone marrow depressants and live virus vaccines

RESPONSE RATES

Melphalan is not curative but can prolong survival of patients with multiple myeloma; it may take 3–12 mo of therapy to evaluate response to the drug; an objective response occurs in 30%–50% of ovarian carcinoma patients taking melphalan alone (combination regimens appear to be more effective); in high-dose regimens, melphalan at doses of 120–200 mg/m^2 is associated with complete remission rates of 30%–50% in patients with myeloma and delayed recurrence of disease when compared with conventional therapy in selected patients

PATIENT MONITORING

CBC, including hemoglobin, platelets, and total and differential leukocyte counts, should be obtained weekly; BUN, serum creatinine, and serum uric acid combinations should be obtained prior to therapy and monthly throughout the course of therapy

NURSING INTERVENTIONS

Monitor treatment tolerance, weight, nutritional status; encourage good oral hygiene; administer antiemetics as necessary; educate patient regarding side effects of melphalan and when to notify the physician; educate patient regarding self-care at home

PATIENT INFORMATION

Avoid use of aspirin and nonsteroidal antiinflammatory agents; oral dose may be taken all at one time and should be given on an empty stomach because food decreases absorption; continue taking melphalan even though you may have some nausea and vomiting; notify the doctor if any signs or symptoms of infection or bleeding develop

FORMULATION

Available as Alkeran (Glaxo-Wellcome, Research Triangle Park, NC) Tablet is supplied in 2-mg bottles of 50 scored tablets; injection form contains a 50-mg single-use vial of melphalan and a 10-mL vial of sterile diluent; should be stored in well-closed, light-resistant container at 15°–30°C. Melphalan should be dispensed in a glass container. Melphalan injection is available in 50-mg glass vials and should be protected from light and stored at 15°–30°C. Melphalan is reconstituted with 10 mL of the supplied sterile diluent. The resulting solution has a concentration of 5 mg/mL of melphalan. The drug should be further diluted in 0.9% sodium chloride injection, USP to a concentration not greater than 0.45 mg/mL and administered over a minimum of 15 min. Complete administration should be accomplished within 60 minutes of reconstitution. The reconstituted solution should not be refrigerated because a precipitate forms

PROCARBAZINE

Procarbazine, a 1-methyl-2-benzyl derivative of hydrazine, is used in combination therapy for the treatment of lymphomas and primary brain cancers. It has very little activity in solid tumors. Its major activity is found in the treatment of Hodgkin's disease. Procarbazine, considered a nonclassic alkylator, is a prodrug that is metabolized to form numerous active intermediates and methylates DNA at O6 of guanine. It acts by inhibiting the incorporation of thymidine, deoxycytidine, formate, adenine, and 4-amino-5-imidazole carboxylamide into DNA, inhibiting RNA synthesis and inhibiting protein synthesis. Studies have shown procarbazine to inhibit mitosis, particularly in the S and G_2 phases, making the drug cell cycle phase specific. The cytotoxic effects of procarbazine are limited to tissues with high rates of cellular proliferation, and these effects are most evident in cells actively synthesizing DNA because O6-methylgaunine lesions are recognized by mismatch repair, resulting in cell death. Procarbazine also has monoamine oxidase–inhibiting properties.

DOSAGE AND ADMINISTRATION

Procarbazine is administered orally. Dosage must be individualized based on clinical and hematologic response, and on patient's body weight. In patients with abnormal fluid retention, the patient's ideal body weight should be used to calculate the dosage

Single agent: 50–200 mg/d for 10–20 d, *or* 50 mg initially, then add 50 mg daily up to a maximum of 300 mg daily, or 2–4 mg/kg/d x 1 wk, then 4–6 mg/kg/d until maximum response is achieved

Maintenance dose: 1–2 mg/kg/d

As component of MOPP therapy for advanced Hodgkin's disease: 100 mg/m^2 on d 1–14 of 28-d cycle (usually given for minimum of 6 cycles or as many cycles as needed to achieve a complete remission plus 2 or 3 additional cycles as consolidation therapy)

Pediatric dose: 50 mg/m^2 qd x 1 wk, then 100 mg/m^2 qd; *pediatric maintenance dose*—50 mg/m^2

SPECIAL PRECAUTIONS

Hypersensitivity to procarbazine; inadequate marrow reserve; G6PD deficiency; pregnant or nursing patients; interrupt therapy if the leukocyte count is reduced to ≤ 4000/mm^3, if the platelet count falls to ≤ 100,000/mm^3, or if hemorrhagic or bleeding tendencies occur

TOXICITIES

Hematologic: bone marrow depression (leukopenia, anemia, thrombocytopenia), pancytopenia, eosinophilia, hemolytic anemia, petechiae, purpura, epistaxis, hemoptysis; **GI:** nausea, vomiting, hepatic dysfunction, jaundice, stomatitis, hematemesis, diarrhea, dysphagia, anorexia, abdominal pain, constipation, dry mouth; **Neurologic:** coma, convulsions, neuropathy, ataxia, paresthesia, nystagmus, headache, dizziness, diminished reflexes, unsteadiness, falling, foot drop, drowsiness, hallucinations, depression, nervousness, confusion, nightmares; **Cardiovascular:** hypotension, tachycardia, syncope; **Respiratory:** pneumonitis, pleural effusion, cough; **Dermatologic:** herpes, dermatitis, pruritus, alopecia, urticaria, flushing; **Miscellaneous:** papilledema, photophobia, diplopia, hematuria, urinary frequency, nocturia, pain, tremors, hearing loss, weakness, fatigue, edema, chills

INDICATIONS

FDA-approved: stage III and IV Hodgkin's disease; clinical studies show activity in non-Hodgkin's lymphomas, mycosis fungoides, brain tumors, small cell lung carcinoma

PHARMACOKINETICS

Absorption: rapidly and nearly completely absorbed from the GI tract; peak plasma concentrations attained within 1 h; **Distribution:** liver, kidneys, intestinal wall, skin; crosses blood–brain barrier and distributes into the cerebrospinal fluid; **Metabolism:** primarily in the liver; **Elimination:** 25%–42% excreted as unchanged drug or as *N*-isopropyl-terephathalmic acid; **Half-life**—10 min

DRUG AND FOOD INTERACTIONS

Barbiturates, antihistamines, opiates, hypotensive agents, phenothiazines, sympathomimetics, local anesthetics, tricyclic antidepressants, and drugs and food with high tyramine content; such as cheese, bananas, tea, coffee, wine, dark beer, cola drinks

RESPONSE RATES

Previously untreated patients with advanced Hodgkin's disease receiving MOPP therapy, 70%–80%; in patients with brain cancer, procarbazine used in combination with CCNU and vincristine improves survival after radiation

PATIENT MONITORING

Bone marrow studies prior to therapy and 2–8 wk after initiation of therapy; hemoglobin, hematocrit, leukocyte and differential counts and reticulocyte and platelet determinations prior to therapy and every 3–4 d thereafter; urinalysis, serum transaminase, serum alkaline phosphatase, BUN obtained prior to therapy and weekly during therapy

NURSING INTERVENTIONS

Monitor treatment tolerance, weight, nutritional status; ensure appropriate lab tests are conducted to monitor for hematologic and hepatic abnormalities

PATIENT INFORMATION

Call physician immediately if intractable nausea or vomiting or fever above 101°C occur; report vomiting episodes that occur soon after taking an oral dose

FORMULATION

Available as Matulane (Roche Laboratories, Nutley, NJ) 50-mg capsules; store in well-closed container at 15°–30°C

STREPTOZOCIN

Streptozocin is an antineoplastic antibiotic produced by *Streptomyces achromogenes*. As an antibiotic, streptozocin has activity against gram-positive and gram-negative bacteria but its cytotoxicity limits its use as an antibiotic. Streptozocin exhibits alkylating action in vivo by decomposing into reactive methylcarbonium ions that methylates DNA at O6 of guanine and exerts its cytotoxic effect by activation of mismatch repair, resulting in apoptosis. Although streptozocin blocks progression of cells into mitosis, it also blocks other sites of the cell cycle and is referred to as cell cycle nonspecific. The presence of D-glucopyranose moiety explains streptozocin's enhanced uptake by pancreatic islet cells. No other alkylating agent contains a sugar moiety.

DOSAGE AND ADMINISTRATION

The usual dose is 500 mg/m²/d for 5 d every 6 wk; single doses exceeding 1.5 g/m² are not recommended due to the increased risk of azotemia; **Dosage adjustment for renal impairment:** patients with a creatinine clearance between 10–50 mL/min should receive 75% of the normal dose; patients with creatinine clearances < 10 mL/min should receive 50% of the normal dose

SPECIAL PRECAUTIONS

Because streptozocin-induced nephrotoxicity may be irreversible and fatal, routine monitoring of renal function is highly recommended; weekly CBCs and liver function tests should be performed; no information available on the use of streptozocin in children; all cytotoxic drugs may be embryotoxic or teratogenic; use with caution in pregnant or nursing patients

(Continued on next page)

INDICATIONS

FDA-approved: Drug of choice for treating pancreatic islet cell carcinoma; clinical studies show activity in malignant carcinoid tumors, lung cancer, squamous cell carcinoma of the oral cavity, synovial sarcoma, adenocarcinoma of the gallbladder, colorectal cancer, malignant Zollinger-Ellison tumors, and Hodgkin's disease

PHARMACOKINETICS

Absorption: oral absorption of streptozocin is poor (< 20%) and the drug is not active when given orally; **Distribution:** protein binding has not been determined; after IV and intraperitoneal administration, streptozocin and its metabolites are rapidly distributed mainly into the liver, kidneys, intestine, and pancreas; although the drug has not been shown to cross the blood–brain barrier, metabolite concentrations in the cerebrospinal fluid equal to the plasma concentrations have been detected; **Metabolism:** extensively metabolized in the liver and kidneys; **Elimination:** biphasic, with an initial half-life of 5 min and a terminal half-life of 35–40 min; in patients with normal renal and hepatic function, approximately 60%–70% of the dose is excreted in the urine as metabolites; 10%–20% of the dose is eliminated unchanged as the parent drug; the drug can also be eliminated in expired air and feces (5% and 1%, respectively)

DRUG INTERACTIONS

Because streptozocin causes a significant amount of nephrotoxicity, the cumulative effect of other nephrotoxic drugs should be avoided; phenytoin has been reported to decrease the cytotoxic effects of streptozocin on beta cells to the pancreas—therefore, concomitant administration of phenytoin and streptozocin when treating pancreatic islet cell carcinoma should be avoided; streptozocin may prolong the elimination half-life of doxorubicin—if used together, the dose of doxorubicin should be decreased

RESPONSE RATES

Response rates of 35%–60% with streptozocin alone and in combination with 5-fluorouracil have been demonstrated in patients with pancreatic islet cell carcinoma; combination therapy may be slightly better than single-agent therapy; when used alone for the palliative treatment of metastatic carcinoid tumor, responses have been partial and of short duration; combination therapy with cyclophosphamide produced evidence of biochemical response and measurable tumor regression in 26% of patients; combination therapy with 5-fluorouracil produced similar responses in 33% of patients

(Continued on next page)

STREPTOZOCIN (Continued)

TOXICITIES

Renal: renal toxicity is the most serious and dose-limiting adverse effect, occurring in approximately 25%–75% of patients; glomerular and renal tubular dysfunction may be manifested by azotemia, anuria, proteinuria, hypophosphatemia, hyperchloremia, and proximal renal tubular acidosis; the first signs of renal abnormalities usually appear as hypophosphatemia and mild proteinuria; increases in BUN and serum creatinine occur later in therapy; histologic changes in the kidneys can occur; the mechanism of streptozocin-induced nephrotoxicity may be the direct effect of the drug and its metabolites on the renal tubular epithelium; some clinicians suggest that adequate hydration may decrease the concentration of the drug and its metabolites in the kidneys and lessen the adverse effect; this is controversial and not clearly established; nephrogenic diabetes insipidus has also been reported; **GI:** severe nausea and vomiting occur in most patients receiving streptozocin— may be dose-limiting and become progressively worse over a 5-d treatment schedule; mild diarrhea may occur; **Hematologic:** mild to moderate myelosuppression is evidenced, with leukocyte and platelet nadirs occurring within 1–2 wk; **Hepatic:** transient and mild increases in serum concentrations of liver enzymes, lactate dehydrogenase or alkaline phosphatase occur in 25% of streptozocin-treated patients; **Metabolic:** hypoglycemia in patients with insulinoma may be severe but transient; hyperglycemia is uncommon in normal and diabetic patients because normal beta cells are usually insensitive to streptozocin's effect; **Local:** streptozocin is considered an irritant and severe necrosis has been reported after extravasation; **Miscellaneous:** confusion, lethargy, depression, and fever

PATIENT MONITORING

Renal function should be assessed in all patients prior to and during therapy; urinalyses and routine serum chemistries should be obtained; attention to BUN, serum creatinine, and electrolyte concentrations should be determined; CBC, including differential leukocyte count and platelet count, should be performed weekly to monitor for neutropenia, thrombocytopenia, and anemia; health care professionals responsible for monitoring patients on streptozocin therapy should be familiar with the broad spectrum of other adverse effects that can occur, albeit less commonly, with this treatment

NURSING INTERVENTIONS

Monitor treatment tolerance, weight, and nutritional status; streptozocin can be administered by rapid IV push or by IV infusion over 15 min–6 h; nausea and vomiting will occur in ≥ 90% of patients—appropriate antiemetics should be administered; wear gloves when administering streptozocin; the drug is considered an irritant and extravasation should be avoided; keep dextrose 50% at the bedside due to the risk of hypoglycemia from sudden release of insulin; test urine for protein and glucose; proteinuria is one of the first signs of renal toxicity

PATIENT INFORMATION

Call the doctor immediately if intractable nausea and vomiting occur, unusual bruising or bleeding occurs, fever above 101°F; avoid people with infections; fluid intake should be increased during therapy with streptozocin to reduce the potential for renal toxicity; diabetic patients should perform intensive glucose monitoring while being treated with streptozocin

FORMULATION

Available as Zanosar (Upjohn Company, Kalamazoo, MI)
1-g vials of powder for injection

TEMOZOLOMIDE

Temozolomide is an imidazotetrazine derivative developed in 1980 after many of its ancestor molecules, discovered in the 1960s, produced profound toxicities. Mitozolomide, the monochloroethyltriazene derivative, demonstrated dose-limiting thrombocytopenia in phase I studies. During phase II trials the recommended and reduced doses continued to be too toxic. The myelosuppression of mitozolomide was determined to be due to the monochloroethyltriazene decomposition. A second generation of imidazotetrazines was explored and temozolomide, the 3-methyl congener, was incorporated in the phase I and II trials. Temozolomide is a prodrug that undergoes ring-opening at physiologic pH to monomethyltriazene (MTIC). Dacarbazine also converts to MTIC by metabolic N-demethylation. The suggested mechanism of action of this nonclassical alkylating agent is probably a methylation reaction at the O^6 position of guanine residues by the reactive species MTIC, with additional alkylation occurring at the N-7 position. Recognition of the O6-methylguanine lesions by mismatch repair enzymes leads to strand breaks, single-strand patches, and induction of apoptosis.

DOSAGE AND ADMINISTRATION

The activity of temozolomide is very schedule dependent. Single bolus doses demonstrated limited clinical activity with various tumor types. The current recommended dose for continued phase II trials is 750–1000 mg/m^2 split over 5 d. The divided dose over 5 d every 4 wk has shown enhanced tumor activity compared with the single-dose regimens. Dose reduction to 500 mg/m^2 may be needed for patients who have been heavily pretreated.

SPECIAL PRECAUTIONS

Myelosuppression is the major dose-limiting toxicity of temozolomide; monitoring for leukopenia and thrombocytopenia should continue throughout therapy; all cytotoxic drugs may be embryotoxic or teratogenic; investigational agents should not be used in pregnant or nursing patients

TOXICITIES

Hematologic: dose-limiting thrombocytopenia (and occasionally leukopenia) occur at approximately 1 g/m^2; patients who have been heavily pretreated with chemotherapy or radiotherapy have a greater risk of myelosuppression; **GI:** mild to moderate nausea and vomiting; **Miscellaneous:** rare alopecia, mild erythematous skin rash, renal toxicity, constipation, and headaches

INDICATIONS

FDA-approved: none; temozolomide is an investigational agent in phase I and II clinical trials. Clinical studies have shown activity in malignant melanoma, recurrent high-grade astrocytomas, mycosis fungoides

PHARMACOKINETICS

Absorption: area under the curve (AUC) increases linearly with increases in dose; when first synthesized, temozolomide was administered by IV infusion over 1 h; owing to the extensive preparation of the IV formulation, oral capsules were developed; temozolomide capsules are rapidly absorbed; oral bioavailability is very good with some studies reporting similar AUC for both IV and oral administration; **Distribution:** peak plasma concentrations of 3.3 to 15.3 µg/mL are reached within 60 m; steady-state volume of distribution is 13 ± 6 L/m^2; cerebrospinal fluid to plasma concentration ratio is 29% ± 8%, therefore achieving adequate penetrating through the blood±brain barrier; there is no accumulation of drug from d 1 to d 5 of therapy; **Metabolism:** limited information available; temozolomide undergoes ring-opening under physiologic pH to monomethytriazene; there is some suggestion of enterohepatic recirculation; **Elimination:** half-life is biexponential with alpha half-life being 1 h and beta-half life of 8–9 h; total body clearance is 32 mL/min/m^2; there is much less interpatient variability than with dacarbazine

DRUG INTERACTIONS

Temozolomide toxicity may be enhanced if given with other myelosuppressive drugs or therapies

RESPONSE RATES

Response rates, both complete and partial, of 17% have been reported in the treatment of metastatic melanoma; varied responses have been reported in patients with high-grade astrocytomas and mycosis fungoides (patient numbers in most trials so far are small)

PATIENT MONITORING

CBC, including differential leukocyte count and platelet count, should be obtained during therapy to monitor for leukopenia and thrombocytopenia; health care professionals responsible for monitoring patients on temozolomide therapy should be familiar with the less common adverse effects that can occur with therapy

NURSING INTERVENTIONS

Monitor treatment tolerance, weight, nutritional status; ensure that appropriate lab tests are conducted to monitor leukopenia and thrombocytopenia; ensure appropriate documentation and notify physician of all adverse effects and patient complaints in patients receiving investigational drugs; ensure that a consent form is signed by the patient to receive investigational drugs; nausea and vomiting are mild to moderate; appropriate antiemetics should be given

PATIENT INFORMATION

Call the doctor immediately if intractable nausea and vomiting occur or if vomiting occurs after taking the temozolomide capsules, unusual bruising and bleeding occurs, or temperature over 101°F occurs; avoid exposure to people with infections

FORMULATION

Available as Temedal (Schering-Plough, Kenilworth, NJ) Hard gelatin capsules containing 20, 50, 100, and 250 mg are available for phase I and II trials; still investigational

THIOTEPA

Thiotepa is a synthetic polyfunctional alkylating agent that also possesses some immunosuppressive activity. Thiotepa interferes with DNA replication and transcription of RNA and ultimately results in the disruption of nucleic acid function. This alkylating agent has been in clinical use for more than 30 years. It can be administered by several different routes and is primarily used as an intravesical instillation for bladder carcinoma. Recently, several studies have investigated the value of thiotepa in high doses to treat several tumor types such as chronic leukemia, Hodgkin's disease, non-Hodgkin's lymphoma, breast and ovarian carcinoma, and melanoma.

DOSAGE AND ADMINISTRATION

Thiotepa can be administered by several different routes including IV, intrapleural, intraperitoneal, intrapericardial, intratumor, intramuscular, intrathecal, and ophthalmic instillation.

Intravesical instillation for superficial bladder tumors: the recommended dose is 30–60 mg in 30 to 60 mL of sterile water instilled by a catheter into the bladder and retained for 2 h; the patient should be repositioned every 15 min for maximum area contact; the treatment course is once a week for 4 wk then once a month for 1 y, as long as the patient remains tumor-free

Intratumor injection: Initial doses of 0.6–0.8 mg/kg administered directly into the tumor; a maintenance dose of 0.07–0.8 mg/kg can be administered every 1–4 wk

Intracavitary and intrapericardial: for intracavitary infusions, doses of 0.6–0.8 mg/kg every week; intrapericardial doses of 15–30 mg have been administered

Conventional doses used for breast, lung, and ovarian cancers, lymphomas and Hodgkin's disease: 0.2 mg/kg IV daily for 5 d repeated every 2–4 wk; or 0.3–0.4 mg/kg IV every 1–4 wk

High dose therapies: 60 to 475 mg/m^2 with or without autologous marrow transplantation; 180 to 1575 mg/m^2 with autologous marrow transplantation

Intrathecal administration: 1 to 10 mg/m^2 once or twice a week as a 1 mg/mL concentration

Ophthalmic instillation: to prevent pterygium recurrence, a 0.05% solution of thiotepa in Ringer's injection instilled into the eye every 3 h during waking hours for 6 to 8 wk postoperatively

SPECIAL PRECAUTIONS

Avoid in patients who have experienced hypersensitivity reactions to the drug; all cytotoxic drugs may be embryotoxic or teratogenic; use with caution in pregnant or nursing patients

(Continued on next page)

INDICATIONS

FDA-approved: Used intravesically in the treatment of superficial tumors of the bladder such as transitional cell carcinoma, papilloma, and carcinoma in situ; clinical studies have shown activity in breast cancer, Hodgkin's disease, non-Hodgkin's lymphoma, chronic leukemias, lung cancer, ovarian cancer, malignant melanoma, and pterygium

PHARMACOKINETICS

Absorption: incompletely absorbed from the GI tract; absorption through serous membranes ranges from 10% to almost 100%; **Distribution:** thiotepa is very lipophilic and penetrates the CNS readily; it is extensively and rapidly distributed to all tissues of the body, exhibiting an average volume of distribution of 0.7 L/kg; it is not known whether thiotepa distributes into breast milk; **Metabolism:** extensively metabolized in the liver; primary active metabolite is trimethylene phosphoramide (TEPA); this metabolite may possess more potent cytotoxic activity than thiotepa; other metabolites may exist but are undefined at this time; **Excretion:** exhibits a biexponential half-life, with an alpha half-life of approximately 10 min and a beta half-life of about 125 min; total clearance ranges from 150–500 mL/h/kg depending on the dose and patient parameters; approximately 60% of the IV dose is excreted in the urine within 24–72 h; TEPA excretion is slower than thiotepa

DRUG INTERACTIONS

The concomitant use of thiotepa and succinylcholine may cause prolonged respirations and apnea; thiotepa inhibits the activity of pseudo-cholinesterase, the enzyme that deactivates succinylcholine; in theory, thiotepa may inhibit the metabolism of other drugs; however, this has not been extensively evaluated in humans

RESPONSE RATES

Complete responses of 38% and partial responses of 24% have been reported in patients with superficial bladder tumors; recurrence rates decrease when thiotepa is used in combination with tumor resection or fulguration; when used as palliative treatment in breast and ovarian carcinomas and in high-dose therapy regimens, response rates of 20%–30% and 30%–50%, respectively, have been reported

(Continued on next page)

THIOTEPA (Continued)

TOXICITIES

Hematologic: leukopenia is the major adverse effect of thiotepa; effects are usually dose-related and cumulative; leukocyte nadir is typically 10–14 d but has been reported to occur at approximately 30 d; manufacturer recommends discontinuing therapy if leukocyte counts fall to 3000/mm^3 and platelet counts fall < 150,000/mm^3; thiotepa can be absorbed through serous membranes—therefore, intracavitary and intravesical instillation can cause systemic hematologic effects; the development of secondary malignancies can occur with thiotepa administration; **GI:** nausea, vomiting, and anorexia occur infrequently at usual doses; high-dose regimens significantly increase the incidence of nausea, vomiting, mucositis, esophagitis, and diarrhea; **CNS:** headache and dizziness with IV administration has been reported; at high doses, CNS toxicity can become dose-limiting; mild to moderate cognitive dysfunction becomes apparent at doses of 1125 mg/m^2; cognitive dysfunction is exhibited by the inability to follow simple commands or perform coordinated tasks; demyelination has been reported; **Dermatologic:** usually absent or mild consisting of allergic reaction type hives, rash, and pruritus; high-dose therapy has been reported to produce a novel skin toxicity described as generalized erythema or a maculopapular, nonpruritic rash associated with dry desquamation; a bronzing of the skin was also noticed several days following therapy; some alopecia has been reported; **Miscellaneous:** intravesical administration can produce lower abdominal pain, vesical irritability, hematuria, and rarely hemorrhagic chemical cystitis; intrathecal administration can be associated with lower extremity weakness and pain; transient elevations (< 10-fold) in liver function tests have been reported with high-dose thiotepa; amenorrhea and impaired spermatogenesis have occurred

PATIENT MONITORING

CBC, including differentia leukocyte count and platelet count, should be performed weekly during therapy and for at least 3 wk after therapy; when treating patients with a high tumor burden, uric acid concentrations should be monitored and allopurinol should be given to decrease the risk of tumor lysis syndrome; a complete neurologic exam should be performed at the beginning and intermittently throughout therapy to evaluate cognitive function; health care professionals responsible for monitoring patients on thiotepa therapy should be familiar with the broad spectrum of other adverse effects that can occur, albeit less commonly, with this treatment

NURSING INTERVENTIONS

Monitor treatment tolerance, weight, and nutritional status; thiotepa is not a vesicant and can be given by several routes—procaine 2% or epinephrine 1:1000, or both, can be mixed with thiotepa and used for local administration; administer antiemetics when appropriate, especially when giving high-dose thiotepa; evaluate cognitive function, coordination, and mental status at each visit

PATIENT INFORMATION

Call the doctor immediately if sore throat, unusual bruising or bleeding, or fever above 101°F occurs; avoid people with infections; do not drink fluids for 8–10 h before bladder installation of thiotepa; hair loss is normal and will grow back after therapy has ended; inform the doctor of any loss of memory or coordination

FORMULATION

Available as Thioplex (Immunex, Seattle, WA) parenteral for injection in a 15-mg vial; each vial also contains 80 mg of sodium chloride and 50 mg of sodium bicarbonate so that following reconstitution with sterile water for injection, solutions of the drug are isotonic; thiotepa sterile lyophilized powder for injection and reconstituted solutions of the drug should be stored at 2–8°C and protected from light; thiotepa powder for injection should be reconstituted with 1.5 mL sterile water for injection to yield a concentration of approximately 10 mg/mL; the reconstituted injection is stable for 8 h at 2–8°C; solutions that are grossly opaque or contain a precipitate should not be used; when intrathecal injections are intended, preservative-free 0.9% sodium chloride should be used; the reconstituted powder can be further diluted in 0.9% sodium chloride, dextrose 5% and water, Ringer's, and lactated Ringer's solutions.

The antimetabolites constitute a large group of anticancer drugs that interfere with metabolic processes vital to the physiology and proliferation of cancer cells. The major classes of the antimetabolites are the antifols, the purine analogues, and the pyrimidine analogues [1–4].

Antimetabolites have been used in cancer treatment since 1948, when Sidney Farber first reported that aminopterin (an antifol related to methotrexate) produced temporary remissions in children with acute lymphoblastic leukemia. The use of methotrexate in women with gestational trophoblastic neoplasia in the late 1950s demonstrated, for the first time, that chemotherapy could cure patients with metastatic cancer. The fluoropyrimidines were the first drugs found to have useful clinical activity in the treatment of gastrointestinal malignancies, and they continue to be important in the management of patients with several common forms of cancer. Insights gained from laboratory studies of the fluoropyrimidines have recently led to the development of new, more effective treatment regimens for advanced colorectal cancer.

Recent years have seen the development of important new antimetabolites, including gemcitabine and the rationally designed 5-FU prodrug, capecitabine. Although modern molecular biology and immunology have opened new frontiers for cancer research, it is clear that antimetabolites will continue to play a major role in cancer treatment for the foreseeable future.

PHARMACOLOGY AND PHARMACOKINETICS

Actively proliferating cancer cells must continually synthesize large quantities of nucleic acids, proteins, lipids, and other vital cellular constituents. Almost all of the antimetabolites in clinical use inhibit the synthesis of purine or pyrimidine nucleotides (needed for DNA synthesis) or directly inhibit the enzymes of DNA replication. Many antimetabolites also interfere with the synthesis of ribonucleotides and RNA, and some antimetabolites (eg, methotrexate) may affect amino acid metabolism and protein synthesis as well (Table 2-1). The effects of a given antimetabolite on different organs, tissues, and cell types can vary greatly due to nuances in cellular metabolism. For example, normal bone marrow is rich in purines, and these purines are actively salvaged and reuti-

lized by normal progenitor cells in the marrow. Therefore, it is not surprising that many purine antimetabolites (eg, thioguanine) are toxic to the bone marrow and particularly effective against malignancies of bone marrow origin (ie, leukemias).

When metabolic pathways for synthesis of vital cellular constituents are blocked by antimetabolites, cancer cells temporarily may stop proliferating (enter a quiescent or noncycling state, a cytostatic effect of treatment). Alternatively, cancer cells that continue to proliferate—even when cellular constituents required for proliferation have been depleted by antimetabolite treatment—can be destroyed (a cytotoxic treatment result). Thus, by interfering with the synthesis of vital cellular constituents, antimetabolites can delay or arrest the growth of cancers.

Antimetabolites also may affect the growth of cancers by other mechanisms. For example, several antimetabolites have been shown to induce terminal differentiation in certain cancer cell lines maintained in vitro. In this process, actively proliferating, poorly differentiated cancer cells acquire the phenotype of mature, differentiated, nonproliferating cells. Antimetabolites also have been shown to trigger apoptosis (or programmed cell death) in some cancer cell lines [5]. Finally, some antimetabolites are known to have effects on the immune system and may alter immune responses to cancer in treated patients.

Table 2-2 describes the route of elimination and elimination half-lives for antimetabolic agents that are marketed in the United States for use in cancer treatment. Table 2-3 lists the FDA-approved cancer treatment indications for these agents.

ADVERSE EFFECTS

Many of the adverse effects of antimetabolite treatment result from suppression of cellular proliferation in mitotically active tissues, such as the bone marrow or gastrointestinal mucosa. Patients treated with these agents commonly experience bone marrow suppression, stomatitis, diarrhea, and hair loss (Table 2-4). As noted previously, however, there are significant metabolic differences among these normal tissues, and the precise pattern and severity of treatment toxicities observed can vary greatly depending on the antimetabolite administered, the schedule of administration, and nutritional and other factors.

Table 2-1. Classes and Mechanisms of Action of Antimetabolites

Generic Name	Class	Primary Pharmacologic Actions
Fluorouracil (5-FU)	Pyrimidine analogue	Thymidylate synthase inhibition; incorporation into RNA
Floxuridine (5-FUdR)	Pyrimidine deoxynucleoside analogue	Thymidylate synthase inhibition
Methotrexate	Antifol	Dihydrofolate reductase inhibition
Leucovorin	Reduced folate (vitamin)	Enhanced thymidylate synthase inhibition (with 5-FU or 5-FUdR); "rescue" from antimetabolic effects of antifols
Hydroxyurea	Synthetic antimetabolite	Ribonucleotide reductase inhibition
Thioguanine (6-TG)	Purine analogue	Inhibition of purine nucleotide biosynthesis; incorporation into DNA
Mercaptopurine (6-MP)	Purine analogue	Inhibition of purine nucleotide biosynthesis
Cytarabine	Pyrimidine deoxynucleoside analogue	Incorporation into DNA; inhibition of DNA synthesis
Pentostatin	Purine deoxynucleoside analogue	Adenosine deaminase inhibitor
Fludarabine phosphate	Purine deoxynucleoside analogue	Ribonucleotide reductase and DNA synthesis inhibition
Cladribine (2-CDA)	Purine deoxynucleoside analogue	Ribonucleotide reductase and DNA synthesis inhibition
Asparaginase	Enzyme	Asparagine (amino acid) depletion
Gemcitabine	Pyrimidine deoxynucleoside analogue	Incorporation into DNA; inhibition of DNA synthesis
Capecitabine	Fluoropyrimidine carbamate A	Prodrug of 5-FU

In addition, many antimetabolites can produce adverse effects that appear to be unrelated to their antiproliferative effects. These effects are more commonly seen at high drug doses and may affect tissues that are not mitotically active. Examples include neurotoxicity seen with high-dose cytosine arabinoside and high-dose methotrexate treatment.

Gonadal function is usually suppressed in patients receiving cytotoxic chemotherapy [6]. Low doses of methotrexate, as used in the treatment of psoriasis, appear to have little effect on gonadal function, but this drug is clearly embryotoxic and teratogenic. Cytosine arabinoside has been shown to produce reversible inhibition of spermatogenesis. With the advent of modern combination chemotherapy regimens, few recent data are available regarding the effects of other individual antimetabolites on gonadal function. Available laboratory and clinical data suggest, however, that the effects of other antimetabolites on gonadal function are less severe and more reversible than, for example, the effects of nitrogen mustard and other DNA alkylating agents.

The administration of antimetabolites in pregnant women deserves special comment. It is sometimes stated that administration of antimetabolites is contraindicated in pregnancy (primarily due to the risk of teratogenesis), whereas other anticancer medications, such as alkylating agents and anthracyclines, may be used with caution. There is, in fact, no laboratory or clinical evidence supporting the concept that antimetabolites *as a class* are more mutagenic or teratogenic than are other cytotoxic anticancer agents. The only antimetabolites known to be significant human teratogens are the antifols (methotrexate, aminopterin, and related compounds). This is consistent with the known teratogenicity of folate deficiency in pregnancy. Clearly, all cytotoxic drugs must be regarded as potentially teratogenic and embryotoxic, and administration of cytotoxic drugs should be avoided in pregnancy whenever possible. However, there is presently no persuasive evidence that antimetabolites other than methotrexate carry a significantly greater risk to the human fetus compared with the risks associated with other classes of cytotoxic drugs.

MECHANISMS OF RESISTANCE

Cancer cells may overcome the cytotoxic and cytostatic effects of antimetabolite chemotherapy by a variety of mechanisms, including allosteric, pathophysiologic, and cell cycle control mechanisms. A comprehensive discussion of all known mechanisms of cancer cell resistance to each of the antimetabolites in clinical use is beyond the scope of this review. Instead, important classes of resistance mechanisms are discussed, using the known mechanisms of resistance to the fluoropyrimidines as examples.

Fluorouracil, the most commonly administered fluoropyrimidine, has several antimetabolic effects on cancer cells, including inhibition of the enzyme thymidylate synthase by the fluorouracil metabolite fluorodeoxyuridine monophosphate (this blocks de novo synthesis of thymidine nucleotides, required for DNA synthesis and repair); misincorporation of fluorodeoxyuridine nucleotides into DNA, in place of thymidine nucleotides (resulting in structural damage to DNA); and interference with RNA synthesis and processing. Inhibition of thymidylate synthase may be the most important mechanism of anticancer action for fluorouracil and other fluoropyrimidines. Inhibition of this enzyme can deplete cellular levels of thymidine nucleotides, which can result in destruction of cancer cells, in the DNA synthetic S phase of the cell cycle.

Cellular levels of vital cellular constituents, such as thymidine nucleotides, are controlled automatically and precisely by a series of allosteric (homeostatic or feedback-control) mechanisms. Inhibition of thymidylate synthase and depletion of cellular thymidine nucleotide levels, as produced by fluorouracil treatment, leads to automatic compensatory increases in the activity of several other key enzymes of

Table 2-2. Pharmacokinetics

Generic Name	Route of Elimination	Elimination Half-Life
Fluorouracil (5-FU)	Metabolic	6–20 min
Floxuridine (5-FUdR)	Metabolic	3–20 min, IV infusion; 70%–90% first-pass clearance, hepatic artery infusion
Methotrexate	Renal	Primary, 3–10 h (low dose) or 10–15 h (high dose)
Leucovorin	Metabolic	Parent compound, 1 h; active 5-methyl metabolite, 4–7 h
Hydroxyurea	Primarily renal	3.5–4.5 h
Thioguanine (6-TG)	Metabolic	25–240 min
Mercaptopurine (6-MP)	Metabolic	90 min
Cytarabine	Metabolic	7–20 min
Pentostatin	Renal	2.5–6.0 h
Fludarabine phosphate	Primarily renal	Active metabolite, 10 h
Cladribine (2-CDA)	Renal	5.7–19.7 h
Asparaginase	Metabolic	8–30 h (IV); 39–49 h (IM)
Gemcitabine	Metabolic	32–94 min (short IV infusion); 245–638 (long IV infusion)
Capecitabine	Metabolic	45 min

Table 2-3. FDA-Approved Indications

Generic Name	Approved Cancer Indications
Fluorouracil (5-FU)	Carcinomas of colon, rectum, breast, stomach, and pancreas
Floxuridine (5-FUdR)	Hepatic arterial infusion, for liver metastases from gastrointestinal adenocarcinomas
Methotrexate	Choriocarcinoma and gestational trophoblastic disease; acute lymphocytic leukemia; meningeal leukemia; breast cancer; squamous head and neck cancers; mycosis fungoides; lung cancer; non-Hodgkin's lymphoma; osteogenic sarcoma
Leucovorin	Advanced colorectal cancer (with 5-FU); "rescue" following high-dose methotrexate; "rescue" following methotrexate overdose; sickle cell painful crises
Hydroxyurea	Ovarian adenocarcinoma; malignant melanoma; chronic myelocytic leukemia; with radiation therapy for squamous head and neck cancers (radiation sensitizer); sickle cell painful crisis
Thioguanine (6-TG)	Acute nonlymphocytic leukemias; chronic myelocytic leukemia (alternative to busulfan)
Mercaptopurine (6-MP)	Acute lymphocytic leukemia; acute nonlymphocytic leukemias
Cytarabine	Acute nonlymphocytic leukemia; acute lyphocytic leukemia; blast phase of chronic myelocytic leukemia; meningeal leukemia
Pentostatin	Hairy cell leukemia
Fludarabine phosphate	Chronic lymphocytic leukemia
Cladribine (2-CDA)	Hairy cell leukemia
Asparaginase	Acute lymphocytic leukemia (induction therapy)
Gemcitabine	Locally advanced or metastatic pancreatic cancer; locally advanced or metastatic non–small cell lung cancer
Capecitabine	Metastatic breast cancer

the de novo and salvage pathways for thymidine nucleotide synthesis. The increased activity of these other enzymes (*eg*, aspartate carbamoyltransferase, ribonucleotide reductase, thymidine kinase) results in production of high levels of the normal substrate for the thymidylate synthase reaction (deoxyuridine monophosphate), which can competitively overcome the inhibition of this enzyme by the fluorouracil metabolite fluorodeoxyuridine monophosphate; and production of more thymidine nucleotides by the thymidine salvage pathway (which uses preformed thymidine), thus bypassing the de novo pathway inhibition produced by fluorouracil.

Cancer cells also exhibit pathophysiologic mechanisms of resistance to antimetabolites. For example, the gene for thymidylate synthase may be amplified in fluorouracil-resistant cancer cells. TS protein content can also increase through accelerated translation. Free TS protein is known to be capable of repressing the translation of its own mRNA through a process known as translational auto regulation. After TS protein is bound to the ternary complex, it is no longer able to suppress its mRNA translation, and thus the rate of new TS protein synthesis increases. The cancer cells may thus produce higher levels of this enzyme, and it becomes much more difficult to adequately inhibit this enzyme with fluorouracil treatment. Alternatively, cancer cells may acquire a mutation in the gene for thymidylate synthase, rendering this enzyme resistant to inhibition by fluorouracil treatment.

Finally, even if thymidine nucleotide levels are successfully depleted by fluorouracil treatment, cancer cells may evade the cytotoxic consequences of thymidine nucleotide depletion via cell cycle control mechanisms. The progression of cells through the cell cycle is regulated tightly by cyclins and other cell-cycle regulatory elements. Cells that are thymidine nucleotide deficient may arrest (stop cycling) at the G_1-S interface and may not proceed into the DNA synthetic S phase of the cell cycle, in which thymidine nucleotide depletion is lethal, until thymidine nucleotide levels are restored.

To make further progress in the use of antimetabolites in cancer treatment, it will be important to fully understand the mechanisms of cancer cell resistance to antimetabolites and to incorporate this understanding in the design of new antimetabolite chemotherapy regimens.

BIOCHEMICAL MODULATION

Biochemical modulation refers to the use of antimetabolites in multidrug regimens that are designed to enhance the efficacy of antimetabolites and overcome known mechanisms of cancer cell resistance to these agents. As noted earlier, laboratory studies of antimetabolites have continued to yield new insights into the mechanisms of action of these drugs and the mechanisms of cancer cell resistance [7]. These laboratory studies have further indicated that certain drug combinations could yield enhanced clinical efficacy in cancer treatment. Fluorouracil and leucovorin combination treatment regimens for colorectal cancer represent the most successful clinical application of biochemical modulation research to date.

Based on studies of the mechanism of thymidylate synthase inhibition by the fluoropyrimidines, Ullman *et al.* [8] first suggested that leucovorin could enhance the efficacy of fluorouracil. Their observations ultimately led to the clinical finding that fluorouracil and leucovorin combination regimens are modestly superior to fluorouracil alone in the treatment of advanced colorectal cancer [9]. The clinical success of this relatively simple biochemical modulation, which modifies only one of the many mechanisms now known to be operative in the resistance of cancer cells to fluorouracil, has stimulated a substantial resurgence in clinical and laboratory biochemical modulation research. More complex drug combination regimens, which target critical metabolic pathways at multiple points, are undergoing laboratory and clinical evaluation at a number of cancer research centers around the world. Whereas these more complex, multidrug regimens can be expected to inhibit the targeted metabolic pathways more effectively, the ultimate clinical success of these regimens will be determined by their degree of selectivity.

SELECTIVITY

Bacterial infections usually are treated easily and successfully because normal host immune defenses efficiently recognize and clear bacteria; bacterial metabolism and human metabolism differ sufficiently to allow for use of selective antimetabolites (antibiotics), which interfere with critical bacterial metabolic pathways but do not have significant adverse effects on the patient. In contrast, cancer cells are immunologically and metabolically very similar to nonmalignant cells of the cancer patient; therefore, selective destruction of cancer cells with systemic chemical or biologic treatment is much more problematic. It is clear, however, that some forms of cancer can be cured with systemic therapy. At least in some patients, selective destruction of cancer cells can be achieved with systemic therapy.

Commonly considered mechanisms for the selective destruction of cancer cells emphasize known or presumed immunologic, metabolic, and kinetic differences between cancer cells and normal cells. Biologic agents with immunomodulating properties have been shown to produce useful antitumor responses in some patients by enhancing immune recognition and destruction of tumor cells (*see* Chapter 4). Antimetabolites are not known to have any therapeutically useful immunomodulatory anticancer activity, although research is continuing into possible roles for combinations of antimetabolites and biologic agents in cancer treatment.

Inherent metabolic differences between cancer cells and nonneoplastic cells may account for some of the selectivity observed with antimetabolites in cancer treatment. For example, useful clinical remissions can sometimes be obtained, with little clinical toxicity, in patients with colorectal cancer who are treated with prolonged continuous infusions of fluorouracil, suggesting that tumor cells sometimes have a greater innate sensitivity to fluorouracil than normal gastrointestinal mucosal cells (or other normal cells). The precise metabolic differences allowing for this selectivity are unclear, but they may relate to toxic effects of imbalances in deoxynucleotide levels that may follow fluorouracil treatment. The expression of thymidine phosphorylase is found to be higher in some tumors than in the surrounding normal tissues, resulting in preferential converting of capecitabine to 5-FU in these tumors. Unfortunately, it appears that cancer cells commonly have (or develop) metabolic capabilities that confer decreased susceptibility to antimetabolites.

Kinetic differences between cancer cells and normal cells may account for much of the clinical selectivity observed with current antimetabolite chemotherapy regimens. Antimetabolites are selectively toxic to proliferating cells and typically produce few toxic effects in nonproliferating cells and tissues. Cancers characteristically exhibit a much higher rate of proliferation than normal cells and tissues even when compared with mitotically active tissues, such as the bone marrow and gastrointestinal mucosa and thus are inherently more susceptible to antimetabolites. Cancers also characteristically exhibit a high rate of cell loss. Normally, cellular proliferation exceeds the rate of cell loss in a

Table 2-4. Antimetabolite Toxicities

Generic Name	Primary Toxic Effects
Fluorouracil	Mucositis, diarrhea, myelosuppression
Floxuridine (5-FUdR)	Chemical hepatitis, sclerosing cholangitis (hepatic arterial infusion)
Methotrexate	Mucositis, diarrhea, myelosuppression
Leucovorin	Increases 5-FU toxicities; decreases methotrexate toxicities
Hydroxyurea	Myelosuppression
Thioguanine (6-TG)	Myelosuppression
Mercaptopurine (6-MP)	Myelosuppression
Cytarabine	Myelosuppression, nausea, vomiting, diarrhea, mucositis; neurotoxicity at high doses
Pentostatin	Nephrotoxicity, neurotoxicity, myelosuppression, immunosuppression
Fludarabine phosphate	Myelosuppression, immunosuppression, neurotoxicity at high doses
Cladribine (2-CDA)	Myelosuppression, fever, immunosuppression
Asparaginase	Hypersensitivity reactions
Gemcitabine	Myelosuppression
Capecitabine	Diarrhea, hand-and-foot syndrome

Table 2-5. Selected New Antimetabolites Under Study in Cancer Treatment

Generic or Common Name	Pharmacologic Actions	Potential Primary Indications
Tomudex	Thymidylate synthase inhibitor	Colorectal cancer
Trimetrexate	Dihydrofolate reductase inhibitor	Colorectal cancer (with fluorouracil and leucovorin)
Edatrexate	Dihydrofolate reductase inhibitor	Breast cancer (with paclitaxel)
S-1	Prodrug of 5-FU combined with a DPD inhibitor	Colorectal cancer

growing tumor. Periodic antimetabolite treatment may serve to alter this balance, leading to stabilization or regression of tumors (until the cancer develops resistance to the antimetabolite treatment regimen).

AREAS OF RESEARCH ACTIVITY

Many research centers are continuing to investigate the biochemical mechanisms of action and resistance of antimetabolite chemotherapy. Clinical studies are beginning to incorporate measures of in vivo biochemical effects of antimetabolite therapy (eg, determining inhibition of a targeted enzyme in a patient's tumor by posttreatment biopsy or using nuclear magnetic resonance spectroscopy to monitor drug uptake and retention in tumors) [10]. This research will clearly enhance our understanding of the failure of current antimetabolite chemotherapy regimens to control cancer growth in many patients and may lead to more effective use of these drugs in new biochemical modulation treatment regimens.

Another area of research activity relates to circadian patterns of cellular metabolic and mitotic activity and the possibility that these patterns may differ between malignant and normal cells. For example, if normal proliferating gastrointestinal cells enter the DNA synthetic S phase primarily in the morning hours, whereas proliferating cells of gastrointestinal malignancies enter the DNA synthetic S phase throughout the day, then it would make sense to administer S-phase–selective antimetabolites to patients with these malignancies at times other than the morning hours [11,12]. Because most antimetabolites have narrow therapeutic indices in cancer treatment, careful attention to details (eg, the timing of administration) may enhance the selectivity of these drugs.

Recently, the molecular basis underlying the cellular uptake of antifolate agents has been elucidated [13]. Two independent transport proteins, the folate receptor and the reduced folate carrier, have been characterized. Knowledge of the presence or absence of these proteins in tumors may be used to develop a more selective treatment program.

REFERENCES

1. Chabner BA, Collins JM (eds): *Cancer Chemotherapy: Principles and Practice.* Philadelphia: JB Lippincott; 1990.

2. Chen AP, Grem JL: Antimetabolites. *Curr Opin Oncol* 1992, 4:1089–1098.

3. Cheson BD: New antimetabolites in the treatment of human malignancies. *Sem Oncol* 1992, 19:695–706.

4. Clarke SJ, Jackman AL, Harrap KR: Antimetabolites in cancer chemotherapy. *Adv Exp Biol Med* 1991, 309A:7–13.

5. Darry MA, Behnke CA, Eastman A: Activation of programmed cell death (apoptosis) by cisplatin, other anticancer drugs, toxins, and hyperthermia. *Biochem Pharmacol* 1990, 40:2353–2362.

6. Averette H, Boike G, Jarrell M: Effects of cancer chemotherapy on gonadal function and reproductive capacity. *CA Cancer J Clin* 1990, 40:199–209.

7. Grem JL, Chu E, Boarman D, *et al.*: Biochemical modulation of fluorouracil with leucovorin and interferon: preclinical and clinical investigations. *Sem Oncol* 1992, 2(suppl 3):36–44.

8. Ullman B, Lee M, Martin DW, Santi DV: Cytotoxicity of 5-fluoro-2′-deoxyuridine: requirement for reduced folate cofactors and antagonism by methotrexate. *Proc Nat Acad Sci U S A* 1978, 75:980–983.

9. Poon MA, O'Connell MJ, Wieand HS, *et al.*: Biochemical modulation of fluorouracil with leucovorin: confirmatory evidence of improved therapeutic efficacy in advanced colorectal cancer. *J Clin Oncol* 1991, 9:1967–1972.

10. Presant C, Wolf W, Albright MJ, *et al.*: Human tumor fluorouracil trapping: Clinical correlations of *in vivo* [19]F nuclear magnetic resonance spectroscopy pharmacokinetics. *J Clin Oncol* 1990, 8:1868–1873.

11. Buchi KN, Moore JG, Hrushesky WJ, *et al.*: Circadian rhythm of cellular proliferation in the human rectal mucosa. *Gastroenterology* 1991, 101:410–415.

12. Von Roemeling R, Hrushesky WJ: Circadian patterning of continuous floxuridine infusion reduces toxicity and allows higher dose intensity in patients with widespread cancer. *J Clin Oncol* 1989, 7:1710–1719.

13. Trippett TM, Bertino JR: Therapeutic strategies targeting proteins that regulate folate and reduced folate transport. *J Chemother* 1999, 11:3–10.

ASPARAGINASE

Asparaginase (or L-asparaginase) is an enzyme that catalyzes the hydrolysis of asparagine (a nonessential amino acid) to aspartic acid and ammonia. Although most normal cells can synthesize all asparagine required for cellular protein synthesis, some cancer cells are dependent on exogenous asparagine to support cellular protein synthesis and proliferation. Asparaginase acts to deplete plasma levels of asparagine, thus depriving susceptible cancer cells of this nutrient. Clinically, asparaginase has useful activity in the treatment of acute lymphocytic leukemia and may have some activity in treatment of lymphomas. Asparaginase also blocks the cytotoxic effects of methotrexate.

The clinical usefulness of asparaginase is limited due to the frequent development of hypersensitivity reactions with repeated courses of treatment. Pegasparaginase, a modified version of asparaginase, is now commercially available for treatment of patients who are hypersensitive to the native form of asparaginase. If necessary, patients hypersensitive to the commercially available formulation can be treated with an investigational one derived from *Erwinia carotovora* (available from the National Cancer Institute for treatment of acute lymphocytic leukemia).

DOSAGE AND ADMINISTRATION

Acute lymphocytic leukemia (in remission-induction combination chemotherapy only; repeated or prolonged use should be avoided):
6000 U/m^2/d (IM injection) for 10 d **or** 500 U/kg (IV) every 10 d **or** 12,000 U/m^2 (IM injection) on d 2, 4, 7, 9, 11, 14
ONCASPAR (pegasparaginase): 2500 IU/m^2 every 14 d IM (preferred) or IV
Pegasparaginase is also approved for use as part of a maintenance regimen

SPECIAL PRECAUTIONS

Hypersensitivity reactions; pregnant and nursing patients

TOXICITIES

Hypersensitivity: urticaria, chills, fever, rash, anaphylaxis
GI: anorexia, nausea, vomiting; elevated serum levels of hepatic enzymes, usually transient; lethal acute hepatic failure (rare); pancreatitis in 5%, with pancreatic insufficiency and hyperglycemia (rarely severe)
Neurologic: headache, lethargy, depression, confusion; obtundation, coma, seizures (rare)
Hematologic: transient myelosuppression (rare)
Miscellaneous: Decreased serum albumin levels; decreased plasma levels of fibrinogen and vitamin K–dependent clotting factors; decreased levels of antithrombin III; proteinuria; renal insufficiency, oliguric renal failure (rare)

INDICATIONS

FDA-approved: acute lymphocytic leukemia (in remission-induction therapy)

PHARMACOKINETICS

Absorption: oral bioavailability very low (administered IM or IV); **Distribution:** plasma volume, little penetration into CSF; **Elimination:** metabolic (degraded by proteolytic enzymes); **Half-life:** 8–30 h (IV); 39–49 h (IM); serum levels of asparagine undetectable within minutes of injection, remain low days after treatment; **Adjustments for organ dysfunction:** unnecessary for renal dysfunction; use with caution in patients with hepatic dysfunction

DRUG INTERACTIONS

Methotrexate; cytarabine; vincristine

RESPONSE RATES

Pediatric ALL (induction phase, combination chemotherapy): complete remission in most patients; cure rate approximately 50%

PATIENT MONITORING

Be prepared for hypersensitivity reactions; monitor vital signs for 1 h following administration; follow-up monitoring of symptoms, hematology, serum chemistry panel, PT, PTT, amylase, glucose

NURSING INTERVENTIONS

Monitor weight, nutritional status; encourage good oral hygiene; give antiemetics, and mouthwashes and other adjuncts as needed for stomatitis

PATIENT INFORMATION

Patient should avoid use of aspirin or nonsteroidal anti-inflammatory agents; call physician if fever or other signs of serious infection develop; maintain good nutrition

FORMULATION

Available as ELSPAR (Merck & Co., West Point, PA) 10-mL vials containing 10,000 IU lyophilized preservative-free E. coli asparaginase. Store at 2°–8°C.
Pegasparaginase is available as ONCASPAR (Rhone-Poulenc-Rorer, Collegeville, PA) 5-mL vials containing 3750 IU preservative-free modified E. coli asparaginase. Stored at 2°–8°C

CLADRIBINE

2-Chlorodeoxyadenosine (2-CDA) or cladribine is a synthetic analogue of the naturally occurring purine nucleoside, deoxyadenosine. Like deoxyadenosine, cladribine is enzymatically converted to active nucleotide metabolites by cellular kinases, and reconverted to the nucleoside parent compound by 5´-nucleotidase. Unlike deoxyadenosine, cladribine is resistant to inactivation by the enzyme adenosine deaminase. Substantial levels of cladribine nucleotides can accumulate in lymphocytes, which have a particularly high ratio of (activating) kinases to (inactivating) 5´-nucleotidase.

The active nucleotide metabolites of cladribine interfere with several vital cellular metabolic processes. Inhibition of ribonucleotide reductase by the triphosphate of cladribine results in depletion and imbalances of cellular deoxyribonucleotide pools. The triphosphate metabolite of cladribine is also an inhibitor of DNA polymerases and can itself be incorporated into DNA. In addition, cells exposed to cladribine exhibit decreased RNA synthesis and an increase in DNA double-strand breaks. Finally, cellular levels of the key cofactor nicotinamide-adenine dinucleotide (NAD) may be depleted, as NAD is consumed in the synthesis of poly (ADP-ribose), which occurs in response to DNA damage. Most of these antimetabolic effects of cladribine are selectively cytotoxic to proliferating cells in the DNA-synthetic S phase of the cell cycle. However, depletion of NAD is cytotoxic to resting cells as well.

In clinical studies cladribine has demonstrated remarkable activity against hairy cell leukemia and substantial activity against other lymphoid malignancies.

DOSAGE AND ADMINISTRATION

Hairy cell leukemia: 0.09 mg/kg/d × 7 d (continuous IV infusion); one course sufficient); **or** 0.12 mg/kg/d × 5 d (IV over 2 h)
Chronic lymphocytic leukemia: 0.05 × 0.2 mg/kg/d × 7 d every 4 wk (continuous IV infusion; repeat up to 4 courses)
Low grade lymphoma: 0.14 mg/kg/d × 5 d (IV over 2 h) every 4 wk

SPECIAL PRECAUTIONS

Pregnant/nursing patients

TOXICITIES

Hematologic: lymphopenia; anemia; neutropenia and thrombocytopenia (mild at low doses; dose-limiting at high doses; may be cumulative); immunosuppression
GI: occasional nausea, vomiting (mild), diarrhea, elevated serum levels of liver enzymes
Miscellaneous: fever; neurotoxicity at high doses

INDICATIONS

FDA-approved: hairy cell leukemia; clinical studies show activity in chronic lymphocytic leukemia, low-grade non-Hodgkin's lymphomas, cutaneous T-cell lymphomas, Waldenström's disease

PHARMACOKINETICS

Absorption: limited data; oral bioavailability may be low and erratic (acid labile); **Distribution:** concentration in cerebrospinal fluid is 25% of that in plasma in patients with CNS disease and exceeds plasma concentrations in patients with meningeal disease; **Elimination:** primarily renal; **Half-life:** 5.7–19.7 h; **Dose adjustments for organ dysfunction:** unknown, use cautiously in patients with renal dysfunction

RESPONSE RATES

Hairy cell leukemia: complete remission rate 75%–85% (relapses are uncommon; 14% at median 33-mo follow-up)
Chronic lymphocytic leukemia, low-grade non-Hodgkin's lymphoma, cutaneous T-cell lymphoma (previously treated): partial remission rates 40%–50%; Waldenström's disease: overall response rate 79% (complete remission rate 10%)

PATIENT MONITORING

Vital signs, symptoms, examination, hematology, serum chemistry panel

NURSING INTERVENTIONS

Monitor weight, nutritional status; encourage good oral hygiene; give antiemetics, and mouthwashes and other adjuncts as needed; administer antipyretics for fever during therapy for hepatocellular carcinoma

PATIENT INFORMATION

Patient should avoid use of aspirin or nonsteroidal anti-inflammatory agents; call physician if fever or other signs of serious infection develop; maintain good nutrition

FORMULATION

Available as LEUSTATIN (Ortho Biotech, Raritan, NJ)
Preservative-free 10-mg vials (1 mg/mL solution). Stored at 2°–8°C and protected from light

CYTARABINE

Cytarabine (cytosine arabinoside or ara-C) acts pharmacologically as a deoxycytidine analogue and has several effects on DNA metabolism. Cellular kinases convert ara-C to active nucleotide metabolites; the triphosphate metabolite (araCTP) inhibits enzymes of DNA synthesis and repair and is incorporated into DNA. Incorporation of araCTP interferes with DNA template function and causes chain termination; this appears to be the primary mechanism of ara-C cytotoxicity. Other antimetabolic and biologic effects of ara-C include inhibition of ribonucleotide reductase and promotion of differentiation of leukemic cells in vitro. Finally, several cytarabine metabolites, including araCDP-choline, araCMP, and araCTP, can inhibit metabolic pathways of glycoprotein and glycolipid synthesis and thus may affect the structure and function of cell membranes.

Deaminases convert ara-C and its active nucleotide metabolites to inactive uracil arabinoside and nucleosides thereof. There is evidence that cells sensitive to the cytotoxic effects of ara-C have higher levels of activating enzymes, or lower levels of inactivating enzymes, than do resistant cells. Pilot studies have suggested that formation and retention of araCTP in leukemic cells may correlate with clinical response to ara-C.

DOSAGE AND ADMINISTRATION

Acute leukemia (usually with anthracycline): 100 mg/m²/d (bolus IV injection) every 12 h × 5–7 d or 100–200 mg/m²/d (continuous IV infusion) × 5–7 d or 3 g/m² (IV infusion over 1 h) every 12 h × 4–8 doses
Leukemic meningitis: 30 mg/m² (intrathecal) repeated every 4 d until negative CSF cytology, then one additional dose

SPECIAL PRECAUTIONS

Patients over 50: severe neurotoxicity, GI toxicity, hepatotoxicity with high-dose ara-C; pregnant and nursing patients

TOXICITIES

Hematologic: neutropenia, thrombocytopenia, anemia (reversible)
GI: anorexia, nausea, vomiting; oral, esophageal, GI mucositis and ulceration (possibly severe, prolonged, with gastrointestinal bleeding); abdominal pain, ileus, diarrhea (possibly severe); reversible intrahepatic cholestasis (common, mild); pancreatitis
Neurologic: neurotoxicity (at intermediate doses); patients with renal dysfunction have a higher incidence of neurotoxicity
Dermatologic: rash
Miscellaneous: fever, conjunctivitis, anaphylaxis (rare)
Intrathecal: nausea, vomiting, fever; paraparesis, paraplegia, leukoencephalopathy (rare)
Intermediate (1 g/m²) **or high-dose** (≥ 3 g/m²): cerebellar dysfunction, dementia, obtundation, coma, seizures, personality changes (usually reversible); severe GI ulceration; pneumatosis cystoides intestinalis and peritonitis; bowel necrosis; jaundice; pulmonary edema; interstitial pneumonitis; hemorrhagic conjunctivitis; severe skin rash with desquamation; alopecia totalis; cardiomyopathy; pancreatitis

INDICATIONS

FDA-approved: remission induction in acute nonlymphocytic leukemia, acute lymphocytic leukemia, blast phase of chronic myelocytic leukemia, meningeal leukemia; clinical studies show activity in non-Hodgkin's lymphomas

PHARMACOKINETICS

Absorption: oral bioavailability very low; **Distribution:** CSF concentration 20%–40% of plasma concentration at steady state); **Elimination:** metabolic (deaminases); **Half-life:** 7–20 min; clearance prolonged with high-dose ara-C; **Adjustments for organ dysfunction:** use intermediate- and high-dose regimens with caution in patients with preexisting hepatic dysfunction or renal insufficiency

DRUG INTERACTIONS

Methotrexate, thioguanine, mercaptopurine, hydroxyurea, thymidine, cisplatin, cyclophosphamide, etoposide, digoxin, gentamicin

RESPONSE RATES

Adult acute nonlymphocytic leukemia (with an anthracycline): complete remission rate 40%–75%, cure rate 5%–15%

PATIENT MONITORING

Vital signs, symptoms (mucositis, abdominal pain, diarrhea), examination, hematology (weekly; daily in leukemia induction therapy), serum chemistry panel

NURSING INTERVENTIONS

Monitor weight, nutritional status; encourage good oral hygiene; give antiemetics; mouthwashes and other adjuncts; and antidiarrheals as needed; evaluate for bacterial etiology if diarrhea is severe

PATIENT INFORMATION

Patient should avoid use of aspirin or other nonsteroidal antiinflammatory agents; call physician if fever or other signs of serious infection develop; avoid excessive sun exposure; maintain good nutrition

FORMULATION

Available as Cytosar-U (Pharmacia & Upjohn Company, Kalamazoo, MI)
100-mg, 500-mg, 1-g, and 2-g vials of cytarabine powder. Stored at 15°–30°C

FLOXURIDINE

Floxuridine (fluorodeoxyuridine or 5-FUDR) is a synthetic analogue of the naturally occurring pyrimidine nucleoside, deoxyuridine. Inhibition of thymidylate synthase (TS) by 5-fluorodeoxyuridine monophosphate (FdUMP), an active metabolite of floxuridine, is believed to be the primary mechanism of anticancer efficacy of this drug. Because 5-FUDR is a direct precursor of FdUMP, this drug may act more selectively as a thymidylate synthase inhibitor than 5-FU (fluorouracil). However, 5-FUDR also can be enzymatically hydrolyzed (to 5-FU). Depending on the precise route and schedule of administration selected, the pharmacologic effects of 5-FUDR may thus closely resemble (or differ from) those observed with fluorouracil administration.

Floxuridine commonly is administered via hepatic arterial infusion to patients who have liver metastases from gastrointestinal malignancies. Compared with 5-FU, 5-FUDR is more water-soluble and more potent, permitting outpatient administration using small, implanted continuous infusion pumps. Also, the high first-pass hepatic metabolism of 5-FUDR results in less systemic exposure and less systemic toxicity. Randomized clinical trials have shown that hepatic arterial 5-FUDR can yield significantly higher objective response rates and a significantly delayed progression of liver metastases compared with systemic fluoropyrimidine treatment.

DOSAGE AND ADMINISTRATION

Hepatic arterial continuous infusion: 0.1–0.6 mg/kg/d × 14 d, repeat every 28 d
IV continuous infusion: 0.1–0.15 mg/kg/d × 14 d, repeat every 28 d
IP administration: 1–2 g/m^2/d × 3 d, repeat every 21 d

SPECIAL PRECAUTIONS

Arterial catheter misplacement, dislodgement and migration; chemical hepatitis; pregnant and nursing patients

TOXICITIES

With hepatic arterial infusions:
Hematologic: neutropenia (rare)
Hepatic: abnormal liver functions, sclerosing cholangitis, acalculous cholecystitis, biliary sclerosis in 8%–21%
Other GI: anorexia (common), nausea, vomiting (mild), oral mucositis (rare), diarrhea; epigastric pain, gastritis, ulcers
Neurologic: headache, confusion, cerebellar ataxia (rare)
Dermatologic: alopecia (rare), dermatitis, pruritus, rash
Cardiovascular: myocardial ischemia (rare), angina
Catheter complications: arterial ischemia, perforation of vessel, dislodgement of catheter, catheter occlusion, thrombosis, infection

INDICATIONS

FDA-approved: hepatic arterial infusion for palliative management of hepatic metastases from gastrointestinal adenocarcinomas

PHARMACOKINETICS

Absorption: oral bioavailability limited, variable; **Distribution:** no data regarding CNS penetration; **Elimination:** metabolized 70%–90% first-pass in liver; **Systemic half-life:** 3–20 min; **Adjustments for organ dysfunction:** reduce dose or hold for abnormal liver function tests

DRUG INTERACTIONS

Leucovorin (increased hepatotoxicity)

RESPONSE RATES

Colorectal cancer with liver metastases: 40%–50%

PATIENT MONITORING

Monitor vital signs, symptoms (abdominal pain, nausea, vomiting, diarrhea—verify hepatic artery catheter placement; mucositis—interrupt treatment); examination; hematology; serum chemistry panel (significant hepatic enzyme elevations—interrupt treatment)

NURSING INTERVENTIONS

Monitor weight, nutritional status; encourage good oral hygiene; give antiemetics; mouthwashes and other adjuncts; antidiarrheals as needed; educate patients on care of vascular access devices and home infusion pumps

PATIENT INFORMATION

Patient should avoid use of aspirin or nonsteroidal anti-inflammatory agents; call physician if any moderate or severe diarrhea, fever, or other signs of serious infection develop; avoid excessive sun exposure; maintain good nutrition

FORMULATION

Available as FUDR (Roche Laboratories, Nutley, NJ) 500-mg vials containing lyophilized powder. Stored at 15°–30°C and protected from light

FLUDARABINE PHOSPHATE

Fludarabine phosphate (2-fluoro-ara-AMP) is a synthetic analogue of the naturally occurring purine nucleotide, deoxyadenosine monophosphate, and is a fluorinated nucleotide analogue of the antiviral agent vidarabine. Compared with vidarabine, the fluorine substitution renders 2-fluoro-ara-AMP relatively resistant to inactivation by the enzyme adenosine deaminase, and the phosphate moiety enhances aqueous solubility. Following intravenous infusion, fludarabine phosphate is rapidly dephosphorylated to 2-fluoro-ara-A; intracellularly, 2-fluoro-ara-A is rephosphorylated to the active triphosphate, 2-fluoro-ara-ATP. This triphosphate metabolite is an inhibitor of several key enzymes in deoxyribonucleotide metabolism and DNA synthesis, including ribonucleotide reductase, DNA polymerase alpha, and DNA primase. Interestingly, fludarabine phosphate also has been shown to stimulate the activity of natural killer cells in in vitro studies.

Fludarabine phosphate has been shown to be effective in the treatment of chronic lymphocytic leukemia and other lymphoid malignancies, but has little or no activity against solid tumors. High doses of this drug can produce profound toxicities, including a distinctive syndrome of progressive neurotoxicity, characterized by delayed onset of progressive encephalopathy with cortical blindness and eventual death. Fortunately, standard doses appear to pose little risk of this catastrophic syndrome, even with repeated dosing.

DOSAGE AND ADMINISTRATION

Chronic lymphocytic leukemia: 25 mg/m^2/d (30-min IV infusion) × 5 consecutive d, repeat at 28-d intervals to maximal response and for three more cycles, then discontinue

SPECIAL PRECAUTIONS

Pregnant and nursing patients

TOXICITIES

Hematologic: neutropenia, thrombocytopenia, autoimmune hemolytic anemia (life threatening and sometimes fatal), transfusion-related graft-versus-host disease during transfer of nonirradiated blood products.
GI: anorexia, nausea, vomiting; stomatitis, diarrhea, GI bleeding (uncommon); abnormal liver function (occasional)
Neurologic: at recommended doses—weakness, agitation, confusion, visual disturbances, coma (rare), peripheral neuropathy; at high doses—delayed dementia, cortical blindness, coma, death (onset 21–60 d after last dose)
Pulmonary: possible increased susceptibility to pneumonia; pulmonary hypersensitivity reactions (dyspnea, cough, interstitial infiltrate)
Flu-like: malaise, fatigue, fever, chills
Miscellaneous: increased frequency of serious opportunistic infections (*Pneumocystis carinii*, *Listeria monocytogenes*, cryptococcus); tumor lysis syndrome (with hyperuricemia, hyperphosphatemia, hypocalcemia, hyperkalemia, urate crystalluria, renal failure); edema; rash; autoimmune hemolytic anemia

INDICATIONS

FDA-approved: chronic lymphocytic leukemia; clinical studies show activity in low-grade non-Hodgkin's lymphomas; macroglobulinemia; mycosis fungoides

PHARMACOKINETICS

Absorption: insufficient data; **Distribution:** insufficient data; **Elimination:** renal; **Half-life:** 10 h; **Adjustments for organ dysfunction:** use with caution in patients with renal insufficiency

DRUG INTERACTIONS

Pentostatin (possibly lethal), dipyridamole

RESPONSE RATES

Chronic lymphocytic leukemia: in previously treated patients, complete response rate 10%–15%, overall response rate 32%–57%; with no prior chemotherapy, complete response rate 33%, overall response rate 79%; **Low-grade non-Hodgkin's lymphomas:** overall response rate 67%

PATIENT MONITORING

Vital signs, symptoms, examination, hematology, serum chemistry panel; bone marrow examination for persistent cytopenias

NURSING INTERVENTIONS

Monitor weight, nutritional status; encourage good oral hygiene; give antiemetics, and mouthwashes and other adjuncts as needed for stomatitis; give antidiarrheals as needed, evaluate for infectious etiology if diarrhea is persistent or severe

PATIENT INFORMATION

Patient should avoid use of aspirin or nonsteroidal anti-inflammatory agents; call physician if fever or other signs of serious infection develop; maintain good nutrition

FORMULATION

Available as FLUDARA (Berlex Laboratories, Richmond, CA)
50-mg vials. Stored at 2°–8°C

FLUOROURACIL

Fluorouracil (5-FU) is a synthetic analogue of the naturally occurring pyrimidine, uracil. Several active metabolites of 5-FU have pharmacologic effects on the synthesis and function of cellular DNA and RNA. Inhibition of thymidylate synthase (TS) by 5-fluorodeoxyuridine monophosphate (FdUMP) is believed to be the primary mechanism of anticancer efficacy of 5-FU. Other active metabolites include 5-fluorouridine triphosphate (FUTP) and 5-fluorodeoxyuridine triphosphate (FdUTP). FUTP is misincorporated into RNA and may affect several aspects of RNA stability and function. Similarly, FdUTP can be misincorporated into cellular DNA (in place of thymidine triphosphate); the level of this misincorporation may be enhanced by the depletion of normal thymidine nucleotides, resulting from thymidylate synthase inhibition by FdUMP. Fluorodeoxyuridine nucleotides that have been misincorporated into DNA are recognized and cleaved by a glycosylase, yielding apyrimidinic sites in the DNA double helix and leading to DNA strand breaks.

Numerous pharmacologic interactions have been observed between 5-FU and other drugs commonly administered to cancer patients. Clinically, leucovorin has been shown to significantly enhance both the toxicity and the anticancer activity of fluorouracil.

DOSAGE AND ADMINISTRATION

Solid tumors: 500 mg/m^2/d (bolus IV injection) × 5 d, repeated at 4–5 wk intervals **or** 1000 mg/m^2/d (continuous IV infusion) × 5 d, repeated every 4 wk **or** 500–600 mg/m^2 (bolus IV injection), repeated weekly × 6 wk **or** 300 mg/m^2/d (continuous IV infusion) × 4 wk or longer
In combination with leucovorin: 5-FU dose usually must be reduced 25%–33%
In combination with irinotecan and leucovorin: 500 mg/in^2 repeated weekly × 4 weeks

SPECIAL PRECAUTIONS

Severe diarrhea (especially in elderly patients and with leucovorin or interferon-α); patients with dihydropyrimidine dehydrogenase deficiency; pregnant and nursing patients

TOXICITIES

Hematologic: neutropenia, occasional thrombocytopenia (reversible)
GI: anorexia, nausea, vomiting (mild); oral, esophageal, GI mucositis and ulceration; diarrhea (sometimes severe), heartburn, taste alterations
Neurologic: cerebellar ataxia (rare) (can be irreversible), obtundation, disorientation, confusion, euphoria, nystagmus, headache; seizures (with leucovorin); acute neurotoxicity with progressive obtundation, hypotension, death (with high doses)
Dermatologic: hand-foot syndrome, rash, dry skin, fissuring, nail changes and loss, photosensitivity, alopecia, hyperpigmentation
Cardiovascular: myocardial ischemia, angina, infarction
Laboratory abnormalities: elevation of alkaline phosphatase, transaminase, and bilirubin (with levamisole, mild and reversible)
Miscellaneous: epistaxis, conjunctivitis, generalized allergic reactions (very rare)

INDICATIONS

FDA-approved: palliative management of carcinomas of the colon, rectum, breast, stomach, and pancreas; clinical studies show activity in head and neck carcinomas; as a radiosensitizer, in the adjuvant treatment of adenocarcinoma of the rectum, esophageal cancer, and head and neck cancer (organ preservation)

PHARMACOKINETICS

Absorption: oral bioavailability low, variable;
Distribution: readily penetrates the CNS and malignant effusions, crosses the placenta; **Elimination:** metabolism (dihydropyrimidine dehydrogenase); **Half-life:** 6–20 min; **Adjustments for hepatic or renal dysfunction:** unnecessary

DRUG INTERACTIONS

Leucovorin, interferon-α, interferon-γ, methotrexate, allopurinol, PALA, uridine, thymidine, dipyridamole, hydroxyurea, levamisole, warfarin

RESPONSE RATES

Colorectal cancer: partial remissions 10%–20%; 30%–40% with leucovorin; **Head and neck squamous cancers:** partial remissions 10%–20%; **Breast cancer:** partial remissions 10%–20%; **Gastric cancer:** partial remissions 10%–15%

PATIENT MONITORING

Vital signs, symptoms (mucositis, diarrhea), examination, hematology, serum chemistry panel

NURSING INTERVENTIONS

Monitor weight, nutritional status; encourage good oral hygiene; give antiemetics as necessary; mouthwashes and other adjuncts for stomatitis; antidiarrheals for mild diarrhea (inform physician); educate on care of central venous access devices and home infusion pumps

PATIENT INFORMATION

Patient should avoid use of aspirin or nonsteroidal antiinflammatory agents. Call physician if any moderate or severe diarrhea, fever, or other signs of serious infection develop. Avoid unprotected sun exposure; maintain good nutrition

FORMULATION

10-mL (50 mg/mL). Stored at 15°–30°C and protected from light. Administer undiluted, or dilute with 5% dextrose in water or 0.9% sodium chloride

GEMCITABINE

Gemcitabine (2'-deoxy-2',2'-difluorocytidine monohydrochloride) is a nucleoside analogue that exhibits cell cycle specificity by affecting cells undergoing DNA synthesis (S-phase) and by blocking the progression of cells through the G_1/S-phase boundary. Gemcitabine is metabolized intracellularly by deoxycytidine kinase to the active forms of diphosphate and triphosphate nucleosides. Gemcitabine diphosphate inhibits ribonucleotide reductase, which catalyzes reactions and generates deoxynucleoside triphosphates for DNA synthesis. The reduction in the intracellular concentration of deoxycytidine triphosphate (dCTP) facilitates the incorporation of gemcitabine triphosphate into DNA. Further chain elongation is terminated after gemcitabine triphosphate and one additional nucleotide are incorporated into the growing DNA strands. DNA polymerase epsilon is unable to remove the incorporated gemcitabine triphosphate.

Gemcitabine is rapidly metabolized to an inactive uridine derivative (dFdU) by cytidine deaminase. However, in comparison with ara-C, gemcitabine has greater membrane permeability and enzyme affinity as well as considerably longer intracellular retention.

DOSAGE AND ADMINISTRATION

Locally advanced or metastatic pancreatic cancer: 1000 mg/m^2 IV over 30 min weekly × 7 wk, followed by 2 wk of rest; then 1000 mg/m^2 IV weekly × 3 every 4 wk

Locally advanced (Stage IIIA or IIIB) or metastatic non–small cell lung cancer: 1000 mg/m^2 IV over 30 minutes on days 1, 8, and 15 of each 28-day cycle with cisplatin 100 mg/m^2 IV on day 1 after the infusion of gemcitabine; 1250 mg/m^2 IV over 30 minutes on days 1 and 8 of each 21-day cycle with cisplatin 100 mg/m^2 IV on day 1 after the infusion of gemcitabine.

SPECIAL PRECAUTIONS

Pregnant and nursing patients

TOXICITIES

Hematologic: anemia, neutropenia, thrombocytopenia
GI: nausea, vomiting (mild), diarrhea, stomatitis, elevation in hepatic transaminases, fatal veno-occlusive disease
Pulmonary: acute interstitial pneumonitis
Cardiovascular: acute myocardial infarction, vasculitis
Dermatologic: rash, radiation recall dermatitis
Miscellaneous: fever, hemolytic uremic syndrome (rare), thrombotic microangiopathy of the kidneys leading to irreversible renal failure, flu-like symptoms, dyspnea, peripheral edema, noncardiogenic pulmonary edema (rare, fatal)

INDICATIONS

FDA-approved: first-line therapy for locally advanced or metastatic pancreatic cancer; first-line therapy (in combination with cisplatin) for inoperable locally advanced (stage IIIA or IIIB) or metastatic (stage IV) non–small cell lung cancer.

PHARMACOKINETICS

Absorption: no data; **Distribution:** Volume of distribution significantly influenced by duration of infusion and gender; clearance influenced by age and gender; **Half-life:** 32–94 min (short IV infusion); 245–638 minutes (long IV infusion); **Adjustment for organ dysfunction:** use with caution in patients with renal dysfunction; dose reduction in patients with elevated bilirubin

RESPONSE RATE

Pancreatic cancer: 22.2% clinical benefit response (defined as a ≥ 50% reduction in pain or analgesic use, improvement in performance status, or ≥ 7% weight gain); non–small cell lung cancer: 26%–33%

PATIENT MONITORING

Vital signs, symptoms, examination, hematology prior to each dose, liver and renal function

NURSING INTERVENTIONS

Monitor weight, nutritional status; encourage good oral hygiene; antidiarrheals as needed; evaluate for bacterial etiology if diarrhea is severe

PATIENT INFORMATION

Patient should avoid use of aspirin or nonsteroidal anti-inflammatory agents during time of neutropenia (may use during flu-like syndrome); call physician if fever or other signs of infection develop

FORMULATION

Available as Gemzar (Eli Lilly and Company, Indianapolis, IN)
200-mg, 1000-mg vials of Gemzar lyophilized powder. Stored at 20°–25°C

HYDROXYUREA

The anticancer effects of hydroxyurea appear to be related to inhibition of ribonucleotide reductase. Clinically, this agent is used primarily in the treatment of chronic myelocytic leukemia and related myeloproliferative disorders. Although hydroxyurea is also approved for use in malignant melanoma and ovarian cancer, currently there is little evidence that this drug has any significant activity in solid tumors. However, potentially synergistic interactions between hydroxyurea and other drugs that affect pyrimidine nucleotide biosynthesis and DNA metabolism (*eg*, methotrexate, the fluoropyrimidines, and cytarabine) have been identified in laboratory studies, and rationally designed combinations of hydroxyurea with other drugs continue to be the subject of numerous clinical investigations. Hydroxyurea can stimulate hemoglobin F production, and it is being investigated as a useful agent in treating sickle cell disease

DOSAGE AND ADMINISTRATION

800–1200 mg/m^2/d PO daily **or** 2000–3200 mg/m^2 PO every 3 d. Dose titrated to response and WBC.

SPECIAL PRECAUTIONS

Pregnant and nursing patients

TOXICITIES

Hematologic: neutropenia (reversible) thrombocytopenia, anemia
GI: anorexia, nausea, vomiting (mild); oral, esophageal, GI mucositis and ulceration; constipation, diarrhea; liver function abnormalities (rarely progressing to jaundice)
Dermatologic: hyperpigmentation, erythema of face and hands, diffuse maculopapular rash, dry skin, thinning of skin, nail changes, alopecia (rare)
lopapular rash, dry skin, thinning of skin, nail changes, alopecia (rare), skin ulcers
Neurologic: headache, drowsiness, dizziness, confusion (mild)
Miscellaneous: transient renal function abnormalities, radiation recall reactions

INDICATIONS

FDA-approved: ovarian adenocarcinoma, malignant melanoma, and chronic myelocytic leukemia; concurrently with radiation therapy for squamous carcinomas of the head and neck; carcinomas of the head and neck, to reduce the frequency of painful crises and to reduce the need for blood transfusions in adult patients with sickle cell anemia with recurrent moderate to severe painful crises (generally at least three during the preceding 12 months); clinical studies show activity in acute nonlymphocytic leukemia and essential thrombocytosis (acute control of dangerously elevated cell counts, pending initiation of standard cytarabine-based treatment regimens); polycythemia vera; as a radiosensitizer, in locally advanced cancer of the uterine cervix

PHARMACOKINETICS

Absorption: high oral availability; **Distribution**: readily penetrates the CNS and malignant effusions (excreted in significant quantities in breast milk); **Elimination**: primarily renal; **Half-life**: 3.5–4.5 hr; **Adjustments for organ dysfunction**: intitial reduced doses to patients with renal dysfunction recommended

DRUG INTERACTIONS

Cytarabine, fluorouracil, methotrexate

RESPONSE RATES

Chronic myelocytic leukemia: reduction of leukocyte count in over 75% of patients

PATIENT MONITORING

Vital signs, symptoms (mucositis, diarrhea), examination, hematology (weekly), serum chemistry panel

NURSING INTERVENTIONS

Monitor weight, nutritional status; encourage good oral hygiene; give antiemetics; mouthwashes and other adjuncts for stomatitis; antidiarrheals as needed

PATIENT INFORMATION

Patient should avoid use of aspirin or nonsteroidal anti-inflammatory agents; call physician if fever or other signs of serious infection develop; avoid excessive sun exposure

FORMULATION

Hydrea, 500-mg capsules; also available as Droxia 200-mg, 300-mg, and 400-mg capsules (Bristol-Myers Oncology Division, Princeton, NJ). Stored at 15°–30°C in a tightly sealed container

LEUCOVORIN

Leucovorin (5-formyl-tetrahydrofolate) is a reduced folate that can be readily transformed to all folates required for cellular metabolism. Thus, it serves as an effective antidote for methotrexate and other antifols and can be used to reduce the adverse effects caused by these drugs. In contrast, leucovorin increases the toxicity and enhances the efficacy of the fluoropyrimidines; the leucovorin metabolite, 5,10-methylene-tetrahydrofolate, enhances the inhibition of the enzyme thymidylate synthase produced by fluorodeoxyuridine monophosphate, an active metabolite of the fluoropyrimidines.

DOSAGE AND ADMINISTRATION

Methotrexate rescue: beginning 24 h after initation of methotrexate therapy, administer leucovorin (dose dependent on regimen) 15 mg IV or PO every 6 h for ~10 doses (until methotrexate level is 0.05 μmol/L). Start rescue no later than 24 h after high-dose methotrexate. Higher leucovorin doses and longer treatement may be required if methotrexate clearance is abnormal (see manufacturer's guidelines). **With fluorouracil** (for colorectal cancer): leucovorin 20 mg/m^2 followed by 425 mg/m^2 fluorouracil **or** leucovorin 200 mg/m^2 followed by 370 mg/m^2 fluorouracil daily for 5 d. Alternate regimen: leucovorin 500 mg/m^2 IV infusion over 2 h with fluorouracil injection (500–600 mg/m^2) at midpoint of leucovorin infusion; repeat weekly for 6 wk.

SPECIAL PRECAUTIONS

Should not be given intrathecally as a rescue for intrathecal methotrexate overdose

TOXICITIES

Allergic: sensitization (possibly)
Neurologic: seizures (with 5-FU)

INDICATIONS

FDA-approved: antidote for overdose of methotrexate or other folic acid antagonists; osteosarcoma (adjuvant chemotherapy, with high-dose methotrexate); advanced colorectal cancer (with 5-FU); clinical studies show activity in advanced breast cancer (with 5-FU)

PHARMACOKINETICS

Absorption: high bioavailability at oral doses up to 40 mg, less at higher doses; **Distribution:** negligible CSF penetration, (approximately 1% of systemic levels); **Elimination:** metabolized and excreted renally; **Half-life:** 1 hr (parent compound) and 4–7 h (active 5-methyl-tetrahydrofolate metabolite); **Adjustments for organ dysfunction:** unnecessary

DRUG INTERACTIONS

Fluoropyrimidines, (including capecitabine), methotrexate, edatrexate, trimetrexate, piritrexim, iododeoxyuridine

RESPONSE RATES

See page on methotrexate; *see* chapter on lower gastrointestinal cancer

PATIENT MONITORING

None required for single-agent leucovorin

NURSING INTERVENTIONS

None required for single-agent leucovorin (see pages on methotrexate and 5-FU for combination therapy)

PATIENT INFORMATION

No specific information required for single-agent leucovorin

FORMULATION

Available from Immunex, Seattle, WA; Wellcovorin (Glaxo Wellcome, Research Triangle Park, NC; Elkins-Sinn, Cherry Hill, NJ; and Roxane Laboratories, Columbus, OH).
5-mg, 10-mg, 15-mg, and 25-mg tablets; 50-mg, 100-mg, and 350-mg vials of cryodessicated powder. Stored at 15°–30°C and protected from light

The information here is provided as guidance only. Prescribers should always consult the manufacturer's current prescribi

49

METHOTREXATE

Methotrexate, a synthetic analogue of folic acid, is a potent inhibitor of dihydrofolate reductase (DHFR), a key enzyme in folate metabolism. Inhibition of DHFR results in depletion of cellular reduced folates and interferes with vital cellular enzymes that require reduced folate cofactors (including enzymes of thymidylate and purine synthesis and amino acid metabolism). Inside the cell, methotrexate is metabolized to active polyglutamate metabolites, which inhibit DHFR and several other cellular enzymes, including enzymes that catalyze formyl transfer reactions in purine biosynthesis. Active polyglutamate metabolites of methotrexate may be retained by cells for long periods of time; hence, the antimetabolic effects of this drug may persist long after circulating levels of methotrexate are undetectable.

Leucovorin can reverse most of the antimetabolic effects produced by methotrexate and thus can rescue both normal and malignant cells from the cytotoxic effects of methotrexate. Used appropriately, leucovorin can enhance the therapeutic index of methotrexate by controlling and limiting the toxicity of higher doses of methotrexate. Pharmacologic interactions may also occur between methotrexate and many other drugs commonly administered to cancer patients. Clinically, the combination of methotrexate and fluorouracil has been extensively evaluated; available data suggest therapeutic synergy for treatment schedules in which fluorouracil administration follows methotrexate administration.

DOSAGE AND ADMINISTRATION

Solid tumors: 30–40 mg/m²/wk (IV infusion) **or** 3–12 g/m² as a 4–6 h (IV infusion) with leucovorin rescue beginning at 6–24 h

Oral regimens: 5–30 mg (total dose) PO, repeated weekly (usually used for psoriasis, rheumatoid arthritis); 2.5–10.0 mg (total dose) PO daily (used for mycosis fungoides)

Intrathecal administration: 10–15 mg/m² (maximum 15 mg); dose according to age (< 1 y, 6 mg; 1 y, 8 mg; 2 y, 10 mg; 3 y or older, 12 mg); repeat administration 1–2 times weekly, until CSF cytology has been negative for malignant cells for 1 wk; consider periodic maintenance therapy. Preservative-free preparations should be used for intrathecal therapy

SPECIAL PRECAUTIONS

Patients with pleural effusions, ascites, impaired renal function (may delay clearance, increase toxicity); pregnant and nursing patients; patients with poor nutritional status; patients on high-dose regimens; recent nitrous oxide anesthesia

TOXICITIES

Hematologic: neutropenia, anemia thrombocytopenia (occasional, reversible)
GI: anorexia, nausea, vomiting, diarrhea; oral, esophageal, GI mucositis and ulceration; transient abnormalities in serum levels of liver enzymes; cirrhosis, hepatic failure (rare)
Neurologic: headache, drowsiness, dizziness; with high doses, acute confusion, obtundation, seizures, encephalopathy, leukoencephalopathy; with intrathecal administration, chronic dementia, acute chemical arachnoiditis (rare, possible severe)
Dermatologic: rash, pruritus, urticaria, pigmentary changes, photosensitivity, alopecia, acne, skin necrosis, exfoliative dermatitis
Pulmonary: interstitial pneumonitis, *Pneumocystis carinii* pneumonia
Cardiovascular: pericarditis, pericardial effusion, hypotension, thromboembolic events
Renal: acute renal failure (especially with high doses), hyperuricemia, alkalinization of urine (pH ≥7) (with high-dose regimen)
Miscellaneous: anaphylaxis (rare), radiation recall, osteopathy, other opportunistic infections, malignant lymphoma (rare), opportunistic infections, malignant lymphoma (rare); soft tissue necrosis and osteonecrosis when given concurrently with radiotherapy

INDICATIONS

FDA-approved: choriocarcinoma and gestational trophoblastic disease, ALL, meningeal leukemia, breast cancer, squamous head and neck cancers, mycosis fungoides, lung cancer, non-Hodgkin's lymphomas, osteogenic sarcoma; clinical studies show activity in carcinoma of the bladder, post-transplantation immunosuppression

PHARMACOKINETICS

Absorption: 60% oral bioavailability (for doses up to 30 mg) significant interindividual variability in pediatric leukemic patients (23%–95%); **Distribution:** 1%–3% penetration into CSF, slow penetrating, slow release from pleural effusions or ascites; **Elimination:** 80%–90% renal; **Half-life:** 3–10 h (at or below 30 mg/m²); 10–15 h (high doses); **Adjustments for renal insufficiency (creatinine clearance < 40 mL/min; or, for high-dose regimens, creatinine clearance < 60 mL/min):** do not administer

DRUG INTERACTIONS

Leucovorin, 5-FU, ara-C, asparaginase, carboxypeptidase, thiopurines, colchicine, nitrous oxide, probenecid, aspirin, NSAID, sulfonamides, triamterene, trimethoprim, pyrimethamine, penicillins, retinoids

RESPONSE RATES

Choriocarcinoma and gestational trophoblastic disease: generally curative; **Pediatric ALL:** response to combination regimens with methotrexate 90%; cured 50%; **Breast cancer:** with cyclophosphamide and 5-FU, 30%–50% remission; **Squamous head and neck cancers:** partial remissions in 30%; **Mycosis fungoides:** complete response rate 40%–50%; **Osteogenic sarcoma:** cure rate of nonmetastatic disease 50%–60% with adjuvant combination therapy

PATIENT MONITORING

Vital signs, symptoms, examination, hematology, serum chemistry panel; with high doses, closely monitor renal function, urine output, urine pH, serum electrolytes, serum methotrexate levels

NURSING INTERVENTIONS

Monitor weight, nutritional status; encourage good oral hygiene; give antiemetics: with high doses, monitor fluid intake and output, assess patient's oral intake and ability to take leucovorin rescue as instructed post-discharge

PATIENT INFORMATION

Patient should avoid use of aspirin or NSAIDs; call physician if moderate or severe adverse effects develop

FORMULATION

Available from (Seattle, WA) and other manufacturers; 50-, 100-, 200-, and 250-mg vials containing 25-mg/mL preservative-free solution; 50-mg and 250-mg vials containing 25-mg/mL preservative-protected solution; 20-mg, 50-mg, and 1-g vials of methotrexate; 2.5-mg tablets. Stored at 15°–30°C and protected from light

MERCAPTOPURINE

Mercaptopurine (6-mercaptopurine or 6-MP) is a thiopurine that has been in clinical use as an antileukemic drug since the 1950s. Mercaptopurine is enzymatically converted to 6-thioinosine monophosphate (6-TIMP) by a purine salvage enzyme, hypoxanthine-guanine phosphoribosyltransferase (HGPRT). Although 6-TIMP is a relatively poor substrate for cellular enzymes and accumulates to significant levels in 6-MP-treated cells, 6-TIMP can be converted to a variety of other metabolites, including the corresponding ribonucleoside and deoxyribonucleoside di- and triphosphates, 6-methylmercaptopurine and its nucleotides, and 6-thioguanine nucleotides. The 6-TIMP metabolite of mercaptopurine inhibits several enzymes important in purine biosynthesis; 6-thiodeoxyguanosine triphosphate formed from 6-MP can be incorporated into DNA and can produce DNA strand breaks; and the many other metabolites of 6-MP produce additional antimetabolic effects. It is not yet clear which mechanisms account for the anticancer activity of mercaptopurine.

Relationships among the thiopurines in clinical use (mercaptopurine, thioguanine, and azathioprine) and genetic polymorphism of thiopurine S-methyltransferase are discussed in the section on thioguanine.

DOSAGE AND ADMINISTRATION

Acute lymphoblastic leukemia: 50–75 mg/m^2/d for 30–36 mo (maintenance chemotherapy, with methotrexate)
Acute nonlymphocytic leukemia: 500 mg/m^2/d IV (using investigational IV formulation) $\times$ 5 d (in induction combination chemotherapy)

SPECIAL PRECAUTIONS

Pregnant and nursing patients; patients receiving allopurinol (reduce doses by 75%)

TOXICITIES

Hematologic: neutropenia, thrombocytopenia, anemia (reversible, dose-related)
GI: anorexia, nausea, vomiting, diarrhea, (mild); oral, esophageal, GI mucositis and ulceration; reversible cholestatic jaundice; hepatic necrosis (rare)
Dermatologic: rash, hyperpigmentation
Miscellaneous: fever, pancreatitis (rare), hematuria and crystalluria with high IV doses, immune hemolytic anemia

INDICATIONS

FDA-approved: acute lymphocytic leukemia, acute nonlymphocytic leukemias; clinical studies show activity in chronic myelocytic leukemia

PHARMACOKINETICS

Absorption: oral bioavailability ($\approx$ 16%), erratic, extensive first-pass metabolism in intestinal mucosa and liver; **Distribution**: no CSF penetration; **Elimination**: via metabolism (xanthine oxidase, other pathways); **Half-life**: 1.5 h; **Adjustments for organ dysfunction**: insufficient data

DRUG INTERACTIONS

Allopurinol, methotrexate, tiazofurin, trimethoprim-sulfamethoxazole, coumadin

RESPONSE RATES

Not applicable (used in maintenance phase treatment following complete remission of pediatric ALL; overall cure rate 50%)

PATIENT MONITORING

Vital signs, symptoms (mucositis, diarrhea), examination, hematology (weekly), serum chemistry panel

NURSING INTERVENTIONS

Monitor weight, nutritional status; encourage good oral hygiene; give antiemetics; mouthwashes and other adjuncts for stomatitis; antidiarrheals as needed

PATIENT INFORMATION

Patient should avoid use of aspirin or nonsteroidal anti-inflammatory agents; call physician if fever or other signs of serious infection develop; avoid excessive sun exposure; maintain good nutrition

FORMULATION

Available as Purinethol, (Glaxo-Wellcome, Research Triangle Park, NC)
50-mg tablets. Stored at 15°–25°C in a dry place.
Investigators with NCI-approved research protocols can obtain investigational tablet (10 mg) and IV formulations from the Pharmaceutical Resources Branch, National Cancer Institute
50-mL vials containing 500-mg mercaptopurine (sodium salt), lyophilized powder. Store unopened vials at room temperature (22°–25°C)

PENTOSTATIN

Pentostatin (2´-deoxycoformycin or DCF) is a purine deoxynucleoside analogue isolated from fermentation cultures of *Streptomyces antibioticus*. Pentostatin is a potent inhibitor of the enzyme adenosine deaminase, which hydrolyzes adenosine to inosine. The pharmacologic actions of pentostatin are believed to be mediated by the accumulation of adenine nucleotides, which can occur when adenosine hydrolysis is blocked. High intracellular levels of deoxyadenosine triphosphate can inhibit the activity of the enzyme ribonucleotide reductase, resulting in depletion of levels of other cellular deoxyribonucleotides. High levels of deoxyadenosine nucleotides can also inhibit the enzyme S-adenosylhomocysteine hydrolase, thus interfering with cellular methylation pathways and causing accumulation of S-adenosylhomocysteine, a toxic metabolite. Cells such as lymphocytes that have low levels of the nucleotide-cleaving enzyme 5´-nucleotidase may be particularly sensitive to these antimetabolic effects of pentostatin. Other known antimetabolic effects of pentostatin include inhibition of RNA synthesis and misincorporation of the triphosphate metabolite of pentostatin into cellular DNA.

In initial phase I studies using high doses of pentostatin, toxicities were frequently observed, with limited evidence of clinical efficacy. However, subsequent research has shown that this agent is highly active against hairy cell leukemia (a B-cell lymphoid neoplasm), has activity in other lymphoid malignancies as well, and can be used safely and effectively at lower doses. Pentostatin is not active in the treatment of solid tumors, and significant immunosuppression occurs as an adverse effect even at low doses of pentostatin.

DOSAGE AND ADMINISTRATION

Hairy cell leukemia: pretreat with allopurinol (300 mg/d) × 7 d. Then pentostatin (4 mg/m^2 IV bolus) every 2 wk until complete response, followed by two additional doses, or to maximum of 12 mo. If no partial response by 6 mo, change to alternate treatment. Adjust dose if creatinine clearance is less than 60 mL/min.

SPECIAL PRECAUTIONS

Opportunistic (*eg, Pneumocystis carinii*) and severe infections
Pregnant/nursing patients

TOXICITIES

Hematologic: lymphopenia (particularly T cells), neutropenia, thrombocytopenia, immunosuppression (possibly severe and prolonged); infectious complications (common, including opportunistic infections)
Neurologic: anxiety, depression, confusion, lethargy, obtundation, coma, seizures, myalgias
Renal: azotemia, acute renal failure, long-term residual impairment (possible)
Dermatologic: rash (possibly severe and increased with continued treatment)
GI: anorexia, nausea, vomiting (not severe), stomatitis, elevations in liver function tests (reversible), diarrhea
Miscellaneous: fever, pneumonitis, myalgias, arthralgias, pleuritis, peritonitis, pericarditis, keratoconjunctivitis, TTP, coughing

INDICATIONS

FDA-approved: untreated or interferon-α–refractory hairy cell leukemia; clinical studies show activity in T- and B-cell lymphomas, acute lymphoblastic leukemia, chronic lymphocytic leukemia, mycosis fungoides, Sézary syndrome, Waldenström's macroglobulinemia; **Possible activity:** multiple myeloma, Hodgkin's lymphomas

PHARMACOKINETICS

Absorption: insufficient data; **Distribution:** insufficient data on CNS penetration; **Elimination:** renal; **Half-life:** 2.5–6 h; **Adjustments for organ dysfunction:** delayed elimination of pentostatin with renal dysfunction; patients should have a creatinine clearance ≥ 60 mL/min

DRUG INTERACTIONS

Fludarabine phosphate, vidarabine, allopurinol

RESPONSE RATES

Hairy cell leukemia (untreated): 68% complete response in blood and marrow plus 5% partial response; **Hairy cell leukemia (refractory to interferon-α):** 58%–85% complete response plus 4%–28% partial response

PATIENT MONITORING

Vital signs, symptoms, examination, hematology, serum chemistry panel; creatinine clearance pretreatment and during treatment; bone marrow examination for persistent cytopenias

NURSING INTERVENTIONS

Monitor weight, nutritional status; encourage good oral hygiene; give antiemetics as necessary; give mouthwashes and other adjuncts as needed for stomatitis; give antidiarrheals as needed; evaluate for infectious etiology if diarrhea is persistent or severe

PATIENT INFORMATION

Patient should avoid use of aspirin or nonsteroidal anti-inflammatory agents; call physician if fever or other signs of serious infection develop; maintain good nutrition

FORMULATION

Available as NIPENT (SuperGen, San Ramon, CA) 10-mg vials of lyophilized powder. Stored at 2°–8°C

THIOGUANINE

Thioguanine (6-thioguanine or 6-TG), a purine analogue, has been in clinical use as an antileukemic drug since the 1950s. Thioguanine is activated to 6-thioguanosine monophosphate by a purine salvage enzyme, hypoxanthine-guanine phosphoribosyltransferase (HGPRT). This ribonucleotide can be phosphorylated further by cellular kinases to generate thioguanosine di- and triphosphates or reduced (via the action of the enzyme ribonucleotide reductase) to generate thioguanine deoxyribonucleotides. Incorporation of thioguanine nucleotides into DNA and RNA is believed to be the principal cytotoxic mechanism of thiopurines.

The thiopurines are active agents in the treatment of acute and chronic leukemias and may have modest activity in the treatment of non-Hodgkin's lymphomas, but they have demonstrated no significant clinical activity against solid tumors. For historic reasons, azathioprine is used as an immunosuppressive, 6-thioguanine is used primarily in treatment of nonlymphocytic leukemias, and 6-mercaptopurine is used primarily in treatment of lymphocytic leukemias. Although clinical comparative studies have not been performed, it is likely that any of these drugs could be used for any of these indications, with comparable results. The only clinically significant pharmacologic difference among these three drugs is that the metabolic elimination of thioguanine is *not* significantly affected by allopurinol; hence, thioguanine doses need not be adjusted in patients receiving allopurinol. Recently, the genetic basis for the phenotypic polymorphism of thiopurine S-methyltransferase (TMPT) has been elucidated. TMPT catalyzes the S-methylation of thiopurines, resulting in reduced formation of the active thioguanine nucleotides. TMPT-deficient patients will accumulate excessive thioguanine nucleotides in hematopoietic tissues and suffer severe hematologic toxicities after receiving standard doses of thiopurines.

DOSAGE AND ADMINISTRATION

Acute leukemia (in combination chemotherapy): 75–200 mg/m^2/d × 5 to 7 d in one or two divided oral doses

SPECIAL PRECAUTIONS

Pregnancy and nursing patients; hepatic impairment

TOXICITIES

Hematologic: neutropenia, thrombocytopenia, anemia (reversible, dose-related)
GI: anorexia, nausea, vomiting (mild), diarrhea; oral, esophageal, GI mucositis and ulceration; cholestatic jaundice
Dermatologic: rash, hyperpigmentation

INDICATIONS

FDA-approved: acute nonlymphocyctic leukemias; chronic myelocyctic leukemia (alternative to busulfan); clinical studies show activity in acute lymphocyctic leukmeia

PHARMACOKINETICS

Absorption: limited oral bioavailability (approximately 30%), highly variable (food intake reduces bioavailability); **Distribution:** does not penetrate CNS; **Elimination:** metabolism (methylation); **Half-life:** 25–240 min; **Adjustments for organ dysfunction:** insufficient data, use with caution in hepatic impairment

DRUG INTERACTIONS

Methotrexate, other antifols, tiazofurin

RESPONSE RATES

Adult acute nonlymphocytic leukemia (with cytosine arabinoside and daunorubicin or doxorubicin): complete remission rate 40%–75%; cure rate 5%–10%

PATIENT MONITORING

Vital signs, symptoms (mucositis, diarrhea), examination, hematology (weekly or daily in leukemia induction therapy), serum chemistry panel

NURSING INTERVENTIONS

Monitor weight, nutritional status; encourage good oral hygiene; give antiemetics; mouthwashes and other adjuncts for stomatitis; antidiarrheals as needed

PATIENT INFORMATION

Patient should avoid use of aspirin or nonsteroidal anti-inflammatory agents; call physician if fever or other signs of serious infection develop; avoid excessive sun exposure; maintain good nutrition

FORMULATIONS

Available as Tabloid (Glaxo Wellcome, Inc., Triangle Research Park, NC).
40-mg tablets. Stored at 15°–25°C in a dry place.
Investigators with NCI-approved research protocols can obtain the investigational IV formulation from the Pharmaceutical Resources Branch, National Cancer Institute.
Investigational IV formulation, 10-mL vials containing 75-mg thioguanine (base), lyophilized powder. Unopened vials are refrigerated (2°–8°C), but are also stable at room temperature (22°–25°C)

CAPECITABINE

Capecitabine is an oral fluoropyrimidine that is enzymatically converted in vivo to 5-fluorouracil (5-FU). On absorption from the gastrointestinal tract, capecitabine is hydrolyzed by a hepatic carboxyesterase to 5'-deoxy-5-fluorocytidine (5'-DFCR), which is subsequently converted to 5'-deoxy-5-fluorouridine (5'-DFUR) by cytidine deaminase. Thymidine phosphorylase then hydrolyzes 5'DFUR to 5-FU. Many tissues throughout the body express thymidine phosphorylase. The expression of this enzyme was found to be higher in some carcinomas that in surrounding normal tissues, which may result in preferential conversion of capecitabine to 5-FU in tumor tissues.

DOSAGE AND ADMINISTRATION

Metastatic breast cancer: 2500 mg/m²/d orally in two divided doses with food for 2 wks followed by a 1-wk rest period, repeated at 3-wk intervals; **Metastatic colorectal cancer:** 2500 mg/m²/d orally in two divided doses with food for 2 wks followed by a 1-wk rest period, repeated at 3-wk intervals

SPECIAL PRECAUTIONS

Severe diarrhea, hand-foot-mouth syndrome, pregnant and nursing mothers

TOXICITIES

Hematologic: neutropenia, thrombocytopenia, anemia; **Gastrointestinal:** diarrhea (sometimes severe), anorexia, nausea, vomiting; stomatitis; dyspepsia; necrotizing enterocolitis (typhlitis); **Neurologic:** paraesthesia, headache, dizziness, insomnia, eye irritation; **Dermatologic:** hand-foot-mouth syndrome; rash, dry skin, fissuring, nail changes and loss, photosensitivity, alopecia, hyperpigmentation; **Cardiovascular:** myocardial ischemia, angina, infarction, arrhythmia, cardiogenic shock, sudden death, electrograph changes; **Laboratory abnormalities:** elevation of bilirubin; **Miscellaneous:** conjunctivitis, generalized allergic reactions (very rare)

INDICATIONS

FDA-approved: treatment of metastatic breast cancer resistant to both paclitaxel and an anthracycline-containing regimen or resistant to paclitaxel and for whom further anthracycline-therapy is not indicated, *eg*, patients who have received cumulative doses of 400 mg/m² of doxorubicin or doxorubicin equivalent. Resistance is defined as progressive disease while on treatment, with or without an initial response, or relapse within 6 months of completing treatment with an anthracycline-containing adjuvant regimen. Clinical studies show activity in colorectal cancer

PHARMACOKINETICS

Absorption: rapidly absorbed from gastrointestinal tract; no data on bioavailability; **Distribution:** binding to plasma proteins is less than 60% and is not concentration-dependent; primarily bound to albumin; **Elimination:** metabolized enzymatically to 5-FU; excretion of intact drug (3%) in urine; **Half-life:** 45 min; **Adjustments for hepatic or renal dysfunction:** use with caution in patients with mild to moderate hepatic or renal dysfunction; discontinue immediately in patients with ≥ grade 2 elevation in bilirubin

DRUG INTERACTIONS

Antacids, warfarin, phenprocoumon, leucovorin

RESPONSE RATES

Breast cancer: partial remissions, 18%–25%; **Colorectal cancer:** 23% (1.3% complete response)

PATIENT MONITORING

Vital signs, symptoms (mucositis, diarrhea), examination, hematology, serum chemistry panel

NURSING INTERVENTIONS

Monitor weight, nutritional status; encourage good oral hygiene; give antiemetics as necessary; mouthwashes and other adjuncts for stomatitis; antidiarrheals for mild diarrhea (inform physician)

PATIENT INFORMATION

Patient should avoid use of aspirin or nonsteroidal anti-inflammatory agents. Call physician if any moderate or severe diarrhea, fever, or other signs of serious infection develop, or if oral intake decreases. Avoid excessive sun exposure; maintain good nutrition

FORMULATION

Available as Xeloda (Roche Laboratories, Nutley, NJ); 150-mg and 500-mg tablets. Stored at 15°–30°C; keep tightly closed

Biologic therapy uses so-called biologic reagents, *ie*, those agents that evoke immune responses, to directly target receptor or signaling pathways, or modify the stroma of the tumor (endothelins, fibroblasts, or macrophages) to elicit tumor regression. The biotherapeutic pharmacopoeia includes recombinant cytokines, some of which possess profound immunomodulatory and antitumor activity, including interleukin-2 (aldesleukin) and interferon-α (IFN-α). Additional cytokines that have been evaluated include tumor necrosis factor-α, interferon-γ, M-CSF, IL-1, IL-4, and IL-12, none of which have been approved for cancer therapy as yet in the United States. Other recombinant proteins, termed colony-stimulating factors (CSF), exert profound effects on hematopoiesis and immune function. They include erythropoietin (epoietin-α), granulocyte-CSF (filgrastim), and granulocyte, macrophage-CSF (sargramostim). Although they do not have direct antitumor activity, these recombinant proteins blunt chemotherapy-induced myelopoietic toxicity, and have become useful adjuvants to bone marrow transplantation and aggressive chemotherapeutic regimens.

Other immunomodulating reagents with demonstrated antitumor activity include bacillus Calmette-Guérin and histamine. Both reagents apparently mediate their antitumor effects through immune modulation. Octreotide is a long-acting octapeptide that mimics the effects of the naturally occurring hormone somatostatin. Its pleiotropic effects include antiproliferative activity against several types of tumor. Additional anticancer biologic reagents, including IL-1, IL-4, IL-6, IL-7, and IL-12, as well as adoptively transferred lymphoid cells, are being evaluated for clinical efficacy but will not be discussed because of their experimental nature.

ALDESLEUKIN

Aldesleukin, or interleukin 2 (IL-2), is a T-cell growth factor that is central to T-cell–mediated immune responses [1,2]. It is a hydrophobic, 15-kD, 133-amino-acid glycoprotein that is elaborated primarily by activated CD4+ T lymphocytes. Its production is regulated at the transcriptional level by signals transduced across the plasma cell membrane when a mature T cell encounters its cognate antigen in concert with secondary signals provided by accessory cells. Aldesleukin is the recombinant protein elaborated by *Escherichia coli* that contain the human IL-2 gene. The cysteine residue at position 125 is substituted in the recombinant product by similar space-occupying amino acids to avoid aggregation and disulfide exchange leading to the accumulation of less active forms. Aldesleukin has been approved for the treatment of patients with metastatic renal cell carcinoma and metastatic malignant melanoma. Aldesleukin has also been used in patients with HIV infection.

Renal Cell Carcinoma

In an update of 255 patients with metastatic renal cell carcinoma treated in a total of seven phase II clinical trials with high-dose aldesleukin (600,000 or 720,000 IU/kg every 8 h IV), an overall response rate of 15% (8% partial and 7% complete responses) has been reported [3,4]. The overall median duration of response was 54.0 months, the median survival for all patients was 16.3 months, and 10% to 20% of patients were estimated to be alive 5 to 10 years following treatment. However, because of the toxicity associated with the administration of high-dose IL-2, other dosing regimens have been evaluated in this disease. Examples of administration of low-dose IL-2 [5], IL-2 by continuous IV [6–9], subcutaneous adminis-

tration [10,11], or in combination with IFN-α with or without 5-fluorouracil [12,13] has resulted in response rates ranging from 14% to 29%. Toxicities associated with these regimens have generally been less severe than those associated with high-dose IL-2. Studies to determine which dosing regimen of IL-2 is optimal for the treatment of patients with metastatic renal cell carcinoma are still inconclusive but are generally most supportive of dose-intensive regimens in patients able to tolerate the toxicity [14].

Melanoma

Recombinant IL-2 has been extensively tested for its effect in the treatment of patients with advanced melanoma. Administered as a single agent, IL-2 induces objective responses in up to 25% of patients with stage IV melanoma [16–19]. This response rate is in the same order as the response rates observed with the most active cytotoxic agents; however, a considerable fraction of IL-2 mediated responses will be long-lasting [20,21], unlike most responses achieved with cytotoxic drugs. Because of its ability to induce durable results, IL-2 has been recently licensed for use in advanced melanoma by the US Food and Drug Administration (FDA).

Various treatment regimens have been used. The four most widely tested regimens include administration of repeated bolus injections every 8 hours for a maximum of 5 days [16], continuous intravenous infusion for 5 days [17], a "decrescendo" schedule of continuous intravenous infusion starting with a high initial dose, which is tapered in a stepwise fashion to a low maintenance dose [18], and intermittent or prolonged subcutaneous applications of a variety of doses. All of these regimens have later been included into combination therapies, but there is no comparative study available with two or more of the different regimens.

Several randomized phase III trials have been performed to assess the role of IL-2 for the treatment of advanced melanoma in combination with various cytotoxic drugs. However, most trials are not yet fully evaluated and have not provided substantial benefit. Clear information from the major trials is expected toward the end of 2001 [22,23].

HIV

Trials of aldesleukin by continuous intravenous or subcutaneous administration (with or without antiviral agents) in patients with HIV have demonstrated reproducible increases in CD4+ T-cell numbers without concomitant increases in viral load [24]. Improved CD4+ T-cell function has also been shown to be positively correlated with administration of aldesleukin as assessed by delayed-type hypersensitivity reactivity. Although these results are encouraging, evidence of a correlation between improved CD4+ T-cell number and function and patient survival remains to be determined.

Although combinations of IL-2 with other agents (*eg*, immune modulators [25]) or the adoptive transfer of dendritic cells continue to be tested, the prolonged response durations of high-dose IL-2 lasting as long as 15 years have yet to be exceeded. Other novel strategies for the use of IL-2 (*eg*, for the treatment of malignant effusions [26], hematologic malignancies [27], or after bone marrow or stem-cell transplantation for hematologic or solid malignancies [28–32]) continue to be tested as well.

MECHANISM OF ACTION

Interleukin 2 plays a central role in T-cell activation. It promotes cell-cycle progression from G1 to S phase and subsequent T-cell proliferation during cell-mediated immune responses. The effects of

IL-2 are mediated through expression of one to three chains of the heterotrimeric receptor (IL-2R). The IL-2 receptor-α chain (IL-2Rα), also referred to as p55, CD25, or Tac, has low affinity for IL-2 (kD $\approx$ 10-8 M) and is not constitutively expressed. The β chain of the IL-2R, or p75, is a 70 to 75 kD, 525 amino acid molecule with intermediate affinity for IL-2 (kD $\approx$ 10-9 M). IL-2Rβ is expressed by monocytes, some mature CD4+ and CD8+ T cells, and large granular lymphocytes (LGL). It is also expressed in concert with IL-2RI on a subset of CD16-NK cells. The high affinity IL-2R (kD $\approx$ 10-11 M) is a noncovalently linked heterotrimer consisting of the α, β, and γ subunits.

Ligation of the high- or the intermediate-affinity IL-2R with IL-2 leads to internalization of the complex and a cascade of genetic events that activates a cell. Large granular lymphocytes proliferate and develop lymphokine-activated killer (LAK) activity. The cytotoxic activity of monocytes and CD8+ T cells is stimulated as well. Activated B cells are induced to proliferate and elaborate secretory rather than membranous IgM. T cells that express the high-affinity IL-2R undergo cell division following exposure to IL-2. The ability of IL-2–stimulated mononuclear cells to elaborate IFN-γ, TNF-α, IL-6, and IL-1 accounts for additional pleiotropic effects. Although IL-2 downregulates the help provided by CD4+ T cells to humoral effector cells in certain models, the net effect of exogenous administration on immune function is stimulatory. The selective antitumor effects seen in some patients treated with aldesleukin are believed to be the result of a cell-mediated immune response. There is compelling evidence derived from both murine models and clinical trials that the antitumor immune response is primarily T-cell mediated.

MECHANISMS OF RESISTANCE

At least 70% of patients with renal cell carcinoma who are treated with IL-2 have no measurable clinical response to therapy. The majority of patients who manifest treatment-related tumor regression eventually develop progressive disease despite retreatment. Although responses have been reported in patients with metastatic melanoma, colorectal carcinoma, ovarian cancer, lymphoma, and lung cancer, these responses have been transient or infrequent. The mechanisms that underlie this apparent escape from immune-mediated tumor regression have not been elucidated. Antigenic heterogeneity within a tumor may allow for the outgrowth of antigenically distinct clones that are not recognized by the immune system. Alternatively, defects in cell trafficking or tumor-cell susceptibility to lysis may develop that lead to unchecked tumor progression. Definition of the mechanisms of resistance await a better understanding of the mechanisms of response [33]. Although antibodies route to IL-2 have been identified in some patients receiving IL-2, especially by the subcutaneous route [34], it does not appear that this causes a change in the effectiveness of IL-2 treatment.

ADVERSE EFFECTS

The supraphysiologic doses of IL-2 that have been used for therapy are associated with myriad side effects, which are most likely mediated by other cytokines (TNF-α in particular). Hematologic toxicity, including anemia requiring transfusion, and thrombocytopenia less than 20,000, have been observed in 60% and about 15% of treatment courses, respectively. Effects on the kidney include oliguria and decreased fractional excretion of sodium associated with rising serum creatinine and blood urea nitrogen in most patients.

These can be managed successfully in most patients with the intravenous administration of volume expanders and dopamine infusions (2–3 μg/kg/min). Renal toxicity resolves in nearly all instances within several days. Cardiovascular toxicity includes increased heart rate, and myocardial depression manifests by decreased ejection fraction. Elevations of adrenocorticotropic hormone, endorphins, growth hormone, prolactin, and glucocorticoids have been observed in treated patients. Some patients develop clinically overt hypothyroidism that requires long-term thyroid hormone replacement therapy. Nearly all patients develop a vascular leak syndrome that is associated with egress of intravascular fluid into the soft tissues, where it remains sequestered until therapy ends. This redistribution of fluid probably contributes to the hypotension observed in most treated patients and can be managed effectively with vigorous fluid resuscitation using volume as crystalloid [35]. The volume of administered fluid is limited in some patients by noncardiogenic pulmonary edema secondary to capillary leak. In these patients, phenylephrine can be used to support the blood pressure in lieu of volume expansion, often while the patient remains in a conventional ward.

INTERFERONS

The interferons include more than 20 antigenically discrete but related immunomodulatory proteins [36,37]. They differ in their physical properties but manifest similar effects on the immune system, albeit to different degrees and with some exceptions. Despite the profound immunomodulatory and antiproliferative effects manifest by the interferons, their use as single agents has been documented to have a survival impact only a few solid tumors [38].

Interferon-α, also referred to as leukocyte interferon, includes more than 23 related subtypes with overlapping activities. These are elaborated primarily by macrophages, large granular lymphocytes, and B cells following exposure to viruses, double-stranded RNA, tumor necrosis factor-α (TNF), and IL-1. Most of the naturally occurring IFN-α subtypes are composed of 166 amino acids and have molecular weights between 18,000 and 20,000. Their structure is that of an α-helix that is stabilized by disulfide bonds between cysteine residues at positions 1, 29, 99, and 139. The IFN-α gene, located on chromosome 9, is constitutively transcribed in some cell types and may confer a degree of protection against viral infection.

Natural IFN-α (Alferon N; Interferon Sciences, Inc., New Brunswick, NJ) is prepared from pooled human leukocytes that have been induced by infection with the avian Sendai virus. The specific composition of this preparation has not been elucidated. Recombinant IFN-α is available in the United States as IFN α-2a (Roferon A; Hoffmann-LaRoche, Nutley, NJ) and IFN α-2b (Inferon A; Schering-Plough, Kenilworth, NJ). These two recombinant cytokines differ from natural IFN-α in that amino acid 44 has been deleted and amino acid 23 has been replaced by lysine (IFN α-2a) or arginine (IFN α-2b).

Interferon β (fibroblast interferon) is a 166-amino-acid glycoprotein that shares 30% homology with IFN-α. The predominant sources of IFN-β in vivo are fibroblasts and epithelial cells. Its production is upregulated by the same stimuli that induce the production of IFN-α. Both IFN-α and IFN-β share a common cell-surface receptor. Unlike most naturally occurring IFN-α subtypes, IFN-β is N-glycosylated, its functional unit is a dimer, its α-helical content is less than 50%, and there is only one molecular species that is encoded by a gene located on chromosome 9. Recombinant IFN β (Betaseron; Berlex Laboratories, Inc., Montville, NJ) is a nonglycosylated analogue in which cysteine has been replaced by serine at position 17 to maintain stability. Its activity is similar to that of the naturally occurring protein. It has not been approved for clinical use in cancer.

Interferon-γ (type II or immune interferon) is a 143-amino-acid glycoprotein that shares little homology to the type I interferons α and β. It is encoded by a gene on chromosome 12 and is made predominantly by CD4+ and CD8+ T cells, NK cells, and macrophages following exposure to antigen, mitogen, or IL-2. The dimeric molecule interacts with a unique, high-affinity, cell-surface receptor that is specific for IFN-γ. There are an estimated 1000 receptors per cell with perhaps higher numbers on some tumor cells. IFN-γ has been approved by the FDA only for the treatment of chronic granulomatous disease. In addition to natural IFN-γ, several recombinant products are available from Genentech (South San Francisco, CA), Biogen Inc. (Cambridge, MA), Schering-Plough, and Amgen Inc. (Thousand Oaks, CA). Differences in the N-terminal sequences and the number of amino acids account for variable pharmacokinetics and bioavailability between these products.

IFN-α has demonstrated activity against many solid and hematologic malignancies. The latter appear to be particularly sensitive. An 80% to 90% response rate has been observed among patients with hairy cell leukemia treated with IFN-α. Complete response in the bone marrow is rare, however, and most patients eventually relapse with the median time to clinically significant hematologic deterioration being 18 to 24 months. Benefits of therapy include a decrease in the incidence of serious infection and a reduced requirement for blood products. Survival appears to be prolonged compared with historical controls.

The hematologic response among patients with chronic myelogenous leukemia who are treated within 1 year of diagnosis is 50% to 70%. Despite an associated 20% complete cytogenetic response rate that appears to be durable, a survival benefit has not been demonstrated. The role of IFN in the treatment of other hematologic malignancies appears to be limited with the exception of essential thrombocythemia in which response rates approaching 80% have been observed.

Adjuvant therapy of melanoma with IFN-α has been approved by the FDA. Kaposi's sarcoma is the only other solid tumor that has been approved by the FDA. The use of high doses (> 20 × 10⁶ U/m²/d) administered intramuscularly or subcutaneously is associated with a response rate of 30% among treated patients without B symptoms and prior opportunistic infection and with CD4+ lymphocyte counts greater than 200. Half of these responses are complete and durable. Several other solid tumors manifest some degree of sensitivity to interferons. These include renal cell carcinoma, malignant melanoma, carcinoid tumor, malignant endocrine pancreatic tumors, basal cell carcinoma, and superficial bladder cancer.

MECHANISM OF ACTION

The interferons have been investigated intensively as anticancer agents because of their pleiotropic effects on immune reactivity, cell differentiation, and the rate of cell proliferation. These effects are mediated through the ligation of cell-surface receptors that are specific for the interferons. About 1000 high-affinity receptors, consisting of two separate chains, are present on most cells and interact with both IFN-α and IFN-β. IFN-γ interacts with a different receptor heterodimer. Following receptor binding, incompletely understood cytoplasmic events ensue that lead to alterations in gene transcription and, as a result, the generation of regulatory enzymes and oncogenes that underlie the biologic effects of IFN.

Interferons retard proliferation of both normal and malignant cells by prolonging all stages of the cell cycle. Some cellular protooncogenes, including c-*myc*, c-*fos*, c-*ras*, and c-*src*, are downregulated, suggesting that this effect is mediated in part at the transcriptional level. The action of growth factors, including platelet-derived growth factor, epidermal growth factor, fibroblast growth factor, insulin, and macrophage-colony stimulating factor is also antagonized. Three interferon-induced enzymes that also could account for the observed antiproliferative effects are 2',5'-oligoadenylate synthetase, protein kinase, and indolamine 2,3 dioxygenase.

Interferons modulate immune reactivity by enhancing target-cell immunogenicity and activating immune effector cells. Major histocompatability complex class I antigen expression is upregulated by all three classes of IFN. The expression of some tumor-associated antigens, such as carcinoembryonic antigen and TAG-72, also is enhanced. These alterations in cell-surface antigen expression are thought to render tumors more susceptible to immune recognition. Direct effects on immune reactivity include enhanced cytotoxic T-cell activity, macrophage and NK-cell activation, induction of B-cell immunoglobulin production, and enhanced NK-cell–mediated antibody-dependent cellular cytotoxicity (ADCC). Effects on cellular differentiation and angiogenesis may contribute indirectly.

MECHANISMS OF RESISTANCE

The clinical responses associated with the use of IFN-α, which are dramatic in some hematologic malignancies, suggest that some neoplastic cells are much more sensitive to IFN than are normal cells. This could be accounted for by antigenic differences that exist between some cancers and normal cells or differences in cell-cycle kinetics. Resistance to IFN is poorly understood. At the cellular level, freshly isolated tumor cells demonstrate a range of sensitivity to IFN that does not correlate with tumor cell type. Resistance in vitro is not necessarily accompanied by changes in the number of cell-surface receptors. A better understanding of resistance awaits elucidation of the mechanisms underlying tumor regression.

ADVERSE EFFECTS

Therapy with IFN-α is usually well tolerated. Fewer than 10% of patients discontinue treatment as a result of severe toxicity. The most common adverse effect is a flu-like syndrome, occurring in as many as 98% of treated patients and consisting of fever (40%–98%), chills (40%–65%), myalgias (30%–75%), headache (20%–70%), malaise (50%–95%), and arthralgias (5%–24%). Fever may be as high as 40°C and occurs within 6 hours of a dose. Chills may be severe. Pretreatment with acetaminophen or nonsteroidal anti-inflammatory drugs can attenuate these toxicities, which become less severe with continued therapy. Adverse hematologic effects are mild and include neutropenia, anemia, and thrombocytopenia. Some patients manifest elevated serum concentrations of AST and ALT. Other gastrointestinal side effects include nausea, vomiting, diarrhea, and a metallic taste. Dyspnea, alopecia, rashes, proteinuria, thyroid dysfunction, and edema also have been reported.

BIOCHEMICAL MODULATION

Synergistic interactions between IFN and other anticancer agents have been well documented [39]. Antiproliferative synergy against transformed cell lines has been demonstrated for IFN-α and IFN-γ. Their immune potentiating effects on NK cells also are enhanced in combination. Synergistic effects also are seen with combinations of IFN-α and IL-2 at lower doses [13,18–23].

IFN-α has been observed to enhance the efficacy of many cancer chemotherapeutics, including 5-FU, cis-platinum, cyclophosphamide, and doxorubicin. This may be a result of altered pharmacokinetics. IFN-α–mediated inhibition of the cytochrome P450 system may delay the metabolism of doxorubicin and cyclophosphamide. The clearance of 5-FU also is inhibited by unknown mechanisms. It is also possible that the antitumor immune response generated by IFN may compliment the pharmacologic tumor debulking characteristic of chemotherapy by eradicating microscopic residual disease.

Melanoma has been reported to respond favorably to IFN-α treatment and has been given in higher dose regimens as an adjuvant following surgical excision of nodal metastatic disease [40–43]. In a randomized controlled study of IFN α-2b in patients with high-risk stage IIb or stage III melanoma, it has been demonstrated that high-dose IFN α-2b significantly prolonged both relapse-free survival and overall survival in comparison with untreated patients [41]. As a result, IFN α-2b has been approved by the FDA for the adjuvant treatment of high-risk melanomas. With IFN-α available, novel application in the combination treatment of malignant neuroendocrine tumors [44] with 5-FU and as a treatment for cutaneous T-cell lymphomas [45] have been proposed. Further applications, particularly in combination with more conventional therapeutics, are forthcoming.

BACILLUS CALMETTE-GUÉRIN

The history of immunotherapy is replete with examples of attempted cancer therapy using agents that were casually observed to augment immunoreactivity. The panoply of agents has included lectins, viable or nonviable bacteria, and bacterial products. No well-executed trials demonstrated any clinical advantage to the use of these agents until recently.

Bacillus Calmette-Guérin (BCG) is a live, attenuated strain of *Mycobacterium bovis* with nonspecific, immunostimulating properties [46]. Intradermal administration of BCG in some animal models has been demonstrated to restore immunocompetence and protect against infection and malignancy. The mechanism responsible for these systemic effects is unknown, although they have been attributed to reticuloendothelial cell activation [46], decreased suppressor cell activity, macrophage and lymphocyte activation.

A number of trials have demonstrated prolonged disease-free survival, prolonged survival, delayed tumor progression, and eradication of carcinoma in situ of the urinary bladder among patients treated with intravesical BCG after transurethral resection (TUR) compared with patients treated with TUR alone [47]. Papillary carcinoma and carcinoma in situ of the bladder seem particularly well suited for local therapy with BCG because of the minimal tumor burden remaining after TUR, the ease of exposing all at-risk surfaces to treatment, the immunocompetence of most patients, and the ease of follow-up evaluation.

MECHANISM OF ACTION

Bacillus Calmette-Guérin is a nonspecific immunostimulant that is believed to exert its antitumor effect through the induction of a DTH-like response. According to this paradigm, tumor cells are destroyed as innocent bystanders, either directly by activated macrophages and lymphoid cells, or indirectly by the local secretion of cytokines. These nonspecific immune effectors represent a reaction to components of the bacillus cell wall. Rare regional responses, which are characterized by regression of some uninjected tumors, suggest that specific antitumor immunity is induced in some treated patients. This, however, has been difficult to prove.

MECHANISMS OF RESISTANCE

Clinical experience has defined criteria that are associated with a low likelihood of response to therapy with BCG. These relate primarily to tumor size and patient immunocompetence. Large tumors are unlikely to regress. The reason for this observed inverse relationship between tumor size and response to therapy is not known; however, tumor vasculature is believed to play a role. This observation has led to the use of intravesical BCG as an adjuvant to transurethral resection of tumors rather than as a primary mode of therapy. It is also applied to the treatment of carcinoma in situ for the same reason.

ADVERSE EFFECTS

The risk of developing toxicity depends in large measure on the integrity of intravesical and systemic immunity. Impairment of either one of these can lead to dissemination of viable organisms and overwhelming mycobacterial infection. Patients who are receiving systemic steroids, bone marrow depressants, or radiation therapy or who have compromised immune systems for any other reason should not be treated. Local factors that predispose to disseminated infection include ongoing urinary tract infection and healing bladder mucosal injury secondary to instrumentation.

Other adverse manifestations of therapy include those related to local effects on the bladder. Urinary symptoms, which include dysuria, frequency, urgency, and decreased bladder capacity, are a result of bladder irritation and usually do not occur until the third course of treatment. Systemic symptoms, including fever, malaise, and chills may be due to hypersensitivity and resolve after 1 to 3 days.

Patients who are immunocompromised at the time of therapy also are unlikely to respond. This is not surprising even in light of our limited understanding of the mechanism of response, which probably involves immune effectors that have been nonspecifically activated by BCG. Commonly encountered causes of immunosuppression in these patients include previous chemotherapy and radiation therapy, use of corticosteroids, poor nutrition, or advanced disease.

LEVAMISOLE

Levamisole is an immunomodulatory drug that initially was developed as an anthelminthic agent [48]. The anthelminthic effect has been shown to be mediated by inhibition of a unique succinate dehydrogenase-fumarate system that serves as a terminal electron acceptor in the generation of adenosine triphosphate. This effectively paralyzes treated worms.

The immunologic effects of levamisole in vitro are protean and include enhancement of polymorphonuclear and mononuclear phagocytosis and chemotaxis. Lymphocyte proliferation in response to mitogens and cytotoxic activity also are enhanced. B-cell and NK-cell function appear to be unaffected. A direct antitumor effect has not been demonstrated [49].

The results of studies designed to evaluate the immunologic effects of levamisole in animals and humans are conflicting and have provided little insight into the design of future clinical trials. In 1989, the North Central Cancer Treatment Group (NCCTG) reported that adjuvant therapy of colorectal cancer with levamisole and 5-FU may be of benefit. This combination was based on the presumption that enhanced immunoreactivity engendered by levamisole would contribute to the minimal effects of 5-FU in eliminating microscopic disease. A subsequent intergroup trial conducted by the Eastern Cooperative Oncology Group, the NCCTG, the Southwest Oncology Group, and the Mayo Clinic corroborated these findings [50]. There was a statistically significant prolongation of disease-free and overall survival among patients with stage III disease who were treated with the combination of levamisole, 50 mg every 8 hours, and 5-FU, 450 mg/m^2/day for 1 year. The observed toxicity was generally that expected with 5-FU. In a final report of this trial [51], 5-year follow-up of 929 patients revealed a 40% reduction in recurrence rate and a 33% reduction in death rate in the group of patients treated with 5-FU and levamisole. These results have been questioned on the basis of the experimental design, which did not include a 5-FU control arm. However, concomitant 5-FU and levamisole represent standard therapy for patients with node-positive colorectal carcinoma who have undergone curative resection.

MECHANISM OF ACTION

Levamisole alone has not consistently demonstrated antitumor activity. It is not known whether levamisole mediates a salutary effect by reversing the immunosuppression associated with 5-FU or whether it biochemically modulates the anticancer activity of 5-FU [52]. Levamisole is a heterocyclic compound that is purported to exert immunomodulatory effects through either its imidazole or thiazol rings. The cytoplasmic or cell-wall targets for this molecule are not known. Neither are the mechanisms by which subsequent biochemical events within the cell are effected. One theory holds that the sulfhydryl group leads to glutathione repletion. Others have suggested that cholinergic-like effects of the imidazole ring underlie the observed enhancement of IL-2–induced T-cell proliferation. It is known that levamisole increases the level of cytoplasmic cGMP and reciprocally decreases levels of cAMP in treated lymphocytes. It may increase the intracellular calcium concentration as well. Decreased cell-membrane adenylate cyclase activity also has been observed. Whether these findings are relevant to the observed immunomodulatory effects is not known.

MECHANISMS OF RESISTANCE

Evasion of a levamisole-induced immune response is one mechanism by which cancer cells may overcome the effects of levamisole and 5-FU. However, clinically exploitable antigenic differences between colon cancer and normal cells have yet to be demonstrated. Resistance also may arise through modulation of the levels of certain vital intracellular constituents. For example, gene duplication or a compensatory increase in the activity of certain enzymes may lead to elevated levels of thymidylate synthetase. This could partially overcome the detrimental effect 5-FU exerts on DNA and RNA synthesis and repair.

ADVERSE EFFECTS

Adverse reactions to levamisole generally are mild. Agranulocytosis, which is usually reversible following discontinuation of treatment, rarely has been reported. This may be accompanied by a flu-like syndrome. Neutropenia, thrombocytopenia, and anemia occur frequently in patients treated with levamisole and 5-FU in combination. Almost all patients treated with levamisole and 5-FU experience toxicity that is otherwise associated with 5-FU alone. Other rare toxicities include rashes, myalgia, arthralgia, and renal failure. Central nervous system toxicity includes confusion, convulsions, hallucinations, impaired concentration, and an encephalopathic syndrome. Fatigue and altered taste sensation also have been reported.

COLONY-STIMULATING FACTORS

The colony-stimulating factors (CSFs), like the interleukins from which they have been arbitrarily distinguished, are cytokines that control hematopoiesis and possess intrinsic immunomodulatory activity. These glycoproteins are elaborated by a variety of cell types, including T cells, B cells, NK cells, granulocytes, macrophages, vascular endothelial cells, smooth muscle cells, and fibroblasts. Some are produced constitutively and probably maintain steady-state levels of circulating cells. Their elaboration can be induced by a variety of physiologic stimuli, including mononuclear cell-derived cytokines, bacterial endotoxin, and hypoxemia.

The CSFs exert their effects at several stages of blood-cell development [53–55]. Multi-CSF (IL-3) and steel factor (*c-kit* ligand) act on the pluripotent stem cell, as do more differentiated cells in multiple lineages. Granulocyte-macrophage-CSF (GM-CSF) acts a little later in blood cell development, probably in concert with IL-3 and steel factor. Monocyte-CSF (M-CSF), granulocyte-CSF (G-CSF), and erythropoietin act on more differentiated cells and are more lineage specific, as their names imply. The picture that has emerged is one characterized by multiple regulatory proteins with overlapping functions that interact with one another within the stromal microenvironment of the bone marrow. Their effects are mediated either directly, through cell surface receptors, or indirectly, through the induction of other cytokines. The outcome is hematopoietic homeostasis that gives way to adaptive increases in the levels of circulating mature and immature cells during periods of stress.

Three CSFs have been approved for clinical use. Erythropoietin (Epoietin-α) is a 166-amino-acid glycoprotein that serves as an obligate growth factor for red blood cell progenitors [56–59]. It is made primarily by peritubular cells within the kidney in response to an oxygen-sensing heme protein. The liver contributes a fraction to the total amount of circulating protein, as well. Under normal conditions the serum level of erythropoietin ranges from 4 to 24 mU/mL. There is an inverse correlation between serum erythropoietin level and hemoglobin concentration below 10.5 g. Levels may rise as high as 10,000 mU/mL in response to profound anemia. A normal response to a specific degree of anemia is difficult to define owing to large variations from the mean that have been observed.

Patients undergoing chemotherapy, radiation therapy, or whose bone marrow is replaced by tumor may develop anemia that is difficult to manage. Some of these patients have lower erythropoietin levels than patients with comparable degrees of iron deficiency anemia, and the inverse correlation between serum hemoglobin concentration and erythropoietin may be attenuated. The administration of epoietin-α between courses of chemotherapy has been observed to reduce the transfusion requirement of some patients, including those with solid tumors, lymphoma, and multiple myeloma [56–59]. Patients whose pretreatment erythropoietin level is greater than 500 mU/mL are unlikely to respond to epoietin-α.

Granulocyte-CSF is a 174 amino acid glycoprotein that is produced by mononuclear phagocytes, endothelial cells, fibroblasts, and neutrophils [60,61]. G-CSF is central to the control of circulating blood neutrophil numbers, during both times of health and infection. G-CSF also has profound effects on mature granulocyte function. Phase III studies have evaluated the efficacy of recombinant G-CSF (filgrastim) in patients with solid tumors who are treated with myelosuppressive chemotherapy. Patients treated with filgrastim have manifested less profound and less persistent neutropenia, decreased incidence of neutropenic fever, and fewer culture-positive infections. This has translated to a decreased use of antibiotics and shorter hospital stays.

Granulocyte-macrophage colony-stimulating factor is a 127-amino-acid protein with a molecular weight that ranges from 18 to 22 kD due to variable glycosylation [62]. It stimulates the growth and differentiation of cells committed to the neutrophil and macrophage lineages. It also synergizes with other CSFs to stimulate multipotential progenitor cells. Randomized, placebo-controlled trials of recombinant GM-CSF (sargramostim) after bone marrow transplantation have revealed shorter periods of neutropenia and fewer infectious complications among treated patients. This has been associated with shorter hospital stays for treated patients.

The availability of reagents that augment the in vivo production of erythrocytes and granulocytes may have profound implications for the palliation and treatment of cancer [63,64]. Anemia associated with malignancy and chemotherapy may be debilitating. Red blood cell transfusion is associated with a small risk of serious infection as well as a variety of immune-mediated transfusion reactions. Many chemotherapeutics also cause life-threatening bone marrow toxicity manifest as granulocytopenia or thrombocytopenia. The risk of infection and bleeding associated with these dose-limiting toxicities is significant, and the impact on treatment efficacy may be substantial [65–68].

MECHANISM OF ACTION

Each of the CSFs mediate their effects by binding to specific cell-surface receptors that share structural characteristics with those of other CSFs and interleukins. High-affinity receptors unique for each growth factor have been identified. Together they constitute the cytokine receptor family, which includes the receptors for erythropoietin, G-CSF, GM-CSF, IL-2J, IL-3, IL-4, IL-5, IL-6, IL-7, prolactin, and growth hormone. All share amino acid sequences that may be functionally important.

Receptor activation leads to the modulation of second messengers, which then initiate a cascade of cytoplasmic events culminating in increased gene transcription. This is probably mediated by nuclear proteins that release cytokine promotors from inhibition. CSF-specific signal transduction pathways remain to be completely defined, but protein kinase C and elevated levels of intracellular calcium are thought to be involved.

The cellular distribution of receptors determines the effect of each CSF. The receptors for GM-CSF are found on pluripotent progenitors as well as on more differentiated cells of the macrophage and granulocyte lineages. This accounts for its effects on many mature lineages, including neutrophils, eosinophils, basophils, macrophages, and Langerhans cells, and its effects on most blast-forming and colony-forming unit precursors. Receptors for erythropoietin and G-CSF are distributed on more mature cells in a lineage-restricted fashion, which accounts for their effects being confined mainly to red blood cells and neutrophils, respectively. Receptors for G- and GM-CSF also are present on endothelial cells. The pleiotropic effects of GM-CSF may be due, in part, to the release of other cytokines.

Effects of filgrastim include decreased transit time of granulocytes from the mitotic to the postmitotic compartment with more rapid release of mature granulocytes from the bone marrow. Mature granulocytes are primed to produce superoxide, and their migration is enhanced. Antibody-dependent cellular cytotoxic activity, IgA-mediated phagocytosis, and release of inflammatory mediators is also augmented. The net effect is to increase the number of mature, circulating granulocytes and to enhance their function.

Sargramostim shares many of these properties with filgrastim. It also enhances the cytotoxic activity of mature eosinophils and macrophages. The macrophages develop tumoricidal activity, as well. The circulating half-life of neutrophils is prolonged. A role for GM-CSF in wound healing is suggested by its augmentation of vascular endothelial cell migration.

ADVERSE EFFECTS

Therapy with filgrastim is rarely associated with clinical toxicity. Mild bone marrow discomfort, which responds to treatment with acetaminophen, occurs in 20% of treated patients. Exacerbation of pre-existing cutaneous inflammatory disorders, including eczema and vasculitis, have been observed. This resolves with discontinuation of filgrastim. Prolonged therapy has been associated with splenomegaly in few patients. This is a result of extramedullary hematopoiesis. Serum uric acid and LDH also may become elevated, reflecting increased cell turnover.

Sargramostim produces dose-dependent toxicities, some of which may be mediated through the release of other cytokines. Side effects seen in patients treated with high doses (1000 μg/m^2) include thrombosis, pleural or pericardial effusion, peripheral edema, headache, and a flu-like syndrome. Lower, clinically effective, doses are better tolerated but may be associated with malaise, anorexia, fever, chills, arthralgias, myalgias, headache, and edema. A first-pass effect, characterized by respiratory distress, has been seen in some patients coincident with the first dose of sargramostim. This may require steroids, if severe, and unrecognized cases may require mechanical ventilation. Induction of cell-surface adhesion molecules on circulating granulocytes by sargramostim or release of cytokines from alveolar macrophages may underlie this toxicity.

Therapy with epoietin-α is well tolerated and is associated with a very low incidence of clinically significant toxicity at therapeutic doses. Pre-existing hypertension may be exacerbated and should be well controlled before instituting therapy. Some patients may experience arthralgias. The propensity for central venous catheters to become occluded by thrombus is increased.

OCTREOTIDE

Octreotide (SMS 201-995) is a long-acting, synthetic octapeptide with pharmacologic actions that mimic those of the naturally occurring, 14-amino-acid hormone somatostatin (SMS 14) [69,70]. Other naturally occurring analogues have been identified, including prosomatostatin (SMS 28) and preprosomatostatins (SMS 128). This family of peptides generally exerts inhibitory effects on a variety of organ systems. It downregulates the release of growth hormone, prolactin, and all gastrointestinal hormones. It inhibits gastric acid secretion, gastrointestinal motility, intestinal absorption, pancreatic secretion, and portal blood flow. The secretion of gastroenteropancreatic peptides, including insulin, vasoactive intestinal peptide, gastrin, and glucagon, also are reduced. Interest in octreotide as an anticancer agent has been stimulated by its documented antiproliferative activity against many tumor cell lines. However, the mechanism underlying this effect has not been fully elucidated.

The half-life of the naturally occurring hormone somatostatin is so ephemeral (3 minutes), it is of no clinical use. The D-amino-acid substitutions of octreotide and other synthetic analogues, such as the octapeptide Somatuline (Ipsen Int., Paris, France), confer resistance to serum peptidases, prolonging their half lives. The half-life of octreotide is about 60 minutes after intravenous administration and 2 hours after subcutaneous injection. Although a formulation for oral use has been developed, its use is limited by very poor bioavailability.

Octreotide acetate has been approved for use as an agent to palliate patients who suffer diarrhea as a result of carcinoid syndrome or VIPoma. It has demonstrated clinical efficacy in the treatment of other hypersecretory disorders, including insulinoma, glucagonoma, Zollinger-Ellison syndrome, acromegaly, and pancreatic ascites. It also has proven to be a useful adjunct in the management of enterocutaneous and pancreaticocutaneous fistulae. Its use as an anticancer agent remains investigational.

MECHANISM OF ACTION

Octreotide exerts its pleiotropic effects through cell-surface receptors that vary in their affinity for different somatostatin analogues. They are widely distributed throughout the body and have been demonstrated on cells that compose the central nervous system, the gastrointestinal tract, the exocrine glands, and the kidneys. These receptors also have been detected in human meningioma, breast carcinoma, and carcinoid tumors.

Octreotide's antiproliferative effects are thought to be mediated in several ways. It inhibits and reduces the levels of several growth factors that have been associated with tumor growth, including epidermal growth factor, platelet-derived growth factor, fibroblast growth factor, transforming growth factor-α, and bombesin. Octreotide also possesses direct antiproliferative effects that are poorly understood. Receptor binding also may be associated with dephosphorylation of cell membrane proteins that are necessary for proliferation. Stimulation of the reticuloendothelial system may be responsible, in part, for the antitumor effects of octreotide that have been observed in murine models.

ADVERSE EFFECTS

The therapeutic index for octreotide is wide, and serious toxicity is unusual. Nausea, diarrhea, and abdominal discomfort have been observed in about 5% to 10% of treated patients. Less common side effects (< 2%) include headache, dizziness, flushing, fatigue, hypoglycemia, and hyperglycemia. There is a risk of cholelithiasis as a result of changes in bile composition and gall bladder contractility, but this has been observed in fewer than 1% of treated patients.

RETINOIDS

Retinoids are a family of structurally and functionally related molecules that exercise a profound effect on cell growth and differentiation [71–75]. This class of compounds includes all-*trans*-retinol (vitamin A), which is obtained primarily through the conversion of dietary precursors, including retinal palmitate and beta-carotene. Conversion occurs within the intestinal lumen and enterocytes, respectively. The conversion of carotenoids to retinol is tightly regulated so that ingestion of excessive amounts of beta-carotene does not produce hypervitaminosis A. Retinol is transported in chylomicrons through intestinal lymph. It is taken up by hepatocytes and transferred to stellate cells within the liver. These cells contain about 80% of the body's store of vitamin A, and they maintain plasma levels at about 2 –M.

Retinol, secreted by stellate cells complexed with a binding protein, is reversibly bound further to transthyretin, a protein that protects vitamin A from loss through glomerular filtration. The mechanism by which target tissues take up retinol remains an enigma. Many of its effects are thought to be mediated by its intracellular conversion to all-*trans*-retinoic acid (tretinoin). Another metabolite of vitamin A with therapeutic potential is 13-*cis*-retinoic acid (isotretinoin).

Retinoids are essential to embryonic development, epithelial cell differentiation, and growth. They may be requisite for immunologic integrity because they have been shown to enhance certain cell-mediated immune responses, augment IL-2–induced LAK-cell generation, and upregulate macrophage phagocytic activity. Vitamin A also plays an important role in vision, reproduction, and hematopoiesis.

Retinoids possess antineoplastic activity and may have some clinical value in the treatment of a variety of malignancies. Transient complete remissions are associated with the use of single-agent tretinoin in most patients with acute promyelocytic leukemia. The role of concomitant chemotherapy remains to be defined. Isotretinoin has induced complete clinical responses in about 50% of patients with basal cell and squamous cell carcinoma of the skin [74]. Tumor regression has been seen less frequently among treated patients with mycosis fungoides.

Retinoids prevent the development of tumors in a variety of animal models. This has led to several chemoprevention trials in patients at high risk for malignancy. Isotretinoin has been associated with a decreased tumor frequency among treated patients with xeroderma pigmentosum. This effect lasted only as long as treatment was continued. Among patients with treated head and neck cancer, isotretinoin is associated with a lower frequency of secondary aerodigestive malignancy. Unfortunately, the incidence of tumor recurrence appears to be unaffected and as many as 33% of patients required discontinuation of therapy due to intolerable toxicity.

MECHANISM OF ACTION

Retinol and retinoic acid are bound within the cell cytoplasm by proteins whose function is unclear. Retinoic acid is then transported to the nucleus, where it is complexed by any of three receptors. These share substantial homology and are members of the steroid-thyroid superfamily of nuclear receptors. Retinoic acid receptor (RAR)-α is widely distributed throughout the body. The distribution of RAR-β is more limited, and RAR-γ is expressed almost exclusively in high levels by epithelial cells of the skin and oral mucosa.

Retinoic acid mediates many of its effects through the induction of gene expression. The RA-RAR complexes bind to specific DNA sequences termed *retinoic acid response elements*. Some of these sequences encode DNA-binding proteins that regulate the transcription of genes encoding proteins that are necessary for cell growth and differentiation. Retinoic acid–responsive genes also include those for epidermal growth factor receptor, vasoactive intestinal peptide receptor, and melanocyte stimulating hormone receptor. Direct effects of retinoic acid include a detergent-like effect on cell membranes that results in decreased membrane stability. Lysosomal membranes also may be disrupted.

Antitumor activity may be mediated by any of several proposed mechanisms. Retinoic acid has been shown to induce cell differentiation. This is evident for some human acute myeloid leukemia, melanoma, neuroblastoma, and teratocarcinoma tumor cell lines. These effects are enhanced by some cytokines, including IFN-α, tumor necrosis factor-α (TNF-α), and G-CSF. Retinoic acid also reverses squamous metaplasia in vitamin A–deficient animals. These observations have served as the basis for chemoprevention trials.

A number of tumor cell lines respond to retinoic acid with growth inhibition. This may be mediated by a direct effect of retinoic acid on the cells or in a paracrine fashion through the induction of transforming growth factor-β (TGF-β) expression. The latter also may be responsible for the induction of apoptosis, which has been associated with the use of retinoic acid. Growth inhibitory effects of retinoic acid are enhanced by IFN-α and IFN-γ.

MECHANISMS OF RESISTANCE

Resistance to the antitumor effects of retinoids is not understood. Some observations suggest that this has a pharmacokinetic basis. Specifically, plasma levels of tretinoin decline during prolonged therapy. This may be a result of homeostatic mechanisms that regulate retinoid metabolism because it is not reversed by dose escalation.

ADVERSE EFFECTS

The spectrum of toxicity differs between tretinoin and isotretinoin. Both are teratogenic, and their use in women who are pregnant or who may become pregnant is contraindicated. It is recommended

that these drugs should not be used in women of childbearing age unless they understand the risks and are capable of following mandatory contraceptive measures. These include the use of effective contraception for 1 month before, during, and after therapy.

The most frequent complication associated with both drugs is cheilitis, which occurs in 90% of treated patients. Xerosis is seen in about 50% of patients. This may be complicated by conjunctivitis, epistaxis, and pruritus. Rash, thinning hair, photosensitivity, and nail changes are seen less frequently. Gastrointestinal morbidity includes nausea and vomiting, which is seen in 20% to 30% of patients. The onset of inflammatory bowel disease has been associated temporally with the use of retinoids, although a cause and effect relationship has not been established. Headache frequently is associated with the use of tretinoin but is uncommon among patients treated with isotretinoin. Other neurologic toxicities are rare and include fatigue, depression, and pseudotumor cerebri. Moderate musculoskeletal symptoms are seen in about 15% of treated patients.

An unusual and potentially fatal complication of therapy with tretinoin has been seen among patients who have acute promyelocytic leukemia. This syndrome includes respiratory distress, fever, pulmonary infiltrates, pleural and pericardial effusions, edema, and myocardial depression. This is almost invariably associated with hyperleukocytosis. Resolution of this syndrome has been associated with the use of dexamethasone, 10 mg intravenously twice daily.

Metabolic effects include hypertriglyceridemia, hepatic transaminasemia, hyperglycemia, hyperuricemia, hypercholesterolemia, and decreased high-density lipoproteins. These effects are reversible on discontinuation of therapy.

NEW AGENTS

As shown in Table 3-1, there are many new agents under evaluation that have yet to be approved by the FDA. This includes the retinoic acid derivatives as well as new cytokines, such as IL-4 [76], IL-6 [77], and IL-12 [78,79]. Anecdotal responses have been observed with all of these agents. New agents under evaluation to support platelets include IL-3 [80], IL-11, and thrombopoietin. Although no antibody preparation has been approved for treatment of cancer, the murine monoclonal antibody 17-1A has demonstrated efficacy as an adjuvant therapy for patients with resected colorectal cancer [81], which needs to be confirmed in prospective studies.

Table 3-1. Agents Being Studied

Agent	Dose/Route	Supplier	Mechanism of Action	Pharmacokinetics (Half-life)
IL-3	1000 µg/m²/d	Immunex	Increase hematopoietic precursors	18.8–52.9 min
IL-4	0.25–5 µg/kg/d SC	Schering-Plough	Enhance immunity; induce apoptosis	8–48 min
IL-10	1–25 µg/kg/d SC	Schering-Plough	Allow emigration of CD8+ cells; inhibit macrophages; prevent apoptosis some cells	60 min
IL-11	Not reported	Genetics Institute	Increased platelet count; gut protection	Not reported
IL-12	10–100 ng/kg/d SC, IV	Genetics Institute, Roche	Antiangiogenesis; enhance immunity	5–8 h
17-1A	100–500 mg	Centocor, Inc.	Antibody-dependent cellular cytotoxicity	8–24 h
PIXY 321			GM-CSF/IL-3 fusion; enhance myelopoiesis	
Transretinoic acid	45 mg/m²/d PO	Immunex Roche	Alone or with IFN-α for the treatment of various malignancies (acute promyelocytic leukemia)	4 h
13-*cis*-retinoic acid	1–3 mg/kg/d PO	Roche	Prevention of second malignancies in patients with previously diagnosed head and neck cancer	10–20 h
Stem cell factor	Not reported	Amgen	Promotes bone marrow reconstitution	Not reported

REFERENCES

1. Rubin JT: Interleukin-2: its biology and clinical application in patients with cancer. *Cancer Invest* 1993, 11:460–472.

2. Lotze MT: Biologic therapy with interleukin-2: preclinical studies. In *The Biologic Therapy of Cancer*, edn 2. Edited by DeVita V, Hellman S, Rosenberg S. Philadelphia: JB Lippincott, 1991:207–234.

3. Fyfe G, Fisher RI, Rosenberg SA, *et al.*: Results of treatment of 255 patients with metastatic renal cell carcinoma who received high-dose recombinant interleukin-2 therapy. *J Clin Oncol* 1995, 13:688–696.

4. Fisher RI, Rosenberg SA, Sznol M, *et al.*: High-dose aldesleukin in renal cell carcinoma: long-term survival update. *Cancer J Sci Am* 1997, 3:S70–S72.

5. Yang JC, Topalian SL, Parkinson D, *et al.*: Randomized comparison of high-dose and low-dose intravenous interleukin-2 for the therapy of metastatic renal cell carcinoma: an interim report. *J Clin Oncol* 1994, 12:1572–1576.

6. West WH, Tauer KW, Yanelli JR, *et al.*: Constant-infusion recombinant interleukin-2 in adoptive immunotherapy of advanced cancer. *N Engl J Med* 1987, 316:898–905.

7. Palmer PA, Vinke J, Evers P, *et al.*: Continuous infusion of recombinant interleukin-2 with or without autologous lymphokine activated killer cells for the treatment of advanced renal cell carcinoma. *Eur J Cancer* 1992, 28A:1038–1044.

8. Gold PJ, Thompson JA, Markowitz DR: Metastatic renal cell carcinoma: long-term survival after therapy with high-dose continuous infusion interleukin-2. *Cancer J Sci Am* 1997, 3:S85–S91.

9. Vlasveld LT, Hekman A, Vyth-Dreese FA, *et al.*: A phase I study of prolonged continuous infusion of low dose recombinant interleukin-2 in melanoma and renal cell cancer, part II: immunological aspects. *Br J Cancer* 1993, 68:559–567.

10. Sleijfer DT, Janssen RA, Buter J, *et al.*: Phase II study of subcutaneous IL-2 in unselected patients with advanced renal cell cancer on an outpatient basis. *J Clin Oncol* 1992, 10:1119–1123.

11. Lissoni P, Barni S, Ardizzoia A, *et al.*: Prognostic factors of the clinical response to subcutaneous immunotherapy with interleukin-2 alone in patients with metastatic renal cell carcinoma. *Oncology* 1994, 51:59–62.

12. Dutcher JP, Atkins M, Fisher R, *et al.*: Interleukin-2-based therapy for metastatic renal cell cancer: the Cytokine Working Group experience, 1989-1997. *Cancer J Sci Am* 1997, 3:S73–S78.

13. Atzpodien J, Lopez JE, Kirchner H, *et al.*: Multi-institutional home therapy trial of recombinant human interleukin-2 and interferon a-2 in progressive metastatic renal cell carcinoma. *J Clin Oncol* 1995, 13:497–501.

14. Yang JC, Rosenberg SA: An ongoing prospective randomized comparison of interleukin-2 regimens for the treatment of metastatic renal cell carcinoma. *Cancer J Sci Am* 1997, 3:S79–S84.

15. Rosenberg SA, Yang JC, Topalian SL, *et al.*: Treatment of 283 consecutive patients with metastatic melanoma or renal cell cancer using high-dose bolus interleukin-2. *JAMA* 1994, 271:907–913.

16. Rosenberg SA: Keynote address: Perspectives on the use of interleukin-2 in cancer treatment. *Cancer J Sci Am* 1997, 3:S2–S6.

17. Legha SS, Gianan MA, Plager C, *et al.*: Evaluation of interleukin-2 administered by continuous infusion in patients with metastatic melanoma. *Cancer* 1996, 77:89–96.

18. Keilholz U, Scheibenbogen C, Tilgen W, *et al.*: Interferon-α and interleukin-2 in the treatment of metastatic melanoma: comparison of two phase II trials. *Cancer* 1993, 72:607–614.

19. Marincola FM, White DE, Wise AP, Rosenberg SA: Combination therapy with interferon α-2a and interleukin-2 for the treatment of metastatic cancer. *J Clin Oncol* 1995, 13:1110–1122.

20. Keilholz U, Scheibembogen C, Möhler T, *et al.*: Addition of dacarbazine or cisplatin to interferon-α/interleukin-2 in metastatic melanoma: toxicity and immunological effects. *Melanoma Res* 1995, 5:283–287.

21. Antoine EC, Benhammouda A, Bernard A, *et al.*: Salpêtrière hospital experience with biochemotherapy in metastatic melanoma. *Cancer J Sci Am* 1997, 3:S16–S21.

22. Keilholz U, Stoter G, Punt CJA, *et al.*: Recombinant interleukin-2-based treatments for advanced melanoma: the experience of the European Organization for Research and Treatment of Cancer Melanoma Cooperative Group. *Cancer J Sci Am* 1997, 3:S22–S28.

23. Thompson JA, Gold PJ, Markowitz DR, *et al.*: Updated analysis of an outpatient chemoimmunotherapy regimen for treating metastatic melanoma. *Cancer J Sci Am* 1997, 3:S29–S34.

24. Kovacs JA, Baseler M, Dewar RJ, *et al.*: Increases in CD4 T lymphocytes with intermittent courses of interleukin 2 in patients with human immunodeficiency virus infection: a preliminary study. *N Engl J Med* 1995, 332:567–575.

25. Holmlund JT, Kopp WC, Wiltrout RH, *et al.*: A phase I clinical trial of glavone-8-acetic acid in combination with interleukin-2. *J Natl Cancer Inst* 1995, 87:134–136.

26. Astoul P, Bertault-Peres P, Durand A, *et al.*: Pharmacokinetics of intrapleural recombinant interleukin-2 in immunotherapy for malignant pleural effusion. *Cancer* 1994, 73:308–313.

27. Fefer A: Interleukin-2 in the treatment of hematologic malignancies. *Cancer J Sci Am* 1997, 3:S35–S36.

28. Mazumder A: Experimental evidence of interleukin-2 activity in bone marrow transplantation. *Cancer J Sci Am* 1997, 3:S37–S42.

29. Meloni G, Vignetti M, Pogliani E, *et al.*: Interleukin-2 therapy in relapsed acute myelogenous leukemia. *Cancer J Sci Am* 1997, 3:S43–S47.

30. Fefer A, Robinson N, Benyunes MC, *et al.*: Interleukin-2 therapy after bone marrow or stem cell transplantation for hematologic malignancies. *Cancer J Sci Am* 1997, 3:S48–S53.

31. van Besien K, Margolin K, Champlin R, *et al.*: Activity of interleukin-2 in non-Hodgkin's lymphoma following transplantation of interleukin-2-activated autologous bone marrow or stem cells. *Cancer J Sci Am* 1997, 3:S54–S58.

32. Slavin S, Nagler A: Cytokine-mediated immunotherapy following autologous bone marrow transplantation in lymphoma and evidence of interleukin-2-induced immunomodulation in allogeneic transplants. *Cancer J Sci Am* 1997, 3:S59–S67.

33. Schwartzentruber DJ: In vitro predictors of clinical response in patients receiving interleukin-2–based immunotherapy. *Curr Opin Oncol* 1993, 5:1055–1058.

34. Scharenberg JGM, Stam AGM, von Blomberg BME, *et al.*: The development of anti-interleukin-2 (IL-2) antibodies in cancer patients treated with recombinant IL-2. *Eur J Cancer* 1994, 30:1804–1809.

35. Pockaj BA, Yang JC, Lotze MT, *et al.*: A prospective randomized trial evaluating colloid versus crystalloid resuscitation in the treatment of the vascular leak syndrome associated with interleukin-2 therapy. *J Immunother* 1994, 15:22–28.

36. DeVita VT, Hellman S, Rosenberg SA: *The Biologic Therapy of Cancer*. Philadelphia: JB Lippincott; 1991.

37. Itri LM: The interferons. *Cancer* 1992, 70:940–945.

38. Wadler S: The role of interferons in the treatment of solid tumors. *Cancer* 1992, 70:949–958.

39. Wadler S, Schwartz EL: Principles in the biomodulation of cytotoxic drugs by interferons. *Semin Oncol* 1992, 19(suppl):45–48.

40. Kirkwood JM: Biologic therapy with interferon-α and J: clinical applications: Melanoma. In *Biologic Therapy of Cancer*, edn 2. Edited by DeVita V, Hellman S, Rosenberg S. Philadelphia: JB Lippincott, 1995:388–410.

41. Kirkwood JM, Strawderman MH, Ernstoff MX, *et al.*: Interferon α-2B adjuvant therapy of high-risk resected cutaneous melanoma: the Eastern Cooperative Oncology Group Trial EST 1684. *J Clin Oncol* 1996, 14:7–17.

42. Cascinelli N, Bufalino R, Morabito A, MacKie R: Results of adjuvant interferon study in WHO melanoma programme. *Lancet* 1994, 343:913–914.

43. Cascinelli N: Evaluation of efficacy of adjuvant rIFNI 2A in melanoma patients with regional node metastases. *Proc ASCO* 1995, 14:410.

44. Andreyev HJN, Scott-Mackie P, Cunningham D, *et al.*: Phase II study of continuous infusion fluorouracil and interferon α-2b in the palliation of malignant neuroendocrine tumors. *J Clin Oncol* 1995, 13:1486–1492.

45. Kuzel TM, Roenigk HH, Samuelson E, *et al.*: Effectiveness of interferon α-2a combined with phototherapy for mycosis fungoides and the Sézary syndrome. *J Clin Oncol* 1995, 13:257–263.

46. Pryor K, Goddard J, Goldstein D, *et al.*: Bacillus Calmette-Guérin (BCG) enhances monocyte- and lymphocyte-mediated bladder tumour cell killing. *Br J Cancer* 1995, 71:801–807.

47. Lamm DL, Blumenstein BA, Crawford ED, *et al.*: A randomized trial of intravesical doxorubicin and immunotherapy with bacille Calmette-Guérin for transitional cell carcinoma of the bladder. *N Engl J Med* 1991, 325:1205–1210.

48. Janssen PAJ: Levamisole as an adjuvant in cancer treatment. *J Clin Pharmacol* 1991, 31:396–400.

49. Stevenson HC, Green I, Hamilton JM, *et al.*: Levamisole: known effects on the immune system, clinical results, and future applications to the treatment of cancer. *J Clin Oncol* 1991, 9:2052–2066.

50. Moertel CG, Fleming TR, MacDonald JS, *et al.*: Levamisole and fluorouracil for adjuvant therapy of resected colon carcinoma. *N Engl J Med* 1990, 322:352–358.

51. Moertel CG, Fleming TR, Macdonald JS, *et al.*: Fluorouracil plus levamisole as effective adjuvant therapy after resection of stage III colon carcinoma: a final report. *Ann Intern Med* 1995, 122:321–326.

52. Schiller JH, Witt PL: Levamisole: clinical and biological effects. *Biol Ther Cancer Updates* 1992, 2:1–14.

53. Crosier PS, Clark SC: Basic biology of the hematopoietic growth factors. *Semin Oncol* 1992, 19:349–361.

54. Brugger W, Rosenthal FM, Kanz L, *et al.*: Clinical role of colony stimulating factors. *Acta Haematol* 1991, 86:138–147.

55. St. Onge J, Jacobson RJ: The role of hematopoietic growth factors in the treatment of neoplastic diseases. *Semin Hematol* 1992, 29(suppl):53–63.

56. Spivak JL: The application of recombinant erythropoietin in anemic patients with cancer. *Semin Oncol* 1992, 19(suppl):25–28.

57. Erslev AJ: The therapeutic role of recombinant erythropoietin in anemic patients with intact endogenous production of erythropoietin. *Semin Oncol* 1992, 19(suppl):14–18.

58. Henry DH, Brooks BJ Jr, Case DC, *et al.*: Recombinant human erythropoietin therapy for anemic cancer patients receiving cisplatin chemotherapy. *Cancer J Sci Am* 1995, 1:252–260.

59. Welch RS, James RD, Wilkinson PM, *et al.*: Recombinant human erythropoietin and platinum-based chemotherapy in advanced ovarian cancer. *Cancer J Sci Am* 1995, 1:261–266.

60. Glaspy JA, Golde DW: Granulocyte colony-stimulating factor (G-CSF): preclinical and clinical studies. *Semin Oncol* 1992, 19:386–394.

61. Gabrilove JL: Granulocyte colony-stimulating factor and granulocyte-macrophage colony-stimulating factor in chemotherapy. *Biol Ther Cancer Updates* 1992, 2:1–11.

62. Demetri GD, Antman KHS: Granulocyte-macrophage colony-stimulating factor (GM-CSF): preclinical and clinical investigations. *Semin Oncol* 1992, 19:362–385.

63. Neidhart JA: Hematopoietic colony-stimulating factors: uses in combination with standard chemotherapeutic regimens and in support of dose intensification. *Cancer* 1992, 70:913–920.

64. Quesenberry PJ: Biomodulation of chemotherapy-induced myelosuppression. *Semin Oncol* 1992, 19(suppl):8–13.

65. Bunn P, Crowley J, Kelly K, *et al.*: Chemoradiotherapy with or without granulocyte-macrophage colony-stimulating factor in the treatment of limited-stage small-cell lung cancer: a prospective Phase III randomized study of the Southwest Oncology Group. *J Clin Oncol* 1995, 13:1632–1641.

66. Rowe JM, Anderson JW, Mazza JJ, *et al.*: A randomized placebo-controlled phase III study of granulocyte-macrophage colony-stimulating factor in adult patients (> 55 to 70 years of age) with acute myelogenous leukemia: a study of the Eastern Cooperative Oncology Group (E1490). *Blood* 1995, 86:457–462.

67. Broxmeyer HE, Benninger L, Patel S, *et al.*: Kinetic response of human marrow myeloid progenitor cell to in vivo treatment of patients with granulocyte colony-stimulating factor is different from the response to treatment with granulocyte-macrophage colony-stimulating factor. *Exp Hematol* 1994, 22:100–106.

68. Grem JL, McAtee N, Murphy R, *et al.*: Phase I and pharmacokinetic study of recombinant human granulocyte-macrophage colony-stimulating factor given in combination with fluorouracil plus calcium leucovorin in metastatic gastrointestinal adenocarcinoma. *J Clin Oncol* 1994, 12:560–568.

69. Evers MB, Parekh D, Townsend CM, *et al.*: Somatostatin and analogues in the treatment of cancer. *Ann Surg* 1991, 213:190–198.

70. Parmar H, Bogden A, Mollard M, *et al.*: Somatostatin and somatostatin analogues in oncology. *Cancer Treat Rev* 1989, 16:95–115.

71. Smith MA, Parkinson DR, Cheson BD, *et al.*: Retinoids in cancer therapy. *J Clin Oncol* 1992, 10:839–864.

72. Hofmann SL: Retinoids: differentiation agents for cancer treatment and prevention. *Am J Med Sci* 1992, 304:202–213.

73. Greenberg ER, Baron JA, Stukel TA: A clinical trial of beta carotene to prevent basal-cell and squamous-cell cancers of the skin. *N Engl J Med* 1990, 323:189–195.

74. Tangrea JA, Edwards BK, Taylor PR: Long-term therapy with low-dose isoretinoin for prevention of basal cell carcinoma: a multicenter clinical trial. *J Natl Cancer Inst* 1992, 84:328–332.

75. Holdener EE, Bollag W: Retinoids. *Curr Opin Oncol* 1993, 5:1059–1066.

76. Lotze MT: Role of IL-4 in the antitumor response in H. In *Interleukin-4*. Edited by Spits H. New York: Raven Press, 1992:237–262.

77. Weber J, Gunn H, Yang J, *et al.*: A phase I trial of intravenous interleukin-6 in patients with advanced cancer. *J Immunother* 1994, 15:292–302.

78. Zeh HJ, Tahara H, Lotze MT: Interleukin-12. In *Cytokine Handbook*. Edited by Thomsom A. London: Academic Press; 1994:342–371.

79. Nastala CL, Edington H, Storkus W, *et al.*: Recombinant interleukin-12 induces tumor regression in murine models: interferon-γ but not nitric oxide dependent effects. *J Immunol* 1994, 153:1697–1706.

80. Kurzrock R, Talpaz M, Estrov Z, *et al.*: Phase I study of recombinant interleukin-3 in patients with bone marrow failure. *J Clin Oncol* 1991, 9:1241–1250.

81. Riethmüller G, Schneider-Gödicke E, Schlimok G, *et al.*: Randomized trial of monoclonal antibody for adjuvant therapy of resected Duke's C colorectal carcinoma. *Lancet* 1994, 343:117–83.

ALDESLEUKIN

Aldesleukin is a highly purified lymphokine produced by genetically engineered *E. coli*. It differs from native IL-2 in that it is not glycosylated, it does not have an N-terminal alanine, and cysteine 125 has been replaced by serine. Aldesleukin possesses the same immunoregulatory capacity as natural IL-2. Some of its effects include T-cell and NK cell activation, the generation of LAK activity, and induction of interferon γ production by macrophages.

The systemic administration of IL-2 to patients with selected malignancies has been associated with tumor regression. IL-2 is potentially active against renal cell carcinoma and metastatic melanoma, with response rates of ~20% [3–23]. Its use with adoptively transferred lymphocytes, chemotherapeutics, other cytokines, and other biologic agents is under investigation.

SPECIAL PRECAUTIONS

Patients should be evaluated carefully for significant cardiac, pulmonary, hepatic, or renal dysfunction prior to therapy. Patients with these impairments are at a very high risk of treatment-limiting morbidity and mortality at the recommended dose of IL-2.

Patients with untreated brain metastases should not receive IL-2 owing to the early onset of treatment-related central nervous system (CNS) toxicity.

Pre-existing infection should be adequately treated prior to therapy.

Reversible renal and hepatic dysfunction is commonly associated with therapy. Concomitant medications should be used with caution.

The effect of IL-2 on fertility is not known. There is no meaningful experience with the use of IL-2 in pregnant women.

IL-2 should be used with caution in patients with gastrointestinal or genitourinary tract bleeding because of the risk of treatment-related thrombocytopenia.

Patients whose tumors encroach on the spinal canal are at risk of spinal cord injury due to IL-2-induced swelling of the tumor.

Patients should not be retreated with IL-2 if they suffered angina or myocardial infarction during initial treatment.

Enhanced cellular immune function may increase the risk of allograft rejection in transplant recipients treated with IL-2.

INDICATIONS

FDA-approved: metastatic renal cell carcinoma and metastatic malignant melanoma; clinical studies show that activity in response rates among patients with metastatic renal cell carcinoma and metastatic melanoma are ~20%; responses also have been observed in patients with non-Hodgkin's lymphoma and colorectal carcinoma

PHARMACOKINETICS

Following a short IV infusion, IL-2 rapidly distributes to the extravascular space with preferential uptake by the liver, kidneys, and lungs; very little IL-2 penetrates the CNS; the serum distribution and elimination half-life are 13 min and 85 min, respectively; IL-2 is cleared from the circulation by glomerular filtration and peritubular extraction; it is metabolized in the cells of the proximal renal tubules with very little bioactive protein appearing in the urine; the mean clearance rate, about 270 mL/min, is not affected by rising serum creatinine

DRUG INTERACTIONS

IL-2 may cause reversible hepatic and renal dysfunction; drugs that are metabolized by either of these routes may require modification of their dosage during IL-2 therapy; for the same reason, nephrotoxic and hepatotoxic drugs should be used with caution; IL-2 has been used concomitantly with TNF, IFN-α, cyclophosphamide, IL-4, radiation therapy, LAK cells, and tumor infiltrating lymphocytes (TILs) to enhance its efficacy. There is no proven benefit to the use of IL-2 in combination with any of these agents over IL-2 alone

RESPONSE RATES

~20% of patients with metastatic renal cell carcinoma who have a good performance status (ECOG 0-1) manifest a partial or complete response to IL-2 therapy; among patients with metastatic melanoma, about 20% of patients respond to therapy; complete responses are durable and may last as long as several years

PATIENT MONITORING

IL-2 must be administered in a hospital where patients can be monitored closely for the development of toxicity; this requires vital signs immediately before each dose and then every 4 h afterward or more frequently depending on the clinical status of the patient; hypotension, tachycardia, and cardiac dysrhythmias are frequent complications of treatment; urine output must be measured and recorded accurately because of the high incidence of oliguria; oxygen saturation should be checked if the patient develops symptoms of hypoxemia; daily or more frequent physical examinations are important to assess patients for capillary leak syndrome, organ hypoperfusion, CNS toxicity, sepsis, pulmonary edema, and stomatitis; blood should be collected at least daily to evaluate renal function, hepatic function, serum magnesium, phosphorus, calcium, electrolytes, CPK, and blood counts; the clinical suspicion of hypothyroidism after therapy should prompt a biochemical evaluation of thyroid function; patients should be transferred to a setting in which they can be closely monitored if they develop hypoxemia, disorientation, or hypotension and oliguria that requires the use of vasopressors

ALDESLEUKIN (Continued)

TOXICITIES

Cardiovascular: both ventricular and supraventricular dysrhythmias have been associated with the use of IL-2. Myocardial infarction has been seen in ~2% of treated patients. Myocarditis also has been described. Hypotension frequently is seen in treated patients and is thought to be due to a capillary leak syndrome

Pulmonary: noncardiogenic pulmonary edema thought to be secondary to a capillary leak syndrome has been observed in most patients. This is accompanied by dyspnea in about 50% of patients and, rarely, reversible respiratory failure. The capillary leak syndrome also may contribute to the development of ascites and pleural effusions that can contribute to shortness of breath

Renal: reversible oliguria occurs in the majority of treated patients and is accompanied by elevations of BUN and creatinine; ~1% of patients require dialysis until their renal function improves

CNS: mental status changes occur in few patients, although the contribution of concomitantly administered psychotropic drugs is unclear; subtle disorientation or impaired cognitive function may precede more profound CNS impairment. This may lead to coma

Dermatologic: pruritus occurs in as many as 50% of patients. Exfoliative dermatitis may occur following treatment; dry skin may be a persistent problem for about 10% of treated patients; hair loss also has been observed

GI: nausea, vomiting, and diarrhea occur in most patients. Stomatitis occurs less frequently; patients rarely may suffer life-threatening intestinal perforation, which requires emergency surgical repair

Musculoskeletal: fewer than 50% of treated patients develop reversible arthralgia and myalgia

Hematologic: anemia, thrombocytopenia, leukopenia, and eosinophilia are common during treatment; rebound lymphocytosis frequently is seen after cessation of IL-2; impaired neutrophil function is associated with an increased incidence of central venous catheter–associated *Staphylococcus aureus* infection

Capillary leak syndrome: this is seen in nearly all treated patients. It is, in part, responsible for hypotension and decreased organ profusion that often occurs. It also is responsible for the development of noncardiogenic pulmonary edema, ascites, pleural effusions, and anasarca.

Miscellaneous: fever and rigors commonly are seen 1–2 h after a dose of IL-2; ~10% of treated patients develop hypothyroidism. Frequent laboratory abnormalities include hypophosphatemia, hypomagnesemia, metabolic acidosis, hepatic transaminasemia, and hyperbilirubinemia.

DOSAGE AND ADMINISTRATION

A dose of 600,000 IU/kg (0.037 mg/kg) is administered intravenously over 15 min every 8 h; each course of therapy consists of 2 cycles, neither one exceeding 14 doses, and administered 7–10 d apart; decisions to withhold doses or terminate a cycle of treatment are made based on the clinical status of the patient; the median number of doses is 20 out of a possible 28; patients who manifest evidence of tumor regression 2 mo after treatment should be retreated if there are no contraindications

NURSING INTERVENTIONS

Dose-limiting toxicities often can be controlled if treated early; patients should be evaluated frequently for nausea, vomiting, diarrhea, and stomatitis; patients should be encouraged to use bicarbonate mouthwash regularly; regular doses of antiemetics and antidiarrheal medications should be initiated coincident with the onset of these toxicities; patients should be evaluated for the onset of rigors 1–2 h after each dose of IL-2; symptomatic treatment includes warm blankets and intravenous meperidine; vital signs and urine output should be monitored closely owing to the frequent occurrence of hypotension, dysrhythmias, and oliguria; a Foley catheter should be placed to accurately monitor urine output, if necessary; patients' mental status should be evaluated regularly; central venous lines should be dressed according to standard protocols; the skin entry site should be monitored for evidence of infection at the time of dressing changes and coincident with the onset of fevers that are not temporally related to doses of IL-2; pruritus is common and can be controlled with diphenhydramine or hydroxyzine

PATIENT INFORMATION

IL-2 may sensitize the skin to solar radiation; patients should be warned to avoid direct sunlight or to wear sunscreen, a hat, long-sleeved shirts, and long pants; patients should refrain from driving until fully recovered; symptoms of hypothyroidism should be reported if they occur; patients should be instructed to use emollients to manage dry skin

PREPARATION AND STORAGE

Each vial contains 22×10^6 IU (1.3 mg) of lyophilized IL-2 with dodecyl sulfate as a solubilizing agent; the contents of each vial should be reconstituted with 1.2 mL of preservative-free, sterile water for injection; when adding the water, it should be directed toward the side of the vial and mix by swirling, not shaking to avoid creating foam; reconstituted in this fashion, each milliliter contains 18×10^6 IU of IL-2; the dose of IL-2 should be diluted with 50 mL of 5% dextrose for injection in a plastic IV administration bag; vials are for single use only; unopened vials and reconstituted drug should be stored at 2°–8°C; once reconstituted, IL-2 should be administered within 48 h

FORMULATIONS

IL-2 is marketed as Proleukin by Chiron Corporation (Emeryville, CA)

BACILLUS CALMETTE-GUÉRIN

Bacillus Calmette-Guérin is a live, attenuated strain of *M. bovis* that has demonstrated efficacy in the treatment of primary or recurrent in situ carcinoma of the urinary bladder. The mechanism of this therapeutic effect is unknown but it is thought to be immune mediated.

SPECIAL PRECAUTIONS

Immunosuppressed patients are at risk of developing systemic mycobacterial sepsis. Patients with ongoing infection should not be treated until the infection is adequately treated.

Urinary tract infection increases the risk of developing disseminated mycobacterial infection and is associated with increased severity of bladder irritation.

Bacillus Calmette-Guérin may sensitize patients to mycobacteria, leading to false-positive PPD reactivity. It may be useful to skin test patients prior to initiating therapy.

Patients with small bladder capacity are at increased risk of developing severe local inflammatory reactions to BCG.

It is not known whether BCG causes fetal harm or is excreted in breast milk.

Patients in whom bladder catheterization was traumatic should have their treatment deferred for 1–2 wk. Similarly, treatments should be delayed 1–2 wk following transurethral resection of bladder tumors.

TOXICITY

Genitourinary: Dysuria, urinary frequency, hematuria, and urinary urgency may occur in as many as 40% of treated patients. Severe reactions occur less frequently. Most bladder toxicity occurs after the third installation, begins within 2 to 4 hours of therapy, and persists for only 1–3 d. Less frequent side effects include bladder cramps, nocturia, passage of urinary debris, and urethritis.

Gastrointestinal: Nausea, vomiting, diarrhea, anorexia, and mild abdominal pain may develop in few treated patients.

Systemic: Systemic side effects are common and include fever, malaise, and chills. These symptoms usually resolve within 3 d.

Miscellaneous: Less frequent side effects include anemia, neutropenia, allergic reactions, systemic infection, hepatitis, and hepatic granuloma.

INDICATIONS

FDA-approved: primary and relapsed carcinoma in situ of the urinary bladder

DRUG INTERACTIONS

Immunosuppressive or myelosuppressive drugs or radiation therapy may abrogate the response to BCG or may predispose treated patients to the development of disseminated BCG infection

RESPONSE RATES

In one study, a complete response rate of 75% was reported. Median time to treatment failure was 48 mo, and median time to death was 2 y; in another study, 75% of treated patients manifested a complete clinical response; after a median follow-up of 4 y, about 40% of them had relapsed and 13% had died of other diseases; two of the former patients responded to another course of treatment

PATIENT MONITORING

Patients should be monitored for symptoms of systemic BCG infection, including fever greater than 39°C, fever greater than 38°C that lasts 2 or more days, severe malaise, and cough; fever, chills, and malaise also may represent hypersensitivity reactions, which may respond to antihistamines; patients should also be monitored for the development of bladder inflammation which can be managed with phenazopyridine, propantheline, or oxybutynin; irritative bladder symptoms may also indicate urinary tract infection, which should be ruled out

NURSING INTERVENTIONS

Bacillus Calmette-Guérin contains a viable, attenuated mycobacteria and should be handled as infectious; all material that comes into contact with BCG should be placed into plastic bags that have been labeled "Infectious Waste" and disposed of accordingly; urine voided within 6 h of treatment should be disinfected with approximately equal volumes of undiluted household bleach for 15 min before flushing; BCG should not be handled by immunocompromised people; health-care personnel should consider wearing gown and gloves while handling BCG; nurses should closely monitor patients for symptoms of bladder irritation, urinary tract infection, and systemic BCG infection, which would include fever and cough

BACILLUS CALMETTE-GUÉRIN (Continued)

DOSAGE AND ADMINISTRATION

Therapy should begin 7–14 d after bladder biopsy or transurethral resection of bladder tumors. One of several published protocols follows [25]. A bladder catheter should be placed in sterile fashion. Reconstituted BCG should be instilled slowly by gravity after the bladder has been drained of all urine. The catheter should then be withdrawn and the patient assisted in lying for 15 min in each of four positions: prone, supine, right side down, and left side down. The patient should try to delay voiding for another hour while up and about. After no more than 2 h, the patient should empty the bladder while seated. Treatment should be delayed at least 1 wk if bladder catheterization is thought to have been traumatic.

Thera-Cys: The contents of three vials (27 mg/vial) reconstituted with the diluent provided and further diluted with 50 mL of sterile, preservative-free saline (53 mL total) are administered for each treatment. This dose should be repeated at 3, 6, 12, 18, and 24 mo.

TICE bacillus Calmette-Guérin: One ampule (50 mg) suspended in 50 mL of sterile, preservative-free saline, should be instilled weekly for 6 wk and then monthly for 6 to 12 mo.

PATIENT INFORMATION

Patients should be instructed to report signs or symptoms of systemic BCG infection and bladder irritation; women should avoid becoming pregnant while being treated; patients should be instructed to disinfect all urine voided within 6 h of treatment

PREPARATION AND STORAGE

Bacillus Calmette-Guérin and its diluent should be protected from light and stored at temperatures between 2° and 8°C; BCG should be administered within 2 h of reconstitution. Thera-Cys is available in vials containing 27 mg ($3.4 \pm 3 \times 10^8$ CFU/vial); BCG should be reconstituted with the accompanying diluent (1 mL/vial); the contents of three vials reconstituted in 3 mL are further diluted with 50 mL of sterile, preservative-free saline prior to administration

TICE BCG is available in 2-mL ampules containing 50 mg ($1–8 \times 10^6$ CFU); the contents of one ampule should be reconstituted with 1 mL of sterile, preservative-free saline and then suspended in an additional 49 mL

FORMULATIONS

TICE bacillus Calmette-Guérin is marketed by Organon, Inc. (West Orange, NJ); Thera-Cys is marketed by Pasteur Mérieux Connaught (Swiftwater, PA); both are freeze-dried suspensions of BCG

The information here is provided as guidance only. Prescribers should always consult the manufacturer's current prescribing information

68

LEVAMISOLE

Levamisole originally was developed as an anthelminthic agent. This effect is mediated by its inhibition of a helminth-specific electron transport system. Levamisole exerts anticholinergic and immunomodulatory activity in humans. Effects on the immune system include enhanced T-cell activation and proliferation, augmented macrophage activity, increased neutrophil chemotaxis, and enhanced antibody formation. Two clinical trials have demonstrated a statistically significant prolongation of disease-free and overall survival among patients who were treated with adjuvant levamisole and 5-FU following resection of Duke's C colon carcinoma. The mechanism of this effect is unknown, and the results of these studies have been questioned owing to the omission of a 5-FU control group.

SPECIAL PRECAUTIONS

Levamisole has been associated with increased plasma levels of phenytoin. Epileptics treated with this drug should have their phenytoin levels closely monitored. The safety of levamisole in pregnant or nursing women has not been established.

TOXICITY

Hematologic: agranulocytosis, which is usually reversible following discontinuation of treatment, has rarely been reported; neutropenia, thrombocytopenia, and anemia occur frequently in patients treated with both levamisole and 5-FU; almost all patients treated with levamisole and 5-FU experience toxicity that is otherwise associated with 5-FU alone

Dermatologic: rashes occur in ~2% of treated patients

Musculoskeletal: myalgia and arthralgia occur in 2% of treated patients

Genitourinary: renal failure is a rare complication of treatment

CNS: these toxicities are rare and include confusion, convulsions, hallucinations, impaired concentration, and an encaphalopathic syndrome

Miscellaneous: a flu-like syndrome may accompany the onset of agranulocytosis

DOSAGE AND ADMINISTRATION

Treatment with levamisole should begin within 7–30 d of surgery, as follows [25]. Levamisole, 50 mg, should be administered orally every 8 h for 3 d. This should be repeated every 14 d. 5-FU should be started concomitantly with a cycle of levamisole between 21–35 d postoperatively. 5-FU should be administered at a dose of 450 mg/m^2/d by rapid IV bolus daily for 5 d. This should be followed after 28 d by weekly doses of 5-FU, 450 mg/m^2/week. Therapy should be continued for 1 y. If mild stomatitis or diarrhea develop during weekly treatment, the next dose of 5-FU should be deferred until these toxicities resolve. If they are moderate to severe, the dose of 5-FU should be reduced by 20% when it is resumed. Other dose modifications of 5-FU should be made according to established protocols. Otherwise the following set of guidelines may be followed:

If WBC = 2500–3500/mm^3, defer 5-FU until WBC > 33,500/mm^3

If WBC < 2500/mm^3, defer 5-FU until WBC > 33,500/mm^3; resume at 80% of the dose if WBC < 2500/mm^3 for ≥10 d, discontinue levamisole

If platelet < 100,000, defer both drugs

INDICATIONS

FDA-approved: use in combination with 5-FU for adjuvant treatment of Duke's C colon cancer following surgical resection

PHARMACOKINETICS

Rapidly absorbed from the GI tract after oral administration; extensively metabolized in the liver, and the metabolites are excreted mainly by the kidneys (70% over 3 d) with lesser amounts appearing in the stool; 5% of the drug appears unchanged in the urine; plasma elimination half-life is 3–4 h; the effect of 5-FU on the pharmacokinetics of levamisole and use in patients with hepatic insufficiency have not been studied

DRUG INTERACTIONS

When used with alcoholic beverages, levamisole may induce a disulfuran-like reaction; coadministration of levamisole and 5-FU has led to an elevation of blood phenytoin levels

RESPONSE RATES

Use of adjuvant levamisole and 5-FU in patients with Duke's C colon cancer has been associated with about a 30% reduction in recurrence rate and death rate; the significance of these results has been questioned in light of the absence of a 5-FU control arm

PATIENT MONITORING

Patients should have a baseline CBC with differential and platelet count, serum electrolytes, and liver function tests performed; perform weekly CBC with differential and platelet count prior to each dose of 5-FU; monitor electrolytes and liver function studies monthly; monitor for mucositis and diarrhea, and modify the dose of 5-FU accordingly; phenytoin levels should be evaluated regularly in patients who take this medication

NURSING INTERVENTIONS

Treatment tolerance, weight, and nutrition should be monitored; patients should be instructed regarding oral hygiene; stomatitis may be managed with a variety of preparations, including combinations of Benadryl (Warner-Lambert, Morris Plains, NJ), a magnesium-based preparation, and viscous lidocaine; oral candidiasis should be ruled out; diarrhea should be treated aggressively, particularly in the aged; hospitalization may be required

PATIENT INFORMATION

Patients should be instructed to immediately report flu-like symptoms; the use of alcohol should be avoided; women should be advised not to become pregnant; nursing should be discontinued

PREPARATION AND STORAGE

Available as 50-mg tablets; should be stored at room temperature

FORMULATIONS

Marketed as Ergamisol (Janssen, Beerse, Belgium)

FILGRASTIM

Granulocyte colony-stimulating factor (G-CSF) is a 174-amino-acid glycoprotein that serves as an obligate factor in maintaining adequate numbers of circulating polymorphonuclear leukocytes (PMN). It targets granulocyte precursors, which are induced to proliferate when G-CSF binds to its cell-surface receptor. PMN chemotaxis, phagocytosis, and intracellular killing through enhanced generation of reactive oxygen intermediates also are augmented.

Filgrastim is the recombinant glycoprotein that has been expressed in *E. coli* containing the human gene. It is well tolerated and has been shown to be of benefit in the setting of chemotherapy-induced neutropenia. Its use after myelosuppressive chemotherapy has been associated with decreases in duration of neutropenia, frequency of infection, incidence of neutropenic fever, and use of antibiotics. Because receptors for G-CSF have been found on small cell lung carcinoma lines, there is a risk that filgrastim may serve as a growth factor for this and other solid tumors. No clinically evident tumor progression has been noted, however.

SPECIAL PRECAUTIONS

Patients with atherosclerotic cardiovascular disease may be at slightly greater risk of myocardial infarction when treated with filgrastim.

Septic patients are at risk of developing adult respiratory distress syndrome due to the pulmonary sequestration of PMN.

The safety of filgrastim in pregnant or nursing women has not been established.

The possibility that filgrastim could serve as a growth factor for any tumor type, particularly myeloid malignancies, has not been excluded unequivocally.

TOXICITY

Hematologic: there is a small risk of excessive leukocytosis (WBC > 100,000/mm^3) associated with therapeutic doses of filgrastim
Cardiovascular: transient decreases in blood pressure rarely may be observed
Musculoskeletal: mild to moderate medullary bone pain may be associated with therapy
Reticuloendothelial: clinically evident splenomegaly has been noted in 3% of patients who are treated chronically with filgrastim
Dermatologic: pre-existing inflammatory conditions, such as eczema or vasculitis, may be exacerbated by therapy
Miscellaneous: reversible, mild elevations of LDH and alkaline phosphatase have been noted

DOSAGE AND ADMINISTRATION

Filgrastim should not be administered during or within 24 h of chemotherapy; a dose of 5 µg/kg/d should be administered as a daily SC or IV injection [25]; the former route may be more effective; doses may be increased incrementally by 5 µg/kg for each chemotherapy cycle depending on the response during the previous cycle; treatment should be continued until the WBC reaches 10,000/mm^3 after the chemotherapy-induced nadir; the duration of therapy will depend on the severity of myelotoxicity; one must be careful to avoid premature termination of treatment based on a frequently observed initial increase in WBC that is due to the release of WBC stores

INDICATIONS

FDA-approved: patients with nonmyeloid malignancies who have severe neutropenia as a consequence of myelosuppressive anticancer drugs

PHARMACOKINETICS

Peak plasma levels of filgrastim are attained within 2–8 h of SC injection; the elimination half-life is about 3.5 h; half-lives are similar for SC or IV administration

DRUG INTERACTIONS

There is a risk that filgrastim could sensitize myeloid progenitors to the toxic effects of chemotherapy by increasing the rate of their proliferation

PATIENT MONITORING

The WBC should be evaluated twice weekly to avoid excessive leukocytosis and assess response to therapy; treatment should be stopped when the WBC reaches 10,000/mm^3 following the expected chemotherapy-induced WBC nadir; platelet counts also should be monitored to not overlook concomitant effects of chemotherapy

NURSING INTERVENTIONS

Patients who can be treated at home require training in the self-administration of filgrastim; they should be instructed in the safe disposal of needles, drug vials, and syringes after each dose

PATIENT INFORMATION

Patients may experience mild bone pain that can be managed with acetaminophen; patients should avoid using aspirin and nonsteroidal anti-inflammatory drugs because thrombocytopenia may accompany chemotherapy; patients should be instructed to discard unused drug and used needles and syringes after each dose

PREPARATION AND STORAGE

Filgrastim is available at a concentration of 300 µg/mL in 1 mL and 1.6 mL single-dose vials; the formulation also contains acetate, mannitol, Tween, and sodium; vials should be stored at 2°–8°C and warmed to room temperature for no more than 6 h prior to use; unused drug and drug left at room temperature for more than 6 h should be discarded; vials should not be agitated

FORMULATIONS

Filgrastim is marketed as Neupogen (Amgen Inc., Thousand Oaks, CA)

The information here is provided as guidance only. Prescribers should always consult the manufacturer's current prescribing information

70

SARGRAMOSTIM

Sargramostim is a 127-amino-acid recombinant, human granulocyte-macrophage-colong-stimulating factor (GM-CSF) that is produced in a yeast expression system. It differs from the natural glycoprotein by the substitution of leucine at amino acid position 23. The carbohydrate moiety also may differ. Sargramostim affects progenitors of multiple lineages, including granulocytes, monocytes, eosinophils, megakaryocytes, and erythrocytes. Its effect on these immature cells requires other CFSs, including erythropoietin. Sargramostim's greatest effect is on lineage-committed granulocyte and monocyte precursors. In addition to increasing the number of circulating PMN and monocytes, it enhances their function.

SPECIAL PRECAUTIONS

Patients with a history of cardiac disease are at slightly increased risk of developing supraventricular dysrhythmias. Dyspnea may occur during infusion of sargramostim. This is thought to be secondary to pulmonary sequestration of granulocytes; therefore, patients with pre-existing hypoxemic lung disease should be treated with caution. Treatment may be associated with fluid retention that could exacerbate pre-existing pericardial effusion, plural effusion, or congestive heart failure. Sargramostim may exacerbate pre-existing hepatic or renal dysfunction. The safety of this drug in pregnant or nursing women has not been established. Use of sargramostim in patients with acute myelocytic leukemia and myelodysplastic syndrome is not recommended due to the risk that it may serve as a growth factor for abnormal myeloid cells. Sargramostim should not be administered within 24 hours of chemotherapy or within 12 hours of radiation therapy. Their concomitant use also is proscribed. The effect of sargramostim on myeloid reconstitution after bone marrow transplantation may be blunted in patients who have previously been treated with intensive chemotherapy or radiation therapy. Patients with excessive myeloid blasts in the bone marrow or peripheral blood (> 10%) should not be treated.

TOXICITY

Cardiovascular: patients with pre-existing heart disease are at risk for the development of supraventricular tachydysrhythmias. These tend to be transient. Fluid retention may exacerbate congestive heart failure and pericardial effusion. Hypotension, flushing, and syncope have been associated with the first dose of sargramostim.
Respiratory: dyspnea may occur as a result of the pulmonary sequestration of granulocytes; this may exacerbate preexisting lung disease.
Immunologic: ~3% of treated patients will develop neutralizing antibodies to sargramostim; the effect this has on hematopoiesis is unknown
Renal: preexisting renal disease may be exacerbated
Hepatic: preexisting liver disease may be exacerbated
Hematologic: reversible thrombocytosis and leukocytosis have occurred
Musculoskeletal: medullary bone pain of mild to moderate severity may be experienced
Gastrointestinal: patient may experience diarrhea
Miscellaneous: a flu-like syndrome may occur, which is characterized by headache, asthenia, fever, and myalgia

DOSAGE AND ADMINISTRATION

Myeloid reconstitution after autologous bone marrow transplantation [25]: 250 µg/m²/d administered as a single, daily 2-h IV infusion for 21 d. Begin treatment 2–4 h after marrow infusion but no less than 24 h after chemotherapy or 12 h after radiation therapy.

Bone marrow transplant failure or engraftment delay [25]: 250 µg/m²/d administered as a single, daily 2-h IV infusion for 14 d. Repeat after 7 d if engraftment has not occurred. A third 14-d course of treatment, 500 µg/m², can be given after 7 d if engraftment still has not occurred. Further therapy, however, would not be useful.

In both case the drug should be discontinued if blast cells appear or disease progression occurs. If severe drug reactions occur, the dose may be decreased or delayed until the reaction abates.

INDICATIONS

FDA-approved: Myeloid reconstitution after autologous bone marrow transplantation, bone marrow transplantation failure, or bone marrow transplant engraftment delay; **Off-label:** myelodysplastic syndrome; HIV-positive patients treated with zidovudine; to decrease the nadir of leukopenia secondary to chemotherapy; to decrease myelosuppression in preleukemic patients; to correct neutropenia in patients with aplastic anemia; and to treat neutropenia in recipients of organ transplants in order to reduce the incidence of damage to the transplanted organ

PHARMACOKINETICS

The serum concentration approaches 23,000 pg/mL after a dose of 250 µg/m² given by a 2-h IV infusion; the α half-life is about 15 min; the β half-life is about 2 h; absorption is good after SC administration with peak serum levels observed about 2 h after injection

DRUG INTERACTIONS

Lithium and corticosteroids may potentiate the myeloproliferative effects of sargramostim

PATIENT MONITORING

To avoid complications of excessive leukocytosis, CBCs should be performed twice weekly; patients with pre-existing renal or hepatic dysfunction should have twice weekly evaluation of renal and hepatic function

NURSING INTERVENTIONS

The flu-like syndrome associated with treatment may be more tolerable if sargramostim is administered in the evening; acetaminophen, given concomitantly, also may be helpful; monitor for evidence of adverse reactions, including flushing, dyspnea, and hypotension

PATIENT INFORMATION

Patients should report signs of fluid retention, including weight gain and edema; patients with preexisting heart or lung disease should be particularly wary of this side effect

PREPARATION AND STORAGE

Sargramostim is available in single-dose vials containing either 250 µg or 500 µg of preservative-free, lyophilized recombinant GM-CSF; this should be reconstituted with 1 mL of preservative-free sterile water for injection; unused drug should be discarded; during reconstitution, the sterile water should be directed at the side of the vial, and the solution should be swirled, not shaken, to avoid foaming; the final dilution should be made with 0.9% sodium chloride for injection if the final concentration is < 10 µg/mL, the final dilution should be made with 0.1% human albumin in sodium chloride; an in-line membrane filter should not be used when infusing the drug; sargramostim should be administered as soon as possible within 6 h of reconstitution; unopened vials and reconstituted drug should be stored at 2°–8°C

FORMULATIONS

Sargramostim is marketed as Leukine (Immunex) and Prokine (Hoechst-Roussel)

EPOIETIN-α (ERYTHROPOIETIN, EPO)

Erythropoietin (epoietin-α) is a 166-amino-acid glycoprotein that is an obligatory growth factor for erythroid progenitors. It is produced predominantly by the kidney in response to decreased tissue oxygen tension as sensed by a heme-like protein in the renal tubules. The recombinant product is made by gene-modified mammalian cells that contain the human gene.

The anemia associated with cancer is thought to be due in part to a blunted response to erythropoietin. This can be overcome to some extent by administering epoietin-α, although it is unclear whether transfusion requirements or quality of life are significantly affected.

SPECIAL PRECAUTIONS

Patients with uncontrolled hypertension should not be treated until their blood pressure is well controlled

Patients with preexisting vascular disease may be at increased risk of thrombotic events

Epoietin-α may exacerbate preexisting porphyria

The safe use of epoietin-α in pregnant or nursing women has not been established

TOXICITY

Epoietin-α is generally well tolerated, even at high doses

Cardiovascular: erythropoietin may exacerbate preexisting hypertension

Musculoskeletal: some patients may experience mild arthralgias

Miscellaneous: there is an increased incidence of thrombosis of venous access devices

DOSAGE AND ADMINISTRATION

Guidelines have been most firmly established for the treatment of anemia associated with chronic renal failure and the use of AZT in HIV-infected patients [25]. Serum iron studies should be assessed prior to starting treatment, and deficits should be corrected with oral iron preparations. Determine the endogenous erythropoietin level. Data suggest that patients whose levels are greater than 500 mU/mL are unlikely to respond to therapy.

For the treatment of cancer-associated or chemotherapy-associated anemia, a dose of 100 U/kg should be administered SC three times a week for 8 wk. The hematocrit should be assessed regularly, and the dose of epoietin-α should be adjusted based on this value.

Epoietin-α is also useful preoperatively for increasing the volume of blood that a patient may store for autologous transfusion. One regimen employs 600 U/kg IV twice weekly for 3 wk. Surgery is then performed about 1 month after phlebotomy.

INDICATIONS

FDA-approved: Anemia associated with chronic renal failure or the use of AZT in HIV-infected patients; **Off-label:** cancer-related or chemotherapy-related anemia; epoietin-α also has been used preoperatively to enhance the volume of donated blood for autologous transfusion

PHARMACOKINETICS

The circulating half-life of epoietin-α is 3–10 h; detectable plasma levels are maintained for at least 24 h after a therapeutic dose; peak serum levels appear between 5 and 24 h after a SC dose

DRUG INTERACTIONS

None

PATIENT MONITORING

Blood pressure should be evaluated regularly because of the risk of hypertension associated with the use epoietin-α; response to therapy should be assessed with twice weekly hematocrits; when the hematocrit surpasses 30%, the dosage should be decreased by a total of 25 U/kg; if the hematocrit approaches or surpasses 36%, doses of epoietin α should be withheld until the value decreases to the target range of 30%–33%; treatment should then be resumed at a dose that is 25 U/kg less than the preceding dose; if the response to 100 U/kg is not satisfactory within 8 wk, the dose can be increased by 50 U/kg to 100 U/kg administered thrice weekly; patients who do not respond to 300 U/kg three times per week over 8 wk are unlikely to respond to higher doses; at this point, other causes of anemia should also be evaluated, such as iron deficiency, bleeding, and hemolysis

Prior to beginning therapy, transferrin saturation, serum iron, total iron binding capacity, and serum ferritin should be assessed; therapy with oral iron preparations should be initiated if iron stores are low; prior to therapy, the endogenous erythropoietin level also should be measured; data suggest that patients with levels > 500 mU/mL are unlikely to respond to treatment

NURSING INTERVENTIONS

Central venous catheters should be well flushed due to the increased risk of thrombosis; the perfusion of the lower legs should be evaluated in patients with significant peripheral vascular disease because of the risk of spontaneous thrombosis; patients who develop arthralgia can be treated with acetaminophen

PATIENT INFORMATION

Patients who are taking concomitant iron should be instructed about the possible side effects of this drug; the incidence of epoietin-α–associated toxicity is very low; patients should understand that arthralgias may be associated with treatment and they can be treated with acetaminophen

PREPARATION AND STORAGE

Epoietin-α is supplied in 1-mL vials containing 2000 U, 3000 U, 4000 U, or 10,000 U; there are 2.5 mg of human albumin per vial and no preservatives; the vials should be stored at 2° to 8°C; vials should not be shaken because this may denature the epoietin-α, rendering it inactive; each vial should be used for 1 dose only, and any unused epoietin-α should be discarded

FORMULATIONS

Epoietin-α is marketed as Epogen (Amgen) and Procrit (Ortho Biotech, Raritan, NJ)

OCTREOTIDE (SOMATOSTATIN ANALOGUE SMS 201-995)

Octreotide is a long-acting somatostatin analogue, the effects of which are pleiotropic and generally inhibitory. Its activity is mediated through binding to widely distributed cell-surface receptors. These have been identified on the cells of some tumor types, suggesting that they may be susceptible to the inhibitory effects of octreotide. Antitumor efficacy also is suggested by its ability to downregulate the activity of myriad growth factors, its direct antiproliferative effects on some tumor-cell lines, and its stimulation of reticuloendothelial activity.

The therapeutic index of octreotide is wide. It has demonstrated activity against some symptoms associated with hypersecretory neuroendocrine tumors. Its inhibitory effects on GI function are useful in the management of enterocutaneous fistulae. Its use in the treatment of cancer, however, remains investigational.

SPECIAL PRECAUTIONS

The half-life of octreotide may be increased in patients with renal dysfunction who require dialysis.

Nursing women and women who are pregnant should use this drug with caution. It is not known whether this drug is excreted in milk. The teratogenic potential in humans has not been investigated adequately.

Diabetics may have to adjust their dose of insulin or sulfonylureas when treated concomitantly with octreotide.

Transplant patients who are taking cyclosporine should be monitored closely. Octreotide has been associated with a decrease in the blood levels of cyclosporine and may have contributed to organ rejection in one patient.

TOXICITY

Gastrointestinal: nausea, diarrhea, or abdominal discomfort may occur in 5%–10% of treated patients; other GI effects, including cholelithiasis, are unusual.
Endocrine: hyperglycemia or hypoglycemia have occurred in ~2% of treated patients; other endocrine effects are unusual.
Soft Tissue: pain at the injection site has occurred in ~5% of treated patients.

DOSAGE AND ADMINISTRATION

SC injection is the preferred route of administration due to its prolonged half life; the initial recommended dosage is 50 µg once or twice daily [25]; dosage adjustment may be required thereafter to achieve control of symptoms; this should be done gradually over several weeks; patients with carcinoid syndrome or VIPoma may be treated more aggressively; daily doses of 200–300 µg given in 2–4 divided doses are recommended during the initial 2 wk of therapy; doses above 450 µg/d usually are not required, although occasional patients have needed doses as high as 1500 µg/d.

INDICATIONS

FDA-approved: Symptomatic treatment of patients with carcinoid syndrome or VIPoma in whom diarrhea, electrolyte abnormalities, and flushing may be improved

PHARMACOKINETICS

Absorption after SC injection is rapid and complete; distribution from plasma occurs quickly with an α half-life of about 10 min; circulating octreotide is bound to lipoprotein and albumin in a concentration-independent manner; elimination half-life is about 100 min, and duration of action may be as long as 12 h; the role of the liver on metabolism of octreotide is unknown; 30% of a dose is excreted unchanged in the urine

DRUG INTERACTIONS

Octreotide has been associated with both hyperglycemia and hypoglycemia; adjustment of the dose of insulin or sulfonylureas may be required; the drug may lower the level of cyclosporine; monitor transplant patients closely

PATIENT MONITORING

Monitor clinical biochemical effects in patients with carcinoid syndrome by measurement of serum serotonin and substance P; monitor urinary 5-hydroxyindole acetic acid (5-HIAA) and thyroid function; patients with VIPoma can be monitored by measurement of serum vasoactive intestinal peptide (VIP); diabetics, in particular, should be monitored for hyperglycemia and hypoglycemia

Fat malabsorption may be exacerbated by octreotide; selected patients should be periodically evaluated with 72-h fecal fat and serum carotene determinations; patients undergoing prolonged therapy should have periodic ultrasound examinations of the gall bladder and biliary tree; transplant patients who are treated with cyclosporine should have their dose carefully evaluated because of the possibility that octreotide may lower serum levels and precipitate organ rejection

NURSING INTERVENTIONS

Patients should be assessed for signs and symptoms of hyperglycemia, hypoglycemia, and hypothyroidism; patients who can be treated at home will require training in the self-administration of octreotide; they should be instructed in the safe disposal of needles, drug vials, and syringes; multiple injections at the same site within short periods of time should be avoided; the drug should not be used if discoloration or particulates develop

PREPARATION AND STORAGE

Octreotide is available in 1-mL ampules that contain either 0.05 mg, 0.1 mg, or 0.5 mg; a patient home starter kit is also available; ampules can be stored at room temperature for the day that they will be used; otherwise, they should be refrigerated at 2°–8°C

FORMULATIONS

Octreotide is marketed as Sandostatin by Novartis (Basel, Switzerland)

RETINOIDS

Retinoids are a family of structurally and functionally related molecules that exercise a profound effect on cell growth and differentiation. This class of compounds includes all-*trans*-retinol (vitamin A); its metabolites, all-*trans*-retinoic acid (tretinoin) and 13-*cis*-retinoic acid (isotretinoin); and beta-carotene. Retinoids possess antineoplastic activity and may have some clinical value in the treatment of acute promyelocytic leukemia, basal cell and squamous cell carcinoma of the skin, and mycosis fungoides. The efficacy of retinoic acid in the treatment of these and other malignancies is being investigated.

Retinoids prevent the development of tumors in a variety of animal models. This has led to several chemoprevention trials in patients at high risk for malignancy. Isotretinoin has been associated with a lower frequency of secondary aerodigestive tumors among patients with surgically treated squamous cell carcinoma of the head and neck.

SPECIAL PRECAUTIONS

Both tretinoin and isotretinoin are teratogenic. Their use in women who are pregnant or who may become pregnant is contraindicated. It is recommended that these drugs should not be used in women of childbearing age unless they understand the risks and are capable of following mandatory contraceptive measures. These include the use of effective contraception for 1 mo before, during, and after therapy.

It is not known whether these drugs are excreted in breast milk. Therefore, their use in nursing mothers is contraindicated.

Patients at risk for hypertriglyceridemia, including those with diabetes mellitus, obesity, increased alcohol intake, and a positive family history, should use these drugs with caution. The effect of treatment on serum lipids should be assessed periodically.

Diabetic patients may require adjustment of their hypoglycemic medications during therapy.

The commercially available formulation of isotretinoin (Accutane; Hoffmann-La Roche Inc.) contains parabens. Patients who are allergic to this drug should not use Accutane.

INDICATIONS
FDA-approved: *Acne vulgaris*

PHARMACOKINETICS
Peak plasma levels of isotretinoin occur about 3 h after an oral dose; in adults with normal renal function, its elimination profile is biphasic with a terminal-phase half-life that varies from 7–40 h; both tretinoin and isotretinoin are metabolized by cytochrome P-450-dependent hydroxylation; they undergo conjugation with glucuronide and are secreted in the bile; ~70% of an oral dose is excreted in the urine and feces in equal proportions; unlike retinol, the metabolites tretinoin and isotretinoin do not accumulate within the liver and cause hepatic damage as a sequelae of prolonged consumption

DRUG INTERACTIONS
Minocycline and tetracycline have been associated with the development of pseudotumor cerebri in patients who are also being treated with retinoic acid; concomitant use of vitamin A should be avoided; topical dermatologics may potentiate the drying effects; ethanol may potentiate the hypertriglyceridemia associated with treatment

PATIENT MONITORING
Women of childbearing age should have a negative serum pregnancy test within 2 wk of beginning therapy; a monthly pregnancy testing should be performed; monitor patients for the development of headache, nausea, vomiting, or visual disturbances—if these symptoms occur, patients should be evaluated for papilledema or ophthalmalogic disorders; a baseline lipid profile should be obtained; this should be repeated once or twice weekly until the lipid response to therapy has been determined, usually 8 wk; other blood tests that should be followed include glucose, liver function studies, uric acid, cholesterol, complete blood counts, and platelet counts

The information here is provided as guidance only. Prescribers should always consult the manufacturer's current prescribing information

74

RETINOIDS (Continued)

TOXICITY

Dermatologic: cheilitis and xerosis occur frequently and may lead to pruritus, conjunctivitis, blepharitis, and epistaxis; thinning of the hair and brittle nails have been reported

GI: dry mouth, nausea, and vomiting are commonly observed; the onset of inflammatory bowel disease has been associated temporally with administration of retinoic acid

Ophthalmic: conjunctivitis occurs in ~40% of treated patients; optic neuritis, corneal opacities, and photophobia occur rarely

CNS: fatigue and headache are uncommon complications of therapy with isotretinoin; these toxicities frequently are associated with the administration of tretinoin; pseudotumor cerebri has occurred during therapy with retinoic acid

Musculoskeletal: moderate musculoskeletal symptoms occur in ~15% of treated patients

Metabolic: reversible hypertriglyceridemia, hyperglycemia, hyperuricemia, and hypercholesterolemia may occur; elevations of AST, ALT, LDH are seen in ~10% of treated patients

DOSAGE AND ADMINISTRATION

Both isotretinoin and tretinoin should be administered orally, preferably with food; the use of these drugs for the treatment and prevention of cancer remains investigational; therefore, the optimal doses have not been defined; clinical responses among patients with acute promyelocytic leukemia have been associated with tretinoin, 45 mg/m^2/d; doses of isotretinoin associated with clinical response among patients with solid tumors have ranged from 1–3 mg/kg/d.

NURSING INTERVENTIONS

Women of childbearing age should be counseled frequently about contraception; two methods of contraception should be used simultaneously unless abstinence is practiced

Decreased night vision may accompany therapy with retinoids; patients should be made aware of this and should be warned to exercise caution when driving at night

Monitor patients for signs and symptoms of inflammatory bowel disease, including abdominal pain, diarrhea, and rectal bleeding; treatment should be discontinued if this occurs; retinoic acid may cause photosensitivity, and patients should be cautioned to avoid significant exposure to the sun and to wear sunscreen

Patients should be instructed not to donate blood for at least 30 d after the discontinuation of therapy owing to the teratogenic potential of retinoic acid

Patients with diabetes mellitus should be made aware that their insulin or antihyperglycemic medications may require adjustment

Patients should be instructed to take their medication with meals and avoid crushing the capsules

Concomitant use of vitamin A supplements and benzoyl peroxide should be avoided

Patients should be instructed to minimize their intake of ethanol

PREPARATION AND STORAGE

Isotretinoin is available as capsules containing either 10, 20, or 30 mg of drug as a suspension in soybean oil; the capsules also contain parabens, EDTA, and glycerin; isotretinoin is photosensitive and should be stored at 15°–30°C in light-resistant containers; the capsules are stable for 2 y after their manufacture

FORMULATIONS

Isotretinoin is marketed as Accutane by Hoffmann-La Roche Inc.; Tretinoin is also made by Hoffmann-La Roche Inc. but is not commercially available

Douglas Yee, David T. Kiang

Hormones play a pivotal role in regulating the growth and development of their target organs. Various hormonal agents have been used in the treatment of tumors originating from these target organs, namely the breast, uterus, ovary, and prostate.

MECHANISM OF ACTION

Estrogens, androgens, and progestins exert their function mainly through their respective receptors. After binding to the receptors in high affinity, the steroids alter the configuration of receptor molecules and make them capable of binding to a segment of DNA template called hormone response element, where they regulate gene transcription and control cellular growth and function [1].

COMPLEX CELLULAR REGULATION UNDER HORMONES

A complex system governs the growth of normal and cancerous cells. Endocrine functions are under tight feedback loops of autoregulation within one type of hormone as well as under interregulation between hormones. The former can best be illustrated using the case of pharmacologic dosages of estrogen that downregulate expression of the estrogen receptors. Regarding interhormonal regulation, estrogens promote the production of progesterone receptor, and progestins, acting through their receptor, can then downregulate the estrogen receptors.

There is also a second level of fine tuning at the site of local microenvironment, in which the cellular functions are mediated through paracrine effects of various growth factors [2]. Estrogen supports the breast cancer growth through an enhanced autocrine production of transforming growth factor-α. Estrogen also increases cellular sensitivity to other mitogens such as the insulin-like growth factors.

Hormonal therapy aims to disrupt these regulatory pathways. Tamoxifen, progestins, and ovariectomy act to reverse the effects of estrogen on growth-factor production. Various modalities of endocrine therapy can be classified arbitrarily as additive, ablative, competitive, and inhibitive (Table 4-1).

APOPTOSIS AS A MECHANISM OF ANTITUMOR EFFECTS

It is well documented that the antitumor effects of many endocrine therapies are mediated through the process of apoptosis (programmed cell death). Deprivation of hormones by orchiectomy or ovariectomy induces apoptosis of tumor cells in prostate and breast cancer, respectively [3]. Both antiestrogen and antiprogestin act through competitive mechanisms to achieve tumor regression through the apoptotic process [4].

TISSUE-SPECIFIC RESPONSE TO TAMOXIFEN

Although the action of tamoxifen in humans is mainly an antiestrogenic effect, tamoxifen also possesses estrogenic effect depending on the type and condition of target tissues. We now understand that the ability of tamoxifen to influence estrogen receptor is cell context dependent [5]. In breast cancer, tamoxifen acts mainly to antagonize estrogen receptor function. In vaginal epithelium, endometrium, and skeletal bones, however, tamoxifen acts like estrogen. This differential function explains why tamoxifen inhibits breast cancer growth while increasing the risk of endometrial cancer. It also explains why tamoxifen, instead of causing osteoporosis, promotes mineral bone formation, as estrogens do. Thus, tamoxifen can be an agonist or antagonist of estrogen receptor-alpha function depending on the cell type. The term *selective estrogen receptor modulator* (SERM) is now used to describe these agents. When breast cancer progresses after an initial response to tamoxifen, a minority of patients can have a response to withdrawal of tamoxifen. In this setting, either tamoxifen itself, or some of its metabolites, may have become agonists for the breast cancer cells.

Tamoxifen may affect cancer cell growth through mechanisms other than the steroid receptor pathway, such as through the protein kinase C system, by inhibition of ornithine decarboxylase and polyamine [6], by suppression of the plasma level of insulin-like growth factor [7], by modulation of the multidrug resistance gene *MDR*, or through antiangiogenesis [8].

INDICATIONS FOR HORMONAL THERAPY

The types of cancers that have shown responses to hormonal agents are listed in Table 4-2. Because the major action of hormones is mediated through steroid receptors, theoretically only receptor-positive tumor cells will respond to this modality of therapy. Indeed, 60% of receptor-positive breast cancers responded to first-line hormonal therapy. Early reports suggested that 10% of estrogen receptor negative breast cancer cells could respond to tamoxifen. However, newer methods used to detect estrogen receptors have shown that in the absence of estrogen receptor expression, the response to tamoxifen is nil. Prostate cancer cells have a high level of expression of androgen receptor and respond to androgen deprivation, either by orchiectomy or by a combination of antiandrogen (flutamide) and a luteinizing hormone–releasing hormone (LH-RH) analogue. The presence of steroid receptors in ovarian and endometrial cancers is less frequent than their presence in breast and prostate cancers. However, even in

Table 4-1. Categories of Current Endocrine Therapy

Additive	Competitive
Estrogens	SERMs
Progestins	Antiandrogens
Androgens	Antiprogestins
Ablative	**Inhibitive**
Ovariectomy	Aromatase inhibitors
LH-RH analogues	LH-RH analogues

Table 4-2. Type of Tumor Subjected to Hormonal Therapy

High Probability of Response (40%–80%)	Low Probability of Response (10%–30%)	Rare Response (< 10%)
Steroid receptor-positive	Endometrial cancer	Steroid receptor-negative
Breast cancer		Prostate cancer
Prostate cancer		Ovarian cancer
Meningioma		Renal cell cancer

receptor-positive tumors, the response of ovarian and uterine cancer to hormonal agents is at best modest or rare.

There is no clear rational basis for treating renal cell cancer or melanoma with hormonal therapy because no genuine steroid receptor has been found in these two types of cancer. Unlike hamster kidney cancer, human renal cell carcinoma is hormonally independent. The estrogen receptors previously reported in melanoma are actually tyrosinase. However, because tamoxifen may bind proteins other than the estrogen receptor, it is possible that tamoxifen could influence other growth regulatory pathways. For example, the response rate of melanoma to combination chemotherapy has been reported in one uncontrolled study to be improved from 10% without tamoxifen to 51% with tamoxifen [9]. However, additional randomized trials have not shown a benefit for tamoxifen with chemotherapy [10].

FLARE FOLLOWING HORMONAL THERAPY

Tumor flare has been observed with every known hormonal therapy. The frequent manifestations are an abrupt increase of bony pain, erythema around skin lesions, and induced hypercalcemia. However, evidence of actual increase of tumor growth is lacking. In some cases, the flare may be a good prognostic sign that the tumor is hormonally responsive. Therefore, by an adequate control of pain or hypercalcemia, a continued use of the hormonal agent may result in tumor regression. This practice is especially important and prudent in the use of LH-RH analogue for prostate cancer, in which an initial increase of the blood androgen level and bone pain is frequently inevitable.

DURATION OF TREATMENT

Because of the cytostatic effects on tumor cells from most hormonal agents, a minimal period of 2 months of continuous treatment is needed to adequately determine the efficacy of these agents.

COMBINED OR SEQUENTIAL USE OF HORMONAL THERAPY

As described earlier, when cancer cell growth is dependent on hormones, there are many ways to interrupt such dependency: by removing or reducing the hormone source or by blocking peripheral conversion of steroids into estrogens, or hormonal action at the receptor site. Therefore, a combined hormone approach makes sense and has been used for treatment of advanced prostate cancer (LH-RH analogue plus flutamide)

[11]. The results of such combination approaches in breast cancer are less convincing; although some data suggest that a combination of tamoxifen plus a LH-RH analogue is superior to tamoxifen alone [12] in the treatment of premenopausal patients with advanced disease. These early results suggest that improved survival may be obtained by combining hormone therapies in breast cancer, although several issues remain unanswered regarding appropriate sequencing of these therapies [13]. Because an initial response to hormone therapy predicts response to a second- or third-line hormonal manipulation, it is recommended that hormone therapy in advanced breast cancer can be used in sequence (Fig. 4-1).

COMBINED HORMONAL THERAPY AND CHEMOTHERAPY

A combination of hormonal therapy and chemotherapy is also logical because these two modalities have different mechanisms of antitumor action and different types of side effects. However, clinical studies around the world have not shown benefit for such a combination, especially in terms of the duration of response or survival in patients with breast cancer [14]. Therefore, for palliative purposes in advanced breast cancer, sequential application of hormonal therapy and chemotherapy to achieve a prolonged control of the disease is advised (Fig. 4-2). It has also been suggested that "hormonal priming" with an estrogen or androgen could enhance subsequent chemotherapeutic responses by placing more cells in S-phase. However, this has not shown to be clinically useful; in fact, in the case of prostate cancer, precipitation of spinal cord compression may be caused by androgen treatment.

NEW DEVELOPMENTS

There is an impressive number of new hormonal agents added in the 2000 roster for the management of malignant diseases. Most of the new agents belong to the category of antiestrogens (toremifene, raloxifene), antiandrogens (bicalutamide, nilutamide), aromatase inhibitors (anastrozole, letrozole), and aromatase inactivator (exemestane). In general, these new agents do not seem to advance the therapeutic indexes; rather a marked improvement is achieved in compliance (eg, once-daily dose) as well as in the reduction of untoward side effects.

In breast cancer, recent studies have shown that anastrazole is therapeutically equivalent to tamoxifen in previously untreated hormone receptor positive breast cancer patients [15,16]. However, fewer thromboembolic effects and less vaginal bleeding was seen in patients receiving anastrozole.

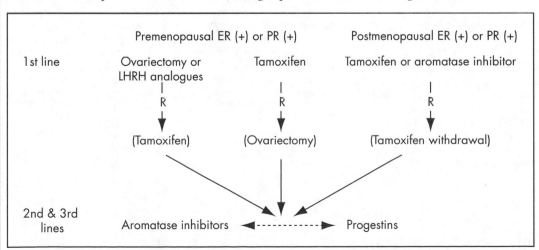

FIGURE 4-1.

Sequential hormonal therapy in advanced breast cancer. ER(+) — estrogen-receptor—positive; PR(+) — progesterone-receptor—positive; R — responders.

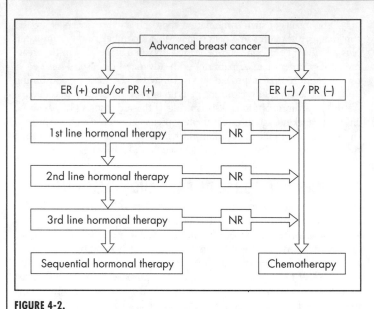

FIGURE 4-2.

Treatment for advanced breast cancer.

These new agents have also provided new options for patients with hormonally responsive disease. For example, patients who initially responded to tamoxifen may respond to an aromatase inhibitor. Given the favorable side effect profile of most hormonal agents, it is advisable to try a second hormonal manipulation in a patient who has previously had a good clinical response.

A major recent thrust is the development of new hormonal agents based on an improved understanding of steroid receptor function. As noted, hormonal agents have different effects on their target tissues in a cell context manner. Once SERMs bind the receptor complex, the receptor undergoes a conformational change that allows the binding of coregulatory proteins. Both coactivators and corepressors have been discovered that significantly influence steroid hormone receptor action. For example, the SERM tamoxifen acts as an estrogen in the uterus, whereas raloxifen does not share this property. Presumably, this differential effect of tamoxifen and raloxifen on the uterus is caused by their ability to induce conformational changes that alter the coregulatory protein binding. In the case of tamoxifen, coactivator proteins (or release of corepressor proteins) are favored and induce gene transcription. Discovery of newer SERMS such as ICI 182,780 (Faslodex, AstraZeneca, Wilmington, DE) appear to be promising agents for treatment of breast cancer. Initial clinical trials suggest that SERMs are not cross-resistant. In animal models and human clinical trials, tamoxifen-resistant tumors may respond to these newer SERMs [17,18]. Thus, development of new hormonal agents for cancer treatment has a promising future.

REFERENCES

1. Baxter JD, Funder JW: Hormone receptors. *N Engl J Med* 1979, 301:1149–1161.

2. Lippman ME, Dickson RB, Bates S, *et al.*: Autocrine and paracrine growth regulation of human breast cancer. *Breast Cancer Res Treat* 1986, 7:59–71.

3. Buttyan R: Genetic response of prostate cells to androgen deprivation: insights into the cellular mechanism of apoptosis. In *Apoptosis: The Molecular Basis of Death*. Edited by Tomei LD, Cope FO. Plainview, NY: Cold Spring Harbor Laboratory Press; 1991:157–173.

4. Bardon S, Vignon F, Montcourrier PHR: Steroid receptor-mediated cytotoxicity of an antiestrogen and an antiprogestin in breast cancer cells. *Cancer Res* 1987, 47:1441–1448.

5. Osborne CK, Zhao H, Fuqua SA: Selective estrogen receptor modulators: structure, function, and clinical use. *J Clin Oncol* 2000, 18:3172–3186.

6. Thomas T, Trend B, Butterfield JR, *et al.*: Regulation of ornithine decarboxylase gene expression in MCF-7 breast cancer cells by anti estrogens. *Cancer Res* 1989, 49:5852–5857.

7. Winston R, Kao PC, Kiang DT: Regulation of insulin-like growth factors by antiestrogen. *Breast Cancer Res Treat* 1994, 31:107–115.

8. Gagliardi A, Collins DC: Inhibition of angiogenesis by antiestrogens. *Cancer Res* 1993, 53:533–535.

9. McClay EF, McClay MET: Tamoxifen: is it useful in the treatment of patients with metastatic melanoma? *J Clin Oncol* 1994, 12:617–626.

10. Creagan ET, Suman VJ, Dalton RJ, *et al.*: Phase III clinical trial of the combination of cisplatin, dacarbazine, and carmustine with or without tamoxifen in patients with advanced malignant melanoma. *J Clin Oncol* 1999, 17:1884–1890.

11. Crawford ED, Eisenberger MA, McLeod DG, *et al.*: A controlled trial of leuprolide with and without flutamide in prostatic carcinoma. *N Engl J Med* 1989, 321:419–424.

12. Klijn JG, Beex LV, Mauriac L, *et al.*: Combined treatment with buserelin and tamoxifen in premenopausal metastatic breast cancer: a randomized study. *J Natl Cancer Inst* 2000, 92:903–911.

13. Davidson NE: Combined endocrine therapy for breast cancer: new life for an old idea? *J Natl Cancer Inst* 2000, 92:859–860.

14. Rausch DJ, Kiang DT: Interaction between endocrine and cytotoxic therapy. In *Endocrine Therapy in Cancer*. Edited by Stoll BA. Basel, Switzerland: Karger; 1988:102–118.

15. Bonneterre J, Thurlimann B, Robertson JF, *et al.*: Anastozole versus tamoxifen as first-line therapy for advanced breast cancer in 668 post-menopausal women: results of the tamoxifen or arimidex randomized group efficacy and tolerability study. *J Clin Oncol* 2000, 18:3748–3757.

16. Nabholtz JM, Buzdar A, Pollak M, *et al.*: Anastrozole is superior to tamoxifen as first-line therapy for advanced breast cancer in post-menopausal women: results of a North American multicenter randomized trial. *J Clin Oncol* 2000, 18:3758–3767.

17. Osborne CK, Coronado-Heinsohn EB, Hilsenbeck SG, *et al.*: Comparison of the effects of a pure steroidal antiestrogen with those of tamoxifen in a model of human breast cancer. *J Natl Cancer Inst* 1995, 87:746–750.

18. Howell A, DeFriend D, Robertson J, *et al.*: Response to a specific antioestrogen (ICI 182780) in tamoxifen-resistant breast cancer. *Lancet* 1995, 345:29–30.

AMINOGLUTETHIMIDE

EFFICACY AND USAGE

Aminoglutethimide has been referred to casually as a medical adrenalectomy. The role of this agent in therapy for breast cancer is attributed to its action as inhibitor of the enzyme aromatase. Aromatase catalyzes the conversion of testosterone to estradiol and the conversion of androstenedione to estrone. This enzyme is present in the adrenal cortex and extraglandular peripheral tissues, including adipose and breast cancer tissues.

DOSAGE AND ADMINISTRATION

250 mg two to four times daily with hydrocortisone 20-mg supplement. Mineralocorticoid replacement (eg, fludrocortisone) may be necessary.

SPECIAL PRECAUTIONS

Given its similarity to the sedative glutethimide, severe sedation may occur especially in elderly patients

TOXICITIES

Side effects are unpredictable and occur in 50% of patients; skin (morbilliform maculopapular) rashes are most common (30%), followed by lethargy and somnolence; thrombocytopenia and leukopenia are less common; others include hypothyroidism, hypotension, and flu-like syndrome

INDICATIONS

FDA-approved: Second- or third-line endocrine therapy for advanced breast cancer in post-menopausal patients. With development of newer aromatase inhibitors for breast cancer (anastrozole, letrozole, exemestane), aminoglutethimide has no advantages for the treatment of breast cancer. However, use as second-line therapy in prostate cancer is still warranted

CONTRAINDICATIONS

History of hypersensitivity to glutethimide

PHARMACOKINETICS

Addition of hydrocortisone is necessary to suppress a reflex rise in ACTH levels, which could act to overcome the blockade in steroid synthesis caused by aminoglutethimide

DRUG INTERACTIONS

Aminoglutethimide binds to cytochrome p450 enzymes and may increase the clearance rate of warfarin, antipyrine, theophylline, digitoxin, and tamoxifen

RESPONSE RATES

Third-line therapy for breast cancer—~30% in patients who previously responded to endocrine therapy

NURSING INTERVENTIONS

Carefully monitor for side effects, especially mental status

PATIENT INFORMATION

Patient should check for skin rashes and drowsiness

AVAILABILITY

Available as Cytadren by Ciba Pharmaceutical Co., Summit, NJ; 250-mg tablets stored in light-protected container at room temperature

ANASTROZOLE

EFFICACY AND USAGE

Anastrozole is a newer nonsteroidal aromatase inhibitor for the treatment of post-menopausal breast cancer. It specifically suppresses the enzyme that converts androgens to estrogens, with no effect on corticosteroid or aldosterone synthesis.

DOSAGE AND ADMINISTRATION

1 mg daily orally

SPECIAL PRECAUTIONS

Anastrozole should not be administered in pregnant woman and should be closely monitored for side effects in patients with impaired liver function

TOXICITIES

The drug is generally well tolerated; the main side effects are gastrointestinal disturbance, headache, hot flashes, and edema; incidence of rashes and central nervous system symptoms (*eg*, lethargy) may occur but much less often than with the first-generation aromatase inhibitors

INDICATIONS

For advanced breast cancer in postmenopausal patients, especially those with estrogen-receptor–positive tumors and a prior history of response to tamoxifen

CONTRAINDICATIONS

None known

PHARMACOKINETICS

Anastrozole is well absorbed and bound to plasma proteins; it is metabolized in liver and excreted mainly through the biliary tract; it reaches the steady-state level at ~7 d with a half-life of 50 h in postmenopausal women

DRUG INTERACTIONS

Although anastrozole inhibits reactions catalyzed by certain P450 enzymes, it does not have known interactions with other drugs

RESPONSE RATES

In patients having prior treatment with tamoxifen for advanced breast cancer, approximately one-third had either an objective response (10%) or stable disease (24%), with an overall median time to progression of 21 wk

NURSING INTERVENTIONS

In patients with poor liver function, the side effects of anastrozole should be closely monitored

PATIENT INFORMATION

In premenopausal patient, pregnancy test should be done prior to receiving anastrozole

AVAILABILITY

Distributed as Arimidex by AstraZeneca Pharmaceuticals, Wilmington, DE., in 1-mg tablets stored in room temperature between 20° to 25°C

The information here is provided as guidance only. Prescribers should always consult the manufacturer's current prescribing information

80

BICALUTAMIDE

EFFICACY AND USAGE

Bicalutamide is a nonsteroidal "pure" antiandrogen used in the treatment of advanced prostate cancer. It competitively binds to androgen receptors and inhibits the action of androgens.

DOSAGE AND ADMINISTRATION

50 mg daily orally

SPECIAL PRECAUTIONS

In patients with moderate to severe hepatic impairment

TOXICITIES

Most common side effects include hot flashes, bone pain, hematuria, and gastrointestinal symptoms (diarrhea)

INDICATIONS

A combination with an LH-RH analogue for the treatment of advanced prostate cancer

CONTRAINDICATIONS

In patients who had a prior history of a hypersensitivity reaction to this drug

PHARMACOKINETICS

Bicalutamide is well absorbed orally and not affected by the food intake; the active component (R-enantiomer) is highly protein bound; it reaches its maximal plasma level by 19 h and a steady-state level by 1 mo. It is metabolized mainly in the liver by glucuronidation and excreted in feces and urine with a half-life of ~6–7 d

DRUG INTERACTIONS

May interact with coumarin at its protein-binding sites

RESPONSE RATES

The response and survival of patients with advanced prostate cancer treated with bicalutamide monotherapy is inferior to that treated with castration; tumors that progress from bicalutamide monotherapy have a high-level amplification of the androgen receptor gene; therefore, bicalutamide should be used in combination with a LH-RH analogue for total androgen blockade; for bicalutamide in combination with LH-RH, the median time to treatment failure in prostate cancer is 97 wk

NURSING INTERVENTIONS

Closely monitor the side effects in patients with impaired liver function; adjust coumarin dosages according the prothrombin time

PATIENT INFORMATION

Bicalutamide should be started simultaneously with an LH-RH analog; it may cause gynecomastia and breast pain

AVAILABILITY

Supplied as Casodex by AstraZenaca Pharmaceuticals, Wilmington, DE; 50-mg tablets stored at room temperature

DIETHYLSTILBESTROL

EFFICACY AND USAGE

Diethylstilbestrol is a synthetic estrogen used for breast cancer and prostate cancer treatment. Because of its dichotomous effects on breast cancer—tumor flare at physiological doses and regression at pharmacologic doses—the dosage for breast cancer should be in the pharmacologic range. On the contrary, the dosage used for prostate cancer should be low in order to prevent cardiovascular complications. The suppression of serum androgens may be measured to document the adequacy of dosage.

DOSAGE AND ADMINISTRATION

Breast cancer: 5 mg three times daily PO
Prostate cancer: 1–3 mg daily PO

SPECIAL PRECAUTIONS

Pregnant patients; patients with poor liver or renal function, congestive heart failure, gallbladder disease, endometrial problems, or history of thrombophlebitis or embolism

TOXICITIES

GI: nausea and vomiting, cholestatic jaundice, and increased gallbladder disease; **Cardiovascular:** exacerbation of congestive heart failure and thromboembolism; **GU:** vaginal bleeding and candidiasis, cystitis-like symptoms; **Metabolic:** hypercalcemia and fluid retention; **CNS:** headache, migraine, and mental depression; **Skin:** pigmentation of nipple and axillae; **Breasts:** gynecomastia in males; **Tumor flare:** 5%–10%

INDICATIONS

FDA-approved: for postmenopausal female patients or male patients with advanced breast cancer and for patients with metastatic prostate cancer

CONTRAINDICATIONS

Pregnancy, active thrombophlebitis, known or suspected estrogen-dependent malignancy

PHARMACOKINETICS

Absorption: relatively complete; **Binding to serum hormone binding globulin:** 40%–50%; **Blood levels:** 0.15–6.0 mg/mL after administration at 1 mg three times daily; **Metabolism:** hepatic biotransformation and biliary excretion

DRUG INTERACTIONS

None directly; however, estrogen decreases the prothrombin time, impairs glucose tolerance, and increases the thyroid-binding globulin

RESPONSE RATES

Approximately 30% of postmenopausal breast cancers and 55%–60% of estrogen receptor–positive cancers will respond; the response rate in male breast cancer is similar to that in female breast cancer; the objective response rate in prostate cancer is ~65%; if subjective pain relief is included as responders, the total response rate could be up to 85%

NURSING INTERVENTIONS

Carefully monitor and document signs and symptoms

PATIENT INFORMATION

Patient should be aware of increased risk of endometrial carcinoma, carcinogenic effects on fetus during pregnancy, and all the potential side effects listed above

AVAILABILITY

No longer available in the United States.

EXEMESTANE

EFFICACY AND USAGE

Exemestane is a steroidal aromatase inactivator for the treatment of post-menopausal breast cancer. It specifically suppresses the enzyme that converts androgens to estrogens, with no effect on corticosteroid or aldosterone synthesis. Compared to anastrazole and letrozole, exemestane binds irreversibly to the aromatase substrate binding site. This causes downregulation of aromatase. It is unclear if this mechanism of action correlates with enhanced clinical response.

DOSAGE AND ADMINISTRATION

25 mg daily orally

SPECIAL PRECAUTIONS

Exemestane should not be administered in pregnant woman and should be closely monitored for side effects in patients with impaired liver function

TOXICITIES

The drug is generally well tolerated; the main side effects are hot flashes, nausea, fatigue, and increased sweating.

INDICATIONS

FDA: Exemestane is approved for the treatment of advanced breast cancer in postmenopausal women whose disease has progressed on tamoxifen.

For advanced breast cancer in postmenopausal patients, especially those with estrogen-receptor–positive tumors and a prior history of response to tamoxifen. Exemestane is also effective for patients who have progressed on anastrazole

PHARMACOKINETICS

Exemestane is well absorbed and bound to plasma proteins; it is metabolized in liver and excreted mainly through the biliary tract. It has a half-life of approximately 24 hours, thus once-daily dosing is appropriate. Steady state levels are achieved in less than a week

DRUG INTERACTIONS

Although exemestane inhibits reactions catalyzed by certain P450 enzymes, it does not have known inter-actions with other drugs

RESPONSE RATES

Early results suggest that first-line treatment of estro-gen receptor positive breast cancer results in an objective response rate at least equivalent, if not better, than tamoxifen. For patients who have progressed on tamoxifen therapy, the objective response rate is about 15% and stable disease is 22%. In this setting, median time to treatment failure is 16 weeks

NURSING INTERVENTIONS

In patients with poor liver function, the side effects of anastrozole should be closely monitored.

FORMULATION

Distributed as Aromasin (Pharmacia, Inc., Peapack, NJ), in 25-mg tablets stored in room temperature between 20° to 25°C

FLUOXYMESTERONE

EFFICACY AND USAGE

Fluoxymesterone is a synthetic steroid hormone used for the treatment of advanced breast cancer. The response rate is lower than that of tamoxifen. It is frequently used as a third-line therapy. The erythropoietic effects may provide a sense of well-being in anemic patients.

DOSAGE AND ADMINISTRATION

10 mg twice daily orally

SPECIAL PRECAUTIONS

Masculinization effects and, occasionally, induced hypercalcemia

TOXICITIES

GU: virilization, amenorrhea, and irregular menstrual periods; GI: nausea, cholestatic jaundice; Hematologic: suppression of clotting factors, and polycythemia; CNS: increased libido, headache, anxiety, aggressiveness, and depression; Skin: acne and hirsutism

INDICATIONS

FDA-approved: advanced breast cancer

CONTRAINDICATIONS

Known hypersensitivity to the drug, suspected prostate cancer, pregnancy, or serious cardiac, hepatic, or renal disease

PHARMACOKINETICS

Absorption: rapid; Biotransformation: in liver; Half-life: 9.2 h; Excretion: 90% in urine after being glucuronidated

DRUG INTERACTIONS

Increases the sensitivity to anticoagulants, decreasing the requirement for insulin and interfering with laboratory testing for thyroid function

RESPONSE RATES

Breast cancer: 15%–25%

NURSING INTERVENTIONS

Monitor and document signs and symptoms

PATIENT INFORMATION

Causes masculinization, hoarseness, acne, and changes in menstrual periods

AVAILABILITY

Distributed as Halotestin by Upjohn Co., Kalamazoo, MI; 2-, 5-, and 10-mg tablets

FLUTAMIDE

EFFICACY AND USAGE

Flutamide is a nonsteroid antiandrogen. It is used in combination with LH-RH analogue for the treatment of metastatic prostate cancer. The drug blocks the androgenic action at its target site.

DOSAGE AND ADMINISTRATION

250 mg every 8 h orally

SPECIAL PRECAUTIONS

Patients with hepatic toxicity with elevation of hepatic transaminases and cholestatic jaundice

TOXICITIES

Most frequent: diarrhea, hot flushes, impotence, and loss of libido; GI—anorexia, nausea, vomiting; Cardiovascular—hypertension and edema; CNS—drowsiness, depression, and anxiety; Hematologic (occasionally)—anemia, leukopenia, thrombocytopenia

INDICATIONS

FDA-approved: advanced prostate cancer

CONTRAINDICATIONS

Liver function impairment

PHARMACOKINETICS

Absorption: it is rapidly orally absorbed; Metabolism: its biologic metabolites reach a maximal plasma level in 2 h and a steady-state level in 9.6 h; Plasma half-life: ~8 h; Excretion: mainly in the urine

DRUG INTERACTIONS

Increased prothrombin time in patients on long-term warfarin

RESPONSE RATES

Flutamide is frequently used in combination with an LH-RH analogue, which suppresses the production of testicular androgens. The overall response rate for the combination therapy is about 70%, and the drug provides a significantly prolonged survival compared with LH-RH alone (36 versus 28 mo)

NURSING INTERVENTIONS

Monitor signs and symptoms

PATIENT INFORMATION

May cause hepatic injury such as cholestatic jaundice and the patient may need more frequent monitoring of prothrombin time while on warfarin

AVAILABILITY

Supplied by Schering Corporation, Kenilworth, NJ, as Eulexin; 125-mg capsules stored at room temperature and protected from heat and moisture

FULVESTRANT

EFFICACY AND USAGE

Fulvestrant is a pure steroidal antiestrogen currently in phase III clinical trials. Unlike other SERMs, Fulvestrant is a pure antiestrogen in all tissues studied. It also causes degradation of the estrogen receptor resulting in a decreased cellular concentration of the receptor. Early clinical trials suggest it is useful in patients who have progressive disease on tamoxifen

DOSAGE AND ADMINISTRATION

250-mg monthly injection

SPECIAL PRECAUTIONS

Fulvestrant should not be administered in pregnant woman and should be closely monitored for side effects in patients with impaired liver function.

TOXICITIES

The side-effect profile of Fulvestrant is not completely known; however, there appears to be no induction of hot flashes, endometrial stimulation, or vaginal dryness.

RESPONSE RATES

Early results suggest that good responses can be obtained in patients who have progressed through tamoxifen, suggesting a lack of cross-resistance

AVAILABILITY

Fulvestrant is currently undergoing phase III clinical trials in the United States. It will be distributed as Faslodex (AstraZeneca, Wilmington, DE)

GOSERELIN ACETATE

Goserelin is a synthetic decapeptide analogue of LH-RH with a much prolonged half-life and 100 times greater potency than that of the natural releasing hormone. Therefore, it downregulates the LH-RH receptors and reduces the release of gonadotropic hormones, which in turn results in a decrease in blood testosterone or estrogen levels. Thus, the functional result of LH-RH analogue therapy is equivalent to medical castration.

DOSAGE AND ADMINISTRATION

A depot dose of 3.6 mg/implant given subcutaneously every 4 wk

SPECIAL PRECAUTIONS

Patients with hypersensitivity to LH-RH; initial exacerbation of symptoms from prostate cancer; pregnant nursing patients

TOXICITIES

Endocrine: sexual dysfunction; gynecomastia, hot flashes, loss of libido, **Respiratory:** bronchitis; **Cardiovascular:** arrhythmias, hypertension; **CNS:** depression, anxiety, headache; **GI:** constipation, diarrhea, dyspepsia

INDICATIONS

FDA-approved: advanced prostate cancer and premenopausal breast cancer

CONTRAINDICATIONS

Pregnant nursing patients
History of hypersensitivity to LH-RH

PHARMACOKINETICS

Absorption: very slow; **Peak blood level:** achieved in 12–15 d following a single dose (3.6-mg) injection; **Action:** following goserelin therapy, the mean serum estradiol or testosterone values fall into the range of castrated level within 2–3 wk; **Elimination:** the drug is excreted through both urine and hepatic metabolism, and there is no drug accumulation on an every-28-d schedule

RESPONSE RATES

Advanced prostate cancer: in combination with flutamide, 70%; **Pre- and perimenopausal receptor-positive breast cancer:** 45%

NURSING INTERVENTIONS

Monitor signs and symptoms

PATIENT INFORMATION

Because of the initial, but transient, surge of blood testosterone level, patient may experience exacerbation of bone pain at metastatic sites of prostate cancer or urethral obstruction; patient may experience hot flushes and sexual dysfunctions

AVAILABILITY

Supplied by AstraZeneca Pharmaceuticals, Wilmington, DE; under the trade name of Zoladex; 3.6-mg disposable syringe device. Stored at room temperature of < 25°C

KETOCONAZOLE

EFFICACY AND USAGE

Ketoconazole is a synthetic imidazole with antifungal action. It inhibits the synthesis of ergosterol, a vital membranous component of fungal cells. Because of its inhibition of testosterone synthesis, ketoconazole is also used for the treatment of advanced prostate cancer.

DOSAGE AND ADMINISTRATION

400 mg every 8 h orally in order to sustain the androgen suppression with hydrocortisone 20 mg po as a supplement

SPECIAL PRECAUTIONS

Patients with hypersensitivity to the drug; at high dosage, decreases the ACTH-induced corticosteroid level

TOXICITIES

Nausea and vomiting can be prominent. Pruitus. Hepatic toxicity and hypersensitivity; in patients treated with 1200 mg daily for prostate cancer, death within 2 wk from unknown mechanism was observed

INDICATIONS

Used for advanced prostate cancer but is not approved by the FDA

CONTRAINDICATIONS

Coadministration with terfenadine, astemizole, cisapride, and oral triazolam

PHARMACOKINETICS

Absorption: rapid; requires gastric acidity; **Peak blood level**: reached within 1–2 h; **Half-life**: biphasic with initial 2 h during the first 10 h then 8 h thereafter; **Plasma binding**: 99% to albumin; **Metabolism**: converts into inactive metabolites; **Excretion**: the major route is via bile; **CNS penetration**: poor

DRUG INTERACTIONS

Inhibits the metabolism of the drugs listed in the Contraindications section above and increases their blood level, resulting in cardiac arrhythmia including ventricular tachycardia; may increase phenytoin serum concentrations; may enhance the anticoagulant effect of warfarin; should not be given concomitantly with rifampin or isoniazid; interacts with cyclosporine and methylprednisolone; concomitant administration with miconazole (another imidazole) may potentiate the hypoglycemia episodes; antacids, anticholinergics, and H_2-blockers reduce the dissolution and absorption of ketoconazole

RESPONSE RATES

Difficult to assess the tumor response rate; most study series included pain relief as response

NURSING INTERVENTIONS

Closely monitor the signs and symptoms and determine the potential interaction with other medications; for overdose: gastric lavage with sodium bicarbonate

PATIENT INFORMATION

Take the medication with a meal and avoid alcohol consumption

AVAILABILITY

Supplied as Nizoral by Janssen Pharmaceutica, Titusville, NJ; 200-mg tablets. Requires acidity for dissolution; store at room temperature

LETROZOLE

EFFICACY AND USAGE

Letrozole is a newer selective and potent aromatase inhibitor. The circulating estrogens decrease by more than 95% within 2 wk of daily doses of letrozole, with no change in aldosterone or clinically significant changes in cortisol levels. It is used for the treatment of advanced breast cancer in postmenopausal patients with disease progression following antiestrogen therapy.

DOSAGE AND ADMINISTRATION

2.5 mg daily orally

SPECIAL PRECAUTIONS

Should not be used in pregnant woman

TOXICITIES

Letrozole is well tolerated; transient thrombocytopenia and elevation of liver transaminases have been reported; other minor side effects are fatigue, nausea, vomiting, musculoskeletal pain, headache, hypertension, dyspnea, hot flashes, and depression

INDICATIONS

Used as a second- and third-line hormonal therapy for advanced breast cancer

CONTRAINDICATIONS

In pregnant woman or patients with known hypersensitivity to this drug

PHARMACOKINETICS

Letrozole is rapidly and completely absorbed through the oral route and reaches a steady-state blood level by 2–6 wk; it is metabolized through the glucuronidation pathway and excreted (90%) in urine with a elimination half-life of 2 d

DRUG INTERACTIONS

None recorded

RESPONSE RATES

Objective response to letrozole as a second- and third-line hormonal therapy in patients with advanced breast cancer are ~24% and ~22%, respectively

NURSING INTERVENTIONS

Monitor the liver function tests in patients with impaired liver function

PATIENT INFORMATION

Be aware of those symptoms that may be derived from estrogen depletion or potential side effects

AVAILABILITY

Distributed as Femara by Novartis Pharmaceuticals Corp., East Hanover, NJ; 2.5-mg tablets stored at room temperature

LEUPROLIDE

EFFICACY AND USAGE

Leuprolide acetate is a synthetic nonapeptide analogue of naturally LH-RH. It desensitizes the LH-RH receptor and reduces the production of gonadotropic hormones. It acts as medical castration in reducing testosterone in males and estrogens in females. It has been used for the treatment of advanced prostate cancer and breast cancer.

DOSAGE AND ADMINISTRATION

7.5-mg depot administered intramuscularly every month or 22.5-mg depot every 3 mo

SPECIAL PRECAUTIONS

Hypersensitivity to the agent and tumor flare may occur owing to an initial surge of blood testosterone or estrogen levels in the beginning of therapy

TOXICITIES

Endocrine: sexual dysfunction; gynecomastia, hot flashes, loss of libido; **Respiratory:** bronchitis; **Cardiovascular:** hot flushes, arrhythmias, hypertension; **CNS:** depression, anxiety, headache; **GI:** constipation, diarrhea, dyspepsia

INDICATIONS

FDA-approved: palliative treatment of advanced prostate cancer and of premenopausal advanced breast cancer

CONTRAINDICATIONS

History of hypersensitivity to the drug
Pregnant nursing patients

PHARMACOKINETICS

Bioavailability: 90%; **Metabolism, distribution, and excretion:** not fully determined

DRUG INTERACTIONS

None reported

RESPONSE RATES

40%–45% response rates have been observed in premenopausal patients with estrogen receptor–positive advanced breast cancer. The response rates of prostate cancer to leuprolide vs leuprolide/flutamide are not significantly different; however, the median survival is in favor of the combination (36 versus 28 mo)

NURSING INTERVENTIONS

Monitor signs and symptoms

PATIENT INFORMATION

Hypersensitivity and sexual dysfunction may occur

AVAILABILITY

Supplied as Lupron depot from TAP Pharmaceuticals, Deerfield, IL; 3.75-mg, 7.5-mg, and 22.5-mg depot formulations for IM injection. Store at room temperature. Protect from freezing. Long-acting implantable forms (Viadur, Alza Pharmaceuticals, Mountain View, CA) are also approved

MEGESTROL ACETATE

EFFICACY AND USAGE

Megestrol acetate is a synthetic progestational drug used in the treatment of advanced breast cancer and endometrial cancer. It is also used to improve anorexia and cachexia in cancer and AIDS patients. Progestins have significant antiestrogenic effect through either the conversion of estradiol to a less active estrone or downregulation of estrogen receptors.

DOSAGE AND ADMINISTRATION

Breast and endometrial cancer: 40 mg tablet four times daily PO; **cachexia/anorexia:** 400–800 mg PO daily

SPECIAL PRECAUTIONS

Weight gain in obese patients; patients with history of thromboembolic episodes

TOXICITIES

In general, the drug is well tolerated; **Endocrine:** breakthrough bleeding, change in menstrual flow; **Metabolic:** weight gain, hypercalcemia; **Cardiovascular:** edema; thromboembolic episodes, hypertension, dyspnea;

GI: nausea, vomiting

INDICATIONS

FDA-approved: advanced breast cancer, endometrial cancer, and cancer-related cachexia

CONTRAINDICATIONS

Early stage of pregnancy

PHARMACOKINETICS

Oral bioavailability: 97%; **Peak plasma levels:** in 2–3 h; **Half-life:** biphasic with a terminal half-life of 15–20 h; **Metabolism:** in liver; **Excretion:** majority in urine

DRUG INTERACTIONS

Decreases the clearance of warfarin

RESPONSE RATES

Approximately 60% of steroid receptor–positive breast cancer respond to megestrol; response rate is higher in tumors with positive progesterone receptors; the response rate in endometrial cancer is ~30%

NURSING INTERVENTIONS

Monitor signs and symptoms

PATIENT INFORMATION

Patient should be aware of the effects of weight gain and thromboembolic episodes and the need to avoid pregnancy. May cause photosensitivity

AVAILABILITY

Supplied as Megace from Bristol-Myers-Squibb Co., Princeton, NJ; 20- and 40-mg tablets to be stored at room temperature. Also available in 40-mg micronized megestrol acetate per milliliter oral suspension with alcohol 0.06% to be stored at < 25°C

MIFEPRISTONE

EFFICACY AND USAGE

Mifepristone is a synthetic derivative of progesterone. It acts as an antiprogestin and antiglucocorticoid. It has anti-tumor effect on rat mammary tumors and human breast cancer and meningioma cell lines. Clinical trials in Europe have shown tumor regression from mifepristone in human breast cancers and unresectable meningioma. It should be noted that about 72% of meningiomas are progesterone-receptor positive.

DOSAGE AND ADMINISTRATION

100 mg to 200 mg twice daily

SPECIAL PRECAUTIONS

Pregnant patients

TOXICITIES

In general, it is well tolerated; **Major side effects:** nausea, anorexia, hot flushes, dizziness, lethargy, gynecomastia in male patients

INDICATIONS

FDA approved for the medical termination of pregnancy through 49 days. Not approved for treatment of cancer or meningioma. However, clinical studies show modest activity in palliative treatment for advanced breast cancer and unresectable meningioma

CONTRAINDICATIONS

Pregnant patients

PHARMACOKINETICS

Half-life: 20 h

DRUG INTERACTIONS

None reported

RESPONSE RATES

Mifepristone showed minimal activity against breast cancer in two small European trials; preliminary results from a recent Canadian phase II study also showed a modest antitumor activity; partial responses observed in only 2 of 22 patients [11]; the response rate for meningioma was reported to be ~30%–40%

NURSING INTERVENTIONS

Monitor and document signs and symptoms

PATIENT INFORMATION

Should not be used in patients who are pregnant or planning for conception

AVAILABILITY

Distributed as Mifiprex (Danco Laboratories, New York, NY), in 200-mg tablets

NILUTAMIDE

EFFICACY AND USAGE
Nilutamide is a nonsteroidal antiandrogen used in conjunction with surgical castration for advance prostate cancer

DOSAGE AND ADMINISTRATION
300 mg daily orally for the first month, then 150 mg daily orally

SPECIAL PRECAUTIONS
Be aware of the untoward side effects mentioned in the Toxicities section

TOXICITIES
Hot flashes, diarrhea, visual disturbance (dark adaptation), interstitial pneumonitis (2% up to 17% in a small study), and hepatitis (1%) with liver function abnormalities; the inhibition of the mitochondrial respiratory chain and adenosine triphosphate formation by nilutamide may contribute to the aforementioned untoward, sometimes serious, toxicities.

INDICATIONS
Nilutamide should be used in combination with castration for metastatic prostate cancer; it should be started simultaneously with castration

CONTRAINDICATIONS
For patients with severe impairment of liver function and respiratory insufficiency or patients with history of hypersensitivities to this drug

PHARMACOKINETICS
Nilutamide is rapidly and completely absorbed through the oral route; ~84% of the drug is bound to plasma proteins; the steady-state plasma concentration is reached within 2–4 wk; the drug is extensively metabolized and mainly excreted through the kidneys; the plasma elimination half-life is ~50–60 h

DRUG INTERACTIONS
Intolerance to ethanol consumption (hot flashes, malaise, and hypotension); interaction with drugs (noticeably, vitamin K antagonists, phenytoin, theophylline, and others) that are metabolized via the P450 system

RESPONSE RATES
Comparing nilutamide/orchiectomy combination therapy with orchiectomy alone, the response rates were 40%–50% vs 24%–33%; progression-free survival was 21 mo vs 15 mo, and overall survival was 37 mo vs 30 mo. The improvement of bone pain and prostate-specific antigen is also in favor of the combination; however, no data is currently available to compare nilutamide with other newer antiandrogen (eg, bicalutamide) in a combination modality with orchiectomy or with LH-RH analog

NURSING INTERVENTIONS
Patient should have a chest radiograph taken before initiation of nilutamide and have liver functions closely monitored; be aware of those drugs that may interact with nilutamide, and monitor the drug level closely

PATIENT INFORMATION
Patients should be aware of possible visual disturbance (delayed adaptation to dark) and should be cautious about driving at night; patients should also be informed about the symptoms of interstitial pneumonitis and potential deterioration of liver functions

AVAILABILITY
Available as Nilandron by Hoechst Marion Roussel, Inc., Kansas City, MO; 50-mg tablets stored at room temperature and protected from light

TAMOXIFEN

EFFICACY AND USAGE

Tamoxifen is a nonsteroidal antiestrogen that exerts its effect on breast cancer by competitively inhibiting the binding of estrogen to estrogen receptors. Tamoxifen has been used in combination with chemotherapeutic agents for cancers other than breast in origin.

DOSAGE AND ADMINISTRATION

20 mg daily orally

SPECIAL PRECAUTIONS

Barrier forms of contraception should be considered in premenopausal patients because tamoxifen may initially induce ovulation; close monitoring of endometrium is required in prolonged use of tamoxifen for early detection of endometrial cancer

TOXICITIES

Vascular: hot flashes, lightheadedness, thromboembolism; **Gynecologic:** vaginal bleeding, altered menses, ovarian cyst, increased incidence of endometrial cancer; **GI:** nausea, vomiting, anorexia; **Metabolic:** hypercalcemia; **CNS:** emotional instability, depression; **Ophthalmologic:** at prolonged high dosage, visual disturbance (macular retinopathy and corneal opacity)

INDICATIONS

FDA-approved: female and male advanced breast cancer; adjuvant therapy after surgical removal of primary breast cancer lesion; in combination with chemotherapy, tamoxifen has been used for other cancer, such as melanoma

CONTRAINDICATIONS

Known hypersensitivity to tamoxifen; pregnant patients

PHARMACOKINETICS

Absorption: well-absorbed; **Plasma peak level:** 4–7 h; **Metabolism:** hydroxylation or N-oxidation to active metabolites; **Half-life:** biphasic, initially 9–12 h, later 7 d; **Excretion:** mainly in the feces

DRUG INTERACTIONS

Tamoxifen is a cytostatic drug that blocks the cell cycle at the late G_1 phase; therefore, it may attenuate cytotoxicity of many chemotherapeutic agents such as 5-fluorouracil and doxorubicin

RESPONSE RATES

When tamoxifen is used as first-line hormonal therapy, ~60% of steroid receptor–positive female and male breast cancers respond

NURSING INTERVENTIONS

Monitor and document signs and symptoms

PATIENT INFORMATION

Barrier form of contraception in premenopausal patients, and frequent gynecologic examination for early detection of endometrial cancer

AVAILABILITY

Supplied as Nolvadex by AstraZeneca Pharmaceuticals, Wilmington, DE, and available in generic form; 10-mg and 20-mg tablets to be stored at room temperature and protected from heat and light

TOREMIFENE

EFFICACY AND USAGE

Toremifene is a newer nonsteroidal antiestrogen used for the treatment of advanced breast cancer in patients with steroid-receptor–positive tumors. It appears to be nearly identical to tamoxifen in action and side effects. However, it has fewer tumorigenic effects in a rodent hepatic model, although this may not be clinically relevant.

DOSAGE AND ADMINISTRATION

60 mg daily orally

SPECIAL PRECAUTIONS

Should be cautious in patients with severe renal and hepatic insufficiency; drug-related hypercalcemia may occur

TOXICITIES

The most common adverse events are hot flashes, nausea, vaginal discharge or bleeding, and dizziness; other minor ones are anorexia, headache, diarrhea, vaginitis, rash, pruritus, depression, and insomnia; thromboembolic events (3%), elevated liver function tests (19%), and hypercalcemia (3%) have also been observed

INDICATIONS

FDA-approved: for the treatment of advanced breast cancer in postmenopausal patients

CONTRAINDICATIONS

Should not be used in pregnant patients

PHARMACOKINETICS

Toremifene is well absorbed after oral administration; the steady state blood level could be reached in 4–6 wk; the drug is mainly metabolized through the cytochrome P450 system in liver and is excreted in feces; the elimination half-life is ~5 d

DRUG INTERACTIONS

May interact with coumarin and cytochrome P450 inducers (phenobarbital, phenytoin) or inhibitors (ketoconazole)

RESPONSE RATES

As a first-line hormonal therapy for estrogen-receptor–positive or unknown advanced breast cancer, the response rates (21%–31%) in various randomized trials are comparable to that of tamoxifen (19%–37%); the time to progression and overall survival are also comparable

NURSING INTERVENTIONS

Monitoring prothrombin time and adjusting the coumarin dosage

PATIENT INFORMATION

Should not be used in pregnant woman

AVAILABILITY

Distributed as Fareston from Schering Corp., Kenilworth, NJ; 60-mg tablets stored at room temperature and protected from heat and light

The information here is provided as guidance only. Prescribers should always consult the manufacturer's current prescribing information

94

The first tubulin-binding drug to be used medicinally was colchicine. Extracted from the plant *Colchicum autumnale*, colchicine was first used by the ancient Egyptians to treat gout. More recently, its capability to block cellular proliferation in metaphase made it a valuable resource in the early studies of mitosis. These studies led to the identification of "tubulins" as "colchicine-binding proteins." The integral role that the tubulins play in chromosomal separation during mitosis has made them attractive targets for antitumor drugs, and the tubulin-targeting class of agents now constitutes a large family of heterogeneous compounds that includes established anticancer drugs such as the vinca alkaloids, taxanes, and estramustine phosphate [1]. Recent clinical successes related to the development of the taxanes has stimulated a search for superior tubulin-targeted compounds so that several structurally and mechanistically unique novel agents are currently undergoing early clinical evaluation [2].

TUBULIN

Tubulins have a central role in eukaryotic biology and are critically important during both cell division and the nonmitotic phases of the cell cycle. To date, the tubulin gene superfamily comprises five different tubulin families (α, β, γ, δ, and ϵ), with the α and β families most prevalent. All are composed of approximately 450 amino acids, they have similar relative molecular masses (50 kD), with about 25% to 30% sequence homology between families. These homologous regions are thought to be involved in GTP binding, although a functional role in GTP hydrolysis has only been described for the β-tubulins. Although highly conserved during vertebrate evolution, these families are structurally and functionally diverse with at least six different isotypes of both α- and β-tubulins present in human cells. These isotypes are encoded by different genes and distinguished by minor differences in amino acid sequences. Further structural diversity is also provided by posttranslational modifications such as phosphorylation and glutamylation. The nature and degree of the functional specificities of the different isotypes remain under investigation.

MICROTUBULES

Microtubules are hollow cylinders composed of tubulin that play diverse and essential roles in eukaryotic cells. During interphase, they serve as tracks on which motor proteins, such as the kinesins, can transport vesicles and other components throughout the cell. Their nonmitotic functions include membrane and intracellular scaffolding, anchorage of subcellular organelles and receptors, cell motility and chemotaxis, cellular adhesion, secretory processes, intracellular transport, and the transmission of receptor signaling [3]. Microtubules are also crucial during both mitosis and meiosis, accurately segregating chromosomes to the two daughter cells by forming a complex superstructure called the mitotic spindle.

Microtubules form by the self-assembly of α- and β-tubulin, a reaction that is initiated in vivo by γ-tubulin complexes at microtubule organizing centers such as the centrosome [4]. Initiation of microtubule formation is also known as microtubule nucleation. Following nucleation, the microtubule-organizing center continues to regulate tubulin polymerization, which results in the formation of tightly linked α β-tubulin heterodimers, the β-subunit of each heterodimer being in contact with the α-subunit of the next. During polymerization, GTP bound to β-tubulin is hydrolyzed to GDP, which can only be re-exchanged for GTP on depolymerization. This noncovalent polymerization of α β-heterodimers is arranged linearly into protofilaments,

and 13 protofilaments associate laterally to form the microtubule, a 25-nm diameter hollow tube. This organization of heterodimers is polarized, resulting in structural and functional kinetic differences at the microtubule ends. This polarization leads to the microtubule having a faster growing end (termed the *plus end*), in which β-tubulin is exposed, and a slower growing end (the *minus end*), which has α-tubulin exposed. Although both ends alternately lengthen or shorten, net elongation occurs at the plus end and net shortening at the minus end. When both of these occur concomitantly, the microtubule is said to be "treadmilling," a phenomenon believed to be critical in the polar movement of chromosomes during anaphase.

Microtubule tubulin polymers exist in an unstable equilibrium with the cellular pool of soluble tubulin, with continuous incorporation of free heterodimers, and simultaneous release of heterodimers into the soluble tubulin pool. The direction of this reaction's equilibrium is influenced by several cofactors including GTP, the ionic environment, the stabilizing microtubule-associated proteins (MAPs) as well as associated destabilizing proteins. This balance between microtubule stabilizing and destabilizing factors is thought to control microtubule polymerization [5]. This dynamic and energy-using process, known as "dynamic instability," is capable of polymerizing, depolymerizing, and moving in the cytoplasm on a time scale of less than 1 second. Although dynamic instability is not completely understood, studies indicate that it is highly regulated, which allows microtubules to adapt spatial arrangements that can change rapidly in response to cellular needs, and to perform mechanical work if required [6].

MITOTIC SPINDLE

Microtubule polymerization during cell division generates the mitotic spindle, a complex and highly regulated superstructure that undertakes chromosome segregation [7]. Classic descriptions of spindle structure originated from the light and electron microscopy features seen during metaphase, during which microtubules are arranged in a symmetric and fusiform structure. The typical mitotic spindle comprises more than 3000 microtubules, which are equally divided between the two half-spindles. Spindle microtubules have a uniform polarity, with the minus end at the poles and the plus ends extending toward the chromosomes or cell periphery. At metaphase, the chromosomes align along the midline, appearing as pairs of sister chromatids linked together only by the centromere, which is connected to the spindle microtubules by the kinetochores, paired disk-like structures that bind 10 to 40 spindle microtubules derived from either pole. The sister chromatids therefore become oriented toward opposite poles, enabling equal DNA segregation during cell division. Each spindle pole contains a centrosome, the specialized organelle responsible for microtubule nucleation.

MECHANISMS OF ACTION

The primary target of tubulin-binding drugs is the mitotic spindle, so that these agents therefore are termed mitotic spindle poisons. However, these compounds are not entirely cell-cycle specific because they also alter important tubulin functions outside cell division. Four main categories of drugs are discussed in this chapter: colchicine and its analogues, the vinca alkaloids, the taxanes, and estramustine. All appear to bind to different parts of tubulin, although a precise binding site has been determined only for the taxanes [8]. Colchicine, its analogues, and the vinca alkaloids all inhibit microtubule assembly by enhancing microtubule depolymerization (*ie*, destabilizing microtubules). This results in depolymerization and an increased soluble tubulin pool. Colchicine and its analogues, however, bind to a different binding site and do not compete for vinca alkaloid binding. The taxanes target a separate site, binding primarily to the amino-terminal 31 amino acids of the β-tubulin subunit. Conversely, they stabilize microtubules against depolymerization by altering the tubulin rate dissociation constants at both ends. Estramustine phosphate inhibits microtubule function by binding to MAPs, as well as to a unique site, on β-tubulin. Estramustine phosphate can both inhibit polymerization and promote stabilization of the microtubule

Despite the apparent differences between the modes of action of the taxanes and the vinca alkaloids, recent results indicate that these compounds have a similar mode of action at substoichiometric concentrations, inhibiting cell proliferation by perturbing microtubule dynamics. These actions generally result in a sustained mitotic blockade at the metaphase–anaphase boundary, which then leads to apoptosis through activation of the caspase cascade. The precise mechanism by which apoptosis is activated has not yet been determined, although genes that regulate apoptosis, such as *p53*, *bcl-2*, *bcl-x*, and *bax* probably determine cell sensitivity to these agents.

DRUG RESISTANCE AND SENSITIVITY

Two main mechanisms of resistance to tubulin-targeted drugs have been described, although their clinical relevance remains under debate [9]. The multidrug resistant (MDR) phenotype, mediated by the 170-kD P-glycoprotein efflux pump encoded by the *mdr1* gene, is the best-characterized resistance mechanism; however, there are other transporter proteins that also confer the MDR phenotype. The P-gycoprotein pump decreases intracellular drug accumulation and retention by actively extruding drug from the cell, which results in varying degrees of cross-resistance to many natural products including colchicine, the vinca alkaloids, the taxanes, the anthracyclines, epipodophylotoxins and actinomycin D. Constitutive overexpression of P-glycoprotein has been observed in many human malignancies, as well as many normal cells such as renal tubular epithelium, colonic mucosa, the blood–brain barrier, and the adrenal medulla. Given that P-glycoprotein is functionally reversible following treatment with various agents (*eg*, verapamil, quinidine, and cyclosporine), much effort has been spent trying to reverse drug resistance through the inhibition of P-glycoprotein. Overall, however, this strategy has been disappointing in clinical settings.

Modifications of microtubule structure resulting in altered microtubule dynamics or altered binding of antitubulin agents are also thought to constitute a significant mechanism of drug resistance. This may occur by gene mutation alone, or combined with posttranslational modifications. Several cell lines resistant to tubulin-binding drugs in vitro have been shown to contain tubulin alterations, in terms of total tubulin content, tubulin polymerization, or tubulin isotype content. Mutant cell lines with taxane resistant "hypostable microtubules" have been identified. These cell lines are conversely sensitive to the vinca alkaloids. β-Tubulin mutations leading to taxane resistance have been related to drug resistance and poor outcomes in patients with non–small cell lung cancer undergoing paclitaxel-based combination chemotherapy [10].

Other mechanisms of resistance to antitubulin targeted drugs have been described. Resistance to the taxanes and vinca alkaloids have been related to alterations in genes, such as *p53*, *bcl-2*, and *bcl-x*, alone or combined with their gene products that influence programmed cell death or apoptosis after significant microtubule disruption. In fact, use of antisense oligonucleotides targeting *bcl-2* is therefore being studied to optimize the cytotoxic response. Overexpression of the MAP τ has also been described in estramustine-resistant cells. Although estramustine can bind to the classical MDR efflux pump, P-glycoprotein–overexpressing cancer cells are not cross-resistant to estramustine. However, drug efflux mechanisms distinct from P-glycoprotein have been described for estramustine.

NOVEL ANTIMICROTUBULE AGENTS

The recent success of the taxanes has led to an intensive search for new chemotypes that work by a similar mechanism of action and have similar binding sites but have higher therapeutic indices. Several natural products that are structurally dissimilar to the taxanes and share their mechanism of action have been identified. These include the epothilones [19]: sarcotidicytins, rhazinilam, discodermolide, and eleutherobin. All are likely substrates for P-glycoprotein to some extent, but most are more potent than the taxanes with regard to actions on tubulin and cytotoxicity. However, other microtubule-stabilizing natural products, such as laulimalide and isolaulimalide, appear to be poor substrates for the P-glycoprotein drug efflux pump.

Several other natural products and semisynthetic antimicrotubule compounds interact with tubulin in the vinca alkaloid–binding or colchicine-binding domains that are in various phases of clinical development. Indanocine is a potent synthetic antimitotic that appears to overcome known mechanisms of drug resistance, targeting the colchicine-binding site on tubulin, whereas the cryptophycins are a family of cyanobacterial macrolides that inhibit microtubule polymerization following binding at the vinca alkaloid–binding site. They are extremely potent antimitotics, and are active against vinca alkaloid–resistant tumors in preclinical studies. In addition, the dolastatins are tubulin-binding oligopeptides with potent cytotoxic activity, noncompetitively inhibiting vinca alkaloid binding to tubulin. Further semisynthetic antimicrotubule compounds, such as the pentafluorophenylsulfonamides that interact with tubulin at the colchicine-binding domain, are currently being evaluated preclinically and in the clinic.

REFERENCES

1. Rowinsky EK, Tolcher AW: Antimicrotubule drugs. In *Cancer, Principles and Practice of Oncology*,edn. 6. Edited by DeVita VT, Jr, Hellman S, Rosenberg SA. Philadelphia: Lippincott-Raven; 2000.
2. Giannakakou P, Sackett D, Fojo T: Tubulin/microtubules: still a promising target for new chemotherapeutic agents. *J Natl Cancer Inst.* 2000, 92:182–183.
3. Jordan A, Wilson L: Microtubules and actin filaments: dynamic targets for cancer chemotherapy. *Curr Opin Cell Biol* 1998, 10:123–130.
4. Nogales E: Structural insights into microtubule function. *Annu Rev Biochem* 2000, 69:277–302.
5. Anderson SSL: Spindle assembly and the art of regulating microtubule dynamics by MAPS and Stathmin/Op18. *Trends Cell Biol* 2000, 10: 261–267.

6. Desai A, Mitchison TJ: Microtubule polymerization dynamics. *Annu Rev Cell Devel Biol* 1997, 13:83–117.

7. Compton DA: Spindle assembly in animal cells. *Annu Rev Biochem* 2000, 69:95–114.

8. Downing KH: Structural basis for the interaction of tubulin with proteins and drugs that affect microtubule function. *Annu Rev Cell Devel Biol* 2000, 16:89–111.

9. Dumontet C, Sikic BI: Mechanisms of action of and resistance to anti-tubulin agents: microtubule dynamics, drug transport, and cell death. *J Clin Oncol* 1999, 17:1061–1070.

10. Monzo M, Rosell R, Sanchez JJ, *et al.:* Paclitaxel resistance in non-small cell lung cancer associated with beta-tubulin mutations. *J Clin Oncol* 1999, 17:1786–1793.

11. Bollag DM, McQueney PA, Zhu J, *et al.:* Epothilones, a new class of microtubule-stabilizing agents with a taxol-like mechanism of action. *Cancer Res* 1995, 55:2325–2333.

The information here is provided as guidance only. Prescribers should always consult the manufacturer's current prescribing information.

97

VINCRISTINE

Vincristine sulfate (VCR) is a plant alkaloid originally derived from the periwinkle *Catharanthus roseus*. The agent, which has a broad antitumor spectrum, is an important component of various curative chemotherapy regimens. Vincristine has a large dimeric structure composed of a dihydroindole nucleus (vindoline) linked by a carbon–carbon bond to an indole nucleus (catharantine). It binds to tubulin, which alters its dynamic instability and inhibiting its polymerization. This leads to mitotic arrest followed by apoptosis.

DOSAGE AND ADMINISTRATION

IV bolus: in doses of up to 1–2 mg/m^2 weekly through rapidly flowing IV infusion at standard adult dose of 1.4 mg/m^2 weekly, and children's dose of 2 mg/m^2 for children who weigh less than 10 kg. Severe neurotoxicity suggests capping restriction of 2 mg, but this restriction largely derives from anecdotal, nonvalidated data, and this practice should be reconsidered. **Prolonged continuous IV infusion:** schedules of VCR have also been studied (0.25–0.5 mg/m^2 /d for 5 days), however, no clear evidence confirms that continuous IV schedules are more advantageous.

SPECIAL PRECAUTIONS

VCR is a potent vesicant. Every precaution must be taken to avoid extravasation. *Never administer SC, IM, IP, or IT. Inadvertent direct IT injection of VCR is invariably fatal.* Underlying comorbid neurologic problems accentuate risk of neurotoxicity. Autonomic neuropathy–derived severe constipation is common, so stool softeners should be considered. With hepatic impairment, VCR dosage should be reduced. A 50% dose reduction is often recommended for patients with serum bilirubin levels between 1.5 and 3 mg/dL; 75% dose reduction if the serum bilirubin level exceeds more than 3 mg/dL. No alteration in dosage is required for renal impairment.

INDICATIONS

Broad antitumor spectrum; important component of combination chemotherapy regimens that commonly produce high remission rates in childhood acute lymphocytic leukemia, Hodgkin's and non-Hodgkin's lymphomas, adult acute lymphoblastic leukemia, Wilms' tumor, Ewing's sarcoma and rhabdomyosarcoma. Curative treatment of poorer prognosis testicular teratoma (BOP-VIP: bleomycin, VBL, and cisplatin, alternating with etoposide, ifosfamide, and cisplatin). Combination regimens in treatment of multiple myeloma, chronic lymphatic leukemia, lymphoblastic crises of chronic myeloid leukemia, sarcoma, and small cell lung carcinoma. Anecdotally, useful in treating several nonmalignant hematologic disorders such as autoimmune thrombocytopenia, hemolytic uremic syndrome, and thrombotic thrombocytopenia purpura

PHARMACOKINETICS

Limited data available; VCR has longest half-life and lowest clearance rate of vinca alkaloids. **Absorption:** not given PO due to poor bioavailability; **Distribution:** high volume of distribution; VCR binds avidly to plasma proteins, platelets, erythrocytes; penetrates poorly into CSF. **Clearance:** mainly hepatic; excretion mainly fecal (70% in 72 h, 40% as multiple metabolites); 12% excreted in urine in first 72 h. Hepatic metabolism mainly by hepatic cytochrome P450 CYP3A. Elimination triphasic, α-phase half-life < 5 min; β- and γ-phase half-lives 50–55 min, 23–85 h, respectively. Long terminal half-life due to extensive tissue binding

DRUG INTERACTIONS

VCR-induced blockade of cellular efflux may enhance intracellular retention of methotrexate. L-asparaginase may reduce VCR hepatic clearance; therefore administer VCR 12–24 h before asparaginase. VCR also reduces serum phenytoin levels and may reduce bioavailability of digoxin. Because of the cytochrome P450 isoenzyme CYP3A in VCR metabolism, inhibitors/inducers of this isoenzyme may alter VCR clearance. Concurrent use of the P450 CYP3A inhibitor erythromycin and the vinca alkaloids, particularly vinblastine, associated with unusually severe toxicity. Conversely, concomitantly administered P450 inducers, such as phenobarbital, may also influence VCR clearance. Interaction between calcium channel blocker nifedipine, which has been used as a P-glycoprotein modulator and VCR has also been observed. P-glycoprotein modulator increases VCR's terminal half-life by 30% with reduced overall clearance. Caution with therapy for AIDS-related Kaposi's sarcoma, when patients are receiving treatment with both zidovudine and VCR; vinca alkaloids may inhibit zidovudine glucuronidation

The information here is provided as guidance only. Prescribers should always consult the manufacturer's current prescribing information

98

VINCRISTINE (Continued)

TOXICITIES

Myelosuppression: with conventional dosing schedules, mild-to-moderate anemia, leukopenia and, thrombocytopenia; **Neurotoxicity:** peripheral neuropathy, the severity of which depends on total administered dose and duration of therapy. Initial symmetric sensory impairment and paresthesias may be followed by neuritic pain, loss of tendon reflexes, ataxia, and motor dysfunction manifested by foot drop, wrist drop, paresis, and paralysis. These symptoms may persist for months after discontinuation of treatment and may not resolve. In adults, after cumulative doses above 5–6 mg, neurologic toxicity invariably becomes apparent. Elderly and patients with antecedent neurologic disorders are more prone to neurotoxicity. Cranial neuropathies (rare); hoarseness, diplopia, nerve deafness, facial pain, palsies, confusion, depression, agitation, insomnia, hypertension, hallucinations, seizures, coma, and the syndrome of inappropriate secretion of antidiuretic hormone (SIADH) have been reported. In addition, visual disturbances, atheosis, ataxia, acute necrotizing myopathy have been observed. Autonomic neuropathy can result in paralytic ileus, urine retention, and postural hypotension. The only consistent methods known to modify or prevent worsening of VCR-induced neurotoxicity are drug discontinuation alone or combined with dose reduction. Coadministration of prophylactic glutamic acid and the adrenocorticotropic hormone ORG 2766 may ameliorate the neurotoxicity of VCR; **Gastrointestinal:** constipation, colicky abdominal pain, nausea, vomiting, diarrhea, oral ulceration, paralytic ileus, intestinal necrosis, and perforation. Severe constipation due to autonomic neuropathy may result in high fecal impaction requiring high enemas. Routine laxative prophylaxis recommended for all patients receiving VCR. Paralytic ileus, more common in pediatric patients, the elderly, patients receiving high-dose therapy (> 2 mg/m^2), and patients with altered hepatic function, usually resolves after conservative treatment; **Genitourinary:** autonomic neuropathy may produce bladder atony leading to polyuria, dysuria, incontinence, and acute retention; **Cardiovascular:** postural hypotension, hypertension, acute cardiac ischemia, nonspecific chest pain, and myocardial infarction; **Endocrine:** SIADH is rare but may result in symptomatic hyponatremia, which may lead to seizures; **Dermatologic:** alopecia in about 20% of patients. Skin rashes are rare. Extravasation is a major risk; take every precaution to avoid. **Other:** fever of unknown origin.

PATIENT MONITORING

Monitor patients before each cycle for neurotoxicity and constipation. Also monitor patient's biochemistry because disease-related deterioration in hepatic function increases risk of VCR toxicity. Electrolytes may also become deranged in VCR-induced SIADH. Therapeutic drug monitoring of phenytoin and digoxin levels recommended in patients taking these concomitant drugs

NURSING INTERVENTIONS

Particular care to avoid extravasation. If extravasation does occur, infusion should be stopped, and site aspirated for any residual drug in the tissue. Application of local heat and SC injection of hyalouronidase circumferentially about site have been recommended to minimize pain and cellulitis. Local and systemic corticosteroid therapy may also be useful. Surgical debridement may need to be considered

PATIENT INFORMATION

Patient must be informed of risk of neurotoxicity and constipation. Prophylactic high-fiber diet or laxative use should be recommended. Women of childbearing age should be advised against pregnancy during therapy

FORMULATION

Available as Oncovin (Eli Lilly and Company, Indianapolis, IN), Vincasar (Pharmacia & Upjohn; Peapack, NJ). VCR is available for injection in 1-, 2- and 5-mL vials containing 1 mg/mL of drug for IV injection only. Stable at room temperature to 1 month; light sensitive so best stored in dark at 2–8°C

VINBLASTINE

Vinblastine sulfate (VBL) is also derived from *Catharanthus roseus*. VBL and VCR differ by an alteration on the vindoline unit that substitutes a CHO moiety for a CH_3 group. As with other vinca alkaloids, VBL alters tubulin dynamic stability, enhances microtubule depolymerization, and prevents tubulin polymerization, thereby leading to mitotic spindle dysfunction, mitotic arrest, and cell death often through apoptosis.

DOSAGE AND ADMINISTRATION

IV bolus: 6 mg/m² usual in combination chemotherapy regimens. Recommended VBL dose is 2.5 mg/m² and 3.7 mg/m² weekly for adults and children, respectively. Administer VBL as bolus, through satisfactorily placed IV cannula, by fast-flowing IV infusion.

SPECIAL PRECAUTIONS

Given substantial interindividual variability in degree of myelosuppression induced by VBL, patient's hematologic profile should always be assessed pretherapy. Because VBL is a potent vesicant, every precaution should be taken to avoid extravasation, which may cause necrosis, cellulitis, and sloughing. If VBL therapy is indicated despite hepatic impairment, dose reduction recommended. Standard guidelines specify 50% reduction for serum bilirubin levels of 1.5–3.0 mg/dL; 75% reduction if serum bilirubin levels exceed 3.0 mg/dL. Dose modifications not required for patients with renal dysfunction.

INDICATIONS

VBL is used in combination regimens to treat both Hodgkin's and non-Hodgkin's lymphoma and germ cell malignancies. A regimen termed PVB (cisplatin, VLB, and bleomycin) was, until recently, standard treatment for advanced testicular carcinoma. However, VBL has generally been replaced by etoposide in this combination, particularly in patients with more favorable disease characteristics because of etoposide's more favorable toxicity profile. Nonetheless, VBL is still frequently used to treat relapsed teratoma (VnIP [VBL, ifosfamide, cisplatin]). For Hodgkin's lymphoma, VBL is often used in combination with doxorubicin, bleomycin, and dacarbazine (ABVD). Regimen is either administered alone or alternated with MOPP (nitrogen mustard, VCR, procarbazine, and prednisone). VBL is also active in carcinomas of the breast, lung, and bladder, as well as in Kaposi's sarcoma, choriocarcinoma, mycosis fungoides, terminal phase of chronic myelogenous leukemia, and histiocytosis X. Infusions of VBL or VBL-loaded platelets have been effective in some cases of refractory autoimmune thrombocytopenia, because of its avidity to platelets

PHARMACOKINETICS

VBL has a similar pharmacokinetic profile to VCR. **Absorption:** poor and erratic, with unpredictable toxicity; not administered orally; **Distribution and clearance:** extensively bound to plasma proteins and tissues at therapeutic levels with poor penetration of the blood-brain barrier. Plasma disposition best fits a triphasic pharmacokinetic model. Its distribution is rapid, with a $T_{1/2\beta}$ of < 5 minutes. Values for $T_{1/2\beta}$ and $T_{1/2\gamma}$ range from 53–99 min and 20–24 h, respectively. VBL more avidly sequestered in the tissues than VCR, with 73% of total administered dose retained in body 6 days after administration. Elimination of VBL primarily hepatic, however, fecal excretion of parent compound is low because highly metabolized. Desacetyl-VBL (vindesine) is the principal hepatic metabolite, as active as the parent compound. Cytochrome P450 CYP3A isoform appears to be the principal enzyme involved in VLB metabolism. Less than 15% of dose administered excreted in urine

DRUG INTERACTIONS

Methotrexate accumulation in tumor cells is enhanced by VBL. L-asparaginase may reduce VBL hepatic clearance. VBL should be given 12–24 h before L-asparaginase. May lower plasma phenytoin levels. Concomitant administration of drugs that inhibit or enhance P450 CYP3A isoenzyme activity may alter VLB elimination, increasing and decreasing risk of toxicity, respectively (see VCR, Drug Interactions)

The information here is provided as guidance only. Prescribers should always consult the manufacturer's current prescribing information

100

VINBLASTINE (Continued)

TOXICITIES

Hematologic: myelosuppression, severity varies widely. Neutropenia is commonest, although thrombocytopenia and anemia also occur. Nadir usually within 4-d, full recovery 7–21 d; **Gastrointestinal:** VBL more likely to cause oral mucositis, stomatitis, and pharyngitis than VCR, as well as nausea and vomiting, diarrhea, anorexia, pain, and hemorrhagic enterocolitis. VBL-induced autonomic neuropathy may also cause constipation, ileus and abdominal pain. **Neurologic:** VBL has lower risk of neurotoxicity than VCR, related to the vindoline ring substitution of the methyl group in VBL for the formyl group in VCR, which effects much longer terminal half-life for VCR, which may be in part responsible for the neurotoxicity, because continuous protracted IV infusion VBL schedules also more likely to impair neuronal function. VBL neurotoxicity, when it occurs, is similar to that of VCR; **Cardiovascular:** hypertension and myocardial and cerebrovascular ischemic events. Raynaud's phenomenon may be a long-standing complication of VBL therapy, may resolve with calcium channel blocker therapy (*eg*, nifedipine); **Pulmonary:** pulmonary toxicity rare, although acute pulmonary edema described. Other pulmonary effects causing dyspnea include acute bronchospasm, acute respiratory distress, and interstitial pulmonary infiltrates. **Dermatologic:** alopecia, usually mild and reversible. Photosensitivity rashes. Potent vesicant may cause severe irritation on contact; **Endocrine:** SIADH and associated hyponatremia; **Miscellaneous:** pain at the tumor site; associated myocardial ischemia.

PATIENT MONITORING

Minimal monitoring is required. Hematologic assessment before each cycle is mandatory. Regular biochemical assessment is recommended. Therapeutic plasma monitoring of interacting drugs (*eg*, phenytoin) is advisable

NURSING INTERVENTIONS

Take adequate precautions to minimize risks of extravasation; use free-flowing IV infusion in a suitably placed venous catheter and flush catheter before and after treatment to ensure patency and complete delivery. If extravasation does occur, discontinue infusion, aspirate any residual drug remaining in the tissues, and apply local heat. Local injection of hyalouronidase 150 mg SC around site may reduce discomfort and possibility of cellulitis

PATIENT INFORMATION

The risks related to myelosuppression need to be explained to the patient, who should be advised to notify physician at first indication of infection. Women of childbearing age should be advised against pregnancy during therapy

FORMULATIONS

Also known commercially as Velban (Eli Lilly and Company, Indianapolis, IN) and Velbe (Eli Lilly, Indianapolis, IN). Supplied in 10-mg vials, either as a lyophilized powder, or in 0.9% NaCl with alcohol preservative at 1 mg/mL. Protect from light and store at 2–8°C. At room temperature, intact vials and reconstituted drug in preservative-containing sodium chloride are stable at least 28 days

VINORELBINE

Generic vinorelbine tartrate (VRL) is a semisynthetic vinca alkaloid derived from VBL by modification of the catharanthine nucleus (5'-norhydroVBL).

DOSAGE AND ADMINISTRATION

Diluted to concentrations between 1.5 and 3.5 mg/mL in 5% dextrose solution or 0.9% saline solution, VRL is usually administered IV either as a slow injection into a running IV infusion or as a short IV infusion over 6–10 min. As single agent, recommended dose is 15–30 mg/m^2 on weekly or biweekly schedule. Although oral administration (80–100 mg/m^2 weekly) is feasible and well tolerated, oral formulation is not yet available.

SPECIAL PRECAUTIONS

Administer through the side port of a fast-flowing IV infusion. Every effort should be taken to minimize the risk of extravasation. Caution in heavily pretreated patients with compromised hemopoietic reserve VRL dosing should be delayed in the presence of an absolute neutrophil count below 1000/ μL. A dose reduction is recommended in patients with impaired hepatic function—a 50% reduction in patients with serum bilirubin levels between 2–3 mg/dL, and a 75% reduction in patients with serum bilirubin levels exceeding 3 mg/dL. Dose reduction is not required in renal dysfunction.

INDICATIONS

VRL is approved in the United States for the treatment of non–small cell lung carcinoma either as a single agent or in combination with cisplatin. Clinically significant activity in patients with metastatic breast carcinoma recurring following initial treatment or as a component of first-line regimens. Active in the treatment of advanced Hodgkin's and non-Hodgkin's lymphomas and epithelial ovarian cancer, which is currently being evaluated

PHARMACOKINETICS

Bioavailability: 43% and 27%, respectively, orally as powder-filled or liquid-filled gelatin capsules. Intraindividual variability in absorption is high, albeit acceptable and generally lower than other vinca alkaloids. VRL exhibits a similar triexponential pharmacokinetic profile to the other vinca alkaloids. After IV administration therapy, a rapid decay in VRL plasma concentrations occurs in the first hour, following which the final elimination phase is slow. The α, β, and γ half-lives have been reported to be less than 5 minutes, 49–168 min, and 18–49 h, respectively. **High plasma protein binding:** 80%–91% of drug is observed. Drug binding to platelets is also high. Only 0.1%–0.20% remains unbound. The high volume of distribution at steady-state (20–75.6 L/kg) reflects its high lipophilicity. VRL achieves higher tissue distribution than the other vinca alkaloids with concentrations in human lung 300-fold higher than plasma levels (13.8-fold higher than for VCR).
Elimination: mainly through hepatic metabolism with 33%–80% excreted in the feces. The cytochrome P450 CYP3A isoenzyme plays a major role in drug metabolism. Urinary excretion accounts for only 16%–30% of drug

DRUG INTERACTIONS

Similar to VCR and VBL. L-asparaginase may decrease hepatic clearance of vinca alkaloids. Concomitant therapy with inhibitors of cytochrome P450 CYP3A may result in severe toxicity due to delayed VRL clearance, whereas coadministration of this isoenzyme with inducers (*eg*, phenytoin) may enhance clearance and reduce anti-tumor activity. Vinca alkaloids may inhibit the glucuronidative metabolism of zidovudine

PATIENT MONITORING

Monitor patient's hematology for myelosuppression before therapy. Modify dose with neutropenia. Hepatic function should also be assessed before each dose because dosage must be reduced with abnormal liver function test results. Therapeutic drug monitoring of concomitant phenytoin levels is advisable

VINORELBINE (Continued)

TOXICITIES

Hematologic: neutropenia, with nadir blood cell counts occurring 7–10 days post-treatment. Recovery is usually complete by day 14. Thrombocytopenia is uncommon. Mild to moderate anemia is frequently observed. Myelosuppression is not cumulative and readily reversible after cessation of treatment. Noncoagulopathy-associated thrombocytosis may occur; **Neurologic:** less neurotoxic than VCR or VBL, but similar to that of the other vinca alkaloids, with a peripheral sensory neuropathy in 7%–31% of patients and an autonomic neuropathy (*eg*, constipation), in as many as 30% of patients. Severe neurotoxicity is uncommon, although paralytic ileus may occur in 2%–3% of patients. During therapy, tumor pain and jaw pain may occur; reversible muscle weakness possible after prolonged treatment; **Gastrointestinal:** commonest GI side effect is constipation. Nausea and vomiting are usually mild. Up to 38% of patients may experience nausea and vomiting, but severe symptoms occur in only 2%–8% of patients. Less than 20% of patients experience nonsevere stomatitis or diarrhea. Oral VRL causes higher risk of GI toxicity; **Dermatologic:** vesicant. Local phlebitis at the injection site and along course of the injected vein is common, with mild erythema, pain, or venous discoloration occurring in as many as 33% of patients. Severe local toxicity is unusual, but more likely when vein not flushed after treatment. A shorter infusion time decreases risk of phlebitis. Alopecia occurs in 10% of patients; hand-foot syndrome has also been reported; **Pulmonary:** dyspnea in approximately 5% of patients. Acute bronchospasm is commonest respiratory toxicity, presumably related to allergic reaction or hypersensitivity phenomenon. Subacute respiratory reaction, characterized by cough, dyspnea, and occasional interstitial infiltrates, which may improve with corticosteroid therapy, after which uncomplicated VRL retreatment has been reported; **Other:** transient and asymptomatic derangement of liver function tests (*eg*, alkaline phosphatase). Pancreatitis may be a rare complication of therapy.

NURSING INTERVENTIONS

Precautions are needed to minimize risks of extravasation. A free-flowing IV infusion in a suitably placed venous catheter should provide a short intravenous infusion. The catheter should be flushed before and after treatment to ensure patency and complete delivery. If extravasation occurs, discontinue infusion, aspirate any residual drug remaining in the tissues, and apply local heat. Local SC injection of 150-mg hyaluronidase around the site may reduce discomfort and possibility of cellulitis

PATIENT INFORMATION

The patient should be informed about risk of neutropenic sepsis and asked to contact physician at first sign of infection, as well as to consume a high-fiber diet and to use a laxative if constipation occurs. Women of childbearing age should be advised against pregnancy during VRL therapy

FORMULATIONS

Available as Navelbine (Glaxo Wellcome Inc., Research Triangle Park, NC), injectable VRL is available as a 1-mL or 5-mL vial of 10 mg/mL. This clear to pale yellow solution must be protected from light and stored at 2–8°C. It is stable at 25°C for up to 72 h if unopened. Once reconstituted, it is stable for up to 24 h in normal light between 5–30°C

PACLITAXEL

Paclitaxel, the prototypical taxane, alters microtubule dynamics, thus stabilizing the microtubule and preventing microtubule disassembly, which blocks cell-cycle progression at the G_2/M junction and induces apoptosis. Paclitaxel was originally isolated from the bark of the pacific yew tree *Taxus brevifolia*. Initially, supply of paclitaxel was limited in development. Now, nearly all clinical supply is currently derived semisynthetically from 10-deacetylbaccatin III and other inactive precursors found in the needles of more abundant and renewable *Taxus* species.

DOSAGE AND ADMINISTRATION

Paclitaxel is usually administered IV at a dose of 175 mg/m^2 over 3 h or 135 mg/m^2 over 24 h every 3 weeks. For the most part, the 24-h schedule is more myelotoxic, and the 3-h schedule more neurotoxic; both schedules approximate similar clinical efficacy. Randomized studies indicate that higher doses increase toxicity but not necessarily clinical efficacy. More protracted schedules have been investigated but no clear evidence confirms any clinical efficacy. Considerable interest exists in a weekly schedule associated with less myelosuppression and similar antitumor activity than the conventional every-3-wk schedule. Weekly treatment at doses below 100 mg/m^2 is well tolerated (generally 80 mg/m^2), and antitumor activity occurs with the weekly schedule in patients who have been previously treated with paclitaxel on the 3-h schedule. Oral administration has been studied, but paclitaxel's oral bioavailability is low. Clinical studies have, however, shown that the concurrent administration of a P-glycoprotein inhibitor (*eg*, cyclosporine) can improve paclitaxel's absorption by blocking both constitutive P-glycoprotein in enterocytes and P450 metabolizing isoenzymes in both enterocytes and hepatic cells, but the clinical relevance of this observation is not known. Intraperitoneal paclitaxel administration has also been shown to be feasible, although abdominal pain precludes administration of doses above 125 mg/m^2. Premedication to minimize the risk of major hypersensitivity reaction to paclitaxel or its polyoxyethylated castor oil (Cremophor EL) vehicle is recommended. Dexamethasone 20 mg PO or IV, 12 and 6 h before treatment, with an H$_1$-histamine antagonist such as diphenhydramine 50 mg IV, and an H$_1$-histamine inhibitor (*eg* ranitidine, 50 mg IV; cimetidine, 300 mg IV; or famotidine, 20 mg IV), 30 min before treatment, has been routinely used. A single dose of dexamethasone administered IV 30 min before therapy with an H$_1$- and H$_2$-histamine antagonist may be as effective in preventing major hypersensitivity reactions.

SPECIAL PRECAUTIONS

Paclitaxel is principally eliminated through hepatic metabolism and biliary excretion. Studies indicate patients with moderate to severe elevations in serum hepatocellular enzymes or bilirubin are at greater risk. Paclitaxel doses must be reduced by at least 50% in patients with moderate or severe hepatic excretory dysfunction (hyperbilirubinemia) and/or significant elevations in hepatic transaminase enzymes. Dose modifications are not required for renal impairment or third-space fluid collections. If paclitaxel is being given in combination with an anthracycline or trastuzamab, cardiac function must be carefully monitored.

INDICATIONS

Most impressive clinical activity has been observed in patients with epithelial ovarian and breast cancers. In the United States and many other countries, paclitaxel initially received regulatory approval for treatment of patients with ovarian and breast cancers only after failure of first-line or subsequent chemotherapy. It subsequently received regulatory approval for patients with advanced breast cancer following failure of combination chemotherapy at relapse or within 6-mo adjuvant chemotherapy. Use in combination with a platinum compound as primary induction therapy in suboptimally debulked stage III or IV ovarian cancer, and as a component of adjuvant chemotherapy following primary local treatment in high-risk patients with early stage breast cancer following primary local treatment, has recently been associated with a clear survival advantage in randomized trials. Paclitaxel has received regulatory approval for second line treatment of AIDS-associated Kaposi's sarcoma, in combination with cisplatin as primary treatment of non–small cell lung cancer, and as a component of adjuvant chemotherapy in high-risk lymph node–positive breast cancer. It provides impressive activity against a broad range of other cancers generally refractory to conventional therapies, including previously treated lymphoma, and small cell lung, head and neck, esophageal, gastric, endometrial, bladder, prostate, and germ cell malignancies

PHARMACOKINETICS

Pharmacokinetics are nonlinear when paclitaxel is administered as a 3-h infusion, with saturable elimination and distribution. Tissue distribution is saturated at lower drug concentrations than elimination. However, implications of paclitaxel's nonlinear pharmacokinetic profile are clinically insignificant at standard doses. Paclitaxel pharmacokinetics follow a triexponential process with $T_{1/2}\alpha$, $T_{1/2}\beta$, and $T_{1/2}\gamma$ of 20 min, 5.8 h, and 10–20 h, respectively. It has a large volume of distribution, with high plasma protein binding (> 95%) and poor penetration into CNS. Clearance is largely hepatic route, with 71% of administered dose excreted into bile to the feces by 5 d as either parent compound or metabolites. Cytochrome P450 mixed function oxidases, in particular isoforms CYP2C8 and CYP3A4, are principally involved drug metabolism. Paclitaxel's hydroxylated metabolites are substantially less active than the parent compound. Renal clearance is less than 14% of administered drug

DRUG INTERACTIONS

Interacts with several cytotoxics. Cisplatin given before 24-h paclitaxel decreases paclitaxel clearance by 33%. The alternate sequence of paclitaxel followed by cisplatin, which has been associated with greater activity in vitro and demonstrated impressive clinical activity in patients with ovarian and non–small cell lung cancers, is therefore recommended. This interaction is not as significant when paclitaxel is administered as 3-h infusion. Combination of paclitaxel and carboplatin results in less thrombocytopenia compared with single agent carboplatin when paclitaxel administered first

PACLITAXEL (Continued)

TOXICITIES

Hypersensitivity reactions: without premedication, incidence of all grades of hypersensitivity phenomena approaches 20%–30%. Severe hypersensitivity reactions usually occur within 10 minutes of treatment during the first cycle. Most reactions resolve with infusion cessation, although occasionally treatment with antihistamines, fluids, and vasopressors is necessary. Although up to 40% of patients develop flushing and rashes, this does not predict the development of more severe reactions. With prophylactic measures, incidence of hypersensitivity reactions is 1%–2%. Safe retreatment of patients who have had major hypersensitivity reactions is usually possible with a substantially lower infusion rate, which is gradually increased, and after treatment with corticosteroids (dexamethasone 20 mg IV every 6 h for 4 doses), although this approach is not always successful; **Myelosuppression:** neutropenia is the principal dose-limiting toxicity of paclitaxel. It begins around day 8 and resolves by day 15–21. The extent of prior therapy is the principal clinical determinant of myelotoxicity, which is not cumulative. Shorter infusions and weekly treatment schedules decrease severity of neutropenia. Severe thrombocytopenia and anemia are rare; **Neurotoxicity:** peripheral, sensory neuropathy, characterized by numbness and paresthesiae, in a glove-and-stocking distribution. There is often symmetric distal loss of sensation carried by both large (proprioception, vibration) and small (temperature, pinprick) fibers, which may begin as soon as 24–72 h after treatment with higher doses, but this usually occurs only after cumulative dosing. Severe neurotoxicity is infrequent. Shorter schedules, particularly those in which paclitaxel is combined with cisplatin or carboplatin, are more likely to cause neurotoxicity. Uncommonly, patients also describe simultaneous onset of perioral numbness, and of symptoms in the arms and legs with diffuse areflexia. Motor and autonomic dysfunction may also occur, particularly in patients with preexisting neuropathies caused by alcoholism and diabetes mellitus. Glutamic acid, amifostine, and pyridoxine have been evaluated in small, uncontrolled studies to ameliorate paclitaxel neurotoxicity, with varying degrees of success. Rarely, optic nerve disturbances with scintillating scotomata may occur. Acute encephalopathy leading to coma and death has been reported after treatment with very high doses (> 600 mg/m^2). **Muscular:** transient myalgia is common at day 2–5 posttreatment; myopathy described with higher doses. Antihistamines have been reported to help prevent acute myalgia; however, narcotics appear to be effective most consistently; **Cardiac:** transient bradycardia in 29% of patients, which does not indicate treatment discontinuation. More serious bradyarrhythmias including third degree heart block have been noted in up to 0.1% of patients. Most episodes have been reversible and uneventful, but more rarely myocardial ischemia/infarction, atrial arrhythmias, and ventricular tachycardia have been described. Paclitaxel was, however, well tolerated in a study of patients with major cardiac risk factors. Routine cardiac monitoring is not usually necessary. Combination therapy with anthracyclines significantly increases risk of congestive cardiac failure. In one study in previously untreated patients with advanced breast cancer treated with escalating doses of paclitaxel (3-h infusion) and doxorubicin 60 mg/m^2 to a cumulative dose of 480 mg/m^2, incidence of cardiotoxicity was significantly higher than expected. This anthracycline dose was predicted to result in less than a 5% incidence of congestive cardiotoxicity; however, incidence of congestive cardiotoxicity in this combination study was 25%. Such incidence was less than 5% when similar patients received identical schedules of paclitaxel and doxorubicin with the cumulative doxorubicin dose not exceeding 360 mg/m^2. Accentuated cardiotoxicity has not been consistently observed with docetaxel suggesting that this is due to a pharmacokinetic interaction.

Dermatologic: alopecia, including bodily hair; phlebitis at administration site; inflammatory reactions at sites of extravasation and in areas of previously irradiated skin (recall reaction); **Other:** nausea, vomiting, and diarrhea are uncommon, mucositis is also rare at clinically relevant doses. Rarely neutropenic enterocolitis, pancreatitis, pneumonitis, and severe hepatotoxicity have been described.

DRUG INTERACTIONS (continued)

When paclitaxel is administered on 24-h infusional schedule before doxorubicin, it reduces doxorubicin clearance by 33%. This sequence-dependent interaction is again not clinically significant with shorter (3-h) paclitaxel schedules. However, paclitaxel, on both short and protracted schedules, enhances cardiotoxic effects of doxorubicin. Therefore, patients receiving both agents in combination generally tolerate lower cumulative doxorubicin doses; incidence of symptomatic cardiotoxicity increasing sharply at cumulative doxorubicin doses exceeding 360 mg/m^2 (see Cardiotoxicity section). Epirubicin clearance is also impaired by paclitaxel but similar cardiotoxic interactions have not been noted. It is thought that these pharmacokinetic interactions are due to competition for hepatic/biliary P-glycoprotein between the polyoxyethylated castor oil in paclitaxel and the anthracyclines, because docetaxel does not alter anthracycline clearance. Taxane is predominantly metabolized by hepatic cytochrome P450 CYP3A4 and CYP2C8 and then excreted in the bile. Concomitant therapy with inducers or inhibitors of these enzymes can theoretically alter paclitaxel pharmacokinetics

PATIENT MONITORING

Patients should be monitored carefully for neutropenia and neurotoxicity. Treatment is usually withheld until recovery of the neutrophil count to above 1500 cells/mm^3 on every-3-week schedules. Dose reduction is required if severe neutropenia is observed. If significant neurotoxicity is observed, a dose reduction or treatment using a more protracted regimen should be considered. If concurrent doxorubicin or Herceptin is being administered, cardiac function should be monitored

NURSING INTERVENTIONS

Observe patients for hypersensitivity reactions during therapy, particularly in the initial administration period. Care against extravasation is important. Avoid the use of polyvinyl chloride (PVC) administration equipment because polyoxyethylated castor oil leaches through such plastic and requires polyethylene-lined administration sets that include an in-line filter with a microporous membrane not larger than 0.22 μm

PATIENT INFORMATION

Inform patient of the risks of neutropenic sepsis and of hypersensitivity reactions. Female patients should be advised to avoid pregnancy during treatment

FORMULATIONS

Paclitaxel is commercially available as Taxol (Bristol-Meyers Squibb, Research Triangle Park, NC), Anzatax (Faulding LMT, Australia) and Onxol (IVAX Corporation, Miami, FL), and is available as a concentrated sterile solution in 5-mL, 16.6-mL, and 50-mL vials containing 6 mg/mL paclitaxel in polyoxyethylated castor oil and dehydrated alcohol. This must be diluted in either 0.9% saline or 5% dextrose to a final concentration of 0.3–1.2 mg/mL. This solution is stable at room temperature for up to 27 hours at room temperature under normal light. Paclitaxel must be diluted and stored in glass or suitable plastic bags (polypropylene or polyolefin) to minimize risk of patient exposure to plasticizers leached from PVC infusion bags or sets

DOCETAXEL/TAXETERE

Docetaxel is a semisynthetic derivative of the readily available taxane precursor 10-deacetyl baccatin III, which is extracted from the needles of the European yew tree, *Taxus baccata*, and other *Taxus* species. Like paclitaxel, this agent alters microtubule dynamics by decreasing microtubule disassembly, stabilizing polymerized tubulin, and promoting microtubule assembly. Docetaxel differs from paclitaxel on the C10 taxane ring position, and on the ester side chain attached at C13. Clinical antitumor activities of the two taxanes are similar, although docetaxel appears to be more potent than paclitaxel with regard to its antimicrotubule effects and cytotoxicity in vitro. However, this does not necessarily translate into enhanced therapeutic efficacy because it may also portend more severe toxicity at identical drug concentrations in vivo. Unlike paclitaxel, docetaxel has linear pharmacokinetics, a longer serum half-life, and longer intracellular retention.

DOSAGE AND ADMINISTRATION

Recommended dosage ranges from 60–100 mg/m^2 given IV over 1 h every 3 wks. However, 75–100 mg/m^2 is commonest dose range in clinical practice. Similar to paclitaxel, weekly treatment has been associated with lower hematologic toxicity than 3 weekly schedules and appears to be well tolerated at 36 mg/m^2/wk.

In patients without hyperbilirubinemia, dose reductions of 25% are recommended with elevated hepatic transaminases (>1.5-fold) and alkaline phosphatase (> 2.5-fold), regardless of whether the elevations are due to hepatic metastases. However, more substantial reductions (50% or greater) may be required for patients who have moderate or severe hepatic excretory dysfunction. Dose modifications are not required for impaired renal function or third-space fluid collections.

Premedication is required, with dexamethasone 8 mg PO twice daily, usually given for 3–5 days starting 1–2 days before treatment to minimize risk of fluid retention and hypersensitivity reactions. H$_1$- and H$_2$-histamine antagonists can also be given IV 30 minutes before docetaxel.

SPECIAL PRECAUTIONS

Severe hypersensitivity reactions are uncommon, with dyspnea, hypotension, and flushing occurring in less than 1% of patients. In patients with impaired liver function, dose reductions recommended. Dose modifications are not required for renal impairment or third-space fluid collections.

INDICATIONS

Impressive antitumor activity in patients with metastatic breast cancer as first-line or salvage treatment, non–small cell lung cancer as first-line or in platinum-refractory disease, and in recurrent or refractory ovarian cancer. Currently approved by the US Food and Drug Administration as second-line treatment following treatment with anthracyclines in patients with metastatic breast cancer. Its role as a component of adjuvant and neoadjuvant chemotherapy following the local treatment of early-stage breast cancer, and of first-line chemotherapy for locally advanced and metastatic non–small cell lung cancer, are being evaluated. Regulatory approval has been granted in many countries for the treatment of patients with locally advanced or metastatic non–small cell lung cancer, because agent has shown a survival advantage when used in the second-line setting following platinum-based therapy. In addition, impressive activity in previously treated patients with carcinomas of the ovary, endometrium, head and neck, esophagus, stomach, urinary bladder, prostate, and small cell lung, as well as lymphomas and other neoplasms. Clinical antitumor spectra for paclitaxel and docetaxel are similar

PHARMACOKINETICS

Linear and are well fit by a three-compartment model. The agent binds avidly to plasma proteins (> 80%–90%) and is widely distributed with a steady-state volume of distribution of 74 L/m^2. Does not cross the blood-brain barrier. Terminal half-life (T$_{1/2\gamma}$) ranges from 10–15 h. It is cleared primarily by hepatic metabolism, with fecal excretion accounting for 70%–80% of drug. Urinary excretion accounts for less than 10%. Cytochrome P450 mixed function oxidases, in particular isoforms CYP3A4 and CYP3A5, are mainly responsible for hepatic metabolism. Principal pharmacokinetic determinants of toxicity are drug exposure and the duration of exposure to biologically relevant plasma concentrations. Docetaxel exhibits a wide interpatient variation in clearance that results in varying degrees of toxicity, perhaps due to variability in CYP3A activity. The measurement of metabolites of substrates of CYP-3A, such as erythromycin in the erythromycin breath test, may predict CYP-3A activity, docetaxel clearance and toxicity

DRUG INTERACTIONS

Interactions with other classes of drugs that can effect the cytochrome P450 system are predicted based on interactions demonstrated for paclitaxel (see Drug Interactions in Paclitaxel section). However, neither significant pharmacokinetic or toxicologic drug-drug interactions between docetaxel and the anthracyclines have been documented, which may reflect differences in taxane formulation and/or potencies that may lead to differences in the number of molecules available for competition for clearance mechanisms with the anthracyclines

DOCETAXEL/TAXETERE (Continued)

TOXICITIES

Hematologic: neutropenia toxicity limits dosage of docetaxel. It is not cumulative and treatment delays due to incomplete recovery of neutrophil counts are unusual. At 100 mg/m^2, using the 1-h schedule, nadir counts are frequently less than 500/μL, which usually occur on day 9 with recovery by days 15–21. The most important predictor of neutropenia is the extent of previous therapy. Severe thrombocytopenia and anemia are infrequent; **Hypersensitivity:** despite not being formulated in polyoxyethylated castor oil, docetaxel caused hypersensitivity reactions in approximately 31% of patients treated without premedication on early trials, which occurred within first few minutes of the initial two courses. Symptoms resolved rapidly with cessation of therapy. Treatment was usually recommenced without adverse effect. Most reactions were minor with flushing, wheezing, chest tightness, anxiety, and lower back pain. Dyspnea, hypotension, and bronchospasm leading to cyanosis were less common. Premedication reduces the risk of hypersensitivity reactions; **Fluid retention:** causes a unique fluid retention syndrome resulting in weight gain, edema, pleural effusions, and ascites, possibly resulting from increased capillary permeability resulting in fluid leakage from vascular compartment. It is not usually a significant problem until a cumulative dose of more than 400-mg/m^2 docetaxel has been administered in the absence of corticosteroid premedication. Premedication with corticosteroids and H$_1$- and H$_2$-histamine antagonists decrease incidence of fluid retention as a function of cumulative dose; **Dermatologic:** alopecia; between 50% and 75% of patients develop an erythematous pruritic maculopapular rash affecting forearms and hands. Premedication decreases rash incidence. Superficial desquamation of the hands and feet and palmar-plantar erythrodysesthesia occur that may respond to oral pyridoxine 50 mg three times daily. Onychodystrophy with brown brittle nails, ridging, onycholysis, and soreness is common. Phlebitis along infusion course and at injection site is occasionally noted, but severe tissue necrosis following extravasation rare; **Neuromuscular:** similar but less marked than with paclitaxel. Mild to moderate peripheral sensory neuropathy predominates, in approximately 40% of chemotherapy-naive patients. Motor effects are less common. Severe toxicity is unusual in the absence of an underlying comorbid neurologic disorder (*eg*, diabetes, alcoholism). Arthralgia and myalgia following treatment are not uncommon but usually short-lived. **Other:** severe lethargy and malaise occur infrequently, particularly in patients who have received large cumulative doses on a weekly basis. Stomatitis more frequent than with paclitaxel. Nausea, vomiting, and diarrhea are uncommon. Little evidence suggests cardiotoxicity.

PATIENT MONITORING

Monitor for fluid retention, neurotoxicity, and myelosuppression and hepatic dysfunction, the later of which may require reduced dosage. Treatment is usually withheld until neutrophil count exceeds 1500 cells/mm^3

NURSING INTERVENTIONS

Observe patient for hypersensitivity reactions, which usually occur in the first two courses within minutes of therapy. Care against extravasation is important, although extravasation reactions do not usually cause necrosis. Avoid infusion sets containing PVC

PATIENT INFORMATION

Advise patient of risk of hypersensitivity reactions, neutropenic sepsis, and fluid retention. Female patients should be advised to avoid pregnancy during treatment

FORMULATIONS

Proprietary name is Taxotere (Aventis Pharmaceuticals, Bridgewater, NJ). Formulated with polysorbate 80 in sterile vials containing 40 mg/mL. Unopened vials should be stored between 2–8°C and protected from light. It is diluted with the supplied sterile diluent containing 13% alcohol to a final premix solution of 10 mg/mL, which is stable for up to 8 h at room temperature and must be diluted in either 0.9% NaCl solution or 5% dextrose solution to achieve a final concentration of 0.3 to 0.9 mg/mL. After preparation, use solution as soon as possible

The information here is provided as guidance only. Prescribers should always consult the manufacturer's current prescribing information.

107

ESTRAMUSTINE PHOSPHATE

Estramustine phosphate was originally designed to accumulate in breast cancer cells bearing estrogen receptors. Composed of a conjugate of the alkylating agent nornitrogen mustard linked to 17β-estradiol, it was designed to target 17β-estradiol receptor-bearing cells. Following tumor cell uptake, degradation of the carbamate ester was to release the alkylating cytotoxic component. However, the agent did not demonstrate an acceptable level of activity in clinical trials in patients with breast carcinoma, and estramustine phosphate was subsequently thought to be inactive. Nevertheless, further studies established that the agent preferentially accumulates in the prostate of the rat and has anticancer activity in this tumor type. This selective accumulation in the prostate is unrelated to estrogen receptors and is mediated by a specific protein found in prostate tissue termed estramustine-binding protein (EMBP). Estramustine phosphate induces tumor cell death by binding to tubulin and MAPs. Its tubulin-binding site is distinct from that of colchicine, the taxanes and vinca alkaloids.

DOSAGE AND ADMINISTRATION

Recommended daily dose is 14 mg/kg/d (600 mg/m^2/d) PO, usually in three to four divided doses, at least 1 h before or 2 h after meals. Continuous oral therapy can be continued for months or years. Short-course administration in combination with taxanes or vinca alkaloids is being investigated.

SPECIAL PRECAUTIONS

Patients with preexisting heart failure are at risk of fluid retention and cardiac decompensation, resulting in left ventricular failure. Patients with known hypercoagulable states should be treated with caution.

TOXICITIES

Gastrointestinal: dose-limiting toxicities include nausea and vomiting, which are not usually severe and can easily be treated and prevented with antiemetics. Rarely cause cessation of therapy; long-term therapy can cause diarrhea.
Other: myelosuppression is rare. Steroidal moiety of compound may cause gynecomastia, fluid retention, thromboembolic complications, and liver dysfunction. Patients with pre-existing comorbid cardiac disease are at risk of developing cardiac failure. Deep venous thrombosis and pulmonary embolism as well as cerebrovascular and coronary thrombotic events have been reported. Transient elevation in hepatic transaminases occurs in approximately 33% of patients.

INDICATIONS

Hormone-refractory metastatic prostatic carcinoma

PHARMACOKINETICS

After oral administration, estramustine phosphate is rapidly dephosphorylated within the GI tract. Bioavailability ranges from 37%–75%. Most absorbed drug is rapidly metabolized to an oxidized isomer, estromustine, which becomes the predominant metabolite detected in plasma. Estromustine concentrations peak 2–4 hours following oral intake, and then decline with a plasma half-life of 14 hours. Estromustine is further metabolized by hydrolysis in the liver, with most drug excreted in feces; less than 1% in urine

DRUG INTERACTIONS

Oral bioavailability significantly impaired by coadministration of calcium-rich foods and calcium-containing antacids. Docetaxel clearance may be decreased in the presence of estramustine phosphate by an as-yet undefined mechanism. If these two agents are to be used in combination, it has been recommended that the docetaxel dose should be reduced

PATIENT MONITORING

Assess patients for fluid retention and thromboembolic events; monitor hepatic function and hematology should be monitored

NURSING INTERVENTIONS

Ensure the patient takes the medication fasted. Assess for fluid retention

PATIENT INFORMATION

Avoid coadministration of calcium rich food (*eg*, milk) and calcium-containing antacids due to impaired estramustine absorption. Patients should take their therapy on an empty stomach, having fasted for 1 hour before or 2 hours after a meal

FORMULATIONS

PO formulation (Emcyt; Pharmacia & Upjohn, Peapack, NJ) is available as white crystals of the disodium salt monohydrate in a capsule containing the equivalent of 140-mg estramustine phosphate. A parenteral formulation being studied because of the variable bioavailability seen when estramustine phosphate is administered PO remains clinically available

The information here is provided as guidance only. Prescribers should always consult the manufacturer's current prescribing information

108

CHAPTER 6: BREAST CANCER
Minetta C. Liu, Marc E. Lippman

EPIDEMIOLOGY AND RISK FACTORS

Breast cancer is the most frequently diagnosed malignancy in women and the second leading cause of cancer-related deaths in the United States, with approximately 183,000 new cases and 41,000 deaths expected in the year 2000 [1]. The incidence of advanced breast cancer and of death from breast cancer have remained fairly stable, but the number of in situ carcinomas and early-stage breast cancers has increased dramatically; as a result, the proportion of women diagnosed with invasive breast cancer who ultimately die of the disease has strikingly declined. This phenomenon most likely results from early detection through routine mammographic screening and advances in systemic therapy. In fact, retrospective analyses have clearly demonstrated an association between the stage of disease at diagnosis and prognosis with the following 5-year survival data: 97% for noninvasive disease; 78% for invasive disease confined to the breast and/or axilla; and 22% for metastatic disease [1].

Major risk factors associated with the development of breast cancer are outlined in Table 6-1. Several represent prolonged exposure to estrogen and include the following: early onset of menarche, late onset of menopause, and prolonged and current use of exogenous estrogen for hormone-replacement therapy in postmenopausal women. Other reproductive risk factors include nulliparity and older age at first pregnancy. Finally, an increased risk of developing breast cancer has also been associated with a personal history of atypical ductal hyperplasia, in situ carcinoma, or invasive breast cancer; advanced age; regular ethanol intake; and exposure to moderate or high doses of ionizing radiation at a young age (especially age < 30).

Familial risk is most likely related to inherited genetic defects and should be suspected in women with a first degree relative (ie, mother, sisters) who developed breast cancer at a young age. For example, if a woman's mother developed breast cancer at an age younger than 40, her relative risk of developing breast cancer is 2.1; if her mother was older than 70 at the time of diagnosis, however, the woman's relative risk of developing breast cancer is 1.5 [2]. Mutations in *BRCA-1* and *BRCA-2* ("breast cancer related genes") have been associated with this hereditary breast cancer syndrome as well as with certain other malignancies; the BRCA-1 syndrome predominantly involves familial cases of breast and ovarian cancer, whereas the BRCA-2 syndrome may include familial cases of prostate cancer, pancreatic cancer, bladder cancer, non-Hodgkin's lymphoma, basal cell carcinoma, and the fallopian tube tumors. Finally, mutations in *p53* and in the phosphatase and tensin homologue (*PTEN*) have also been associated with increased breast cancer risk, specifically in relation to Li-Fraumeni syndrome and Cowden disease, respectively [3].

RECOMMENDATIONS FOR SCREENING

Several randomized trials have demonstrated that breast cancer screening in women over age 40 can reduce the incidence of breast cancer–related mortality. Two such studies are the Health Insurance Plan of New York Randomized Clinical Trial (HIP Trial), which randomized women to screening with both mammography and clinical breast examination versus usual care, and the Swedish Two-County Study, which compared single-view mammography with no mammography; screening was found to reduce the number of breast cancer deaths by 23% [4] and 32% [5], respectively. On the basis of these and other large trials, the American Cancer Society (ACS), National Cancer Institute (NCI), and American College of Radiology (ACR) now recommend that women begin routine screening with mammograms and clinical breast examinations in their 40s; the NCI recommends that screening be performed in 1- or 2-year intervals, but the ACS and ACR specify annual screening [6]. None of these guidelines offers an upper age limit for screening. In addition, those women at an increased risk for breast cancer because of a suggestive family history, a known genetic mutation, or a high-risk assessment score require increased surveillance and should consult their physicians about when to initiate breast cancer screening with mammography and clinical breast examinations.

Much debate has taken place about the value of screening women in certain age groups, specifically women between the ages of 40 and 49 (a group relatively underrepresented in the randomized trials) and women over the age of 70 (a group essentially excluded from participation in the randomized trials). The primary concern with women younger than 50 is that many will have screening mammograms and only a few isolated patients will have a positive finding. In addition, increased breast tissue density can decrease the sensitivity of mammography and thus lead to a significant number of false-negative studies. Current investigations into various new methods of breast imaging—including digital full field mammography, magnetic resonance mammography, high-resolution CT, electrical impedance imaging, light scanning, and infrared imaging—may ultimately eliminate this latter concern. In contrast, issues regarding the need for breast cancer screening in women over age 70 relate to cost-effectiveness in a population with likely comorbidities. Given the increasing estimated life span for women and high incidence of breast cancer in this age group, however, it seems appropriate to determine the value of breast cancer screening on a case-by-case basis with special attention to the individual woman's overall health and performance status. If she is a candidate for local therapy with surgery and/or radiation, she should be considered an appropriate candidate for screening as well.

DIAGNOSIS, STAGING, AND PROGNOSIS

Suspicious findings on a screening mammogram include the following: foci of spiculated architectural distortion, poorly circumscribed masses with variable x-ray attenuation, and clusters of pleomorphic intraparenchymal microcalcifications. These, as well as any suspicious palpable breast mass, require further evaluation with diagnostic

---

Table 6-1. Risk Factors for the Development of Breast Cancer

Reproductive factors
  Early menarche
  Late onset of menopause
  Prolonged and current use of exogenous estrogens
  Nulliparity
  Older age at first pregnancy
Nonreproductive factors
  Advanced age
  Personal history of atypical ductal hyperplasia or in situ carcinoma
  Personal history of invasive breast cancer
  Family history of breast cancer
  Positive genetic testing for the BRCA-1 or BRCA-2 mutation
  Regular alcohol intake
  Exposure to ionizing radiation at a young age

---

mammograms using magnification and/or spot compression views. If a mass is suspected on either physical examination or mammogram, a breast ultrasound or fine needle aspiration may be performed to differentiate a solid lesion from a fluid-filled cyst. Correlative radiographic studies such as dynamic magnetic resonance imaging with gadolinium, positron-emission tomography, and radionuclide scans using ^{99m}Tc may prove to be helpful in distinguishing benign from malignant lesions in the future, but they currently remain investigational. Therefore, a suspicious breast mass still requires an initial histopathologic evaluation, and this can be achieved in one of four ways. Fine-needle aspiration is the least invasive method, but its sensitivity and specificity depend greatly on good technique and the availability of a practiced cytopathologist; its utility is also limited by the inability to differentiate in situ from invasive carcinoma [7]. Other means of obtaining tissue for histopathologic diagnosis include core needle biopsies, excisional biopsies, and incisional biopsies. Ultimately, the selection of biopsy technique is at the discretion of the surgeon and the patient depending on the exact clinical situation.

After malignancy has been confirmed, the exact tumor-node-metastasis (TNM) stage [8] should be determined (Table 6-2). An accurate assessment of tumor size requires complete excision of the breast lesion either by wide local excision (lumpectomy) or by partial or complete mastectomy. Two special situations, however, deserve mention. First, if more than one primary breast tumor is present, the official T stage is based on the size of the larger lesion only. Second, tumor that is identified on core needle biopsies only is considered TX disease because of the inability to determine size accurately. Note that although the overall TNM classification for breast cancer has remained constant for the past several years, the revised classification does differ from previous versions with the addition of a T0 (no evidence of a primary tumor) and a T1mic (microinvasion of 0.1 cm or less in greatest dimension) stage.

Lymph node status is traditionally obtained by dissection of level I and level II axillary lymph nodes, although undissected internal mammary lymph nodes are positive in up to 9.9% of patients with negative axillary lymph nodes [9]. To limit the extent of upper extremity lymphedema, numbness, pain, and weakness associated with the full axillary dissection, there has been growing interest in the concept of a sentinel lymph node biopsy. This procedure requires surgical expertise and uses lymphatic mapping with a radiolabeled colloid and/or blue dye to identify the first lymph node(s) that drain the primary tumor. With a skilled surgeon accustomed to performing the procedure, the sentinel node is successfully identified in over 90% of the cases and reflects the presence or absence of axillary lymph node metastases almost 100% of the time [10]. This level of accuracy is attainable, however, only when use of the sentinel lymph node biopsy is restricted to the appropriate patient population; that is, when it is not performed on patients with clinically positive lymph nodes, tumors larger than 5 cm, locally advanced breast cancer, multicentric disease, recent treatment with neoadjuvant chemotherapy, or a history of previous surgery in the axillary region.

A metastatic work-up completes the full staging assessment. The current standard of care requires a full physical examination, chest radiograph, and routine blood tests including a complete blood cell count and full hepatic panel. Other studies, such as abdominal imaging and nuclear medicine bone scans, are left to the discretion of the treating oncologist on the basis of each patient's symptoms and clinical presentation. Taken together, the tumor size, lymph node status, and presence/absence of distant metastases provide the strongest indicator of a patient's prognosis. Tumor grade, the presence/absence

of lymphovascular involvement, hormone receptor status, and Her-2/neu status are other well-established predictors of the risk of recurrence and/or death from breast cancer and should therefore be reported by the pathologist for all tumors. The true prognostic value of other parameters such as DNA ploidy, S phase content, and Ki-67 staining remains to be determined [11].

PROLIFERATIVE BREAST LESIONS AND IN SITU CARCINOMA

Certain benign breast lesions are thought to have premalignant potential and therefore warrant intervention or close follow-up. These lesions can be divided into two subgroups: proliferative lesions without atypia, which includes moderate to florid ductal hyperplasia of the usual type, intraductal papillomas, sclerosing adenosis, and fibroadenomas; and atypical hyperplasia, which includes both the lobular and ductal variants [12,13]. The theory is that there is a progression from usual hyperplasia to atypical hyperplasia to in situ carcinoma and then to frank invasive carcinoma. Support for this model of breast cancer development derives from a prospective study that followed a large population of women with benign breast lesions. After prolonged follow-up, the authors concluded that the relative risk of developing breast cancer was 1.0 to 2.0 for women who had proliferative lesions without atypia and 4.0 to 5.0 for women with atypical lobular or ductal hyperplasia [12,14].

In situ carcinomas are premalignant breast lesions because they lack the ability to penetrate the basement membrane, invade the surrounding stroma, and metastasize. Lobular carcinoma in situ (LCIS) is not commonly associated with specific clinical signs or radiographic changes and therefore is typically discovered as an incidental finding on breast biopsy. An important distinction from other breast lesions is the observation that LCIS is frequently multicentric (ie, characterized by multiple foci that are present in more than one quadrant of the breast) and/or bilateral. Although it does not always progress to cancer, LCIS is associated with up to a tenfold risk of progressing to ipsilateral or contralateral invasive breast cancer—a risk that appears to persist indefinitely [15]. Interestingly, LCIS is more often associated with the development of infiltrating ductal carcinoma than with infiltrating lobular carcinoma. No official guidelines exist regarding the management of this lesion, but chemoprophylaxis with tamoxifen or bilateral prophylactic mastectomies should be recommended for breast cancer prevention. There is no role for local treatment with complete surgical excision or breast irradiation in cases of pure LCIS.

Ductal carcinoma in situ (DCIS) can present as an incidental biopsy finding or in association with a palpable breast mass or pathologic nipple discharge. With the widespread use of breast cancer screening, it is now more commonly diagnosed by the detection of suspicious microcalcifications on routine mammography [16]. The acronym DCIS actually applies to a heterogeneous group of lesions with different cytologic features and prognostic significance. The most aggressive of these lesions is characterized by comedo-type architecture, prominent areas of central luminal necrosis, and cells with a high nuclear grade and mitotic index [17]. Various classification schemes exist for DCIS, but the high degree of interobserver variability makes routine use of these systems very difficult. Nonetheless, DCIS is considered to have high malignant potential and thus require treatment. Simple mastectomy, for example, results in cure rates of close to 100% for all subtypes [16]. Of note, there is no indication for axillary lymph node sampling in patients with

DCIS, except in cases of a large primary lesion in which complete exclusion of an invasive component is often not possible.

The advent of breast conserving therapy for invasive disease ultimately led to interest in its use for DCIS as well. (For the simplicity of discussion here, use of the term *lumpectomy* in reference to DCIS refers to a wide local excision that removes all suspicious clinical findings and radiographic microcalcifications.) No randomized trials directly comparing mastectomy to lumpectomy have been performed, but large, prospective, randomized trials have investigated the following modalities of breast conserving therapy: use of lumpectomy alone versus lumpectomy followed by breast irradiation [18], and use of lumpectomy followed by breast irradiation versus lumpectomy followed by breast irradiation and preventative therapy with tamoxifen [19]. Essentially, the risk of recurrent breast disease—whether intraductal or invasive—decreases significantly with lumpectomy/radiation and more so with lumpectomy/radiation/tamoxifen in certain subpopulations of patients with higher risk lesions. Factors indicative of high recurrence rates include large tumor size, the presence of close surgical margins, and documentation of high-grade histology [20]. Survival, conversely, does not appear to improve with the addition of radiation or radiation and tamoxifen; one must keep in mind, however, that the data are inconclusive with respect to overall survival because the studies were not sufficiently powered to detect small survival benefits in a population in which virtually all patients are expected to be cured. Therefore, although the in-breast recurrence rates are higher with all variants of breast conserving therapy than with mastectomy, breast conservation is still an acceptable alternative for patients who are made fully aware of its potential risks and benefits—including the need for a salvage mastectomy on disease recurrence.

CHEMOPREVENTION

Long-term tamoxifen administration has been shown to prevent breast cancer development in mouse models [21], and women who received tamoxifen as adjuvant therapy for early stage breast cancer have been shown to have a lower incidence of second primary breast cancers [22]. These laboratory and clinical observations, coupled with the relatively low incidence of treatment-related toxicities, have prompted interest in the use of tamoxifen in breast cancer prevention for high-risk women. The largest prospective, randomized clinical trial performed to date that attempts to answer this question is the National Surgical Adjuvant Breast and Bowel Project's (NSABP) P-1 Breast Cancer Prevention Trial [23]. This trial randomized over 13,000 women with a high risk of developing breast cancer to receive either tamoxifen 20 mg daily or placebo for 5 years. The results reported after an average of 48 months of follow-up indicate that tamoxifen decreased the risk of both invasive and noninvasive breast cancer by approximately 50% in all age groups studied. Subgroup analysis revealed that women with a history of LCIS or atypical hyperplasia derived the greatest benefit from chemoprevention, with a 56% and 86% reduction in the risk of developing breast cancer, respectively. Importantly, a histopathologic review revealed that tamoxifen selectively decreased the number of estrogen receptor–positive tumors and had little to no effect on the number of estrogen receptor–negative tumors. These positive data have prompted the initiation of the NSABP P-2 Trial, which compares the efficacy of raloxifene—a newer selective estrogen receptor modulator that reportedly lacks tamoxifen's association with endometrial cancer—to tamoxifen as a chemopreventive agent for postmenopausal women at high risk of developing breast cancer.

Of note, two European trials also investigated tamoxifen in breast cancer prevention: the Royal Marsden Trial [24], which randomized only those women with a positive family history of breast cancer; and the Italian Chemoprevention Trial [25], which randomized only

---

Table 6-2. American Joint Committee Staging Guidelines for Breast Cancer [8]

T — Primary Tumor

TX	Primary tumor cannot be assessed
T0	No evidence of primary tumor
Tis	Carcinoma in situ: intraductal carcinoma, lobular carcinoma in situ, or Paget's disease of the nipple with no tumor
T1	Tumor 2 cm or less in greatest dimension:
	T1mic: microinvasion 0.1 cm or less in greatest dimension
	T1a: tumor > 0.1 but not > 0.5 cm in greatest dimension
	T1b: tumor > 0.5 but not > 1.0 cm in greatest dimension
	T1c: tumor > 1.0 but not > 2.0 in greatest dimension
T2	Tumor > 2.0 cm but not > 5.0 in greatest dimension
T3	Tumor > 5.0 cm in greatest dimension
T4	Tumor of any size with direct extension to (a) chest wall or (b) skin, only as described below:
	T4a: extension to chest wall
	T4b: edema (including peau d'orange) or ulceration of the skin of the breast or satellite skin nodules confined to the same breast
	T4c: both (T4a and T4b)
	T4d: inflammatory carcinoma

N — Regional Lymph Nodes

NX	Regional lymph nodes cannot be assessed (eg, previously removed)
N0	No regional lymph node metastasis
N1	Metastasis to moveable ipsilateral axillary lymph node(s)
N2	Metastasis to ipsilateral axillary lymph nodes fixed to one another or to other structures
N3	Metastasis to ipsilateral internal mammary lymph node(s)

M — Distant Metastasis

MX	Distant metastasis cannot be assessed
M0	No distant metastasis
M1	Distant metastasis (includes metastasis to ipsilateral supraclavicular lymph node[s])

Stage Grouping

Stage 0	Tis	N0	M0
Stage 1	T1	N0	M0
Stage IIA	T0	N1	M0
	T1	N1	M0
	T2	N0	M0
Stage IIB	T2	N1	M0
	T3	N0	M0
Stage IIIA	T0	N2	M0
	T1	N2	M0
	T2	N2	M0
	T3	N1	M0
	T3	N2	M0
Stage IIIB	T4	Any N	M0
	Any T	N3	M0
Stage IV	Any T	Any N	M1

---

those women who had undergone a hysterectomy (with or without concurrent bilateral oophorectomy), irrespective of their breast cancer risk. These two studies failed to demonstrate any risk reduction between the treatment and control groups, but they were both marked by a relatively low number of breast cancer events and a relatively high rate of patient noncompliance in comparison with the NSABP P-1 trial. These observations suggest that neither the Royal Marsden Trial nor the Italian Chemoprevention Trial are adequate to definitively prove or disprove the efficacy of tamoxifen as a chemopreventive agent.

LOCAL THERAPY FOR EARLY-STAGE DISEASE

Management of the breast and axillary region has evolved from William Halsted's method of radical resection to the modified radical mastectomy to breast conserving therapy. Current options for managing the primary tumor include mastectomy (with or without reconstruction) and breast conserving surgery followed by radiation therapy. Seven prospective, randomized clinical trials involving women with stage I and II disease have demonstrated that survival is equivalent with these two methods of treatment. These findings were also substantiated in a published meta-analysis [26]. Ultimately, the decision about which local intervention is appropriate for a particular patient depends on the patient's preferences about breast conservation and cosmesis. As a result, the size of the tumor, the location of the lesion, and the patient's breast size are often determinants in deciding whether to proceed with a lumpectomy or mastectomy. Finally, surgical staging of the axilla is necessary whether patients opt for mastectomy or lumpectomy with radiation; not only is lymph node status important in determining the patient's prognosis and the need for adjuvant systemic therapy, but some evidence also suggests that regional control of the axilla may have a positive impact on the rate of distant metastases and overall survival [27]. For patients with early-stage breast cancer and a breast surgeon experienced with the technique, a sentinel lymph node biopsy is a potential alternative to the full axillary dissection.

The rate of in-breast recurrences with conservative breast surgery and adjuvant whole breast radiation is relatively low, although factors such as youth, a positive family history, the presence of an extensive intraductal component, involved or close surgical margins, multiple primary tumors, and diffuse microcalcifications on mammogram are somewhat predictive of an increased risk of recurrence and argue against the use of breast-conserving therapy. No formal investigations have been made about the role of chest wall and regional lymph node irradiation in breast conservation, but data from studies of adjuvant radiotherapy to the chest wall and regional lymph nodes following mastectomy indicate a benefit for a subpopulation of patients. In fact, postoperative radiation has been shown to decrease the rate of local-regional recurrence in certain high-risk patients, namely those with four or more positive axillary lymph nodes, obvious extracapsular nodal extension, close or involved deep margins of resection, and large tumor size [26]. In addition, a few trials have demonstrated a survival advantage in patients treated with mastectomy and postoperative radiotherapy, but only after prolonged (ie, ≥ 10 years) follow-up [28–30]; the data are not sufficiently persuasive, however, and additional trials and analyses are currently ongoing with special attention to the possibility that the survival benefit observed with additional radiotherapy may be offset by the potential morbidity and mortality associated with radiation-induced cardiopulmonary complications.

ADJUVANT SYSTEMIC THERAPY FOR OPERABLE DISEASE

With local therapy alone, the risk of recurrence and death from breast cancer is approximately 30% in women with node-negative disease and 75% in women with node-positive disease. These statistics reflect distant micrometastases that are present but undetected at the time of diagnosis. The only potential means by which to eradicate these micrometastases is the administration of systemic therapy, preferably when the tumor burden is minimal. This concept has been a driving force behind the evolution of adjuvant chemotherapy and endocrine therapy over the past three decades. Although results from randomized trials and meta-analyses clearly indicate that all patients with early-stage breast cancer derive a statistically significant survival benefit from systemic therapy, the degree of benefit varies among different groups of patients; moreover, this degree of benefit depends on the patient's age and axillary lymph node status as well as on the various histopathologic and biochemical characteristics of the tumor itself. It is the responsibility of medical oncologists to advise their patients of the relative benefits of adjuvant therapy and help them make an informed decision in light of the potential toxicities associated with the individual agents recommended.

Important concepts about the role of systemic therapy in early stage breast cancer have been introduced as a result of the meta-analyses published by the Early Breast Cancer Trialists' Collaborative Group (EBCTCG) [22,31–34], each of which presents a thorough, systematic overview of the major randomized trials investigating some aspect of adjuvant therapy for early stage breast cancer. The most noteworthy conclusions are summarized below.

Adjuvant Chemotherapy

The EBCTCG overviews published in 1992 [32] and 1998 [34] are based on randomized trials representing a variety of chemotherapeutic regimens. Nonetheless, combination chemotherapy was clearly more effective than monotherapy in terms of both disease-free and overall survival rates. In addition, comparisons between longer and shorter treatments revealed no significant advantage to extending chemotherapy beyond 6 months. Focusing on the use of adjuvant chemotherapy overall, the analysis revealed that adjuvant systemic therapy can improve 10-year survival for women with early-stage breast cancer—a conclusion substantiated by the results of such individual, large, randomized trials as the NSABP B-13 [35] and the Intergroup INT-0011 studies [36]. Proportional benefits were greater for women younger than 50 years old than for women between the ages of 50 and 69, which translated into a 7% to 11% and a 2% to 3% absolute improvement in 10-year survival, respectively; patients older than 70 years old were not represented in these studies. Subgroup analysis also revealed that although a 30% to 40% proportional risk reduction was observed for women with both node-positive and node-negative disease, the absolute risk reduction at 10 years was much lower for women in the latter group. Taken together, these findings suggest that a group of post-menopausal women with node-negative breast cancer may be at a sufficiently low-risk to preclude adjuvant chemotherapy because the potential risks outweigh the small benefits of proceeding with treatment.

The most highly represented drug regimen in the EBCTCG meta-analyses was cyclophosphamide/methotrexate/5-FU (CMF)—either alone or in combination with other chemotherapeutic agents. A few studies compared CMF or one of its variants with an anthracycline-containing regimen. With relatively short-term follow-up, those patients who received either doxorubicin or epirubicin as part of their adjuvant treatment demonstrated greater proportional reductions in both recurrence and mortality [34]; of note, most of the patients randomized were under 50 years of age. The largest direct comparison of an anthracycline regimen versus CMF, however, revealed only marginal benefits in both disease-free and overall survival when high-risk, node-negative patients were randomized to receive either cyclophosphamide/doxorubicin/5-FU (CAF) or CMF [37]. In addition, no significant difference was found in the rates of breast cancer recurrence or mortality in either the NSABP B-15 study [38] or the recent NSABP B-23 study [39], both of which compare four cycles of doxorubicin/cyclophosphamide (AC) with six cycles of CMF in women with estrogen receptor–negative, node-negative breast cancer. Although it is not clear that AC is truly more efficacious than CMF in the adjuvant setting, persuasive evidence suggests that anthracycline-responsiveness is a function of Her-2/neu overexpression [40]. Nonetheless, AC has a shorter treatment course (12 weeks versus 18 to 24 weeks for CMF) and requires fewer physician visits, making it the more appealing adjuvant systemic chemotherapy regimen.

Taxanes are cytotoxic agents that promote microtubule assembly and stabilize tubulin formation. Most importantly, they appear to lack cross-resistance with the anthracyclines [41]. Paclitaxel was initially shown to be highly effective as a single agent in the treatment of metastatic breast cancer with overall response rates of up to 60% in minimally pretreated patients [42,43] and 20% to 40% in heavily pretreated patients [44]. Subsequent investigations have established its role in the adjuvant setting as well, particularly in those patients with high-risk disease [45] who now receive paclitaxel in conjunction with either AC or CMF. Additional randomized clinical trials are currently under way to substantiate these findings and determine the optimal dose and schedule of paclitaxel and its related drug, docetaxel. The Cancer and Leukemia Group B (CALGB), for example, is conducting a randomized study comparing concurrent AC to concurrent doxorubicin/paclitaxel (AT), but the results of this trial will not be available for several more years.

In addition to the development of novel agents, interest is growing in the concept of increasing dose intensity to overcome drug resistance. This is accomplished by increasing dose *density*—the amount of drug administered per unit of time—without necessarily increasing the total drug dose. Randomized trials have applied this approach to the administration of AC in primary breast cancer by combining a standard regimen of doxorubicin with escalating doses of cyclophosphamide [46,47], and by combining a standard regimen of cyclophosphamide with escalating doses of doxorubicin [45]. Thus far, no significant survival advantage has been demonstrated with either regimen. Ongoing studies now focus on adjuvant chemotherapy protocols with decreased dosing intervals as opposed to increased total dose, working on the hypothesis that more frequent drug administration minimizes the tumor growth period and thus increases treatment efficacy against micrometastatic disease; the CALGB, for example, is comparing sequential, every 2-week therapy with doxorubicin, paclitaxel, and cyclophosphamide versus concurrent AC followed by paclitaxel in different treatment intervals. Finally, the ultimate means by which to increase dose intensity is with myeloablative doses of chemotherapy with hematopoietic stem cell support (*ie*, autologous bone marrow transplantation or autologous peripheral blood stem-cell rescue). No conclusive evidence exists to support this approach, but the current trials of high-dose chemotherapy are relatively small and may not be powered to detect a small but clinically relevant improvement in overall survival.

The current standard of care for operable breast cancer involves the administration of adjuvant chemotherapy following definitive breast surgery. Arguments in favor of using neoadjuvant chemotherapy in early-stage breast cancer, however, are provocative. First, it allows for an early in vivo assessment of treatment efficacy; the presence of significant residual disease after the administration of neoadjuvant therapy is likely to indicate tumor resistance to a particular regimen, suggesting that the patient is at a higher risk of recurrence and should therefore receive additional or alternative chemotherapeutic agents. Second, early treatment may prevent the development of resistant clones that would otherwise proliferate if chemotherapy were delayed until after surgery. Finally, preoperative treatment may allow some women with large tumors the option of breast conservation rather than mastectomy. These potential advantages to neoadjuvant therapy must be weighed against the likely disadvantages, including the potential for downstaging axillary lymph node status (which would overestimate prognosis in node-positive patients who become node-negative after chemotherapy) and the need to rely on a fine needle aspirate or core needle biopsy for the initial diagnosis. The NSABP investigated these possibilities in a large clinical trial in which women with operable breast cancer were randomized to post-operative AC versus preoperative AC [48]. No detectable difference was found in disease-free survival, distant disease-free survival, or overall survival, but 80% of the women did achieve a significant decrease in tumor size with neoadjuvant chemotherapy; this resulted in an increase in the number of patients managed with breast conserving surgery. Longer follow-up is necessary to assess whether or not any significant differences exist in the rate of local recurrence.

Adjuvant Hormonal Therapy

Estrogen manipulation, accomplished with oophorectomy, ovarian ablation through irradiation, adrenalectomy, or hypophysectomy, is the oldest treatment for breast cancer. This ultimately evolved into the development of various hormonal agents, including estrogens, antiestrogens, progestins, antiprogestins, androgens, antiandrogens, aromatase inhibitors, and gonadotropin-releasing hormone analogues. Most studies have focused on the use of these therapies in the metastatic setting, but those agents that have shown efficacy in advanced disease have been tried in patients with early-stage breast cancer as well. Tamoxifen, a selective estrogen receptor modulator with both estrogen antagonist and estrogen agonist properties, has been studied the most extensively thus far in this regard.

In addition to their analyses of adjuvant chemotherapy, the EBCTCG published an overview of adjuvant tamoxifen in the treatment of early-stage breast cancer [22]. Tamoxifen was shown to decrease recurrence rates (a 10-year proportional reduction of 47% with 5 years' use) and improve survival (a 10-year proportional reduction of 26% with 5 years' use) in patients with estrogen receptor–positive or estrogen receptor–unknown tumors; no clear benefit was seen in women with estrogen receptor–negative tumors, and evidence from other studies suggests that tamoxifen may have detrimental effects in this population of women [37]. Importantly, the same degree of benefit was seen in all women regardless of age, and the proportional reductions in recurrence and mortality were similar regardless of nodal status. Although statistically significant proportional reductions were seen with 1, 2, and 5 years of therapy with tamoxifen, a longer duration of therapy was associated with greater proportional reductions in recurrence and less so in mortality. Notably, the survival benefits appear to persist for several years even after the completion of therapy. Direct comparisons of 2 versus 5 years of adjuvant tamoxifen in postmenopausal women have helped to substantiate this finding [49,50]. The next logical assumption is that treatment beyond 5 years is more efficacious, but randomized trials have failed to demonstrate a survival advantage in continuing tamoxifen for 10 as opposed to 5 years in both node-negative [51] and node-positive patients [52].

The association between adjuvant ovarian ablation and increased survival in premenopausal women with both node-negative and node-positive, early-stage breast cancer has been clearly established [32,33]. Traditionally, ovarian ablation was achieved by either oophorectomy or irradiation. More recent studies focus on ovarian suppression using luteinizing hormone-releasing hormone (LHRH) analogues. One agent, goserelin, has already demonstrated comparable efficacy to ovarian ablation in advanced breast cancer [53], and at least one study has shown equivalent recurrence and overall survival rates between premenopausal patients treated with ovarian ablation and those treated with standard chemotherapy for early-stage breast cancer [54]. Several large, randomized, multicenter trials are currently under way to evaluate the use of adjuvant LHRH analogues in place of or in conjunction with adjuvant chemotherapy and/or

tamoxifen in the treatment of women with early-stage breast cancer [55]. Endpoints of these studies include treatment efficacy (eg, rates of disease-free survival and overall survival) as well as relative toxicities. With respect to the latter, concern remains about the potential long-term effects of goserelin on premenopausal women, including decreased bone mineral density and worsening of the blood lipid profile. Preliminary data published in abstract form indicate that goserelin may improve the time to relapse but does not have a significant impact on overall survival [56,57]. Long-term follow-up, however, is necessary before any final conclusions can be made and ovarian suppression can be considered standard practice.

Conclusions

The treatment of early stage breast cancer involves a multidisciplinary approach with contributions from surgeons, radiation oncologists, and medical oncologists. The timing of chemotherapy and radiation was previously debated, but at least one randomized study of women undergoing breast conserving therapy has shown that the rate of distant recurrences—and thus possibly the rate of overall survival—is lower if adjuvant chemotherapy is administered before radiation [58]. In terms of endocrine therapy, no definitive data support the initiation of tamoxifen at a specific time in relation to chemotherapy or radiation. Many groups, however, advocate the use of chemotherapy and then radiation before tamoxifen to avoid any potential for additive toxicities; nonetheless, several clinical trials have begun chemotherapy and tamoxifen or radiation and tamoxifen simultaneously without obvious detrimental effects.

Adjuvant therapy was initially restricted to patients with node-positive disease, but conclusive evidence supports its value in the management of most subgroups of breast cancer patients. In some cases, however, the degree of benefit in terms of disease-free and overall survival may not outweigh the potential for toxicities. In addition, it appears that chemotherapy and endocrine therapy have independent benefits with respect to disease-free survival and overall survival. General guidelines exist by which systemic treatment options are stratified according to patient group (Table 6-3), but the decision to proceed with chemotherapy and/or endocrine therapy often requires a detailed discussion between patient and oncologist. Variables to consider include such prognostic factors as menopausal status, tumor size, axillary lymph node status, and tumor histologic grade. Predictive factors—indicators of response to therapy—would also be helpful in selecting treatment regimens, but these are lacking. Other than the associations between estrogen receptor positivity and responsiveness to endocrine therapy and between Her-2/neu status and responsiveness to trastuzumab, there are currently no true predictors of response to therapy.

THERAPY FOR LOCALLY ADVANCED DISEASE

Locally advanced breast cancer describes tumors larger than 5 cm with involvement of axillary lymph nodes, tumors of any size with matted axillary lymph nodes, tumors of any size with involvement of the internal mammary lymph nodes or the supraclavicular lymph nodes, and tumors of any size with associated skin or chest wall involvement. *Inflammatory breast cancer* describes a subset of locally advanced tumors characterized by diffuse erythema, edema (*peau d'orange*), and ridging of the skin; tumor emboli within the dermal lymphatics are often seen on histopathologic evaluation, but their presence is not diagnostic. In general, this advanced stage of disease is associated with a high risk of relapse and poor prognosis. Traditionally, patients with

Table 6-3A. Guidelines for Adjuvant Systemic Therapy in Premenopausal Women

Stage of Disease	Hormonal Therapy	Chemotherapy
Node-negative		
Hormone receptor negative		
≤ 1 cm tumors with grade 1 histology	-	-
1–2 cm tumors with grade 1–2 histology	-	+
≥ 2 cm tumors or grade 3 histology	-	+
Hormone receptor positive		
≤ 1 cm tumors with grade 1 histology	±	-
1–2 cm tumors with grade 1–2 histology	+	±
≥ 2 cm tumors or grade 3 histology	+	+
Node-positive		
Hormone receptor negative	-	+
Hormone receptor positive	+	+

Table 6-3B. Guidelines for Adjuvant Systemic Therapy in Postmenopausal Women

Stage of Disease	Hormonal Therapy	Chemotherapy
Node-negative		
Hormone receptor negative		
≤ 1 cm tumors with grade 1 histology	-	-
1–2 cm tumors with grade 1–2 histology	-	±
≥ 2 cm tumors or grade 3 histology	-	+
Hormone receptor positive		
≤ 1 cm tumors with grade 1 histology	±	-
1–2 cm tumors with grade 1–2 histology	+	±
≥ 2 cm tumors or grade 3 histology	+	±
Node-positive		
Hormone receptor negative	-	+
Hormone receptor positive	+	+

- indicates treatment not recommended; + indicates treatment strongly recommended; ± indicates treatment should be considered.

locally advanced breast cancer were treated with local therapy alone. Despite improvements in local control with combined surgery and radiation, however, overall survival remained unchanged [59]. This was especially true for patients considered inoperable because of skin ulceration, edema, fixation, and/or inflammatory changes (ie, stage IIIB disease), which predict for an extremely poor prognosis. Significant improvements in local recurrence rates and overall survival were not achieved until the inclusion of systemic therapy in the treatment plan. The current standard of care for women with locally advanced breast cancer now entails a multidisciplinary approach that includes systemic therapy, surgery, and radiation.

Some of the same principles discussed with regard to neoadjuvant chemotherapy in early-stage breast cancer also apply to its role in locally advanced disease. In addition, breast conservation in patients with locally advanced disease should be considered only with documentation of an excellent response to neoadjuvant therapy, resolution of associated cutaneous and chest wall abnormalities, unicentric disease, and no obvious intramammary lymph node involvement. In terms of the concern that preoperative therapy will downstage the axilla and remove an important source of prognostic information, prospective studies of neoadjuvant chemotherapy followed by modified radical mastectomy in locally advanced breast cancer indicate that the prognostic importance of axillary lymph node status is maintained [60]; in fact, patients with residual lymph nodes despite the administration of preoperative chemotherapy are considered to have a poorer prognosis such that the addition of adjuvant chemotherapy is warranted. In addition, patients with locally advanced breast cancer—particularly stage IIIB disease—are often considered poor operative candidates at the time of diagnosis, so neoadjuvant chemotherapy is really the best (and sometimes only) treatment option. Although objective response rates associated with neoadjuvant therapy can be dramatic, ranging from 50% to 90% [61], there is only indirect evidence of an improvement in overall survival when compared with data from the studies of postoperative chemotherapy. Nonetheless, neoadjuvant chemotherapy with or without adjuvant therapy remains the treatment of choice for advanced disease.

The optimal type, scheduling, and duration of chemotherapy have not yet been defined. Most clinical trials in the United States have used regimens that include various combinations of doxorubicin, cyclophosphamide, and paclitaxel either concurrently or sequentially. In addition, clinical experience has revealed that the duration of neoadjuvant therapy that is necessary in order to achieve a maximum tumor response varies anywhere between 3 and 10 cycles; this observation supports the concept of individualizing treatment for each patient according to tumor response and her tolerance for drug-related toxicities. As with adjuvant chemotherapy for early-stage disease, great interest exists in the concept of dose intensification through the administration of high-dose chemotherapy with hematopoietic stem cell transplantation, but no evidence supports this treatment approach. Finally, several small studies have shown some benefit from primary hormonal therapy [61]; this may be the most appropriate option for elderly women with estrogen receptor–positive disease.

Most of the information about the treatment of locally advanced breast cancer has been derived from indirect comparisons of the results obtained from small, single institution, single arm studies. Multicenter, prospective, randomized trials are needed before any definitive conclusions can be made with respect to improvements in overall survival with neoadjuvant chemotherapy and/or the multimodality treatment approach. In the meantime, most women with locally advanced breast cancer are likely to receive preoperative therapy followed by definitive breast surgery (a modified radical mastectomy or a wide local excision with axillary lymph node dissection), adjuvant chemohormonal therapy (particularly if the response to neoadjuvant therapy was minimal), and radiation to the chest wall, surrounding skin, surrounding soft tissues, regional lymph nodes, and residual breast tissue. Specific treatment regimens, however, need to be determined for each individual patient on the basis of her response to each phase of therapy.

MANAGEMENT OF METASTATIC DISEASE

The treatment goals in metastatic breast cancer are to prolong survival and maintain quality of life. The biology of this disease is so heterogeneous that actual survival ranges from weeks to years despite a median survival of 18 to 24 months [62]. Complete cure is unlikely, but between 5% and 10% of women may achieve durable remissions of at least 10 years. Several systemic treatment options exist, and the decision on how to proceed requires much consideration in terms of tumor burden, rate of disease progression, degree of disease-related symptoms, and impact on quality of life. An asymptomatic patient with minimal disease and a good performance status, for example, may be a candidate for close observation as opposed to aggressive therapy with its associated toxicities. In contrast, a patient with rapidly progressive, multiorgan disease is more likely to opt for immediate treatment to control the malignancy promptly.

Chemotherapy

Systemic chemotherapy is indicated for patients with hormone refractory disease and for patients with a short disease-free interval, widespread visceral metastases, symptomatic disease, and poorly differentiated, estrogen receptor–negative tumors. Patients with metastatic disease are often treated with combination chemotherapy, which can yield response rates of 45% to 80% [63] in previously untreated patients. Monotherapy with certain agents, however, can often result in comparable response rates and improvements in overall survival without additive toxicities. In addition, patients often become more and more refractory to treatment with each chemotherapeutic exposure—a fact that ultimately translates into decreased benefit and increased risk. Few direct comparisons have been made between the different agents, but indirect comparisons indicate a trend toward equivalent benefits. Efforts to improve treatment efficacy include investigations into dose density through either an escalation in total dose or a decrease in dosing interval, and ongoing clinical trials with various drug regimens continue in an effort to define the optimal dose and schedule.

The anthracyclines and taxanes are the most active agents in the treatment of breast cancer. Patients who did not receive one or both of these agents as adjuvant therapy should therefore receive one or both of these agents early in their treatment for metastatic disease. Doxorubicin is the most widely used anthracycline in the United States, either alone or in combination with cyclophosphamide and 5-FU (CAF); epirubicin and mitoxantrone have also been incorporated into various regimens. A major concern about anthracyclines is their association with dose-dependent cardiomyopathy and the potential for severe congestive heart failure. The cumulative dose of doxorubicin used in the adjuvant setting is rarely associated with this entity; however, cumulative doses in excess of 450 mg/m^2, as might be achieved in the metastatic setting, are worrisome. Mechanisms by which to circumvent the potential for cardiotoxicity include the development of liposomal formulations of doxorubicin [64] and the development of cardioprotective agents such as dexrazoxane [65], both of which are indicated when the total dose of doxorubicin approaches 450 mg/m². Paclitaxel is highly active in the treatment of metastatic breast cancer with overall response rates of up to 60% in minimally pretreated patients [42,43] and 20% to 40% in heavily pretreated patients [44]. The same is true for docetaxel, although clinical trials are ongoing. This group of agents shows activity in anthracycline-naive and anthracycline-resistant tumors with a median survival of 8 to 12 months when used as monotherapy [66]. All patients with metastatic disease, therefore, should receive a taxane early in the course of treatment for metastatic disease—either alone or in combination with another active drug (eg, doxorubicin, trastuzumab).

If the disease progresses despite treatment with both an anthracycline and a taxane, there are several alternatives for additional treatment. Of the newer cytotoxic agents, vinorelbine has shown the most promise as an alternative first- or second-line agent with substantial antitumor activity in breast cancer [67]. Other evidence shows that gemcitabine has activity in metastatic disease, warranting several investigations of its value as a single agent [68] and in combination with anthracyclines [69]. Etoposide, an agent with known activity in several malignancies including breast cancer, is another treatment option—especially in light of its oral bioavailability [70]. In addition, 5-FU has long been used in the oral and intravenous forms of CMF, and recent evidence suggests that a low-dose continuous infusion of 5-FU has significant activity even in those patients whose tumors have become resistant to treatment with bolus administration of the drug [71]. The inconvenience of continuous intravenous infusions, however, ultimately prompted the development of orally bioavailable fluoropyrimidines. Capecitabine, a 5-FU prodrug, was the first such agent developed, and it has demonstrated significant antitumor activity even in heavily pretreated patients; in fact, it is the only approved treatment for patients with disease refractory to both anthracyclines and taxanes [72]. There is also interest in the co-administration of oral 5-FU and an inhibitor of dihydropyrimidine dehydrogenase (the enzyme chiefly responsible for 5-FU catabolism); this combined approach has had some success in Japan and is currently under investigation in the United States.

Endocrine Therapy

Endocrine therapy is typically used in the treatment of patients with estrogen and/or progesterone receptor–positive tumors, a history of previous response to endocrine therapy, a long disease-free interval, and/or isolated bony or soft tissue disease with minimal symptoms. Response rates in metastatic disease can range from 30% to 70% depending on whether the tumor is positive for one or both of the hormone receptors. Tamoxifen remains first-line therapy for all stages of breast cancer. The choice of hormonal therapy after or in place of tamoxifen then varies according to the patient's menopausal status and the toxicity profile of each particular agent. Newer agents have been developed and some are already approved for use in metastatic breast cancer. Overall, these agents appear to have similar response rates despite varying mechanisms or activity and associated toxicities (Table 6-4). As breast cancer progresses and develops drug resistance, endocrine therapies should therefore be given sequentially—from those of least to greatest toxicity.

The ovary serves as the primary source of estrogens in premenopausal women. Second-line hormonal therapy therefore consists of either ovarian ablation (through oophorectomy or pelvic irradiation) or medical ovarian suppression. The latter is equivalent to oophorectomy, has the potential to be reversible, and can be

achieved through the use of LHRH analogues. Goserelin is the most widely used, but buserelin and leuprolide have also been studied with equivalent results. Interest also exists in the concurrent administration of goserelin and tamoxifen. A meta-analysis of four studies [73] reveals that the combination yields modest improvements in disease-free survival and overall survival; toxicities are additive, however, and

Table 6-4. Commonly Used Hormonal Agents

Class	Agent	Dosage	Potential Toxicities
Antiestrogens	Tamoxifen	20 mg PO QD	Hot flashes; vaginal discharge; amenorrhea or dysmenorrhea; thromboembolism; endometrial cancer; drug-induced cataracts; nausea; diarrhea; transaminitis; weight gain; rash; fatigue; depression; thrombocytopenia
	Toremifene	60 mg PO QD	Nausea; hot flashes; vaginal discharge; hepatotoxicity; thromboembolism; endometrial hyperplasia; drug-induced cataracts; dizziness; cardiotoxicity
Aromatase inhibitors	Anastrozole	1 mg PO QD	Nausea; diarrhea or constipation; hot flashes; peripheral edema; cough, dyspnea; asthenia; headache, dizziness; bone pain, pelvic pain; dry mouth; thromboembolism; weight gain
	Letrozole	25 mg PO QD	Nausea; peripheral edema; bone pain; hot flashes; diarrhea or constipation; headache, dizziness; cough, dyspnea; weight gain; abnormal vaginal bleeding; thromboembolism; rash; fatigue; anxiety, depression
	Exemestane	25 mg PO QD	Hot flashes; nausea; fatigue; weight gain
Progestins	Megestrol acetate	40 mg PO QID	Weight gain, change in appetite; thromboembolism; asthenia; abnormal vaginal bleeding; decreased libido; maculopapular rash; hypertension; nausea; diarrhea or constipation; insomnia; urinary frequency; cardiotoxicity
LHRH analogues	Goserelin	3.6 mg SQ Qmo	Thromboembolism; bone pain; hot flashes; amenorrhea; asthenia; decreased libido; diarrhea or constipation; depression; headache; weight gain; anemia

each patient must consider whether the potential for increased hot flashes, loss of libido, and vaginal dryness is worth the potential for a small benefit in survival.

In postmenopausal women, the major sources of estrogen production are fat and muscle because the ovaries have ceased to function. Circulating estrogen levels are relatively low, rendering this population of patients particularly susceptible to the effects of antiestrogens (tamoxifen, toremifene, droloxifene, raloxifene, faslodex). Other endocrine therapies block the peripheral conversion of androgens; this can be achieved through the use of nonselective aromatase inhibitors (eg, anastrozole, letrozole, aminoglutethimide), selective aromatase inhibitors (eg, exemestane, formestane), and progestins (eg, megestrol acetate, medroxyprogesterone acetate). Currently, the aromatase inhibitors are considered second-line therapy, and the progestins are considered third-line therapy. This distinction is the result of randomized trials comparing anastrozole with megestrol acetate [74], letrozole to megestrol acetate [75], and exemestane with megestrol acetate [76]. Anastrozole was comparable to megestrol acetate in terms of disease-free survival, but both letrozole and exemestane were shown to significantly increase the time to progression. Added benefits of the aromatase inhibitors are a decreased incidence of both weight gain and nausea/vomiting, not inconsiderable in light of the need for daily administration. Given these findings, the aromatase inhibitors are now being compared to the current standard of care. A clinical trial comparing anastrozole versus tamoxifen versus anastrozole plus tamoxifen in postmenopausal women has completed accrual, but it will be several years before any mature results can be obtained.

Tamoxifen's success has prompted the development of other antiestrogens. Toremifene was approved by the Food and Drug Administration for the treatment of metastatic breast cancer in postmenopausal women, but evidence suggests that it has cross-resistance to and is no more efficacious than tamoxifen [77]. Raloxifene was recently studied in the Multiple Outcomes of Raloxifene Evaluation (MORE) trial [78], which demonstrated a lower incidence of breast cancer among women randomized to receive raloxifene; this, in turn, prompted the initiation of the NSABP P-2 trial, which will compare the preventative effects of tamoxifen and raloxifene in women at high risk of developing breast cancer. Toremifene and raloxifene, of note, are selective estrogen receptor modulators—a term used to describe agents with mixed estrogen antagonist and agonist properties. Pure antiestrogens, such as faslodex, are also in development and are currently being evaluated in clinical trials [79].

Targeting Signal Transduction Pathways
Approximately 30% of breast cancers overexpress human epidermal growth factor receptor-2 (also referred to as c-erb-B2 or Her-2/neu), a member of the tyrosine kinase family of growth factor receptors. This glycoprotein receptor plays a key role in the intracellular signaling process for growth stimulation, and Her-2/neu overexpression is associated clinically with accelerated tumor growth, increased frequency of metastases, and decreased survival [80]. Early evidence suggests that tumors with strong Her-2/neu positivity by immunohistochemistry are less responsive to endocrine therapy [81] and CMF chemotherapy [82] but more responsive to regimens that include an anthracycline [83] or taxane [84]. Trastuzumab is a humanized monoclonal antibody that binds tightly to the extracellular domain of the Her-2/neu receptor, blocks transmission of the growth signal, and inhibits the growth of tumor cells overexpressing Her-2/neu. Initial phase II trials revealed an overall response rate of 15% for trastuzumab monotherapy [85]. A subsequent randomized trial then compared chemotherapy (AC or paclitaxel) with and without trastuzumab, and there was a statistically significant increase in both overall response (62% vs 36.2%) and overall survival (25.4 vs 20.9 months) in favor of chemotherapy plus trastuzumab [86,87]. These results suggest that the monoclonal antibody enhances the antitumor effects of the respective chemotherapeutic agents; note, however, that an increased incidence of cardiotoxicity was noted in the group that received AC plus trastuzumab, such that this combination of agents is not currently recommended.

Trastuzumab is indicated for use in patients with metastatic breast cancer characterized by Her-2/neu overexpression. It is often started either alone or in combination with a taxane upon the diagnosis of metastatic disease, but no set guidelines exist for the initiation or termination of treatment with this agent. Further investigations are necessary before any recommendations can be made with regard to its use in the adjuvant setting and with Her-2/neu negative tumors.

NEW TREATMENT STRATEGIES
Exciting innovations in the treatment of breast cancer have occurred over the past several years. Not only are there newer chemotherapeutic agents and alternative strategies for the scheduling of drug administration, but there are entirely new therapeutic approaches as well. Advances in molecular and cellular biology have allowed for the identification of proteins that are uniquely expressed or overexpressed by tumor cells and for an understanding of the molecular basis of tumor development, growth, invasion, and metastasis. This knowledge has led to the development of therapies directed against specific cell surface antigens and/or specific intracellular signaling pathways in an effort to return cellular growth, differentiation, and proliferation back to its "normal" state. Mechanisms by which to achieve these ends include the use of monoclonal or polyclonal antibodies

Table 6-5. New Treatment Strategies

Modulate drug resistance
  Valspodar (PSC 833)
  Dexverapamil
Inhibit p53-mediated signal transduction
  Farnesyl protein transferase inhibitors
  MAP kinase inhibitors
Inhibit growth factor receptor activity
  Epidermal growth factor receptor inhibitors (eg, C225, Iressa)
  Her-2/new inhibitors (eg, trastuzumab)
Inhibit angiogenesis
  Vascular endothelial growth factor inhibitors (eg, bevacizumab)
  TNP-470
  Thalidomide
Inhibit tumor invasion and metastasis
  Matrix metalloproteinase inhibitors (eg, Marimastat)
  Bisphosphonates (eg, clodronate)
Immunomodulation
  Vaccine administration (active immunotherapy with the MUC1 and human IL-2 antigens)
  Autologous bone marrow transplantation with IL-2–activated stem cells
Modulate apoptosis
  bcl-2 antisense oligonucleotides (eg, G3139)
  Retinamide
  Telomerase inhibitors

(*eg*, trastuzumab against the Her-2/neu receptor, C225 against the epidermal growth factor receptor), vaccines (*eg*, p53 vaccine, MUC1 vaccine), gene therapy, and antisense therapy. Selected examples of these translational treatment strategies are provided in Table 6-5, and the number of new agents entering the clinical trial phase is increasing rapidly.

REFERENCES

1. Greenlee RT, Murray T, Bolden S, *et al.*: Cancer statistics, 2000. *CA Cancer J Clin* 2000, 50:7–33.

2. Colditz GA, Willett WC, Hunter DJ, *et al.*: Family history, age, and risk of breast cancer. *JAMA* 1993, 270:338–343.

3. Ellisen LW, Haber DA: Hereditary breast cancer. *Annu Rev Med* 1998, 49:425–436.

4. Shapiro S: Periodic screening for breast cancer: the HIP Randomized Controlled Trial (Health Insurance Plan). *J Natl Cancer Inst Monogr* 1997, 22:27–30.

5. Tabar L, Vitak B, Chen HH, *et al.*: The Swedish Two-County Trial twenty years later: updated mortality results with new insights for long-term follow-up. *Radiol Clinic North Am* 2000, 38:625–651.

6. Jardines L, Haffty BG, Theriault RL, *et al.*: Breast cancer overview: risk factors, screening, genetic testing, and prevention. In *Cancer Management: A Multidisciplinary Approach*. Edited by Pazdur R, Coia LR, Hoskins WJ, *et al.*: PRR: Melville; 2000:135–157.

7. The uniform approach to breast fine-needle aspiration biopsy: NIH Consensus Development Conference. *Am J Surg* 1997, 174:371–385.

8. Breast. In *American Joint Committee on Cancer's AJCC Cancer Staging Manual*. Edited by Fleming ID, Cooper JS, Henson DE, *et al.*: Philadelphia: Lippincott–Raven; 1997:171–180.

9. Morrow M, Foster RS, Jr.: Staging of breast cancer: a new rationale for internal mammary node biopsy. *Arch Surg* 1981, 116:748–751.

10. Giuliano AE, Jones RC, Brennan M, *et al.*: Sentinel lymphadenectomy in breast cancer. *J Clin Oncol* 1997, 15:2345–2350.

11. Isaacs C, Stearns V, Hayes DF: New prognostic factors for breast cancer recurrence. Submitted for publication.

12. Dupont WD, Page DL: Risk factors for breast cancer in women with proliferative breast disease. *N Engl J Med* 1985, 312:146–151.

13. Dupont WD, Page DL, Parl FF, *et al.*: Long-term risk of breast cancer in women with fibroadenoma. *N Engl J Med* 1994, 331:10–15.

14. Page DL, Dupont WD, Rogers LW, *et al.*: Atypical hyperplastic lesions of the female breast: a long-term follow-up study. *Cancer* 1985, 55:2698–2708.

15. Rosen PP, Kosloff C, Lieberman PH, *et al.*: Lobular carcinoma in situ of the breast: detailed analysis of 99 patients with average follow-up of 24 years. *Am J Surg Pathol* 1978, 2:225–251.

16. Winchester DP, Jeske JM, Goldschmidt RA: The diagnosis and management of ductal carcinoma in situ of the breast. *CA Cancer J Clin* 2000, 50:184–200.

17. Simpson JF, Page DL: The role of pathology in premalignancy and as a guide for treatment and prognosis in breast cancer. *Semin Oncol* 1996, 23:428–435.

18. Fisher B, Dignam J, Wolmark N, *et al.*: Lumpectomy and radiation therapy for the treatment of intraductal breast cancer: findings from the National Surgical Adjuvant Breast and Bowel Project B-17. *J Clin Oncol* 1998, 16:441–452.

19. Fisher B, Dignam J, Wolmark N, *et al.*: Tamoxifen in treatment of intraductal breast cancer: National Surgical Adjuvant Breast and Bowel Project B-24 randomised controlled trial. *Lancet* 1999, 353:1993–2000.

20. Silverstein MJ, Lagios MD, Craig PH, *et al.*: A prognostic index for ductal carcinoma in situ of the breast. *Cancer* 1996, 77:2267–2274.

21. Jordan VC, Lababidi MK, Langen-Fahey S: Suppression of mouse mammary tumorigenesis by long-term Tamoxifen therapy. *J Natl Cancer Inst* 1991, 83:492–496.

22. Early Breast Cancer Trialists' Collaborative Group: Tamoxifen for early breast cancer: an overview of the randomised trials. *Lancet* 1998, 351:1451–1467.

23. Fisher B, Costantino JP, Wickerham DL, *et al.*: Tamoxifen for prevention of breast cancer: report of the National Surgical Adjuvant Breast and Bowel Project P-1 Study. *J Natl Cancer Inst* 1998, 90:1371–1388.

24. Powles T, Eeles R, Ashley S, *et al.*: Interim analysis of the incidence of breast cancer in the Royal Marsden Hospital tamoxifen randomized chemoprevention trial. *Lancet* 1998, 352:98–101.

25. Veronesi U, Maisonneuve P, Costa A, *et al.*: Prevention of breast cancer with tamoxifen: preliminary findings from the Italian randomised trial among hysterectomised women (Italian Tamoxifen Prevention Study). *Lancet* 1998, 352:93–97.

26. Early Breast Cancer Trialists' Collaborative Group: Effects of radiotherapy and surgery in early breast cancer: an overview of the randomised trials. *N Engl J Med* 1995, 333:1444–1455.

27. Blichert-Toft M: Axillary surgery in breast cancer management: background, incidence and extent of nodal spread, extent of surgery and accurate axillary staging, surgical procedures. *Acta Oncol* 2000, 39:269–275.

28. Ragaz J, Jackson SM, Le N, *et al.*: Adjuvant radiotherapy and chemotherapy in node-positive premenopausal women with breast cancer. *N Engl J Med* 1997, 337:956–962.

29. Overgaard M, Hansen PS, Overgaard J, *et al.*: Postoperative radiotherapy in high-risk premenopausal women with breast cancer who receive adjuvant chemotherapy. *N Engl J Med* 1997, 337:949–955.

30. Overgaard M, Jensen MB, Overgaard J, *et al.*: Postoperative radiotherapy in high-risk postmenopausal breast-cancer patients given adjuvant Tamoxifen: Danish Breast Cancer Cooperative Group DBCG 82c randomized trial. *Lancet* 1999, 353:1641–1648.

31. Early Breast Cancer Trialists' Collaborative Group: Effects of adjuvant tamoxifen and of cytotoxic therapy on mortality in early breast cancer: an overview of 61 randomised trials among 28,296 women. *N Engl J Med* 1988, 319:1681–1692.

32. Early Breast Cancer Trialists' Collaborative Group: Systematic treatment of early breast cancer by hormonal, cytotoxic, or immune therapy: 133 randomised trials involving 31,000 recurrences and 24,000 deaths among 75,000 women. *Lancet* 1992, 339:1–15, 71–85.

33. Early Breast Cancer Trialists' Collaborative Group: Ovarian ablation in early breast cancer: overview of the randomised trials. *Lancet* 1996, 348:1189–1196.

34. Early Breast Cancer Trialists' Collaborative Group: Polychemotherapy for early breast cancer: an overview of the randomised trials. *Lancet* 1998, 352:930–942.

35. Fisher B, Dignam J, Mamounas EP, *et al.*: Sequential methotrexate and fluorouracil for the treatment of node-negative breast cancer patients with estrogen receptor–negative tumors: eight-year results from National Surgical Adjuvant Breast and Bowel Project (NSABP) B-13 and first report of findings from NSABP B-19 comparing methotrexate and fluorouracil with conventional cyclophosphamide, methotrexate, and fluorouracil. *J Clin Oncol* 1996, 14:1982–1992.

36. Mansour EG, Gray R, Shatila AH, *et al.*: Survival advantage of adjuvant chemotherapy in high-risk node-negative breast cancer: ten-year analysis—an intergroup study. *J Clin Oncol* 1998, 16:3486–3492.

37. Hutchins L, Green S, Ravdin P, *et al.*: CMF vs CAF with and without tamoxifen in high-risk node-negative breast cancer patients and a natural history follow-up study in low-risk node-negative patients: first results of Intergroup Trial INT 0102. *Proc Am Soc Clin Oncol* 1998, 17:1a.

38. Fisher B, Brown AM, Dimitrov NV, *et al.*: Two months of doxorubicin-cyclophosphamide with and without interval reinduction therapy compared with 6 months of cyclophosphamide, methotrexate, and fluorouracil in positive-node breast cancer patients with tamoxifen-nonresponsive tumors: Results from the National Surgical Adjuvant Breast and Bowel project B-15. *J Clin Oncol* 1990, 8:1483–1496.

39. Fisher B, Anderson S, Wolmark N, *et al.*: Chemotherapy with or without Tamoxifen for patients with ER-negative breast cancer and negative nodes: results from NSABP B23. *Proc Am Soc Clin Oncol* 2000, 19:72a.

40. Paik S, Bryant J, Park C, *et al.*: erbB-2 and response to doxorubicin in patients with axillary lymph node-positive, hormone receptor-negative breast cancer. *J Natl Cancer Inst* 1998, 90:1361–1370.

41. Seidman AD, Reichman BS, Crown JP, *et al.*: Paclitaxel as second and subsequent therapy for metastatic breast cancer: activity independent of prior anthracycline response. *J Clin Oncol* 1995, 13:1152–1159.

42. Holmes FA, Walters RS, Theriault RL, *et al.*: Phase II trial of Taxol, an active drug in the treatment of metastatic breast cancer. *J Natl Cancer Inst* 1991, 83:1797–1805.

43. Reichman BS, Seidman AD, Crown JD, *et al.*: Paclitaxel and recombinant human granulocyte colony-stimulating factor as initial chemotherapy for metastatic breast cancer. *J Clin Oncol* 1993, 11:1943–1951.

44. Seidman AD, Tiersten A, Hudis C, *et al.*: Phase II trial of paclitaxel by 3-hour infusion as initial and salvage chemotherapy for metastatic breast cancer. *J Clin Oncol* 1995, 13:2575–2581.

45. Henderson IC, Berry D, Demetri G, *et al.*: Improved disease free (DFS) and overall survival (OS) from the addition of sequential paclitaxel (T) but not from the escalation of doxorubicin (A) dose level in the adjuvant chemotherapy of patients (pts) with node-positive primary breast cancer (bc). *Proc Am Soc Clin Oncol* 1998, 17:390a.

46. Fisher B, Anderson S, Wickerham DL, *et al.*: Increased intensification and total dose of cyclophosphamide in a doxorubicin-cyclophosphamide regimen for the treatment of primary breast cancer: findings from National Surgical Adjuvant Breast and Bowel Project B-22. *J Clin Oncol* 1997, 15:1858–1869.

47. Fisher B, Anderson S, DeCillis A, *et al.*: Further evaluation of intensified and increased total dose of cyclophosphamide for the treatment of primary breast cancer: findings from National Surgical Adjuvant Breast and Bowel Project B-25. *J Clin Oncol* 1999, 17:3374–3388.

48. Fisher B, Bryant J, Wolmark N, *et al.*: Effect of preoperative chemotherapy on the outcome of women with operable breast cancer. *J Clin Oncol* 1998, 16:2672–2685.

49. Rutqvist LE, Hatschek T, Ryden S, *et al.* (Swedish Breast Cancer Cooperative Group): Randomized trial of two versus five years of adjuvant tamoxifen for postmenopausal early stage breast cancer. *J Natl Cancer Inst* 1996, 88:1543–1549.

50. Current Trials Working Party of the Cancer Research Campaign Breast Cancer Trials Group: Preliminary results from the Cancer Research Campaign Trial evaluating tamoxifen duration in women aged fifty years or older with breast cancer. *J Natl Cancer Inst* 1996, 88:1834–1839.

51. Fisher B, Dignam J, Bryant J, *et al.*: Five versus more than five years of tamoxifen therapy for breast cancer patients with negative lymph nodes and estrogen receptor-positive tumors. *J Natl Cancer Inst* 1996, 88:1529–1542.

52. Stewart HJ, Forrest AP, Everington D, *et al.*: Randomised comparison of 5 years of adjuvant tamoxifen with continuous therapy for operable breast cancer: the Scottish Cancer Trials Breast Group. *Br J Cancer* 1996, 74:297–299.

53. Taylor CW, Green S, Dalton WS, *et al.*: Multicenter randomized clinical trial of goserelin versus surgical ovariectomy in premenopausal patients with receptor-positive metastatic breast cancer: an Intergroup study. *J Clin Oncol* 1998, 16:994–999.

54. Scottish Cancer Trials Breast Group and ICRF Breast Unit–Guy's Hospital London: Adjuvant ovarian ablation versus CMF chemotherapy in premenopausal women with pathological stage II breast carcinoma: the Scottish trial. *Lancet* 1993, 341:1293–1298.

55. Kaufmann M: Luteinizing hormone-releasing hormone analogues in early breast cancer: updated status of ongoing clinical trials. *Br J Cancer* 1998, 78 (suppl 4):9–11.

56. Davidson N, O'Neill A, Vukov A, *et al.*: Effect of chemohormonal therapy in premenopausal, node (+), receptor (+) breast cancer: an Eastern Cooperative Oncology Group phase III Intergroup trial (E5188, INT–0101). *Proc Am Soc Clin Oncol* 1999, 18:67a.

57. Rutqvist LE: Zoladex and tamoxifen as adjuvant therapy in premenopausal breast cancer: a randomised trial by the Cancer Research Campaign (CRC) Breast Cancer Trials Group, the Stockholm Breast Cancer Study Group, the South-East Sweden Breast Cancer Group and the Gruppo Interdisciplinare Valutazione Interventi in Oncologia (GIVIO). *Proc Am Soc Clin Oncol* 1999, 18:67a.

58. Recht A, Come SE, Henderson IC, *et al.*: The sequencing of chemotherapy and radiation therapy after conservative surgery for early–stage breast cancer. *N Engl J Med* 1996, 334:1356–1361.

59. Hortobagyi GN, Buzdar AU. Locally advanced breast cancer: a review including the MD Anderson experience. In *High-Risk Breast Cancer*. Edited by Rajaz J, Ariel IM: Berlin: Springer-Verlag; 1991:382.

60. McCready DR, Hortobagyi GN, Kau SW, *et al.*: The prognostic significance of lymph node metastases after preoperative chemotherapy for locally advanced breast cancer. *Arch Surg* 1989, 124:21–25.

61. Esteva FJ, Hortobagyi GN: Locally advanced breast cancer. *Hematol Oncol Clin North Am* 1999, 13:457–472.

62. Greenberg P, Hortobagyi G, Smith T, *et al.*: Long-term follow-up of patients with complete remission following combination chemotherapy for metastatic breast cancer. *J Clin Oncol* 1996, 14:2197–2205.

63. Dickson RB, Lippman ME: Cancer of the breast. In *Cancer: Principles and Practice of Oncology*. Edited by DeVita VT, Hellman S, Rosenberg SA. Philadelphia: Lippincott–Raven Publishers; 1997:1541–1616.

64. Ranson M, Carmichael J, O'Byrne K, *et al.*: Treatment of advanced breast cancer with sterically stabilized liposomal doxorubicin: results of a multicenter phase II trial. *J Clin Oncol* 1997, 15:3185–3191.

65. Swain S, Whaley F, Gerber M, *et al.*: Cardioprotection with dexrazoxane for doxorubicin-containing therapy in advanced breast cancer. *J Clin Oncol* 1997, 15:1318–1332.

66. Nabholtz JM, Senn HJ, Bezwoda WR, *et al.*: Prospective randomized trial of docetaxel versus mitomycin plus vinblastine in patients with metastatic breast cancer progressing despite previous anthracycline-containing chemotherapy (304 study group). *J Clin Oncol* 1999, 17:1413–1424.

67. Weber BL, Vogel C, Jones S, *et al.*: Intravenous vinorelbine as first-line and second-line therapy in advanced breast cancer. *J Clin Oncol* 1995, 13:2722–2730.

68. Carmichael J, Possinger K, Phillip P, *et al.*: Advanced breast cancer: a phase II trial with gemcitabine. *J Clin Oncol* 1995, 13:2731–2736.

69. Garcia-Conde J, LLuch A, Perez-Manga G, *et al.*: Gemcitabine + doxorubicin in advanced breast cancer: final results from an early phase II study. *Proc Am Soc Clin Oncol* 1997, 16:515a.

70. Neskovic-Konstantinovic ZB, Bosnjak SM, Radulovic SS, *et al.*: Daily oral etoposide in metastatic breast cancer. *Anticancer Drugs* 1996, 7:543–547.

71. Cameron DA, Gabra H, Leonard RC: Continuous 5-fluorouracil in the treatment of breast cancer. *Br J Cancer* 1994, 70:120–124.

72. Blum JL: Xeloda in the treatment of metastatic breast cancer. *Oncology* 1999, 57:16–20.

73. Klijn JGM, Blarney RW, Boccardo F, *et al.*: Combination LHRH–agonist plus tamoxifen treatment is superior to medical castration alone in premenopausal metastatic breast cancer. *Breast Cancer Res Treat* 1998, 50:227.

74. Buzdar A, Jonat W, Howell A, *et al.*: Anastrozole, a potent and selective aromatase inhibitor, versus megestrol acetate in postmenopausal women with advanced breast cancer: results of overview analysis of two phase III trials. *J Clin Oncol* 1996, 14:2000–2011.

75. Dombernowsky P, Smith I, Falkson G, *et al.*: Letrozole, a new oral aromatase inhibitor for advanced breast cancer: Double-blind randomized trial showing a dose effect and improved efficacy and tolerability compared with megestrol acetate. *J Clin Oncol* 1998, 16:453–461.

76. Kaufmann M, Bajetta E, Dirix LY, *et al.*: Exemestane is superior to megestrol acetate after tamoxifen failure in postmenopausal women with advanced breast cancer: results of a phase III randomized double-blind trial. (The Exemestane Study Group). *J Clin Oncol* 2000, 18:1399–1411.

77. Hayes DF, Van Zyl JA, Hacking A, *et al.*: Randomized comparison of tamoxifen and two separate doses of toremifene in postmenopausal patients with metastatic breast cancer. *J Clin Oncol* 1995, 13:2556–2566.

78. Ettinger B, Black DM, Mitlak BH, *et al.*: Reduction of vertebral fracture risk in postmenopausal women with osteoporosis treated with raloxifene: results from a 3-year randomized clinical trial. (Multiple Outcomes of Raloxifene Evaluation (MORE) Investigators). *JAMA* 1999, 282:637–645.

79. Howell A, Osborne CK, Morris C, *et al.*: ICI 182,780 (faslodex): development of a novel, "pure" antiestrogen. *Cancer* 2000, 89:817–825.

80. Slamon DJ, Clark GM, Wong SG, *et al.*: Human breast cancer: correlation of relapse and survival with amplification of HER–2/neu oncogene. *Science* 1987, 235:177–182.

81. Carlomagno C, Perrone F, Gallo C, *et al.*: c-erb-B2 overexpression decreases the benefit of adjuvant tamoxifen in early-stage breast cancer without axillary lymph node metastases. *J Clin Oncol* 1996, 14:2702–2708.

82. Gusterson BA, Belber RD, Goldhirsch A, *et al.*: Prognostic importance of c-erb-B2 expression in breast cancer. *J Clin Oncol* 1992, 10:1049–1056.

83. Muss HB, Thor AD, Berry DA, *et al.*: c-erb-B2 expression and response to adjuvant therapy in women with node-positive breast cancer. *N Engl J Med* 1994, 330:1260–1266.

84. Gianni L: Future directions of paclitaxel-based therapy of breast cancer. *Semin Oncol* 1997, 24(Suppl 17):91–96.

85. Cobleigh MA, Vogel CL, Tripathy D, *et al.*: Multinational study of the efficacy and safety of humanized anti-HER2 monoclonal antibody in women who have HER2 overexpressing metastatic breast cancer that has progressed after chemotherapy for metastatic disease. *J Clin Oncol* 1999, 37:2639–2648.

86. Slamon D, Leyland-Jones B, Shak S, *et al.*: Addition of Herceptin (humanized anti–Her2 antibody) to first line chemotherapy for Her2 overexpressing metastatic breast cancer (Her2+/MBC) markedly increases anticancer activity: a randomized, multinational controlled phase III trial. *Proc Am Soc Clin Oncol* 1998, 17:98a.

87. Norton L, Slamon D, Leyland-Jones B, *et al.*: Overall survival (OS) advantage to simultaneous chemotherapy (CRx) plus the humanized anti–Her2 monoclonal antibody Herceptin (H) in Her2-overexpressing (Her2+) metastatic breast cancer (MBC). *Proc Am Soc Clin Oncol* 1999, 18:127a.

CMF
(Cyclophosphamide, methotrexate, and 5-fluorouracil)

Cyclophosphamide is an alkylating agent that inhibits DNA replication. Methotrexate is a folate antimetabolite that inhibits dihydrofolate reductase and the subsequent generation of thymidine that is necessary for DNA synthesis. 5-Fluorouracil (5-FU) is a pyrimidine antimetabolite that blocks the methylation of deoxyuridylate to thymidylate, thus inhibiting the synthesis of both DNA and RNA. This chemotherapeutic regimen was used most frequently in the initial randomized trials of adjuvant chemotherapy.

DOSAGE AND SCHEDULING
ORAL CYCLOPHOSPHAMIDE REGIMEN (28-DAY CYCLES; 6 CYCLES FOR ADJUVANT THERAPY)

	Day 1–14
Cyclo 100 mg/m² PO QD d 1–14	(continuous d 1–14)
MTX 40 mg/m² IV, d 1, 8	d 1, 8
5-FU 600 mg/m² IV, d 1, 8	d 1, 8

Day: 1 2 3 4 5 6 7 8 9 10 11 12 13 14

IV CYCLOPHOSPHAMIDE REGIMEN (21-DAY CYCLES; 6 CYCLES FOR ADJUVANT THERAPY)

Cyclo 600 mg/m² IV d 1	d 1, 22
MTX 40 mg/m² IV d 1	d 1, 22
5-FU 600 mg/m² IV d 1	d 1, 22
CBC, electrolytes, Cr, LFT	d 1, 22

Day: 1 2 3 4 5 6 7 8 9 10 11 12 13 14 15 16 17 18 19 20 21 22

DOSAGE MODIFICATIONS: Delay treatment for an ANC < 1000/mm³ or a platelet count < 50,000/mm³ on day 1; 50% dose reduction of all agents if the ANC remains at 1000–1500/mm³ and the platelet count remains at 50,000–75,000/mm³ despite a delay in treatment. 25% dose reduction of MTX for a creatinine clearance < 25 cc/min.

RECENT EXPERIENCES AND RESPONSE RATES

Study	Evaluable Patients, n	Dosage/Schedule	Response for Metastatic Disease, %
Valagussa et al., Proc Am Soc Clin Oncol 1983, 2:111	53	C 100 mg/m² PO d 1–14 M 40 mg/m² IV d 1, 8 F 600 mg/m² IV d 1, 8 q 4 wk	53
Canellos et al., Cancer 1976, 38: 1882-1886	93	C 100 mg/m² PO d 1–14 M 60 mg/m² IV d 1, 8 F 600 mg/m² IV d 1,8 q 4 wk	53
Muss et al., Arch Int Med 1977, 137: 1711-1714	38	C 10 mg/kg IV d 1, 5 mg/kg IV d 15 then q 7 d M 0.2 mg/kg IV d 1, 0.1 mg/kg IV d 15 then q 7 d F 12 mg/kg IV d 1, 10 mg/kg d 15 then q 7 d	34
Aisner et al., J Clin Oncol 1987, 5: 1523-1533	99	C 100 mg/m² PO d 1–14 M 40 mg/m² IV d 1, 8 F 500 mg/m² IV d 1, 8 q 4 wk	37
Creech et al., Cancer 1975 35:1101-1107	46	C 50 mg/m² PO d 1–14 M 25 mg/m² IV d 1, 8 F 500 mg/m² IV d 1, 8 q 4 wk	46
DeLena et al., Tumori 1998, 74:57	62	C 600 mg/m² IV d 1 M 40 mg/m² IV d 1 5-FU 600 mg/m² IV d 1 q 3 wk	42

CANDIDATES FOR TREATMENT
Adjuvant therapy for early stage breast cancer, particularly when use of an anthracycline is contraindicated; treatment of metastatic disease in patients with aggressive visceral disease or hormone-refractory breast cancer

SPECIAL PRECAUTIONS
Enhanced leukopenia and skin toxicity with extensive radiation therapy

ALTERNATIVE THERAPIES
AC or CAF combination chemotherapy in the adjuvant setting; CAF or single-agent doxorubicin for metastatic disease

TOXICITIES
Cyclophosphamide: nausea, vomiting, anorexia, fatigue, leukopenia, thrombocytopenia, alopecia, hyperpigmentation of the skin and nails, gonadal dysfunction; hemorrhagic cystitis, interstitial pneumonitis and pulmonary fibrosis, hepatitis, renal tubular acidosis, syndrome of inappropriate antidiuretic hormone secretion (rare); **methotrexate:** nausea, vomiting, anorexia, diarrhea, stomatitis, fatigue, leukopenia, thrombocytopenia, dermatitis, photosensitivity, hepatitis; interstitial pneumonitis, acute tubular necrosis (rare); **5-fluorouracil:** nausea, vomiting, anorexia, diarrhea, abdominal cramps, stomatitis, leukopenia, anemia, alopecia, dermatitis, hyperpigmentation of the skin and nails, photosensitivity, increased lacrimation; myocardial infarction, stroke (rare)

DRUG INTERACTIONS
Cyclophosphamide: phenobarbital, allopurinol; **methotrexate:** nonsteroidal anti-inflammatory agents, sulfa drugs, phenytoin, nonabsorbable antibiotics used for sterilization of the gastrointestinal tract, warfarin; **5-fluorouracil:** interferon, leucovorin

NURSING INTERVENTIONS
Monitor blood counts, renal function, and hepatic function prior to drug administration; use appropriate antiemetics for a regimen with moderate emetogenic potential

PATIENT INFORMATION
High fluid intake of 1 to 2 L is required for the duration of treatment with oral cyclophosphamide and for 24 hours after intravenous administration of the drug. Patients must immediately report episodes of chest pain, shortness of breath, severe mucositis, persistent nausea/vomiting/diarrhea, abdominal cramps, and signs of infection (eg, fever, chills, sweats, cough, dysuria)

CAF
(Cyclophosphamide, doxorubicin, and 5-fluorouracil)

Cyclophosphamide is an alkylating agent that inhibits DNA replication. Doxorubicin is an anthracycline antibiotic that intercalates between DNA base pairs and inhibits topoisomerase II, thus inhibiting DNA synthesis. 5-Fluorouracil (5-FU) is a pyrimidine antimetabolite that blocks the methylation of deoxyuridylate to thymidylate, thus inhibiting the synthesis of both DNA and RNA. No definitive evidence confirms that CAF is superior to CMF, and toxicity tends to be greater with anthracycline-containing regimens. Nonetheless, the superior efficacy of single agent doxorubicin in the metastatic setting has prompted the widespread use of CAF in recent years.

DOSAGE AND SCHEDULING

ORAL CYCLOPHOSPHAMIDE REGIMEN (28-DAY CYCLES; 6 CYCLES FOR ADJUVANT THERAPY)

Cyclo 100 mg/m^2 PO QD d 1–14	███████████████████████████████													
Doxo 30 mg/m^2 IV, d 1,8	■							■						
5-FU 500 mg/m^2 IV, d 1,8	■							■						
CBC, electrolytes, Cr, LFT	□							□						
Day	1	2	3	4	5	6	7	8	9	10	11	12	13	14

28-Day cycles; 6 cycles for adjuvant therapy

IV CYCLOPHOSPHAMIDE REGIMEN (21-DAY CYCLES; 6 CYCLES FOR ADJUVANT THERAPY)

Cyclo 500 mg/m^2 IV d 1	■																				■	
Doxo 50 mg/m^2 IV d 1	■																				■	
5-FU 500 mg/m^2 IV d 1	■																				■	
CBC, electrolytes, Cr, LFT	□																				□	
Day	1	2	3	4	5	6	7	8	9	10	11	12	13	14	15	16	17	18	19	20	21	22

DOSAGE MODIFICATIONS: *Delay treatment for an ANC < 1000/mm^3 or a platelet count < 50,000/mm^3 on day 1; 50% dose reduction of all agents if the ANC remains at 1000–1500/mm^3 and the platelet count remains at 50,000–75,000/mm^3 despite a delay in treatment. 50% dose reduction of doxorubicin for a bilirubin of 1.5–3 mg/dL; 75% dose reduction of doxorubicin for a bilirubin > 3 mg/dL. Termination of treatment should be considered upon the development of any signs or symptoms of congestive heart failure.*

RECENT EXPERIENCES AND RESPONSE RATES

Study	Evaluable Patients, n	Dosage/Schedule	Response for Metastatic Disease, %
Kardinal et al., Breast Cancer Res Treat 1983 3:365–372	116	C 100mg/m^2 PO d 1-14 A 25 mg/m^2 IV d 1,8 F 500 mg/m^2 IV d 1,8 q 4 wk	51
Tranum et al., Cancer 1978, 41:2078–2083	105	C 400 mg/m^2 IV d 1 A 40 mg/m^2 IV d 1 F 400 mg/m^2 IV d 1,8 q 3 wk	49
Smalley et al., Cancer 1977, 40:625-632	59	C 500 mg/m^2 IV d 1 A 50 mg/m^2 IV d 1 F 500 mg/m^2 IV d 1 q 3 wk	64
Tormey et al., Cancer Clin Trials 1979, 2:247–256	46	C 100 mg/m^2 PO d 1-14 A 30 mg/m^2 IV d 1,8 F 500 mg/m^2 IV d 1,8 q 4 wk	52
Vogel et al., J Clin Oncol 1984, 2:643–651	66	C 500 mg/m^2 IV d 1 A 50 mg/m^2 IV d 1 F 500 mg/m^2 IV d 1 q 3 wk	29
Bull et al., Cancer 1978, 41:1649–1657	38	C 100 mg/m^2 PO d 1-14 A 30 mg/m^2 IV d 1,8 F 500 mg/m^2 IV d 1,8 q 4 wk	82

CANDIDATES FOR TREATMENT:
Adjuvant therapy for early stage breast cancer; neoadjuvant therapy for locally advanced disease; treatment of metastatic disease in patients with aggressive visceral disease or hormone-refractory breast cancer

SPECIAL PRECAUTIONS
Doxorubicin-associated cardiomyopathy with cumulative doses in excess of 450 mg/m^2, particularly with recent breast irradiation; vesicant extravasation with the potential for tissue necrosis from doxorubicin, requiring administration through a large peripheral or central vein

ALTERNATIVE THERAPIES
AC or CMF combination chemotherapy in the adjuvant setting; CMF or single-agent doxorubicin for metastatic disease

TOXICITIES
Cyclophosphamide: nausea, vomiting, anorexia, fatigue, leukopenia, thrombocytopenia, alopecia, hyperpigmentation of the skin and nails, gonadal dysfunction; hemorrhagic cystitis, interstitial pneumonitis and pulmonary fibrosis, hepatitis, renal tubular acidosis, syndrome of inappropriate antidiuretic hormone secretion (rare); **doxorubicin:** nausea, vomiting, anorexia, fatigue, mucositis, leukopenia, anemia, thrombocytopenia, alopecia, hyperpigmentation of the skin and nails, tissue necrosis with drug extravasation; cardiotoxicity (with high cumulative doses); **5-fluorouracil:** nausea, vomiting, anorexia, diarrhea, abdominal cramps, stomatitis, leukopenia, anemia, alopecia, dermatitis, hyperpigmentation of the skin and nails, photosensitivity, increased lacrimation; myocardial infarction, stroke (rare)

DRUG INTERACTIONS
Cyclophosphamide: phenobarbital, allopurinol; **doxorubicin:** cyclophosphamide, mercaptopurine, digoxin, barbiturates; **5-fluorouracil:** interferon, leucovorin

NURSING INTERVENTIONS
Monitor blood counts, renal function, and hepatic function prior to drug administration; use appropriate antiemetics for a regimen with high emetogenic potential

PATIENT INFORMATION
High fluid intake of 1 to 2 L is required for the duration of treatment with oral cyclophosphamide and for 24 hours after intravenous administration of the drug. Patients must immediately report episodes of chest pain, shortness of breath, severe mucositis, persistent nausea/vomiting/diarrhea, abdominal cramps, signs of infection (*eg*, fever, chills, sweats, cough, dysuria), and pain or erythema at the injection site

AC
(Doxorubicin and cyclophosphamide)

Cyclophosphamide is an alkylating agent that inhibits DNA replication. Doxorubicin is an anthracycline antibiotic that intercalates between DNA base pairs and inhibits topoisomerase II, thus inhibiting DNA synthesis. No definitive evidence confirms that AC is superior to CMF, and toxicity tends to be greater with anthracycline-containing regimens. Nonetheless, the superior efficacy of single-agent doxorubicin in the metastatic setting and the shorter treatment course (compared with CMF and CAF) have prompted the widespread use of AC in recent years—particularly in the adjuvant therapy of premenopausal women with estrogen receptor–negative disease.

DOSAGE AND SCHEDULING (28-DAY CYCLES; 6 CYCLES FOR ADJUVANT THERAPY)

	Day 1																				Day 22
Cyclo 600 mg/m^2 IV d 1	■																				■
Doxo 60 mg/m^2 IV d 1	■																				■
CBC, electrolytes, Cr, LFT	□																				□
Day	1 2 3 4 5 6 7 8 9 10 11 12 13 14 15 16 17 18 19 20 21 22																				

DOSAGE MODIFICATIONS: *Delay treatment for an ANC < 1000/mm^3 or a platelet count < 50,000/mm^3 on day 1; 50% dose reduction of all agents if the ANC remains at 1000–1500/mm^3 and the platelet count remains at 50,000–75,000/mm^3 despite a delay in treatment. 50% dose reduction of doxorubicin for a bilirubin of 1.5–3 mg/dL; 75% dose reduction of doxorubicin for a bilirubin > 3 mg/dL. Termination of treatment should be considered upon the development of any signs or symptoms of congestive heart failure.*

RECENT EXPERIENCE AND RESPONSE RATES

Study	Evaluable Patients, n	Dosage/Schedule	3-Y Disease-Free Survival, %
Fisher *et al.*, *J Clin Oncol* 1990, 8.1483-1496	535	Doxo 60 mg/m^2 IV d 1 Cyclo 600 mg/m^2 IV d 1 q 3 wk	68

CANDIDATES FOR TREATMENT

Adjuvant therapy for early stage breast cancer; treatment of metastatic disease in patients with aggressive visceral disease or hormone-refractory breast cancer

SPECIAL PRECAUTIONS

Doxorubicin-associated cardiomyopathy with cumulative doses in excess of 450 mg/m^2, particularly with recent breast irradiation; vesicant extravasation with the potential for tissue necrosis from doxorubicin, requiring administration through a large peripheral or central vein

ALTERNATIVE THERAPIES

CMF or CAF combination chemotherapy in the adjuvant setting; CMF, CAF, or single-agent doxorubicin for metastatic disease

TOXICITIES

Doxorubicin: nausea, vomiting, anorexia, fatigue, mucositis, leukopenia, anemia, thrombocytopenia, alopecia, hyperpigmentation of the skin and nails, tissue necrosis with drug extravasation; cardiotoxicity (with high cumulative doses); **cyclophosphamide:** nausea, vomiting, anorexia, fatigue, leukopenia, thrombocytopenia, alopecia, hyperpigmentation of the skin and nails, gonadal dysfunction; hemorrhagic cystitis, interstitial pneumonitis and pulmonary fibrosis, hepatitis, renal tubular acidosis, syndrome of inappropriate antidiuretic hormone secretion (rare)

DRUG INTERACTIONS

Doxorubicin: cyclophosphamide, mercaptopurine, digoxin, barbiturates; **cyclophosphamide:** phenobarbital, allopurinol

NURSING INTERVENTIONS

Monitor blood counts, renal function, and hepatic function prior to drug administration; use appropriate antiemetics for a regimen with high emetogenic potential

PATIENT INFORMATION

High fluid intake of 1 to 2 L is required for 24 hours after intravenous administration of the drug. Patients must immediately report episodes of chest pain, shortness of breath, severe mucositis, persistent nausea/vomiting/diarrhea, abdominal cramps, signs of infection (*eg*, fever, chills, sweats, cough, dysuria), and pain or erythema at the injection site

PACLITAXEL

Paclitaxel stabilizes microtubules by promoting the polymerization of tubulin and by binding to preformed tubulin oligomers and polymers. Initial studies in patients with metastatic breast cancer demonstrated excellent overall response rates. Subsequent investigations then established this agent's role in the adjuvant setting as well, particularly in those patients with high-risk disease who would otherwise receive only AC or CMF.

DOSAGE AND SCHEDULING (21-DAY CYCLES; 4 CYCLES FOR ADJUVANT THERAPY)

PREMEDICATE WITH DEXAMETHASONE 20 MG PO 12 H AND 6 H PRIOR TO INFUSION (DOSE OF DEXAMETHASONE MAY BE DECREASED WITH SUBSEQUENT CYCLES AS TOLERATED); PREMEDICATE WITH DEXAMETHASONE 20 MG IV, CIMETIDINE 300 MG IV, AND DIPHENHYDRAMINE 50 MG IV 30 MIN PRIOR TO DRUG INFUSION (DOSE OF DEXAMETHASONE MAY BE DECREASED WITH SUBSEQUENT CYCLES AS TOLERATED)

Paclitaxel 175 mg/m² IV over 3 h	■																					■	
CBC, electrolytes, Cr, LFT	□																					□	
Day	1	2	3	4	5	6	7	8	9	10	11	12	13	14	15	16	17	18	19	20	21	22	

DOSAGE MODIFICATIONS: *Delay treatment for an ANC < 1000/mm³ or a platelet count < 50,000/mm³ on the day of treatment; 20% dose reduction if the ANC remains < 500/mm³ for 7 consecutive days. A dose reduction should accompany any evidence of hepatic dysfunction (AST or ALT > 1.5 × normal; elevated total bilirubin; alkaline phosphatase > 2.5 × normal). A dose reduction or termination of treatment should also be considered in patients who develop a persistent peripheral neuropathy.*

DOSAGE AND SCHEDULING (WEEKLY ADMINISTRATION; FOR METASTATIC DISEASE ONLY)

PREMEDICATE WITH DEXAMETHASONE 20 MG PO 12 H AND 6 H PRIOR TO INFUSION (DOSE OF DEXAMETHASONE MAY BE DECREASED WITH SUBSEQUENT CYCLES AS TOLERATED); PREMEDICATE WITH DEXAMETHASONE 20 MG IV, CIMETIDINE 300 MG IV, AND DIPHENHYDRAMINE 50 MG IV 30 MIN PRIOR TO DRUG INFUSION (DOSE OF DEXAMETHASONE MAY BE DECREASED WITH SUBSEQUENT CYCLES AS TOLERATED)

Paclitaxel 80–100 mg/m² IV over 1 h weekly	■							■							■							■	
CBC weekly before treatment	□							□							□							□	
Electrolytes, Cr, LFT	□																					□	
Day	1	2	3	4	5	6	7	8	9	10	11	12	13	14	15	16	17	18	19	20	21	22	

DOSAGE MODIFICATIONS: *Delay treatment for an ANC < 1000/mm³ or a platelet count < 50,000/mm³ on the day of treatment; 20% dose reduction if the ANC remains < 500/mm³ for 7 consecutive days. A dose reduction should accompany any evidence of hepatic dysfunction (AST or ALT > 1.5 × normal; elevated total bilirubin; alkaline phosphatase > 2.5 × normal). A dose reduction or termination of treatment should also be considered in patients who develop a persistent peripheral neuropathy. Note that the optimal schedule for weekly paclitaxel has not yet been determined, and some consideration should be given to cyclic as opposed to strict weekly therapy (eg, treatment on day 1 and 8 in 21-day cycles).*

RECENT EXPERIENCES AND RESPONSE RATES

Study	Evaluable Patients, n	Dosage/Schedule (Every 3 wk)	Response for Metastatic Disease, %
Abrams *et al.*, *J Clin Oncol* 1995, 13:2056	172	175 mg/m² IV over 24 h	23
Nabholtz *et al.*, *J Clin Oncol* 1996, 14:1858	227	135 mg/m² IV over 3 h	22
Nabholtz *et al.*, *J Clin Oncol* 1996, 14:1858	223	175 mg/m² IV over 3 h	29
Seidman *et al.*, *J Clin Oncol* 1995, 13:1152	76	200–250 mg/m² IV over 24 h	33
Sledge *et al.*, *Proc Am Soc Clin Oncol* 1997, 16:1a	266	175 mg/m² IV over 24 h	33
Seidman *et al.*, *J Clin Oncol* 1998, 16:3353	36	Paclitaxel 100 mg/m² IV weekly	53

CANDIDATES FOR TREATMENT

Adjuvant therapy following the administration of AC for high-risk, early-stage breast cancer; treatment of metastatic disease in patients who have already received an anthracycline and who have aggressive visceral disease or hormone-refractory breast cancer

SPECIAL PRECAUTIONS

Hypersensitivity reaction, which can be prevented with the appropriate premedications; vesicant extravasation with the potential for tissue necrosis, requiring administration through a large peripheral or central vein; enhanced toxicity with prior or concomitant radiation therapy

ALTERNATIVE THERAPIES

Single-agent therapy with docetaxel or vinorelbine

TOXICITIES

Nausea, vomiting, diarrhea, anorexia, fatigue, mucositis, leukopenia, anemia, thrombocytopenia, alopecia, myalgias, arthralgias, asthenia, sensory peripheral neuropathy, hypersensitivity reaction; hepatitis, cardiac arrhythmias, peripheral motor neuropathy, ataxia (rare)

DRUG INTERACTIONS

Ketoconazole, erythromycin

NURSING INTERVENTIONS

Monitor blood counts, renal function, and hepatic function prior to drug administration; use appropriate antiemetics for a regimen with moderately low emetogenic potential; ensure that the proper premedications are administered; monitor closely for signs and symptoms of hypersensitivity during drug infusion; manage hypersensitivity reactions appropriately by discontinuing the drug infusion and administering epinephrine, intravenous fluids, antihistamines, and/or corticosteroids as needed

PATIENT INFORMATION

Patients must immediately report episodes of chest pain, shortness of breath, severe mucositis, persistent nausea/vomiting/diarrhea, abdominal cramps, signs of infection (*eg*, fever, chills, sweats, cough, dysuria), and pain or erythema at the injection site

DOCETAXEL

Docetaxel is a semisynthetic analogue of paclitaxel. It, too, stabilizes microtubules by promoting the polymerization of tubulin and by binding to preformed tubulin oligomers and polymers. Initial studies in patients with metastatic breast cancer demonstrated response rates comparable with those of paclitaxel.

DOSAGE AND SCHEDULING (21-DAY CYCLES; 4 CYCLES FOR ADJUVANT THERAPY)

PREMEDICATE WITH DEXAMETHASONE 8 MG PO BID FOR 3 D, BEGINNING 1 D PRIOR TO INFUSION (DOSE OF DEXAMETHASONE MAY BE DECREASED WITH SUBSEQUENT CYCLES AS TOLERATED)

	1	2	3	4	5	6	7	8	9	10	11	12	13	14	15	16	17	18	19	20	21	22
Docetaxel 60–100 mg/m² IV over 1 h d 1	■																					■
CBC, electrolytes, Cr, LFT	□																					□
Day	1	2	3	4	5	6	7	8	9	10	11	12	13	14	15	16	17	18	19	20	21	22

DOSAGE MODIFICATIONS: Delay treatment for an ANC < 1000/mm³ or a platelet count < 50,000/mm³ on the day of treatment; 20% dose reduction if the ANC remains < 500/mm³ for 7 consecutive days. A dose reduction should accompany any evidence of hepatic dysfunction (AST or ALT > 1.5 × normal; elevated total bilirubin; alkaline phosphatase > 2.5 × normal). A dose reduction or termination of treatment should also be considered in patients who develop severe fluid retention, a persistent peripheral neuropathy, or an extensive cutaneous reaction.

DOSAGE AND SCHEDULING (WEEKLY ADMINISTRATION; FOR METASTATIC DISEASE ONLY)

PREMEDICATE WITH DEXAMETHASONE 8 MG PO BID FOR 3 D, BEGINNING 1 D PRIOR TO INFUSION (DOSE OF DEXAMETHASONE MAY BE DECREASED WITH SUBSEQUENT CYCLES AS TOLERATED)

	1	2	3	4	5	6	7	8	9	10	11	12	13	14	15	16	17	18	19	20	21	22
Docetaxel 40 mg/m² IV over 1 h weekly	■							■							■							■
CBC weekly before treatment	□							□							□							□
Electrolytes, Cr, LFT	□																					□
Day	1	2	3	4	5	6	7	8	9	10	11	12	13	14	15	16	17	18	19	20	21	22

DOSAGE MODIFICATIONS: Delay treatment for an ANC < 1000/mm³ or a platelet count < 50,000/mm³ on the day of treatment; 25% dose reduction if the ANC remains < 500/mm³ for 7 consecutive d. A dose reduction should accompany any evidence of hepatic dysfunction (AST or ALT > 1.5 × normal; elevated total bilirubin; alkaline phosphatase > 2.5 × normal). A dose reduction or termination of treatment should also be considered in patients who develop severe fluid retention, a persistent peripheral neuropathy, or an extensive cutaneous reaction. Note that the optimal schedule for weekly docetaxel has not yet been determined, and some consideration should be given to cyclic as opposed to strict weekly therapy (eg, treatment on day 1 and 8 in 21-day cycles).

RECENT EXPERIENCES AND RESPONSE RATES

Study	Evaluable Patients, n	Dosage/Schedule	Response for Metastatic Disease, %
Chevallier et al., J Clin Oncol 1995, 13:314	31	100 mg/m² IV over 1 h q 3 wk	68
Dieras et al., Br J Cancer 1996, 74:650	31	75 mg/m² IV over 1 h q 3 wk	52
Hudis et al., J Clin Oncol 1996, 14:58	37	100 mg/m² IV over 1 h q 3 wk	64
Ravdin et al., J Clin Oncol 1995, 13:2879	35	100 mg/m² IV over 1 h q 3 wk	58
Piccart et al., Eur J Cancer 1994, 30A(suppl 2):24	52	50 mg/m² IV over 1 h, d 1, 8	33
Chan et al., J Clin Oncol 1999, 17:2341.	161	100 mg/m² IV q 3 wk	48
Salminen et al., J Clin Oncol 1999, 17:1127.	31	100 mg/m2 IV q 3 wk	48
Burstein et al., J Clin Oncol 2000, 18:1212.	29	40 mg/m² IV weekly × 6 Q 8 wk	41

CANDIDATES FOR TREATMENT

Treatment of metastatic disease in patients who have already received an anthracycline and who have aggressive visceral disease or hormone-refractory breast cancer

SPECIAL PRECAUTIONS

Hypersensitivity reaction and fluid retention, which can be prevented with the appropriate premedications; vesicant extravasation with the potential for tissue necrosis, requiring administration through a large peripheral or central vein; enhanced toxicity with prior or concomitant radiation therapy

ALTERNATIVE THERAPIES

Single-agent therapy with paclitaxel or vinorelbine

TOXICITIES

Nausea, vomiting, diarrhea, fatigue, mucositis, leukopenia, anemia, thrombocytopenia, alopecia, maculopapular rash, nail changes, myalgias, arthralgias, asthenia, fluid retention/peripheral edema, sensory peripheral neuropathy, hypersensitivity reaction; bradycardia, hypotension, peripheral motor neuropathy (rare)

DRUG INTERACTIONS

Cyclosporine, terfenadine, ketoconazole, erythromycin

NURSING INTERVENTIONS

Monitor blood counts, renal function, and hepatic function prior to drug administration; use appropriate antiemetics for a regimen with moderate emetogenic potential; ensure that the proper premedications are administered, monitor closely for signs and symptoms of hypersensitivity during drug infusion; manage hypersensitivity reactions appropriately by discontinuing the drug infusion and administering epinephrine, intravenous fluids, antihistamines, and/or corticosteroids as needed

PATIENT INFORMATION

Patients must immediately report episodes of chest pain, shortness of breath, severe mucositis, persistent nausea/vomiting/diarrhea, abdominal cramps, signs of infection (eg, fever, chills, sweats, cough, dysuria), and pain or erythema at the injection site

TRASTUZUMAB

Trastuzumab is a humanized monoclonal antibody that binds tightly to the extracellular domain of the Her-2/neu receptor, blocks transmission of the growth signal, and thus inhibits the growth of tumor cells overexpressing Her-2/neu. Clinical trials have demonstrated treatment efficacy for trastuzumab alone and in combination with chemotherapeutic agents in the setting of metastatic disease.

DOSAGE AND SCHEDULING
PREMEDICATE WITH ACETAMINOPHEN 650 MG PO AND DIPHENHYDRAMINE 50 MG PO 30 MIN PRIOR TO DRUG INFUSION

Trastuzumab 4 mg/kg IV over 90 min for the initial loading dose, then 2 mg/kg IV over 30 min weekly	■						■							■								■
CBC, electrolytes, Cr, LFT	☐																					☐
Day	1 2 3 4 5 6 7 8 9 10 11 12 13 14 15 16 17 18 19 20 21 22																					

DOSAGE MODIFICATIONS: *No formal recommendations.*

RECENT EXPERIENCES AND RESPONSE RATES

Study	Evaluable Patients, *n*	Dosage/Schedule	Response for Metastatic Disease, %
Cobleigh *et al., J Clin Oncol* 1999, 17:2639.	222	Trastuzumab 4 mg/kg IV loading dose then 2 mg/kg IV over 30 min weekly	15
Slamon *et al., Proc Am Soc Clin Oncol* 1998, 17:98a.	235	Trastuzumab 4 mg/kg IV loading dose then 2 mg/kg IV over 30 min weekly; Paclitaxel 175 mg/m^2 IV over 3 h q 3 wk	38

CANDIDATES FOR TREATMENT
Treatment of metastatic disease in patients whose tumors overexpress Her-2/neu

SPECIAL PRECAUTIONS
Allergic-type reaction may be decreased; increased risk of cardiotoxicity, especially if given with an anthracycline

ALTERNATIVE THERAPIES
Combination therapy with either paclitaxel or vinorelbine

TOXICITIES
Nausea, vomiting, diarrhea, rash, asthenia, headache, rhinitis, infusion reaction; leukopenia, paresthesias, cardiotoxicity, pulmonary toxicity (rare)

DRUG INTERACTIONS
None reported

NURSING INTERVENTIONS
Monitor blood counts prior to drug administration; use appropriate antiemetics for a regimen with low emetogenic potential; ensure that the proper premedications are administered; monitor closely for signs and symptoms of an infusion reaction and treat appropriately with acetaminophen, diphenhydramine, and/or meperidine as needed

PATIENT INFORMATION
Patients must immediately report episodes of chest pain, shortness of breath, persistent nausea/vomiting/diarrhea, abdominal cramps, and signs of infection (*eg,* fever, chills, sweats, cough, dysuria)

VINORELBINE

Vinorelbine is a semisynthetic vinca alkaloid that binds to tubulin and depolymerizes microtubules, resulting in mitotic inhibition. Recent studies indicate that this agent has substantial antitumor activity in the treatment of breast cancer.

DOSAGE AND SCHEDULING

Vinorelbine 25–30 mg/m² IV over 15 min weekly	■	■	■	■
CBC weekly before treatment	□	□	□	□
Electrolytes, Cr, LFT	□			□
Day	1 2 3 4 5	6 7 8 9 10 11 12 13	14 15 16 17 18 19	20 21 22

DOSAGE MODIFICATIONS: *Delay treatment for an ANC < 1000/mm³ or a platelet count < 50,000/mm³ on the day of treatment; 50% dose reduction if the ANC remains at 1000–1500/mm³. 50% dose reduction for a bilirubin of 1.5–3 mg/dL; 75% dose reduction for a bilirubin > 3 mg/dL. Note that the optimal schedule for weekly vinorelbine has not yet been determined, and some consideration should be given to cyclic as opposed to strict weekly therapy (eg, treatment on days 1 and 8 in 21-day cycles).*

RECENT EXPERIENCES AND RESPONSE RATES

Study	Evaluable Patients, n	Dose	Response for Metastatic Disease, %
Terenziani et al., Breast Cancer Res Treat 1996, 39:285.	57	30 mg/m² IV d 1, 8 q 3 wk	47
Weber et al., J Clin Oncol 1995, 13:2722.	107	30 mg/m² IV weekly	34
Garcia-Conde et al., Ann Oncol 1994:854.	54	25 mg/m² IV weekly with growth factor support	41
Nistico et al., Breast Cancer Res Treat 2000, 59:223.	40	25 mg/m² IV weekly with growth factor support	52

CANDIDATES FOR TREATMENT

Treatment of metastatic disease in patients who have already received an anthracycline and a taxane and who have aggressive visceral disease or hormone-refractory breast cancer

SPECIAL PRECAUTIONS

Vesicant extravasation with the potential for tissue necrosis, requiring administration through a large peripheral or central vein

ALTERNATIVE THERAPIES

Capecitabine, paclitaxel, docetaxel

TOXICITIES:

Nausea, vomiting, diarrhea, constipation, leukopenia, anemia, alopecia, rash, chemical phlebitis, asthenia, peripheral sensory neuropathy, generalized pain; hepatitis, cough, jaw pain (rare)

DRUG INTERACTIONS

None reported

NURSING INTERVENTIONS

Monitor blood counts, renal function, and hepatic function prior to drug administration; use appropriate antiemetics for a regimen with low emetogenic potential; use warm compresses to manage extravasation

PATIENT INFORMATION

Patients must immediately report episodes of persistent diarrhea, abdominal cramps, signs of infection (*eg*, fever, chills, sweats, cough, dysuria), and pain or erythema at the injection site

CAPECITABINE

Capecitabine is an orally administered prodrug of 5-fluorouracil that blocks the methylation of deoxyuridylate to thymidylate, thus inhibiting the synthesis of both DNA and RNA. It has demonstrated significant antitumor activity, even in heavily pretreated patients. Currently, capecitabine is the only approved treatment in the United States for patients with disease refractory to both anthracyclines and taxanes.

DOSAGE AND SCHEDULING (21-DAY CYCLES)

Capecitabine 2500 mg/m^2 PO QD in two divided doses d1–14	▄▄▄▄▄▄▄▄▄▄▄▄			
CBC weekly starting on d 1	☐	☐	☐	☐
Electrolytes, Cr, LFT	☐			☐
Day	1 2 3 4 5 6 7 8 9 10 11 12 13 14 15 16 17 18 19 20 21 22			

DOSAGE MODIFICATIONS: *Immediately terminate the treatment cycle with the development of major toxicity. Dose reductions for subsequent cycles are specified according to the grade of toxicity.*

RECENT EXPERIENCES AND RESPONSE RATES

Study	Evaluable Patients, *n*	Dose	Response for Metastatic Disease, %
Blum *et al.*, *J Clin Oncol* 1999, 17:485.	162	2500 mg/m^2 PO QD in two divided doses d1–14 q 3 wk	20
O'Shaughnessy *et al.*, *Proc Am Soc Clin Oncol* 1998, 17:103a.	62	2500 mg/m^2 PO QD in two divided doses d1–14 q 3 wk	25

CANDIDATES FOR TREATMENT

Treatment of metastatic disease in patients who have already received an anthracycline and a taxane and who have aggressive visceral disease or hormone-refractory breast cancer

SPECIAL PRECAUTIONS

Severe diarrhea requires aggressive fluid and electrolyte replacement; hand-foot syndrome requires pristine local care

ALTERNATIVE THERAPIES

Vinorelbine

TOXICITIES

Nausea, vomiting, anorexia, diarrhea, constipation, abdominal discomfort, stomatitis, fatigue, lymphopenia, anemia, thrombocytopenia, paresthesias, hand-foot syndrome, dermatitis, hyperbilirubinemia; cardiotoxicity, peripheral edema, ocular irritation (rare)

DRUG INTERACTIONS

Antacids

NURSING INTERVENTIONS

Monitor blood counts, renal function, and hepatic function prior to each treatment cycle

PATIENT INFORMATION

Patients must immediately report episodes of persistent nausea/vomiting/diarrhea, abdominal cramps, palmar and/or plantar pain and erythema, and signs of infection (*eg*, fever, chills, sweats, cough, dysuria). Capecitabine should be taken with food

ETOPOSIDE

Etoposide (VP-16) is a topoisomerase II inhibitor that produces single-stranded breaks in DNA. It has known activity in several malignancies—including breast cancer—and is a particularly good treatment option in terms of its oral bioavailability.

DOSAGE AND SCHEDULING (28-DAY CYCLES)

Etoposide 50 mg/m² PO QD d 1–21	████████████████████					
CBC weekly starting on d 1	☐	☐	☐	☐	☐	
Electrolytes, Cr, LFT	☐				☐	
Day	1 2 3 4 5 6 7 8 9 10 11 12 13 14 15 16 17 18 19 20 21 22 23 24 25 26 27 28 29					

DOSAGE MODIFICATIONS: Delay treatment for an ANC < 1000/mm³ or a platelet count < 50,000/mm³ on day 1; 50% dose reduction if the ANC remains at 1000–1500/mm³ despite a delay in treatment. 50% dose reduction for a bilirubin of 1.5–3 mg/dL; 75% dose reduction for a bilirubin > 3 mg/dL. 25% dose reduction for a creatinine clearance < 50 mL/min.

RECENT EXPERIENCES AND RESPONSE RATES

Study	Evaluable Patients, n	Dose	Response for Metastatic Disease, %
Bontenbal et al., Breast Cancer Res Treat 1995, 34:185–189.	27	50 mg/m² PO QD d 1–21 q 4 wk	10
Saphner et al., Am J Clin Oncol 2000, 23:258.	30	50 mg/m² PO QD d 1–21 q 4 wk	30
Neskovic-Konstantinovic et al., Anticancer Drugs 1996, 7:543.	21	50 mg/m² PO QD d 1–21 q 4 wk	33

CANDIDATES FOR TREATMENT

Treatment of metastatic disease in patients who have already received an anthracycline and a taxane and who have aggressive visceral disease or hormone-refractory breast cancer

SPECIAL PRECAUTIONS

None

ALTERNATIVE THERAPIES

Capecitabine

TOXICITIES

Nausea, vomiting, anorexia, diarrhea, stomatitis, fatigue, leukopenia, anemia, thrombocytopenia, alopecia; dermatitis, peripheral neuropathy, hepatitis, allergic reaction (rare)

DRUG INTERACTIONS

Cyclosporine

NURSING INTERVENTIONS

Monitor blood counts, renal function, and hepatic function prior to each treatment cycle

PATIENT INFORMATION

Patients must immediately report episodes of persistent nausea/vomiting/diarrhea, abdominal cramps, and signs of infection (eg, fever, chills, sweats, cough, dysuria); capsules should be stored in refrigerator (do not freeze)

Malignancies of the upper gastrointestinal (GI) tract pose substantial challenges for therapy (Tables 7-1 and 7-2). Surgery remains the only known therapeutic method for this group of diseases; however, 5-year survival rates continue to be low even after definitive resection. Such results have stimulated interest in alternate and combined forms of management for these malignancies. Experience with chemotherapy and radiation therapy is growing. This chapter compares various therapeutic approaches within each disease group and highlights selected chemotherapy regimens that either are in common use or have unique applications in upper GI tract cancer.

ESOPHAGEAL CANCER

In 2001, 12,500 new cases of esophageal carcinoma are expected in the United States; men will have more than a twofold increase in risk compared with that of women. For unknown reasons, incidence of adenocarcinoma of the esophagus is increasing at a rate faster than that of nearly any other cancer. Overall 5-year survival rates have never exceeded 12% [1]. Locoregional or systemic spread of disease is often attributed to the lack of anatomic barriers to dissemination. The esophagus does not have a serosa to provide a natural defense for local invasion and is rich in submucosal lymphatics, which probably allow longitudinal spread from the primary site. Autopsy findings from patients who have recently undergone surgery for squamous cell carcinoma of the esophagus have demonstrated a high incidence of unsuspected early metastatic disease.

Patients with esophageal cancer usually present with dysphagia. Diagnosis is made with a contrast study alone, or combined with endoscopy. Staging evaluation consists of a CT scan of the chest and abdomen, in addition to endoscopic ultrasound. Fine needle aspirates should be performed on suspicious cervical or periumbilical adenopathy, and a bone scan should be done if symptoms of bone pain are present. Bronchoscopy should also be performed on patients with proximal lesions at risk of tracheobronchial fistula. Based on the staging evaluation and the patient's general state of health, a treatment protocol is designed (Table 7-3, Fig. 7-1). Patients with dysphagia whose disease is deemed unresectable often benefit from a percutaneous gastrostomy tube for alimentation during further therapy. This is not recommended for the surgical candidate, because the stomach is the primary conduit used to replace the esophagus. Patients who are surgical candidates can be staged further with laparoscopy, and a feeding jejunostomy may be placed at that time for alimentation during neoadjuvant therapy prior to surgery [2].

Therapy for Advanced Disease

Single-agent chemotherapy is now rarely used for advanced disease. Agents with adequate activity include bleomycin, mitomycin C, doxorubicin, cisplatin, carboplatin, plant alkaloids, 5-fluorouracil, lomustine, ifosfamide, mitoguazone, methotrexate, and the relatively newer agents paclitaxel and vindesine. Paclitaxel as a single agent has been reported to produce a response rate of 34% and 28% in patients with adenocarcinoma and squamous cell carcinoma, respectively [3]. The best response rates are achieved with a combination of chemotherapeutic agents, however, there have been no randomized trials comparing and thus confirming the superiority of combination regimens over single agent therapy. The most commonly used combination chemotherapy regimen is 5-fluorouracil (5-FU) and cisplatin, which can produce an objective response rate as high as 42%. Other agents in cisplatin-containing combinations have included etoposide, epirubicin and protracted infusion 5-FU, and interferon with 5-FU. These combinations have shown encouraging response rates of up to 65% [4–6]. Cisplatin and irinotecan have recently been used in conjunction to produce objective responses of 57% associated with median survival of 14.6 months and diminished dysphagia in 90% of treated patients [7].

Therapy for Locally Unresectable Disease

Perhaps the most vigorously tested role of combination chemotherapy in esophageal cancer has been in the multimodal management of local or regional disease. In the past, radiation therapy had been the mainstay of therapy as palliation for patients who were believed to have disease that could not be resected with reasonable chance for cure (T4, M1 disease) (Table 7-3). Relief of dysphagia in these patients is excellent, with reported palliative responses of up to 80%.

Table 7-1. Risk Factors for Cancers of the Upper Gastrointestinal Tract

Esophagus	*Pancreas*
Exposure to nitrosomines	Cigarette smoking
Cigarette smoking	Exposure to beta-naphthylamine, benzidine
Excessive alcohol use	Chronic pancreatitis
Lye ingestion	Family history
Achalasia	
Barrett's mucosa	*Liver*
Tylosis	Hepatitis B carrier state
Infection with transforming viruses (HPV, HSV, CMV, EBV)	Chronic liver disease (chronic active hepatitis, cirrhosis)
Plummer-Vinson syndrome	Exposure to mycotoxin, ionizing radiation, steroid hormones, arsenic
Mycotoxin	*Bile Ducts*
	Sclerosing cholangitis
Stomach	Parasitic infections
Achlorhydria	Use of steroid hormones
Helicobacter pylori infection	
Previous gastrectomy, Billroth II procedures	
Family history	

CMV—cytomegalovirus; EBV—Epstein-Barr virus; HPV—human papillomavirus; HSV—herpes simplex virus.

Table 7-2. General Guidelines for Prevention and Early Detection of Cancers of the Upper Gastrointestinal Tract

Prevention	Early Detection
Avoid cigarette smoking	Esophagus
Use alcohol in moderation	Annual upper gastrointestinal endoscopy in patients with known Barrett's mucosa, tylosis, or history of caustic esophageal injury
Eat a low-fat diet, rich in fresh fruit and vegetables	
Avoid exposure to occupational toxins	Hepatoma
Immunize against infectious hepatitis	Periodic α-fetoprotein measurement and liver ultrasound for patients with chronic liver disease
Avoid unnecessary use of steroid hormones	

However, even a small change in tumor size can lead to marked improvement in swallowing function, which results from decreased resistance to flow; this may explain why the high palliative rate observed with radiation therapy alone has not resulted in significant changes in median survival. Various studies have assessed the safety, feasibility, and regression rates of combination chemotherapy and radiation for patients with locally unresectable disease. The mainstay of drug therapy in this setting has been 5-FU combined with other radiation-sensitizing drugs, such as cisplatin or mitomycin. Pilot experiences with this approach showed encouragingly high 2-year survival rates and, in some cases, durable complete responses were observed. One such approach in the treatment of patients with

adenocarcinoma of the esophagus and gastroesophageal junction involved a combination of 5-FU and mitomycin in addition to radiation therapy as definitive treatment. Complete response in 7 of 8 patients with T1 and T2 disease and a median relapse-free survival of 10 months were observed. Studies such as these led the Radiation Therapy Oncology Group (RTOG), the Southwest Oncology Group (SWOG), and the North Central Cancer Treatment Group (NCCTG) to conduct a randomized trial [8] comparing a combination of fluorouracil (1000 mg/m^2 by continuous infusion daily for 4 days) and cisplatin (75 mg/m^2 on day 1) plus 50 Gy of radiation therapy to 64 Gy of radiation therapy alone in patients with epidermoid carcinoma or adenocarcinoma of the thoracic esophagus. As might be expected, severe and life-threatening side effects (predominantly mucositis and myelosuppression) were seen more frequently in patients treated with combined-modality therapy. One patient in the combined-modality group died from complications of renal and bone marrow failure, and many were not able to complete the full chemotherapeutic course. A 5-year follow-up for all patients showed a median survival of 14 months and an overall survival of 26% in the combined treatment group; whereas the median survival was 9.3 months with no patient alive at 5 years in the group tested with radiation alone [9]. Actuarial incidence of local failure as the first site of failure was also significantly decreased in the combined-modality group (45% vs 68%; $P = 0.0123$). The randomizing protocol was closed early due to these positive results; after this, an additional 50 patients were treated with combined therapy. The 5-year mortality for this group was 14% [10]. These survival results have also been suggested by a recently published, broad-based practice survey [11].

Neoadjuvant Therapy

Numerous randomized clinical trials have shown that neither radiation nor chemotherapy are of benefit when used alone prior to surgery [12,13]; however, the combination of the two has shown promising results. Early studies used 5-FU as a common denominator in induction chemotherapy as a single agent [14], in combination with cisplatin or mitomycin C, or as a multiagent regimen [15]. Although these trials varied in their study populations with respect to the proportion of epidermoid carcinomas to adenocarcinomas and with respect to presenting stage of disease, these reports were notable for the documentation of complete responses with eradication of pathologic evidence of disease. Naunheim *et al.* [16] reported an overall median survival of 23 months; in the report by Forastiere *et al.* [15], the median survival time was 29 months, and 34% of the patients were alive at 5 years. In both studies, the complete histologic response rate was over 20%. These encouraging results led to several phase three investigations. Urba *et al.* [17] randomized 100 patients—75% with adenocarcinoma, 25% with squamous carcinoma—to surgery alone versus cisplatin, 5-FU, vinblastine, and 45-Gy radiation followed by surgery. The group receiving neoadjuvant therapy had a 3-year survival of 32% compared with the control group's 15% survival. This result was of borderline statistical significance with a *P* value of 0.07. A recent report updating this trial has found no statistically significant survival difference [18]. In patients with esophageal adenocarcinoma, a prospective randomized trial performed by Walsh *et al.* [19] clearly showed the superiority of combined modality therapy—2 courses of 5-FU and cisplatin with 40 Gy of radiotherapy followed by surgery—compared with surgery alone. The overall survival rates at 3 years were 32% and 6%, respectively. This study has been criti-

Table 7-3 TNM Staging Criteria for Esophageal Cancer

Staging	Criteria
TX	Primary tumor cannot be assessed
T0	No evidence of primary tumor
Tis	Carcinoma in situ
T1	Tumor invades lamina propria or submucosa
T2	Tumor invades muscularis propria
T3	Tumor invades adventitia
T4	Tumor invades adjacent structures
NX	Regional lymph nodes cannot be assessed
N0	No regional lymph node metastasis
N1	Regional lymph node metastasis
MX	Distant metastasis cannot be assessed
M0	No distant metastasis
M1	Distant metastasis
Tumors of the lower thoracic esophagus:	
M1a	Metastasis in celiac lymph nodes
M1b	Other distant metastasis
Tumors of the midthoracic esophagus:	
M1a	Not applicable
M1b	Nonregional lymph nodes and/or other distant metastasis
Tumors of the upper thoracic esophagus:	
M1a	Metastasis in cervical nodes
M1b	Other distant metastasis

Stage	TNM
0	Tis, N0, M0
I	T1, N0, M0
IIA	T2, N0, M0
	T3, N0, M0
IIB	T1, N1, M0
	T2, N1, M0
III	T3, N1, M0
	T4, any N, M0
IV	Any T, any N, M1
IVA	Any T, any N, M1a
IVB	Any T, any N, M1b

cized, because the survival rate of those receiving surgery alone seems unusually low. Randomized trials with squamous cell cancer have not shown a clear-cut benefit. In one multicenter randomized trial, Bossett *et al.* found improved disease-free survival and survival free of local disease, but no overall survival benefit between the groups receiving multimodal therapy and those receiving surgery alone [20]. Notably, however, cisplatin was the only chemotherapeutic agent used in the combined treatment arm in this latter study. Law *et al.* [21] more recently reported no survival benefit using cisplatin, 5-FU, and 40Gy in addition to surgery for squamous cell cancer. Many had hoped that the present controversy would be clarified by CALGB C9781, a phase III trial comparing neoadjuvant therapy to surgery alone, but unfortunately this trial has recently closed because of lack of accrual.

Preoperative strategies can be associated with a high toxicity profile, primarily from myelosuppression and esophagitis. For instance, Adelstein *et al.* [22] studied 5-FU and cisplatin chemotherapy in combination with accelerated fractionation radiation and found a perioperative mortality of 18%. Because of the toxicity of preoperative chemoradiotherapy and its unproven efficacy in phase III trials, both physicians and patients should weigh the benefits and side effects when electing treatment. Despite this, recent well-designed phase II trials demonstrate 2-year survival as high as 60% and minimal morbidity with multimodal therapy [23]. Many physicians believe combined preoperative chemoradiotherapy should be considered in patients with clinical evidence of stage III disease (Fig 7-1).

Palliative Therapy

As already mentioned, combined chemoradiation is very good at relieving the symptoms of obstruction. Unfortunately this usually takes 4 to 6 weeks to occur. Patients with severe obstruction who are at risk for aspiration can benefit from physical methods of maintaining esophageal patency while awaiting the benefits of chemoradiation. A recent study indicates that dilatation alone provides adequate palliation in this group compared to dilatation and neodymium-yttrium-aluminum-garnet (Nd-YAG) laser therapy [24]. Endoscopic laser therapy and endoluminal radiation can be employed in patients whose dysphagia has not been lessened with chemoradiation. Expansile metal stents are particularly good for refractory obstruction or tracheoesophageal fistulas with an overall success rate of 90% [25]. These stents result in fewer complications compared with older plastic prostheses [26].

STOMACH CANCER

In 2001, approximately 21,700 new cases of stomach cancer will be diagnosed in United States, and an estimated 12,800 people will die of this disease [1]. Cancer of the stomach appears to be decreasing in incidence. The explanation for this perplexing change in incidence is not known; however, some have attributed the decrease to the common practice of adding ascorbic acid as a food preservative, which decreases gastric pH and limits endogenous nitrosamine production by bacteria in the upper GI tract. A link between gastric cancer and *Helicobacter pylori* infections as a risk factor has been described [27,28]. The overall 5-year survival rate for affected patients remains low at approximately 21% [1]. Because the presenting symptoms of stomach cancer tend to be extremely vague, most patients are diagnosed with extensive local involvement or regional lymph node metastases, which explains in part the poor 5-year survival rate following surgery (Table 7-4). The staging work-up is similar to that used in esophageal cancer including endoscopy, endoscopic ultrasound, and abdominal CT.

Therapy for Locoregional Disease

Perhaps no topic in gastric cancer has received as much focus as the role of the extended lymphadenectomy. This aggressive surgical technique is embraced in Japan where stage-specific survival is significantly higher than that reported in Western series. There are now three randomized trials comparing D1 (removal of local draining lymph nodes) and D2 (removal of the next level of draining nodes) dissections in Western countries. Increased morbidity has been shown with the larger dissection but not increased survival [29–32]. For these reasons, D1 rather than D2 lymph node dissections have been accepted as standard cancer operations in the West.

The Southwest Oncology Group has reviewed findings in 453 patients who underwent resection for gastric adenocarcinoma and demonstrated that a D0 dissection (an inadequate cancer operation) is what was performed in more than half of the cases [33]. This group has now gone on to demonstrate in a recent phase III randomized trial that postoperative combined radiation and chemotherapy improves disease-free survival, and overall survival in patients who have undergone resection of gastric adenocarcinoma [34]. The 557 patients who had undergone resection with curative intent and demonstrated no sign of metastasis, were randomized to either treatment (with 5-FU, leucovorin, and 45 Gy of radiation) or observation. Nodal metastases were present in 85% of pathologic specimens. Therapy resulted in mortality in 1%, grade 3 toxicity in 32%, and grade 4 toxicity in 41% of patients treated. At a median of 3.3 years

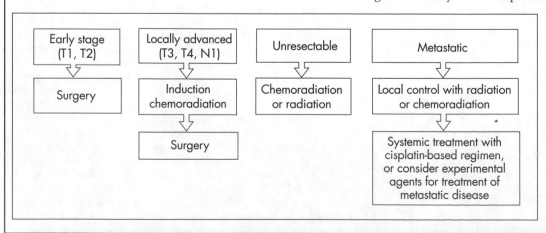

FIGURE 7-1.

Treatment strategies for esophageal and esphagogastric cancer.

Table 7-4. TNM Staging Criteria for Gastric Cancer

Staging	Criteria
TX	Primary tumor cannot be assessed
T0	No evidence of primary tumor
Tis	Carcinoma in situ: intraepithelial tumor without invasion of the lamina propria
T1	Tumor invades lamina propria or submucosa
T2	Tumor invades muscularis propria or subserosa
T3	Tumor penetrates serosa (visceral peritoneum) without invasion of adjacent structures
T4	Tumor invades adjacent structures
NX	Regional lymph node(s) cannot be assessed
N0	No regional lymph node metastasis
N1	Metastasis in 1–6 regional lymph nodes
N2	Metastasis in 7–15 regional lymph nodes
N3	Metastasis in > 15 regional lymph nodes
MX	Distant metastasis cannot be assessed
M0	No distant metastasis
M1	Distant metastasis

Stage	TNM
0	Tis, N0, M0
IA	T1, N0, M0
IB	T1, N1, M0
	T2, N0, M0
II	T1, N2, M0
	T2, N1, M0
	T3, N0, M0
IIIA	T2, N2, M0
	T3, N1, M0
	T4, N0, M0
IIIB	T3, N2, M0
IV	T4, N1, M0
	T1, N3, M0
	T2, N3, M0
	T3, N3, M0
	T4, N2, M0
	T4, N3, M0
	Any T, any N, M1

of follow-up, 3-year disease free survival is 49% in treated patients compared with 32% in the control group (*P*=0.001). Overall survival is 49% and 32%, respectively (*P*=0.003). Although this is a powerful result and will probably quickly dictate the standard of care, there are those who criticize the study [35] stating perhaps the effect of the adjuvant therapy was to increase the survival from that obtained with an inadequate D0 dissection to that documented for D1 resections in the past [30].

Before the appearance of this more recent analysis, results for adjuvant therapy in the United States had been poor. A meta-analysis involving 11 randomized trials had concluded that postoperative adjuvant therapy did not appear to be useful [36].

Previous disappointing results with postoperative adjuvant chemotherapy spawned attempts at improving surgical outcome with preoperative chemotherapy. Several studies are noteworthy in this regard. EAP has been tested preoperatively in patients with advanced locoregional disease (*eg*, those positive lymph nodes, T3 or T4 primary lesions) [37,38]. EAP therapy was continued until patients achieved a maximum response to therapy, at which point resection was attempted. The objective response rate to preoperative EAP was 70%, including a 21% complete response rate. Twenty patients subsequently underwent resection. At a median follow-up of 20 months, the relapse rate was 60% at a median survival time of 18 months. The high complete remission rate with the EAP regimen could not be confirmed in a more recent multi-institutional trial reported by Ajani *et al.* [39] involving early stage gastric cancers. Ajani [48] *et al.* also evaluated the preoperative response rate and resectability following administration of etoposide, 5-FU, and cisplatin. In that study, 24% of the patients had major preoperative responses to chemotherapy, including two complete responses. The resection rate was 72%, and with a median follow-up of 25 months the median survival was 15 months. Safran *et al.* [41,42] evaluated the combination of paclitaxel with concurrent radiation therapy for locally advanced gastric cancer and determined a response rate of 70% in patients with evaluable disease. Of these patients, 30% subsequently underwent resection. Another approach incorporated postoperative intraperitoneal therapy with fluorouracil and cisplatin in addition to preoperative FAMTX. For patients who underwent curative resection in this study, the median survival was 31 months; peritoneal failure was seen in 16% of the patients, with acceptable levels of toxicity [41,42]. More recently, Ajani *et al.* [43] administered 5-FU, interferon, and cisplatin to 30 patients before scheduled surgery. Only half these patients could tolerate the planned five cycles. Clinical response was seen in 34% and complete response in 7%. Complete R0 resection was performed in 83%, producing a median

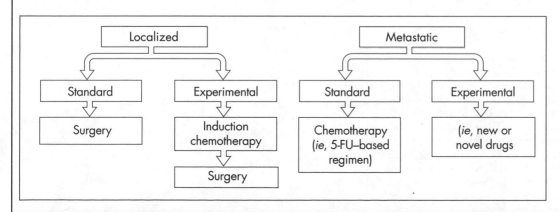

FIGURE 7-2.

Treatment strategies for gastric cancer.

survival of 30 months. These early reports require confirmation in larger randomized trials before these approaches can be accepted as standard management for gastric cancer (Fig. 7-2).

Therapy for Advanced Disease

Both single-agent and combination chemotherapy have been widely tested in advanced metastatic gastric cancer. More active agents in the past have included 5-FU, trimetrexate, mitomycin C, hydroxyurea, epirubicin, and carmustine, the partial response rates of which vary from 18% to 30%. Combination chemotherapy with these and other marginally active agents appears to produce higher objective response rates higher than those seen with single agents. More recently, promising results have been seen with newer drug combinations involving the taxanes [44] and irinotecan. Single-institution trials have reported objective response rates as high as 53% [45]. Recently, irinotecan in combination with cisplatin has shown objective responses in 42% to 57% of patients with acceptable toxicity and complete remission in 2% [46]. Docetaxel has been used in a multicenter trial in conjunction with cisplatin inducing complete responses in 4%, partial responses in 52% and a median survival of 9 months. Hematologic toxicities were the most severe, but 78% of patients were able to receive treatment as planned [47]. Murad et al. [48] treated 29 patients with paclitaxel and 5-FU to achieve objective responses in 65% including complete responses in 24%. Of these patients, 3 had pathologic complete response confirmed at laparotomy. Toxicity was low and easily managed. Median survival was 12 months with a 2-year survival rate of 20%. In 45 patients, paclitaxel in combination with 5-FU and cisplatin produced complete responses in 11%, partial responses in 40%, and a median survival of 9 months. Treatment was reasonably well tolerated and had to be modified in only 17% [49]. Another study used paclitaxel, etoposide, and cisplatin in 25 patients with advanced disease. Three of these patients had complete pathologic responses documented by laparotomy; 19 had partial responses [50].

Higher objective response rates did not hold up in phase III trials with past regimens, and to date, no single combination chemotherapy program tested in prospective randomized trials has shown a statistically significant improvement in median survival compared with those found in other regimens.

Various multiagent regimens with activity against gastric cancer are available. Unfortunately, it is not yet clear whether any specific regimen can improve median survival compared with results accruing from the best single-agent or other combination regimens. Further phase III trials are needed to clarify the role of combination chemotherapy in advanced metastatic gastric cancer.

PANCREATIC CANCER

Adenocarcinoma

Adenocarcinoma of the pancreas represents the fifth most common cause of cancer-related death in US men. An estimated 29,200 cases may be expected to occur in 2001. Incidence of the disease approximately equals the age-adjusted mortality rate, which underscoring the aggressive nature of this malignancy [1] (Table 7-5). In large studies, only 5% to 22% of presenting patients have resectable tumors. Unfortunately, even successful resection is associated with a low 5-year survival rate, ranging from 3.5% to 19%. Lesions in the body and tail of the pancreas present at an advanced stage with nonspecific symptoms. Lesions of the head and neck of the pancreas present at an earlier stage typically with painless jaundice. A spiral

CT scan demonstrating a resectable mass in the absence of distant metastasis is the only staging necessary before surgery. A diagnosis based on tissue samples is only necessary to plan medical therapy for unresectable lesions. Patients with unresectable adenocarcinomas of the pancreas confined to the pancreas often undergo palliative surgery or biliary stent placement for relief of jaundice in addition to prophylactic duodenal bypass procedures to prevent obstruction (observed in 10% of patients). Chemotherapy can add to both quantity and quality of life in advanced pancreatic cancer, although the benefit could be limited to selected patients [51].

Therapy for Locoregional Disease

The role of chemotherapy in the management of pancreatic carcinoma is best understood in the context of combined-modality treatment for the adjuvant therapy of pancreatic carcinoma after resection or in the management of locally unresectable lesions. The GITSG reported a better than twofold increase in the 2-year actuarial survival (46% and 43% vs 18%) for patients treated with a combination of 5-FU and split-course radiation therapy following resection, compared with resection alone. In addition, the GITSG demonstrated an almost twofold increase in median survival in patients with unresectable disease treated with 5-FU plus split-course radiation,

Table 7-5. TNM Staging Criteria for Pancreatic Cancer

Staging	Criteria
TX	Primary tumor cannot be assessed
T0	No evidence of primary tumor
Tis	In situ carcinoma
T1	Tumor limited to the pancreas ≤ 2 cm or less in greatest dimension
T2	Tumor limited to the pancreas > 2 cm in greatest dimension
T3	Tumor extends directly into any of the following: duodenum, bile duct, peripancreatic tissues
T4	Tumor extends directly into any of the following: stomach, spleen, colon, adjacent large vessels
NX	Regional lymph nodes cannot be assessed
N0	No regional lymph node metastasis
N1	Regional lymph node metastasis
pN1a	Metastasis in a single regional lymph node
pN1b	Metastasis in multiple regional lymph nodes
MX	Distant metastasis cannot be assessed
M0	No distant metastasis
M1	Distant metastasis

Stage	TNM
0	Tis, N0, M0
I	T1, N0, M0
	T2, N0, M0
II	T3, N0, M0
III	T1, N1, M0
	T2, N1, M0
	T3, N1, M0
IVA	T4, any N, M0
IVB	Any T, any N, M1

compared with high-dose radiation therapy alone. Intraoperative radiotherapy and interstitial brachytherapy have been employed rather than external beam radiotherapy but neither technique has demonstrated improved survival. Bolus 5-FU has also been studied in combination with intraoperative radiation therapy and with brachytherapy, although randomized trials are not available to determine the role of 5-FU in this clinical setting. Protracted-infusion 5-FU combined with radiation has shown similar activity to bolus 5-FU and radiotherapy but with less toxicity [52]. Taxol in combination with radiotherapy has shown some promise in preliminary trials [53]. In a recent phase II trial using 5-FU, leucovorin, and cisplatin in conjunction with radiotherapy in 38 patients with locally unresectable disease, Kornek *et al.* [54] achieved 1- and 2-year survivals of 53% and 18%, respectively, without surgery. At present, RTOG 97-04, a large randomized phase III trial, is addressing the efficacy of postoperative infusional 5-FU and radiation coupled with repeating cycles of either infusional 5-FU or gemcitabine [55]. RTOG 98-12 is a phase II trial coupling radiation (50 Gy) with weekly paclitaxel (50/m^2) in the treatment of unresectable disease [54].

Neoadjuvant Therapy

Early reports of neoadjuvant therapy used standard fractionation radiation therapy 5000cGy over 5.5 weeks with concomitant 5-FU, and one third of patients treated required hospital admission for GI toxicity [56]. Many newer approaches employ rapid fractionation delivering therapy over 2 weeks totaling 30 Gy with 300 cGy per fraction being delivered 5 days a week. Preliminary results suggest that neoadjuvant regimens can be delivered at this point without increasing the morbidity and mortality of subsequent surgical resections [57,58], and may in fact decrease the rate of pancreatic fistula [59]. Spitz *et al.* [60] reviewed the outcome of preoperative or postoperative chemoradiation and showed that preoperative chemoradiation could be delivered over a shorter time period without causing a delay in surgery. Planned postoperative therapy resulted in one quarter of eligible patients who remained untreated because of prolonged recovery or perioperative complications following surgery. Unfortunately, no survival benefit has yet been shown with this approach.

Prophylactic preoperative irradiation of the liver has been advocated as this is a common site of metastasis, but this can be related with life threatening toxicities [61].

Currently, an active area of investigation involves the use of preoperative chemotherapy and radiation to improve the opportunities for complete resection. Hoffman *et al.* [62] have reported on the preoperative regimen of 5-FU, mitomycin C, and local radiation; they observed a resection rate of 32%. Staley *et al.* [63] have reported a resection rate of 61% after preoperative chemoradiation with a median survival of 19 months and 4 year actuarial survival rate of 19%. More recent efforts have attempted to downstage disease that was deemed unresectable by radiologic evaluation or previous surgery. Brunner *et al.* [64]. treated 27 unresectable patients with conformal radiation (50.4 Gy), 5-FU, and gemcitabine; after restaging, 60% were explored and a standard Whipple procedure was performed with negative margins on 37%. Resected patients had a 2-year survival of 50% as opposed to 6% in the unresected group.

Therapy for Advanced Disease

Use of chemotherapy for patients with widespread metastatic disease has been extremely disappointing. There appears to be no highly active single agent and virtually all approved chemotherapy drugs have now been tested. 5-FU may have activity as a single agent; for instance, a phase II trial using 5-FU and more optimal biochemical modulation with leucovorin demonstrated a modest response rate of 7% and a median survival of 6.2 months [65]. Gemcitabine has been compared to 5-FU in a phase III trial. This study demonstrated a superior median survival of 5.7 months for gemcitabine compared with 4.4 months for 5-FU and also demonstrated improved relief of symptoms with gemcitabine. Due to its palliative potential, gemcitabine, as a single agent should be considered for unresectable pancreatic adenocarcinoma [66,67]. Recently, fixed-dose rate gemcitabine (using a dose-intense regimen) has been shown to have a better median survival than high-dose gemcitabine using a standard infusing schedule [68].

Combination chemotherapy regimens have, in some cases, demonstrated improved objective response rates. However, randomized trials with popular regimens such as FAM and streptozocin, mitomycin C, and 5-FU (SMF) have failed to demonstrate superiority of any single regimen. It seems clear that either new drugs or novel therapeutic approaches for pancreatic adenocarcinoma are desperately needed (Fig. 7-3) [69,70].

Islet Cell Carcinoma

Another important subgroup of pancreatic tumors includes islet cell tumors. These include malignant insulinoma, gastrinoma, vasoactive intestinal polypeptide-secreting tumor (VIPoma), glucagonoma, and somatostatinoma. It is important to recognize these lesions histologi-

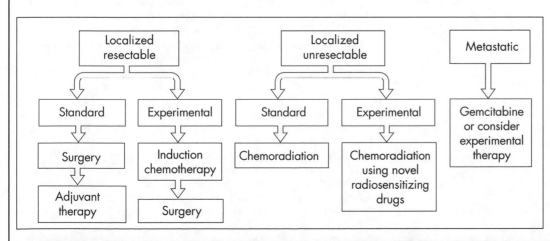

FIGURE 7-3.

Treatment strategies for pancreas cancer.

cally because the natural history and management of these pancreatic tumors are different.

Many islet cell tumors produce fascinating and distinctive syndromes related to secretory hormones. These tumors are often indolent in their growth; management is often directed at palliation of the associated symptoms. Treatment may include surgical reduction of tumor bulk, up to and including total orthotopic liver transplantation, hepatic artery occlusion for symptomatic metastatic disease, and specific end-organ blockade of the hormonal system. Examples of the latter would include omeprazole, an inhibitor of the parietal cell hydrogen pump, is more effective than H-2 blockers in the management of symptomatic gastrinomas. Octreotide, a somatostatin analogue now available in a long-acting preparation, has shown beneficial effect on tumor growth with stabilization of the disease as the most favorable response [71]. Octreotide is also helpful in palliating symptoms in patients with islet-cell carcinomas depending upon the cell type.

In the past, chemotherapy was reserved as a therapy of last resort in patients with these indolent tumors. Active drugs have included streptozocin, doxorubicin, chlorozotocin, and dacarbazine. A randomized trial was conducted showing superiority of streptozocin and doxorubicin over streptozocin plus 5-FU or single-agent chlorozotocin [72]. In this trial, the combination of streptozocin

and doxorubicin produced an improved response rate over the other two arms (69% vs 45% and 30%, respectively) and a significant survival advantage (median survival, 2.2 years vs 1.4 years and 1.4 years, respectively). These results may justify the use of this therapy as an initial approach in some patients. Chemoembolization also appears to be an effective alternative for patients with liver metastases of neuroendocrine origin. Ruszniewski *et al.*, in various studies [73–76], have reported that hepatic artery chemoembolization with iodized oil and doxorubicin can provide symptom control and tumor regression or stabilization in up to 80% of carcinoid tumors and gastrinomas.

HEPATIC CANCER

Hepatocellular carcinoma (HCC) is the most prevalent cancer in the world. About 16,200 new cases are anticipated to occur in the United States in 2001 [1]. Any form of chronic liver injury and cirrhosis predisposes to the development of this malignancy. Worldwide, the most common risk factor is chronic viral hepatitis; in the United States, other causes of chronic liver disease, such as cirrhosis related to alcoholism, are also important risk factors. Regardless of the etiology, the only known curative modality for hepatoma is surgical resection.

Patients with liver disease should be monitored for the development of hepatoma with serum alpha-fetoprotein (AFP) levels and ultrasound examinations. When suspicions are raised, dynamic CT and magnetic resonance imaging (MRI) should be performed. Without elevated serum AFP levels, fine needle aspiration may be required to diagnose radiologically indistinct lesions.

Therapy for Locoregional Disease

The patient's degree of cirrhosis and the anatomic location of tumor determine if partial hepatectomy can be performed. Even at high volume centers specializing in the procedure, operative mortality has been shown to increase from 1% to 14% in the presence of cirrhosis [77]. For this reason, resection is reserved for patients with Child's A liver function. Multiple lesions do not preclude resection. Intraductal tumors causing obstructive jaundice can be successfully resected. In this situation, it is important to distinguish obstruction from underlying liver disease as the cause of the patient's jaundice. Patients with unresectable disease because of severe underlying liver disease, anatomic location of tumor, or the presence of distant metastases have an extremely poor prognoses (Tables 7-6 and 7-7).

Total hepatectomy followed by orthotopic liver transplantation is a sensible strategy to treat patients with cirrhosis and cancer, and experience is growing with this approach. As expected, the best results have been recorded in patients who had small HCC discovered incidentally at transplantation performed for liver failure [78]. Lesions smaller than 5 cm treated by transplantation have a significantly better prognosis, and, because organs are scarce, transplantation for HCC is usually limited to this setting. Mazzaferro *et al.* [79] have reported liver transplantation as an effective treatment for small, unresectable, hepatocellular carcinoma in patients with cirrhosis, with 4-year recurrence-free survival of 83%.

Administration of an acyclic retinoid, polyprenoic acid has been shown to reduce the incidence of recurrence of new hepatomas after surgical resection or percutaneous injection of ethanol [80–82]. Aggressive adjuvant chemotherapy protocols aimed at improving outcome following transplantation have been designed for hepatoma [83,84] (Figs. 7-4 and 7-5).

Table 7-6. TNM Staging for Biliary Cancer	
Staging	**Criteria**
TX	Primary tumor cannot be assessed
T0	No evidence of primary tumor
Tis	Carcinoma in situ
T1	Tumor invades subepithelial connective tissue or fibromuscular layer
T1a	Tumor invades subepithelial connective tissue
T1b	Tumor invades fibromuscular layer
T2	Tumor invades perifibromuscular connective tissue
T3	Tumor invades adjacent structures: liver, pancreas, duodenum, gallbladder, colon, stomach
NX	Regional lymph nodes cannot be assessed
N0	No regional lymph node metastasis
N1	Metastasis in cystic duct, pericholedochal and/or hilar lymph nodes (*ie*, in the hepatoduodenal ligament)
N2	Metastasis in peripancreatic (head only), periduodenal, periportal, celiac, and/or superior mesenteric and/or posterior pancreaticoduodenal lymph nodes
MX	Distant metastasis cannot be assessed
M0	No distant metastasis
M1	Distant metastasis

Stage	**TNM**
0	Tis, N0, M0
I	T1, N0, M0
II	T2, N0, M0
III	T1, N1, M0
	T1, N2, M0
	T2, N1, M0
	T2, N2, M0
IVA	T3, any N, M0
IVB	Any T, any N, M1

Chemotherapy that is directed through the hepatic artery has also been used to treat disease isolated to the liver. This can be done by percutaneous approach with chemoembolization, or with catheter placement at laparotomy. Using catheter directed fluorodeoxyuridine (FUDR), mitomycin, and subcutaneous interferon alfa, therapeutic responses in six of 10 patients with HCC have been reported [85].

Ablative techniques include ethanol injection, cryotherapy, and radiofrequency therapy. Percutaneous ethanol injection is a very effective technique for treating small hepatomas [86–88]. Cryoablation has been shown to be a safe and effective technique of destroying large HCCs by freezing. It is performed during laparotomy for lesions not amenable to surgical resection [89]. Radiofrequency ablation destroys tumor by heat; it can be performed on large or small tumors through percutaneous, laparoscopic, or open approaches [90].

Therapy for Advanced Disease

Use of systemic chemotherapy in the management of unresectable or metastatic hepatoma has been extremely disappointing. Cisplatin, 5-FU, mitomycin have all been used with little success [91,92]. Although doxorubicin is often considered to be an active

single agent in hepatoma, the objective response rate to this agent is low and therapy with doxorubicin probably does not influence group survival when compared with no antitumor therapy.

BILIARY CANCER

Carcinoma of the gallbladder is often discovered as an incidental finding at surgery. If the disease is confined to the mucosa, cholecystectomy is curative. Unfortunately, advanced local and regional disease is usually present and the overall 5-year survival rate is less than 5%. The prognosis for patients with carcinoma of the distal bile duct is more optimistic, with an average 5-year survival after radical pancreaticoduodenectomy of approximately 40%. However, proximal bile duct carcinomas and hilar cholangiocarcinomas are much more difficult to treat surgically. In bile duct carcinomas, a favorable outcome is mainly determined by curative resection in the absence of lymph nodes metastases [93]. To achieve this a major liver resection with extensive nodal dissection is often required. The operative mortality with this aggressive approach has now fallen below 10% in experienced centers, and median survival rates at 24 months (as opposed to those at 6 months) are being achieved [94].

Therapy for Locoregional Disease

Many researchers have examined the use of external beam radiation in unresectable biliary cancer; no clear benefit has yet been demonstrated. Slightly more encouraging results have been achieved with intraoperative radiation and biliary bypass. In some cases, palliation and disease control can be achieved with brachytherapy using Iridium 192 placed through a biliary drainage catheter.

Therapy for Advanced Disease

The role of systemic chemotherapy in unresectable metastatic biliary tract cancers has also not been well defined. Because of the low incidence of these diseases, associated medical complications, and poor performance status of affected patients, few patients are referred for clinical trials. A recent review of the use of chemotherapy in the treatment of bile duct cancer suggests that possible active agents include 5-FU and mitomycin C either as single agents or in combination therapy with doxorubicin (FAM) or a combination of 5-FU and interferon [95]. Phase II studies with docetaxel have been disappointing [96]. Taxol as a single agent appears to be ineffective.

Table 7-7. TNM Staging Criteria for Hepatocellular Carcinoma

Staging	Criteria
TX	Primary tumor cannot be assessed
T0	No evidence of primary tumor
T1	Solitary tumor ≤ 2 cm in greatest dimension without vascular invasion
T2	Solitary tumor ≤ 2 cm in greatest dimension with vascular invasion, or multiple tumors limited to one lobe, none more than 2 cm in greatest dimension without vascular invasion, or a solitary tumor > 2 cm in greatest dimension without vascular invasion.
T3	Solitary tumor > 2 cm in greatest dimension with vascular invasion, or multiple tumors limited to one lobe, none > 2 cm in greatest dimension, with vascular invasion, or multiple tumors limited to one lobe, any > 2 cm in greatest dimension, with or without vascular invasion
T4	Multiple tumors in more than one lobe or tumor(s) involve(s) a major branch of the portal or hepatic vein(s) or invasion of adjacent organs other than the gallbladder or perforation of the visceral peritoneum
NX	Regional lymph nodes cannot be assessed
N0	No regional lymph node metastasis
N1	Regional lymph node metastasis
MX	Distant metastasis cannot be assessed
M0	No distant metastasis
M1	Distant metastasis

Stage	TNM
I	T1, N0, M0
II	T2, N0, M0
IIIA	T3, N0, M0
IIIB	T1, N1, M0
	T2, N1, M0
	T3, N1, M0
IVA	T4, any N, M0
IVB	Any T, any N, M1

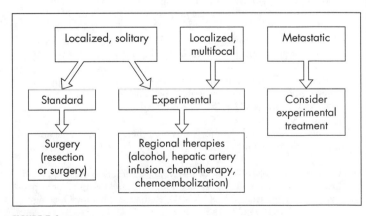

FIGURE 7-4.
Treatment strategies for hepatoma.

Combination of taxanes and other agents waits future testing [97]. In addition, hepatic artery infusion chemotherapy with agents such as 5-FU, fluorodeoxyuridine, and doxorubicin have been studied in small numbers in patients, and objective partial responses have been reported.

Newer techniques, such as conformal radiation (which spares uninvolved liver), have permitted studies of combined chemother-apy and radiation in hepatobiliary cancers. Robertson *et al.* [98] studied hepatic artery infusion of fluorodeoxyuridine and concur-rent conformal radiation in localized hepatobiliary cancer and observed a high response to treatment, with a median survival of 19 months. Although modest progress is being made in hepatobiliary cancer, a concerted effort to better understand the role of chemotherapy in these diseases is needed.

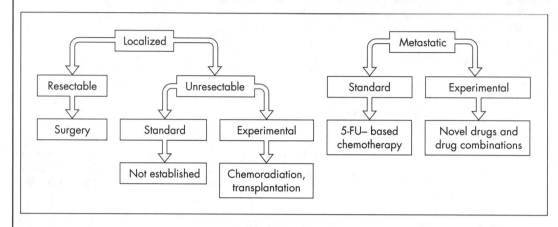

FIGURE 7-5.

Treatment strategies for gallbladder and cholangiocarcinoma.

REFERENCES

1. Greenlee RT, *et al.*: *Cancer Facts and Figures 2001*. American Cancer Society; 2001.

2. Heath EI, Kaufman HS, Talamini MA, *et al.*: The role of laparoscopy in preoperative staging of esophageal cancer. *Surg Endosc* 2000, 14:495–499.

3. Kelsen D, Ajani J, Ilson D, *et al.*: A phase II trial of paclitaxel (Taxol) in advanced esophageal cancer: preliminary report. *Semin Oncol* 1994, 21(Suppl. 8):44–48.

4. Spiridonidis CH, Laufman LR, Jones JJ, *et al.*: A phase II evaluation of high dose cisplatin and etoposide in patients with advanced esophageal adenocarcinoma. *Cancer* 1996, 78:2070–2077.

5. Bamias A, Hill ME, Cunningham D, *et al.*: Epirubicin, cisplatin, and protracted venous infusion of 5-fluorouracil for esophagogastric adeno-carcinoma: response, toxicity, quality of life, and survival. *Cancer* 1996, 77:1978–1985.

6. Wadler S, Haynes H, Beitler JJ, *et al.*: Phase II clinical trial with 5-fluorouracil, recombinant interferon alpha-2b, and cisplatin for patients with metastatic or regionally advanced carcinoma of the esophagus. *Cancer* 1996, 78:30–34.

7. Ilson DH, Saltz L, Enzinger P, *et al.*: Phase II trial of weekly irinote-can plus cisplatin in advanced esophageal cancer. *J Clin Oncol* 1999, 17:3270–3275.

8. Herskovic A, *et al.*: Combined chemotherapy and radiotherapy compared with radiotherapy alone in patients with cancer of the esophagus. *N Engl J Med* 1992, 326:1593–1598.

9. al-Sarraf M, Herskovic A, Leichman L, *et al.*: Progress report of combined chemoradiotherapy versus radiotherapy alone in patients with esophageal cancer: an intergroup study. *J Clin Oncol* 1997, 15:277–284.

10. Cooper JS, Guo MD, Herskovic A, *et al.*: Chemoradiotherapy of locally advanced esophageal cancer: long-term follow-up of a prospec-tive randomized trial (RTOG 85-01). Radiation Therapy Oncology Group. *JAMA* 1999, 281:1623–1627.

11. Coia LR, Minsky BD, Berkey BA, *et al.*: Outcome of patients receiv-ing radiation for cancer of the esophagus: results of the 1992–1994 Patterns of Care Study. *J Clin Oncol* 2000, 18:455–462.

12. Arnott SJ, *et al.*: Preoperative radiotherapy in esophageal carcinoma: a meta-analysis using individual patient data (Oesophageal Cancer Collaborative Group). *Int J Radiat Oncol Biol Phys* 1998, 41:579–583.

13. Kelsen DP, Ginsberg R, Pajak TF, *et al.*: Chemotherapy followed by surgery compared with surgery alone for localized esophageal cancer. *N Engl J Med* 1998, 339:1979–1984.

14. Urba SG, Orringer MB, Perez-Tamayo C, *et al.*: Concurrent preoper-ative chemotherapy and radiation therapy in localized esophageal adenocarcinoma. *Cancer* 1992, 69:285–291.

15. Forastiere AA, Orringer MB, Perez-Tamayo C, *et al.*: Preoperative chemoradiation followed by transhiatal esophagectomy for carcinoma of the esophagus: final report. *J Clin Oncol* 1993, 11:1118–1123.

16. Naunheim KS, Petruska P, Roy TS, *et al.*: Preoperative chemotherapy and radiotherapy for esophageal carcinoma [with discussion]. *J Thorac Cardiovasc Surg* 1992, 103:887–895.

17. Urba S, *et al.*: A randomized trial comparing surgery to preoperative concomitant chemoradiation plus surgery in patients with resectable esophageal cancer: updated analysis. *Proc Am Soc Clin Oncol* 1997, 16:277.

18. Urba S, *et al.*: Randomized trial of preoperative chemoradiation versus surgery alone in patients with locoregional esophageal carcinoma. *J Clin Oncol 2001, 19:305–313*.

19. Walsh TN, Noonan N, Hollywood D, *et al.*: A comparison of multi-modal therapy and surgery for esophageal adenocarcinoma. *N Engl J Med* 1996, 335:462–467.

20. Bosset JF, Gignoux M, Triboulet JP, *et al.*: Chemoradiotherapy followed by surgery compared with surgery alone in squamous-cell cancer of the esophagus. *N Engl J Med* 1997, 337:161–167.

21. Law S, *et al.*: Preoperative chemoradiation for squamous cell esophageal cancer: a prospective randomized trial. *Can J Gastroenterol* 1998, 12:56.

22. Adelstein DJ, Rice TW, Becker M, et al.: Use of concurrent chemotherapy, accelerated fractionation radiation, and surgery for patients with esophageal carcinoma. *Cancer* 1997, 80:1011–1020.

23. Heath EI, Burtness BA, Heitmiller RF, et al.: Phase II evaluation of preoperative chemoradiation and postoperative adjuvant chemotherapy for squamous cell and adenocarcinoma of the esophagus. *J Clin Oncol* 2000, 18:868–876.

24. Anand BS, Saeed ZA, Michaletz PA, et al.: A randomized comparison of dilatation alone versus dilatation plus laser in patients receiving chemotherapy and external beam radiation for esophageal carcinoma. *Dig Dis Sci* 1998, 43:2255–2260.

25. Reed CE: Endoscopic palliation of esophageal carcinoma. *Chest Surg Clin North Am* 1994, 4:155–172.

26. Knyrim K, Wagner HJ, Bethge N, et al.: A controlled trial of an expansile metal stent for palliation of esophageal obstruction due to inoperable cancer. *N Engl J Med* 1993. 329:1302–1307.

27. Parsonnet J, Friedman GD, Vandersteen DP, et al.: Helicobacter pylori infection and the risk of gastric carcinoma. *N Engl J Med* 1991, 325:1127–1131.

28. Parsonnet J, Friedman GD, Orentreich N, Vogelman H: Risk for gastric cancer in people with CagA positive or CagA negative *Helicobacter pylori* infection. *Gut* 1997, 40:297–301.

29. Bonenkamp JJ, Songun I, Hermans J, et al.: Randomised comparison of morbidity after D1 and D2 dissection for gastric cancer in 996 Dutch patients. *Lancet* 1995, 345:745–748.

30. Bonenkamp JJ, Hermans J, Sasako M, et al.: Extended lymph-node dissection for gastric cancer. Dutch Gastric Cancer Group. *N Engl J Med* 1999, 340:908–914.

31. Cuschieri A, Weeden S, Fielding J, et al.: Patient survival after D1 and D2 resections for gastric cancer: long- term results of the MRC randomized surgical trial. Surgical Co-operative Group, *Br J Cancer* 1999, 79:1522–1530.

32. Cuschieri A, Fayers P, Fielding J, et al.: Postoperative morbidity and mortality after D1 and D2 resections for gastric cancer: Preliminary results of the MRC randomised controlled surgical trial. The Surgical Cooperative Group. *Lancet* 1996, 347:995–999.

33. Estes NC, MacDonald JS, Touijer K, et al.: Inadequate documentation and resection for gastric cancer in the United States: a preliminary report. *Am Surg* 1998, 64:680–685.

34. Macdonald JS, et al.: Postoperative combined radiation and chemotherapy improves disease-free survival and overall survival in resected adenocarcinoma of the stomach and GE Junction. *Proc Am Soc Clin Oncol* 2000, 19:????.

35. Kelsen DP: Postoperative adjuvant chemoradiation therapy for patients with resected gastric cancer: intergroup 116. *J Clin Oncol* 2000, 18(Suppl):32S–34S.

36. Hermans J, Bonenkamp JJ, Boon MC, et al.: Adjuvant therapy after curative resection for gastric cancer: Meta- analysis of randomized trials. *J Clin Oncol* 1993, 11:1441–1447.

37. Wilke H, Stahl M, Fink U, et al.: Preoperative chemotherapy for unresectable gastric cancer. *World J Surg* 1995, 19:210–215.

38. Wilke H, Meyer HJ, Fink U: Preoperative chemotherapy in gastric cancer. *Recent Results Cancer Res* 1996, 142:237–248.

39. Ajani JA, Mayer RJ, Ota DM, et al.: Preoperative and postoperative combination chemotherapy for potentially resectable gastric carcinoma. *J Natl Cancer Inst* 1993, 85:1839–1844.

40. Ajani JA, Ota DM, Jessup JM, et al.: Resectable gastric carcinoma. An evaluation of preoperative and postoperative chemotherapy. *Cancer* 1991, 68:1501–1506.

41. Safran H, King TP, Choy H, et al.: Paclitaxel and concurrent radiation for locally advanced pancreatic carcinoma. *Front Biosci* 1998, 3:E204–E206.

42. Safran H, et al.: Paclitaxel and concurrent radiation for locally advanced pancreatic and gastric cancer: a phase I study. *J Clin Oncol* 1997, 15:901–907.

43. Ajani JA, Mansfield PF, Lynch PM, et al.: Enhanced staging and all chemotherapy preoperatively in patients with potentially resectable gastric carcinoma. *J Clin Oncol* 1999, 17:2403–2411.

44. Choy H: Taxanes in combined-modality therapy for solid tumors. *Oncology (Huntingt)* 1999, 13(Suppl. 5):23–38.

45. Karpeh MS, Brennan MF: Gastric carcinoma [review]. *Ann Surg Oncol* 1998, 5:650–656.

46. Buku N, Ohtsu A, Shimada Y, et al.: Phase II study of a combination of irinotecan and cisplatin against metastatic gastric cancer. *J Clin Oncol*, 1999, 17:319–323.

47. Roth AD, Maibach R, Martinelli G, et al.: Docetaxel (Taxotere)-cisplatin (TC): An effective drug combination in gastric carcinoma. Swiss Group for Clinical Cancer Research (SAKK), and the European Institute of Oncology (EIO). *Ann Oncol* 2000, 11:301–306.

48. Murad AM, Petroianu A, Guimaraes RC, et al.: Phase II trial of the combination of paclitaxel and 5-fluorouracil in the treatment of advanced gastric cancer: a novel, safe, and effective regimen. *Am J Clin Oncol* 1999, 22:580–586.

49. Kollmannsberger C, Quietzsch D, Haag C, et al.: A phase II study of paclitaxel, weekly, 24-hour continuous infusion 5- fluorouracil, folinic acid and cisplatin in patients with advanced gastric cancer. *Br J Cancer* 2000, 83:458–462.

50. Lokich JJ, Sonneborn H, Anderson NR, et al.: Combined paclitaxel, cisplatin, and etoposide for patients with previously untreated esophageal and gastroesophageal carcinomas. *Cancer* 1999, 85:2347–2351.

51. Glimelius B, Hoffman K, Sjoden PO, et al.: Chemotherapy improves survival and quality of life in advanced pancreatic and biliary cancer. *Ann Oncol* 1996, 7:593–600.

52. Ishii H, Okada S, Tokuuye K, et al.: Protracted 5-fluorouracil infusion with concurrent radiotherapy as a treatment for locally advanced pancreatic carcinoma. *Cancer* 1997, 79:1516–1520.

53. Safran H, Akerman P, Cioffi W, et al.: Paclitaxel and concurrent radiation therapy for locally advanced adenocarcinomas of the pancreas, stomach, and gastroesophageal junction. *Semin Radiat Oncol* 1999, 9(Suppl. 1):53–57.

54. Kornek GV, et al.: Treatment of unresectable, locally advanced pancreatic adenocarcinoma with combined radiochemotherapy with 5-fluorouracil, leucovorin and cisplatin. British Journal of *Cancer* 2000, 82:98–103.

55. Rich TA: Chemoradiation for pancreatic and biliary cancer: current status of RTOG studies [review]. *Ann Oncol* 1999, 10(Suppl. 4):231–233.

56. Evans DB, Rich TA, Byrd DR, et al.: Preoperative chemoradiation and pancreaticoduodenectomy for adenocarcinoma of the pancreas. *Arch Surg* 1992, 127:1335–1339.

57. Miller AR, et al.: Neoadjuvant chemoradiation for adenocarcinoma of the pancreas [review]. *Surg Oncol Clin North Am* 1998, 7:183–197.

58. Breslin TM, et al.: Neoadjuvant chemoradiation for adenocarcinoma of the pancreas. *Front Biosci* 1998, 3:E193–E203.

59. Evans DB, et al.: Preoperative chemoradiation strategies for localized adenocarcinoma of the pancreas. *J Hepatobil Pancreat Surg* 1998, 5:242–250.

60. Spitz FR, Abbruzzese JL, Lee JE, et al.: Preoperative and postoperative chemoradiation strategies in patients treated with pancreaticoduodenectomy for adenocarcinoma of the pancreas. *J Clin Oncol* 1997, 15:928–937.

61. Evans DB, Abbruzzese JL, Cleary KR, *et al.*: Preoperative chemoradiation for adenocarcinoma of the pancreas: Excessive toxicity of prophylactic hepatic irradiation. *Int J Radiat Oncol Biol Phys* 1995, 33:913–918.

62. Hoffman JP, Weese JL, Solin LJ, *et al.*: A pilot study of preoperative chemoradiation for patients with localized adenocarcinoma of the pancreas [with discussion]. *Am J Surg* 1995, 169:71–78.

63. Staley CA, Lee JE, Cleary KR, *et al.*: Preoperative chemoradiation, pancreaticoduodenectomy, and intraoperative radiation therapy for adenocarcinoma of the pancreatic head [with discussion]. *Am J Surg* 1996, 171:118–125.

64. Brunner TB, *et al.*: Preoperative chemoradiation in locally advanced pancreatic carcinoma: a phase II study. *Onkologie* 2000, 23:436–442.

65. DeCaprio JA, Mayer RJ, Gonin R, Arbuck SG: Fluorouracil and high-dose leucovorin in previously untreated patients with advanced adenocarcinoma of the pancreas: results of a phase II trial. *J Clin Oncol* 1991, 9:2128–2133.

66. Burris HA, Moore MJ, Andersen J, *et al.*: Improvements in survival and clinical benefit with gemcitabine as first-line therapy for patients with advanced pancreas cancer: a randomized trial. *J Clin Oncol* 1997, 15:2403–2413.

67. Au E: Clinical update of gemcitabine in pancreas cancer [review]. *Gan to Kagaku Ryoho [Japanese Journal of Cancer & Chemotherapy]* 2000, 27(Suppl. 2):469–473.

68. Tempero M, *et al.*: Randomized phase II trial of dose intense gemcitabine by standard infusion vs. fixed dose rate in metastatic pancreatic adenocarcinoma. *Am Soc Clin Oncol* 1999, 18:273.

69. van der Schelling GP, Jeekel J: Palliative chemotherapy and radiotherapy for pancreatic cancer: is It worthwhile?. [Review] *World J Surg* 1999, 23:950–953.

70. Cascinu S, Graziano F, Catalano G: Chemotherapy for advanced pancreatic cancer: It may no longer be ignored [review]. *Ann Oncol* 1999, 10:105–109.

71. Arnold R, Frank M, Kajdan U: Management of gastroenteropancreatic endocrine tumors: the place of somatostatin analogues. *Digestion* 1994, 55(Suppl.3):107–113.

72. Moertel CG, Lefkopoulo M, Lipsitz S, *et al.*: Streptozocin-doxorubicin, streptozocin-fluorouracil or chlorozotocin in the treatment of advanced islet-cell carcinoma. *N Engl J Med* 1992, 326:519–523.

73. Ruszniewski P, Rougier P, Roche A, *et al.*: Hepatic arterial chemoembolization in patients with liver metastases of endocrine tumors: a prospective phase II study in 24 patients. *Cancer* 1993, 71:2624–2630.

74. Dominguez S, Denys A, Madeira I, *et al.*: Hepatic arterial chemoembolization in the management of advanced digestive endocrine tumours. *Ital J Gastroenterol Hepatol* 1999, 31(Suppl.2):S213–S215.

75. Dominguez S, *et al.*: Hepatic arterial chemoembolization with streptozotocin in patients with metastatic digestive endocrine tumours. *Eur J Gastroenterol Hepatol* 2000, 12:151–157.

76. Ruszniewski P, Malka D: Hepatic arterial chemoembolization in the management of advanced digestive endocrine tumors. *Digestion* 2000, 62(Suppl.1):79–83.

77. Vauthey JN, Klimstra D, Franceschi D, *et al.*: Factors affecting long-term outcome after hepatic resection for hepatocellular carcinoma [with discussion]. *Am J Surg* 1995, 169:28–35.

78. Haug CE, Jenkins RL, Rohrer RJ, *et al.*: Liver transplantation for primary hepatic cancer. *Transplantation* 1992, 53:376–382.

79. Mazzaferro V, Regalia E, Doci R, *et al.*: Liver transplantation for the treatment of small hepatocellular carcinomas in patients with cirrhosis [see comments]. *N Engl J Med* 1996, 334:693–699.

80. Muto Y, Moriwaki H, Saito A: Prevention of second primary tumors by an acyclic retinoid in patients with hepatocellular carcinoma. *N Engl J Med* 1999, 340:1046–1047.

81. Muto Y, Moriwaki H, Ninomiya M, *et al.*: Prevention of second primary tumors by an acyclic retinoid, polyprenoic acid, in patients with hepatocellular carcinoma. *Digestion* 1998, 59(Suppl.2):89–91.

82. Muto Y, *et al.*: Prevention of second primary tumors by an acyclic retinoid, polyprenoic acid, in patients with hepatocellular carcinoma. Hepatoma Prevention Study Group. *N Engl J Med* 1996, 334:1561–1567.

83. Holman M, Harrison D, Stewart A, *et al.*: Neoadjuvant chemotherapy and orthotopic liver transplantation for hepatocellular carcinoma. *NJ Med* 1995, 92:519–522.

84. Stone MJ, Klintmalm GB, Polter D, *et al.*: Neoadjuvant chemotherapy and liver transplantation for hepatocellular carcinoma: a pilot study in 20 patients. *Gastroenterology* 1993, 104:196–202.

85. Atiq OT, Kemeny N, Niedzwiecki D, Botet J: Treatment of unresectable primary liver cancer with intrahepatic fluorodeoxyuridine and mitomycin C through an implantable pump. *Cancer* 1992, 69:920–924.

86. Orlando A, D'Antoni A, Camma C, *et al.*: Treatment of small hepatocellular carcinoma with percutaneous ethanol injection: a validated prognostic model. *Am J Gastroenterol* 2000, 95:2921–2927.

87. Bartolozzi C, Lencioni R: Ethanol injection for the treatment of hepatic tumours. *Eur Radiol* 1996, 6:682–696.

88. Livraghi T, Giorgio A, Marin G, *et al.*: Hepatocellular carcinoma and cirrhosis in 746 patients: Long-term results of percutaneous ethanol injection. *Radiology* 1995, 197:101–108.

89. Onik GM, Atkinson D, Zemel R, Weaver ML: Cryosurgery of liver cancer. *Semin Surg Oncol* 1993, 9:309–317.

90. McGahan JP, *et al.*: Radiofrequency ablation of the liver: Current status. *Am J Radiol* 2001, 176:3–16.

91. Farmer DG, Busuttil RW: The role of multimodal therapy in the treatment of hepatocellular carcinoma. *Cancer* 1994, 73:2669–2670.

92. Farmer DG, Rosove MH, Shaked A, Busuttil RW: Current treatment modalities for hepatocellular carcinoma. *Ann Surg* 1994, 219:236–247.

93. Klempnauer J, Ridder GJ, von Wasielewski R, *et al.*: Resectional surgery of hilar cholangiocarcinoma: a multivariate analysis of prognostic factors. *J Clin Oncol* 1997, 15:947–954.

94. Baer HU, Stain SC, Dennison AR, *et al.*: Improvements in survival by aggressive resections of hilar cholangiocarcinoma. *Ann Surg* 1993, 217:20–207.

95. Patt YZ, Jones DV, Hoque A, *et al.*: Phase II trial of intravenous fluorouracil and subcutaneous interferon alfa-2b for biliary tract cancer. *J Clin Oncol* 1996, 14:2311–2315.

96. Pazdur R, Royce ME, Rodriguez GI, *et al.*: Phase II trial of docetaxel for cholangiocarcinoma. *Am J Clin Oncol* 1999, 22:78–81.

97. Jones DV, Lozano R, Hoque A, *et al.*: Phase II study of paclitaxel therapy for unresectable biliary tree carcinomas. *J Clin Oncol* 1996, 14:2306–2310.

98. Robertson JM, Lawrence TS, Dworzanin LM, *et al.*: Treatment of primary hepatobiliary cancers with conformal radiation therapy and regional chemotherapy. *J Clin Oncol* 1993, 11:1286–1293.

STREPTOZOCIN AND DOXORUBICIN

Streptozocin is a methyl nitrosourea produced by the fermentation of *Streptomyces archromogenes*. It decomposes spontaneously to generate alkylating and carbamoylating moieties, and alkylation is thought to be its principal mechanism of antitumor activity. Streptozocin is capable of transferring methyl groups to DNA but cannot form cross-links.

Doxorubicin is an antitumor antibiotic agent with an extremely wide spectrum of activity. It does not have a single mechanism of cytotoxicity but can produce cellular dysfunction and death by multiple means. Two of its most important mechanisms of cytotoxicity include intercalation among DNA base pairs and generation of toxic intracellular free radicals. These actions can cause single- and double-stranded DNA breaks, which in turn lead to inhibition of RNA and protein synthesis and defective mitoses.

DOSAGE AND SCHEDULING

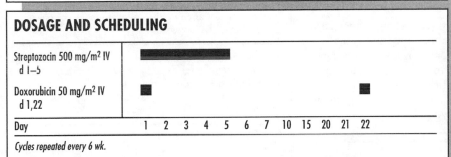

Streptozocin 500 mg/m² IV d 1–5													
Doxorubicin 50 mg/m² IV d 1,22													
Day	1	2	3	4	5	6	7	10	15	20	21	22	

Cycles repeated every 6 wk.

PRIOR TO THERAPY: *CBC and platelets, liver chemistry, BUN, creatinine. Baseline estimates of cardiac ejection fraction.*

RECENT EXPERIENCE AND RESPONSE RATES

Study	Evaluable Patients, *n*	Dosage and Scheduling	Any Regression/ Complete Regression, %	Median Duration of Regression, *mo*
Moertel *et al.*, N Engl J Med 1992, 326:519–523	36	Streptozocin 500 mg/m²/d × 5 Doxorubicin 50 mg/m²/d; days 1 and 22	69/14	22
	33	Chlorozotocin, 150 mg/m² every 7 wk	30/6	21
	33	Streptozocin 500 mg/m²/d × 5 5-FU 400 mg/m²/d × 5 (repeat every 6 wk)	45/4	13

CANDIDATES FOR TREATMENT
Patients with metastatic islet cell tumors

SPECIAL PRECAUTIONS
Patients with preexisting renal or heart disease

ALTERNATIVE THERAPY
Chlorozotocin, dacarbazine

TOXICITIES
Streptozocin: renal toxicity (azotemia, anuria, hypophosphatemia, glycosuria, renal tubular acidosis), severe nausea and vomiting possible; mild-to-moderate abnormalities of glucose tolerance (hypoglycemia); hepatic toxicity and myelosuppression possible (usually mild); **Doxorubicin:** bone marrow suppression, anorexia, nausea and vomiting, alopecia, possible cardiotoxicity

DRUG INTERACTIONS
Streptozocin: none known; **Doxorubicin:** digoxin (suspected)

NURSING INTERVENTIONS
Monitor blood counts, liver function, pulmonary function, cardiac function; administer appropriate antiemetics to avoid severe nausea and vomiting; avoid extravasation; can cause severe necrosis

PATIENT INFORMATION
Myelosuppression may occur; call physician if signs and symptoms of infection develop; call physician if injection site becomes painful, red, or swollen; possible red-colored urine for 1–2 d after treatment; nausea and vomiting may occur; hair loss likely.

EAP

Etoposide, Doxorubicin, and Cisplatin

Etoposide is a semisynthetic derivative of podophyllotoxin. Its mechanism of cytotoxic action involves the inhibition of the nuclear enzyme topoisomerase II. This enzyme has the ability to disentangle topologically intertwined DNA helices, cleave double-stranded DNA, and then covalently bond to DNA to form DNA–topoisomerase II complexes. The cleaved DNA is then reunited after a second duplex DNA has passed through. Etoposide is believed to stabilize the DNA–topoisomerase II complex and prevent rejoining of the double-stranded DNA.

Doxorubicin is an antitumor antibiotic agent with an extremely wide spectrum of activity. It does not have a single mechanism of cytotoxicity but can produce cellular dysfunction and death by multiple means. Two of its most important mechanisms of cytotoxicity include intercalation among DNA base pairs and generation of toxic intracellular free radicals. These actions can cause single- and double-stranded DNA breaks, which in turn lead to inhibition of RNA and protein synthesis and defective mitoses.

Cisplatin is activated intracellularly to generate a positively charged aquated complex. This complex functions similarly to a bifunctional alkylating agent by interacting with the nucleophilic sites on DNA, RNA, and protein, producing intrastrand links and cross-links. These reactions alter the DNA template and inhibit DNA synthesis. Cisplatin lacks cell-cycle specificity.

Combination therapy with these drugs is based on in vitro and in vivo experimental data that have suggested synergistic cytotoxicity.

CANDIDATES FOR TREATMENT

Patients with advanced locoregional or metastatic gastric cancer prior to surgery

SPECIAL PRECAUTIONS

Patients with cardiac dysfunction or renal dysfunction

ALTERNATIVE THERAPIES

ELF or 5-FU, cisplatin, and etoposide for neoadjuvant therapy; FAM, FAMTX, or ELF for metastatic disease

TOXICITIES

Drug combination: severe myelosuppression (leukopenia, anemia, thrombocytopenia); **cisplatin:** renal toxicity, alopecia

DRUG INTERACTIONS

Etoposide: synergistic in vitro with cytarabine, cyclophosphamide, carmustine, vincristine, cisplatin, hydroxyurea, 5-FU, methotrexate, verapamil; **Doxorubicin:** digoxin (suspected)

NURSING INTERVENTIONS

Monitor blood counts, liver function, cardiac function, renal function, electrolytes; administer doxorubicin with caution—an extravasant; give adequate antiemetics and maintain adequate hydration; hypotension may occur with rapid administration of etoposide

PATIENT INFORMATION

Myelosuppression common; call physician if signs and symptoms of infection develop; call physician if injection site becomes painful, red, or swollen; possible red-colored urine for 1–2 d after treatment; nausea and vomiting may occur; hair loss likely

DOSAGE AND SCHEDULING

	Day 1	2	3	4	5	6	7	8	9	10
Etoposide 120 mg/m² IV d 4,5,6				■	■	■				
Doxorubicin 20 mg/m² IV d 1,7	■						■			
Cisplatin 40 mg/m² IV d 2,8		■						■		

Cycles repeated every 3–4 wk

PRIOR TO THERAPY: *CBC and platelets, liver chemistries, BUN, creatinine, electrolytes. Baseline estimates of cardiac ejection fraction using a gated pool scan may be useful in some patients.*

RECENT EXPERIENCES AND RESPONSE RATES

Study	Evaluable Patients, n	Dosage and Scheduling	CR/PR	Median Duration of Survival, mo
Lerner et al., J Clin Oncol 1992, 10:536–540	36	Etoposide 120 mg/m²/d days 4,5,6 Doxorubicin 20 mg/m²/d days 1,7 Cisplatin 40 mg/m²/d days 2,8	3/9 (33%)	7.5
Kelsen et al., J Clin Oncol 1992, 10:541–548	30	Etoposide 120 mg/m²/d days 4,5,6 Doxorubicin 20 mg/m²/d days 1,7 Cisplatin 40 mg/m²/d days 2,8	0/6 (20%)	6.1
Preusser et al., J Clin Oncol 1989, 7:1310–1317	67	Etoposide 120 mg/m²/d days 4,5,6 Doxorubicin 20 mg/m²/d days 1,7 Cisplatin 40 mg/m²/d days 2,8	14/29 (64%)	9.0
Wilke et al., Sem Oncol 1990, 17:61–70	145	Etoposide 120 mg/m²/d days 4,5,6 Doxorubicin 20 mg/m²/d days 1,7 Cisplatin 40 mg/m²/d days 2,8	22/61 (57%)	—

FAMTX
5-Fluorouracil, Doxorubicin, Methotrexate, and Leucovorin

5-Fluorouracil (5-FU) is a fluorinated uracil analogue that is metabolized intracellularly to its active forms, fluorouridine triphosphate (FUTP) and fluorodeoxyuridine monophosphate (FdUMP). FdUMP inhibits the enzyme, thymidylate synthetase, which is necessary for DNA synthesis. Another mechanism of cytotoxicity involves the false incorporation of 5-FUTP into RNA, causing transcription errors.

Doxorubicin is an antitumor antibiotic agent with an extremely wide spectrum of activity. It does not have a single mechanism of cytotoxicity, but can produce cellular dysfunction and death by multiple means. Two of its most important mechanisms of cytotoxicity include intercalation among DNA base pairs and generation of toxic intracellular free radicals. These actions can cause single- and double-stranded DNA breaks, which in turn lead to inhibition of RNA and protein synthesis and defective mitoses.

Methotrexate is an antifolate antimetabolite that exerts its primary cytotoxic effect during the S phase. Methotrexate is actively transported across the cell membrane where it binds to its target enzyme, dihydrofolate reductase (DHFR). This enzyme is essential for regenerating the oxidized folates produced during thymidine synthesis to their active forms. In the absence of unbound DHFR, thymidylate and purine biosynthesis can no longer occur.

Leucovorin, also known as folinic acid, is the active, chemically reduced derivative of folic acid, which is involved as a cofactor for one-carbon transfer reactions in the biosynthesis of purines and pyrimidines. It is a potent antidote for the hematopoietic and reticuloendothelial effects of folic acid antagonists because it is easily converted to tetrahydrofolic acid derivatives. Leucovorin also acts as a biochemical modulator of 5-FU by enhancing the ability of 5-FU to bind and then block the action of thymidylate synthetase.

CANDIDATES FOR TREATMENT
Patients with metastatic gastric cancer

SPECIAL PRECAUTIONS
Patients with cardiac dysfunction, renal dysfunction, any third-space fluid collection or ascites, pleural effusion, seroma

ALTERNATIVE THERAPIES
EAP, FAM, ELF, 5-FU (with or without leucovorin)

TOXICITIES
Drug combination: myelosuppression, mucositis, alopecia, **5-FU:** diarrhea; **Methotrexate:** renal toxicity, pulmonary fibrosis

DRUG INTERACTIONS
5-FU: leucovorin, methotrexate, interferon α, dipyridamole, allopurinol, thymidine; **Doxorubicin:** digoxin (suspected); **Methotrexate:** salicylates, sulfonamides, tetracycline, phenylbutazone, chloramphenicol, phenytoin, probenecid, NSAIDs, L-asparaginase, vincristine, etoposide, 5-FU

NURSING INTERVENTIONS
Monitor blood counts, renal function; patient must have normal renal function, adequate hydration, and urine alkalinization prior to high-dose methotrexate administration; monitor use of all NSAIDs (can enhance methotrexate toxicity); investigate and report pulmonary symptoms (such as dry nonproductive cough); monitor for ascites or other third-space fluid collection (can enhance methotrexate toxicity); give antiemetics as necessary; monitor hepatic function; administer doxorubicin with caution—an extravasant; monitor methotrexate levels.

PATIENT INFORMATION
Myelosuppression can occur; call physician if signs and symptoms of infection develop (fever, chills, flu-like symptoms); oral mucositis and diarrhea possible; hair loss likely; call physician if injection site becomes painful, red, or swollen; possible red-colored urine for 1–2 d after treatment; maintain adequate hydration.

DOSAGE AND SCHEDULING

5-FU 1500 mg/m^2 IV d 1
Doxorubicin 30 mg/m^2 IV d 15
Methotrexate 1500 mg/m^2 IV d 1
Leucovorin 15 mg/m^2 PO every 6 h d 2,3

| Day | 1 | 2 | 3 | 4 | 5 | 6 | 7 | 8 | 9 | 10 | 11 | 12 | 13 | 14 | 15 |

Cycles repeated every 4 wk.

PRIOR TO THERAPY: *CBC and platelets, liver chemistries, BUN, creatinine. Baseline estimates of cardiac ejection fraction using a gated pool scan may be useful in some patients.*

RECENT EXPERIENCES AND RESPONSE RATES

Study	Evaluable Patients, *n*	Dosage and Scheduling	CR/PR	Median Duration of Survival, *mo*
Kelsen *et al., J Clin Oncol* 1992, 10:541–548	30	5-FU 1.5 g/m^2/d day 1 Doxorubicin 30 mg/m^2/d day 15 Methotrexate 1.5 g/m^2/d day 1 Leucovorin 15 mg/m^2 PO every 6 h × 3 days starting day 2	3/7 (33%)	7.3
Wils *et al., J Clin Oncol* 1991, 9:827–831	81	5-FU 1.5 g/m^2/d day 1 Doxorubicin 30 mg/m^2/d day 15 Methotrexate 1.5 g/m^2/d day 1 Leucovorin 15 mg/m^2 PO every 6 h × 48 h starting day 2	5/28 (41%)	10.5
Wils *et al., J Clin Oncol* 1986, 4:1799–1803	67	5-FU 1.5 g/m^2/d day 1 Doxorubicin 30 mg/m^2/d day 15 Methotrexate 1.5 g/m^2/d day 1 Leucovorin 15 mg/m^2 PO every 6 h × 48 h starting day 2	9/13 (33%)	6.0

ELF
Etoposide, Leucovorin, and 5-Fluorouracil

Etoposide is a semisynthetic derivative of podophyllotoxin. Its mechanism of cytotoxic action involves the inhibition of the nuclear enzyme topoisomerase II. This enzyme has the ability to disentangle topologically intertwined DNA helices, cleave double-stranded DNA, and then covalently bond to DNA to form DNA–topoisomerase II complexes. The cleaved DNA is then reunited after a second duplex DNA has passed through. Etoposide is believed to stabilize the DNA–topoisomerase II complex and prevent rejoining of the double-stranded DNA.

Leucovorin, also known as folinic acid, is an active, chemically reduced derivative of folic acid. Reduction by the enzyme dihydrofolate reductase is not required for leucovorin to participate in reactions that use folates as a source of one-carbon moieties. Leucovorin also acts as a biochemical modulator of 5-fluorouracil by enhancing the ability of 5-FU to bind and then block the action of thymidylate synthetase.

5-FU is a fluorinated uracil analogue that is metabolized intracellularly to its active forms, fluorouridine triphosphate (FUTP) and fluorodeoxyuridine monophosphate (FdUMP). FdUMP inhibits the enzyme, thymidylate synthetase, which is necessary for DNA synthesis. Another mechanism of cytotoxicity involves the false incorporation of 5-FUTP into RNA, causing transcription errors.

Etoposide and 5-fluorouracil are both active agents in gastric carcinoma. In combination, they act synergistically and are not cross-resistant in vitro or in vivo.

Leucovorin contributes to the synergism of this regimen by enhancing the cytotoxicity of 5-FU by increasing its ability to bind and then block the action of thymidylate synthetase.

CANDIDATES FOR TREATMENT
Patients with metastatic or advanced locoregional gastric cancer, especially for elderly or high-risk patients

SPECIAL PRECAUTIONS
None noteworthy

ALTERNATIVE THERAPIES
EAP, FAMTX, FAM, 5-FU (with or without leucovorin)

TOXICITIES
Myelosuppression, possible mucositis, diarrhea

DRUG INTERACTIONS:
Etoposide: synergistic in vitro with cytarabine, cyclophosphamide, carmustine, vincristine, cisplatin, hydroxyurea, 5-FU, methotrexate, verapamil; **Leucovorin:** 5-fluorouracil; **5-FU:** leucovorin, methotrexate, interferon α, dipyridamole, allopurinol, thymidine

NURSING INTERVENTIONS
Monitor blood counts; administer etoposide slowly over 45 to 60 minutes or longer (hypotension can occur if given too rapidly)

PATIENT INFORMATION
Oral mucositis may occur; skin reactions possible; call physician if diarrhea develops

DOSAGE AND SCHEDULING

Etoposide 120 mg/m² IV d 1,2,3	▬▬▬															
Leucovorin 300 mg/m² IV d 1,2,3	▬▬▬															
5-FU 500 mg/m² IV d 1,2,3	▬▬▬															
Day	1	2	3	4	5	6	7	8	9	10	11	12	13	14	15	

PRIOR TO THERAPY: CBC and platelets.

RECENT EXPERIENCES AND RESPONSE RATES

Study	Evaluable Patients, n	Dosage and Scheduling	CR/PR	Median Duration of Survival, mo
Preusser et al., Sem Oncol 1990, 17:61–70	51	Etoposide 120 mg/m²/d days 1,2,3 Leucovorin 300 mg/m²/d days 1,2,3 5-FU 500 mg/m²/d days 1,2,3	8/16 (53%)	11.0
Wilke et al., Invest New Drugs 1990, 8:65–70	33	Etoposide 120 mg/m²/d days 1,2,3 Leucovorin 300 mg/m²/d days 1,2,3 5-FU 500 mg/m²/d days 1,2,3	4/12 (48%)	10.5

FAM
5-Fluorouracil, Doxorubicin, and Mitomycin C

5-Fluorouracil is a fluorinated uracil analogue that is metabolized intracellularly to its active forms, fluorouridine triphosphate (FUTP) and fluorodeoxyuridine monophosphate (FdUMP). FdUMP inhibits the enzyme, thymidylate synthetase, which is necessary for DNA synthesis. Another mechanism of cytotoxicity involves the false incorporation of 5-FUTP into RNA, causing transcription errors.

Doxorubicin is an antitumor antibiotic agent with an extremely wide spectrum of activity. It does not have a single mechanism of cytotoxicity but can produce cellular dysfunction and death by multiple means. Its two most important mechanisms of cytotoxicity include intercalation among DNA base pairs and generation of toxic intracellular free radicals. These actions can cause single- and double-stranded DNA breaks, which in turn lead to inhibition of RNA and protein synthesis and defective mitoses.

Mitomycin C contains both quinoline and aziridine ring structures, allowing it to exert antitumor activity by two different mechanisms. Reduction of the quinoline ring by one electron transfer allows for free radical reactions similar to those seen with the anthracyclines. The aziridine ring functions as an alkylator producing DNA cross-links.

DOSAGE AND SCHEDULING

	1	2	3	4	5	6	7	8	9	10	11	12	13	14
5-FU 600 mg/m² IV d 1 of wk 1,2,5,6	▮	▮			▮	▮								
Doxorubicin 30 mg/m² d 1 of wk 1,5	▮				▮									
Mitomycin C 10 mg/m² IV d 1 of wk 1	▮													
Week	1	2	3	4	5	6	7	8	9	10	11	12	13	14

Cycles repeated every 6 wk.

PRIOR TO THERAPY: *CBC, platelets, liver chemistries. Baseline estimates of cardiac ejection fraction using a gated pool scan may be useful in some patients. Pulmonary function tests may be useful in selected patients.*

RECENT EXPERIENCES AND RESPONSE RATES

Study	Evaluable Patients, n	Dosage and Scheduling	CR/PR	Median Duration of Response, mo
MacDonald et al., Ann Intern Med 1980, 93:533–536	62	5-FU 600 mg/m²/d days 1,8,29,36 Doxorubicin 30 mg/m²/d days 1,29 Mitomycin C 10 mg/m²/d day 1	0/26 (42%)	9
Brian et al., Oncology 1989, 46:83–87	43	5-FU 600 mg/m²/d days 1,8,29,36 Doxorubicin 30 mg/m²/d days 1,29 Mitomycin C 10 mg/m²/d day 1	0/18 (42%)	7
Arbuck et al., Cancer 1990, 65:2442–2445	26	Leucovorin 500 mg/m²/d IV over 2 h days 1,8,29,36 5-FU 600 mg/m²/d IVP 1 h after leucovorin, days 1,8,29,36 Doxorubicin 30 mg/m²/d day 1,29 Mitomycin C 10 mg/m²/d day 1	1/9 (38%)	6

CANDIDATES FOR TREATMENT
Patients with metastatic gastric cancer

SPECIAL PRECAUTIONS
Patients with preexisting heart disease or pulmonary dysfunction

ALTERNATIVE THERAPIES
EAP, FAMTX, ELF, 5-FU (with or without leucovorin)

TOXICITIES
Drug combination: cumulative bone marrow suppression, including enhanced leukopenia and thrombocytopenia, alopecia, anorexia, nausea and vomiting; **Doxorubicin:** congestive cardiomyopathy, **Mitomycin C:** hemolytic anemia-like syndrome, pulmonary fibrosis

DRUG INTERACTIONS
5-FU: leucovorin, methotrexate, interferon-α, dipyridamole, allopurinol, thymidine; **Doxorubicin:** digoxin (suspected); **Mitomycin C:** none

NURSING INTERVENTIONS
Monitor blood counts, liver function, pulmonary function, cardiac function; administer doxorubicin and mitomycin C with great caution—extravasation injury can be extremely severe.

PATIENT INFORMATION
Myelosuppression common; call physician if signs and symptoms of infection develop; call physician if area around site of injection becomes painful, red, or swollen; oral mucositis and diarrhea may occur; call physician if diarrhea persists; skin reactions possible; possible red-colored urine for 1–2 d after treatment.

5-FLUOROURACIL AND RADIATION THERAPY

5-Fluorouracil is a fluorinated uracil analogue that is metabolized intracellularly to its active forms, fluorouridine triphosphate (FUTP) and fluorodeoxyuridine monophosphate (FdUMP). FdUMP inhibits the enzyme, thymidylate synthetase, which is necessary for DNA synthesis. Another mechanism of cytotoxicity involves the false incorporation of 5-FUTP into RNA, causing transcription errors.

When 5-FU is combined with radiation, enhancement of radiation effects is observed. It is known that 5-FU can significantly affect the slope of the radiation therapy survival curve when present in cytotoxic concentrations. The mechanism of this effect is unknown but may involve incorporation into DNA or RNA and cell-cycle effects. Inhibition of sublethal damage repair does not seem to play a role.

DOSAGE AND SCHEDULING

5-FU: 500 mg/m^2/d × 3 d every 2 wk × 2, then 500 mg/m^2 every wk for a total of 2 y of therapy—weekly doses begin 1 mo after radiation therapy is complete;
Radiation: 2000 cGy over 5 d × 2 courses; 2-wk separation between doses

RECENT EXPERIENCES AND RESPONSE RATES

Study	Evaluable Patients, n	Dosage and Scheduling	Median Duration of Survival, mo	2-y Actuarial Survival, %
GI Tumor Study Group, *Arch Surg* 1985, 120:899–903	21	5-FU 500 mg/m^2/d x 3 days q 2 wk x 2; then 500 mg/m^2/wk starting 1 month after radiation therapy complete Plus Radiation 2000 rads/5 d x 2 (2-wk separation between doses)	21.0	43
	22	No treatment—control group	10.9	18
GI Tumor Study Group, *Cancer* 1987, 59:2006–2010	30	5-FU 500 mg/m^2/d x 3 days q 2 wk x 2; then 500 mg/m^2/wk starting 1 month after radiation therapy complete Plus Radiation 2000 rads/5 d x 2 (2-wk separation between doses)	18.0	46

Chemotherapy was continued on a weekly schedule for 2 y of therapy.

CANDIDATES FOR TREATMENT

Patients with locally unresectable pancreatic cancer or with pancreatic cancer causing severe back pain from retroperitoneal extension of disease

SPECIAL PRECAUTIONS

None noteworthy

ALTERNATIVE THERAPIES

Radiation therapy alone, chemotherapy

TOXICITIES

Mucositis, diarrhea, myelosuppression, anorexia, nausea, vomiting, diarrhea, skin irritation

DRUG INTERACTIONS

5-FU: leucovorin, methotrexate, interferon-α, dipyridamole, allopurinol, thymidine

NURSING INTERVENTIONS

Monitor blood counts; inform patients of possible skin reactions, diarrhea, mucositis

PATIENT INFORMATION

Possible nausea, vomiting, anorexia, oral mucositis, skin reactions, diarrhea

CISPLATIN, 5-FLUOROURACIL, AND RADIATION THERAPY

Cisplatin is activated intracellularly to generate a positively charged aquated complex. This complex functions similarly to a bifunctional alkylating agent by interacting with the nucleophilic sites on DNA, RNA, and protein, producing intrastrand links and cross-links. These reactions alter the DNA template and inhibit DNA synthesis. Cisplatin lacks cell-cycle specificity.

5-Fluorouracil is a fluorinated uracil analogue that is metabolized intracellularly to its active forms, fluorouridine triphosphate (FUTP) and fluorode-oxyuridine monophosphate (FdUMP). FdUMP inhibits the enzyme, thymidylate synthetase, which is necessary for DNA synthesis. Another mechanism of cytotoxicity involves the false incorporation of 5-FUTP into RNA, causing transcription errors.

Both cisplatin and 5-FU, as single agents, are moderately active against esophageal carcinoma. When used in combination with radiation therapy, a radiation-enhancing effect is seen. Ideally, this multimodality approach would enhance the effects of radiation on local tumors and the systemic drug therapy would reduce the chance of distant micrometastases.

DOSAGE AND SCHEDULING

5-FU 1000 mg/m^2/d by continuous infusion every day × 5 d
Cisplatin 70–100 mg/m^2, d 1 only

PRIOR TO THERAPY: *CBC, platelets, electrolytes, BUN, creatinine.*

RECENT EXPERIENCES AND RESPONSE RATES

Study	Evaluable Patients, n	Dosage and Scheduling	Median Duration of Survival, mo	Survival Rates, % 12 mo	Survival Rates, % 24 mo
Patients with Localized Disease					
Herskovic et al., N Engl J Med 1992, 326:1593–1598	121	5-FU 1000 mg/m^2/d × 4 days continuous infusion Cisplatin 75 mg/m^2 day 1 only Radiation 5000 cGy/5 wk	12.5	50	38
		Radiation alone, 6400 cGy/6.4 wk	8.9	33	10
Seitz et al., Cancer 1990, 66:214–219		5-FU 1000 mg/m^2/d × 5 d continuous infusion Cisplatin 70 mg/m^2/d day 2 only Radiation 20 cGy/5 d	17.0	—	41
Presurgical Chemotherapy Regimen					
Walsh et al., N Engl J Med 1996, 335:462–467.	48	5-FU 15 mg/kg/d IV over 16 h daily × 5 d, wk 1 and 6 Cisplatin 75 mg/m^2 IV over 8 h ×1 dose on d 7, wk 1 and 6 Radiation 40 cGy in 15 fractions (d 1–5, 8–12, 15–19)	16.0	52	37

	Evaluable Patients, n	Dosage and Scheduling	CR/PR	Response Rate, %
Patients with Metastatic Disease and Control of Primary Tumor				
Debesi et al., Cancer Treat Rep 1986, 70:909–910	37	5-FU 1000 mg/m^2/d × 5 d continuous infusion Cisplatin 100 mg/m^2 day 1 only Allopurinol 600 mg daily day -2 to +5	3/10	35
Kies et al., Cancer 1987, 60:2156–2160	26	5-FU 1000 mg/m^2/d × 5 d continuous infusion Cisplatin 100 mg/m^2/d day 1 only	3/8	42

CANDIDATES FOR TREATMENT

Patients with esophageal carcinoma

SPECIAL PRECAUTIONS

Patients with renal dysfunction

ALTERNATIVE THERAPIES

Preoperative: 5-FU and mitomycin C; 5-FU, vinblastine, and cisplatin plus radiation; cisplatin and bleomycin with or without vindesine; cisplatin and 5-FU; etoposide, cisplatin, and 5-FU; etoposide, doxorubicin, and cisplatin; **Inoperable or metastatic disease:** cisplatin and bleomycin with or without vindesine; cisplatin, methotrexate, and bleomycin

TOXICITIES:

Cisplatin: myelosuppression, nausea, vomiting, renal dysfunction, possible ototoxicity, possible neurotoxicity; **5-FU:** myelosuppression, mucositis, diarrhea; **Chemotherapy plus radiation therapy:** enhanced myelosuppression, severe esophagitis or stomatitis, nausea, vomiting, anorexia, diarrhea, possible ototoxicity, possible neurotoxicity

DRUG INTERACTIONS

5-FU: leucovorin, methotrexate, interferon alpha, dipyridamole, allopurinol, thymidine; **Cisplatin:** none

NURSING INTERVENTIONS

Monitor blood counts, renal function, electrolytes; inform patients of possible skin reactions; give adequate amounts of antiemetics before and after cisplatin therapy; maintain adequate hydration; use diuretics as indicated

PATIENT INFORMATION

Oral mucositis and severe esophagitis may occur; myelosuppression is likely; call physician if signs of infection or diarrhea develop; call physician if hearing loss occurs; nausea and vomiting possible (possibly protracted); skin reactions possible, taste changes (metallic) possible.

5-FLUOROURACIL, RECOMBINANT INTERFERON-α-2B, AND CISPLATIN

Cisplatin is activated intracellularly to generate a positively charged aquated complex. This complex functions similarly to a bifunctional alkylating agent by interacting with the nucleophilic sites on DNA, RNA, and protein, producing intrastrand links and cross-links. These reactions alter the DNA template and inhibit DNA synthesis. Cisplatin lacks cell-cycle specificity.

5-Fluorouracil is a fluorinated uracil analogue that is metabolized intracellularly to its active forms, fluorouridine triphosphate (FUTP) and fluorodeoxyuridine monophosphate (FdUMP). FdUMP inhibits the enzyme thymidylate synthetase, which is necessary for DNA synthesis. Another mechanism of cytotoxicity involves the false incorporation of 5-FUTP into RNA, causing transcription errors.

Biochemical modulation with recombinant interferon-α (IFN-α) has been shown to augment the cytotoxicity of both 5-Fluorouracil and Cisplatin in vitro and may be a viable strategy in the treatment of esophageal carcinoma.

CANDIDATES FOR TREATMENT

Patients with regionally advanced or metastatic esophageal carcinoma

SPECIAL PRECAUTIONS

Patients with renal dysfunction

ALTERNATIVE THERAPIES

Cisplatin and bleomycin with or without vindesine, cisplatin and 5-FU, cisplatin and etoposide, methotrexate, and bleomycin

TOXICITIES

Myelosuppression, primarily thrombocytopenia, fatigue, neurologic toxicities, mucositis, diarrhea

DRUG INTERACTIONS

5-FU: leucovorin, methotrexate, dipyridamole, allopurinol, thymidine; IFN: cisplatin, and 5-FU (augments cytotoxicity)

NURSING INTERVENTIONS

Monitor blood counts, renal function, electrolytes; inform patients of possible skin reactions; give adequate antiemetics and maintain adequate hydration during cisplatin administration

PATIENT INFORMATION

Possible nausea, vomiting, anorexia, oral mucositis, diarrhea. Call physician if signs of infection or diarrhea develop. Possible neurologic toxicities include dizziness and gait disturbances

DOSAGE AND SCHEDULING

	Day 1 2 3 4 5 6 7 8 9 10 11 12 13 14 15 16 17 18 19 20 21 22
Interferon-α-2b 10 MU SQ weekly on d 1,3,5	▪ ▪ ▪ (continue weekly on d 1,3,5)
Cisplatin 100 mg/m^2 IV d 1	▪
Cisplatin 25 mg/m^2 IV weekly	▪ (d15) ▪ (d22)
Fluorouracil 750 mg/m^2/d IV	▪ ▪ ▪ ▪ ▪ ▪ (d15) ▪ (d22)
GM-CSF 5 µg/kg SQ 5 X/wk	▪ ▪ ▪ ▪ ▪ ▪ ▪ ▪ ▪ ▪ ▪

GM-CSF—granulocyte–macrophage colony-stimulating factor.

SEQUENCE OF ADMINISTRATION: IFN-α → cisplatin → 5-FU with cisplatin administered immediately after IFN-α.
5-FU is administered at 750 mg/m^2 daily for 5 d beginning on d 1, then at 750 mg/m^2 every wk beginning on d 15.
Cisplatin is administered at 100 mg/m^2 over 2 h on d 1, then at 25 mg/m^2 every wk (immediately before the 5-FU bolus) beginning on d 15.
IFN-alpha is administered at 10 MU SQ each wk on d 1 (immediately before the cisplatin), then on d 3 and 5.
GM-CSF is administered at 5 µg/kg SQ on d 7–13, then on d 2–5 each wk beginning the day after chemotherapy.

PRIOR TO THERAPY: CBC, platelets, electrolytes, BUN, creatinine, liver function.

RECENT EXPERIENCES AND RESPONSE RATES

Study	Evaluable Patients, *n*	Dosage and Scheduling	CR/ PR	Response Rate, %
Wadler et al., Cancer 1996, 78:30–34	23	5-FU 750 mg/m^2/d×5 d, then 750 mg/m^2 q wk beginning d 15 Cisplatin 100 mg/m^2 IV d 1, then 25 mg/m^2 weekly beginning d 15 IFN-α(Intron) 10 MU SQ on d 1,3,5	1/14	65
Kelsen et al., J Clin Oncol 1992, 10:269–274.	37	5-FU 750 mg/m^2/d×5 d, continuous IV infusion 5-FU 750 mg/m^2 once weekly IVP beginning on d 12 IFN-α (Roferon-A) 9 MU SQ 3X/wk	1/9	27
Wadler et al., Cancer 1993, 71:1726–1730 .	20	5-FU 750 mg/m^2/d×5 d, continuous IV infusion 5-FU 750 mg/m^2 once weekly IVP IFN-α (Roferon-A) 9 MU SQ 3X/wk	2/3	25
Ilson et al., Cancer 1995, 75:2197–2202	26	5-FU 750 mg/m^2/d×5 d, continuous IV infusion q 28 d Cisplatin 100 mg/m^2 IV d 1, q 28 d X 3, then q 56 d IFN-α (Roferon-A) 3 MU SQ daily on d 1–28	2/13	50

HIGH-DOSE CISPLATIN AND ETOPOSIDE

Etoposide is a semisynthetic derivative of podophyllotoxin. Its mechanism of cytotoxic action involves the inhibition of the nuclear enzyme topoisomerase II. This enzyme has the ability to disentangle topologically intertwined DNA helices, cleave double-stranded DNA, and then covalently bond to DNA to form DNA–topoisomerase II complexes. The cleaved DNA is then reunited after a second duplex DNA has passed through. Etoposide is believed to stabilize the DNA–topoisomerase II complex and prevent rejoining of the double-stranded DNA.

Cisplatin is activated intracellularly to generate a positively charged aquated complex. This complex functions similarly to a bifunctional alkylating agent by interacting with the nucleophilic sites on DNA, RNA, and protein, producing intrastrand links and cross-links. These reactions alter the DNA template and inhibit DNA synthesis. Cisplatin lacks cell-cycle specificity.

Combination therapy with these drugs is based on in vitro and in vivo experimental data that have suggested synergistic cytotoxicity.

CANDIDATES FOR TREATMENT

Patients with unresectable or metastatic esophageal adenocarcinoma

SPECIAL PRECAUTIONS

Patients with renal dysfunction and patients with both renal and hepatic dysfunction

ALTERNATIVE THERAPIES

5-Fluorouracil and interferon, 5-Fluorouracil, interferon, and cisplatin

TOXICITIES

Neutropenia, thrombocytopenia, nausea and vomiting, peripheral sensory neuropathy, renal dysfunction, ototoxicity

DRUG INTERACTIONS

Cisplatin: interferon; Etoposide: synergistic in vitro with cytarabine, cyclophosphamide, carmustine, vincristine, cisplatin, hydroxyurea, 5-FU, methotrexate, verapamil

NURSING INTERVENTIONS

Monitor blood counts, renal function, electrolytes; give adequate amounts of antiemetics; maintain adequate hydration; use diuretics as indicated

PATIENT INFORMATION

Myelosuppression is likely; call physician if signs of infection develop. Nausea and vomiting (possibly protracted) and taste changes (metallic) may occur. Inform physician if hearing loss occurs

DOSAGE AND SCHEDULING

Cisplatin 30 mg/m²/d days 1–5	■	■	■	■	■
Etoposide 60 mg/m²/d days 1–5	■	■	■	■	■
Day	1	2	3	4	5

Cycles repeated q 21 d for a total of 3 cycles.

DOSAGE MODIFICATIONS: Patients > 70 y of age are given reduced doses of cisplatin and etoposide. Patients with responding metastatic disease were given one additional cycle of chemotherapy. Patients with locoregional disease received radiation 1.8 Gy daily, 5 d/wk for a total dose of 41.4 Gy. 5-FU is administered by continuous infusion at 300 mg/m2/d for the duration of radiation.

PRIOR TO THERAPY: CBC, platelets, BUN, creatinine, electrolytes, liver chemistries.

RECENT EXPERIENCES AND RESPONSE RATES

Study	Evaluable Patients, n	Dosage and Scheduling	CR/PR	Response Rate, %
Spiridonidis et al., Cancer 1996, 77:2070–2077	24	Cisplatin 30 mg/m²/d × 5 d IV over 1 h Etoposide 60 mg/m²/d × 5 d IV over 2 h (3 cycles of cisplatin/etoposide followed by 5-FU and radiation in patients with locoregional disease)	5/8	54
Kelsen et al., J Clin Oncol 1992, 10:269–274	37	5-FU 750 mg/m²/d × 5 d, continuous IV infusion 5-FU 750 mg/m² once weekly IVP beginning on d 12 IFN-α (Roferon-A) 9 MU SQ 3×/wk	1/9	27
Ilson et al., Cancer 1995, 75:2197–2202	26	5-FU 750 mg/m²/d × 5 d, continuous IV infusion q 28 d Cisplatin 100 mg/m² IV d 1 q 28 d × 3, then q 56 d IFN-α (Roferon-A) 3 MU SQ daily d 1–28	2/13	50
Wadler et al., Cancer 1996, 78:30–34	23	5-FU 750 mg/m²/d × 5 d, then 750 mg/m² every wk beginning d 15 Cisplatin 100 mg/m² IV d 1, then 25 mg/m² weekly beginning d 15 IFN-α (Intron) 10 MU SQ d 1,3,5	1/14	65

COLORECTAL CANCER

Cancers arising in the large bowel are the third most common type of cancer in men and women in the United States. Approximately 130,000 new cases will be diagnosed in the year 2000, and about 56,000 cancer deaths are expected [1]. Recently, the incidence of colorectal cancer appears to be declining by about 2% per year, which may reflect the combined results of screening, polyp removal, and prevention of polyp transformation to invasive cancer. The survival of patients with resectable colorectal cancer is also improving, and is most likely due to earlier diagnosis, improvements in surgical technique, and the impact of adjuvant therapy. Finally, the prognosis of patients with metastatic colorectal cancer is also improving due to systemic combination therapy with irinotecan and leucovorin-modulated fluorouracil, and in selected cases, regional management of metastatic disease confined to the liver.

About 72% of new cases originate in the colon (defined as the segment of the large bowel proximal to the peritoneal reflection). The remaining new cases arise in the rectum. During the past 25 years, a shift in location of tumors has been observed, with a decrease in the percentage of tumors arising in the rectum and descending colon cases, and an increasing incidence of tumors arising in the proximal colon. Adenocarcinomas account for the vast majority (> 90%) of large bowel cancers, whereas carcinoid tumors account for most of the remaining malignant neoplasms. Rarely, primary lymphomas, melanomas, and sarcomas of the large bowel are reported.

Etiology and Risk Factors

The average age at diagnosis is 60 to 65 years, but the incidence per 100,000 patients at risk increases with age, from eight per 100,000 at 40 years, to 150 per 100,000 at 60 years, to 500 per 100,000 at 80 years. The cumulative risk of developing colorectal cancer is about

6% by the ninth decade in the United States. About 75% of colorectal cancer cases occur in individuals 50 years of age or older with no obvious excess risk factors (so-called sporadic cancer) (Fig. 8-1) [2]. The remaining cases occur in high-risk populations, which includes individuals with a family history of colorectal cancer in close relatives in the absence of known genetic predispositions, hereditary nonpolyposis coli (HNPCC; Lynch syndromes I and II), familial adenomatous polyposis (FAP), and inflammatory bowel disease (IBD) [3,4]. Families with HNPCC have been found to have mutations in at least five different genes involved in DNA nucleotide mismatch repair (chromosome location): *MSH2* (2p), *MSH6* (2p), *HMLH1* (3p), *PMS1* (2q), and *PMS2* (7p). FAP and its variants, including Gardener's syndrome, attenuated adenomatous polyposis, and hereditary flat adenoma syndrome, are associated with mutations in the *APC* gene (chromosome 5q) that result in a truncated protein product. Extremely rare hereditary syndromes include Peutz-Jeghers (*LKB1* gene, 19p3.3) and juvenile polyposis (*SMAD4/DPC4*, 19q). In patients with IBD, cancers arise in areas of chronically inflamed epithelium, and the duration and extent of involvement are two independent risk factors. For patients with extensive ulcerative and Crohn's colitis, the risk of developing colon cancer begins to increase above age-matched controls after 7 to 10 years of disease. Cancers associated with IBD do not arise from adenomatous polyps, but rather from dysplastic epithelium that is generally indistinguishable from nondysplastic adjacent epithelium. Therefore, multiple random biopsies are needed for surveillance, with the risk for sampling error.

In asymptomatic people at normal risk, the 1997 American Gastroenterological Association recommendations for screening are as follows. For the general population, annual guaiac-based fecal blood tests should begin at age 50. Low-risk individuals should have a flexible sigmoidoscopy at age 50 with a complete colonoscopy if a polyp is found. Sigmoidoscopy should be performed every 3 to 5 years if the initial study is negative. All polyps should be removed when detected and examined pathologically, because removal of adenomatous polyps may reduce the risk of subsequent colorectal cancer. Follow-up colonoscopy is recommended at 3 years for those patients who had either multiple adenomas, an adenoma larger than 0.5 cm, or a family history of colorectal cancer. If an adenoma is detected at the first follow-up colonoscopy, subsequent follow-up should be scheduled for 3 years unless the adenoma is a single small tubular polyp 0.5 cm or smaller (follow-up at 5 years). If no adenoma is detected at first follow-up, then subsequent colonoscopy can be done 5 years later. For high-risk populations, screening needs to be initiated at a much earlier age, and must be repeated more frequently.

Two recent studies screened a large cohort of asymptomatic patients aged 50 years or older with colonoscopy. Both studies showed that about half of the asymptomatic colon cancers or polyps associated with a high risk of cancer in the proximal colon had no distal adenomas, and thus would have been missed by sigmoidoscopy alone [6,7]. Therefore, the current screening recommendations may not be sufficient.

Progression of adenomatous polyps to large bowel adenocarcinoma is clearly documented, and the molecular genetic events that lead from mucosal proliferation to carcinogenesis have been well described [3,8]. The risk for malignant conversion of polyps is related to polyp size, number, and histology. Polyps less than 1 cm have approximately a 1% chance of containing a malignant focus. Risk for malignancy increases from 5% to 10% for polyps 1 to 2 cm in diameter, and from 20% to 50% for those greater than 2 cm. In addition to the additive risk of multiple polyps (each of which has an

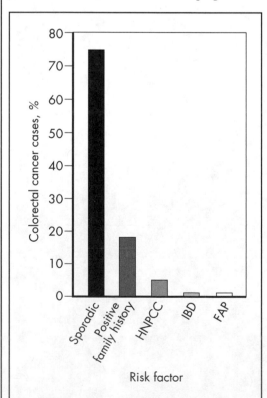

FIGURE 8-1.

Incidence of predisposing risk factors at diagnosis in patients with colorectal cancer. About three quarters of patients diagnosed with colorectal cancer have no obvious predisposing risk factors (ie, sporadic), whereas 25% occur in high-risk populations. FAP—familial adenomatous polyposis; HNPCC—hereditary nonpolyposis coli; IBD—inflammatory bowel disease.

independent chance of neoplastic transformation), a colonic epithelium in which multiple polyps develop shows increasing tendency for neoplasia with increasing numbers of polyps. Whether this is due to increased exposure to environmental factors, an intrinsic genetic susceptibility, or both is unclear. Information from the National Polyp Study suggests that it takes about 10 years for transformation of the smallest polyps into cancer, whereas an average of 5.5 years is required for transformation of a large polyp (> 1 cm) [8].

A standardized classification of adenomatous polyps by histologic type has not been agreed on. However, tubular adenomas are the most common histologic type of adenomatous polyps (75% to 85%), and less than 5% of these will contain foci of cancer. Tubulovillous (10% to 15% of adenomas) or villous adenomas (5% to 10% of adenomas) show malignant features in 20% and 40% of polyps, respectively.

Molecular genetic abnormalities commonly seen in sporadic colorectal cancer involve either activation of certain oncogenes, such as K-*ras*, or inactivation/loss of functional tumor suppressor genes, such as *APC*, *DCC* (deleted in colon cancer, gene found on 18q), and p53 (gene found on 17p) [2,3,4, 9]. About 10% to 13% of sporadic colorectal cancers exhibit the phenotype of microsatellite instability (generally due to hypermethylation of the *hMLH1* gene leading to gene silencing).

Diets high in total fat, protein, and calories and low in calcium and folate are associated with an increased risk of colorectal cancer [10]. However, dietary supplementation with cereal fiber, or diets high in fiber, fruits, and vegetables and low in fat have not reduced the rate of adenoma recurrence over a 3- to 4-year period. In patients with FAP, nonsteroidal anti-inflammatory drugs (NSAIDS) can prevent adenoma formation or cause adenomatous polyps to regress. Case-control studies in normal risk populations also suggest a lower risk of colorectal cancer with regular use of aspirin or other NSAIDs. Cigarette smoking has been associated with an increased tendency to form adenomas and develop colorectal cancer.

Staging and Prognosis

The most reproducible prognostic indicator for large bowel cancers is operative staging [11]. Table 8-1 is a brief summary of the tumor, node, metastasis system, which has been standardized by the Union Internationale Contre Cancer (UICC) and the American Joint Commission on Cancer (AJCC) [11]. Stage I tumors have partial bowel invasion with extension to the muscularis propria and no lymph node involvement or distant metastatic disease (old staging: Dukes' A or Modified Astler-Coller A and B1). Stage II tumors

invade through the thickness of the bowel wall and may extend to adjacent structures, but show no further tumor involvement (old staging: Dukes B or Modified Astler-Coller B2 and B3). Lymph node involvement without metastatic disease defines stage III (old staging: Duke's C or Modified Astler-Coller C1- C3). The presence of distant metastases is described as stage IV (old staging: Dukes' D).

The approximate distribution of patients at the time of diagnosis will be 15% with stage I tumor, 20% to 30% stage II, 30% to 40% stage III, and 20% to 25% stage IV. Excluding the stage IV patients, who rarely can be cured, the remaining three quarters of people have a tumor that may be approached with curative intent resection. Patients with stage I disease have an excellent prognosis (≥ 90% survival at 5 years). The natural history following surgery alone for colon cancer in the control arms of several randomized trials assessing the worth of various adjuvant chemotherapy strategies is shown in Table 8-2 according to stage of disease [12–16].

Surgical Considerations

Even if a malignant focus is found, local removal may be curative if there is no invasion beyond the mucosa. Surgical resection of the bowel segment containing the tumor, the adjacent mesentery, and the regional lymph nodes remains the primary therapy for colorectal cancer. Adjuvant chemotherapy with 5-fluorouracil (5-FU) and leucovorin decreases the risk for recurrence and improves survival rates in node-positive (stage III) patients with colon primaries [15,17,18,19], and has now supplanted adjuvant therapy with 5-FU and levamisole. Conflicting evidence exists pertaining to the benefit of adjuvant chemotherapy in patients with stage II colon cancer; because these patients have a much better prognosis than node-positive patients, the absolute benefit appears to be small. Bowel obstruction, perforation, direct extension of tumor to adjacent structure (T3), aneuploid DNA content, high S-phase fraction, or deletion of 18q are associated with a higher risk of recurrence in stage II disease.

For patients with rectal cancer, postoperative adjuvant chemotherapy and pelvic radiation has been shown to decrease local failure rate for patients with either bowel wall penetration by tumor (stage II) and in those with positive nodes (stage III) [20,21].

Table 8-1. TNM Staging of Colon and Rectal Cancer

Stage	TNM	Criteria
0	Tis, N0, M0	Carcinoma in situ
I	T1, N0, M0	Tumor invades submucosa
	T2, N0, M0	Tumor invades muscularis propria
II	T3, N0, M0	Tumor invades through muscularis propria into the subserosa, or into nonperitonealized pericolic or perirectal tissues
	T4, N0, M0	Tumor directly invades other organs or structures and/or perforates visceral peritoneum
III	Any T, N1, M0	Metastasis in 1 to 3 regional lymph nodes
	Any T, N2, M0	Metastasis to 4 or more regional lymph nodes
IV	Any T, any N, M1	Distant metastasis

Table 8-2. Survival of Colon Cancer Patients with Surgery Alone: Data from Randomized Trials

Trial	Stage	Recurrence-free Survival, %	Overall Survival, %
Intergroup 0035 [20,21]	II	7 y: 71	7 y: 72
	III	7 y: 44	7 y: 46.7
NSABP C-01 [22]	II, III	5 y: 51	5 y: 59
NCCTG [23]	High-risk II, III	5 y: 58	5 y: 63
IMPACT [24]	II	3 y: 76	3 y: 90
	III	3 y: 44	3 y: 54
Meta-analysis: portal vein [25]	All stages	5 y: not reported	5 y: 57.1
	I, II		70.5
	III		46.9

IMPACT — International Multicentre Pooled Analysis of Colon Cancer Trials; NCCTG — North Central Cancer Treatment Group; NSABP — National Surgical Adjuvant Breast and Bowel Project.

Surveillance Guidelines for Detection of Recurrent Colorectal Cancer

The American Society of Clinical Oncology's surveillance guidelines recommend the taking of a clinical history and physical examination every 3 to 6 months for the first three years, and annually thereafter [22]. All patients should have a colonoscopy to document a cancer- and polyp-free colon. Routine annual colonoscopies are not recommended for all patients, and the data are considered sufficient to recommend colonoscopy every 3 to 5 years to detect new cancers and polyps. If resection of liver metastases would be clinically indicated, it is recommended that postopoerative serum CEA testing be performed every 2 to 3 months in patients with stage II or III disease for at least 2 years after diagnosis. An elevated carcinoembryonic antigen (CEA) level should be confirmed by repeat testing; if elevated, further evaluation for metastatic disease is warranted. The cost and intensity of follow-up must be guided by the patient's ability and willingness to undertake aggressive treatment of any recurrent disease. Anastomotic or local-regional recurrences should be completely resected. Surgical resection of isolated metastases in the liver can lead to 5-year disease-free survival of about 20% [23].

Preoperative Radiation Therapy for Rectal Cancer

Preoperative radiation therapy for patients with resectable tumors is considered standard in Europe, but not in North America [24,25]. Potential advantages of preoperative radiation include the maintained vascularity of the tumor tissue, which may render it more radiosensitive. In addition, surgical adhesions that may retain normal loops of bowel in a radiation port have not formed. Potential disadvantages include possible tumor progression prior to the definitive surgical procedure. Further, in the absence of full surgical staging, a proportion of patients with stage I or IV disease will inappropriately receive radiation. Others contend that the full extent of tumor may be best defined and marked for radiation planning at the time of surgery, and that effective surgical techniques exist for excluding the small bowel from a radiation port. Randomized trials in North America attempting to compare preoperative versus postoperative adjuvant chemoirradiation closed prematurely due to poor patient accrual. Preoperative chemoirradiation has been used in patients with unresectable tumors; reduction in tumor size may allow subsequent surgery with curative intent.

Adjuvant Therapy

For stage III colon cancer primaries, bolus 5-FU with leucovorin is the current standard for adjuvant therapy [15,17,18,19]. Several dose schedules of 5-FU + leucovorin have been tested in randomized trials: bolus 5-FU with leucovorin at 425/20 mg/m^2 or 370/200 mg/m^2 daily for 5 days every 4 weeks, or 500 mg/m^2 5-FU given at the midpoint of a 2-hour infusion of 500 mg/m^2 leucovorin weekly for 6 of 8 weeks. The duration of therapy has ranged from 6 to 12 months. Results from intergroup study 0089 indicate that six cycles of the monthly schedule of 5-FU + low-dose leucovorin and four cycles of the weekly for 6 weeks schedule have comparable efficacy in terms of 5-year disease-free survival (59% and 59%) and overall survival (66% and 65%) [19]. The ongoing National Surgical Breast and Bowel Project protocol C-07 is evaluating three cycles of the weekly for 6 of 8 weeks schedule of 5-FU + high-dose leucovorin alone or with oxaliplatin, whereas a North American intergroup trial is evaluating the worth of adding irinotecan to 5-FU + leucovorin. The long-term results of these two pivotal trials will not be known for several years.

For rectal cancer, standard therapy in the United States consists of 5-FU chemotherapy in combination with pelvic irradiation. Such therapy has reduced pelvic recurrences to 8% to 12% of patients; systemic relapse is also reduced, and overall survival is improved, with 50% to 60% alive at 5 years [20,21]. A standard regimen involves two monthly cycles of bolus 5-FU 500 mg/m^2 given on days 1 to 5 prior to 5-FU + radiation (45 Gy in 25 fractions). A 540-cGy boost is given to the entire tumor bed, the adjacent lymph nodes, and the 2 cm of adjacent tissue; however, the perineum is excluded after 45 Gy in patients undergoing abdominoperineal resection. A second boost of 360 cGy can be given to a smaller field in patients with good displacement of the small bowel out of the field. One month after completing the radiation, two more cycles of bolus 5-FU, 450 mg/m^2 on days 1 to 5, are given. Maturing results from an intergroup trial will define the potential benefit of adding leucovorin to bolus 5-FU on this schedule [26]. Two schedules of 5-FU delivery during the course of radiation therapy have been compared: bolus 5-FU (500 mg/m^2 IV for 3 days during weeks 1 and 5 of radiation) or a prolonged infusion schedule (225 mg/m^2/d throughout radiation). At 4 years, patients who received concurrent infusional 5-FU had significantly higher disease-free survival (63% vs 53%; $P = 0.01$) and overall survival (70% vs 60%; $P = 0.005$) [20]. The benefit for prolonged infusion of 5-FU as a radiation sensitizer must be weighed against the costs and morbidity of the requirement for an infusion pump and a central venous device.

Radiation therapy to anatomically fixed areas of the colon outside the rectum (ie, the cecum, the splenic, and the hepatic flexures), may be incorporated into a multimodality, adjuvant regimen for T4 or node-positive tumors in an attempt to reduce local relapse. Mature results from a phase III study comparing 5-FU + levamisole alone or with adjuvant radiation therapy in patients with resected, high-risk colon cancer (T4, or T3N1-2) will define the benefit of radiation in this setting.

Therapy for Advanced Disease

In the past, there was controversy regarding the benefit of treating asymptomatic patients with metastatic colorectal cancer. However, data from several randomized prospective trials indicates that initiating chemotherapy at the time of diagnosis of metastatic disease relieves anxiety, prolongs the time before symptoms appear, and increases survival [27–29]. These trials confirm that chemotherapy with a 5-FU–based regimen is worthwhile compared with best supportive care in good-performance-status patients with metastatic disease.

A meta-analysis of randomized clinical trials in metastatic colorectal cancer comparing intravenous bolus 5-FU with or without leucovorin modulation revealed a collective response rate of 11% for 5-FU alone and 23% for 5-FU and leucovorin, without an impact on survival [30]. The two most widely used schedules are a 5-day bolus regimen repeated every 4 weeks and a weekly regimen administered for 6-week cycles separated by 2-week rests. Stomatitis and myelosuppression are more commonly associated with the former schedule, whereas diarrhea is typically dose-limiting with the weekly schedule. Randomized clinical trials in both advanced disease and the adjuvant setting suggest that these two schedules of bolus 5-FU + leucovorin are therapeutically equivalent [19,30].

A meta-analysis of eight randomized trials comparing modulation of 5-FU by methotrexate ± leucovorin rescue showed a doubling of the response rate compared with 5-FU alone (19% vs 10%; $P < 0.0001$); the median survival was also higher with methotrexate + 5-FU (10.7 vs 9.1 months; $P = 0.024$) [31]. However, modulation of 5-FU with other agents such as interferon, dipyridamole, N-phosphonacetyl-l-aspartate (PALA), and hydroxyurea has not shown an improvement in response rate, time to progression, or survival in randomized trials.

A meta-analysis of six randomized trials comparing 5-FU given by either continuous infusion or bolus injection demonstrated superiority of infusional 5-FU in terms of response rate (22.5% vs 13.6%; P = 0.002) and survival (median 12.1 vs. 11.3 months; P = 0.04) [32]. Palmar-plantar erythrodysesthesia occurs significantly more often with infusional 5-FU, whereas hematologic toxicity is more frequent with bolus 5-FU [33].

There are various infusional 5-FU schedules. Protracted low-dose infusions can either be given continuously until toxicity supervenes, or for 28 of 35 days [34]. Intermittent high-dose infusions of 5-FU are also frequently used: three such regimens include weekly 24-hour infusion alone or with leucovorin modulation [34–36], a weekly 48-hour infusion [37], and an every-2-week regimen of mixed bolus and infusional 5-FU modulated by leucovorin (de Gramont regimen) [38]. Phase III clinical trials comparing each of these high-dose weekly or every other week infusional schedules with monthly bolus 5-FU and low-dose leucovorin have shown an improvement in response rate, time to treatment failure, and reduced toxicity in favor of the infusional arm [36,37,38].

Irinotecan has activity when used as the initial therapy for metastatic colorectal cancer, and also in patients whose disease has progressed on 5-FU therapy. Randomized trials have shown that irinotecan is superior to either best supportive care or infusional 5-FU in patients with disease progression on 5-FU [39,40]. Two schedules of irinotecan are commonly used: either weekly for 4 of 6 weeks, or once every 3 weeks.

Recently, two randomized trials demonstrated that the combination of irinotecan, 5-FU, and leucovorin was associated with a significant improvement in response rate, time to progression, and survival compared with 5-FU + leucovorin alone [41,42]. Irinotecan has received approval of the US Food and Drug Administration to be used as a component of first-line therapy for patients with metastatic colorectal cancer on either of two schedules: weekly for 4 of 6 weeks (Saltz regimen) or every 2 weeks (Douillard regimen).

Capecitabine is a 5-FU prodrug with good oral bioavailability; on systemic absorption, it undergoes three sequential enzymatic reactions before 5-FU is released. The last step in the metabolic activation is mediated by thymidine phosphorylase. Phase II studies indicate that capecitabine has activity in advanced colorectal cancer, and randomized trials in metastatic colorectal cancer suggest equivalent activity when compared with monthly IV bolus 5-FU given with low-dose leucovorin [43]. Ftorafur is another 5-FU prodrug that can be administered orally. UFT is uracil combined with ftorafur in a molar ratio of 4:1. Ftorafur can be converted to 5-FU through both cytoplasmic enzymes and oxidative metabolism. Uracil serves as a competitive inhibitor of dihydropyrimidine dehydrogenase, the enzyme that governs the rate-limiting catabolism of 5-FU to dihydrofluorouracil. Thus, uracil is used to increase the availability of enzymatically generated 5-FU. UFT is active as first-line therapy for patients with advanced colorectal cancer. Randomized trials comparing oral UFT 300 mg/m^2 + LV 90 mg given in three divided doses daily for 28 of 35 days, versus monthly IV bolus 5-FU and low-dose leucovorin suggest equivalent activity [44].

Oxaliplatin, a platinum compound with a trans-L-diamino-cyclohexane moiety, has a distinct spectrum of activity compared to cisplatin, and retains activity against tumors that are defective in nucleotide mismatch repair and some cisplatin-resistant tumors. These distinguishing features have been attributed to the ability of the DACH-moiety of oxaliplatin to form bulkier DNA adducts that are more difficult to repair. Oxaliplatin has single-agent activity when used as either first-line or second-line therapy for metastatic colorectal cancer. An intriguing clinical observation is that the addition of oxaliplatin to a 5-FU + leucovorin regimen on which patients have documented disease progression may result in further tumor shrinkage or disease stabilization [45]. Phase III trials conducted in France suggest an advantage of oxaliplatin given in combination with infusional 5-FU + leucovorin regimens in terms of response rate and time to disease progression [46]. However, because no survival advantage was seen, oxaliplatin did not receive US Food and Drug Administration approval for use as initial therapy for patients with metastatic colorectal cancer. Ongoing clinical trials with oxaliplatin combined with 5-FU–based regimens are establishing its potential value as salvage therapy for patients in whom prior irinotecan and 5-FU + leucovorin fails. For first-line therapy of patients with metastatic colorectal cancer, an intergroup trial is comparing both the Saltz regimen (weekly irinotecan given with bolus 5-FU + leucovorin) and the de Gramont regimen (oxaliplatin plus mixed bolus and infusional 5-FU + leucovorin) versus irinotecan combined with oxaliplatin.

Regional therapy to the liver in patients with metastatic colorectal cancer confined to the liver using continuous hepatic arterial infusion of fluorodeoxyuridine or 5-FU has been under evaluation for several decades. In general, significantly higher response rates and improvements in time to hepatic disease progression have been achieved with regional therapy compared to intravenous therapy with 5-FU or fluorodeoxyuridine. However, this approach has not improved overall survival when compared with systemic therapy alone, and is associated with additional cost and toxicities, such as biliary sclerosis. A meta-analysis of seven randomized trials indicated a tripling of the response rate (41% vs 14%; $P < 10^{-10}$) [47]. There was a trend for greater median survival with regional therapy versus systemic intravenous therapy (16 vs 12 months; P = 0.14), but the difference was significant only seen when data were included from two trials that allowed delay in the start of intravenous chemotherapy until symptoms developed. Some patients with colorectal cancer with metastases confined to the liver whose disease has progressed on prior systemic therapy can achieve a partial response with hepatic arterial infusion of fluorodeoxyuridine. A current area of interest is the use of regional therapy alone or in combination with intravenous chemotherapy as adjuvant therapy for patients who have undergone successful resection of hepatic metastases [48].

Management of Treatment-Related Toxicity

With bolus 5-FU therapy, measures should be taken to reduce oral mucositis and to treat the diarrhea. A good oral hygiene program is essential. Because the plasma half-life of 5-FU is short (8 to 12 minutes), stomatitis may be markedly reduced in severity with oral cryotherapy (ie, holding ice chips or an iced slurry in the mouth before, during, and for 30 minutes after bolus injection). Routine antidiarrheal preparations, such as diphenoxylate hydrochloride with atropine sulfate (Lomotil; GD Searle & Co., Chicago, IL), loperamide hydrochloride (Imodium; McNeil Consumer Healthcare, Fort Washington, PA) or tincture of opium, are usually adequate to control drug-induced diarrhea of mild to moderate severity [49]. Diarrhea may be cholera-like in intensity and life-threatening, particularly with bolus schedules. With the daily for 5 days schedule of bolus 5-FU + leucovorin, diarrhea typically begins after all doses have been given. With weekly 5-FU + leucovorin, patients must be questioned carefully about any change in stool frequency or consistency before the administration of each dose; chemotherapy must be withheld if stools are loose or have increased in number over baseline. Management of severe diarrhea requires early, vigorous parenteral replacement of fluids and electrolytes. Subcutaneous injections of octreotide (Sandosatin; Novartis Pharmaceuticals Corp., East Hanover, NJ), 100 to 150 µg three times daily, may reduce or completely ablate the diarrhea within 24 to 72 hours. Disruption of the integrity of the intestinal mucosa may permit access of bacteria into the bloodstream. If the patient has concurrent neutropenia, institution of antibiotic therapy providing coverage against enteric organisms should be considered if fever develops or the patient's clinical condition deteriorates.

Irinotecan is associated with both two forms of diarrhea, early and delayed, which appear to have different mechanisms. Early diarrhea (occurring during or within 24 hours of drug administration) may be accompanied by cholinergic symptoms including abdominal cramping from hyperperistalsis, flushing, diaphoresis, lacrimation, increased salivation, and miosis. These cholinergic symptoms can be treated or prevented with atropine. Delayed diarrhea should be treated promptly, and high-dose loperamide therapy appears to be effective [49]. As described earlier for 5-FU–associated diarrhea, aggressive fluid resuscitation should be provided in the event of dehydration. Clinical studies are ongoing to assess the worth of long-acting somatostatin analogue to ameliorate irinotecan-associated diarrhea.

Infusional 5-FU regimens require the use of indwelling central venous access devices and a portable infusion pump. Catheter-associated thrombosis is an undesirable consequence of this approach. Prophylaxis with low-dose warfarin (1 mg orally daily) can reduce the incidence of catheter-associated thrombosis.

ANAL CANCER

Anal cancer is defined by cancers arising in the anal canal from the anorectal ring to the anal verge. The lining of the proximal anal canal is columnar epithelium, whereas the distal anal canal comprises stratified squamous epithelium. The dentate line is the transition zone between the proximal and distal anal canal. Anal cancer is an uncommon tumor, but the overall risk of anal cancer is rising due to an association with sexually transmitted disease [50]. Keratinizing squamous cell carcinomas are the predominant histology; typically they occur distal to the dentate line. Nonkeratinizing tumors (also referred to as transitional cell tumors) occur proximal to the dentate line. The natural history and prognosis of keratinizing and nonkeratinizing tumors is similar. Adenocarcinomas arising from anal glands or fistulae formation are rare, but appear to behave like rectal adenocarcinomas. Most of the tumor morbidity and mortality is associated with uncontrolled locoregional disease. Regional lymph node involvement generally occurs prior to spread to distant organs, and the pattern of lymphatic drainage depends on the primary tumor location. For distal cancers arising below the dentate line, the arterial supply is provided by the inferior and middle rectal arteries, venous drainage is systemic through the inferior rectal vein, and lymphatic drainage occurs most commonly through the inguinal nodes. For tumors arising proximal to the dentate line, the superior and middle rectal arteries provide the arterial supply; venous drainage is through the superior rectal vein to the portal vein, and lymphatic drainage predominantly flows to pelvic and periaortic nodes. Radical surgery has been replaced in anal cancers with chemoradiation therapy and limited sphincter-sparing resections.

Etiology and Risk Factors

In the United States, about 3400 cases of anal cancer are expected in the year 2000 [1]. The average age at diagnosis is older than 60 years. Strong risk factors include sexually transmitted diseases, particularly human papilloma virus and condylomata acuminata, a history of receptive anal intercourse, more than 10 sexual partners, immunosuppression related to organ transplantation, and, in women, a history of cervical, vulvar, or vaginal cancer [50–52]. HIV-positive patients are much more likely to have anal human papillomavirus infection. Cigarette smoking has been suggested to be another risk factor.

Staging and Prognosis

Staging based on the TNM system (Table 8-3) includes stage 0 for carcinoma in situ, stage I for tumors up to 2 cm in diameter with negative nodes, and stage II for tumors 2 to 5 cm (T2) or more than 5 cm (T3) in diameter with negative nodes [53]. Tumors of any size that extend into adjacent pelvic or peritoneal structures are T4. Stage III designates involvement of regional nodes or a T4 tumor, and is subdivided into IIIA and IIIB. Systemic metastases define stage IV disease. Early-stage lesions (0–I) have 5-year survival rates of 80% or greater. Historically, the presence of any nodal metastases, even with small tumors, confers about a 50% or worse 5-year survival rate. Locally invasive tumors, distant metastatic disease, and recurrent cancers are associated with a 7- to 12-month median survival rate. The major prognostic indicators are tumor size (< 2 cm versus all others), degree of differentiation, (well versus poorly differentiated), and site of origin (anal canal versus anal margin).

Treatment Strategy

Initial diagnostic evaluation includes anorectal digital examination and palpation of inguinal nodes as well as direct visualization with anoscopy and proctoscopy. Suspicious lesions and enlarged lymph nodes should be biopsied, but an inguinal node dissection is not useful. Concurrent benign anal pathology, such as fissures or fistulas, are commonly present. These may mask the malignant process; after a 2-week trial of appropriate analgesics and topical therapy, a malignant cause for persistent symptoms should be pursued. It is essential in the primary diagnosis and management of perianal complaints to re-evaluate after no more than 2 to 4 weeks. If a presumed benign condition has not responded markedly to treatment by that time, it must be biopsied or evaluated under anesthesia.

Table 8-3. Staging in Anal Cancer

Stage	TNM	Criteria
0	Tis, N0, M0	Carcinoma in situ
I	T1, N0, M0	Tumor < 2 cm
II	T2-3, N0, M0	Tumor 2–5 cm
IIIA	T1-3, N1, M0	Tumor spread to perirectal lymph nodes
	T4, N0, M0	Tumor spread to adjacent organs
IIIB	T4, N1, M0	Tumor spread to both adjacent organs, perirectal nodes; tumor
	Any T, N2, M0	spread to unilateral internal iliac, inguinal nodes, or both,
	Any T, N3, M0	spread to perirectal, inguinal nodes and/or bilateral internal iliac and/or inguinal nodes
IV	Any T, any N, M1	Distant lymph node metastases within abdomen or to other organs

Therapy for Primary Disease

Very early lesions of the anal margin and distal anal canal may be treated with wide local resection and skin graft. T0 to T1 lesions are found infrequently, and make up only about 10% of all tumors. Historically, abdominal-perineal resection (APR) is curative in up to half of all patients, but has now been relegated to the role of salvage therapy after an initial attempt at cure with sphincter-sparing radiation or chemoradiation therapy. Radiation therapy in doses of 60 Gy may achieve cure in more than half of all cases, but subsequent APR may be required for recurrent disease or the management of late sequelae of radiation fibrosis including proctitis, ulcers, stenosis, and necrosis.

Nonrandomized trials suggested that chemotherapy with mitomycin C and 5-FU given concurrently with radiation doses to about 50 Gy had less long-term toxicity than would be expected with higher doses of radiation given alone, but seemed to be equally efficacious in terms of local-regional control and survival. Two randomized clinical trials compared radiation therapy alone or in combination with 5-FU and mitomycin [54,55]. In these trials, 5-FU was given either as a 96-hour infusion (1000 mg/m^2/d) or a 120-hour infusion (750 mg/m^2/d) during the first and final week of radiation (45 Gy), and a single dose of mitomycin C was given (12 to 15 mg/m^2 day 1). Response was assessed 6 weeks after radiation. A radiation boost was given for patients with a partial or complete response, whereas surgery was performed for patients whose tumor had a poor response. Both trials demonstrated a significant improvement in local-regional control, and significantly fewer patients required abdominal-perineal resection (Table 8-4). Although no significant difference in overall survival was seen, the excellent local-regional control, and the ability to avoid radical surgery with colostomy has established chemoradiation as the best option for patients with anal cancer.

A randomized trial conducted by the Eastern Cooperative and Radiation Therapy Oncology Groups questioned whether the dose of mitomycin C could be omitted in an effort to reduce toxicity. With the addition of mitomycin C, local-regional control at 4 years was significantly improved (16% vs 34% failure), as was colostomy-free survival (71% vs 59%), and disease-free survival (76% vs 51%) [56]. A nonsignificant survival advantage was also observed with the mitomycin-C–containing arm (76% vs 67%). For patients with residual tumor at biopsy 6 weeks after initial therapy, additional chemoradiation with cisplatin, 5-FU, and 9 Gy radiation rendered half of the patients disease-free. Thus, abdominal-perineal resection is needed only for patients in whom primary and salvage chemoradiation fails, and in those who develop recurrent disease.

Issues that are currently being addressed in ongoing randomized trials include the value of induction chemotherapy with bolus cisplatin and 5-FU given by 96-hour infusion prior to chemoradiation, and definition of the optimal radiation dose.

Surveillance after Primary Therapy

Follow-up after treatment of the cancer includes careful examination of local-regional structures every 3 months for the first 2 to 3 years, then every 6 months for an additional 3 to 5 years. There are currently no evidence-based guidelines to recommend routine radiographic imaging or blood chemistry studies.

Only 10% and 17% of patients treated with combined chemotherapy and radiation therapy in two randomized trials developed distant metastases, most commonly in the liver; most of these patients also had local-regional recurrence [54,55]. These observations suggest that surveillance for distant metastatic disease in the absence of symptoms is likely to be a low-yield endeavor.

Immunocompromised Patients

The randomized trials that have evaluated primary chemoradiation of anal cancer have not included HIV-positive patients. Therefore, recommendations for therapy of the increasing number of patients with anal cancer who are HIV positive are not based on firm evidence. The available data suggest that combined chemotherapy plus radiation can be successfully used in HIV-positive patients with anal cancer, but the toxicity may be greater, particularly in patients whose CD4 counts are low, and when the total radiation dose exceeds 30 Gy [57,58].

Therapy for Advanced Disease

Because of its rarity, there are no established regimens to treat metastatic squamous cell cancer. Based on analogy with the efficacy of chemotherapy agents for squamous cell cancers arising in other sites, single-agent therapy with platinum analogues, taxanes, gemcitabine, and methotrexate may be considered. The potential benefit of multi- versus single-agent palliative therapy in this setting is unknown.

Table 8-4. Combined Chemotherapy and Radiation for Anal Cancer: Results from Three Randomized Trials

Cooperative Group	Trial Design and Patients Randomized (*n*)	Patients Assessable, *n*	Local-regional Failure, %	Colostomy-free Survival, %	Overall Survival, %
UK [83]	RT vs RT + 5-FU + mitomycin C (585)	562	3 y: 61 vs 36	See footnote*	3 y: 58 vs 65
		279			
		283			
EORTC [84]	RT vs RT + 5-FU + mitomycin C (110)	103	5 y: ~50 vs ~32	5 y: ~40 vs ~72	5 y: ~54 vs ~58
		52			
		51			
RTOG/ECOG [85]	RT + 5-FU vs RT + 5-FU + mitomycin C (310)	291	4 y: 34 vs 16	4 y: 59 vs 71	4 y: 67 vs 76
		145			
		146			

*In this trial, 41% of patients receiving radiation alone underwent subsequent abdominal-perineal resection, colostomy formation, or failed to have a preoperative colostomy closed, compared with 24% of patients receiving chemoirradiation.

ECOG — Eastern Cooperative Oncology Group; EORTC — European Organization for Research and Treatment of Cancer; 5-FU — 5-fluorouracil; RTOG — Radiation Therapy Oncology Group.

REFERENCES

1. Greenlee RT, Murray T, Bolden S, *et al.*: Cancer statistics, 2000. *Ca Cancer J Clin* 2000, 50:7–33.

2. Midgley R, Kerr D: Colorectal cancer. *Lancet* 1999, 353:391–399.

3. Kinzler KW, Vogelstein B: Lessons from hereditary colorectal cancer. *Cell* 1996, 87:159–170.

4. Aaltonen LA: Hereditary intestinal cancer. *Sem Cancer Biol* 2000, 10:289–298.

5. Winawer SJ, Fletcher RH, Miller L, *et al.*: Colorectal cancer screening: clinical guidelines and rationale. *Gastroenterology* 1997, 112:594–642. (Published errata appears in *Gastroenterology* 1997, 112:1060; *Gastroenterology* 1998, 114:625.]

6. Lieberman DA, Weiss DG, Bond JH, *et al.*: Use of colonoscopy to screen asymptomatic adults for colorectal cancer. *N Engl J Med* 2000, 343:162–168.

7. Imperiale TF, Wagner DR, Lin CY, *et al.*: Risk of advanced proximal neoplasms in asymptomatic adults according to the distal colorectal findings. *N Engl J Med* 2000, 343:169–174.

8. Winawer SJ, Zauber AG, Ho MN, *et al.*: Prevention of colorectal cancer by colonoscopic polypectomy: The National Polyp Study Workgroup. *N Engl J Med* 1993, 329:1977–1981.

9. Kennedy EP, Hamilton SR: Genetics of colorectal cancer. *Sem Surg Oncol* 1998, 15:126–130.

10. Jänne PA, Mayer RJ: Chemoprevention of colorectal cancer. *N Engl J Med* 2000, 342:1960–1968.

11. American Joint Committee on Cancer: Colon and Rectum. In *AJCC Cancer Staging Manual*, edn 5. Philadelphia: Lippincott-Raven; 1997:83–90.

12. Moertel CG, Fleming TR, Macdonald JS, *et al.*: Fluorouracil plus levamisole as effective adjuvant therapy after resection of stage III colon carcinoma: a final report. *Ann Intern Med* 1995, 122:321–326.

13. Moertel CG, Fleming TR, Macdonald JS, *et al.*: Fluorouracil plus levamisole as adjuvant therapy for stage II/Duke's B2 colon cancer. *J Clin Oncol* 1995, 13:2936–2943.

14. Wolmark N, Fisher B, Rockette H, *et al.*: Postoperative adjuvant chemotherapy of BCG for colon cancer: results from NSABP protocol C-01. *J Natl Cancer Inst* 1988, 80:30–36.

15. O'Connell MJ, Mailliard JA, Kahn MJ, *et al.*: Controlled trial of fluorouracil and low-dose leucovorin given for 6 months as postoperative adjuvant therapy for colon cancer. *J Clin Oncol* 1997, 15:246–250.

16. Liver Infusion Meta-analysis Group: Portal vein chemotherapy for colorectal cancer: a meta-analysis of 4000 patients in 10 studies. *J Natl Cancer Inst* 1997, 89:497–505.

17. Wolmark N, Rockette H, Fisher B, *et al.*: The benefit of leucovorin-modulated fluorouracil as postoperative adjuvant therapy for primary colon cancer: results from National Surgical Adjuvant Breast and Bowel Project Protocol C-03. *J Clin Oncol* 1993, 10:1879–1887.

18. Wolmark N, Rockette H, Mamounas E, *et al.*: Clinical trial to assess the relative efficacy of fluorouracil and leucovorin, fluorouracil and levamisole, and fluorouracil, leucovorin and levamisole in patients with Duke's B and C carcinoma of the colon: results from National Adjuvant Breast and Bowel Project protocol C-04. *J Clin Oncol* 1999, 17:3553–3559.

19. Haller DG, Catalano PJ, Macdonald JS, *et al.*: Fluorouracil, leucovorin and levamisole adjuvant therapy for colon cancer: five-year year final report of INT-0089 [abstract]. *Proc Am Soc Clin Oncol* 1998, 17:265.

20. O'Connell MJ, Martenson JA, Wieand HS, *et al.*: Improving adjuvant therapy for rectal cancer by combining protracted infusion fluorouracil with radiation therapy after curative surgery. *N Engl J Med* 1994, 33:502–507.

21. Wolmark NH, Wieand S, Hyams DM: Randomized trial of postoperative adjuvant chemotherapy with or without radiotherapy for carcinoma of the rectum: National Surgical Adjuvant Breast and Bowel Project protocol R-02. *J Natl Cancer Inst* 2000, 92:388–396.

22. Desch CE, Benson AB III, Smith TJ, *et al.*: Recommended colorectal cancer surveillance guidelines by the American Society of Clinical Oncology. *J Clin Oncol* 1999, 17:1312–1321.

23. Steele G, Bleday R, Mayer RJ, *et al.*: A prospective evaluation of hepatic resection for colorectal carcinoma metastases to the liver: Gastrointestinal Tumor Study Group Protocol 6584. *J Clin Oncol* 1991, 9:1105–1112.

24. Swedish Rectal Cancer Trial: Improved survival with preoperative radiotherapy in resectable rectal cancer. *N Engl J Med* 1997, 336:980–987.

25. Francois Y, Nemoz J, Baulieux J, *et al.*: Influence of the interval between preoperative radiation therapy and surgery on downstaging and on the rate of sphincter-sparing surgery for rectal cancer: the Lyon R90-01 randomized trial. *J Clin Oncol* 1999, 17:2396–2402.

26. Tepper JE, O'Connell MJ, Petroni GR, *et al.*: Adjuvant post-operative fluorouracil-modulated chemotherapy combined with pelvic radiation therapy for rectal cancer: initial results of intergroup 0114. *J Clin Oncol* 1997, 15:2030–2039.

27. Earlam S, Glover L, Davies M, *et al.*: Effect of regional and systemic fluorinated pyrimidine chemotherapy on quality of life in colorectal metastasis patients. *J Clin Oncol* 1997, 15:2022–2029.

28. Nordic Gastrointestinal Tumor Adjuvant Therapy Group: Expectancy of primary chemotherapy in patients with advanced asymptomatic colorectal cancer: a randomized trial. *J Clin Oncol* 1992, 10:904–911.

29. Scheithauser W, Rosen H, Kornek G-V, *et al.*: Randomized comparison of combination chemotherapy plus supportive care with supportive care alone in patients with metastatic colorectal cancer. *Br Med J* 1993, 306:752–755.

30. Advanced Colorectal Cancer Meta-analysis Project: Modulation of fluorouracil by leucovorin in patients with advanced colorectal cancer: evidence in terms of response rate. *J Clin Oncol* 1992, 10:896–903.

31. Advanced Colorectal Cancer Meta-Analysis Project: Meta-analysis of randomized trials testing the biochemical modulation of fluorouracil by methotrexate in metastatic colorectal cancer. *J Clin Oncol* 1994, 12:960–969.

32. Meta-Analysis Group In Cancer: Efficacy of intravenous continuous infusion of fluorouracil compared with bolus administration in advanced colorectal cancer. *J Clin Oncol* 1998, 16:301–308.

33. Meta-Analysis Group In Cancer: Toxicity of fluorouracil in patients with advanced colorectal cancer: effect of administration schedule and prognostic factors. *J Clin Oncol* 1998, 16:3537–3541.

34. Leichman CG, Fleming TR, Muggia FM, *et al.*: Phase II study of fluorouracil and its modulation in advanced colorectal cancer: a Southwest Oncology Group Study. *J Clin Oncol* 1995, 131:1303–1311.

35. Köhne CH, Schoffski P, Wilke H, *et al.*: Effective biomodulation by leucovorin of high-dose infusion fluorouracil given as a weekly 24-hour infusion: results of a randomized trial in patients with advanced colorectal cancer. *J Clin Oncol* 1998, 16:418–426.

36. Schmöll HJ, Köhne CH, Lorenz M, *et al.*: Weekly 24 h infusion of high-dose 5-fluorouracil with or without folinic acid vs. bolus 5-FU/FA (NCCTG/Mayo) in advanced colorectal cancer: a randomized Phase III trial of the EORTC, GITCCG and the AIO [abstract]. *Proc Am Soc Clin Oncol* 2000, 19:241.

38. Aranda E, Diaz-Rubio E, Cervantes A, *et al.*: Randomized trial comparing monthly low-dose leucovorin and fluorouracil bolus with weekly high-dose 48-hour continuous-infusion fluorouracil for advanced colorectal cancer: a Spanish Cooperative Group for Gastrointestinal Tumor Therapy (TTD) study. *Ann Oncol* 1998, 9:727–731.

39. de Gramont A, Bosset JF, Milan C, *et al.*: Randomized trial comparing monthly low-dose leucovorin and fluorouracil bolus with bimonthly high-dose leucovorin and fluorouracil bolus plus continuous infusion for advanced colorectal cancer: a French intergroup study. *J Clin Oncol* 1997, 15:808–815.

40. Cunningham D, Pyrhonen S, James RD, *et al.*: Randomised trial of irinotecan plus supportive care versus supportive care alone after fluorouracil failure for patients with metastatic colorectal cancer. *Lancet* 1998, 352:1413–1418.

41. Rougier P, Van Cutsem E, Bajetta E, *et al.*: Randomised trial of irinotecan versus fluorouracil by continuous infusion after fluorouracil failure in patients with metastatic colorectal cancer. *Lancet* 1998, 352:1407–1412. [published erratum appears in Lancet 1998, 352:1634]

41. Douillard JY, Cunningham D, Roth AD, *et al.*: Irinotecan combined with fluorouracil compared with fluorouracil alone as first-line treatment for metastatic colorectal cancer: a multicentre randomised trial. *Lancet* 2000, 355:1041–1047.

42. Saltz LB, Cox JV, Blanke C, *et al.*: Irinotecan plus fluorouracil and leucovorin for metastatic colorectal cancer. *N Engl J Med* 2000, 343:905–914.

43. Cox JV, Pazdur R, Thibault A, *et al.*: A phase III trial of Xeloda (capecitabine) in previously untreated advanced/metastatic colorectal cancer [abstract]. *Proc Am Soc Clin Oncol* 1999, 18:265.

44. Pazdur R, Douillard J-Y, Skillings JR, *et al.*: Multicenter phase III study of 5-fluorouracil or UFT in combination with leucovorin in patients with metastatic colorectal cancer [abstract]. *Proc Am Soc Clin Oncol* 1999, 18:263.

45. Andre T, Bensmaine MA, Louvet C, *et al.*: Multicenter phase II study of bimonthly high-dose leucovorin, fluorouracil infusion, and oxaliplatin for metastatic colorectal cancer resistant to the same leucovorin and fluorouracil regimen. *J Clin Oncol* 1999, 17:3560–3568.

46. de Gramont A, Figer A, Seymour M, *et al.*: Leucovorin and fluorouracil with or without oxaliplatin as first-line treatment in advanced colorectal cancer. *J Clin Oncol* 2000, 18:2938–2947.

47. Meta-Analysis Group in Cancer: Reappraisal of hepatic arterial infusion in the treatment of nonresectable liver metastases from colorectal cancer. *J Natl Cancer Inst* 1996, 88:252–258.

48. Kemeny N, Huang Y, Cohen AM, *et al.*: Hepatic arterial infusion of chemotherapy after resection of hepatic metastases from colorectal cancer. *N Engl J Med* 1999, 341:2039–2048.

49. Wadler S, Benson AB III, Engelking C, *et al.*: Recommended guidelines for the treatment of chemotherapy-induced diarrhea. *J Clin Oncol* 1998, 16:3169–3178.

50. Ryan DP, Compton CC, Meyer RJ: Carcinoma of the anal canal. *N Engl J Med* 2000, 342:792–800.

51. Frisch M, Glimelius B, van den Brule AJC, *et al.*: Sexually transmitted infection as a cause of anal cancer. *N Engl J Med* 1997, 337:1350–1358.

52. Arends MJ, Benton EC, McLaren KM, *et al.*: Renal allograft recipients with high susceptibility to cutaneous malignancy have an increased prevalence of human papillomavirus DNA in skin tumors and a greater risk of anogenital malignancy. *Br J Cancer* 1997, 75:722–728.

53. American Joint Committee on Cancer: Anal Cancer. In *AJCC Cancer Staging Manual*, edn 5. Philadelphia: Lippincott-Raven; 1997:91–95.

54. UKCCCR Anal Cancer Trial Working Party: Epidermoid anal cancer: results from the UKCCCR randomized trial of radiotherapy alone versus radiotherapy, 5-fluorouracil and mitomycin C. *Lancet* 1996, 348:1049–1054.

55. Bartelink H, Roelofsen F, Eschwege F, *et al.*: Concomitant radiotherapy and chemotherapy is superior to radiotherapy alone in the treatment of locally advanced anal cancer: results of a phase III randomized trial of the European Organization for Research and Treatment of Cancer Radiotherapy and Gastrointestinal Cooperative Groups. *J Clin Oncol* 1997, 15:2040–2049.

56. Flam M, John M, Pajack TF, *et al.*: Role of mitomycin in combination with fluorouracil and radiotherapy, and of salvage chemoradiation in the definitive nonsurgical treatment of epidermoid carcinoma of the anal canal: results of a phase III randomized intergroup study. *J Clin Oncol* 1996, 14:2527–2539.

57. Peddada AV, Smith DE, Rao AR, *et al.*: Chemotherapy and low-dose radiotherapy in the treatment of HIV-infected patients with carcinoma of the anal canal. *Int J Radiat Oncol Biol Phys* 1997, 37:1101–1105.

58. Hoffman R, Welton ML, Klencke B, *et al.*: The significance of pretreatment CD4 count on the outcome and treatment tolerance of HIV-positive patients with anal cancer. *Int J Radiat Oncol Biol Phys* 1999, 44:127–131.

BOLUS 5-FU AND LEUCOVORIN

DOSAGE AND SCHEDULING

Leucovorin 20 mg/m^2 IV bolus	■	■	■	■	■
Leucovorin + 5-FU 425 mg/m^2 IV bolus daily for 5 d q 4 wk	■	■	■	■	■
Day	1	2	3	4	5

DOSAGE AND SCHEDULING

Leucovorin 500 mg/m^2 IV over 2 h	■	■	■	■	■	■		
5-FU* 500–600 mg/m^2 IV bolus at 1 h of leucovorin infusion; repeat weekly for 6 of 8 wk	■	■	■	■	■	■		
Week	1	2	3	4	5	6	7	8

Adjuvant therapy, 500 mg/m^2; metastatic disease, 600 mg/m^2

CANDIDATES FOR TREATMENT
Patients with colorectal cancer

SPECIAL PRECAUTIONS
Pregnant and nursing patients

ALTERNATIVE THERAPY
Other 5-FU–based regimens

TOXICITIES
Myelosuppression, mucositis, diarrhea

DRUG INTERACTIONS
5-FU: allopurinol, cimetidine, folinic acid, methrotrexate, thymidine

PATIENT INFORMATION
Patient should report diarrhea > 3 × d, soreness in mouth, difficulty swallowing, rash, fever. Patient should be informed of possible skin reactions. Use of oral cryotherapy may reduce severity of mucositis

CONTINUOUS IV 5-FU

5-FU is a fluorine-substituted uracil that blocks the methylation reaction of deoxyuridylic acid to thymidylic acid, interfering with DNA synthesis. Direct incorporation of fluoropyrimidine nucleotide into DNA and RNA also occurs. With continuous daily infusion, the activity and toxicity profiles are different than those seen with bolus therapy. The mechanism responsible for these differences is not completely understood.

DOSAGE AND SCHEDULING: PROLONGED INFUSION

5-FU 300 mg/m²/24 h via ambulatory infusion pump daily for 28 of 25 d	■■■■■■■	■■■■■■■	■■■■■■■	■■■■■■■	
With concurrent radiation: 5-FU 225 mg/m²/24 h via ambulatory infusion pump throughout radiation	■■■■■■■	■■■■■■■	■■■■■■■	■■■■■■■	■■■■■■■
Day	1–7	8–14	15–21	22–28	29–35

DOSAGE AND SCHEDULING: DE GRAMONT REGIMEN

Leucovorin 200 mg/m² IV over 2 h	■	■	■	■
5-FU 400 mg/m² IV bolus followed by 600 mg/m²/22h; repeat daily for 2 d every 2 wk	■→■	■→■	■→■	■→■
Day	1	2	15	16

RECENT EXPERIENCES AND RESPONSE RATES: DE GRAMONT REGIMEN

Study	Evaluable Patients, n	Response Rate, %	Median Progression-free Survival, mo	Median Survival, mo
de Gramont et al., J Clin Oncol 1997, 15:808–815.	217 (first line)	32.6 (n = 175)	6.4	14.3

DOSAGE AND SCHEDULING: WEEKLY HIGH-DOSE 24-HOUR INFUSION

Leucovorin 500 mg/m²/2 h IV	■	■	■	■
5-FU 2600 mg/m²/24 h IV; repeat weekly	■	■	■	■
Week	1	2	3	4

RECENT EXPERIENCES AND RESPONSE RATES: WEEKLY HIGH-DOSE 24-HOUR INFUSION

Study	Evaluable Patients, n	Response Rate, %	Median Progression-free Survival, mo	Median Survival, mo
Köhne et al., J Clin Oncol 1998, 16:418–426.	91	44	7.1	16.6

CANDIDATES FOR TREATMENT
Patients with colorectal cancer

SPECIAL PRECAUTIONS
Pregnant and nursing patients

ALTERNATIVE THERAPY
Other 5-FU–based regimens

TOXICITIES
Myelosuppression and mucositis are *less* severe, palmar-plantar erythrodysesthesia (possibly dose-limiting); loss of appetite, diarrhea, abdominal cramps, difficulty with coordination, mouth sores, dry skin or nose, splitting fingernails, metallic taste, watery eyes, nausea, vomiting, temporary alopecia, leukopenia leading to anemia, photosensitivity, skin rash, hyperpigmentation, local tissue irritation if drug extravasation occurs

DRUG INTERACTIONS
5-FU: allopurinol, cimetidine, folinic acid, methotrexate, thymidine

NURSING INTERVENTIONS
Instruct patient in care of semipermanent IV access and ambulatory pump; assess patient performance and mental status; monitor weight, encourage adequate fluid, caloric, and protein intake; give antiemetics, antidiarrheals, food supplements as necessary; monitor blood counts and liver function

PATIENT INFORMATION
Patient should report diarrhea > 3 ×/d, soreness in mouth, difficulty swallowing, rash, fever. Patient should be informed of possible skin reactions.

IRINOTECAN

DOSAGE AND SCHEDULING

Irinotecan 350 mg/m^2/90 min every 3 wk	■			■		
Irinotecan 125 mg/m^2/90 min weekly for 4 of 6 wk	■	■	■	■		
Week	1	2	3	4	5	6

RECENT EXPERIENCES AND RESPONSE RATES

Study	Evaluable Patients, n	Regimen	Response Rate, %	Median Survival, mo
Saltz et al., N Engl J Med 2000, 343:905–9145	226 (first line)	Weekly	18	12.0
Rougier et al., Lancet 1998, 352:1407–1412	133 (prior 5-FU)	q 3 wk	4.5	10.8
Cunningham et al., Lancet 1998, 352:1413–1418.	189 (prior 5-FU)	q 3 wk	Not reported	9.2

CANDIDATES FOR TREATMENT
Patients with colorectal cancer whose disease has progressed on 5-FU therapy

SPECIAL PRECAUTIONS
Pregnant and nursing patients; impaired hepatic function

ALTERNATIVE THERAPIES
Infusional 5-FU in patients with prior bolus 5-FU

TOXICITIES
Early diarrhea; delayed diarrhea; myelosuppression; nausea and vomiting

DRUG INTERACTIONS
Prior pelvic/abdominal irradiation increases risk of myelosuppression

NURSING INTERVENTIONS
Atropine can relieve early diarrhea

PATIENT INFORMATION
Loperamide 4 mg orally at the first onset of delayed diarrhea, then 2 mg every 2 h until the patient is diarrhea-free for at least 12 h. During the night, the patient can take 4 mg every 4 h.

IRINOTECAN, 5-FU, AND LEUCOVORIN

DOSAGE AND SCHEDULING

Irinotecan 125 mg/m²/90 min IV	■	■	■	■		
Leucovorin 20 mg/m² IV bolus	■	■	■	■		
5-FU 500 mg/m² IV bolus; repeat weekly for 4 of 6 wk	■	■	■	■		
Week	1	2	3	4	5	6

RECENT EXPERIENCES AND RESPONSE RATES

Study	Evaluable Patients, n	Regimen	Response Rate, %	Median Progression-free Survival, mo	Median Survival, mo
Saltz et al., N Engl J Med 2000, 343:905–914	231	Irinotecan + 5-FU + leucovorin	39; P< 0.001	7.0; P = 0.004	14.8; P = 0.04
	226	5-FU + LV (Mayo)	21	4.3	12.6
Douillard et al., Lancet 2000, 355:1041–1047	198	Irinotecan + 5-FU + leucovorin	34.8; P=0.005	6.7; P < 0.001	17.4; P=0.031
	187	5-FU + leucovorin (de Gramont)	21.9	4.4	14.1

CANDIDATES FOR TREATMENT
Initial therapy for metastatic colorectal cancer

SPECIAL PRECAUTIONS
Pregnant and nursing patients; impaired hepatic function

ALTERNATIVE THERAPIES
Other 5-FU–based regimens

TOXICITIES
Early and late diarrhea, myelosuppression, nausea and vomiting, mucositis

DRUG INTERACTIONS
Prior pelvic/abdominal irradiation may increase risk of myelosuppression with irinotecan; 5-FU: allopurinol, cimetidine, folinic acid, methrotrexate, thymidine

PATIENT INFORMATION
Loperamide 4 mg orally at the first onset of delayed diarrhea, then 2 mg every 2 h until the patient is diarrhea-free for at least 12 h

COMBINED MODALITY THERAPY FOR ANAL CANCER

DOSAGE AND SCHEDULING (US INTERGROUP TRIAL): PRIMARY THERAPY

	1	2	3	4	5
5-FU 1000 mg/m²/24 h for 96 h	■■■■				■■■■
Mitomycin C 10 mg/m² IV day 1	■				■
Radiotherapy 45 Gy days 1–5	■■■■■	■■■■■	■■■■■	■■■■■	■■■■■
Week	1	2	3	4	5

DOSAGE AND SCHEDULING: SALVAGE THERAPY

	1
5-FU 1000 mg/m²/24 h for 96 h	■■■■
Cisplatin 100 mg/m²/6 h IV day 2	■
Radiotherapy 9 Gy days 1–5	■■■■■
Week	1

CANDIDATES FOR TREATMENT
Patients with primary anal cancer

SPECIAL PRECAUTIONS
Immunocompromised patients; pregnant and nursing patients; avoid in patients with pre-existing cytopenias

ALTERNATIVE THERAPIES
Radiation therapy alone or less effective

TOXICITIES
Diarrhea, cutaneous, myelosuppression

DRUG INTERACTIONS
5-FU: allopurinol, cimetidine, folinic acid, methrotrexate, thymidine

NURSING INTERVENTIONS
Mitomycin is a vesicant, and should be given through a free-flowing IV

PATIENT INFORMATION
Severe local skin reactions may occur

Roger Stupp, Everett E. Vokes

ETIOLOGY AND RISK FACTORS

Cancers of the head and neck comprise approximately 5% of malignancies in the United States [1]. Incidence is higher in African Americans and in all men but the rate is declining in white men. Tobacco and alcohol are the two major risk factors. Increasing tobacco consumption is responsible for a rising incidence of head and neck cancer in women. Tobacco chewing is a common risk factor in Asia that results in a high incidence of head and neck cancer in parts of the Far East. Although alcohol and tobacco are independent risk factors, together they produce an often a synergistic potentiation of the carcinogenic risk [2].

Other possible risk factors include nutritional deficiencies, poor orodental care, an immunocompromised state, and a genetic disposition (Table 9-1). Exposure to wood dust, nickel scraps, or textile fibers is associated with adenocarcinoma of the paranasal sinuses. Nasopharyngeal carcinoma is associated with Epstein-Barr-Virus (EBV) and is endemic in some regions of North Africa and Asia [3,4]. An increased incidence of oral cancer with chronic infection of herpes virus and Papillomavirus is suggested. Genetic factors may account for increased susceptibility. Mutations of the *p53* tumor suppressor gene and other genes are frequent [5]. Head and neck cancer is typically an environmentally induced disease and avoidance of the risk factors is the best prevention. Patients at risk should receive a regular physical examination, careful inspection of the oral cavity, discussion with the patient about changes in eating habits, and early referral for laryngoscopy if hoarseness or other symptoms persist (Table 9-2).

STAGING AND PROGNOSIS

Head and neck cancer comprises a heterogeneous group of cancers originating from different primary localizations. Squamous cell carcinoma is the commonest histologic type in adults. Other histologic diagnoses include adenocarcinoma, adenoid cystic carcinoma, mucoepidermoid carcinoma and undifferentiated carcinoma of the nasopharynx type. Lymphoma, Hodgkin's disease, sarcoma, and melanoma may all arise in the head and neck and must therefore be distinguished. Metastases of lung cancer or gastrointestinal neoplasms may present primarily in the neck. Treatment depends on localization, resectability, and histology. For squamous cell carcinoma, local and regional extension determines the stage and prognosis.

Tumor staging depends on the exact anatomic localization of the tumor. Lesions considered to be T1 and T2 are small primary tumors, whereas T3 and T4 lesions are locally advanced, with T4 invading surrounding structures (*eg*, bone, cartilage, skin). Regional lymph nodes are staged uniformly for all anatomic sites as N1 to N3 according to increasing size and number of nodes (Table 9-3). Stages I and II represent T1N0 and T2N0 lesions, respectively, whereas stages III and IV represent locally advanced disease (T3, T4) and regional involvement (N1–N3). Distant metastases are present in 10% of patients at diagnosis and are included in stage IV. Lungs, bones, and liver are the most commonly involved sites [6]. Most patients (60%) have locoregionally advanced disease (T3 and T4 or N1–N3) at presentation and die of locoregional disease, indicating the inability of currently available therapy to produce cure consistently. Nodal neck involvement appears to be the most important prognostic factor (Table 9-4). Up to 25% of the patients with advanced squamous cell carcinoma relapse with distant metastases, and autopsy series suggest 40% to 50% of the patients to have occult metastatic disease. Less than 30% of patients with locally advanced disease are cured with surgery and radiation therapy alone, but cure may be achieved in more patients with combined modality treatment. In early stage disease, cure rates vary from 60% to 90%. Laryngeal cancer appears to have a somewhat better prognosis than other tumor sites. Poor tissue vascularization and hoarseness as symptoms leading to early diagnosis may be contributing factors to higher cure rates in larynx cancer.

Nasopharyngeal Cancer and Epstein-Barr Virus

Nasopharyngeal cancer with a distinct undifferentiated or lymphoepithelial histology must be considered separately from cancer in the nasopharynx with squamous cell histology. Surgical

---

Table 9-1. Risk Factors

Tobacco	Smokeless tobacco (chewing)
Alcohol	Malnutrition
Poor orodental care	Mechanical irritation
Genetic susceptibility	Viruses: Epstein–Barr virus, herpes simplex virus, human papilloma virus
Occupational exposure: wood dust, textile fibers, nickel, cadmium, radium	

Table 9-2. Prevention and Early Detection

Prevention	Early Detection (Patients at Risk)
Avoid alcohol	Yearly physical examination with special attention to the upper aerodigestive tract and neck
Avoid smoking	Digital examination of oral cavity
Avoid combination of alcohol and smoking	Refer to ear, nose, and throat specialist for unexplained symptoms lasting > 4 weeks
Discontinue risk factor exposure after diagnosis: reduction of risk of second malignancy	Leukoplakia as possible early sign of transformation: biopsy and frequent follow-up necessary
Participation in chemoprevention trials (*see* Table 9-6)	

Table 9-3. TNM Staging and Survival

	5-y Survival		N0	N1	N2	N3
Stage I	75%–90%	T1				
Stage II	40%–70%	T2				
Stage III	20%–50%	T3				
Stage IV	<10%–30%	T4		(any M1)		

Stages I and II	Early stage	N0	no lymph node involved
T3N0, T1-2, N1	Intermediate stage	N1	single ipsilateral lymph node, <3 cm
T3, T4 and N1-3, M0	Locoregionally advanced	N2	nodes > 3–6 cm
Advanced		N2a	single node, ipsilateral
		N2b	multiple nodes, ipsilateral
		N2c	multiple nodes, bilateral or contralateral
		N3	lymph node > 6 cm

---

accessibility is difficult and because of its hidden location, the cancer causes few symptoms. Most patients present with an advanced stage of disease, nodal involvement, and frequently distant metastases. Undifferentiated carcinoma of the nasopharynx is one of the commonest tumor types in Southeast Asia. A strong etiologic association has been found for EBV infection [4]. Activation of the viral genome may be caused by frequent consumption of salted fish or nitrosamines. EBV genome and viral protein expression can be detected in most nasopharyngeal tumors. Nasopharyngeal cancer is exquisitely sensitive to both radiation and chemotherapy, suggesting the usefulness of a combined modality treatment. In a randomized trial, three cycles of BEC chemotherapy (bleomycin, epirubicin, cisplatin) followed by radiation were compared with radiotherapy alone [7]. Despite an excess in toxic deaths in the experimental arm, which correlated with the experience of the treating center, a significantly improved disease-free survival rate with induction

chemotherapy was observed. In a randomized intergroup trial, concomitant chemoradiotherapy with cisplatin followed by adjuvant chemotherapy with cisplatin and 5-fluorouracil (5-FU) was compared with standard radiotherapy (RT). This trial was closed early after an interim analysis showed a significantly improved outcome for the combined modality treatment (3-year survival 76% versus 46% with RT and radiation and concomitant chemotherapy, respectively, *P*<0.001) [8]. Similarly, a randomized trial from Hong Kong reported improved local control with concomitant cisplatin chemotherapy (40 mg/m2 weekly) and radiotherapy [9]. In the light of these results, all patients should be treated with chemotherapy and radiation. Repeated cycles of systemically active chemotherapy are needed because of an elevated risk of distant metastases.

Salivary Gland Cancer

Salivary gland cancers are different form squamous carcinomas of the head and neck. Histologically, these are commonly adenocarcinomas, adenoid cystic carcinomas [10], or mucoepidermoid carcinomas. Low-grade histologies tend to recur locoregionally with a natural history over many years, whereas high-grade tumors frequently invade adjacent muscle, bone, and nerves. Management of these tumors affecting primarily elderly patients is mainly surgical; adenoid cystic carcinoma is sensitive to radiation. Chemotherapy for recurrent or metastatic disease commonly includes an anthracycline-containing regimen (*eg*, CAP [cyclophosphamide, doxorubicin, cisplatin] or FAP [5-FU, doxorubicin, cisplatin]).

TREATMENT STRATEGY

Stage is the main determinant factor when deciding on a treatment strategy for an individual patient (Fig. 9-1) [11]. Patients are best evaluated jointly by a head and neck surgeon, a radiation therapist,

Table 9-4. Prognostic Factors

	Comment
Nodal involvement, N-stage	Most important prognostic factor: N0 better than N+
Extracapsular spread	Tendency for recurrence in the neck and distant metastases
Tumor size	
Histologic differentiation	Salivary gland cancer only
Hypopharynx	Commonly advanced with poor outcome
Larynx	Overall prognostically better, potential for organ preservation with induction chemotherapy
Nasopharynx	Chemosensitive tumor, tendency for distant metastases, median survival 4–5 y, late relapses frequent

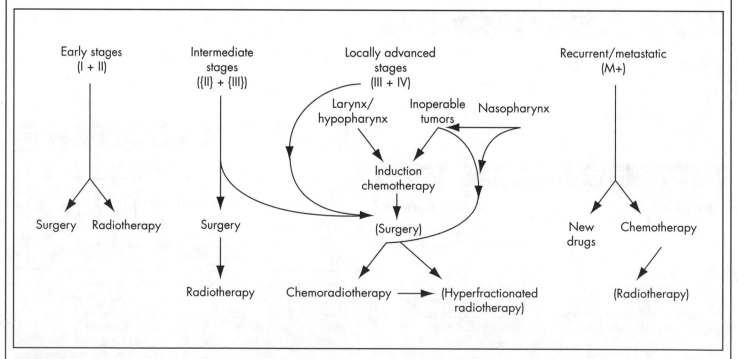

FIGURE 9-1.

Treatment strategies for head and neck cancer. (*Adapted from* Stupp and Vokes [11].)

and a medical oncologist. In addition, an experienced radiologist, an oral surgeon, a nutritionist, and a social worker are often valuable resources when determining an overall treatment strategy.

Early stage cancers can usually be cured with surgery, RT, or a combination of both. In the frequently locally advanced stages, a multimodal approach is necessary for optimal patient care. Local control can be improved by concomitant chemoradiotherapy. Organ preservation with sequential or concomitant chemo- and radiation therapy can be an important goal for compliant patients. Surgery is then reserved to patients failing to respond or with recurrent disease. For patients who cannot comply with a lengthy and intensive treatment and regular follow-up, radical surgery remains the treatment of choice. Patients with recurrent or metastatic disease, are candidates for palliative chemotherapy [12].

Early-stage Disease

Early stage tumors (T1 + T2) can be cured with surgery combined with RT or with RT alone in 60% to 90% of cases. If surgery is performed, it frequently includes elective dissection of the regional lymph nodes. This procedure allows more accurate pathologic staging with important prognostic and therapeutic implications. In more than 50% of cases, the pathologic stage will be higher than the clinical stage. Newer radiologic procedures (eg, ultrasound, computer tomography, magnetic resonance imaging, positron emission tomography) also have an increasing role in the staging of this disease.

A similar outcome in early stage disease can be achieved with radiation therapy. Primary RT may allow for organ preservation and may be an alternative to surgery in patients with serious underlying morbidities (eg, chronic obstructive pulmonary disease, coronary artery disease, or liver cirrhosis). Radiation therapy is a lengthy process over 6 to 7 weeks with mucositis, xerostomia, and loss of taste as the major secondary effects. This modality should only be chosen for reliable and compliant patients. For early-stage laryngeal cancer, RT therapy is often the first choice; laser resection and partial laryngectomy may be alternative treatments.

Locally Advanced Disease

Up to 70% of patients initially present with locally advanced disease (stage III + IV) and many patients' disease does recur locally or regionally. In locally advanced disease, bimodal therapy with surgery followed by RT has been the standard treatment for the last 3 decades in patients with resectable disease. This approach resulted in low cure rates of less than 20% to 30%. Depending on localization and size of the primary, surgery may lead to impaired or lost organ function, muscle atrophy, and disfigurement. New strategies have been developed to improve cure rates and overall survival. Multimodal therapy, with concomitant chemoradiotherapy, improves locoregional control and survival; induction chemotherapy allows for organ preservation in patients with advanced laryngeal and hypopharyngeal tumors. Combined modality therapy must now be considered the standard approach for most patients with locally advanced head and neck carcinomas.

Induction Chemotherapy

Rationale

Early use of chemotherapy as induction or neoadjuvant treatment has the theoretical advantage of an intact vascular bed (before surgery, with improved delivery of chemotherapy) and early control of systemic micrometastases [13]. With improved control of locoregional disease, the latter may be important for long-term survival.

Induction chemotherapy might also facilitate surgery or allow for organ preservation. Chemosensitive tumors with a better prognosis may be identified. Conversely, delaying surgery might result in only incomplete resectability because of tumor progression. Patients who respond may subsequently refuse the planned surgery or RT and thus miss the opportunity for cure. Finally, induction chemotherapy prolongs the overall treatment duration by another 3 months and increases toxicity and raises cost with no proven overall benefit to overall survival. Induction chemotherapy should be restricted to patients with laryngeal and hypopharyngeal carcinoma that aims at organ preservation and to inoperable patients. Neoadjuvant chemotherapy to facilitate subsequent surgery should not be given.

Induction chemotherapy with cisplatin and 5-FU results in complete response rates of 20% to 50% and a overall response rate of 80% to 100%. Responding patients do survive longer, but this mainly reflects patient selection. Most investigators administer three to four cycles of induction chemotherapy [14].

Randomized Trials

Although induction chemotherapy with cisplatin and 5-FU results in high response rates, this has not translated into a significant survival advantage in six conclusive randomized trials [14–19]. However, a reduction in distant metastasis was demonstrated, which suggests systemic activity against early micrometastatic disease [14,15,20]. Improved survival was shown for primarily inoperable patients after induction chemotherapy followed by radiation [14]. A survival advantage was also shown by subset analysis for patients with oral cancer and N2-disease after induction and adjuvant chemotherapy [21].

Organ Preservation

Organ preservation has been a primary endpoint of two randomized trials [15,19]. Patients with larynx cancer [15] and pyriform sinus cancer [19] were treated with three cycles of induction chemotherapy with cisplatin and 5-FU, patients who responded then received definitive radiation. Surgery was restricted to unresponsive [14] or incompletely responsive [18] patients, and as salvage treatment in patients with residual disease after radiation or with recurrent disease. For laryngeal primaries, organ preservation at 3 years was 64%, for hypopharyngeal primaries, the 3-year estimates of survival with a functional larynx was 42%. The feasibility of organ preservation has also been shown for nonlaryngeal sites [22]. The European Organization for the Research and Treatment of Cancer (EORTC) is conducting a randomized trial comparing alternating chemoradiotherapy with induction chemotherapy followed by radiation. Organ preservation in resectable hypopharyngeal and laryngeal cancer is the major endpoint.

Concomitant Chemoradiotherapy

Concepts and Rationale

High response rates and consistently decreased incidence of distant metastases underline the efficacy of chemotherapy in the treatment of squamous cell head and neck cancer. Use of chemotherapy as a radiation sensitizer is well established. The goal of concomitant chemoradiotherapy is to administer both treatment modalities at an optimal dose and schedule simultaneously within a short time. Overall three different, but similar, concepts have been investigated:

1. Standard and uninterrupted radiation with simultaneous low-dose single agent chemotherapy with a pure radiosensitizing objective.

2. Modified radiation therapy schedule with planned treatment breaks and simultaneous, intensified (at systemically active doses) combination chemotherapy
3. Rapidly alternating sequenced therapy with radiation and combination chemotherapy.

The rationale for concomitant chemotherapy and RT has been reviewed extensively [23,24]. Concomitant chemotherapy may eradicate radiation resistant tumor cells, presumably by making the tumor cells more susceptible to radiation. Further, chemotherapy may eliminate micrometastatic disease outside the radiation field (spatial cooperation). Although concomitant chemoradiotherapy enhances treatment efficacy, it also adds significant toxicity. Mucositis, neutropenia, and infections can be severe and occasionally life-threatening complications [25,26]. Nevertheless, concomitant intensive chemoradiotherapy is the treatment of choice for most patients with advanced head and neck cancer. Because of increased acute toxicities, these treatments should be administered by an experienced and multidisciplinary team. Most patients require close follow-up and supportive care (*eg*, percutaneous endoscopic gastrostomy).

Randomized Trials

Many well-conducted randomized trials were published in the past few years, all suggesting improved locoregional control or prolonged survival with concomitant chemoradiotherapy. 5-FU has been widely used with concomitant radiation [27]. In a placebo-controlled trial, 5-FU (1200 mg/m^2 continuous infusion, days1 to 3) was added to standard RT on weeks 1 and 3. The 2-year survival with 5-FU was 63% versus 50% (P=0.076) without chemotherapy [28]. There was no impact on the incidence of distant metastases. In an earlier trial, 5-FU bolus (250 mg/m^2) every other day was comparable with hyperfractionated twice daily radiotherapy (2 × 1.1 Gy) and significantly superior to standard RT alone. Median survival was 85, 84, and 38 months, respectively. Prolonged survival was also shown for cisplatin (50 mg/wk) and standard radiation versus RT alone. The 2-year survival rates were 75% versus 44% (P<0.05) [29]. The combination of cisplatin (12 mg/m^2, days 1 to 5) and 5-FU (600 mg/m^2, days 1 to 5) during the 1st and 6th weeks of hyperfractionated radiotherapy was compared with twice daily hyperfractionated (125 cGy twice daily) RT alone, suggesting an improved 3-year survival (28% vs 15%, P=0.06) and a decreased incidence of distant metastases [30].

In a large randomized multicenter trial concomitant, split course chemoradiotherapy with cisplatin and 5-FU was compared with sequential chemotherapy (induction) followed by radiation. Locoregional control was improved in the concomitant arm; however, an excess death rate due to complications in the concomitant chemoradiotherapy arm emphasize the increase in toxicity and necessity of center experience [25]. Intergroup 0126 compared standard RT (2 Gy/d, 70 Gy) with the same RT and concomitant cisplatin (100 mg/m^2, days 1, 22, and 43) and with split-course RT and three cycles of concomitant cisplatin (75 mg/m^2) and 5-FU (1000 mg/m^2 continuous infusion, days 1 to 4) chemotherapy [31]. Improved survival was seen with the concomitant administration of chemotherapy and uninterrupted standard RT. However, split-course radiation and a more intensive combination chemotherapy regimen did not improve survival rates, possibly due to unnecessarily long delays of RT, whereas only 10% of patients underwent the planned surgery. Intensive chemoradiotherapy regimens are required to improve both local control and distant failure rate [32–36].

In a randomized trial, rapidly alternating chemoradiotherapy with cisplatin/bolus 5-FU was compared with standard RT [37]. Of 157 patients with advanced, unresectable head and neck cancer, 41% of the patients treated with combined modalities survived at 3 years but only 23% in the RT alone treatment group (P<0.05). Recent and ongoing trials attempt to improve response and overall outcome by using hyperfractionated radiation therapy with chemotherapy [39] or accelerated RT with concomitant combination chemotherapy and amifostine as a cytoprotective agent [39]. Promise has also been suggested by the addition of an antiepidermal growth factor (EGF)-receptor monoclonal antibody to radiation [40,41] A prospective randomized trial is ongoing.

Hyperfractionated Radiotherapy

Concepts and Rationale

Altered fractionation schemes have been extensively evaluated in head and neck cancer [42]. Shortening the time interval between doses reduces tumor repopulation. Simple hyperfractionation (smaller dose per fraction) leads to better tumor control with less late toxicity, allowing for administration of higher total doses. Accelerated hyperfractionated radiation delivers higher radiation doses per treatment time. Increased treatment intensity however leads to more acute toxicity.

Randomized Trials

Despite several randomized trials a benefit of hyperfractionation has only been demonstrated in a few studies [43–46]. Possibly the increased acute toxicity with accelerated treatment regimes lead to more treatment interruptions, thus loosing the gained benefit. In a randomized trial reported by Sanchiz and coworkers [45] in 1990 hyperfractionated (64 fractions of 1.1 Gy, 2 fractions/d) was equivalent to chemoradiation (30 × 2 Gy, + 5-FU every other day), but significantly superior to conventional radiotherapy alone. Pinto *et al.* [46] reported improved locoregional control and survival for patients with unresectable stage III and IV oropharyngeal cancer treated with hyperfractionated RT. Two early EORTC trials suggest an improved local control with hyperfractionated radiation [43,44]. However, the RTOG could not demonstrate a benefit with hyperfractionation [47]. The randomized continuous hyperfractionated

Table 9-5. Current Treatment Regimens

	Response Rates[†]
Methotrexate 40–60 mg/m^2 IV weekly	10%–29%
Cisplatin 100 mg/m^2 iv every 3–4 wk	15%–27%
Cisplatin 100 mg/m^2 + 5-FU 800–1000 mg/daily as continuous infusion for 4–5 d, repeat every 3–4 wk*	30%–80%
Carboplatin 300–400 mg/m^2 + 5-FU 800–1000 mg/m^2 daily as continuous infusion for 4–5 d, repeat every 3–4 wk	20%–25%
Cisplatin 100 mg/m^2 + 5-FU 600–800 mg/m^2 with leucovorin (PFL) daily as continuous infusion for 4–5 d, repeat every 3–4 wk*	15%–90%
Docetaxel 100 mg/m2 IV every 3 wk	21%–43
Paclitaxel 135–175 mg/m^2 over 3–24 h every 3–4 wk	30%–40%
Docetaxel 75 mg/m2 + cisplatin 75 mg/m2 + 5-FU 750 mg/m2 daily as continuous infusion for 5 d, repeat every 3 wk	—
Cisplatin, 5-FU, hydroxyurea and concomitant radiation*	70%–80%

*See separate listing later in this chapter.
†Range for untreated and recurrent disease.

accelerated radiotherapy trial (CHART) giving three daily fractions (3 × 1.50 Gy) for 12 days continuously also could not confirm an earlier impression of improved locoregional control [48].

Recently, the first results of a large randomized RTOG trial were reported [49]. Over 1100 patients were randomized between standard once daily RT, or hyperfractionated RT (2 × 1.2 Gy, 81.6 Gy for 7 weeks), or accelerated split course RT (2 × 1.6 Gy/67.2 Gy for 8 weeks including a planned 2-week rest) and accelerated RT with concomitant boost 1 x 1.8 Gy + 1 × 1.5 Gy boost in the afternoon of the last 2.5 weeks, 72 Gy/6 weeks). Locoregional control rates were 46% and 47.5% for the standard fractionation and accelerated split-course RT, respectively, compared with 54.4% and 54.5% with hyperfractionation and accelerated concomitant boost RT (P=0.05). An increased incidence of grade III acute toxicity or higher was observed in all three experimental treatment arms (35% with standard fractionation, compared with 2) 55%, 3) 50%, and 4) 59% with altered fractionation). No significant difference was observed in the incidence of late effects.

The French GORTEC study conducted a randomized trial on 268 patients with locally advanced inoperable head and neck cancer [50]. Standard once daily RT (70 Gy in 7 weeks) was compared with accelerated RT (2 Gy twice daily, 62 to 64 Gy in 3 weeks). Acute toxicity was substantial and prolonged in the accelerated treatment; however, no difference was seen in late toxicity. Both locoregional control (58% vs 34% at 2 years; P=0.01) and overall survival (2-year survival: 38% vs 25%; P=0.13) were improved with the accelerated arm. This regimen is now compared with concomitant radiochemotherapy.

Adjuvant Radiotherapy

Primary treatment of head and neck cancer frequently involves primary surgery followed by postoperative radiotherapy. Indications for adjuvant radiation include involved or close surgical margins, perineural involvement, advanced primary tumor (T3 or T4), advanced nodal stage (N2 or N3) or lymph node involvement with extracapsular spread. Two similar randomized trials by the RTOG and EORTC of postoperative RT with or without concomitant chemotherapy (cisplatin 100 mg x 3 doses) have been completed and first results are expected in 2001.

Recurrent or Metastatic Disease

Chemotherapy has traditionally been used only in recurrent or metastatic disease [11,51]. In this setting, the following drugs have been found effective: methotrexate, cisplatin, carboplatin, 5-FU, bleomycin, mitomycin C, cyclophosphamide, doxorubicin, and hydroxyurea. More recently paclitaxel [52], docetaxel [53–55], gemcitabine [56], vinorelbine [57,58], topotecan, and MTA [59] have shown activity (Table 9-5). Response rates as single agents are 10% to 30% with a short response duration of only 2 to 6 months.

A combination of cisplatin and 5-FU has frequently been used for recurrent disease with response rates of 30% to 40 %. In a randomized trial, the response rate for the combination was 32%, compared with 13% for single agent 5-FU and 17% for cisplatin [60]. Despite this increased response rate, an improved survival rate could not been demonstrated. Another randomized trial compared cisplatin/5-FU and carboplatin/5-FU with methotrexate [61]. Response rates were 32%, 21%, and 10%, respectively. Median response durations was only 4.2, 5.1, and 4.1 months, respectively, and no difference in overall survival was observed. This combination increased toxicity—nausea and vomiting, nephrotoxicity, and ototoxicity. Patients receiving 5-FU experienced significant mucositis. Patients with a poor performance status usually tolerate chemotherapy less well and are more prone to complications. Because of the lack of a survival advantage, some investigators still consider single-agent methotrexate as standard chemotherapy despite its low response rates. Paclitaxel has shown promise in phase II trials [52]; however, a randomized phase II study comparing two schedules of paclitaxel and weekly methotrexate was unable to suggest a higher activity with the newer agent [62]. Combining a taxane with cisplatin and 5-FU is feasible [63,64] and will be further explored in a randomized EORTC trial.

CHEMOPREVENTION
Leukoplakia

Oral leukoplakia is a recognized premalignant condition, which can lead to invasive squamous cell carcinoma. Thus, 13-cis-retinoic acid has been shown efficacious in reversing this precancerous condition (Table 9-6) [65]. The response rate was 67% with a clinical complete response of 54% and a histologic response of 38%. In the high

Table 9-6. Current Cooperative Group Trials

Group	Patient Selection	Treatment	Remarks
Intergroup	Larynx, resectable, stage III/IV (not T1 or T4)	Radiotherapy vs cisplatin/RT vs induction CT-RT	Goal: larynx preservation NCI high priority trial
Intergroup	Resectable, stage III/IV	Surgery + RT vs surgery + RT/cisplatin	
ECOG/Intergroup	Unresectable head and neck cancer	Cisplatin/RT vs PF + split course RT vs standard RT	
SAKK	Most sites, stage III/IV locoregionally advanced	Hyperfractionated RT vs hyperfract RT/cisplatin	
EORTC	Early stage oral cavity; larynx and lung cancer	Postoperative RT vs postoperative RT/cisplatin	
England	Most sites, stage III/IV locoregionally advanced	CHART vs conventional RT	
Intergroup/RTOG	T1N0, T2N0 oral cavity, pharynx, larynx	Isotretinoin vs placebo	Chemoprevention
ECOG/NCCTG	T1N0, T2N0 head and neck cancer	Isotretinoin vs placebo	Chemoprevention
SWOG	T1N0, T2N0 head and neck cancer	Beta-carotene vs placebo	Chemoprevention
Euroscan/EORTC	Early stage oral cavity; larynx and lung cancer	N-acetylcystein vs retinylpalmitat vs N-acetylc. + R.-palmitat bs observation only	Chemoprevention: accrual complete, first results expected by 1997

CHART—Continous hyperfractionated, accelerated radiation therapy; CT—chemotherapy; ECOG—Eastern Cooperative Oncology Group; EORTC—European Organisation for Research and Treatment of Cancer; NCCTG—Northern California Cancer Treatment Group; RT—radiotherapy; RTOG—Radiation Therapy Oncology Group; SAKK—Swiss Group for Clinical Cancer Research.

HEAD AND NECK CANCER

Table 9-7. Chemoprevention Trails With 13-*cis* Retinoic Acid

	Evaluable Patients, *n*	Regimen	Response Rates
Oral Leucoplakia			
Induction–3 mo	24	*cis*-RA 1–2 mg/kg	16 (67%)
(Hong *et al.* [65])	20	Placebo	2 (10%)
			(*P*=0.0002)
			Progression
Maintenance–9 mo	26	*cis*-RA 0.5 mg/kg	2 (8%)
(Lippman *et al.* [66])	33	Beta-carotene	16 (55%)
			(*P*<0.001)
Second Malignancies			**Second Primary**
Maintenance–12 mo	49	*cis*-RA 50–100 mg/m²	2 (4%)
(Hong *et al.* [60])	51	Placebo	12 (24%)

dosages used (1 to 2 mg/kg), the retinoic acid has significant toxicity, particularly dry and peeling skin, facial erythema, cheilitis (79%), hypertriglyceridemia (71%), conjunctivitis (54%), as well as headaches, fatigue, anorexia, and pruritus. After discontinuing therapy, a high incidence of relapse after a few month is noted and low dose (0.5 mg/kg/d) maintenance therapy may be required [66]. Over 9 months, only 8% of the patients receiving maintenance therapy with low dose retinoic acid progressed, compared to a control group treated with β-carotene, in which 55% of the patients had progression [66].

Second Malignancies

In the first 2 to 3 years, local recurrence is the commonest site of relapse. In subsequent years, a higher percentage of patients present with secondary malignancies (*eg*, a second head and neck cancer, or lung cancer). Regular monitoring and follow-up should focus on other potential disease sites. Instructions and support to avoid further risk factor exposure (smoking, alcohol) are needed. Hong *et al.* showed that the incidence of second primary tumors can be markedly reduced by a daily high-dose (50 to 100 mg/m[RL3]²) of 13-cis retinoic acid (Table 9-6). However, this therapy does not prevent recurrence of the original tumor [67,68]. Large chemoprevention trials have all been negative to date [68–70].

REFERENCES

1. Vokes EE, Weichselbaum RR, Lippman SM, *et al.*: Medical progress: Head and neck cancer. *N Engl J Med* 1993, 328:184–194.

2. Spitz MR: Epidemiology and risk factors for head and neck cancer. *Semin Oncol* 1994, 21:281–288.

3. Fandi A, Altun M, Azli N, *et al.*: Nasopharyngeal cancer: epidemiology, staging, and treatment. *Semin Oncol* 1994, 21:382–397.

4. Vokes EE, Liebowitz DN, Weichselbaum RR: Nasopharyngeal carcinoma. *Lancet* 1997, 350:1087–1091.

5. Li X, Lee NK, Ye YW, *et al.*: Allelic loss at chromosomes 3p, 8p, 13q, and 17p associated with poor prognosis in head and neck cancer. *J Natl Cancer Inst* 1994, 86:1524–1529.

6. Calhoun KH, Fulmer P, Weiss R, *et al.*: Distant metastases from head and neck squamous cell carcinomas. *Laryngoscope* 1994, 04:1199–1205.

7. Cvitkovic E, Eschwege F, Rahal M, *et al.*: Preliminary results of a randomized trial comparing neoadjuvant chemotherapy (cisplatin, epirubicin, bleomycin) plus radiotherapy vs. radiotherapy alone in stage IV (≤ N2, M0) undifferentiated nasopharyngeal carcinoma: a positive effect on progression–free survival. *Int J Radiat Oncol Biol Phys* 1996, 35:463–469.

8. Al–Sarraf M, LeBlanc M, Shanker Giri PG, *et al.*: Chemoradiotherapy versus radiotherapy in patients with advanced nasopharyngeal cancer: phase III randomized Intergroup study 0099. *J Clin Oncol* 1998, 16:1310–1317.

9. Chan A, Teo P, Ngan R, *et al.*: A phase III randomized trial comparing concurrent chemotherapy–radiotherapy with radiotherapy alone in locoregionally advanced nasopharyngeal carcinoma [abstract 1637]. *Proc Am Soc Clin Oncol* 2000, 19:415a.

10. Kim KH, Sung MW, Chung PS, *et al.*: Adenoid cystic carcinoma of the head and neck. *Arch Otolaryngol Head Neck Surg* 1994, 20:721–726.

11. Stupp R, Vokes E: Kopf– und Halstumoren. In *Therapiekonzepte Onkologie*, edn 3. Edited by Seeber S, Schütte S. Berlin and Heidelberg: Springer; 1998:436–475.

12. Browman GP, Cronin L: Standard chemotherapy in squamous cell head and neck cancer: what we have learned from randomized trials. *Semin Oncol* 1994, 21:311–319.

13. Forastiere AA: Randomized trials of induction chemotherapy: a critical review. *Hematol Oncol Clin North Am* 1991, 5:725–736.

14. Paccagnella A, Orlando A, Marchiori C, *et al.*: Phase III trial of initial chemotherapy in stage III or IV head and neck cancers: a study by the Gruppo di Studio sui Tumori della Testa e del Collo. *J Natl Cancer Inst* 1994, 86:265–272.

15. The Department of Veterans Affairs Laryngeal Cancer Study Group: Induction chemotherapy plus radiation compared with surgery plus radiation in patients with advanced laryngeal cancer. *N Engl J Med* 1991, 324:1685–1690.

16. Laramore GE, Scott CB, Al–Sarraf M, *et al.*: Adjuvant chemotherapy for resectable squamous cell carcinomas of the head and neck: report on intergroup study 0034. *Int J Radiat Oncol Biol Phys* 1992, 23:705–713.

17. Schuller DE, Metch B, Mattox D, *et al.*: Prospective chemotherapy in advanced head and neck cancer: final report of the Southwest Oncology Group. *Laryngoscope* 1988, 98:1205–1211.

18. Head and Neck Contracts Program: Adjuvant chemotherapy for advanced head and neck squamous carcinoma: final report. *Cancer* 1987, 60:301–311.

19. Lefebvre J, Chevalier D, Luboinski B, , *et al.* for the EORTC Head and Neck Cooperative Group: larynx preservation in pyriform sinus cancer. Preliminary results of a European Organization for Research and Treatment of Cancer phase III trial. *J Natl Cancer Inst* 1996, 88:890–899.

20. Schuller DE, Stein DW, Metch B: Analysis of treatment failure patterns: a Southwest Oncology Group Study. *Arch Otolaryngol Head Neck Surg* 1989, 115:834–836.

21. Jacobs C, Makuch R: Efficacy of adjuvant chemotherapy for patients with resectable head and neck cancer: a subset analysis of the Head and Neck Contracts Program. *J Clin Oncol* 1990, 8:838–847.

22. Urba SG, Forastiere AA, Wolf GT, *et al.*: Intensive induction chemotherapy and radiation for organ preservation in patients with advanced resectable head and neck carcinoma. *J Clin Oncol* 1994, 12:946–953.

23. Stupp R, Weichselbaum RR, Vokes EE: Combined modality therapy of head and neck cancer. *Semin Oncol* 1994, 21:349–358.

24. Vokes EE, Weichselbaum RR: Concomitant chemoradiotherapy: rationale and clinical experience in patients with solid tumors. *J Clin Oncol* 1990, 8:911–934.

25. Denham JW, Abbott RL: Concurrent cisplatin, infusional fluorouracil, and conventionally fractionated radiation therapy in head and neck cancer: Dose-limiting mucosal toxicity. *J Clin Oncol* 1991, 9:458–463.

26. Taylor SG, Murthy AK, Vannetzel JM, *et al.*: Randomized comparison of neoadjuvant cisplatin and fluorouracil infusion followed by radiation versus concomitant treatment in advanced head and neck cancer. *J Clin Oncol* 1994, 12:385–395.

27. Stupp R, Vokes EE: 5-fluorouracil plus radiation for head and neck cancer. *J Infus Chemother* 1995, 5:55–60.

28. Browman GP, Cripps C, Hodson DI, *et al.*: Placebo-coontrolled randomized trial of infusional fluorouracil during standard radiotherapy in locally advanced head and neck cancer. *J Clin Oncol* 1994, 12:2648–2653.

29. Bachaud JM, David JM, Boussin G, *et al.*: Combined postoperative radiotherapy and weekly cisplatin infusion for locally advanced squamous cell carcinoma of the head and neck: preliminary report of a randomized trial. *Int J Radiat Oncol Biol Phys* 1991, 20:243–246.

30. Brizel D, Albers M, Fisher S, *et al.*: Hyperfractionated irradiation with or without concurrent chemotherapy for locally advanced head and neck cancer. *N Engl J Med* 1998, 338:1798–1804.

31. Adelstein D, Adams G, Li Y, *et al.*: A phase III comparison of standard radiation therapy (RT) versus RT plus concurrent cisplatin (DDP) versus split-course RT plus concurrent DDP and 5-Fluorouracil in patients with unresectable squamous cell head and neck cancer: an Intergroup study [abstract 1624]. *Proc Am Soc Clin Oncol* 2000, 19:411a.

32. Vokes EE, Haraf DJ, Mick R, *et al.*: Concomitant chemoradiotherapy for intermediate stage head and neck cancer [abstract 909]. *Proc Am Soc Clin Oncol* 1994, 13:282.

33. Haraf DJ, Kies M, Rademaker AW, *et al.*: Radiation therapy with concomitant hydroxyurea and fluorouracil in stage II and III head and neck cancer. *J Clin Oncol* 1999, 17:638–644.

34. Kies MS, Haraf DJ, Mittal B, *et al.*: Intensive combined therapy with C-DDP, 5-FU, hydroxyurea, and bid radiation (C-FHX) for stage IV squamous cancer (SCC) of the head and neck (meeting abstract #886). *Proc Annu Meet Am Soc Clin Oncol* 1996, 15:314.

35. Brockstein B, Haraf D, Stenson K, *et al.*: A phase I study of concomitant chemoradiotherapy with paclitaxel, 5-FU, and hydroxyurea with granulocyte colony stimulating factor support for patients with poor prognosis cancer of the head and neck. *J Clin Oncol* 1998, 16:735–744.

36. Brockstein B, Haraf D, MK, Stenson K, *et al.*: Distant metastases after concomitant chemoradiotherapy for head and neck cancer: risk is dependent upon pretreatment lymph node stage [abstract 1635]. *Proc Am Soc Clin Oncol* 2000, 19:414a.

37. Merlano M, Vitale V, Rosso R, *et al.*: Treatment of advanced squamous cell carcinoma of the head and neck with alternating chemotherapy and radiotherapy. *N Engl J Med* 1992, 327:1115–1121.

38. Leyvraz S, Pasche P, Bauer J, *et al.*: Rapidly alternating chemotherapy and hyperfractionated radiotherapy in the management of locally advanced head and neck carcinoma: four-year results of a phase I/II study. *J Clin Oncol* 1994, 12:1876–1885.

39. Ozsahin M, Kütter J, Martinet S, *et al.*: Promising results using weekly concomitant boost accelerated radiotherapy and concomitant full-dose chemotherapy in locally advanced squamous cell carcinoma of the head and neck [abstract 389]. 5th International Conference on Head and Neck Cancer. Program and Abstracts Book 2000, 164.

40. Baselga J, Pfister D, Cooper MR, *et al.*: Phase I studies of anti-epidermal growth factor receptor chimeric antibody C225 alone and in combination with cisplatin. *J Clin Oncol* 2000, 18:904–914.

41. Ezekiel M, Bonner J, Robert F, *et al.*: Phase I trial of chimerized anti-epidermal growth factor receptor (anti-EGFr) antibody in combination with either once-daily or twice-daily irradiation for locally advanced head and neck malignancies [abstract 1501]. 1999, 18:388a.

42. Beck-Bornholdt HP, Dubben HH, Liertz-Petersen C, *et al.*: Hyperfractionation: where do we stand? *Radiother Oncol* 1997, 43:1–21.

43. Horiot JC, Bontemps P, Begg AC, *et al.*: Hyperfractionated and accelerated radiotherapy in head and neck cancer: Results of the EORTC trials and impact on clinical practice. *Bull Cancer Radiother* 1996, 83:314–320.

44. Horiot JC, Le Fur R, N'Guyen T, *et al.*: Hyperfractionation versus conventional fractionation in oropharyngeal carcinoma: Final analysis of a randomized trial of the EORTC cooperative group of radiotherapy. *Radiother Oncol* 1992, 25:231–241.

45. Sanchiz F, Milla A, Torner J, *et al.*: Single fraction per day versus two fractions per day versus radiochemotherapy in the treatment of head and neck cancer. *Int J Radiat Oncol Biol Phys* 1990, 19:1347–1350.

46. Pinto L, Canary P, Araujo C, *et al.*: Prospective randomized trial comparing hyperfractionated versus conventional radiotherapy in stages III and IV oropharyngeal carcinoma. *Int J Radiat Oncol Biol Phys* 1991, 21:557–562.

47. Marcial VA, Pajak TF, Chu C, *et al.*: Hyperfractionated photon radiation therapy in the treatment of advanced squamous cell carcinoma of the oral cavity, pharynx, larynx, and sinuses, using radiation therapy as the only planned modality: preliminary report by the Radiation Therapy Oncology Group (RTOG). *Int J Radiat Oncol Biol Phys* 1987, 13:41–47.

48. Saunders MI, Dische S, Barrett A, *et al.* on behalf of the CHART steering committee: randomised multicentre trials of CHART vs conventional radiotherapy in head and neck and non-small-cell lung cancer. An interim report. *Br J Cancer* 1996, 73:1455–1462.

49. Fu KK, Pajak TF, Trotti A, *et al.*: A Radiation Therapy Oncology Group (RTOG) phase III randomized study to compare hyperfractionation and two variants of accelerated fractionation to standard fractionation radiotherapy for head and neck squamous cell carcinomas: first report of RTOG 9003. *Int J Radiat Oncol Biol Phys* 2000, 48:7–16.

50. Bourhis J, Lapeyre M, Rives M, *et al.*: Very accelerated radiotherapy in HNSCC: Results of the Gortec 94-02 randomized trial [abstract 1627]. *Proc Am Soc Clin Oncol* 2000, 19:412a.

51. Gebbia V, Agostara B, Callari A, *et al.*: Head and neck carcinoma with distant metastases: a retrospective analysis of 44 cases treated with cisplatin-based chemotherapeutic regimens. *Anticancer Res* 1993, 13:1129–1131.

52. Forastiere AA: Paclitaxel (Taxol) for the treatment of head and neck cancer. *Semin Oncol* 1994, 21:49–52.

53. Catimel G, Verweij J, Mattijssen V, *et al.*: Docetaxel (Taxotere): An active drug for the treatment of patients with advanced squamous cell carcinoma of the head and neck. *Ann Oncol* 1994, 5:533–537.

54. Dreyfuss AI, Clark JR, Norris CM, *et al.*: Docetaxel: an active drug for squamous cell carcinoma of the head and neck. *J Clin Oncol* 1996, 14:1672–1678.

55. Couteau C, Chouaki N, Leyvraz S, *et al.*: A phase II study of docetaxel in patients with metastatic squamous cell carcinoma of the head and neck. *Br J Cancer* 1999, 81:547–562.

56. Catimel G, Vermorken JB, Clavel M, *et al.*: A phase II study of Gemcitabine (LY 188011) in patients with advanced squamous cell carcinoma of the head and neck. *Ann Oncol* 1994, 5:543–547.

57. Gebbia V, Testa A, Valenza R, *et al.*: A pilot study of vinorelbine on a weekly schedule in recurrent and/or metastatic squamous cell carcinoma of the head and neck. *Eur J Cancer* 1993, 29a:1358–1359.

58. Testolin A, Recher G, Cristoferi V, *et al.*: Vinorelbine in pre-treated advanced head and neck squamous cell carcinoma: a phase II study. *Invest New Drugs* 1994, 12:231–234.

59. Pivot X, Raymond E, Laguerre B, *et al.*: MTA (LY231514, a multitargeted antifolate) in recurrent, locally advanced or metastatic squamous cell carcinoma of the head and neck [abstract 165]. 5th International Conference on Head and Neck Cancer: Program and Abstract Book:2000, 165 [abstract #165], 2000.

60. Jacobs C, Lyman G, Velez Garcia E, *et al.*: A phase III randomized study comparing cisplatin and fluorouracil as single agents and in combination for advanced squamous cell carcinoma of the head and neck. *J Clin Oncol* 1992, 10:257–263.

61. Forastiere AA, Metch B, Schuller DE, *et al.*: Randomized comparison of cisplatin plus fluorouracil and carboplatin plus fluorouracil versus methotrexate in advanced squamous-cell carcinoma of the head and neck: a Southwest Oncology Group study. *J Clin Oncol* 1992, 10:1245–1251.

62. Vermorken J, Catimel G, De Mulder P, *et al.* for the EORTC Head and Neck Cancer Cooperative Group: randomized phase II trial of weekly methotrexate (MTX) versus two schedules of triweekly paclitaxel (Taxol) in patients with metastatic or recurrent squamous cell carcinoma of the head and neck (SCCHN) [abstract #1527]. *Proc Am Soc Clin Oncol* 1999, 18:395a.

63. Colevas AD, Norris CM, Tishler RB, *et al.*: Phase II trial of docetaxel, cisplatin, fluorouracil, and leucovorin as induction for squamous cell carcinoma of the head and neck [see comments]. *J Clin Oncol* 1999, 17:3503–3511.

64. Posner MR, Glisson B, Frenette G, *et al.*: Multicenter phase I–II trial of docetaxel, cisplatin, and fluorouracil induction chemotherapy for patients with locally advanced squamous cell cancer of the head and neck. *J Clin Oncol* 2001, 19:1096–1104.

65. Hong WK, Endicott J, Itri LM, *et al.*: 13-cis-retinoic acid in the treatment of oral leukoplakia. *N Engl J Med* 1986, 315:1501–1505.

66. Lippman SM, Batsakis JG, Toth BB, *et al.*: Comparison of low-dose isotretinoin with beta carotene to prevent oral carcinogenesis. *N Engl J Med* 1993, 328:15–20.

67. Hong WK, Lippman SM, Itri LM, *et al.*: Prevention of second primary tumors with isotretinoin in squamous-cell carcinoma of the head and neck. *N Engl J Med* 1990, 323:795–801.

68. Papadimitrakopoulou VA, Hong WK, Lee JS, *et al.*: Low-dose isotretinoin versus beta-carotene to prevent oral carcinogenesis: long-term follow-up. *J Natl Cancer Inst* 1997, 89:257–258.

69. van Zandwijk N, Dalesio O, Pastorino U, *et al.*: EUROSCAN, a randomized trial of vitamin A and N-acetylcysteine in patients with head and neck cancer or lung cancer: for the European Organization for Research and Treatment of Cancer Head and Neck and Lung Cancer Cooperative Groups [see comments]. *J Natl Cancer Inst* 2000, 92:977–986.

70. Bolla M, Laplanche A, Lefur R, *et al.*: Prevention of second primary tumours with a second generation retinoid in squamous cell carcinoma of oral cavity and oropharynx: long term follow-up [letter]. *Eur J Cancer* 1996, 32A:375–376.

CISPLATIN AND 5-FLUOROURACIL (±DOCETAXEL)

Platinum compounds are complex molecules, which covalently bind to DNA and also interact with proteins. Two available agents in this class, cisplatin and carboplatin, have a different toxicity profile. Carboplatin produces lower renal toxicity, but myelosuppression and especially thrombocytopenia can be marked. Response rates as a single agent are approximately 30% for cisplatin and 20% for carboplatin.

The antimetabolite 5-flourouracil (5-FU) is commonly used in many combination regimens and as a single agent. This pyrimidine analogue interferes with DNA and RNA synthesis by binding to thymidylate synthase, or it is incorporated into RNA as a false messenger. In head and neck cancer, 5-FU alone has not commonly been used, but single agent response rates of 15% have been reported. The response rate depends on dosage and schedule. A randomized trial has shown that continuous infusion therapy over 4 to 5 days is superior to IV bolus administration (when given in combination with cisplatin) in recurrent disease.

Combining the two agents improves overall response rate and objective responses up to 40%, with 15% complete responses reported in recurrent disease. However, randomized trials have failed to demonstrate improved survival using this combination, compared with single-agent chemotherapy.

Two taxanes, paclitaxel and docetaxel, have demonstrated single-agent activity in patients with recurrent head and neck cancer. Integration of docetaxel in combination chemotherapy regimens with cisplatin with and without 5-FU is feasible and has demonstrated encouraging responses. Randomized trials assessing the real value of these newer agents are ongoing.

CANDIDATES FOR TREATMENT

Recurrent or metastatic disease; locally advanced advanced laryngeal and hypopharynx cancer for organ preservation

SPECIAL PRECAUTIONS

Hydration for 6–12 h before and after cisplatin administration; antiemetic prophylaxis during initial 48 h after cisplatin administration

ALTERNATIVE THERAPIES

Methotrexate, carboplatin and 5-FU, cisplatin or 5-FU (single agent), paclitaxel

TOXICITIES

Cisplatin: highly emetogenic, nephrotoxicity, cumulative ototoxicity, metallic taste in mouth; late chronic neuropathy (up to 40% of patients); myelosuppression (nadir after approx 10 d); electrolyte wasting (K, Mg); **5-FU**: mucositis, diarrhea, increased liver enzymes

DRUG INTERACTIONS

Cisplatin: antimetabolites, nephrotoxic agents (*eg*, aminoglycoside); **5-FU**: leucovorin, interferon, dipyridamole

RECENT EXPERIENCE AND RESPONSE RATES

Study	Evaluable Patients, *n*	Regimen	Response Rates/Survival
Recurrent disease			
Clavel *et al.*/*EORTC Ann Oncol* 1994, 5:521–526	116	cDDP 100 mg/m² x 1 + 5-FU 1000 mg/m2 x 4 d ci	CR=1.7%, RR=31%; TTP 17 wk
	127	cDDP 50 mg/m², d 4; methotrexate 40 mg/m², d 1, 8; bleomycin 10 mg + vincristine 2 mg, d 1, 8, 15	CR=9.5%, RR=34%; TTP 19 wk, median survival for all 365 patients: 29 wk
	122; mainly recurrent, no prior chemotherapy	cDDP 50 mg/m², d 1, 8	CR=2.5%, RR=15%; TTP 12 wk
Jacobs *et al. J Clin Oncol* 1992, 10:257–263	79, eval. 63	cDDP 100 mg/m² x 1 + 5-FU 1000 mg/m² x 4 d ci	CR=5, PR=20; RR=32%; surv. > 9 mo: 40
	83, eval. 80	cDDP 100 mg/m² x 1	CR=3, PR=11; RR=17%; surv. > 9 mo: 24
	83, eval. 75; recurrent or metastatic	5-FU 1000 mg/m² x 4 d	CR=2, PR=9; RR=13%; surv. > 9 mo: 27
Forastiere *et al.* (SWOG), *J Clin Oncol* 1992, 10:1245–1251	87; randomized	cDDP 100 mg/m² + 5-FU 1000 mg/m² x 4 d ci	RR=32%; surv. 6.6 mo
	86	Carboplatin 300 mg/m² + 5-FU 1000 mg/m² x 4 d ci	RR=21% (ns); surv. 5.0 mo
	88; recurrent or metastatic	MTX 40 mg/m2 IV every week	RR=10%; surv. 5.6 mo
Kish *et al. Cancer* 1985 56:2740–2744	18; randomized	cDDP 100 mg/m² + 5-FU 600 mg/m² bolus d 1 + 8	CR=2, PR=2; RR=20%
	20; locally adv. + recurrent	cDDP 100 mg/m² + 5-FU 1000 mg/m² x 4 d ci	CR=4, PR=9; RR=72%

Continued

CISPLATIN AND 5-FLUOROURACIL (±DOCETAXEL) (Continued)

RECENT EXPERIENCE AND RESPONSE RATES Continued

Study	Evaluable Patients, n	Regimen	Response Rates/Survival
No prior therapy/induction chemotherapy			
Posner et al. J Clin Oncol 2001, 19:1096–1104	43	Docetaxel 75 mg/m², cDDP 100 mg/m² + 5-FU 1000 mg/m² × 4 d ci, + antibiotics	CR 17, PR 23, RR 93%
Schrijvers et al., Proc Am Soc Clin Oncol 1999, 18:394a.	45	Docetaxel 75 mg/m², cDDP 75 mg/m² + 5-FU 750 mg/m² × 5 d ci	Dose-finding study
Paccanella et al. J Natl Cancer Inst 1994, 86:265–272	118	cDDP 100 mg/m² x 1 + 5-FU 1000mg/m², d 1–5 ci x 4 cycles, followed by (surgery) + XRT 200 cGy/1 x d versus	CR=31, PR=55, RR=80%; 2-y survival: 37; inop. pts, 2-y survival: 30; distant mets: 9 at 2 y
	119; locally advanced	(Surgery) + XRT 200 cGy/1 x d	CR=67 (56%); 2 y survival: 29; inop. pts, 2-y survival: 19; distant mets: 32 at 2 y
Veterans Affairs Larynx Cancer Study Group. N Engl J Med 1991, 324:1685–1690	166	cDDP 100 mg/m² x 1 + 5-FU 1000mg/m², d 1–5 ci, x 3 cycles, followed by XRT 200 cGy/1 x d ± salvage surgery versus	CR=31, RR=54%; distant mets: 11%
	166	surgery + XRT 200 cGy/1 x d	Larynx preservation: 64%; distant mets: 17%
de Andres et al., J Clin Oncol 1995, 13:1493–1500	49 **versus** 46 (stage IV/M0)	cDDP 100 mg/m² × 1 + 5-FU 1000 mg/m², d 1–5 ci × three cycles, followed by XRT 200 cGY/1 × d or surgery **versus** CBDCA 400 mg/m² × 1 + 5-FU 1000 mg/m², d 1–5 ci, × 3 cycles, followed by XRT 200 cGY/1 × d or surgery	3 y: 48% actuarial
	advanced larynx; 51, neoadjuvant and adjuvant	Grade III/IV: mucositis 4%, thrombopenia 0%; RR 92%, CR 27%; 5-y survival 49% **versus** Grade III/IV: mucositis 21%, thrombopenia 15%; RR 92%, CR 27%; 5-y survival 25%; also, early termination and superiority of control arm	
Vokes et al. J Clin Oncol 1991, 9:1376–1384		cDDP 100 mg/m² x 1, 5-FU 1000 mg/m² x 5 d ci	CR=22 (43%); pCR=24%; PR=24 (47%); RR=90%

NURSING INTERVENTIONS

Agents can be administered by a peripheral venous access. Extravasation causes local irritation; monitor fluid status; watch for dehydration and overhydration; do not administer cisplatin if urine output <100 mL/h over the last 4 h prior to start; monitor electrolytes including magnesium and start supplements early

PATIENT INFORMATION

Patient may experience delayed nausea/vomiting with cisplatin; antiemetic must be available at all times; contact physician immediately for fevers (neutropenia possible), bleeding (thrombocytopenia rare), and diarrhea (electrolyte wasting, dehydration).

DOSAGE AND SCHEDULING

Cisplatin 100 mg/m² IV over 2–6 h: d 1	■									
5-FU 1000 mg/m²/d IV continuous infusion for 4–5 d	████████████									
CBC, platelets: d 1, 5, 10	☐				☐					
Na, K, Mg, BUN, Crea: d 1, 3, 5, 10	☐		☐		☐					☐
SGOT, SGPT, alk. Phos, Albumin: d 1	☐									
Day	1	2	3	4	5	6	7	8	9	10

Repeat every 3–4 wk.

CR—complete response; pCR—pathologic complete response; PR—partial response.

Dosage Modifications: For impaired renal function, reduce cDDP to 75% for creatinine clearance of 50–75 mL/min, to < 50% for clearance of 25–50 mL\min. Do not administer if clearance < 25 mL/min. For grade III mucositis, decrease 5-FU to 80% (eg, administer 4 d only).

CONCOMITANT CHEMORADIOTHERAPY WITH SINGLE-AGENT 5-FLUOROURACIL OR CISPLATIN

Cisplatin and 5-fluorouracil (5-FU) are known for their radiosensitizing effects. The mechanism of this interaction is not completely known. Theoretically, several mechanisms have been postulated. Ideally both, the chemotherapeutic agent and the radiation must have independent antitumor activity. Acting against different sites of the tumor cell, they enhance each other by inhibiting tumor cell recovery from sublethal damage. They have additive cytotoxicity and prevent tumor resistance. Because radiation therapy is cell-cycle specific, the chemotherapy may synchronize and block the tumor cells in S phase and, thus, make them more radiosensitive. Decreased tumor bulk may improve drug delivery to the remaining tumor cells.

Cisplatin causes direct DNA damage by intrastrand crosslinks and breaks. It acts mainly with synergistic cytotoxicity by inhibiting DNA repair from sublethal cell damage.

5-FU is either incorporated into RNA or binds to thymidylate synthase and, thus, inhibits DNA synthesis. Synergy with radiation has been shown in several in vitro studies in which subtherapeutic doses of radiation or 5-FU were not able to induce cell death, but the combination showed increased cytotoxicity. The mechanism of this interaction remains unclear; possibly the cells become more sensitive to the radiation by modification of the cell kinetics.

CANDIDATES FOR TREATMENT

Patients with locally advanced squamous cell carcinoma of the head and neck, recurrent unresectable disease for locoregional control; patients who are candidates for postoperative radiotherapy

TOXICITIES

Mucositis, weight loss, myelosuppression, renal insufficiency (with cisplatin), nausea and vomiting

NURSING INTERVENTIONS

Good oral hygiene with nonalcoholic antiseptic mouthwashes (4 x d); fungal prophylaxis with nystatin mouthwash or clotrimazole troches; watch nutritional status (if insufficient, suggest feeding tube)

PATIENT INFORMATION

Patient should be aware of mucositis potential; mouth care needs to be emphasized; encourage good and regular nutrition and fluid intake.

RECENT EXPERIENCES AND RESPONSE RATES

Study	Evaluable Patients, n	Regimen	Response Rates	Survival
Brizel et al., N Engl J Med 1998, 328:1798–1804.	56	cDDP 12 mg/m^2 × 5+5-FU 600 mg/m^2/d × 5 week 1 + 6 and RT (125 cGY bid, 70 Gy) **versus**	—	3 y: 55% Mucositis grade III/IV: 77%
	60	RT (125 cGY bid, 75 Gy)		3 y: 34% ($P = 0.07$); mucositis grade III/IV: 75%
Al-Sarraf (RTOG 88-24): Int J Radiat Oncol Biol Phys 1997, 37:777–782	52	Cisplatin 200 mg/m^2; d 1, 22, 43; + RT qd (30 X 2 Gy)	postoperative RT	3-y: 48% (actuarial)
Bachaud et al.: Int J Radiat Oncol Biol Phys 1991, 20:243–246	39	Cisplatin 50 mg/wk + RT qd **versus**	postoperative RT	2-y: 75%
	44	RT qd		2-y: 44% ($P < 0.05$)
Glicksman et al.: Int J Radiat Oncol Biol Phys 1994, 30:1043–1050	101	Cisplatin 20 mg/m^2, d1-4, wk 1 & 3 + RT qd	pathologic CR of operated patients: 82%	3-y: 78% (other causes of death excluded) actuarial 9-y: 49%
Jeremic et al.: Radiother Oncol 1997, 43:29–37	53	Carboplatin 25 mg/m^2 qd + RT qd (35 × 2 Gy) **versus**	CR 68%, PR 17%	Median: 30 mo, 2 y: 55%
	53	Cisplatin 6 mg/m^2 qd + RT qd (35 × 2 Gy) **versus**	CR 72%, PR 9%	Median: 32 mo, 2 y: 58%
	53	RT qd (35 × 2 Gy)	CR 38%, PR 21%	Median: 16 mo, 2 y: 35%
Browman et al.: J Clin Oncol 1994, 12: 2648–2653	87	Placebo infusion + XRT 200 cGy/d **versus**	CR 49 (56%)	24 mo: 50%
	88	5-FU 1200 mg/m^2/d × 3 d ci, wk 1 & 3, + concomitant XRT 200 cGy/d	CR 60 (68%)	24 mo: 63%
Sanchiz et al.: Int J Radiat Oncol Biol Phys 1990, 19:1347–1350	306	5-FU 250 mg/m^2 qod + RT 2.0 Gy qd **versus**	CR 96%	Median: 85 mo
	292	RT 1.1 Gy bid **versus**	CR 90%	Median: 84 mo
	294	RT 2.0 Gy qd	CR 68%	Median: 38 mo

CONCOMITANT CHEMORADIOTHERAPY WITH SINGLE-AGENT 5-FLUOROURACIL OR CISPLATIN (Continued)

DOSAGE AND SCHEDULING

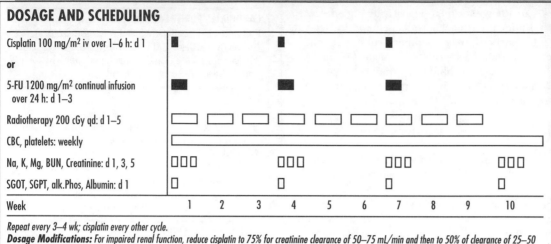

	Week 1	2	3	4	5	6	7	8	9	10
Cisplatin 100 mg/m² iv over 1–6 h: d 1	■			■			■			
or										
5-FU 1200 mg/m² continual infusion over 24 h: d 1–3	■			■			■			
Radiotherapy 200 cGy qd: d 1–5	(continuous weekly blocks across weeks 1–10)									
CBC, platelets: weekly	(continuous across weeks 1–10)									
Na, K, Mg, BUN, Creatinine: d 1, 3, 5	□□□			□□□			□□□			□□□
SGOT, SGPT, alk.Phos, Albumin: d 1	□			□			□			□

Repeat every 3–4 wk; cisplatin every other cycle.
Dosage Modifications: *For impaired renal function, reduce cisplatin to 75% for creatinine clearance of 50–75 mL/min and then to 50% of clearance of 25–50 min. Do not administer if clearance < 25 mL/min. Avoid cisplatin in patients who are hearing impaired. For grade III mucositis, decrease 5-FU to 80%.*

CONCOMITANT SPLIT-COURSE CHEMORADIO-THERAPY (WEEK ON/WEEK OFF)
5-Fluorouracil, Hydroxyurea ± Cisplatin

5-Fluorouracil, hydroxyurea, cisplatin (cDDP), and paclitaxel are known for their radiosensitizing effects, although the mechanism of this interaction remains incompletely understood. Several theoretical mechanisms have been postulated. Ideally both, the chemotherapeutic agent and the radiation therapy must have independent antitumor activity. Acting against different sites of the tumor cell, they enhance each other by inhibiting tumor cell recovery from sublethal damage. They have additive cytotoxicity and prevent tumor resistance. Given that radiation therapy is cell-cycle specific, chemotherapy may synchronize and block the tumor cells in S phase and thus render them more radiosensitive. Decreased tumor bulk may improve drug delivery to remaining tumor cells. These drugs have been used as single agents with simultaneous radiation therapy for various malignant diseases.

Concomitant radiation therapy with full-dose chemotherapy significantly increases toxicities. Severe mucositis is common and most patients require placement of a feeding tube. For regeneration of the normal tissues, this approach requires scheduled rest periods.

Cisplatin directly damages DNA by intrastrand crosslinks and breaks. It acts mainly with synergistic cytotoxicity by inhibiting DNA repair from sublethal cell damage.

5-fluorouracil (5-FU) is either incorporated into RNA or binds to thymidylate synthase and thus inhibits DNA synthesis. Synergy with radiation has been shown in several in vitro studies, where subtherapeutic doses of radiation or 5-FU could not induce cell death, but the combination showed increased cytotoxicity. The mechanism of this interaction remains unclear; possibly the cells become more sensitive to the radiation by modification of the cell kinetics.

Hydroxyurea (HU) inhibits ribonucleotide reductase specifically in the S-phase. It alters the cell kinetics by inhibiting entry into the radioresistant S-phase. Hydroxyurea as a antimetabolite inhibits DNA synthesis or repair. Although it has single-agent activity in head and neck cancer, it is rarely used other than as a radiosensitizer.

Paclitaxel stabilizes the mitotic spindle tubules, causing cell cycle arrest in the radiation-sensitive G_2/M-phase of the cell cycle. Prolonged exposure appears to increase radiosensitizing properties. Paclitaxel has single-agent activity against head and neck cancer.

CANDIDATES FOR TREATMENT
Patients with locally advanced and recurrent squamous cell carcinoma of the head and neck

TOXICITIES
Severe mucositis, weight loss (forced feeding commonly necessary), nausea, vomiting

NURSING INTERVENTIONS
Good oral hygiene with nonalcoholic antiseptic mouthwashes (4 ×/d); fungal prophylaxis with nystatin mouthwash or clotrimazole troches; insufficient food and fluid intake commonly requires feeding tube

PATIENT INFORMATION
Patient should be aware of mucositis potential; mouth care needs to be emphasized

CONCOMITANT SPLIT-COURSE CHEMORADIO-THERAPY (WEEK ON/WEEK OFF) (Continued)
5-Fluorouracil, Hydroxyurea ± Cisplatin

RECENT EXPERIENCES AND RESPONSE RATES

Study	Evaluable Patients, n	Regimen	Response Rates	Survival/Remarks, %
Vokes et al. J Clin Oncol 1994, 12:2351–2359	17 (recurrent)	CDDP 100 mg/m², d 1 + 5-FU 800 mg/m², d 1–5 + HU 1000 mg bid plus concomitant XRT 200 cGy/1 × d ± G-CSF	CR=11 (64%) RR=76%	Median survival: 12 mo Median TTF: 8 mo
	28 (no prior therapy)		CR=21 (75%) RR=89%	Median survival: 12 mo Median TTF: not reached
Taylor et al. J Clin Oncol 1994, 12:385–395	107 vs.	CDDP 100 mg/m², d 1 + 5-FU 1000 mg/m²/d, d 1-5 ci × 3 cycles followed by XRT (seq)	CR=50 (47%) PR=28 (26%) RR=73%	Marked differences in response rates depending on treatment institution; significantly improved local control with concomitant therapy
	107 (locally advanced)	CDDP 60 mg/m², d1 +5-FU 800 mg/m²/d, d 1–5 ci plus concomitant XRT 200 cGy/1× d, every other week	CR=52 (49%) PR=41 (38%) RR=87	
Adelstein et al./ECOG J Clin Oncol 1993, 11:2136–2142	52 (locally advanced)	CDDP 75 mg/m² × 1 + 5-FU 1000 mg/m² × 4 d ci plus concomitant XRT 200 cGy qd × 15 (3000 cGy total), followed by chemotherapy only × 1 cycle and subsequently the same chemoradiotherapy	CR=77%	4-y survival: 49%
Adelstein et al. Cancer 1990, 65:1685–1691	24 (simultaneous therapy) vs.	CDDP 75 mg/m² × 1 + 5-FU 1000 mg/m² × 4 d ci (repeat chemo on d 28) plus concomitant XRT 200 cGy qd × 15 (3000 cGy total), possibly surgery and repeat above	CR=16, PR=8 RR=100%	Neutropenia grade IV: 10 (42%), one toxic death; trend for improved overall survival with simultaneous therapy
	24 (sequential therapy)	CDDP 100 mg/m² × 1 + 5-FU 1000 mg/m² × 5 d ci × 3 cycles, followed by possible surgery and RT 6000 cGy total	CR=7, PR=13 RR=83%	Neutropenia grade IV: 14 (58%), two toxic deaths
Weppelmann et al. Int J Radiat Oncol Bio Phys 1992, 22:1051–1056	21 (evaluated 20) Recurrent or metastatic, after previous surgery and radiation	5-FU 300 mg/m² × 5 d ci + HU > 1500 mg/m² qd × 5 d + XRT 200 cGy qd × 5 d every other week	CR=9, PR=6, RR=75%	1-y survival: 56%
Wendt et al. J Clin Oncol 1989, 7:471–476	59 (locally advanced)	CDDP 60 mg/m² × 1 + 5-FU 350 mg/m² × 4 d ci + LV 50 mg/m² × 4 d ci plus concomitant XRT 180 cGy qd × 11 d	CR=48 (81%) PR=11 (19%) RR=100%	
Brockstein et al. Ann Oncol 2000, 11:721–728	54 (prior chemo: 25)	Paclitaxel 100 mg/m², d 1 + 5-FU 600 mg/m2, d 1-5 ci + HU 500 mg bid plus concomitant XRT 150 cGy/once daily or 150 cGy/twice daily	2-Y survival=45%	Phase dose-finding study

CDDP—cisplatin; ci—continuous infusion; CR—complete response rate; 5-FU—5-Fluorouracil; HU—hydroxyurea; PR—partial response rate; RR—overall response rate; XRT—external radiation therapy.

DOSAGE AND SCHEDULING

	Day													
	1	2	3	4	5	6	7	8	9	10	11	12	13	1
Cisplatin 100 mg/m² IV over 2–6 h: d 1	■													■
Paclitaxel 100 mg/m²/d IV over 1 h; d 1	■													
5-FU 1000 mg/m²/d IV continuous infusion for 5 d	▬▬▬▬▬▬▬													■
Hydroxyurea 1000 mg PO bid x 11 doses, first dose 12 h before RT, d 1–6	▬▬▬▬▬▬▬													■
Radiotherapy 200 cGy qd, d 1–5	▬▬▬▬▬▬▬													■
CBC, platelets: d 1, 5	□			□										□
Na, K, Mg, BUN, Crea: d 1, 3, 5	□		□		□									□
SGOT, SGPT, alk Phos, albumin: d 1	□													□

Repeat every 2 wk : cisplatin every other cycle.

ALTERNATING CHEMORADIOTHERAPY

A conceptually similar approach to concomitant chemoradiotherapy is to alternate chemotherapy administration and radiation rapidly. Again, sublethally damaged cells may be eliminated by the other modality. Although radiation is a locoregional treatment, chemotherapy acts systemically. Because of nonsimultaneous administration of treatment modalities, overall toxicity and tolerability may be reduced somewhat, thus allowing for more intensive chemotherapy. This approach is currently being further tested in a randomized EORTC trial, comparing sequential induction chemotherapy followed by radiation with alternating chemotherapy.

CANDIDATES FOR TREATMENT

Patients with locally advanced squamous cell carcinoma of the head and neck, those seeking organ preservation of resectable disease, and those with inoperable disease

TOXICITIES

Severe mucositis, weight loss (forced feeding commonly necessary)

NURSING INTERVENTIONS

Good oral hygiene with nonalcoholic antiseptic mouthwashes (4 times per day), fungal prophylaxis with nystatin mouthwash or clotrimazole troches; insufficient food and fluid intake commonly requires feeding tube

PATIENT INFORMATION

Patient should be aware of potential for mucositis; meticulous mouth care must be emphasized to patients

RECENT EXPERIENCES AND RESPONSE RATES

Study	Evaluable patients, n	Regimen	Response Rates	Survival
Leyvraz et al., J Clin Oncol 1994, 12:1876–1885.	91 (locally advanced)	cDDP 80–100 mg/m², d 1 + 5-FU 1000 mg/m², d 1–4, ci ± vindesine alternating with hyperfractionated radiotherapy 200 cGY/3 times per day	CR 69%; RR 96%	Median survival: 24 mo; 64% organ preservation
Merlano et al., N Engl J Med 1992, 327:115–121.	80 (locally advanced, unresectable)	cDDP 20 mg/m² × 5 d + 5-FU 200 mg/m² × 5 d bolus alternating with XRT 200 cGY × 5 d × 2 wk	CR 43%; PR 29%	3-y survival: 41%; P < 0.05
		vs.		
	77	XRT 200 cGY QD (70 Gy total)	CR 22%; PR 43%	3-y survival: 23%

DOSAGE AND SCHEDULING

Cisplatin 100 mg/m² IV over 2–6 h: d 1	▥			▥			▥			▥		
5-FU 200 mg/m², bolus d 1–5 or 5-FU 800 mg/m² ci d 1–5	▥ ■ or			▥ ■ or			▥ ■ or			▥ ■ or		
Radiotherapy 200 cGY QD × 10 d		▥	▥		▥	▥		▥	▥			
CBC, platelets: d 1,5	XX	XX	XX	XX	XX	XX	XX	XX	XX	XX	XX	XX
Na, K, Mg, BUN, Crea: d 1, 3, 5	XXX	X	X	XXX	X	X	XXX	X	X	XXX	X	X
SGOT, SGPT, alk, phos, albumin: d 1	X			X			X			X		
Week	1	2	3	4	5	6	7	8	9	10	11	12

DOSAGE MODIFICATIONS: For impaired renal function, reduce cDDP to 75% for creatinine clearance of 50–75 mL/min, to < 50% for clearance of 25–50 mL/min. Do not administer if clearance < 25 mL/min. For grade III mucositis, decrease 5-FU to 80% (eg, administer 4 d only).

Lung cancer is the leading cause of cancer-related mortality in both men and women in the United States, accounting for more than 28% of all cancer deaths in 2000. The estimated number of new cases of lung cancer in 2000 is 164,100 with an estimated 156,900 lung cancer deaths [1]. Lung cancer is the third most common cancer type in the United States after prostate and breast cancer but more Americans die from this dreaded disease than from breast cancer, prostate cancer, and colorectal cancer combined because of the low 14% cure rate [1]. This low rate can be ascribed almost exclusively to the high propensity for metastatic spread, lack of effective screening measures, and inability of systemic therapy to cure metastatic disease. Most patients present with inoperable stage III disease or with metastasis to distant organs (stage IV) [2]. Patients with stage IV disease are rarely cured with previous chemotherapeutic approaches [2]. A small minority of patients, between 15% and 25%, with advanced regional disease stage III with either small cell lung cancer (SCLC) or non-small cell lung cancer (NSCLC) may be cured with intensive combined-modality approaches. Surgery cures 10% to 80% of operable cases depending on stage [2]. Because most patients develop systemic disease, chemotherapy is indicated for a high percentage of patients. Chemotherapeutic options have improved considerably in recent years with more effective and less toxic regimens now available. Chemotherapy improves symptoms, quality of life, and survival of lung cancer patients.

ETIOLOGY AND RISK FACTORS

Most lung cancers are caused by carcinogens and tumor promoters derived from cigarette smoking (Table 10-1). Overall, the relative risk of developing lung cancer is increased about 13-fold by active smoking and about 1.5-fold by long-term passive exposure to cigarette smoke [2]. There appears to be a dose-response relationship between the lung cancer death rate and the total amount (often expressed in "cigarette pack years") of cigarette smoke, such that the risk increases 60- to 70-fold for a man or woman smoking two packs a day for 20 years compared with findings in a nonsmoker. Conversely, the chance of developing lung cancer decreases with cessation of smoking but never returns to the level of the nonsmoker [3]. For this reason, more than half of all lung cancer diagnosis is the United States are now in former smokers [4].

Cigarette smoking is more common in blacks than whites. In 1993, 32% of American blacks and 27% of whites were smokers, although whites smoked more cigarettes per day. The greatest differences in smoking was seen between educational groups with a 36% incidence in those with less than a high school education compared

with 14% among college graduates [5]. Many countries have launched programs to decrease tobacco use and to educate the public. These programs include legislative activity (eg, smoke-free areas, banning of tobacco advertisements), educational activities through mass media and schools, and interventional approaches targeted to groups at highest risk for developing tobacco-related cancer. The greatest impact on decreased smoking habits appears to be the stigma placed on smokers by society. These activities have reduced the percentage of the US population who smoke from a high of about 50% to about 25%. Linkage of cigarette smoking to lung cancer and other diseases has resulted in a decrease in tobacco use among men. As a result, a modest decrease in the death rate due to lung cancer has occurred among US men. Unfortunately, the rate of lung cancer among US women continues to rise largely due to their continued use of cigarettes. Young women continue to take up the habit of cigarette smoking more rapidly than their male counterparts. This observation suggests that the death rate due to lung cancer will continue to increase in US women for many years to come.

A small minority of lung cancer cases may be caused by exposure to other carcinogens [2]. Increases in lung cancer risk accompany exposure to carcinogens such as asbestos, radon, bis(chloromethyl) ether, polycyclic aromatic hydrocarbons, chromium, nickel, and inorganic arsenic compounds. The association with occupational exposure to these agents appear to be independent of cigarette smoking [6]. However, exposure to both increases the risk of lung cancer in an exponential manner.

PATHOLOGY

Four major cell types make up 95% of all primary lung neoplasms [7,8]. These are SCLC, squamous (epidermoid) carcinoma, adenocarcinoma (including bronchoalveolar) and large cell (undifferentiated) carcinoma (Table 10-2). The latter three cell types are often

Table 10-1. Lung Cancer Etiology*

Cause	Percentage
Active tobacco smoking	85
Current smoking	35
Former smoking	50
Passive tobacco exposure	3
Radon	3
Other environmental factors (eg, asbestos, arsenic, chloromethyl ether)	0.1–3.0

*Data from Schottenfeld [6] and Fraumeni et al. [7].

Table 10-2. Lung Cancer Pathology*

Cell type	Frequency, %	Features
Non–small cell lung cancer Squamous	35	Central location; more common in males; less metastases; associated with hypercalcemia, clubbing, hypertrophic pulmonary osteoarthropathy
Adenocarcinoma (includes broncholveolar)	35	Peripheral in location; equal frequency in both sexes; associated with scars; metastatic potential common; most common type in nonsmokers; hypercoagulable states; associated with filtered cigarettes
Large cell	10	Peripheral in location; equal frequency in both sexes; anaplastic; undifferentiated metastatic potential
Small cell lung cancer	20	Central location; strong relationship with smoking; associated with neuroendocrine features, paraneoplastic syndromes; metastasizes widely; most sensitive to chemotherapy and radiotherapy

*Data from Travis et al. [8].

lumped together and referred to as NSCLC. The remaining 5% include carcinoids, bronchial gland tumors, and mesotheliomas. The various cell types have different natural histories and responses to therapy, and thus a correct histologic diagnosis by an experienced pathologist is the first step to correct treatment. Major treatment decisions are made on the basis of the crucial distinction between histologic classification of a tumor as SCLC or NSCLC. Therapy is discussed separately here for SCLC and NSCLC. With regards to chemotherapy, all NSCLC cases are considered together because no evidence confirms that specific therapies ought be based on cell type.

Squamous cell carcinoma (SCC), at one time, was the most frequent of all lung cancers. SCC arises most frequently in proximal segmental bronchi and is preceded by squamous metaplasia. Because of its central location and ability to exfoliate, squamous cancers can be detected by cytologic examination in an early stage. With further growth, SCC invades the basement membrane and extends into the bronchial lumen, producing obstruction with resultant atelectasis or pneumonia. These tumors tend to be slow growing so that it is estimated that up to 3 or 4 years are required from the development of in situ carcinoma to a clinically apparent tumor. Histologically, the SCC tumor is composed of sheets of epithelial cells, which may be well or poorly differentiated. Most well-differentiated tumors demonstrate keratin pearls.

Adenocarcinoma has become the most frequent lung cancer histology in North America, accounting for about 35% to 40% of all cases of lung cancer. Most such tumors are peripheral in origin, arising from alveolar surface epithelium or bronchial mucosal glands. They also can arise from peripheral scar tumors. Adenocarcinoma appears to have a worse prognosis for operable stages than SCC because of its propensity for early metastases. Histologically, these tumors form glands and produce mucin. Bronchoalveolar carcinoma is a distinct clinicopathologic type of adenocarcinoma. This tumor appears to arise from type II pneumocytes, growing along alveolar septa by lepidic growth, and showing little if any desmoplastic or glandular change. They can present in three different fashions: a solitary peripheral nodule, multifocal disease, or a rapidly progressive pneumonic form that appears to spread from lobe to lobe ultimately encompassing both lungs.

Large cell carcinoma is the least common of all NSCLC tumor types, accounting for about 15% of all lung cancers. Most are located peripherally and are similar to adenocarcinomas in prognosis.

SCLCs have both biologic and clinical differences from NSCLC tumors. Biologically, SCLCs have neuroendocrine features, which lead to frequent endocrine and neurologic paraneoplastic syndromes. SCLCs also have more rapid growth and a greater propensity for early metastatic spread [9]. More than 90% of patients with SCLC have mediastinal lymph node metastases and more than two thirds of cases have distant organ metastases at the time of diagnosis. SCLC has the most aggressive clinical course of any type of pulmonary tumor, with median survival from diagnosis of only 2 to 4 months without treatment. Because of its propensity for distant metastases, localized forms of treatment (*eg*, radiotherapy or surgical resection) rarely produce long-term survival [9]. SCLCs are more sensitive to chemotherapy than NSCLCs and chemotherapy represents the cornerstone of therapy.

EARLY DETECTION AND SCREENING

No method has been established as effective in early detection or screening for lung cancer [10]. Annual chest radiographs or routine sputum cytology examinations, or a combination of both, were studied in large scale trials because they were thought to be useful as screening and early detection strategies to reduce lung cancer mortality [11–15]. The Mayo Lung Project (MLP), a randomized, controlled trial that was conducted between 1971 and 1983, observed no reduction in lung cancer mortality with an intense regimen of chest radiographs and sputum cytology. Recent data on an extended median follow-up of 20.5 years of the MLP continues to demonstrate no decrease in lung cancer mortality rate [16]. Similar results have been obtained in other studies. Thus, these trials did not prove a screening role for either sputum or chest radiographs. Subsequently, the American Cancer Society, the National Cancer Institute, and other organizations resolved that large scale radiologic and cytologic screening for lung cancer could not be justified [17]. These studies lacked the power to exclude a useful role for chest radiographs and thus, the Prostate, Lung, Colorectal and Ovarian (PLCO) cancer study is currently examining the role of annual chest radiographs. Although standard sputum cytology may not be sufficiently sensitive for a routine screening examination, it remains as an excellent diagnostic test for smokers with symptoms.

The new generation of spiral computed tomography (SCT) scanners has led to faster image acquisition times with more data being captured and lower radiation exposure [18]. In the Early Lung Cancer Action Project, Henschke *et al.* demonstrated low-dose SCT was superior to chest radiograph in the detection of early or resectable lung cancers [19]. A strong correlation was found between lesion size and likelihood of cancer, with a greater percentage of lung cancers' being detected by SCT (2.7%) compared with (0.7%) by chest radiographs [19]. Of those lung cancers detected by SCT, 96% were resectable and 85% were stage I. Although the rate of false-positive findings at baseline screening was high, the annual report screening showed much lower rates [19]. Thus, it appears that SCT scans can detect early lung cancers better than chest radiographs. It also detects many nonmalignant nodules that are expensive to evaluate, but it is not certain that it will reduce lung cancer–related mortality. Additional studies are necessary before it can be adopted as a routine screening measure.

PREVENTION OF LUNG CANCER

That between 85% and 87% of lung cancers are caused by active tobacco smoking makes primary prevention an essential element of any prevention strategy. Worldwide efforts to limit tobacco usage have been relatively ineffective. In the United States, the percentage of adult smokers declined progressively from the time of the Surgeon General's report on the association between tobacco smoke and lung cancer in 1964 until 1998 when about 24.1% of the population were active smokers [20]. Unfortunately, over the past several years, the percentage of smokers has ceased to decline and may even have increased slightly. Education and public awareness can aid in preventing individuals from starting smoking and thus becoming addicted to nicotine. Other efforts are aimed at helping smokers quit. Smoking cessation efforts including physician and nurse advice and nicotine replacement therapy may increase the rate of successful quitting. Although the minority of smokers (< 10%) are able to stop smoking successfully for 1 year or more in their first attempt, more than half have been able to stop with the assistance of health professionals [21].

The risk of lung cancer declines within 1 or 2 years after the cessation of smoking and continues to decline through at least 15 years but never reaches that of a nonsmoker [3]. Consequently, about half of the lung cancers now diagnosed in the United States are in former smokers [4]. Thus, secondary preventive measures such as chemoprevention must be considered as well. Epidemiologic evidence has supported a protective association between the consumption of large amounts of carrots and yellow and green leafy vegetables, rich in vitamin A and β-carotene, and the risk of lung cancer [22]. These compounds have relatively little toxicity when given in therapeutic doses and have been the first agents studied for the secondary prevention of lung cancer.

Two large randomized prevention studies were completed during 1990s, the α-tocopherol, β-carotene study (ATBC) in Finland and the β-carotene and retinol efficacy trial (CARET) in the United States. Surprisingly, both studies confirmed the increased risk of lung cancer in the group taking β-carotene [23,24]. A more recent strategy has been to study chemoprevention agents on patients with early stage aerodigestive cancers treated for cure. This represents a group with the highest risk of developing new primary lung cancers. A US Intergroup study randomized patients with completely resected stage I lung cancer to 13-*cis*-retinoic acid or placebo for 3 years. This trial showed no reduction in the rate of second primary cancers, and the rates were somewhat higher in smokers who received the 13-*cis*-retinoic acid [25]. Similarly, a European study randomized patients with resected early-stage lung cancer and head and neck cancer to placebo, retinyl palmitate, or *N*-acetyl cysteine or both agents for 2 years. There was no benefit in survival, event-free survival, or second primary tumors for patients with head and neck cancer or with lung cancer. Most of these patients were previous or current smokers [26]. The effects of selenium, nonsteroidal anti-inflammatory agents, and diets high in fresh fruits and vegetables are currently under study.

STAGING AND PROGNOSIS

The most important prognostic factors for lung cancer are the stage, the patient's performance status, and the amount of weight loss before diagnosis of lung cancer. The staging classification for NSCLC was recently modified and the current classification is shown in Table 10-3 [27]. The primary tumor is indicated by the T stage, which goes from the smallest lesion (< 3 cm) (T1), to the most extensive lesion with invasion of the mediastinum and great vessels, extensive pleural involvement with pleural effusion, or satellite lesions within the same lobe of the lung (T4). Regional lymph node metastases may be uninvolved (N0), involve hilar or peribronchial nodes (N1), ipsilateral mediastinal nodes (N2), or may be extensively involved including high paratracheal, supraclavicular, or contralateral nodes (N3). Distant spread to other organs indicates metastatic involvement (M1). The T, N, and M designations are then used to divide patients into stages. As shown in Table 10-3, survival rates decline as the stage increases, with a 5-year survival rate of about 67% for pathologic stage IA compared with 1% for stage IV disease.

The stage of disease is based on a combination of clinical (physical examination, radiologic, and laboratory studies) and pathologic (biopsy of lymph nodes, bronchoscopy, mediastinoscopy or other type of thoracotomy) studies. For asymptomatic patients, a complete history and physical examination, a chest radiograph and CT scan of the chest and upper abdomen to include the liver and adrenals, complete blood count, and blood chemistry are usually all that is required to determine the clinical stage. Additional studies such as magnetic resonance imaging (MRI) scans of the brain or bone scans are only indicated if there is a question of metastatic spread based on patient's symptoms, signs, or laboratory data. Evaluation should include questions regarding weight loss, focal skeletal pain, chest pain, seizures, syncope, extensive weakness, headache, and mental status changes. CT scans of the chest can provide an accurate assessment of the size of lymph nodes in the mediastinum but lymph node size is a poor predictor of cancer involvement. Thus, mediastinoscopy with biopsy of these nodes is indicated in most cases for adequate staging of nodal status. Whole-body positron-emission tomography (PET) scanning is a new imaging modality that has recently been demonstrated to be more accurate than conventional imaging methods in the staging of NSCLC [28]. It is more effective than CT in evaluating the mediastinum, with reported sensitivity of 91% and specificity of 86%—with the corresponding values of CT being 75% and 66%, respectively [28]. In a randomized trial PET scanning was shown to reduce the costs of evaluating and treating early stage lung cancer patients because it reduces the rate of "futile" thoracotomy. HICFA has approved payments for PET scanning to stage early lung cancer patients and its routine use will increase in frequency.

SCLC is classified as either limited or extensive stage [9]. Limited stage disease is confined to the hemithorax of origin, the mediastinum, or the supraclavicular lymph nodes, which is encompassable within a "tolerable" radiotherapy port. Radiation therapy cannot be delivered to an entire hemithorax. Therefore, patients with malignant pleural effusions as well as with distant metastases are included in the classification of extensive stage disease.

Performance status describes the functional ability of patients to carry out their usual daily activity. It is usually scored from 0 to 4 using the Eastern Cooperative Oncology Group (ECOG) or from 0% to 100% using the Karnofsky scale. Patients with decreased activity have a poorer prognosis and more toxicity after therapy [29]. Similarly, the degree of weight loss also correlates with a shorter survival [30]. In SCLC, other prognostic factors in addition to stage and performance status include lactate dehydrogenase (LDH) levels and gender. Patients with performance status of 0 or 1, a normal LDH level, and female gender have a better prognosis [9].

THERAPY FOR SMALL CELL LUNG CANCER

Small cell lung cancer accounts for 15% to 25% of the total lung cancer cases in the United States, with the number of cases in 2000 estimated at 34,300. At time of diagnosis, 65% to 70% of patients with SCLC present with extensive disease—metastasis beyond the ipsilateral lung and regional lymph nodes [2,9]. The remaining 30% to 35% of the cases present with limited stage SCLC; disease confined to one lung, the mediastinum, and ipsilateral or contralateral supraclavicular lymph nodes or both—that can be encompassed in a tolerable radiation port. SCLC has distinct histologic, clinical, and biologic features including high response rates to chemotherapy and radiation therapy, high propensity for metastases, neuroendocrine features, and paraneoplastic syndromes [9]. SCLC in general carries a poor prognosis. When untreated, the median survival time after diagnosis is only 2 to 4 months. With first-line multiagent chemotherapy, response rates approximate 80% to 90%, with complete response in 10% to 50% of patients, depending on disease stage [9]. Survival improved to a median 8 to 12 months for extensive stage and 14 to 20 months for limited stage. Chemotherapy is the cornerstone of therapy for all patients with concurrent radiation for those with limited stage and with surgery for the sure stage I patient.

Limited-Stage Small-Cell Lung Cancer

Patients with limited-stage SCLC are currently treated with concurrent chemotherapy and chest irradiation. This bimodal therapy was shown to be superior to either modality alone, resulting in increased complete response rate, decreased local recurrence, and improved survival [31–39]. A recent meta-analysis of 13 randomized trials showed a modest but significant 14% reduction in the relative mortality rate of patients receiving combined-modality therapy, with 14% of patients alive after 3 years compared with 9% in the chemotherapy-only group [31,32]. Patients receiving chemotherapy and chest irradiation experienced greater toxicity, but the gain in response and survival is thought to outweigh the increased toxicity in most instances.

The most widely used chemotherapy regimen for combined modality approach is etoposide and cisplatin (EP) (Table 10-4) [33–37]. EP is the standard chemotherapy regimen for SCLC. It replaced the cyclophosphamide, doxorubicin, vincristine (CAV) regimen of the 1970s and the cyclophosphamide, doxorubicin, etoposide (CEA) regimen of the early 1980s largely because it was less toxic and more convenient [38]. New chemotherapy combinations are currently under investigation.

Optimal timing of concurrent radiotherapy remains somewhat undefined. The earlier studies by the National Cancer Institute of Canada (NCIC) supported the early administration of thoracic radiotherapy [39,40]. In one NCIC trial, Murray *et al.* demonstrated that progression-free survival ($P = 0.036$) and overall survival ($P = 0.008$) were superior by starting radiotherapy concurrent and early in the course of chemotherapy [39]. A subsequent phase-III randomized trial from the Japan Clinical Oncology Group also favored the early concurrent treatment approach [41]. This group compared an early concurrent (C) schedule with conventional consolidative sequential (S) radiotherapy after platinum-etoposide therapy.

Table 10-3. Staging Classification of Lung Cancer

Primary tumor (T)

TX: primary tumor cannot be assessed, or tumor is proven by the presence of malignant cells in sputum or bronchial washings but not visualized by imaging or bronchoscopy

T0: No evidence of primary tumor

Tis: Carcinoma in situ

T1: Tumor that is ≤ 3.0 cm in greatest diameter and surrounded by lung or visceral pleura, without evidence of invasion more proximal than the lobar bronchus (ie, not in the main bronchus)

T2: Tumor with any of the following features of size or extent:

> 3.0 cm in greatest dimension

Involving the main bronchus, > 2.0 cm or more distal to the carina

Invading the visceral pleura

Associated with atelectasis or obstructive pneumonitis that extends to the hilar region but does not involve the entire lung

T3: Tumor of any size with direct extension to the chest wall (including superior sulcus tumors), diaphragm, mediastinal pleura, parietal pericardium; tumor in the main bronchus < 2.0 cm distal to the carina but without involvement of the carina; associated atelectasis or obstructive pneumonitis of the entire lung

T4: Tumor of any size that invades any of the following: mediastinum, heart, great vessels, trachea, esophagus, vertebral body, carina; or tumor with a malignant pleural or pericardial effusion or with satellite tumor nodule(s) within the ipsilateral primary-tumor lobe of the lung

Nodal involvement (N)

NX: Regional lymph nodes cannot be assessed

N0: No regional lymph node metastasis

N1: Metastasis in ipsilateral peribronchial and/or ipsilateral hilar lymph nodes, including direct extension

N2: Metastasis in ipsilateral mediastinal and/or subcarinal lymph nodes

N3: Metastasis in contralateral mediastinal, contralateral hilar, ipsilateral or contralateral scalene, or supraclavicular lymph nodes

Distant metastasis (M)

MX: Presence of distant metastasis cannot be assessed

M0: No distant metastasis

M1: Distant metastasis (beyond the ipsilateral supraclavicular nodes)

Staging	TNM	5-y Survival, %
Stage 0	Tis, N0, M0	0
StageIA	T1, N0, M0	67
Stage IB	T2, N0, M0	57
Stage IIA	T1, N1, M0	34
Stage IIB	T2, N1, M0	24
Stage IIB	T3, N0, M0	22
Stage IIIA	T3, N1, M0	9
Stage IIIA	T1–3, N2, M0	13
Stage IIIB	T4, any N, M0	7
Stage IIIB	any T, N3, M0	3

Although the response rates were not significantly different between the two arms (97.4% for arm C, 90.4% for arm S), the median survival time favored arm C (27.2 months versus 19.5 months). The overall survival rates at 2 and 3 years were significantly superior in the concurrent treatment arm (55.3% vs 35.4%) and (30.9% vs 20.7%), respectively (*P* = 0.057). Thus, these studies support the evidence that starting radiotherapy concurrent and early in the course of chemotherapy is most beneficial for long-term survival of patients with limited-stage SCLC.

Increasing the frequency of delivery of the radiotherapy by giving it twice daily in fractions that are one half (hyperfractionated) or more than the usual daily dose accelerated hyperfractionated radiotherapy (AHRT) has also been evaluated. A randomized intergroup trial showed that the AHRT approach produced a significant improvement in local control and a small improvement in survival, but also it increased toxicity [37]. The 5-year survival rates increased from 16% to 26% in the AHRT arm. It is not known whether increasing the once-daily therapy to biologically equivalent doses (*eg*, 65 Gy) would produce the same result. In practice either the twice-daily fractionation or a higher total dose with once-daily therapy should be chosen for good risk patients. More recent studies adjusted the radiotherapy component by reducing volumes through using ports designed by CT scans and by using postchemotherapy volumes or shrinking fields. These studies suggest volume reductions have reduced toxicity without adversely affecting outcome. Unfortunately, patients with limited-stage SCLC who receive combined modality therapy still have a high relapse rate at both local and distant sites [42].

Based on these and other related data, it can be concluded that four to six cycles of platinum/etoposide plus a course of radiotherapy (given either once or twice daily beginning with cycle 1 of chemotherapy) is an appropriate therapy for patients with limited-stage SCLC.

For the rare stage IA patient without nodal involvement or distant metastases (T1 N0; T2 N0), surgery followed by chemother-

apy with or without radiotherapy appears to be a reasonable treatment option [9,43]. Cure rates exceeding 60% are reported in these instances. For stage IB, II, and III disease, surgery in addition to chemotherapy and radiotherapy failed to improve outcome [44].

Extensive-Stage Small-Cell Lung Cancer

Several combinations of chemotherapeutic agents have been used over the past 20 to 30 years to manage SCLC [9]. In the 1970s and in the early part of the 1980s, the CAV combination was the most commonly used therapeutic regimen for both limited- and extensive-stage disease. In the latter, CAV demonstrated overall response rates of 55% to 65%, complete response rates of 10% to 15%, and a small number of 5-year survivors (1% to 5%) were also observed [45,46]. However, a relatively high rate of grade 4 myelosuppression, pulmonary toxicity, and neuropathy were noted with the CAV regimen. Furthermore, failure to respond to CAV meant, in general, poor response to second-line chemotherapy—usually less than 10% overall response with a dismal survival of 8 to 12 weeks. It was obvious then that the search for new combination drug regimens active in SCLC was crucial.

The EP is a combination regimen demonstrating significant activity in SCLC. It was originally developed in the early 1980s as a salvage treatment for CAV-refractory SCLC [47]. The EP regimen demonstrated a response rate of 50% on patients who relapsed after induction therapy with CAV [47]. A subsequent study showed that the EP regimen used after CAV induction demonstrated significant improvement in survival compared with CAV alone [48]. Another study reported data on the use of EP as a first-line therapy in a small cohort of patients with both extensive- and limited-stage SCLC who were not candidates to receive induction therapy with the CAV regimen due to underlying cardiac history. An overall response rate of 86% (43% complete response [CR], 43% partial response [PR]) was reported with an increased median duration of response and survival time [49].

Table 10-4. Combined Chemotherapy with Cisplatin Plus Etoposide and Thoracic Radiotherapy in Limited-Stage Small Cell Lung Cancer

Study	Chemotherapy Dosage Schedule, *mg/m²*	Chest Radiotherapy	CR, %	PR, %	MS, *mo*	2-Y Survival, %	Comments
McCracken [33]	cDDP: 50 iv, d 1+8,29+36,57+64 E: 50 iv, d 1–5,29–33,57–61 V: 1.4 iv, d 15,22,43,50	45 Gy concurrent, 180 cGy/fr OD, 25 fr, d 1–25	56	27	17.5	45	Every 4 wk × 3 cycles; PCI 30 Gy; consolidation with V,M,E alternating with A,Cy
Turrisi [34]	cDDP: 60 iv, d 1 E: 120 iv, d 4,6,8	45 Gy concurrent, 150 cGy/fr BID × 30 fr d 1–21	78	18	20	36	Every 3 wk × 2 cycles, PCI 30 Gy obligat; consolidation with PE alternating CAV 6 cycles
Johnson [35]	cDDP: 30 iv, d 1–3 E: 120 iv, d 1–3	45 Gy alternating, 150 cGy/fr BID × 30 fr d8–12,29–33,50–54	59	38	18	44	Every 3 wk × 4 cycles, PCI optional, consolidation with Cy/E
Johnson [36]	cDDP: 80 iv, d 1 E: 80 iv, d 1–3	45 Gy concurrent, 150 cGy/fr BID × 30 fr d 6–24	74	22	21.3	43	Every 4 wk × 4 cycles, PCI optional, consolidation with CAV × 4 cycles or individualized chemotherapy
Turrisi [37]	cDDP: 60 iv, d 1 E:120 iv, d 1–3	45 Gy, concurrent 180 cGY/fr OD × 30 fr d 1–41	46	35.2	19 (8-y md-fu)	41.7 (2 y) 16 (5 y)	Every 3 wk × 4 cycles, PCI for patients in CR
	cDDP: 60 iv, d 1 E: 120 iv, d 1–3	150 cGy/fr BID × 30 fr d 1–20	52.7	29.1	23 (8-y md-fu)	44.3 (2 y) 26 (5 y)	

BID—twice daily; cDDP—cisplatin; CR—complete response; Cy—cyclophosphamide; E—etoposide; fr—fraction; LD—limited stage disease; M—methotrexate; OD—once daily; PCI—prophylactic cranial irradiation; V—vincristine.

SCLC is highly sensitive to combination chemotherapy with high initial response rates. However, the number and duration of these responses remain limited because of the emergence of drug-resistant clones of tumor cells. The mathematical model of Goldie and Coldman [50] focuses on development of tumor cell drug resistance. It predicts that the optimal use of chemotherapeutic agents in malignant disease will involve the simultaneous use of all active agents early in the disease process. However, realization of this model is prevented due to the presence of agents with similar toxicities—mainly myelosuppression. To decrease the odds of appearance of multiply resistant tumor clones, the next best option, theoretically, would be alternation of non–cross-resistant combination agents. On this basis, the alternating CAV/EP regimens were developed and tested. In the first NCIC study, significantly higher response rate, progression-free survival, and overall survival were obtained with the alternating chemotherapy regimen. Subsequently, the Southeastern Study Group conducted a phase III trial composed of three induction treatment arms: arm 1: EP alone; arm 2: CAV alone; and arm 3: the alternating regimen (CAV/PE) [45]. No significant differences were shown in treatment outcome for any arm of the study in terms of response rate, complete response rate, or median survival. Myelosuppression was the dose-limiting toxicity for all patients, with incident leukopenia/granulocytopenia higher in those treated with CAV or alternating therapy (CAV/EP). The conclusion was that the combination regimens EP and CAV were equally effective induction therapies in extensive SCLC and that alternating therapy provided no therapeutic advantage compared with use of either of the individual regimens alone [45]. In a similar phase III study by the Japanese, Fukuoka et al. [46] reported results that slightly favored the alternating chemotherapy (CAV/PE) over the individual regimens of CAV and PE in a cohort of patients with both limited- and extensive-stage SCLC. In this study, the response rates/complete response rates for the PE, CAV/PE, CAV were similar: 78%/14%, 76%/16%, and 55%/15%, respectively. Survival was also equivalent except in a subset analysis of limited disease where the alternating regimen was preferred [46]. The conclusion from these studies is that any of these combinations could be used. Four cycles of PE were most convenient and least toxic.

Attempts to enhance efficacy of CAV or EP regimens by increasing dosage or increasing frequency of drug delivery have largely been unsuccessful. Individual randomized trials comparing standard-dose CAV with dose-intensified CAV and comparing standard-dose EP with dose-intensified EP revealed enhanced toxicity without improving survival [51,52]. In another randomized trial, granulocyte-colony stimulating factor (G-CSF) was used to allow the increase of the dose of the standard-drug regimen [53]. However, despite improved dose intensity allowed by the addition of G-CSF to the treatment regimen, this study failed to demonstrate improvement in response rate or survival. G-CSF ought not be included in regimens for limited-stage disease that include concurrent radiation therapy, however. These growth factors have been associated with significant high-grade thrombocytopenia and other toxicities when used in combination with radiation therapy [9].

Increasing dose intensity by increasing frequency of drug delivery led to the testing of weekly regimens. In the early 1990s, Murray et al. [54] combined four of the most active drugs against SCLC, cisplatin, vincristine, doxorubicin, and etoposide, creating the weekly CODE regimen [54]. The regimen was designed to double the dose intensity of these drugs compared with the standard alternating regimen of CVA/EP for extensive stage SCLC. Results of this pilot study prompted design of an Intergroup Phase III trial of CODE versus CAV/EP for extensive stage SCLC to compare CODE plus thoracic irradiation with CAV/EP in the treatment of extensive-stage SCLC [55]. The response rate with the CODE regimen (87%) was significantly higher than with the CAV/EP regimen (70%). Conversely, no significant difference was observed on progression-free survival (median of 0.66 years on both arms) and overall survival (medium, 0.98 years for CODE and 0.91 years for CAV/EP). Of concern was the percentage of toxic deaths associated with the CODE arm (8.2%) compared with that (0.9%) on the CAV/EP arm. Murray et al. concluded from this randomized trial that although the response rate with CODE was higher than CAV/EP, progression-free and overall survival were not significantly improved. Moreover, because the CODE regimen-related mortality rate was unacceptably high compared with that of the CAV/EP regimen, CODE is not recommended for treatment of extensive stage SCLC [55]. This randomized trial failed to show any advantage of increasing the frequency and intensity of drug delivery compared with standard regimens.

Activity of carboplatin in SCLC was recognized some time after cisplatin became a standard agent. Carboplatin has the advantage of producing less nephrotoxicity, ototoxicity, neuropathy, nausea, vomiting, and it is easier to administer. Two randomized trials showed carboplatin to be equivalent in efficacy and less toxic compared with cisplatin [56,57]. Therefore, the etoposide/carboplatin combination regimen is often used by oncologists today.

MAINTENANCE THERAPY

Some debate continues about the optimal number of chemotherapy cycles and the role of maintenance therapy. Three large randomized trials showed that time to progression was longer in the groups receiving maintenance chemotherapy, but no differences in survival rates were found [58–61]. Toxicity was higher in patients receiving the maintenance therapy. At present, both continued exposure to the toxic chemotherapy and the fact that patients whose disease progresses under maintenance chemotherapy tend to do poorly under salvage treatment make the discontinuation of chemotherapy after four to six cycles a preferred approach. Subsequent randomized trials using the biologic agent interferon [62] and a new chemotherapeutic agent, topotecan [63], have also failed to show any improvement in survival with maintenance therapy even though on the latter study, topotecan did prolong time to progression.

THERAPY FOR OLDER PATIENTS AND THOSE IN POOR PHYSICAL CONDITION

Many older patients have several comorbid conditions in addition to SCLC, especially with a long-term history of smoking. Several studies showed that single-agent oral etoposide (VP-16) is well tolerated by this patient population, and that response and survival rates are similar to those reported in younger and healthier patients. However, randomized trials comparing oral VP-16 with standard combination regimens showed that the combination regimens produce better quality of life and longer survival without increased toxicity [64,65]. Therefore, standard chemotherapy combinations are the preferred treatment for those with a poorer prognosis.

NEW AGENTS

Unfortunately, most SCLC patients relapse and die from progressive disease. Extensive-stage SCLC patients who receive chemotherapy have a 5-year survival rate of only 1%. Thus, it has been reasonable to study new agents in untreated extensive-stage SCLC patients. In many trials in which ineffective agents are studied in previously untreated patients, those study subjects receiving the more ineffective agent have a worse outcome than those receiving standard therapy. In most studies reviewed, however, patients were crossed over to standard treatment regimens after 6 weeks if no response was seen. With this study design, no negative survival impact of the new agent was identified [58].

Several chemotherapy agents with novel mechanisms of action have become available over the past 10 years. These include the taxanes (paclitaxel, docetaxel), the topoisomerase-I-targeting agents (irinotecan and topotecan), the synthetic vinca alkaloid (vinorelbine), and a novel antimetabolite (gemcitabine). These drugs have demonstrated significant activity as single agents in SCLC [66].

Irinotecan (CPT-11) is a water-soluble derivative of camptothecin, a potent inhibitor of DNA topoisomerase-I that has demonstrated activity in phase II trial conducted by Masuda et al. in refractory or relapsed SCLC [67]. The objective response rate was 47% with a median duration of response of 58 days. Dose-limiting toxicities included leukopenia and diarrhea. The conclusion was that CPT-11 was an active agent against refractory/relapsed SCLC. On the basis of the reported synergistic activity of the combination of cisplatin and irinotecan in SCLC, the West Japan Thoracic Oncology Group (WJTOC) conducted a phase II study of this combination regimen in patients with previously untreated SCLC [68]. The investigators reported an overall response rate of 84% (29% CR). Of the 40 patients with limited-stage disease, the overall response rate, median response duration, and median survival were 83% (30% CR), 8.0 months, and 14.3 months, respectively. For the 35 patients with extensive-stage parameters, the findings were 86% (29% CR), 6.6 months, and 13 months, respectively [68]. Toxicities associated with this combination regimen were also neutropenia, leukopenia, and diarrhea. These encouraging results led to a phase-III trial comparing the irinotecan/cisplatin-regimen (IP) with the standard VP-16/cisplatin-regimen (EP) recently reported by Noda et al. [69]. The overall response rate in the IP-arm was 83% (3% CR, 81% PR) versus 68% (9% CR, 58% PR) in the EP-arm. The reported median overall survival (OS)/median progression-free survival (PFS) favored IP with OS/PFS of 390 days/209 days. Myelosuppression was more prominent in the EP-arm and diarrhea was reported only in the IP-arm. Noda et al. [69] proposed that the irinotecan/cisplatin regimen should be considered a new standard treatment for extensive-stage SCLC because of the superior results with IP ($P>0.01$). Because this is the only randomized trial comparing EP with IP, IP can be considered an acceptable therapy and is added to the standard therapies given later in this chapter. However, unless other studies confirm its superiority, this regimen should be considered as only one of several acceptable therapies.

Topotecan is another semisynthetic water soluble analogue of camptothecin that shares similar activity with the other topoisomerase-I inhibitor, irinotecan. Both these drugs stabilize a covalent DNA topoisomerase I complex to yield enzyme-linked DNA single-strand breaks [70]. The recommended starting dose of topotecan as a single agent is 1.5 mg/m^2 [70]. Schiller et al. [71] reported an objective response rate, median response duration, and overall median survival of 39% (no CR), 4.8 months, and 10 months, respectively. This study confirmed the activity of single-agent topotecan in previously untreated SCLC patients.

A phase II study involving patients with refractory and sensitive SCLC was conducted by Ardizzoni et al. [72]. Refractory patients are those that never responded to first-line therapy or who responded but whose disease progressed within 3 months from the end of treatment. These patients rarely respond to second-line therapy [72]. The sensitive patient population is defined as those who responded to first-line therapy and relapsed after treatment-free interval of 3 or more months. These patients have a reasonable chance of responding to second-line chemotherapy. Those authors reported an overall response rate of 6.4% and 37.8%, a median survival of 4.7 months and 6.9 months in the refractory and sensitive groups, respectively. Overall median duration of response was 7.6 months. These data stimulated a subsequent phase III trial conducted by von Pawel et al. [73] comparing CAV versus topotecan (1.5 mg/m^2) in patients with SCLC who had relapsed at least 60 days after completion of first-line therapy. These authors reported equivalent response rates of 24.3%/18.3%, median progression-free survival of 13.3 weeks/12.3 weeks, and median survival of 25 weeks/24.7 weeks, for the topotecan/CAV regimens, respectively. None of these latter reported parameters demonstrated any statistical significance. Relief of patient's symptoms was more frequent with topotecan. They concluded that topotecan was at least as effective as CAV in the treatment of patients with recurrent SCLC and produced improvement in various symptoms to a greater degree.

Other novel agents with broad-spectrum activity that have shown activity in SCLC are the two taxanes: paclitaxel (Taxol) and docetaxel (Taxotere). In a phase II study by ECOG of paclitaxel in patients with extensive stage SCLC, Ettinger et al. [74] reported an overall response rate of 34%. Nonresponders or partial responders subsequently received salvage chemotherapy with EP. In a similar phase II study by the North American Cancer Treatment Group, Kirschling et al. [75] reported an overall response rate of 53%. However, the response duration was short (median, 3.4 months). These authors concluded that paclitaxel was indeed an active agent in SCLC and thus attractive for use in combination regimens. The European Organization for Research and Treatment of Cancer (EORTC) reported that docetaxel at a dose of 100 mg/m^2 led to an objective response rate of 25% among 28 patients, most of whom had received prior therapy. Of their patients, however, 90% developed grade 4 neutropenia, and a significant minority of the patients developed clinically significant pulmonary effusion, ascites, and edema [76]. Thus, both taxanes have activity.

The activity of single-agent paclitaxel in SCLC stimulated researchers at the University of Colorado Cancer Center to conduct a phase I study of the triple therapy cisplatin/etoposide/paclitaxel in patients with extensive stage SCLC [77]. Kelly et al. reported response, median survival, and 1-year survival rates of 83%, 10 months, and 39%, respectively. These authors concluded that paclitaxel could be added safely to full doses of cisplatin and etoposide with encouraging efficacy and acceptable toxicity. G-CSF, however, was required to ameliorate the high rate of grade 4 neutropenia. In a subsequent phase II trial conducted by SWOG, the cisplatin/etoposide/paclitaxel regimen reproduced the encouraging results with objective response, median survival, and 1-year survival rates of 56%, 11 months, and 43%, respectively [78]. These data have provided the foundation for the ongoing randomized Intergroup trial comparing the cisplatin/etoposide/paclitaxel regimen of SWOG-9705 with the standard platinum/etoposide (PE) regimen in patients with extensive-stage SCLC with optimal Karnofsky Performance scores (KPS).

In a study from Greece, Mavroudis *et al.* [79] reported data on a randomized trial comparing TEP with EP in a small cohort of patients with limited- and extensive-stage SCLC. The outcome (survival and response) was not improved in the three-drug combination. The study was closed early due to the increased number of toxic deaths in the cisplatin/etoposide/paclitaxel treatment arm. Therefore, at the present time, due to the limited number of patients, this and other triple combinations must remain experimental unless the ongoing large randomized Intergroup trial demonstrates an overall benefit.

PROPHYLACTIC CRANIAL IRRADIATION

Because of the high frequency of brain metastases in SCLC, prophylactic cranial irradiation (PCI) was evaluated and shown to reduce metastases of the central nervous system (CNS). Its effects on prolongation of survival was debated until a meta-analysis of all randomized trials was reported in 1999 [80]. An initial retrospective review of seven studies in which patients had been randomized to PCI versus no PCI while in complete remission after standard induction therapy, neuropsychological impairment was reported in 76% and 15% of these patients, respectively [9]. Other studies have shown no significant difference in long-term neuropsychologic function among those patients randomized to PCI- and control-arm. These studies suggest that further studies on the optimal dose and schedule of PCI are needed but that it can be offered to patients with a good response to induction therapy. The Prophylactic Cranial Irradiation Overview Collaborative Group reported a 5.4% increase in the rate of survival at 3 years in favor of the treatment group (15.3% in the control group vs 20.7% in the treatment group) [80]. The treatment group was also demonstrated to have a higher rate of disease-free survival and a decrease in the cumulative index of brain metastasis. The meta-analysis also reported a significant trend to a greater decrease in the risk of brain metastasis with larger doses of radiation. Finally, a significant trend toward a decrease in the risk of brain metastasis was observed with earlier administration of PCI after initiation of induction chemotherapy. The conclusion this meta-analysis reached is that PCI does indeed improve the overall survival and disease-free survival of patients with SCLC who have achieved a complete remission after standard induction therapy [80].

THERAPY FOR NON–SMALL CELL LUNG CANCER

Treatment of Stages I and II Non–Small Cell Lung Cancer

Surgery is the primary therapy for patients with stage I and II NSCLC, with the goal of removing the entire tumor with negative resection margins [2]. Assessment of lung function by simple spirometry remains one of the most important determinants of operability. In general, an FEV_1 (forced expiratory volume of 1 s) of at least 2.0 L (< 60% of predicted value), a maximum voluntary ventilatory capacity of more than 50%, or a diffusing capacity of carbon monoxide of more than 60% means that a patient likely has the pulmonary reserve to tolerate a pneumonectomy or lesser resection. For those who do not meet these criteria, smoking cessation, pulmonary rehabilitation, and intensive preoperative respiratory therapies can help. Patients continuing to have poor pulmonary function tests after these measures can still undergo resection if a postoperative predictive FEV_1 of more than 40% or 800 mL is obtained. Most often this requires a lobectomy or a pneumonectomy [2]. The latter is required in only a few cases. When the tumor is centrally located or extends into several lobes, it can only be removed in its entirety by pneumonectomy. Lesser resection, such as wedge resection, segmental resection, or sleeve lobectomy should be reserved for patients with compromised pulmonary function who could not tolerate a lobectomy. This was shown in an LCSG study in T1N0 NSCLC comparing limited resection with lobectomy. In this study, a higher local recurrence rate and shorter survival were noted in the limited resection group [81]. Chest wall resection and sleeve resection may be performed for T3 lesions. Sleeve resections are performed for tumors near the carina where a distal bronchus from an uninvolved lobe is sewn into the carina after resection.

Surgical therapy provides excellent results with cure rates exceeding 65% only for stage IA (T1, N0, M0) NSCLC [2,27]. No convincing evidence confirms that any adjuvant therapy including immunotherapy, radiotherapy, or chemotherapy improves survival for these patients. Because most of these patients are cured by surgery, it is probably best to reserve further study of adjuvant chemotherapy until such adjuvant therapy shows value in NSCLC patients at higher risk of relapse. However, stage I lung cancer patients resected for cure have a high risk of developing second primary tumors that exceeds the risk of disease recurrence. Because of this, patients should be encouraged to stop smoking. These patients also serve as excellent subjects for chemoprevention studies.

Most patients with stage IB to IIIA NSCLC have disease recurrence after surgical therapy and most such recurrences are in distant sites [82]. Postoperative radiation therapy in stage IB-IIIA NSCLC has been found to reduce the rate of local recurrence but has no benefit in overall survival [82,83]. A randomized trial by the LCSG investigating the efficacy of postoperative mediastinal irradiation in completely resected squamous cell carcinoma of the lung demonstrated a reduction in local recurrence (41% to 3%), but this improvement did not translate into a survival benefit because most of the failures were distant [83]. Meta-analysis of all randomized trials of post-operative radiotherapy (PORT) showed a worsening of survival with a 21% increase in the hazard of death and a 7% decrease in the 2-year survival rate [84]. This detrimental effect was more pronounced for patients with stage I/II, N0-N1 disease, whereas for stage IIIA(N2) disease, no clear evidence confirmed any adverse effect [84]. This study has been criticized because many older studies used cobalt radiotherapy and larger ports. Nonetheless, there are no positive randomized trials so that radiotherapy should be considered judiciously in select patients until a randomized trial shows some benefit.

The earliest studies of postoperative adjuvant chemotherapy used alkylating agents alone or in combination [85]. These studies showed no benefit for postoperative chemotherapy and in several studies, including the one given here, survival was actually shortened. Meta-analysis of all postoperative adjuvant studies with alkylating agent–based therapy confirmed an increased hazard ratio for death and a shortened survival [85]. These therapies were also relatively toxic; these findings led to considerable pessimism for the role of adjuvant chemotherapy.

After cisplatin-based chemotherapy was shown to have activity in advanced NSCLC, it was evaluated as postoperative therapy in resected patients. Many trials used the CAP regimen consisting of cyclophosphamide, adriamycin, and low-dose cisplatin (40 mg/m²). Postoperative compliance was often poor. Some of these studies showed survival advantages for the chemotherapy, whereas others did not [82]. Meta-analysis showed that the cisplatin therapy was associated with an absolute increase of 5% in the 5-year survival rate, which was a 13% reduction in the hazard rate of death [85]. Given the small number of patients in these studies, this survival increase was of borderline statistical significance. Physicians in the United Kingdom were surveyed after being shown these data and fewer than 5% indicated that they would recommend chemotherapy for their patients. In contrast, when such data were explained to patients, more than 90% wished to be offered chemotherapy and more than 50% wanted chemotherapy if it would improve the cure rate by 1%. Fortunately, we now have many ongoing randomized trials investigating the role of postoperative adjuvant therapy (including superior chemotherapeutic agents with lower toxicity profile) for early-stage resectable NSCLC.

A phase II trial conducted by the Bimodality Lung Oncology Team (BLOT) demonstrated that induction chemotherapy followed by surgery produces high response rates and is safe/feasible in early-stage NSCLC [86]. The BLOT study evaluated two cycles of neoadjuvant paclitaxel and carboplatin (PC) and with three additional cycles of PC given to patients undergoing complete resection. The objective response rate to neoadjuvant chemotherapy was 56%, the complete resection rate was 86%, the pathologic complete response was 6%, with an estimated 1-year survival rate of 85% for all patients. The median survival was not reached with a projected 4-year survival rate of 65%. In a French randomized phase III trial, Depierre et al. [87] demonstrated that neoadjuvant chemotherapy offers survival advantage in resectable NSCLC. Patients with resectable stage I, II, and IIIA NSCLC were randomized to undergo direct surgery or to two cycles of neoadjuvant mitomycin, ifosfamide, and cisplatin (MIC). Two additional cycles of MIC were administered postoperatively for those who obtained objective response. Postoperative thoracic radiotherapy was given to all pT3 or pN2 patients in both arms of the study. The initial pathologic response rate was 64% (11% CR; 53% PR). Initial survival data favored the induction chemotherapy arm but the differences did not reach statistical significance. The median survival was 26 months and 36 months for the surgery group and neoadjuvant chemotherapy group, respectively; the 1-, 2-, and 3-year survival rates were 73%, 52%, 41% and 77%, 59%, and 49% for each group, respectively. Although these are promising data, larger randomized trials using neoadjuvant or adjuvant chemotherapy are required to determine the role of this treatment approach in the routine treatment of early-stage NSCLC. Fortunately, randomized trials of neoadjuvant chemotherapy are available in the United States and Europe, and patients should be considered for these trials.

Treatment of Stage IIIA-N2 Non–Small Cell Lung Cancer

The 5-year survival rates for patients with clinical stage IIIA-N2 NSCLC treated with surgery alone is poor (10% to 15%). Postoperative radiotherapy improves local control but fails to improve survival [84]. The poor survival rate and high rate of distant relapse made studies of preoperative chemotherapy logical. Phase II studies of such an approach provided encouraging results. Typical results from some studies are summarized in Table 10-5. The Memorial Sloan-Kettering Cancer Center evaluated two or three cycles of neoadjuvant mitomycin, vinblastine, and cisplatin chemotherapy [88]. The objective response rate to chemotherapy was 77%, the complete resection rate was 78%, the pathologic complete response rate was 14%, and for all the patients, the 5-year survival rate was 17%. Nearly all the 5-year survivors were in the subgroup of patients undergoing complete resection. This subset had a 5-year survival of 26%. A group in Toronto using the same chemotherapy regimen reported a 71% response rate and a 51% complete resection rate [89]. The median survival rate was 21.3 months. The 5-year survival rates were encouraging (< 20%).

A large phase II trial by the CALGB evaluated 74 patients with stage IIIA NSCLC treated with two cycles of vinblastine/cisplatin before complete resection, followed by chest irradiation in patients who had incomplete resection or no response to chemotherapy [90] (see Table 10-5). The objective response plus stable disease rate was 88%. In the study, 86% of patients were treated with surgery and 36% had complete resection. The 3-year overall survival rate was 23%, with median survivals of 20.9 months in patients undergoing complete resection and 17.8 months in those with incomplete resection compared with 8.5 months in patients whose tumors were not resected. A SWOG phase II study was done to assess the feasibility of concurrent chemotherapy and irradiation followed by surgery in locally advanced NSCLC [91]. This study reported 85% resectability for the stage IIIA (N2) group and 80% resectability for the IIIB group (see Table 10-5). The 2- and 3-year survival rates were 37% and 27%, respectively. The 6-year outcome from this SWOG trial was recently reported by Albain et al. [92]. The long-term survival levels at 20% and was still identical for patients with both bulky IIIA(N2) and IIIB tumors treated with trimodality therapy. Those authors also reported that nearly 50% of patients with T4 N0-1 tumors survived 6 years after resection of stable disease. Furthermore, they concurred that clearance of mediastinal nodal involvement remains the strongest favorable outcome predictor for those patients with initial N2/N3 disease [92].

Encouraging results of these phase II neoadjuvant studies led to two prospective phase III randomized trials using neoadjuvant cisplatin-based chemotherapy. In the Spanish trial, Rosell et al. [93,94] compared the chemotherapy regimen of cisplatin/ifosfamide/mitomycin C for three cycles followed by surgery versus surgery alone. The median survival of (26 vs 8 months) and the 3-year survival of (25% vs 0%) favored the chemotherapy arm. In the MD Anderson Cancer Center study, Roth et al. compared preoperative chemotherapy with cisplatin/cyclophosphamide/etoposide for three cycles followed by surgery versus surgery alone [95,96]. Postoperative chemotherapy was also administered and postoperative radiotherapy was allowed at the discretion of the physician. Results again favored the chemotherapy arm with an improved median survival of 64 vs 11 months and 3-year survival of (56% vs 15%). Both these studies had a small number of patients (60 in each study). Further accrual was appropriately halted based on ethical considerations due to the highly statistically significant improvement in

Table 10-5. Selected Phase II Neoadjuvant Results in IIIA Non–Small Cell Lung Cancer

Study	Treatment	Patients, n	Response rate, %	Median Survival, mo	Percent Survival*
MSKCC [88]	MVP	136	77	19	17 (5)
Toronto [89]	MVP	55	71	21	20 (5)
CALGB [90]	VP	74	88†	20.9	33 (3)
SWOG [91,92]	EP + RT	75	88†	13	20 (6) – IIA
					22 (6) – IIIB

*Percent of patients alive at year indicated in parentheses.
†Includes stable disease and responders.
CALGB—Cancer and Leukemia Group B; EP—etoposide, cisplatin; MSKCC—Memorial Sloan-Kettering Cancer Center; MVP—mitomycin, vinblastine, cisplatin; RT—radiation therapy; SWOG—Southwest Oncology Group; VP—vinblastine, cisplatin.

survival associated with the chemotherapy arm. Recent data on the 7-year follow-up of patients enrolled in both of these randomized studies revealed that the increase in survival conferred by perioperative chemotherapy was maintained during the period of extended observation [94,96]. Many physicians concluded that these studies showed that single modality surgical therapy for preoperatively defined N2 disease could no longer be justified.

The optimal combined therapy approach remains undefined. Excellent results have been achieved with chemotherapy plus surgery, with chemotherapy plus radiotherapy, and with all three modalities. Future randomized trials are necessary to clarify the optimal approach. The North American Intergroup trial in stage III disease (INT-0139) is currently comparing concurrent induction chemotherapy/radiotherapy with chemotherapy/radiotherapy followed by surgical resection. This study is targeting primarily stage IIIa-N2 patients and requires pathologic documentation of N2 involvement [97].

A major remaining controversy is whether preoperative therapy (chemotherapy or chemotherapy/radiotherapy) should now be considered the standard of care in stage IIIA disease. Experts consider that the two major subsets of stage III disease must be considered as separate entities. For unresectable, stage IIIA-bulky-N2 or IIIB disease, surgery after chemotherapy/radiotherapy has not been proven to be superior to chemotherapy/radiotherapy alone and thus cannot be considered the standard of care [97]. The INT-0139 trial is currently addressing this question. Conversely, long-term survival data reported in both the Rosell *et al.* and Roth *et al.* landmark studies supports consideration of preoperative therapy in selected patients with stage IIIA-disease. Patients with minimal stage IIIA disease that is technically resectable appear to be the ideal population to benefit from preoperative therapy, assuming the multimodality team involved is experienced in this approach and works in a collaborative manner to maximize the efficacy and minimize potential toxicities.

TREATMENT OF STAGE IIIB NON–SMALL CELL LUNG CANCER

Radiotherapy was the primary therapy for stage IIIB NSCLC for many years because it alleviated symptoms and because between 5% and 10% of patients survived at 5-years [2]. Survival of patients with locally advanced, unresectable NSCLC treated with radiotherapy is poor with a median survival of only 9 to 10 months. The addition of chemotherapy was tested to evaluate its ability to improve local control and eliminate or delay the emergence of metastatic disease. Multiple randomized trials of radiotherapy alone versus radiotherapy plus chemotherapy have been completed, most of which showed survival advantage for the combined approach (Table 10-6).

The CALGB, using sequential chemotherapy-radiotherapy, compared two cycles of cisplatin and vinblastine induction chemotherapy followed by chest irradiation with radiotherapy alone in patients with stage III NSCLC [98] (see Table 10-6). The median survival rates were 13.8 months and 9.7 months for the combined modality and the radiotherapy group alone, respectively (*P* = 0.0066). Survival rates at 2 and 3 years were 24% and 23%, and 14% and 11%, respectively. After more than 7 years of follow-up, long-term survival remained greater for the chemotherapy/radiotherapy group (5-year survival rate of 17% vs 6%) [99]. The superiority of this combined regimen was confirmed by a subsequent RTOG study that compared standard radiation therapy with induction chemotherapy of cisplatin and vinblastine followed by radiation therapy with twice-daily radiation therapy in unresectable NSCLC patients [100].

The combined modality arm was statistically superior to the other two treatment arms (median and 1-year survival of 13.8 months and 60% compared with 11.4 months and 46% in the standard arm and 12.3 months and 51% in the hyperfractionated arm).

A French group compared the effects of standard radiotherapy alone (arm 1) with those of sequential chemotherapy-radiotherapy (arm 2) in unresectable NSCLC [101] (see Table 10-6). Patients in arm 2 received three cycles of vindesine, cyclophosphamide, cisplatin, and lomustine (VCPC), with three additional cycles of VCPC administered after radiotherapy to patients with stable disease. The objective response rates were 35% (20% CR) and 31% (16% CR) for patients on arms 1 and 2, respectively. The rate of distant metastases at 2 years was 64% in the radiotherapy group compared with 43% in the combined modality group (*P*< 0.001). The combined modality therapy was associated with significant improvement in length of survival (median survival, 12 months versus 10 months) and reduced incidence of distant disease.

A concurrent combined-modality approach was evaluated in an EORTC phase III trial in inoperable, nonmetastatic NSCLC. This study compared split-course radiation therapy alone with split-course radiation therapy combined with cisplatin, given either weekly or daily [102] (see Table 10-6). Survival significantly improved in the combination group compared with the findings in the radiotherapy only group (*P* = 0.009). Also noted was improved local control in the daily cisplatin/radiotherapy group (*P* = 0.003), suggesting that this schedule results in maximal radiation enhancement.

A randomized study of hyperfractionated radiation therapy with or without concurrent chemotherapy of carboplatin and etoposide in stage III NSCLC was conducted by Jeremic *et al.* [103]. The median and 3-year survival rates were significantly better for the chemotherapy groups (13 months, 16% in the high-dose carboplatin arm versus 18 months and 23% in the low-dose carboplatin arm vs 8 months, 6.6% in the radiation only arm). There was a higher incidence of acute and/or late high-grade toxicity in the combined groups; even so no patients died as a result of treatment-related toxicity. A subsequent study was performed by the same group comparing hyperfractionated radiation therapy with or without concurrent low-dose daily carboplatin (50 mg) and etoposide (50 mg). A significantly longer survival time was found in the group receiving both radiation and chemotherapy (median survival of 22 months versus 14 months and 4-year survival rates of 23% versus 9%) [104].

Meta-analysis of 14 randomized trials of combination therapy and radiotherapy alone in locally advanced, unresectable NSCLC was subsequently done [105]. Compared with radiotherapy alone, combined chemotherapy/radiotherapy reduced the risk for death by 12% at 1 year, 13% by 2 years, and 17% by 3 years. When considered separately, trials of concurrent and sequential chemotherapy yielded similar treatment effects. The addition of chemotherapy to radiotherapy was associated with a 10% to 20% decrease in the risk for death. When the analysis was restricted only to the trials in which cisplatin was used as part of the chemotherapy regimen, the results were similar. Any absolute benefit should be balanced against the increased toxicity associated with the addition of chemotherapy. A UK study showed an improved quality of life when chemotherapy was added to radiation therapy on patients with localized disease [106]. Meta-analysis showed that the combination of chemotherapy and radiotherapy, either concurrently or sequentially, had a positive effect on survival and quality of life. The optimal approach, however, needs to be further delineated.

The West Japan Lung Cancer Group data on a randomized trial comparing concurrent versus sequential thoracic radiotherapy in combination with mitomycin, vindesine, and cisplatin in unresectable stage III NSCLC [107] are listed in Table 10-6. This group demonstrated a significantly better response rate and survival with the concurrent chemoradiotherapy regimen compared with sequential therapy. A response rate of 84% versus 66% ($P = 0.0002$) and a median survival of 16.5 months versus 13.3 months ($P = 0.03998$) were reported for the concurrent and sequential arms, respectively. The 2-, 3-, 4-, and 5-year survival rates were also superior for the concurrent group (34.6%, 22.3%, 16.9%, and 15.8%, respectively) compared with findings in the sequential group (27.4%, 14.7%, 10.1%, and 8.9%, respectively). A similar randomized trial by RTOG compared two concurrent cisplatin-based chemotherapy and thoracic radiotherapy regimens with a standard sequential chemotherapy (cisplatin and vindesine) combined with radiotherapy approach [108]. With a median follow-up of 40 months, the data revealed a significantly improved median survival time of 17 months for the concurrent therapy arm compared with 14.6 months for the sequential therapy arm [108] (see Table 10-6). It appears then that in good performance status patients with unresectable stage III NSCLC, the concurrent approach of chemoradiation therapy yields significantly increased response and enhanced median survival rates when compared with the sequential approach.

THERAPY OF STAGE IV NON–SMALL CELL LUNG CANCER

Until the last several years, considerable pessimism endured about the role of chemotherapy in advanced NSCLC [109,110]. No agent consistently produced objective responses in more than 20% of patients, and no evidence showed that chemotherapy prolonged the survival of these patients. During the 1980s, several randomized trials compared cisplatin-based chemotherapy combinations with best supportive care (BSC). All these studies showed superior survival results with the cisplatin therapy but this difference was not always statistically significant. Meta-analysis showed a highly statistically significant survival advantage for patients receiving cisplatin-based therapy. However, the survival advantage was modest [85]. A randomized study by the CNCI showed a median survival of 33

weeks in patients treated with chemotherapy compared with 17 weeks in patients treated with BSC (109). The 1-year survival rate more than doubled from 10% to over 20% and symptoms improved in responding patients. In the meta-analysis, cisplatin-based combinations significantly improved median survival by about 2 months with a 10% (from 10% to 20%) increase in the percentage of patients alive at 1 year [85]. Combination chemotherapy also improved quality of life and palliated symptoms. A UK study showed that chemotherapy (mitomycin, ifosfamide, and cisplatin) significantly improved quality of life in addition to median survival compared with standard treatment in inoperable NSCLC of both stages III and IV [106].

As discussed regarding SCLC, six novel chemotherapy agents demonstrated significant activity in the treatment of NSCLC. The low response rate and survival benefits from older standard platinum-based regimens (eg, etoposide/cisplatin) made the discovery of these more effective agents imperative. During the 1990s, a series of Phase I/II clinical trials of these novel agents alone or in combination with a platinum-containing agent (Table 10-7) were conducted. The single agent and its combination with a platinum agent demonstrated superior overall response rates and survival gains compared with standard therapy [110,111]. Two randomized trials comparing single-agent paclitaxel and docetaxel to best supportive care showed significantly improved survival with the taxane and a reduction in the hazard of death of more than 30%, which is superior to the 26% reduction from cisplatin-based therapies [112,113]. Two other randomized trials, conducted to compared the combination vinorelbine or gemcitabine plus cisplatin with single-agent cisplatin, both confirmed the superiority of the combination regimen [114,115]. This led to two subsequent randomized studies comparing the old standard cisplatin/etoposide (ECOG) or tenoposide/cisplatin (EORTC) with paclitaxel/cisplatin. The reported data favored the paclitaxel/cisplatin arm with superior overall response rate and median survival (ECOG trial) [116] but no significant difference in median survival between the arms on the (EORTC trial) [117]. These optimal results standardized a novel agent plus platinum combination regimen as primary treatment regimen for patients with advanced-stage NSCLC [110,111].

Table 10-6. Randomized Trials of Sequential or Concurrent Chemotherapy and Radiation Therapy

Study	Patients, n	Type	CT + RT Schedule	Median Survival (CT + RT vs RT Alone)	2-Y Survival (CT + RT vs RT Alone)
Dillman et al. [98,99]	155	Sequential	P/Vb × 2 + 60 Gy/6 wk	13.8 vs 9.7	24 vs 14 (2 y)
					23 vs 11 (3 y)
					17 vs 6 (5 y)
Sause et al. [100]	452	Sequential	P/Vb × 2 + 60 Gy/6 wk	13.8 vs 11.4	30 vs 19
LeChevalier et al. [101]	353	Sequential	VCPC × 3 + 65 Gy/5.5 wk + VCP × 3	12 vs 10	21 vs 14
Schaake-Koning et al. [102]	308	Concurrent	P + 30 Gy/2 wk + 25 Gy/2 wk (split)	13 vs 12	25 vs 13
Takada et al. [107]	314	Concurrent	MVP + 28 Gy/3 wk followed by 28 Gy/3 wk	16.5	34.6
		Sequential	MVP followed by 56 Gy	13.3	27.4
Curran et al. [108]	611	Concurrent	PV/60 Gy (start d 1–Qd)	17.0*	NR
		Sequential	PV– 60 Gy (start d 50)	14.6*	NR
		Concurrent (BID-RT)	P+E(po)/69.6 Gy (start d1–BID)	15.6*	NR

*Preliminary results.
CBDCA + VP16—carboplatin 50 mg/m^2 and VP16 50 mg daily; MVP—mitomycin 8 mg/m^2 d1,29; vinblastine 3 mg/m^2 d1,8,29,36; cisplatin 80 mg/m^2 d1,29; P—cisplatin 30 mg/m^2 every wk × 4 or 6 mg/m^2 every d × 20; VCPC—vindesine 1.5 mg/m^2 d1,2; lomustine 50 mg/m^2 d2 and 25 mg/m^2 d3, cyclophosphamide 200 mg/m^2 d2,4.

SWOG subsequently conducted the first randomized trial comparing two novel agents plus cisplatin combinations [118] (Table 10-9). Patients were randomized to vinorelbine/cisplatin or to paclitaxel/carboplatin. The overall response rate (28% versus 25%), median survival time (8 months on both treatment arms), and 1-year survival rates (36% versus 38%) were nearly identical. Both regimens were well tolerated. Either combination regimen was then recommended by SWOG for treatment of advanced-stage NSCLC. A subsequent four-arm randomized phase III trial conducted by ECOG compared three two-drug combinations with results in a cisplatin/paclitaxel control arm (119) (see Table 10-8). Patients were randomized to cisplatin/paclitaxel, cisplatin/gemcitabine, cisplatin/docetaxel, and to carboplatin/paclitaxel. Neither the median survival (7.8, 8.1, 7.4, and 8.2 months, respectively); overall response rates (21.3%, 21%, 17.3%, and 15.3%, respectively) nor the 1-year survival rates (31%, 36%, 31%, and 35%, respectively) were significantly different in any of the four arms. Overall toxicity was similar in each treatment arm, except for a higher grade 3 or 4 thrombocytopenia and anemia rate in the cisplatin/gemcitabine arm compared with the control arm ($P = 0.05$). The carboplatin/paclitaxel combination had significantly less grade 4 to 5 toxicity. Therefore, all these combination regimens are currently recommended for treatment by ECOG for advanced-stage NSCLC.

Three-Drug Regimen (Triple Therapy) in Non–Small-Cell Combination Therapy

SWOG-9805 and ECOG-1594 established five acceptable novel-agent/platinum combinations for the treatment of advanced NSCLC [118,119]. The next approach is how to use these new agents in future trials to improve survival rates in these patients. An established approach has been the addition of a second novel agent to the new double combinations. Although three-drug regimens have not consistently demonstrated superiority over two-drug regimens, introduction of a novel agent has been a reasonable approach, especially because of the low toxicity profiles of these new agents. Several phase I/II trials have been conducted with three-drug combination. The triple combination of paclitaxel/carboplatin/gemcitabine demonstrated response rates that ranged from 21% to 64%. Median survivals were 7.5 and 9.4 months with 1-year survivals of 32% and 45% (110). Another triplet that has been explored in phase I trials is the docetaxel/carboplatin/gemcitabine triplet. In a small study ($n = $ 45 patients) an objective response rate of 51%, median survival of 13.5 months, and 1-year survival rate of 46% were obtained.

Although this regimen appears active, the toxicity profile showed high rates of grade 3 or 4 neutropenia, thrombocytopenia, and neuropathy in 47%, 29%, and 22% of the patients, respectively. A third triple combination of vinorelbine/cisplatin/gemcitabine has also been evaluated in multiple phase I/II trials with an average response rate of 50% and encouraging median survival times of 12.5 and 14 months reported [110]. The impressive 1-year survival rate of 55% reported in one of the trials that had an acceptable toxicity profile is rather encouraging. The fourth triple combination that has undergone multiple phase I/II trials is vinorelbine/ifosfamide/gemcitabine. A response rate of 53% was reported on the two available studies [110]. One of these trials reported a median survival of 10.2 months, with a 46% 1-year survival rate [110].

The elevated response rates, prolonged survival time, and acceptable toxicity profiles reported with these triple combinations promulgated three small phase III randomized trials. An American study compared paclitaxel 225 mg/m^2/carboplatin (area under the curve [AUC] = 6) [PC] with paclitaxel 200 mg/m^2/carboplatin (AUC 5)/gemcitabine 1000 g/m$^{[2]}$. Their preliminary data on 83 patients revealed overall response rates of 36% and 59% for the PC and PCG arms, respectively ($P = 0.4$) [120]. Actuarial median survival times were 7.6 months (PC) and 12.4 months (PCG) ($P = 0.33$) [120]. Two similarly underpowered, randomized trials were conducted by the Southern Italy Cooperative Oncology Group (SICOG). In the

Table 10-7. Phase II Studies of New Drugs Plus Cisplatin or Carboplatin*

Agent	Patients, n	Total CR + PR, %	Median Survival, wk*	1-Y Survival, %*
Vinorelbine + cisplatin	328	135 (41)	38	35–40
Paclitaxel + cisplatin	286	121 (42)	42	36
Paclitaxel + carboplatin	333	137 (46)	38	40
Docetaxel + cisplatin	255	88 (35)	35	58
Gemcitabine + cisplatin	245	114 (47)	57	61
Irinotecan + cisplatin	185	81 (44)	34	NR
Topotecan + cisplatin	22	3 (22)	32	26

*Data from Rapp et al. [109] and Bunn and Kelly [110].
CR—complete response; NR—not reported; PR—partial response.

Table 10-8. Randomized Trials of New Drug Combinations

Study	Regimen	Patients, n	Response Rate, %	Median Survival, mo	1-Y Survival, mo
SWOG [114]	cDDP: 100 mg/m^2 every 3 wk; V; 25 mg/m^2 weekly × 3	214	25	8	33
	cDDP: 100 mg/m^2 every 4 wk	218	10	6	12
SWOG-9805 [118]	P: 225 mg/m^2 over 3 h; C: (AUC = 6) d1; V: 25 mg/m^2 weekly; C: 100 mg/m^2 every 3 wk	207	27	8	36
		201	27	8	33
ECOG-1594 [119]	P: 135 mg/m^2 over 24 h d1; C: 75 mg/m^2 d2 every 3 wk	292	21.3	7.8	31
	C: 100 mg/m^2 d1 every 4 wk; G: 1000 mg/m^2 d1,8,15	288	21	8.1	36
	C: 75 mg/m^2 d 1 every 3 wk; D: 75 mg/m^2 d1	293	17.3	7.4	31
	C: (AUC = 6) d 1 every 3 wk; P: 225 mg/m^2 over 3 h d 1	290	15.3	8.2	35

C—carboplatin; cDDP—cisplatin; D—docetaxel; ECOG—Eastern Cooperative Oncology Group; G—gemcitabine; P—paclitaxel; SWOG—Southwestern Oncology Group; V—vinorelbine.

first study, SICOG compared cisplatin/gemcitabine/vinorelbine with cisplatin/vinorelbine and to cisplatin/gemcitabine. This study revealed median survival and 1-year projected survival rates of 12.8 months, 45%, 8.8 months, 35%, and 10.5 months, 40% for the PGV, PV, and PG arms, respectively [121]. The second SICOG trial compared the two triple combinations cisplatin/gemcitabine/vinorelbine (PGV) and cisplatin/gemcitabine/paclitaxel (PGT) with the double-therapy cisplatin/gemcitabine (PG). Those authors reported response, median survival, 1- and 2-year survival rates of: 44%/12.8 months/47%/15%, 48%/12.8 months/46%/12%, and 28%/9.5 months/39%/9% for the PGV, PGT, and PG arms, respectively [122]. Although the preliminary results of these randomized trials are encouraging, the apparent high toxicity profile and small size are of concern.

An alternative approach to these combination therapies is the sequential use of these drug combinations to decrease the odds of overlapping toxicity between the agents [110]. A pilot study by Edelman et al. [123] demonstrated the feasibility and tolerability of this approach. In this trial, patients were given three cycles of gemcitabine/carboplatin followed by three cycles of paclitaxel. In all, 37 patients were enrolled in this trial of whom 32 were evaluable for response. The overall response rate, median survival time, and 1-year survival rate were 31%, 9.8 months, and 35%, respectively. Grade 4 neutropenia and thrombocytopenia were reported in 21% and 19% of patients, respectively. Another pilot study evaluated three cycles of vinorelbine/cisplatin followed by three cycles of docetaxel. The results with these regimens were similar to those of the gemcitabine/carboplatin followed by paclitaxel combination.

In conclusion, triple-drug regimens in NSCLC appear to be associated with a greater overall response rate, median survival time, and 1-year overall survival compared with the standard two-drug regimen combining a novel agent plus cisplatin. However, the toxicity profile is a major concern, in that essentially all triple therapies are associated with greater hematologic toxicity. Although these results are encouraging, large randomized phase III trials are necessary before the routine use of such triple therapy is adopted.

Non–Platinum Double-Therapy in Advanced-Stage Non–Small Cell Lung Cancer

Cisplatin is a highly toxic and inconvenient agent and the development of non-platinum combinations could reduce overall toxicity and increase convenience. Therefore, a series of phase I/II trials of two new drugs have been conducted. The gemcitabine/paclitaxel regimen's response rates ranged from 30% to 47% with three studies reporting median survival times of 4.9, 7.3, and 9.7 months, respectively. A 1-year survival rate of 26% was reported for the first trial [124]. This treatment regimen was well tolerated with minimal hematologic toxicities. Owing to its low toxicity profile, a subsequent phase III randomized trial was conducted by the Hellenic Cooperative Oncology Group (HeCOG) [125]. This trial compared the standard paclitaxel/carboplatin regimen (PC) with paclitaxel/gemcitabine (PG). The overall response rate, median survival time, and 1-year survival rates were 28.7%, 10.7 months, 41.3% for the PC arm and 36.5%, 12.3 months, 51.3% for the PG arm, respectively. These results indicated that both have similar activity profile and toxicity in patients with advanced-stage NSCLC. The EORTC is currently comparing paclitaxel/cisplatin with gemcitabine/cisplatin and with paclitaxel/gemcitabine [110].

Combined docetaxel/gemcitabine was evaluated by Georgoulias et al. [126] in a phase II trial. This group reported an overall response

rate, median survival time, and 1-year survival rate of 38%, 13 months, and 51%, respectively. The Greek group subsequently conducted a randomized phase II trial comparing DG double therapy with the standard DC regimen [127]. They reported rates, median survival, and 1-year survival rates of 34%, 9.5 months, and 38% for the DG arm and 32%, 10 months, and 42% for the DC arm, respectively. The grade 3 or 4 toxicity rates were significantly higher in the cisplatin arm. Thus, DG double therapy appears to be similar but better tolerated than the DC regimen.

Docetaxel/irinotecan double therapy has also undergone phase II evaluation. Takeda et al. [128] reported a response rate of 34% with median survival and 1-year survival of 9.8 months and 38%, respectively. A subsequent randomized phase III trial conducted by the West Japan Thoracic Oncology Group [129] compared standard DC double therapy with a docetaxel/irinotecan (DI) combination. The reported response rates and median survival were 40.9% and 8.5 months for the DC arm and 35% and 9.8 months for the DI arm, respectively. No statistical interarm difference was found. Thus, DC double therapy has a comparable activity and toxicity profile when compared with DI.

Gemcitabine/vinorelbine double therapy demonstrated response rates in the range of 19% to 73% with two studies revealing median survivals of 9 and 12 months, respectively. Grade 3 and 4 hematologic toxicity was often reported on these trials [110]. Two randomized phase III trials are currently being conducted. A German group is comparing gemcitabine/vinorelbine with triple gemcitabine/vinorelbine/cisplatin therapy, and an Italian group is randomizing patients to either gemcitabine/vinorelbine, gemcitabine/cisplatin, or vinorelbine/cisplatin.

In conclusion, non–platinum-containing double therapy appears to have an activity and toxicity profile similar to that of the current standard cisplatin-containing regimens. However, larger phase III-randomized trials are needed to confirm these preliminary findings. Therefore, these non-platinum double therapies should not become standard first-line therapy for advanced-stage NSCLC in general oncology practice.

Second-Line Chemotherapy for Refractory and Relapsed Non–Small Cell Lung Cancer

Before these new agents were introduced into the treatment of advanced NSCLC, no therapy had been proven to improve survival of NSCLC patients in the second-line setting. This situation has now changed because docetaxel has been proven to improve survival in this regard. Two randomized studies of second-line docetaxel in patients previously treated with cisplatin-based chemotherapy showed a survival advantage for the taxane arm. In the TAX 320 study [130], patients were randomized to either docetaxel 100 mg/m^2 (D100 arm) or 75 mg/m^2 (D75 arm) versus a control regimen of vinorelbine or ifosfamide. Those authors reported significantly different response rates in the docetaxel arms (10.8% with D100 and 6.7% with D75) compared with 0.8% with the control arm. The patients in the docetaxel arms also had a longer time to progression ($P = 0.046$) and longer progression-free survival ($P = 0.005$). The best survival data were obtained in the D75 arm, in which 32% of the patients were alive at 1 year, compared with 21% and 19% in the D100 and control arms, respectively ($P = 0.025$). In a subsequent multicenter international randomized phase-III trial conducted by Shepherd et al. [131], patients with similar characteristics were randomized to receive either D100, D75, or BSC. The overall response rate of 7.1% in this trial was similar to that obtained in the TAX 320 trial. The median survival and overall 1 year survival rates were significantly different for the docetaxel patients of 7.0 months and 29% compared with 4.6 months and 19% for BSC patients. Survival data were again significantly better for the D75 patients compared with the BSC patients with reported median and 1-year survival of 7.5 months and 37% and 4.6 months and 11%, respectively. In conclusion, single-agent docetaxel improves survival of NSCLC patients in the second-line setting. Docetaxel 75 mg/m² every 21 days appears to be the optimal dose and has been approved by the U.S. Food and Drug Administration for use in this setting.

First-Line Therapy in Older Patients with Advanced Non–Small Cell Lung Cancer

Older patients with advanced NSCLC are often unsuitable for cisplatin-based chemotherapy. Therefore, clinical investigators have devoted great efforts to identifying optimal and less toxic chemotherapeutic regimens for such patients with advanced NSCLC. Two agents that have been explored in several trials of elderly patients with NSCLC are vinorelbine and gemcitabine.

In a phase II study of single agent vinorelbine, Gridelli *et al.* [132] reported a response rate of 23%, with high rates of symptom regression and improvement in performance status in elderly people with advanced NSCLC. Vinorelbine, as a single agent, was well-tolerated by this patient population. The Elderly Lung Cancer Vinorelbine Italian Study (ELVIS) Group conducted a multicenter randomized study to compare the efficacy of single-agent vinorelbine to supportive care alone in terms of quality of life and survival in older patients with advanced NSCLC [133]. In this trial, vinorelbine prolonged survival and had a positive impact on quality of life compared with supportive care. The median survival increased from 21 to 28 weeks (*P* = 0.03) in patients receiving vinorelbine, with survival rates at 6 and 12 months of 41% and 14% and of 55% and 32% for the control and vinorelbine arms, respectively. The patients treated with vinorelbine also scored better than the control arm on quality of life functional scales. They also reported reduced lung cancer–related symptoms.

A subsequent randomized phase III trial conducted by the Southern Italy Cooperative Oncology Group compared the impact on survival and quality of life of the gemcitabine/vinorelbine combination with that of single-agent vinorelbine in elderly people with advanced NSCLC [134]. The combination arm was associated with significantly better survival (median survival time, 7.3 months) in comparison with the single agent vinorelbine arm (median survival time, 4.5 months). The reported overall response rates were 22% and 15% for the combination and vinorelbine arms, respectively. In addition, the quality of life score worsened on 60% of the patients in the vinorelbine arm versus 40% of patients in the gemcitabine/vinorelbine arm. The superior results obtained with this novel combination therapy are rather encouraging, particularly because no significantly different toxicity profile was observed between the two arms.

In conclusion, vinorelbine and gemcitabine have each demonstrated optimal activity and toxicity profile in older patients with advanced NSCLC. The results of the ELVIS trial are convincing enough, and in clinical practice single-agent therapy or even the double-agent therapy should be considered as the first therapeutic option when discussing treatment options with older patients with advanced NSCLC.

COST-BENEFIT ANALYSIS

Compared with the 16- or 17-week median survival of patients who received BSC, patients treated with new agents alone or in combination have median survival of about 39 to 48 weeks, a gain of about 26 weeks. Chemotherapy, especially with the new agents, is expensive. Because they prolong survival, the costs per year of life gained can be determined and compared with those found with other medical therapies. In a Canadian study, the survival benefit of 8 weeks in favor of patients receiving CAP chemotherapy was associated with an economic saving of $620.97 when compared with BSC [135]. This translated into a savings of $4035 per year of life gained. The VP arm, etoposide, and high-dose inpatient-administered cisplatin, resulted in a mean survival benefit of 12.8 weeks and an increased cost of $2378 per patient, translating to $9664 per added year of life. The VP arm resulted in both increased costs and increased survival when compared to BSC. It was, therefore, less economically favorable than CAP but the costs associated with its use remain acceptable when compared with the benefits. Evans, using a model of lung cancer diagnosis and treatment by disease stage and cell type, examined the cost-effectiveness of common chemotherapy regimens compared with BSC (136). Cisplatin and etoposide saved $1461 per patient compared with costs related to BSC. Newer chemotherapeutic regimens were compared with etoposide and cisplatin as the standard regimen. Cisplatin and vinorelbine cost $8566/life year saved, gemcitabine and cisplatin $10,963, and paclitaxel and cisplatin $12,116. Thus, the cost of chemotherapy for advanced NSCLC, although expensive, is well within the range of other accepted medical therapies and will be much lower when generic agents become available.

CONCLUSIONS

Chemotherapy is a major component of therapy for both SCLC and NSCLC patients. Completely resected stage I NSCLC patients have a high risk of developing second primary tumors and should be encouraged to stop smoking as well as being considered for screening and chemoprevention studies. For resectable NSCLC, stage IB, IIA and IIB NSCLC patients, randomized trials with preoperative or postoperative chemotherapy should be considered. In this setting, postoperative cisplatin therapy showed a 13% reduction in the hazard rate of death, translating into a 5% absolute increase in 5-year survival. In addition, preoperative cisplatin therapy reduced the hazard rate of death by 23%, which led to a 10% improvement in 5-year survival. However, these studies were limited by small size and lack of significance (*P* = 0.08). Inasmuch as modern chemotherapy regimens are markedly superior to both low-dose and high-dose cisplatin combinations, it is likely that they will further increase the cure rate when given preoperatively in these NSCLC patients.

For patients with stage III disease, chemotherapy improves survival in both stage IIIB patients when added to radiotherapy and stage IIIA patients when added to surgery. In stage IIIA N2, single modality therapy is not sufficient. Randomized trials have shown that combined chemotherapy and radiotherapy is superior to either modality alone in both SCLC and in NSCLC. Chemotherapy plus surgery has also been shown to be superior to surgery alone in stage IIIA NSCLC. It remains unclear which combination is better: chemotherapy + radiotherapy, chemotherapy + surgery, or all three in combination. In stage III SCLC, the combination of chemotherapy + radiotherapy + surgery was not found to be superior to chemotherapy + radiotherapy. In stage III NSCLC, this question is currently being addressed in a randomized intergroup study. For stage IIIB NSCLC patients, combined chemotherapy and radiotherapy approaches are favored over either modality alone with median survivals of 14 to 16 months and 5-year survival rates between 15% and 20%.

Meta-analyses of randomized trials showed that chemotherapy prolongs the survival of patients with stage III and stage IV SCLC and NSCLC. In extensive stage SCLC, chemotherapy improves median survival from 2 months to about 9 to 10 months. In NSCLC, newer agent–based chemotherapy improves survival from 4 months to about 10 months and 1-year survival from 10% to between 40% and 50%. These therapies also improve patients' quality of life and their cost is similar to that of other accepted medical therapies. The guidelines of lung cancer therapy of the American Society of Clinical Oncology reflect the contribution of chemotherapy to prolonging the survival of these patients [137]. Thus, it is reasonable to offer chemotherapy to advanced NSCLC patients with good performance status.

REFERENCES

1. Parker SL, Tong T, Bolden S, *et al.*: Cancer statistics, 2000. *Cancer J Clin* 47:5–27, 2000

2. Ginsberg RJ, Vokes EE, Raben A: Non–small cell lung cancer. In *Cancer. Principles and Practice of Oncology*, edn 5. Edited by DeVita VT, Hellman S, Rosenberg SA. Philadelphia: Lippincott–Raven; 1997:858–911, 1997.

3. Okene JK, Kuller LH, Svendsen KH, *et al.*: The relationship of smoking cessation to coronary artery disease and lung cancer in the multiple risk factor intervention trial (MRFIT). *Am J Public Health* 1990, 80:954–958.

4. Strauss G, DeCamp M, Dibiccaro E, *et al.*: Lung cancer diagnosis is being made with increasing frequency in former cigarette smokers [abstract]. *Proc Am Soc Clin Oncol* 14:A1106, 1995.

5. *Cancer facts and figures, 1996*. American Cancer Society; 1996.

6. Schottenfeld D: Epidemiology of lung cancer in lung cancer. In *Principles and Practice*. Edited by Pass HI, Mitchell JB, Johnson DH, *et al.*. Philadelphia: Lippincott-Raven; 1996:305–321.

7. Fraumeni JF, et al. Lung and pleura. In *Cancer Epidemiology and Prevention*. Edited by Schottenfeld D, Fraumeni JF. Philadelphia: WB Saunders; 1982:564–670.

8. Travis WD, James L, Mackey B: Classification, histology, cytology and electron microscopy. In *Lung Cancer: Principles and Practice*. Edited by Pass HI, Mitchell JB, Johnson DH, *et al.* Philadelphia: Lippincott-Raven Publishers; 1996:361–395.

9. Cook R, Miller Y, Bunn PA: Small cell lung cancer: etiology, biology, clinical features, staging and treatment. *Curr Probl Cancer* 1993, 17:69–144.

10. Berlin NI, Buncher CR, Fontana RS, *et al.*: National Cancer Institute Cooperative Lung Cancer Detection Program: results of initial screen (prevalence) early lung cancer detection. Introduction. *Am Rev Respir Dis* 1984, 130:545–549.

11. Shaw GL: Screening for lung cancer. In *Lung Cancer*. Edited by Johnson BE, Johnson DH. New York: Wiley-Liss; 1995:55–72.

12. Early Lung Cancer Cooperative Study Group: Early lung cancer detection: summary and conclusions. *Am Rev Respir Dis* 1984, 130:565–570.

13. Flehinger BJ, Melamed MR, Zaman MB, *et al.*: Early lung cancer detection: Results of the initial (prevalence) radiologic and cytologic screening in the Memorial Sloan Kettering Study. *Am Rev Respir Dis* 1984, 130:555–560.

14. Fontana RS, Sanderson DR, Taylor WF, *et al.*: Early lung cancer detection: Results of the initial (prevalence) radiologic and cytologic screening in the Mayo Clinic Study. *Am Rev Respir Dis* 1984, 130:561–565.

15. Frost JK, Ball WC Jr, Levin ML, *et al.*: Early lung cancer detection: results of the initial (prevalence) radiologic and cytologic screening in the Johns Hopkins Study. *Am Rev Respir Dis* 1984, 130:549–554.

16. Marcus PM, Bergstralh EJ, Fagerstrom RM, *et al.*: Lung cancer mortality in the Mayo Lung Project: Impact of extended follow-up. *J Natl Cancer Inst* 2000, 92:1308–1316.

17. Eddy DM: Screening for lung cancer. *Ann Intern Med* 1989, 111:232–237.

18. Karp D, Mulshine J, Henschke C, *et al.*: Non–small-cell lung cancer: screening, new imaging and prevention. *Am Soc Clin Oncol* Educational Book; 587–501, 2000.

19. Henschke C, McCauley D, *et al.*: Early Lung Cancer Action Project: overall design and findings from baseline screening. *Lancet* 1999, 354: 99–105.

20. US Centers for Disease Control and Prevention: cigarette smoking among adults: United States, 1998. *MMWR Morb Mortal Wkly Rep* 2000, 49:981–884.

21. Hunt RD, Dale LC, Frederickson PA, *et al.*: Nicotine patch therapy for smoking cessation combined with physician advice and nurse followup. *JAMA* 1994, 27:595–600.

22. Kvale G, Bjelke E, Gart JJ: Dietary habits and lung cancer risk. *Int J Cancer* 1983, 31:397–405.

23. The Alpha–Tocopherol, Beta Carotene Cancer Prevention Study Group: the effect of vitamin E and beta carotene on the incidence of lung cancer and other cancers in male smokers. *N Engl J Med* 1994, 330:1029–1035.

24. Omenn GS, Goodman GE, Thornquist MD, *et al.*: Risk factors for lung cancer and for intervention effects in CARET, the Beta-Carotene and Retinol Efficacy Trial. *J Nat Cancer Inst* 1996, 88:1550–1559.

25. Hong WK; Personal communication: November, 2000.

26. Van Zandwijk N, Dalesio O, Pastorino U, deVries N, *et al.*: EUROSCAN, a randomized trial of vitamin A and N–acetylcysteine in patients with head and neck cancer or lung cancer. *J Nat Cancer Inst* 2000, 92:977–986.

27. Mountain CF. Revisions in the international system for staging lung cancer. *Chest* 1997, 111:1710–1717.

28. Pieterman RM, Van Putten J, Meuzelaar JJ, *et al.*: Preoperative staging of non-small-cell-lung cancer with positron-emission tomography. *N Engl J Med* 2000, 343: 254–261.

29. O'Connell JP, Kris MG, Gralla RJ, *et al.*: Frequency and prognostic importance of pretreatment clinical characteristics in patients with advanced non-small cell lung cancer treated with combination chemotherapy. *J Clin Oncol* 1986, 4:1604–1614.

30. DeWys WD, Begg C, Lavin PT, *et al.*: Prognostic effect of weight loss prior to chemotherapy in cancer patients. *Am J Med* 69:491–497, 1980.

31. Warde P, Payne D: Does thoracic irradiation improve survival and local control in limited-stage small-cell carcinoma of the lung? A meta-analysis. *J Clin Oncol* 1992, 10:890–895.

32. Pignon JP, Arriagada R, Ihde CE, *et al.*: A meta-analysis of thoracic irradiation for small cell lung cancer. *N Engl J Med* 1992, 327:1618–1624.

33. McCracken JD, Janaki LM, Crowley JJ, *et al.*: Concurrent chemotherapy/radiotherapy for limited small-cell lung carcinoma: a Southwest Oncology Group Study. *J Clin Oncol* 1990, 8:892–898.

34. Turrisi AT, Wagner H, Glover B, *et al.*: Limited small cell lung cancer (LSCLC): concurrent BID thoracic radiotherapy (TRT) with platinum-etoposide (PE): An ECOG study [abstract]. *Proc Am Soc Clin Oncol* 1990, 9:A887.

35. Johnson DH, Turrisi AT, Chang AY, et al.: Alternating chemotherapy at twice-daily thoracic radiotherapy in limited-stage small-cell lung cancer: a pilot study of the Eastern Cooperative Oncology Group. *J Clin Oncol* 1993, 11:879–884.

36. Johnson BE, Bridges JD, Sobczeck M, et al.: Patients with limited-stage small-cell lung cancer treated with concurrent twice-daily chest radiotherapy and etoposide/cisplatin followed by cyclophosphamide, doxorubicin, and vincristine. *J Clin Oncol* 1996, 14:806–813.

37. Turrisi AT 3rd, Kim K, Blum R, et al.: Twice-daily compared to once-daily thoracic radiotherapy in limited small-cell lung cancer treated concurrently with cisplatin and etoposide. *N Engl J Med* 1999, 340:265–271.

38. Albain KS, Crowley JJ, LeBlanc M, Livingstone RB: Determinants of improved outcome in small-cell lung cancer: An analysis of 2850 patient Southwest Oncology Group data base. *J Clin Oncol* 1990, 8:1563–1547.

39. Murray N, Coy P, Peter JL, et al.: Importance of timing for thoracic irradiation in the combined modality treatment of limited-stage small-cell lung cancer. *J Clin Oncol* 1993, 11:336–344.

40. Murray N, Coldman C: The relationship between thoracic irradiation timing and long–term survival in combined modality therapy of limited stage small-cell lung cancer [abstract]. *Proc Am Soc Clin Oncol* 1995, 14:A1099.

41. Goto K, Nishiwaki Y, Takada M, et al.: Final results of a phase III study of concurrent versus sequential thoracic radiotherapy (TRT) in combination with cisplatin (P) and etoposide (E) for limited-stage small cell lung cancer (LD–SCLC): The Japan Clinical Oncology Group (JCOG) Study [abstract 1805]. *Proc Am Clin Oncol* 1999, 18:468a.

42. Janaki L, Rector D, Turrisi AT, et al.: Patterns of failure and second malignancies from SWOG 8269: Concurrent cisplatin, etoposide, vincristine, and once daily radiotherapy for the treatment of limited small-cell lung cancer [abstract A1096]. *Proc Am Soc Clin Oncol* 1994, 13

43. Shepherd FA, Ginsberg RJ, Evans WK, et al.: Surgical treatment for limited small-cell lung cancer. *J Thorac Cardiovasc Surg* 1991, 101:385–393.

44. Lad T, Piantandosi S, Thomas P, et al.: A prospective randomized trial to determine the benefit of surgical resection of residual disease following response of small-cell lung cancer to combination therapy. Chest 1994, 106 (suppl):S320–S323.

45. Roth B, Johnson DH, Einhorn L, et al.: randomized study of cyclophosphamide, doxorubicin, and vincristine versus etoposide and cisplatin versus alternation of these regimens in extensive small-cell lung cancer: a phase III trial of the Southeastern Cancer Study Group. *J Clin Oncol* 1992, 10:282–291.

46. Fukuoka M, Furuse K, Saijo N, et al.: Randomized trial of cyclophosphamide, doxorubicin, and vincristine versus cisplatin and etoposide versus alternation of these regimens in small-cell lung cancer. *J Natl Cancer Inst* 1991, 83:855–861.

47. Evans W, Osoba D, Feld R, et al.: Etoposide (VP-16) and cisplatin: An effective treatment for relapse in small cell lung cancer. *J Clin Oncol* 1985, 3:65–71.

48. Einhorn L, Crawford J, Birch R, et al.: Cisplatin plus etoposide consolidation following cyclophosphamide, doxorubicin, and vincristine in limited small-cell lung cancer. *J Clin Oncol* 1988, 6:451–456.

49. Evans WK, Shepherd FA, Feld R, et al.: VP-16 and cisplatin as first-line therapy for small–cell lung cancer. *J Clin Oncol* 1985, 3:1471–1477.

50. Goldie JH, Coldman AJ: A mathematical model for relating the drug sensitivity of tumors to their spontaneous mutation role. *Cancer* 1979, 63:1727–1733.

51. Johnson DH, Einhorn LH, Birch R, et al.: A randomized comparison of high-dose versus conventional dose cyclophosphamide, doxorubicin and vincristine for extensive-stage small cell lung cancer: A phase III trial of the Southeastern Cancer Study Group. *J Clin Oncol* 1987, 5:1731–1738.

52. Ihde DC, Johnson BE, Mulshine JL, et al.: Randomized trial of high dose versus standard dose etoposide and cisplatin in extensive stage small cell lung cancer. *J Clin Oncol* 1994, 12:2022–2034.

53. Crawford J, Ozer H, Stoller R, et al.: Reduction by granulocyte colony–stimulating factor of fever and neutropenia induced by chemotherapy in patients with small cell lung cancer. *N Engl J Med* 1991, 235:164–170.

54. Murray N, Shah A, Osoba D, et al.: Intensive weekly chemotherapy for the treatment of extensive-stage small-cell lung cancer. *J Clin Oncol* 1991, 90:1632–1638.

55. Murray N, Livingston R, Shephard F, et al.: Randomized study of CODE versus alternating CAV/EP for extensive-stage small-cell lung cancer: An intergroup study of the National Cancer Institute of Canada Clinical Trial Group and the Southwest Oncology Group. *J Clin Oncol* 1999, 17:2300–2308.

56. Wolf M, Drings P, Hans K, et al.: Alternating chemotherapy with adriamycin/ifosfamide/vincristine (AIO) and either cisplatin/etoposide (PE) or carboplatin/etoposide (CE) in small cell lung cancer (SCLC) [abstract A527]. *Lung Cancer* 1991, 7(Suppl)

57. Skarlos DV, Samantas E, Kosmidis P, et al.: Randomized comparisons of etoposide-cisplatin versus etoposide-carboplatin and irradiation in small cell lung cancer. A Hellenic Cooperative Oncology Group Study. *Ann Oncol* 1994, 5:601–607.

58. Bunn PA, Cullen M, Fukuola M, et al.: Chemotherapy in small cell lung cancer. A Consensus report of the International Association for the Study of Lung Cancer Workshop. *Lung Cancer* 1989, 5:127–134.

59. Giaccone G, Dalesio O, McVie GJ, et al.: Maintenance chemotherapy in small cell lung cancer: Long term results of a randomized trial. *J Clin Oncol* 1993, 11:1230–1240.

60. Spiro SG, Souhami RL, Geddes DM, et al.: Duration of chemotherapy in small cell lung cancer: a Cancer Research Campaign trial. *Br J Cancer* 1989, 58:578–583.

61. Bleehan NM, Fayers PM, Girling DJ, et al.: Controlled trials of twelve versus six courses of chemotherapy in small cell lung cancer. *Br J Cancer* 1989, 59:584–590.

62. Kelly K, Crowley JJ, Bunn PA, et al.: Role of recombinant interferon alpha-2a maintenance in patients with limited-stage small-cell lung cancer responding to concurrent chemoradiation: a Southwest Oncology Group study. *J Clin Oncol* 1995, 13:2924–2930.

63. Johnson DH, Adak S, Schiller JH, et al.: Topotecan (T) vs observation (OB) following cisplatin (P) plus etoposide (E) in extensive stage small cell lung cancer (ES SCLC) (E7593): A phase III trial of the Eastern Cooperative Oncology Group (ECOG) [abstract 1886]. *Proc Am Soc Clin Oncol* 2000, 19:482a.

64. Harper PG, Underhill C, Ruiz de Elvira MC, et al.: A randomized study of oral etoposide versus combination chemotherapy in poor prognosis small cell lung cancer. *J Clin Oncol* 1996, 14:1750.

65. Clark PI, Thatcher N, Lallenand G, et al.: Updated results of a randomized trial confirm that oral etoposide alone is inadequate palliative chemotherapy for small cell lung cancer (SCLC). *Lancet* 1996, 348:563–566.

66. Kelly K: New chemotherapeutic agents for small cell lung cancer—review. *Chest* 2000, 117 (Suppl 1):156S–162S.

67. Masuda N, Fukuoka M, Kusunoki Y, et al.: CPT-11: a new derivative of camptothecin for the treatment of refractory or relapsed small-cell lung cancer. *J Clin Oncol* 1992, 10:1225–1229.

68. Kudoh S, Fujiwara Y, Takada Y, *et al.*: Phase II study of irinotecan combined with cisplatin in patients with previously untreated small-cell lung cancer. *J Clin Oncol* 1998, 16:1068–1074.

69. Noda K, Nishiwaki Y, Kawahara M, Negoro S, *et al.*: Randomized phase III study of irinotecan (CPT-11) and cisplatin versus etoposide and cisplatin in extensive–disease small–cell lung cancer: Japan Clinical Oncology Group study (JCOG-9511) [abstract 1887]. *Proc Am Soc Clin Oncol* 2000, 19: 483a.

70. Rowinsky E, Grochow L, Hendricks C, *et al.*: Phase I and pharmacologic study of topotecan: A novel topoisomerase Inhibitor. *J Clin Oncol* 1992, 10:647–656.

71. Schiller J, Kim K, Hutson P, *et al.*: Phase II study of topotecan in patients with extensive–stage small–cell carcinoma of the lung: an Eastern Cooperative Oncology Group Trial. *J Clin Oncol* 1996, 14:2345–2352.

72. Ardizzoni A, Hansen H, Dombernowsky P, *et al.*: Topotecan, a new active drug in the second-line treatment of small-cell lung cancer: A phase II study in patients with refractory and sensitive disease. *J Clin Oncol* 1997, 15:2090–2096.

73. Von Powel J, Schiller J, Shepherd F, *et al.*: Topotecan versus cyclophosphamide, doxorubicin, and vincristine for the treatment of recurrent small–cell lung cancer. *J Clin Oncol* 1999, 17:658–667.

74. Ettinger D, Finkelstein D, Sarma R, *et al.*: Phase II study of paclitaxel in patients with extensive-disease small-cell lung cancer: an Eastern Cooperative Oncology Group Study. *J Clin Oncol* 1995, 13:1430–1435.

75. Kirschling RJ, Grill JP, Jett JR, *et al.*: Paclitaxel and G-CSF in previously untreated patients with extensive stage small-cell lung cancer: a phase II study of the North Central Cancer Treatment Group. *Am J Clin Oncol* 1999, 22:517–522.

76. Bunn PA, Jr.: Future directions in therapeutic approaches for small cell lung cancer. *Semin Oncol* 1996, 23(Suppl 16):136–138.

77. Kelly K, Pan Z, Wood ME, Bunn PA Jr.: A phase I study of paclitaxel, etoposide, and cisplatin in extensive-stage small cell lung cancer. *Clin Cancer Res* 1999, 5:3419–3424.

78. Kelly K, Bunn P, Lovato L, *et al.*: Final results from Southwest Oncology Group Trial 9705: a Phase II Trial of cisplatin, etoposide, and paclitaxel, with G-CSF in untreated patients with extensive-stage small cell lung cancer [abstract 1923]. *Proc Am Soc Clin Oncol* 2000, 19:492a.

79. Mavroudis D, Papadakis E, Veslemes M, *et al.*: A multicenter randomized phase III study comparing paclitaxel-cisplatin-etoposide versus cisplatin-etoposide as front-line treatment in patients with small cell lung cancer [abstract 1894]. *Proc Am Soc Clin Oncol* 2000, 19:484a.

80. Auperin A, Arriagada R, Pignon J, *et al.*: Prophylactic cranial irradiation for patients with small–cell lung cancer in complete remission. *N Engl J Med* 1999, 341:476–484.

81. Ginsberg RJ, Rubinstein L: The comparison of limited resection to lobectomy for T1N0 non-small cell lung cancer. *Chest* 1994, 106:318S–319S.

82. Bunn PA, Jr.: The treatment of non-small cell lung cancer: Current perspectives and controversies, future directions. *Semin Oncol* 1994, 21 (suppl 6):49–59.

83. Weisenburger JH, Lung Cancer Study Group. Effects of postoperative mediastinal radiation on completely resected stage II and stage III epidermoid carcinoma of the lung. *N Engl J Med* 1986, 315:1377.

84. Postoperative radiotherapy for NSCLC. Port Meta-analysis Trialists Group. *Cochrane Database Syst Rev* 2000, CD002142.

85. Non-Small Cell Lung Cancer Collaborative Group: Chemotherapy in non-small cell lung cancer: a meta-analysis using updated data on individual patients from 52 randomized clinical trials. *BMJ* 1995, 311:899–909.

86. Pisters K, Ginsberg R, Bunn PA, *et al.*: Induction chemotherapy before surgery for early–stage lung cancer; a novel approach. *J Thorac Cardiovasc Surg* 2000, 119:429–439.

87. Depierre A, Milleron B, Moro D, *et al.*: Phase-III trial of neo-adjuvant chemotherapy in resectable stage-I (except T1N0), II, IIIA NSCLC: The French experience [abstract 1792]. *Proc ASCO* 1999, 18:465a.

88. Martini N, Kris M, Flehinger B, *et al.*: Preoperative chemotherapy for stage IIIA (N2) lung cancer: The Sloan Kettering experience with 136 patients. *Ann Thorac Surg* 1993, 55:1365–1374.

89. Burkes R, Ginsberg, Shepherd F, *et al.*: Induction chemotherapy with mitomycin C, vindesine and cisplatin for stage III unresectable non-small cell lung cancer: results of the Toronto phase II trial. *J Clin Oncol* 1992, 10:580–586.

90. Sugarbaker DJ, Herndon J, Kohman LJ, *et al.*: Results of Cancer and Leukemia Group B Protocol 8935: Multiinstitutional phase II trimodality trial for stage IIIA (N2) NSCLC. *J Thorac Cardiovasc Surg* 1995, 109:473–485.

91. Albain KS, Rusch V, Crowley J, *et al.*: Concurrent cisplatin/etoposide plus chest radiotherapy followed by surgery for stages IIIA and IIIB non-small cell lung cancer: Mature results of Southwest Oncology Group phase II study 8805. *J Clin Oncol* 1995, 13:1880–1892.

92. Albain K, Rusch V, *et al.*: Long-term survival after concurrent cisplatin/etoposide (PE) plus chest radiotherapy (RT) followed by surgery in bulky stage–IIIA(N2) and IIIB NSCLC; 6-year outcome from SWOG-8805 [abstract 1801]. *Proc ASCO* 1999, 18:467a.

93. Rosell R, Gomez-Codina J, Camps C, *et al.*: A randomized trial comparing preoperative chemotherapy plus surgery with surgery alone in patients with non-small cell lung cancer. *N Engl J Med* 1994, 330:153–158.

94. Rosell R, Gomez-Codina J, Camps C, *et al.*: Preresectional chemotherapy in stage IIIA non-small-cell lung cancer: a 7-year assessment of a randomized controlled trial. *Lung Cancer* 1999, 47:07–14.

95. Roth JAB, Fossella F, Komaki R, *et al.*: A randomized trial comparing perioperative chemotherapy and surgery with surgery alone in resectable stage IIIA non-small cell lung cancer. *J Natl Cancer Inst* 1992, 86:673–680.

96. Roth J, Atkinson EN, Fossella F, *et al.*: Long-term follow-up of patients enrolled in a randomized trial comparing perioperative chemotherapy and surgery with surgery alone in resectable stage IIIA non-small-cell lung cancer. *Lung Cancer* 1998, 21:1–6.

97. Gandara D, Leigh B, Vallieres E, *et al.*: Preoperative chemotherapy in stage III non-small-cell lung cancer: Long-term outcome. *Lung Cancer* 1999, 26:3–6.

98. Dillman RO, Seagren SL, Herndon J, *et al.*: A randomized trial of induction chemotherapy plus high-dose radiation versus radiation alone in stage III non-small cell lung cancer. *N Engl J Med* 1990, 323:940–945.

99. Dillman RO, Herndin J, Seagren SL, *et al.*: Improved survival in stage III non-small cell lung cancer: seven year follow-up of cancer and leukemia group B (CALGB) 8433 trial. *J Natl Cancer Inst* 1996, 88:1210–1215.

100. Sause WT, Scott C, Taylor S, *et al.*: Radiation Therapy Oncology Group (RTOG) 88-08 and Eastern Cooperative Oncology Group (ECOG) 4588: Preliminary results of a phase III trial in regionally advanced, unresectable non-small cell lung cancer. *J Natl Cancer Inst* 1995, 87:198–205.

101. Le Chevalier T, Arriagada R, Quiox E, *et al.*: Radiotherapy alone versus combined chemotherapy and radiotherapy in nonresectable non-small cell lung cancer: First analysis of a randomized trial in 353 patients. *J Natl Cancer Inst* 1991, 83:417–423.

102. Schaake-Koning C, Van Den Bogert W, Dalesio O, *et al.*: Effects of concomitant cisplatin and radiotherapy in inoperable non-small cell lung cancer. *N Engl J Med* 1992, 326:524–530.

103. Jeremic B, Shibamoto Y, Acinovic L, et al.: Randomized trial of hyperfractionated radiation therapy with or without concurrent chemotherapy for stage III non-small cell lung cancer. *J Clin Oncol* 1995, 13:452–458.

104. Jeremic B, Shibamoto Y, Acinovic L, et al.: Hyperfractionated radiation therapy with or without concurrent low dose daily carboplatin/etoposide for stage III non-small cell lung cancer: a randomized study. *J Clin Oncol* 1996, 14:1065–1070.

105. Pritchard RS, Anthony SP: Chemotherapy plus radiotherapy compared with radiotherapy alone in the treatment of locally advanced, unresectable, NSCLC: a meta-analysis. *Ann Intern Med* 1996, 125:723–729.

106. Cullen MH, Billingham LJ, Woodroffe CM, et al.: Mitomycin, ifosfamide and cisplatin (MIC) in unresectable non-small cell lung cancer: Effects on survival and quality of life. *J Clin Oncol* 1999, 17:3188–3194.

107. Takada Y, Furuse K, Fukuoka YH, et al.: A randomized phase III study of concurrent versus sequential thoracic radiotherapy (TRT) in combination with mitomycin, vindesine, and cisplatin in unresectable stage III non-small cell lung cancer (NSCLC) [abstract]. *Lung Cancer* 1997, 18 (suppl 1):A294.

108. Curran WJ, Scott C, Langer C, et al.: Phase III comparison of sequential vs concurrent chemotherapy for PTS with unresectable stage III non-small cell lung cancer (NSCLC): Initial report of Radiation Therapy Oncology Group (RTOG) 9410 [abstract 1891]. *Proc Am Soc Clin Oncol* 2000, 19:484a.

109. Rapp E, Pater JL, Willan A, et al.: Chemotherapy can prolong survival in patients with advanced non-small cell lung cancer: report of a Canadian multi-center randomized trial. *J Clin Oncol* 1988, 6:663–641.

110. Bunn PA, Jr, Kelly K: New chemotherapeutic agents prolong survival and improve quality of life in non-small cell lung cancer: a review of the literature and future directions. *Clin Cancer Res* 1998, 4:1087–1100.

111. Kelly K: Future directions for new cytotoxic agents in the treatment of advanced-stage non-small-cell lung cancer. *Am Soc Clin Oncol Educational Book.* 2000, 357–367.

112. Thatcher N, Ranson M, Anderson H, et al.: Phase-III study of paclitaxel versus supportive care in inoperative NSCLC [abstract 40]. *Ann Oncol* 1998, 9:1.

113. Roszkowski K: Taxotere versus best supportive care in chemonaive patients with unresectable NSCLC: Final results of the phase-III study [abstract]. *Eur J Cancer* 1999, 35: 246.

114. Wozniak AJ, Crowley JJ, Balcerzak SP, et al.: Randomized trial comparing cisplatin with cisplatin plus vinorelbine in the treatment of advanced non-small-cell lung cancer: A Southwest Oncology Group Study. *J Clin Oncol* 1998, 16:2459–2465.

115. Sandler A, Nemunaitis J, Deham C, et al.: Phase III trial of gemcitabine plus cisplatin versus cisplatin alone in patients with locally advanced or metastatic non-small-cell lung cancer. *J Clin Oncol* 2000, 18:122–130.

116. Bonomi P, Kim K, Fairclough D, et al.: Comparison of survival and quality of life in advanced non–small–cell lung cancer patients treated with two dose levels of paclitaxel combined with cisplatin versus etoposide with cisplatin: Results of an Eastern Cooperative Oncology Group Trial. *J Clin Oncol* 2000, 18:623–631.

117. Giaccone G, Postmus P, Debruyne C, et al.: Final results of an EORTC phase III study of paclitaxel vs teniposide, in combination with cisplatin, in advanced NSCLC [abstract 1653]. *Proc Am Soc Clin Oncol* 1997, 16:460a.

118. Kelly K, Crowley J, Bunn PA, et al.: A randomized phase III trial of paclitaxel plus carboplatin (PC) versus vinorelbine plus cisplatin (VC) in untreated advanced non-small-cell lung cancer (NSCLC): Southwest Oncology Group (SWOG) Trial [abstract 1777]. *Proc Am Soc Clin Oncol* 1999, 18:461a.

119. Schiller JH, Harrington D, Sandler A, et al.: A randomized phase III trial of four chemotherapy regimens in advanced non-small-cell lung cancer (NSCLC)—(ECOG-1594) [abstract 2]. *Proc Am Soc Clin Oncol* 2000, 19:1a.

120. Hussein A, Birch R, Waller J, et al.: preliminary results of a randomized study comparing paclitaxel and carboplatin (PC) with or without gemcitabine (G) in newly diagnosed non small cell lung cancer (NSCLC) [abstract 1973]. *Proc Am Soc Clin Oncol* 2000, 19:504a.

121. Comella P, Frasci G, Panza N, et al.: Randomized trial comparing cisplatin, gemcitabine, and vinorelbine with either cisplatin and gemcitabine or cisplatin and vinorelbine in advanced non-small-cell lung cancer: interim analysis of a phase III trial of the Southern Italy Cooperative Oncology Group. *J Clin Oncol* 2000, 18:1451–1457.

122. Comella G, Comella P, Frasci G, et al.: Cisplatin-gemcitabine, vs. cisplatin-gemcitabine-vinorelbine, vs. cisplatin-gemcitabine-paclitaxel in advanced non-small-cell lung cancer. First-Stage Analysis of Southern Italy Cooperative Oncology Group (SICOG) phase III trial [abstract 1933]. *Proc Am Soc Clin Oncol* 2000, 19:494a.

123. Edelman MJ, Gandara DR, Lau D, et al.: Sequential chemotherapy in non-small cell lung cancer (NSCLC): Carboplatin and gemcitabine followed by paclitaxel [abstract 2603]. *Proc Am Soc Clin Oncol* 2000, 19:525a.

124. Bhatia S, Ng E, Ansari R, et al.: A phase II study of paclitaxel (P) and gemcitabine (G) in patients with advanced non small cell lung cancer—a Hoosier Oncology Group study [abstract 2091]. *Proc Am Soc Clin Oncol* 2000, 19: 532a.

125. Kosmidis PA, Bacoyiannis C, Mylonakis N, et al.: A randomized phase III trial of paclitaxel plus carboplatin versus paclitaxel plus gemcitabine in advanced non small cell lung cancer (NSCLC) [abstract 1908]: a preliminary analysis. *Proc Am Soc Clin Oncol* 2000, 19:488a.

126. Georgoulias V, Kouroussis C, Androulakis N, et al.: Front-line Treatment of advanced non-small-cell lung cancer with docetaxel and gemcitabine: a Multicenter phase II trial. *J Clin Oncol* 1999, 17:914–920.

127. Georgoulias V, Papadakis E, Alexopoulos A, et al.: Docetaxel plus cisplatin versus docetaxel plus gemcitabine chemotherapy in advanced non-small cell lung cancer: a preliminary analysis of a multicenter randomized phase II trial [abstract 1778]. *Proc Am Soc Clin Oncol* 1999, 18:461a.

128. Takeda K, Negoro S, Masuda N, et al.: Phase I study of docetaxel (Doc) and irinotecan (CPT-11) for previously untreated advanced non-small cell lung cancer (NSCLC) [abstract 2019]. *Proc Am Soc Clin Oncol* 1999, 18:524a.

129. Takeda K, Yamamoto N, Negoro S, et al.: Randomized phase III study of docetaxel (DOC) plus cisplatin (CDDP) versus DOC plus irinotecan in advanced non-small-cell lung cancer (NSCLC): A West Japan Thoracic Oncology Group (WJTOG) Study [abstract 1944]. *Proc Am Soc Clin Oncol* 2000, 19:497a.

130. Fossella F, DeVore R, Kerr R, et al.: Randomized phase-III trial of docetaxel versus vinorelbine or ifosfamide in patients with advanced non-small-cell lung cancer previously treated with platinum containing chemotherapy regimens. *J Clin Oncol* 2000, 18:2354–2362.

131. Shephard F, Dancey J, Ramlou R, et al.: Prospective randomized trial of docetaxel versus best supportive care in patients with non–small–cell lung cancer previously treated with platinum-based chemotherapy. *J Clin Oncol* 2000, 8:2095–2103.

132. Gridelli C, Perrone F, Gallo C, *et al.*: Vinorelbine is well tolerated and active in the treatment of elderly patients with advanced non-small cell lung cancer. A two-stage phase–II study. *Eur J Cancer* 1997, 33:392–397.

133. Gridelli C, Perrone F, Gallo C, *et al.*: Effects of vinorelbine on quality of life and survival of elderly patients with advanced NSCLC— - The Elderly Lung Cancer Vinorelbine Italian Study (ELVIS) group. *J Natl Cancer Inst* 1999, 91:66–72.

134. Frasci G, Lorusso V, Panze N, *et al.*: Gemcitabine + vinorelbine (GV) yields better survival than vinorelbine alone in elderly NSCLC patients—final analysis of a Southern Italy Cooperative Oncology Group (SICOG) Phase-III Trial [abstract 1895]. *Proc Am Soc Clin Oncol* 2000, 485a.

135. Jaakkimainen L, Goodwin PJ, Pater J, *et al.*: Counting the costs of chemotherapy in a National Cancer Institute of Canada randomized trial in non-small-cell lung cancer. *J Clin Oncol* 1990, 8:1301–1309.

136. Evans WK: Treatment of NSCLC with chemotherapy is controversial because of low response and high cost. *Lung Cancer* 1997, 18(Suppl 2):117–118.

137. Clinical practice guidelines for the treatment of unresectable non-small-cell lung cancer. *J Clin Oncol* 1997, 15:2996–3018.

138. Joos G, Pinson P, Renterghem, *et al.*: Randomized study comparing vincristine, Adriamycin, cyclophosphamide (VAC) to carboplatin, etoposide (CE) in previously untreated small cell lung cancer (SCLC) [abstract 1812]. *Proc Am Soc Clin Oncol* 1999, 18:470a.

139. Ettinger DS: The role of carboplatin in the treatment of small-cell lung cancer. *Oncology (Huntingt)* 1998, 12(suppl 2):36–43.

140. Okamoto H, Watanabe K, Nishiwaki Y, *et al.*: Phase II study of area under the plasma-concentration-versus-time curve-based carboplatin plus standard-dose intravenous etoposide in elderly patients with small-cell lung cancer. *J Clin Oncol* 1999, 17:3540–3545.

141. Hainsworth JD, Gray JR, Stroup SL, *et al.*: Paclitaxel, carboplatin, and extended-scheduled etoposide in the treatment of small-cell lung cancer: comparison of sequential phase II trials using different dose-intensities. *J Clin Oncol* 1997, 15:3464–3470.

CISPLATIN AND ETOPOSIDE IN SMALL CELL LUNG CANCER

Cisplatin, a platinum analogue, is one of the most active antineoplastic agents for lung cancer. It inhibits DNA synthesis by producing intrastrand and interstrand crosslinks, similar to bifunctional alkylating agents. Etoposide exerts its effect on DNA by forming a complex with DNA and the DNA-unwinding enzyme topo-isomerase II, which causes strand breakage. The combination of cisplatin and etoposide (PE) is currently considered to be one of the most active drug combinations for small cell lung cancer, reaching response rates up to 90% of patients with complete remissions in up to 50% [48]. In limited-stage disease, PE combined with chest irradiation has been shown to improve local control and median survival. In fact, a concurrent application of chemotherapy and radiotherapy is preferred by most centers (*see* Table 10-4) [33-37].

CANDIDATES FOR TREATMENT

Small cell lung cancer: limited-stage disease concurrent with, alternated with, or followed by chest irradiation; extensive-stage disease

SPECIAL PRECAUTIONS

Patients with renal dysfunction and impaired hearing function

ALTERNATIVE THERAPIES

Carboplatin and etoposide; irinotecan and cisplatin; new drugs such as taxanes, topotecan, gemcitabine and irinotecan as a single agents or in combination with a platinum compound (experimental)

TOXICITIES

Myelosuppression, nausea, vomiting, nephrotoxicity with electrolyte wasting, neurotoxicity (peripheral neuropathy), auditory impairment, hypotension, hypersensitivity (including anaphylactic reactions), mucositis, diarrhea, alopecia, asthenia

DRUG INTERACTIONS

Cisplatin: other nephro- and ototoxic drugs (*eg*, aminoglycosides, furosemide); **Etoposide:** not known

NURSING INTERVENTIONS

Hypersensitivity: anaphylactic reactions have been documented with both agents; diphenhydramine and epinephrine should be readily available as well as a crash cart; **Myelosuppression:** monitor blood counts; inquire about symptoms of infection, bleeding, and anemia; **Nausea and vomiting:** give antiemetics before chemotherapy and as needed; assess for delayed nausea and vomiting; **Nephrotoxicity:** monitor renal function indices (serum creatinine, blood urea nitrogen, creatinine clearance) and electrolytes (especially magnesium and calcium); encourage adequate oral and intravenous hydration as well as high urine flow during therapy; **Neurotoxicity:** assess for weakness and numbness of legs, feet, arms, and hands; **Hypotension:** usually attributed to fast infusion rate of etoposide (due to vehicle); stop infusion and give supportive care; restart infusion at slower rate or consider change to etoposide phosphate; **Local:** venous spasm and occasionally phlebitis

PATIENT INFORMATION

Drink plenty of fluids and urinate frequently; report immediately symptoms of infection (fever, chills, sore throat), unusual bleeding, bruising, breathing problems, upset stomach, numbness, and tingling; maintain good nutrition and exercise; report any nausea or vomiting

CARBOPLATIN AND ETOPOSIDE IN SMALL CELL LUNG CANCER

Carboplatin, a platinum analogue like cisplatin, inhibits DNA synthesis by causing irreversible intra- and interstrand crosslinks. Carboplatin is highly effective in small cell lung cancer as a single agent. Etoposide, a topoisomerase II inhibitor, produces irreversible strand breakage. In two randomized studies, the combination of carboplatin and etoposide was shown to be as active but less toxic than the combination of cisplatin and etoposide in patients with limited- and extensive-stage disease [56,57]. Another randomized study comparing CE with cyclophosphamide/adriamycin/vincristine (CAV) concluded that CE and CAV were equally effective; with the CE arm's being better tolerated and offering a survival advantage to patients with extensive-stage disease [138]. Nonhematologic forms of toxicity such as neuropathy, renal toxicity, asthenia, nausea, and vomiting compare favorably with those found with the platinum/etoposide (PE) regimen. Therefore, CE (intravenous or perioral) is frequently used in older patients with poor performance status and extensive stage disease showing a remarkable response rate and survival [140]. Furthermore, when paclitaxel is combined with CE, the combination's toxicity profile remains tolerable [141]. Several randomized trials are currently comparing this triple therapy with standard CE combination in extensive stage SCLC.

CANDIDATES FOR TREATMENT

Small cell lung cancer: limited-stage disease with chest irradiation and extensive-stage disease; elderly patients

SPECIAL PRECAUTIONS

Treatment delay and transfusions may be mandatory due to myelosuppression. In case of impaired renal function, consult drug instruction form or consider use of Calvert formula (in which the total dose is in mg, area under the curve [AUC] = 4–5, and GFR is the glomerular filtration rate [use creatinine clearance]):

Total Dose = AUC $\times$ (GFR + 25)

ALTERNATIVE THERAPIES

Carboplatin and etoposide; irinotecan and cisplatin; new drugs (*eg*, the taxanes, topotecan, gemcitabine, and irinotecan) as single agents or in combination with a platinum compound (experimental)

TOXICITIES

Myelosuppression, nausea, vomiting, alopecia, mucositis, infection, peripheral neuropathy, hypotension, hypersensitivity (including anaphylactic reactions), anorexia, mild renal toxicity

DRUG INTERACTIONS

Other nephro- or ototoxic drugs (*eg*, aminoglycosides, furosemide)

NURSING INTERVENTIONS

Hypersensitivity: anaphylactic reactions have been documented with both agents; diphenhydramine and epinephrine should be readily available as well as crash cart; **Myelosuppression:** monitor blood counts; inquire about symptoms of infection, bleeding, and anemia; **Nausea, vomiting:** give antiemetics before chemotherapy and as needed; **Nephrotoxicity:** monitor renal function indices (serum creatinine, blood urea nitrogen) and magnesium; **Neurotoxicity:** assess for weakness and numbness of legs, feet, arms, and hands; **Hypotension:** usually attributed to fast infusion rate of etoposide (due to vehicle); stop infusion and give supportive care; restart infusion at slower rate or consider change to etoposide phosphate; **Local:** venous spasm and occasionally phlebitis

CARBOPLATIN AND ETOPOSIDE IN SMALL CELL LUNG CANCER (Continued)

RANDOMIZED TRIALS COMPARING CARBOPLATIN AND ETOPOSIDE WITH CISPLATIN-CONTAINING REGIMENS IN LIMITED AND EXTENSIVE-STAGE SMALL CELL LUNG CANCER

Study	Patients, n	Dosage Schedule, mg/m²	CR,%		PR, %		RR, %	Median Survival, mo	Comments
			LD	ED	LD	ED			
Wolf [56]	129	A/I/V alternating with	20	17	53	34	—	12.0 (LD)	q 4 wk× 4 cycles; chest RT for LD
		C: 300 IV, d1						9.3 (ED)	
		E: 120 IV, d1–3							
		vs.							
	133	A/I/V alternating with	22	14	56	36	—	14.3 (LD)	
		cDDP: 90 IV, d 1						9.3 (ED)	
		E: 150 IV, d 1–3							
Skarlos [57]	72	C: 300 IV, d1	37	19	49	48	—	11.8 (LD/ED)	q 3 wk × 6 cycles, chest RT for LD, PCI if complete remission
		E: 100 IV, d 1–3							
		vs.							
		cDDP: 50 IV, d 1,2							
	71	E: 100 IV, d 1–3	44	10	29	40	—	12.5 (LD/ED)	
Joos [138]	93	V:1.4 IV, d 1 q 3 wk	—	—	—	—	81 (LD)	11.7 (LD)	q 3 wk × 6 cycles
		A: 50 IV, d1 q 3 wk					50 (ED)	6.4 (ED)	
		C: 1000 IV, d 1 q 3 wk							
		vs.							
		C: 100 IV, d 1 q 3 wk					77 (LD)	14.0 (LD)	
	102	E: 120 IV, d1–3 q 4 wk	—	—	—	—	67 (ED)	8.4 (ED)	q 4 wk × 3 cycles

A—doxorubicin (adriamycin); C—carboplatin; cDDP—cisplatin; CR—complete response; Cy—cyclophosphamide; E—etoposide; ED—extensive stage disease; I—ifosfamide; IV—intravenously; LD—limited stage disease; NR—not reported; PCI—prophylactic cranial irradiation; PO—per oral; PR—partial response; q—cycle length; RT—radiotherapy; V—vincristine.

NONRANDOMIZED CARBOPLATIN/ETOPOSIDE TRIALS IN LIMITED AND EXTENSIVE STAGE SMALL CELL LUNG CANCER

Study	Patients, n	Dosage Schedule, mg/m²	RR (LD + ED), %	Median Survival, %	Comments
Ettinger [139]	NR	C: single agent	60	NR	Previously untreated
			17	NR	Previously untreated
Okamoto [140]	36	C: AUC = 5 IV, d1	75	11.6 (LD)	q 3 wk × 4 cycles
		E: 100 IV, d 1–3		10.1 (ED)	
Hainsworth [141]	72	P: 200 IV, d1	91	NR (LD)	Chest RT for LD with cycle 3 and 4
		C: AUC = 5 IV, d1	98 (LD)	10.0 (ED)	
		E: 50/100 IV, qod, d 1–10	84 (ED)		

C—carboplatin; E—etoposide; ED—extensive stage disease; IV—intravenous; LD—limited stage disease; NR—not reported; q—cycle length; RR—overall response rate.

The information here is provided as guidance only. Prescribers should always consult the manufacturer's current prescribing information

198

IRINOTECAN AND CISPLATIN IN SMALL CELL LUNG CANCER

Irinotecan (CPT-11) is a unique, water-soluble, semisynthetic analogue of the alkaloid camptothecin, derived from the *Camptotheca acuminata* tree. It inhibits topoisomerase I, which is an enzyme with swivel-like enzymatic activity that may be required for the elongation phase of DNA replication and RNA transcription. Irinotecan induces protein-linked DNA single-strand breaks that depend on topoisomerase I content in the cell. Inhibition of topoisomerase I activity damages DNA, which leads to cell death. Irinotecan has shown activity as a single agent against SCLC. It has also been demonstrated to have in vitro synergistic activity with cisplatin against SCLC. In a randomized phase III trial by the Japan Clinical Oncology Group, combined irinotecan/cisplatin (IP) was compared with etoposide/cisplatin (EP) in patients with extensive-stage SCLC [69]. The study demonstrated the IP arm was significantly superior to the EP arm with response rate and median survival of 83%/13 mo and 68%/9.6 mo, respectively.

CANDIDATES FOR TREATMENT
Patients with extensive-stage SCLC

SPECIAL PRECAUTIONS
Patients with renal dysfunction and impaired hearing function

ALTERNATIVE THERAPIES
Cisplatin/etoposide, carboplatin/etoposide, or paclitaxel, docetaxel, gemcitabine, topotecan, and irinotecan as single agents

TOXICITIES
Myelosuppression, diarrhea, nausea, vomiting, nephrotoxicity with electrolyte wasting, neurotoxicity (peripheral neuropathy), auditory impairment, alopecia

DRUG INTERACTIONS
Cisplatin: other nephrotoxic and ototoxic drugs

NURSING INTERVENTIONS
Hypersensitivity: anaphylactic reactions have been documented with cisplatin so that diphenhydramine and epinephrine should be readily available; **Myelosuppression:** associated with both drugs, monitor blood counts, inquire about symptoms of infection, bleeding and anemia; **Diarrhea:** particularly associated with irinotecan, inquire about diarrhea, loperamide 1 or 2 tablets every 2 hours until diarrhea resolved, check electrolytes, blood urea nitrogen (BUN)/creatinine (Cr) clearance levels; **Nausea/vomiting:** give antiemetics before chemotherapy and as needed; **Nephrotoxicity:** monitor renal function indices (serum creatinine, BUN, Cr clearance), monitor electrolytes, especially magnesium and calcium, encourage PO and IV hydration as well as high levels of urine flow during therapy; **Neurotoxicity:** assess for weakness and numbness of legs, feet, arms, and hands

PATIENT INFORMATION
Drink plenty of fluids; report immediately symptoms of infection (fever, chills, sore throat), unusual bleeding, bruising and breathing problems; report frequency of diarrhea; report nausea/vomiting

The information here is provided as guidance only. Prescribers should always consult the manufacturer's current prescribing information.

199

PACLITAXEL AND CISPLATIN IN NON–SMALL CELL LUNG CANCER

Paclitaxel is a unique diterpene anticancer agent derived from the bark of the *Taxus brevifola* tree. It exerts its antitumor effect by stabilizing microtubules, rendering them resistant to disassembly. This differs from the other antimicrotubule agents like the vinca alkaloids, which induce microtubule disassembly. Two initial phase II studies of paclitaxel as 24-h infusions showed a response rate of 22% among the 49 patients with an improved median survival of ~40 wk. Subsequent studies in combination with cisplatin ensued. The Eastern Cooperative Oncology Group did a randomized study comparing low-and high-dose paclitaxel with cisplatin to the standard regimen of cisplatin and etoposide [116]. Both the paclitaxel arms showed a higher response rate (26.5% and 32.1% vs 12.0%) and better 1-y survival rates. The European Organization for Research in Cancer Therapy did a randomized study using a short infusion of paclitaxel and cisplatin compared with teniposide and cisplatin [117]. This study showed a higher response rate (44% vs 30%), reduced toxicity, and improved quality of life in patients receiving paclitaxel. Survival was similar in both treatment groups. Southwestern Oncology Group (SWOG)-9805 and ECOG-1594 have both demonstrated the superior activity of this double therapy in the treatment of advanced stage NSCLC [118,119].

RECENT EXPERIENCES AND RESPONSE RATES

Study	Patients, n	Chemotherapy Dosage Schedule, mg/m²	Response Rate, %	Median Survival, mo	1-Y Survival, %	Comments
Bonomi [116]	201	P: 135 IC over 24 h d1	27	27	10.3	Phase III study every 3 wk
		C: 75 d1				
		or				
	196	P: 250 IV over 24 h d1 + GCSF 5 µg/kg SQ d3–10	32	32	10.8	
		C: 75 d1				
Giaccone [117]	154	P: 175 IV over 3 h d1	44	44	9.7	Phase III study every 3 wk
		C: 80 IV d1				

C—cisplatin; P—paclitaxel.

CANDIDATES FOR TREATMENT
Patients with stage III and stage IV disease as well as preoperatively in resectable early-stage disease

SPECIAL PRECAUTIONS
Patients with renal dysfunction; a history of cardiac toxicity should caution the caregiver

ALTERNATIVE THERAPIES
Carboplatin/paclitaxel, cisplatin/vinorelbine, cisplatin/gemcitabine, carboplatin/gemcitabine, cisplatin/docetaxel, or vinorelbine, gemcitabine, and paclitaxel as single agents

TOXICITIES
Paclitaxel: myelosuppression (almost exclusively neutropenia; thrombocytopenia is rare), neurotoxicity (peripheral neuropathy, seizures), gastrointestinal (nausea, vomiting, diarrhea, mucositis, neutropenic enterocolitis), cardiac (arrhythmia, ventricular tachycardia, myocardial infarction, bradycardia), anaphylactic and urticarial reactions, and alopecia and radiation pneumonitis (when administered concomitantly with radiation); **Cisplatin:** gastrointestinal (nausea, vomiting, anorexia), renal toxicity (with an elevation of blood urea nitrogen, creatinine, serum uric acid, impairment of endogenous creatinine clearance, and renal tubular damage), ototoxicity (with hearing loss that initially is in the high-frequency range and tinnitus), peripheral neuropathy, and hyperuricemia; anaphylactic-like reactions (*eg*, facial edema, bronchoconstriction, tachycardia, and hypotension) may occur; myelosuppression often with delayed erythrosuppression is expected; electrolyte disturbances (*eg*, hypomagnesemia and/or hypocalcemia) can occur, resulting in tetany or seizures; subsequent courses should not be given until serum creatinine returns to normal if elevated

DRUG INTERACTION
Agents that are nephrotoxic should be given with caution

NURSING INTERVENTIONS
Hypersensitivity: give premedications for prevention of allergic reactions to paclitaxel (dexamethasone, diphenhydramine, and cimetidine); **Myelosuppression:** monitor blood counts; inquire about symptoms of infection, bleeding, and anemia; **Nausea, vomiting:** give antiemetics before chemotherapy and as needed; **Nephrotoxicity:** monitor renal function indices (serum creatinine, blood urea nitrogen), monitor magnesium, give adequate hydration; **Neurotoxicity:** assess for weakness and numbness of legs, feet, arms, and hands

PATIENT INFORMATION
Patient should drink plenty of fluids and urinate frequently; report prolonged upset stomach and symptoms of infection (fever, chills, sore throat) or neurotoxicity (numbness and tingling sensation of hands or toes); report nausea/vomiting

PACLITAXEL AND CARBOPLATIN IN NON–SMALL CELL LUNG CANCER

Due to a higher incidence of peripheral neuropathy associated with the cisplatin-paclitaxel combination, several trials combining carboplatin with paclitaxel (either as a 24-h or 3-h infusion) have been initiated. It appears that short infusion schedules of paclitaxel have similar degrees of efficacy as compared with 24-h infusion schedules. Shorter infusion schedules result in less myelosuppression, and neuropathy becomes dose limiting. The Southwestern Oncology Group (SWOG) conducted a study comparing carboplatin and paclitaxel with cisplatin and vinorelbine [118]; and the Eastern Cooperative Oncology Group (ECOG) conducted a 4-arm study comparing docetaxel/cisplatin with paclitaxel/cisplatin to paclitaxel/carboplatin to gemcitabine/cisplatin [119]. All novel-agent/platinum combinations studied revealed similar results. Thus, SWOG-9805 and ECOG-1594 have established five acceptable novel-agent/platinum combinations for treatment of advanced NSCLC.

RECENT EXPERIENCES AND RESPONSE RATES

Study	Patients, n	Chemotherapy	RR, %	MS, mo	1-Y Survival, %
SWOG-9805	207	P, 225 mg/m² over 3 h	27	8	36
		C: (AUC = 6) d1			
		vs.			
	201	V: 25 mg/m² weekly	27	8	33
		C: 100 mg/m² d 1			
ECOG-1594	292	P: 135 mg/m² over 24 h d1	21.3	7.8	31
		C: 75 mg/m² d2 q 3 wk			
	288	C: 100 mg/m² d1 q 4 wk	21	8.1	36
		G: 100 mg/m² d 1,8,15			
	293	C: 75 mg/m² d1 q 3 wk	17.3	7.4	31
		D: 75 mg/m² d1			
	290	C: (AUC = 6) d1 q 3 wk	15.3	8.2	35
		P: 225 mg/m² over 3 h d1			

C—cisplatin; D—docetaxel; G—gemcitabine; P—paclitaxel; V—vinorelbine.

CANDIDATES FOR TREATMENT

Patients with stage III and IV disease who have been untreated or refractory to other regimens

SPECIAL PRECAUTIONS

Patients with renal dysfunction; a history of cardiac toxicity should caution the caregiver

ALTERNATIVE THERAPIES

Cisplatin/paclitaxel, carboplatin/paclitaxel, cisplatin/vinorelbine, cisplatin/gemcitabine, cisplatin /docetaxel, carboplatin/gemcitabine; or single agent vinorelbine, gemcitabine, and paclitaxel

TOXICITIES

Carboplatin: myelosuppression, nausea, vomiting, and loss of appetite are common; rare toxicities include gross hematuria, hyponatremia, ageusia, allergic reaction, peripheral neuropathy, veno-occlusive disease, liver and kidney damage, hearing loss, dizziness, and blurred vision; **Paclitaxel:** myelosuppression (almost exclusively neutropenia; thrombocytopenia is rare), neurotoxicity (peripheral neuropathy, seizures), gastrointestinal (nausea, vomiting, diarrhea, mucositis, neutropenic enterocolitis), cardiac (arrhythmia, ventricular tachycardia, myocardial infarction, bradycardia), anaphylactic and urticarial reactions, and alopecia and radiation pneumonitis (when administered concomitantly with radiation)

DRUG INTERACTIONS

None known

NURSING INTERVENTION

Hypersensitivity: give premedications for prevention of allergic reactions to paclitaxel (dexamethasone, diphenhydramine, and cimetidine); **Myelosuppression:** monitor blood counts; inquire about symptoms of infection, bleeding, and anemia; **Nausea, vomiting:** give antiemetics before chemotherapy and as needed; **Nephrotoxicity:** monitor renal function indices (serum creatinine, blood urea nitrogen) and magnesium; give adequate hydration; **Neurotoxicity:** assess for weakness and numbness of legs, feet, arms, and hands

PATIENT INFORMATION

Patient should drink plenty of fluids and urinate frequently; report prolonged upset stomach and irregularities in heart rhythm, and symptoms of infection (fever, chills, sore throat) or neurotoxicity (tingling or numbness of hands and toes)

VINORELBINE AND CISPLATIN IN NON–SMALL CELL LUNG CANCER

Vinorelbine is a unique semisynthetic vinca alkaloid. Its mechanism of action is similar to the other vinca alkaloids in that it is an inhibitor of microtubule assembly. It binds to tubulin, resulting in disruption of the mitotic spindle apparatus during metaphase. Vinorelbine has a lesser effect on axonal microtubules, and because neurotoxicity of vinca alkaloids is postulated to derive from damage to axonal microtubules, a more favorable therapeutic index of vinorelbine has been postulated. Preclinical studies with vinorelbine indicate activity against several tumor cell lines representing leukemia, small, and non–small cell lung cancer, breast and colon cancer, and melanoma. Vinorelbine was later demonstrated to have significant activity in previously untreated NSCLC patients (see Table 10-7). SWOG-9805 established the navelbine/cisplatin combination as one of the current standard treatment of advanced NSCLC [118].

CANDIDATES FOR TREATMENT

Preoperative resectable stage II–IIIA as well as stage IIIB and IV disease

SPECIAL PRECAUTIONS

Patients with renal dysfunction; a history of peripheral neuropathy should caution the caregiver

ALTERNATIVE THERAPIES

Carboplatin/paclitaxel, cisplatin/paclitaxel, cisplatin/gemcitabine, carboplatin/gemcitabine, cisplatin/docetaxel; or vinorelbine, paclitaxel, and gemcitabine as single agents

TOXICITIES

Vinorelbine: myelosuppression with neutropenia and leukopenia are the most frequent dose-limiting toxicities (thrombocytopenia is rare; however, thrombocytosis is fairly common); mild to moderate constipation and decreased deep tendon reflexes are the most frequent occurring neurotoxicities; paresthesias occur infrequently; foot drop, peripheral neuropathy, and paralytic ileus have also been observed; mild to moderate nausea and vomiting occur in ~50% of patients; phlebitis characterized by erythema and tenderness extending over the palpable length of the infused vein has been associated with intravenous vinorelbine; mild to moderate alopecia has occurred and is related to duration of treatment; allergic reactions, fatigue, inappropriate antidiuretic hormone syndrome, hemorrhagic cystis, and insomnia have been reported

DRUG INTERACTIONS

None known

NURSING INTERVENTIONS

Myelosuppression: monitor blood counts; ask for symptoms of infection, bleeding, and anemia; **Nausea, vomiting:** give antiemetics before chemotherapy and as needed; **Nephrotoxicity:** monitor renal function indices (serum creatinine, blood urea nitrogen) and magnesium; give adequate hydration; **Neurotoxicity:** assess for weakness and numbness of legs, feet, arms, and hands.

RECENT EXPERIENCES AND RESPONSE RATES

Study group	Patients, n	Chemotherapy Dosage Schedule, mg/m²	Response Rate, %	Median Survival, wk	1-y Survival, %	Comments
Depierre [132]	116	CDDP: 80 IV every 3 wk V: 30 weekly	43.0	32	NR	Phase III study with patients treated a minimum of 6 wk
Berthaud [133]	32	CDDP: 120 IV every 4–6 wk V: 30 weekly	33.0	44	NR	Phase I–II study
Frontini [134]	74	CDDP: 80 IV d 1 V: 25 IV d 1, 8	56.7	52	NR	Phase II study with regimen every 3 wk for 3 cycles
Wozniak [107]	195	CDDP: 100 IV every 3 wk V: 25 mg/m2/wk × 3	25.0	28	33	Phase III study that showed a better 1-y survival rate of this combination compared with CDDP alone
LeChevalier [101]	206	CDDP: 120 mg/m2 IV d 1, 28 then every 6 wk V: 30 mg/m2/wk × 6 then every 2 wk	30.0	40	35	Phase III study comparing this regimen with vinorelbine alone and with cisplatin and vindesine; it showed higher response and 1-y survival rates with a major difference in survival in stage IV patients

CDDP—cisplatin; V—vinorelbine.

GEMCITABINE AND CISPLATIN IN NON–SMALL CELL LUNG CANCER

Gemcitabine is a new deoxycytidine analogue related to cytosine arabinoside (Ara-C) that has been found to have considerable activity in NSCLC. Several phase II trials using gemcitabine in advanced, untreated NSCLC patients showed an overall response rate of 20% among 332 patients (see Table 10-7). The impressive low toxicity profile of gemcitabine adds to its appeal in combining it with other active agents such as cisplatin. Several phase II studies in combination with cisplatin have reported an overall response rate of 47% with an average median survival of 57 weeks and 1-year survival rate of 61% (see Table 10-8). ECOG-1594 has established the gemcitabine/platinum combination one of the current standard treatment for advanced stage NSCLC [119].

RECENT EXPERIENCES AND RESPONSE RATES

Study	Patients, n	Chemotherapy Dosage Schedule	Response Rate, %	Median Survival, wk	1-y Overall Survival, %	Comments
Manegold et al. [135]	66	G: 1000 mg/m² /wk × 3 wk	18.2	15.3	29	Phase III study every 4 wk for a minimum of 6 cycles
Perng et al. [136]	26	G: 1250 mg/m² /wk × 3 wk	19.2	37.0	38	Phase III study every 4 wk
Einhorn et al. [137]	27	G: 1000 mg/m² /wk × 3 wk CDDP: 100 mg/m² d 1	37.0	33.6	37	Every 4 wk
Abratt et al. [138]	50	G: 1000 mg/m² /wk × 3 wk CDDP: 100 mg/m² d 15	52.0	42.0	61	Every 4 wk
Anton et al. [139]	40	G: 1250 mg/m² /wk × 3 wk CDDP: 100 mg/m² d 15	47.5	10.4	35	Every 4 wk
Shepherd et al. [140]	39	G: 1250 mg/m² /wk × 3 wk CDDP: 30 mg/m² weekly × 3 wk	26.0	26.0	NR	Every 4 wk
Lopez-Cabrezio et al. [110]	65	G: 1250 mg/m² d 1, 8 CDDP: 100 mg/m² d 1	49.0	NR	NR	Every 4 wk; a higher response rate compared with EP
Gonzalez-Baron et al. [141]	51	G: 1200 mg/m² /wk × 3 wk CDDP: 100 mg/m² d 1	43.0	NR	NR	Every 4 wk

CDDP—cisplatin; EP—etoposide and cisplatin; G—gemcitabine; NR—not reported.

CANDIDATES FOR TREATMENT
Patients refractory to standard chemotherapy; patients with stage III and stage IV NSCLC

SPECIAL PRECAUTIONS
Patients with renal dysfunction and impaired liver function

ALTERNATIVE THERAPIES
Etoposide and paclitaxel, etoposide and carboplatin, carboplatin and paclitaxel, cisplatin and vinorelbine, vinorelbine alone, or gemcitabine alone

TOXICITIES
Gemcitabine: myelosuppression is the dose-limiting toxicity; thrombocytopenia occurs occasionally, but thrombocytosis is also reported; abnormalities in liver transaminase enzymes can occur; nausea and vomiting occurs in two thirds of patients; mild proteinuria and hematuria can be present but is not associated with any change in serum creatinine or blood urea nitrogen; a rash is seen in 25% of patients and is associated with pruritus in ~10% of patients; other reported toxicities include a flu-like syndrome, mild to moderate peripheral edema, pulmonary edema, and rarely facial edema

DRUG INTERACTION
Cisplatin with other nephro- or ototoxic drugs

NURSING INTERVENTIONS
Myelosuppression: monitor blood counts; inquire about symptoms of infection, bleeding, and anemia; **Nausea, vomiting:** give antiemetics before chemotherapy and as needed; **Nephrotoxicity:** monitor renal function indices (serum creatinine, blood urea nitrogen) and magnesium; give adequate hydration; **Neurotoxicity:** assess for weakness and numbness of legs, feet, arms, and hands

PATIENT INFORMATION
Patients should drink plenty of fluids and urinate frequently; report prolonged upset stomach, symptoms of infection (fever, chills, sore throat), and unusual bleeding or bruising; report nausea/vomiting

DOCETAXEL AND CISPLATIN IN NON–SMALL CELL LUNG CANCER

Docetaxel (taxotere) is synthesized from the extracts of the leaves of *Taxus baccata*. It enhances microtubule assembly and inhibits the depolymerization of tubulin. As with paclitaxel, this can lead to bundles of microtubules in the cell, leading to an inability of the cell to divide. The cell cycle is halted in M-phase. In initial clinical studies, taxotere produced clinical responses in patients with breast cancer, ovarian cancer, NSCLC, and pancreatic cancer. Single-agent docetaxel has produced response rate of 26% and a 1-year survival rate of 52% in patients with advanced NSCLC (see Table 10-7). Phase II trials of the docetaxel/cisplatin doublet in NSCLC have demonstrated response, median survival, and 1-year survival rates of 35%, 35 weeks, and 58%, respectively (see Table 10-8). ECOG-1594 demonstrated docetaxel/cisplatin double therapy to be equivalent in efficacy to cisplatin/paclitaxel, cisplatin/gemcitabine, and carboplatin/paclitaxel [119].

CANDIDATES FOR TREATMENT
Patients with stage IIIB or IV NSCLC

SPECIAL PRECAUTIONS
Patients with renal dysfunction; previous reactions to the taxanes

ALTERNATIVE THERAPY
Cisplatin/paclitaxel, carboplatin/paclitaxel, cisplatin/vinorelbine, cisplatin/gemcitabine, carboplatin/gemcitabine; or vinorelbine, gemcitabine, and paclitaxel as single agents

TOXICITIES
Docetaxel: dose-limiting neutropenia; thrombocytopenia noted but less frequent anaphylactic reactions consistent with dyspnea, rash, anxiety noted in a few patients on the first course of treatment. After pretreatment with diphenhydramine and dexamethasone, patients have been able to be treated without difficulty. Other toxicities include phlebitis and alopecia. Pleural effusions and peripheral edema have both been reported. Premedication with dexamethasone as well as the modification of the treatment regimen to lower weekly doses or a maximum dose of 75 mg/m^2 every 3 weeks have decreased the incidence of fluid retention

NURSING INTERVENTIONS
Myelosuppression: monitor blood counts and ask for symptoms of infection, bleeding, and anemia; **Nausea/vomiting:** give antiemetics before chemotherapy and as needed; **Nephrotoxicity:** monitor renal function indices (serum creatinine, BUN), monitor magnesium, give adequate hydration; **Neurotoxicity:** assess for weakness and numbness of legs, feet, arms, and hands; **Fluid retention:** make sure the patient has been premedicated with dexamethasone before docetaxel infusion

CHAPTER 11: MELANOMA AND OTHER TUMORS OF THE SKIN

Michael T. Lotze, John M. Kirkwood

The most commonly occurring human neoplasms are those arising in the skin. The nonmelanoma neoplasms are chiefly squamous and basal cell carcinomas that evolve slowly, generally permitting early recognition and cure by local. Less often, radiation and topical chemotherapeutic approaches are used. Melanoma is a less common but more aggressive cutaneous neoplasm that in up to 15% of patients, has a considerably more lethal progression pattern, involving regional and distant sites. Recently, new biologic therapies capable of preventing relapse after surgical excision and leading to sustained regression in patients with metastatic disease have been identified. Melanoma less frequently arises in a variety of noncutaneous sites, including the mucosae and subungual areas of the toes and fingers and the uveal tract of the eye. Indeed ocular melanoma is the most lethal tumor of the eye in adults. The incidence of melanoma has risen more rapidly than any other solid tumor. Approximately 45,000 patients develop melanoma annually, with one in 75 white patients expected to be at risk for developing melanoma in their lifetime at the beginning of this millennium [1]. Interestingly, the increase appears to be primarily in thin melanomas, those most readily cured with simple excision [2]. The following chapter will deal solely with cutaneous melanoma and basal and squamous cell carcinomas, the predominant skin cancers that confront the clinician.

MELANOMA

Melanoma is a fascinating tumor with well-described patterns of genetic predisposition in 10% of cases, a clear association with episodic ultraviolet exposure, and strong evidence of host immune response that can be enhanced to treat the disease in many patients. Spontaneous regression is observed in < 1% of patients, and as many as 10% of patients may develop metastases without a known primary. Although the incidence of melanoma increases with age, young adults and even children may develop this tumor. Surgical excision of the primary lesion remains the mainstay of treatment for localized melanoma. New techniques of isotopic and dye localization of lymphatic drainage allows selective lymph node dissection to acquire prognostic information. Its role in enhancing outcome is now being tested in prospective clinical trials. Biologic therapy using alpha interferon in patients with regional metastatic spread has recently been confirmed to prolong life and increase apparent cures in patients with this disease.

ETIOLOGY AND RISK FACTORS

Evidence for an inherited predisposition to melanoma comes from observations that a family history of this disease is a risk factor for melanoma, especially in association with a characteristic precursor lesion termed the dysplastic nevus. Genes localized on chromosomes 1, 6, 7, and 10 appear to be important, especially the region associated with cell cycle inhibition including products of the p16/INK4A locus. The p16 gene encodes a cell cycle regulatory protein that also enhances the risk for pancreatic cancer [2–4]. Ten percent of all melanoma is associated with a family history, and in this setting, those individuals with the dysplastic nevus syndrome, a precursor lesion, have increased risk of melanoma. With dysplastic nevi and two cases of melanoma in a family, the risk of developing melanoma approaches 100% at 70 years of age [5]. Dysplastic nevi are suspected precursors in 25% to 40% of sporadic cases, but the molecular and

immunologic features of progression from normal nevi to atypical and frankly malignant melanocytic lesions are being identified. Early evidence suggests that alterations in growth factors and their receptors, as well as vascularization and the presence of integrins and adhesion molecules, are important [6]. Congenital melanocytic nevi are precursors related to a small subset of melanoma in the population at large. Apart from the presence of dysplastic nevi, the risk for primary melanoma is directly related to the total number of all moles. With a personal history of melanoma, the presence of atypical nevi increases eight-fold the risk of a second primary melanoma [7].

Ultraviolet exposure clearly plays a role in development of melanoma [8]. Evidence to support this notion is found in the topographic distribution of cutaneous melanoma, which is directly related to sun exposure. The incidence of melanoma is associated with latitude and the intensity of solar exposure among susceptible populations. Fair-skinned, light-complected individuals who have migrated to Australia and New Zealand are at particularly high risk because of the local intensity of solar radiation, the regional thinning of the ozone layer, and the constitutional susceptibility of this population. In melanoma found to arise in the background of an atypical/dysplastic nevus, the neoplastic component most frequently arises in the junctional rather than the dermal component. Educational programs designed to modify the population's behavior in relation to sun exposure have been developed and been notably effective [9].

The evidence for host immune reactivity to melanoma includes the frequent observation of regression in both acquired nevi and, on rare occasion, melanoma. Aside from these risk factors, a variety of other conditions associated with immunodeficiency are also associated with increased risk of melanoma and include ataxia telangiectasia, chronic lymphocytic leukemia, Hodgkin's disease, immunosuppression for organ transplantation, AIDS, and treatment with nucleoside analogues (Table 11-1) [10,11]. Histologic evidence supporting a role of the immune response in melanoma includes the frequent finding of lymphocytic infiltrates in primary lesions and dysplastic nevi, which are diminished (if present at all) in metastatic lesions. Melanoma is responsive to many biologic therapies, including interferon (IFN)-α and interleukin (IL)-2 (see Treatment section). Serologic and/or cellular reactivity to melanoma has been detected in a significant fraction of patients. An increasing number of protein peptide antigens recognized by cloned T cells [12] and ganglioside tumor antigens identified by serologic detection will enable measurement of host response to these tumor antigens in relationship with vaccination and other therapies and will facilitate establishment of their therapeutic roles (Table 11-2).

CLINICAL AND PATHOLOGIC APPEARANCE

The clinical characteristics of melanoma have been well described. These include the "ABCDE" criteria of asymmetry, border variation, color variation, diameter greater than 4 mm, and evolution or change noted by the patient or by a friend or family member. Bleeding and ulceration are findings that clinically suggest a poor prognosis. Evolution in the characteristics of a lesion should prompt investigation and possible biopsy. The various gradations of progression in human melanoma involve a series of morphologic and histopathologic steps: 1) an acquired melanocytic nevus, 2) melanocytic nevus with various degrees of architectural and cytologic atypia (dysplasia), 3) radial growth phase primary melanoma, 4) vertical growth phase primary, 5) regional lymph node metastatic melanoma, and 6) distant hematogenous metastatic melanoma. Often a patient can give a clear-cut history of progression from a pigmented lesion appearing as a nevus to the appearance of surface irregularity or ulceration associated with a vertical growth phase melanoma. A variety of morphologic types of melanoma can be distinguished: 1) superficial spreading (flat) melanoma, 2) nodular melanoma, 3) lentigo maligna melanoma, 4) acral lentiginous (including subungual) melanoma, and 5) ocular melanoma. However, with the availability of microstaging for tumor depth in the past 25 years, their prognostic importance is no longer as great.

DIAGNOSIS, PROGNOSIS, AND STAGING

The treatment of melanoma varies according to disease stage as defined by the American Joint Commission on Cancer (AJCC) staging system (Tables 11-3, 11-4) which is currently in revision. Previously, melanoma [13] was simply divided into three general prognostic subgroups: 1) local disease, for which surgical therapy is the predominant therapy; 2) regional disease, for which adjuvant IFN-α therapy has recently entered standard clinical practice and selective lymph node sampling is in current evaluation; and 3) systemic disease, for which a variety of experimental chemotherapeutic and immunologic approaches exist. None of the treatments for metastatic disease have been proven to prolong survival. In the AJCC staging system, stage I and II encompass localized disease of low- and intermediate/high-recurrence risk, stage III encompasses lymph nodal disease, and stage IV represents distant metastatic disease. In stage III, the most important factors relating to local- and distant-recurrence risk are the presence or absence of extranodal/extracapsular extension and the number of lymph nodes involved. The AJCC staging system revisions would incorporate such factors as ulceration

in the primary and node number involved for regional disease. These are widely accepted prognostic factors not formally included in the current AJCC classification [13].

A workup for primary melanoma includes a physical examination with attention to skin pigmentation, including the presence of hypopigmentation. This may reflect obliterated primary site or paraneoplastic vitiligo-like destruction of the normal pigment cells in the skin. If a patient presents with nodal or metastatic disease in the absence of an obvious primary tumor, it is important to examine the less obvious potential noncutaneous sites of melanoma, including mucosal surfaces and the uveal tract of the eye. A chest radiograph and liver function test for the lactate dehydrogenase enzyme are performed to detect signs of occult metastatic disease in these two major organs, although neither is highly sensitive. More intensive protocols may specify computer tomography or magnetic resonance imaging to evaluate the head, chest, and abdomen to identify with greater sensitivity (although with less specificity) the potential site of metastasis. Follow-up for primary melanoma [14] has recently been defined. Based on the hazard ratio for recurrence, the following surveillance schedules are recommended in addition to patient education for detection of recurrence: 1) stage I, annually; 2) stage II, every 6 months for years 1,2 and annually thereafter; 3) stage III, every 3 months for year 1, every 4 months for year 2, and every 6 months for years 3–5; 4) past year 6, all patients should have annual surveillance, due to the risk of late recurrence and/or metachronous multiple primaries.

The recognition of primary melanoma and its precursor lesions (including dysplastic nevi) depends on awareness of change in pigmented lesions. Photographic evaluation is useful in providing a reference frame for follow-up of skin lesions in patients with particularly numerous or varied lesions. Excisional surgical or punch biopsy is required to evaluate lesions suspected of being melanoma. Patients with regional lymphadenopathy in the absence of evidence of systemic spread are best treated with regional lymphadenectomy. Patients without regional lymphadenopathy who have primary tumors of intermediate-risk (AJCC stage II) are potential candidates for the evaluation of regional lymph nodes if they would be considered for further systemic adjuvant therapy, as follows. Previously, lymphadenectomy was performed electively for the drainage basin at greatest risk defined according to the anatomic location of the primary. However, this method of determination has been found to be erroneous in up to 30% of cases. Scintigraphic and dye methods have been developed to more precisely ascertain the exact drainage of melanoma and other tumors, allowing sentinel node biopsy and selective lymphadenectomy for diagnostic and possibly therapeutic purposes [15].

Elective lymphadenectomy has shown no survival benefit in any of several large randomized controlled trials, and the therapeutic value of selective lymph node dissection is currently under study. Selective

Table 11-1. Risk factors of melanoma and nonmelanoma skin cancers

Risk factor	Lifetime risk	Cancer type
Sun exposure	1%–2% (in whites)	Melanoma & SCC/BCC
Light complexion (skin that tans poorly or burns easily)	1%–2%	Melanoma & SCC/BCC
Cigarette smoking	1%–2%	SCC
Human papillomavirus (HPV 16, 18)	ND	SCC/BCC
Arsenic	ND	SCC/BCC
Polycyclic aromatic hydrocarbons	ND	SCC/BCC
Xeroderma pigmentosum (autosomal recessive)	2%–100%	Melanoma & SCC/BCC
Basal-cell nevus syndrome (autosomal dominant)	1%–5%	SCC/BCC
Albinism (autosomal recessive)	1%–5%	SCC/BCC
Epidermodysplasia verruciformis (autosomal recessive)	1%–5%	SCC/BCC
Acquired immunodeficiency syndrome	5%	Melanoma & SCC/BCC
Chronic wounds and scars	ND	SCC/BCC
Chronic immunosuppression	5%	SCC
Familial Syndromes (including atypical nevi) — p16 and p53 mutations	2%–5%	Melanoma & SCC/BCC
Multiple nevi (especially > 50 y of age)	2–12 times	Melanoma

BCC—basal cell carcinoma; ND—not determined; SCC—squamous cell carcinoma

Table 11-2. Antigens of human melanoma defined by T cell and antibody response

Cancer–testis antigens	Differentiation antigens
MAGE 1, 3	Tyrosinase (internal, leader)
BAGE, GAGE, RAGE	gp100 (HMB-45) (multiple, both mutated and native)
NY ESO-1	Melan-A/MART-1 (multiple)
	TP1/gp75
	TRP2/dopachrome tautomerase

lymphadenectomy offers greater precision and lower morbidity for staging of regional lymph nodes than elective full regional lymphadenectomy. This procedure, coupled with availability of an effective adjuvant IFN-α therapy now available (*see* Treatment section), is becoming more widely adopted in the treatment of melanoma. The presence of distant metastasis limits therapeutic options and outcome for patients. Suspected metastatic sites of tumor are reasonable to document by needle biopsy or only with serial radiological follow-up when a change of therapy is not an issue.

Prognostic factors predictive of survival include microstage of disease as defined by tumor thickness (Breslow depth) and, less importantly, skin layer penetration (Clark level) (Table 11-3). Mitotic rate, ulceration, and the presence of satellites are prognostically important histologic factors (Table 11-4). Younger patients, females, and patients with extremity lesions fare better than older

males and those with truncal tumors. Although T-cell infiltrate is a factor associated with improved prognosis, expression of the class II MHC molecules (DR, DP, DQ) has been associated with poorer prognosis. The loss of class I MHC expression is recognized as a factor relevant to the evasion of immune recognition.

TREATMENT

The surgical treatment of primary melanoma has been studied for many years now. Consensus from a number of published studies indicates that a wide local excision should be performed for lesions deeper than 1.0 mm; 2-cm margins have recently been demonstrated to be equivalent to 4-cm margins in a prospective randomized trial for primary tumors of 1–4 mm Breslow depth [16]. Therapeutic lymphadenectomy is indicated for manifest, regional lymph node

Table 11-3. AJCC TNM Classification System for Melanoma

Current 1992	Current 1992	Proposed 2000	
T stage			
T0	Tis	Tis	
T1	< 0.76	< 1.0	A: no ulceration
			B: ulceration or level IV or V
T2	0.76–1.5	1–2	A: no ulceration
T3	1.5–4.0	2–4	B: ulceration
T4	> 4	> 4	
N stage			
N1	1	One lymph node	A: Micrometastasis
			B: Macrometastasis
N2	2–4	2–3 lymph nodes	A: Micrometastasis
			B: Macrometastasis
			C: In-transit disease without positive nodes
N3	≥ 5	≥ 4 metastatic lymph nodes, matted nodes, ulcerated melanoma and metastatic lymph node(s) or nodal disease and in-transit or satellite lesions	
M stage			
M1	Any systemic metastasis	Any systemic metastasis	A: Distant skin, soft tissue or nodal metastases
			B: Pulmonary metastases
			C: All other visceral involvement or any melanoma patient with elevated blood levels of LDH

Table 11-4. AJCC TMN Stage Grouping for Cutaneous Melanoma

Pathologic Stage	T	N	M	Clinical Stage	T	N	M
0	Tis	N0	M0	0	Tis	N0	M0
IA	T1a	N0	M0	IA	T1a	N0	M0
IB	T1b	N0	M0	IB	T1b	N0	M0
	T2a	N0	M0		T2a	N0	M0
IIA	T2b	N0	M0	IIA	T2b	N0	M0
	T3a	N0	M0		T3a	N0	M0
IIB	T3b	N0	M0	IIB	T3b	N0	M0
	T4a	N0	M0		T4a	N0	M0
IIC	T4b	N0	M0	IIC	T4b	N0	M0
IIIA	T1–4a	N1a	M0	IIIA	Any T1–4a	N1b	M0
IIIB	T1–4a	N1b	M0	IIIB	Any T1–4a	N2b	M0
	T1–4a	N2a	M0				
IIIC	Any T	N2b, N2c	M0	IIIC	Any T	N2c	M0
	Any T	N3	M0		Any T	N3	M0
IV	Any T	Any N	M1	IV	Any T	Any N	M1

metastases in the absence of distant disease. Prophylactic regional lymph node dissection has not been demonstrated to be of value in prolonging survival or time to relapse in any of a number of large, randomized controlled studies. Selective regional lymphadenectomy performed after scintigraphic and dye-lymphographic identification of the sentinel draining lymph node(s) offers improved prognostic precision as noted above, and its therapeutic role is currently under study in the Multicenter Selective Lymphadenectomy Trial. Limited cutaneous or nodal tumor resection has a role in palliation of symptomatic mass lesions without any demonstrable impact on survival. Patients with isolated visceral metastatic brain disease or with gastrointestinal tract tumors may obtain significant benefit from resection of limited metastatic disease, especially following long disease-free intervals or with disease that has a long doubling time on serial radiologic follow up. In general, resection of metastases of lung, liver, and other abdominal viscera is of little advantage [17,18] but has been promoted for selected patients with limited disease without other options.

Radiation therapy is an alternative palliative modality for inoperable visceral metastatic sites, particularly those occurring within the bone and brain. In high-dose fractions given for metastatic brain disease, steroid premedication should be used to limit edema, which may exacerbate symptoms or provoke hemorrhage. Bleeding into brain metastases is particularly frequent in patients with melanoma. Intensive local irradiation using a stereotactic delivery in special multibeam units (gamma-knife therapy) appears to be useful for treatment of patients with unresectable, isolated, or a limited number of small (< 2.5 cm) lesions [19]. Whole-brain radiotherapy has been used to reduce the size and risk of bleeding from brain metastases. Recent studies to evaluate its role in conjunction with stereotactic radiation therapy demonstrate little additive benefit.

Dacarbazine (dimethyl triazeno imidazole carboxamide or DTIC) and interleukin-2 (IL-2) are the only FDA-approved therapeutic agents for treatment of metastatic melanoma in the United States. Complete and partial responses with dacarbazine alone or combined with cisplatin and IL2/IFN-α occur in 13% to 20% of patients, with a mean duration of response that is 5 to 7 months [20–22]. Response to DTIC has been correlated with disease limited to soft tissues and female gender. Dacarbazine requires hepatic transformation to its active intermediate, whereas temozolomide, a newer fully absorbed oral prodrug, shows a wider distribution in the body (including central nervous system) and spontaneously transforms into the same active intermediate as for dacarbazine. To date, no benefit has been demonstrated for adjuvant chemotherapy with dacarbazine alone or in combination with other chemotherapeutic or hormonal agents. Patients presenting with asymptomatic or minimally symptomatic metastatic melanoma can reasonably be offered a variety of investigational treatment programs. Combination chemotherapy historically has been associated with increased toxicity that outweighs the minimal gains in response rate obtained using a variety of different protocols. Early studies of dacarbazine with tamoxifen appeared to have been of benefit for subjects in one randomized trial, whereas dacarbazine and IFN-α2 showed benefit in another. Unfortunately, larger multicenter studies of these two combinations conducted in the Eastern Cooperative Oncology Group (ECOG) (E3690) have shown no survival benefit for either combination or for all three agents together over dacarbazine alone [23]. A considerable degree of interest and enthusiasm was raised in a series of reports of uncontrolled trials using the four-agent combination of dacarbazine, bischlorethylnitrosourea (BCNU), cisplatin, and tamoxifen, which is known as the Dartmouth regimen [24]. Careful controlled studies of

the National Cancer Institute-Canada have dismissed the previous suggestion of benefit from tamoxifen in this combination [22], and a recently concluded trial [25] of the ECOG and Memorial-Sloan Kettering Cancer Center (MSKCC) (M91-140) showed no benefit of the Dartmouth combination when compared with dacarbazine. High-dose chemotherapy with bone marrow rescue using melphalan, thiotepa, or BCNU have achieved improved short-term responses but not durable complete remissions or overall survival benefit.

IFN-α treatment is associated with response in 16% to 22% of a collected series of patients with metastatic melanoma [26]. Treatment achieves durable complete remissions in one third of responders. Response is associated with soft tissue or pulmonary sites and is higher in smaller-bulk disease. A variety of combinations with chemotherapy have been investigated with contradictory results, which may be due to the dose and sequence of agents used. IL-2 (a T-cell growth factor employed since 1984 in the treatment of patients with melanoma [27–30]) has achieved a response rate of up to 20% with a subset of patients who experience durable complete response. Treatment with IL-2 (recently approved by the FDA for treatment of metastatic melanoma and renal cell cancer) requires high doses for induction of response. Associated vascular leak syndrome, hypotension, myocardial infarction, and renal failure has tempered the application of this modality.

Other cytokines (including IL-1, -4, -12, tumor necrosis factor [TNF], and IL-18) have attractive rationale but as yet have not been demonstrated to be valuable for the treatment of melanoma. Significant interest in vaccines has existed in the field of melanoma for many years, and a variety of vaccines have been tested, but none has yet shown evidence of an increase in survival in properly controlled trials [15,31]. Adoptive immunotherapy with transfer of cellular reagents (including tumor infiltrating lymphocytes, lymphokine-activated killer cells with IL-2 or dendritic cells) have been shown to induce response rates of 30% to 50% in limited series. Their role singly or in combination with IL-2 remains to be demonstrated. Gene therapy that introduces cytokine genes or costimulatory molecules such as CD80 (B7.1) into tumors are currently undergoing evaluation at a number of centers [32].

Isolated limb perfusion using melphalan has been applied for many years and has gone through a resurgence of interest in combination with TNF-α administered by perfusion with and without IFN-α administered systemically [33,34]. Recent results from a randomized study comparing melphalan alone with the combination performed at the NCI have not shown improved outcome with the combination overall, although there is a suggestion that it may be superior for patients with extensive disease (> 10 lesions). Similarly a randomized study showed no clear benefit to the addition of gamma interferon [34]. There is currently no convincing evidence to apply it as an adjuvant therapy.

The risk factors predicting outcome in the setting of metastatic disease have recently been analyzed [14, 18, 35–37]. Independent variables predicting survival include 1) initial site of the metastases (patients with distant cutaneous, nodal, and gastrointestinal disease fare better than those presenting with lung disease, which is better than other visceral sites), 2) disease-free interval prior to distant metastases, and 3) stage of disease preceding distant metastases. In long-term survivors, prior immunotherapy, younger age and female gender tended to be correlated with improved survival. A significant difference was the ability of the long-term surviving patients to have all metastatic disease resected or a complete or partial response with initial chemotherapy or immunotherapy. Multivariate analysis [18] of a recent series of ECOG trial patients with metastatic disease has shown independent prognostic roles for blood lactic dehydrogenase, alkaline phosphatase and platelet levels. These factors could be considered in the design of future trials in the setting of metastatic disease.

ADJUVANT THERAPY

The staging of melanoma by classical tumor-node-metastasis (TNM) and AJCC systems is detailed in Table 11-3. In AJCC staging (the current standard), primary melanomas deeper than 0.76 mm (T2) without associated metastatic involvement of regional lymph nodes (N0) are defined as stage IB, whereas melanomas deeper than 1.50 mm (T3) in the absence of lymphadenopathy are defined as stage IIA. Those deeper than 4.0 mm (T4) and free of clinically apparent regional nodal involvement or other signs of metastasis are defined as stage IIB, with a risk that approaches that of patients with clinical manifestations of regional lymph node metastasis, which is defined as stage IIIA (N1). The prognostic subclassification of nodal involvement has previously been formally defined by node size (>3 cm), but it is widely recognized that the prognosis for node-positive patients is better quantified by the number of tumor-involved lymph nodes. Patients with distant metastasis beyond the regional draining nodal group (M1) are defined as stage IV. These disease groupings contrast to the three classical staging groups of primary disease (old stage I), regional nodal involvement (old stage II), and distant metastases (old stage III). Newer systems, incorporating the presence of ulceration and satellite involvement in the prognostication of localized disease and the number of involved nodes for patients in stage III, have been proposed and are expected to be assimilated into the AJCC system [14].

High risk of relapse, generally exceeding 50% in the first 2 years of follow-up, is associated with AJCC stage III melanoma (the pres-

ence of regional lymph node metastasis) or stage IIB disease with deep invasion at the site of the primary lesion > 4 mm. These have ominous prognostic significance. For this reason, patients in these prognostic groups have been widely considered for new therapies (ranging from chemotherapy to biologicals), including interferons, cytokines, antibodies, and tumor vaccines.

Extensive literature has been published detailing the results of multiple randomized controlled trials of chemotherapy and chemotherapy with older biologicals (eg, the crude microbial immunostimulants bacille Calmette–Guérin [BCG], *Corynebacterium parvum*, and OK 432 [38]. These studies failed to yield consistent evidence of benefit to support further investigation of these regimens (based largely on the drug dacarbazine). Chemical immunomodulators and the antihelminthic agent levamisole have also been intensively investigated, with controversial results that have not led to regulatory approval or clinical use of levamisole as adjuvant therapy outside Canada [39,40].

The largest and most positive literature for adjuvant therapy surrounds IFN-α2, which has been tested in high-risk groups of patients with resected stage III and IIB melanoma [41]. The E1684 study showed the first significant benefit of adjuvant therapy, both in terms of survival rate and relapse-free interval. The ECOG high-dose regimen, which employed intravenous office therapy (20 MU/m2/d, 5 d/wk for 4 wk) followed by subcutaneous patient-administered therapy (10 MU/m2d three times weekly for 11 mo) with IFN-α2b, has significantly prolonged relapse-free survival ($P = 0.002$) and overall survival ($P = 0.023$) of patients treated within 56 days of surgery. This agent has been approved by the FDA as the first and only agent capable of preventing relapse and death in high-risk melanoma. The toxicity of treatment at the maximally tolerable dosages employed in the study were significant, and severe toxicity was noted in a majority of

Table 11-5. Summary of Current Cooperative Group Trials for Adjuvant Therapy of High- and Intermediate-Risk Melanoma as Defined by 2001 AJCC Staging System

Disease Stage	Risk Category	5-y Estimated Relapse/Mortality, %	Experimental Arm	Reference Arm (Standard)
Stage IIa	Low to intermediate	25–40	—	—
ECOG E1697 (Intergroup ECOG/NCI-C)	—	—	Induction mo 1 only (HDI 20 MU/m2/d × 5/7d/wk × 4 wk)	Observation
Stage IIB—IIA	Intermediate risk disease	50	—	—
ECOG E1601 (Intergroup US proposed, 2001)	—	—	Induction mo 1 only (HDI 20 MU/m2/d × 5/7d/wk × 4 wk)	HDI (E1684 regimen × 1 y)
Stage IIIB—C	High risk	75	—	—
SWOG S0008 (Intergroup US)	—	—	Chemobiotherapy × 3 cycles with CVD—IL-2 + IFN-α2b	HDI (E1684 regimen × 1 y)
Stage IIIC—IV (resected)	Very high risk	90	—	—
ECOG E4697 Intergroup	—	—	GM-CSF, CG-CSF + multiepitope peptide	Observation*
—	—	—	Vaccine** or multiepitope peptide vaccine**	—
Stage IIIA, B, C	High risk	—	—	—
EORTC 18991	—	—	PEG-IFN-α2b weekly for 5 y	Observation†

*Placebo for granulocyte-macrophage colony-stimulating factor (GM-CSF) for HLA-A2 negative; placebo for GM-CSF, or multiepitope peptide vaccine, or both for HLA-A2 positive.
**Patients who are HLA-A2 positive on major histocompatibility class I typing.
†Europe and Australia only (not the United States or Canada).
AJCC—American Joint Committee on Cancer; CVD—cisplatin, vinblastine, dacarbazine; ECOG—Eastern Cooperative Oncology Group; EORTC—European Organization for Research and Treatment of Cancer; HDI—hexamethylene diisocyanate; IFN—interferon; PEG—polyethylene glycol; SWOG—Southwestern Oncology Group.

patients at least once during therapy. However, the regimen was given entirely in the outpatient setting, and (with dose modification for these dose-limiting constitutional [50%], hematologic [24%], or hepatic [15%] toxicities) 74% of patients without relapse continued on treatment through the full year [41].

The quality of life during and following this therapy has been evaluated since 1984 in the ECOG. Adjuvant therapy for resected stage IIB-III AJCC disease using the foregoing intravenous and subcutaneous high-dose regimen showed benefit (even accounting for toxicity), significantly prolonged survival (2.8 to 3.8 years), and improved by 40% the fraction of patients who never relapsed at a mature median follow-up of 7 years. This adjuvant regimen approved by the FDA for use in high-risk postoperative patients has been assessed for cost efficacy and shows figures comparable with accepted adjuvant chemotherapy in breast and colorectal cancer [41–43]. Alternative IFN regimens seeking to obtain similar benefit with lower dosages or shorter intervals of treatment have been pursued. None of these has yet demonstrated significant impact on relapse-free or overall survival rates. A randomized prospective trial comparing high dose IFN alpha with lower doses and a third obser-

vation arm have confirmed the value of high dose IFN as an adjuvant therapy with an increase in relapse-free survival [44]. Shorter intramuscular regimens given for 3 months at 20 MU/m^2 are less effective. Adjuvant radiation therapy to the area of extracapsular nodal disease may provide local benefit [45] but has not been rigorously studied.

A variety of vaccines have been developed and tested for melanoma, ranging from the whole-cell vaccines administered with either the immunostimulant BCG, or a detoxified Lipid A derivative (Detox; Corixa Corporation, Hamilton, MT). The results obtained by these investigators in a randomized controlled trial performed by the Southwestern Oncology Group (S9035) have recently been reported. This trial tested the efficacy of a commercially produced allogeneic tumor cell vaccine (Melacine; Corixa Corporation, Hamilton, MT) in more than 600 patients accrued over the past 7 years with resected stage II primary melanoma. The results of this trial revealed no significant improvement in relapse-free survival unless a secondary intention to treat analysis was performed. In this instance modest improvements were noted. A larger multicenter trial of Newcastle disease virus melanoma oncolysate is the largest multi-

Table 11-6. Recent Trials on Therapy for Melanoma

Trial Author or Group and Therapy	Subjects with Particular Stage, n (Total Number in Trial)	Overall Survival	Relapse-Free Survival Benefit	Subjects, n (total)	Overall Survival	Relapse-Free Survival	Comments
Intermediate Risk AJCC II				**High Risk AJCC III**			
Creagan: NCCTG 837052 HDI* 3 mo vs OBS	160 (262)	Negative	Negative	102 (262)	Negative	Positive (Cox *P2* = 0.03)	Retrospective subset analysis of interest
Kirkwood: E1684 HDI 1 y vs OBS	31 (287)	Negative	Negative	249 (287)	Positive	Positive	First benefit in both OS and RFS in a properly conducted RCT: *P* = 0.02–0.004
Kirkwood: E1690 HDI 1 y or LDI† 2 y vs OBS	112 or 160 (642)	—	—	480 (642)	Negative	Positive	Confirmation of RFS but not OS benefit, perhaps due to removal of requirement for ELND in T4, and systematic crossover from OBS to IFN
Kirkwood: E1694 HDI 1 y vs GMK vaccine	220 (880)	Positive	Positive	660 (880)	Positive	Positive	Second RCT positive for OS and RFS: IFN at high dosage for 1 y vs vaccine GM2 *P* = 0.02–0.0005
Cascinelli: WHO 16 LDI 3 y vs OBS	—	—	—	440 (440)	Negative	Negative	
Pehamberger (Austrian) LDI 18 mo vs OBS	311	Negative	Positive	NA	—	Negative	
Grob (French) LDI 12 mo vs OBS	499	Negative	Positive	NA	—		
McKie (Scottish) LDI 6 mo vs OBS	99	Negative	Positive	—	—		
Eggermont: EORTC 18952 IDI(A)‡ IDI(B)§	380 (1418) A=12 mo B=24 mo	Negative Negative	Negative Positive	1040 (1400)	Negative Negative		Overall impact DMFI 1 y NS 2 y 0.074, 0.059–94, 0.03 marginal 0.07 for RFS, no impact (yet) reported on survival MFUT 1.6 y

*20 MU/m^2 IV QD 5/7 d/wk ×4 followed by 10 MU/m^2 SC TIW × 48 wk.
†3 MU QD or TIW.
‡10 MU QD or TIW.
§5 MU QD or TIW.
AJCC—American Joint Committee on Cancer; HDI—hexamethylene diisocyanate; IFN—interferon; NA—not applicable;
NS—not significant; OS—overall survival; RCT—randomized controlled trial; RFS—relapse-free survival.

center controlled trial of vaccine therapy in the literature, and it is negative [46].

Vaccine therapies designed to induce antibody reactive with the gangliosides of melanoma (GM2, GD2) have been tested in controlled phase II-III single-institution trials at MSKCC. Initial vaccines employed the older immunostimulant BCG; a trend to prolonged relapse-free survival was observed among vaccinated patients with high titers of antibody against GM2 (IgM). The unbalanced presence of native antibody in the unvaccinated control population (9%), and the limited size of this phase III trial (122 patients) resulted in findings that are not significant, despite a trend to benefit from this GM2/BCG vaccine. Recently, a modified commercial vaccine composed of GM2 coupled to keyhole-limpet hemocyanin administered with the potent immunologic adjuvant QS-21 has given higher and more durable titers of antibodies IgM and IgG against GM2 (GMK, Progenics Inc., Tarrytown, NJ). This agent has been evaluated in an intergroup phase III trial (E1694) that commenced in 1996 and accrued 880subjects through 1999. This phase III trial showed highly significant superiority of high-dose IFN-α2 over the GMK vaccine (P = 0.0015 for relapse; P = 0.009 for survival) reaffirming the current standard E1684 regimen of IFN. The potential for synergistic and additive (or, on the other hand, antagonistic) effects of IFN given concurrently with or directly following the initiation of this vaccine has recently been reported by ECOG in a study of GM2 vaccination versus GM2 with IFN (or GM2 followed after a month of vaccination by IFN). This trial (E2696) demonstrating the efficacy of high-dose IFN [59] has also shown superior relapse-free survival for recipients of IFN, adding a fourth trial to the literature.

CELLULAR IMMUNITY

During the past several years, a number of studies have been conducted on the autologous CD4 and CD8 T-cell-mediated response to human melanoma [12]. The emerging picture indicates that melanomas express multiple T-cell-defined epitopes, some of which are unique to a given tumor and reflect mutations, whereas others are shared by allogeneic melanomas of patients who are of similar HLA type. These epitopes represent short (9–10) amino acid peptides derived from tumor-associated antigens that are recognized by the CD8+ T cells in the context of major histocompatibility complex (MHC) class I antigens of the host antigen-presenting cell. A classification of antigens defined by T-cell recognition in human cancers includes three categories: 1) differentiation or lineage antigens (chiefly associated with the process of melanization and pigment formation in melanoma); 2) cancer testis antigens, referring to a series of melanoma antigens (MAGE 1,2,3; NY-ESO-1; and HO-MEL-40) specified by X-linked genes and expressed only in cancers of a range of organs as well as normal testis (and ovary); and 3) a group of antigens found to result from mutation of normal gene products [1]. Clinical trials evaluating representatives of these classes of peptide vaccines are underway at many centers in the U.S. and Europe with surprising early successes.

The most exciting new prospect for the specific vaccine therapy of melanoma may lie in the use of the peptide epitopes or whole protein recognized by the host T cell. T-cell recognition occurs in conjunction with the presenting MHC molecules of the host, with restrictions that to date have limited the application of these vaccine approaches. The genes encoding these targets have been cloned by investigators in the US and Europe over the past several years [12],

and alternative strategies using the whole proteins (or DNA encoding these antigens) may obviate the difficulties associated with MHC-restricted recognition of peptide antigens. These peptides, proteins, and complimentary DNA vaccines are currently undergoing testing in clinical trials. The use of macrophage derived dendritic cells (DC) are also quite promising. Animal studies using synthetic [47] or stripped [48] peptides pulsed onto DC and administered in the setting of advanced tumors potently inhibited tumor growth. DC can be generated easily from peripheral blood monocytes [49] particularly in association with interferon alpha and this may in part explain its utility in clinical trials alone. Nestle [50] studied 30 patients with melanoma in which peptide or tumor pulsed DCs were administered. Patients of HLA serotype HLA-A1 were treated with appropriate peptides derived from the MAGE-1 and MAGE-3 antigens; those who were HLA-A2+ were treated with peptides from Melan-A/MART-1, gp100 and tyrosinase; and those who expressed HLA-B44 received treatment with peptides derived from MAGE 3 and tyrosinase. Clinical responses were noted in 27% (eight of 30) of patients, including three CRs and five PRs. A University of Pittsburgh Cancer Institute trial initiated in 1996 has also shown encouraging evidence of activity in 23 patients. The first developed a complete remission and remained free of disease for more than 20 months prior to recurrence in which surgical excision again made her tumor free. Another patient on this study attained a CR sustained now for over 4 years, and one third had a transient PR.

OCULAR MELANOMA

Arising from the pigmented epithelium of the choroid, ocular melanoma is associated with visual disturbances at presentation and rarely with metastatic disease. The usual clinical treatment is either enucleation or radiotherapy, which are being compared in a formal trial by the collaborators of the Ocular Melanoma Study Committee with the support of the National Eye Institute and the NCI. Photodynamic therapy has been tested with an apparent improved response rate [51]. The risk of metastasis varies with the histologic type and size of these tumors as well as their location in the eye. Prognosis is directly related to presence of cyclin D1 and p53 mutations [52] and neovasculature. Historically, metastases occur most frequently in the liver but have been well documented in bone, skin, lung, and a variety of other tissues. Hepatic metastases from ocular melanoma are unusually resistant to systemic chemotherapy or immunotherapy. Remarkably, even the 10% to 20% response rate observed with cutaneous melanoma is not observed. Recent trials evaluating regional isolated intra-arterial perfusion chemotherapy with melphalan have suggested transient benefit [53].

NONMELANOMA SKIN CANCERS

The most frequent tumors in the white population are nonmelanoma skin tumors [54]. More than 500,000 new cases of basal cell carcinoma and 100,000 cases of squamous cell carcinomas occur each year. The incidence has increased by 65% since 1980, probably due to increased sun exposure [1]. Most of the tumors occur on skin exposed to the sun, and there is clearly a relationship between latitude, cumulative solar exposure, and incidence of these tumors. Deaths due to these tumors are extremely infrequent, allowing most cancer protocols treating tumors at other sites to permit these as preceding malignancies. Approximately 1500 deaths occur each year due largely to squamous cell carcinoma (about one in 500 patients). This death rate is approximately one fourth of that due to melanoma. There are multiple risk factors associated with these nonmelanoma skin cancers (Table 11-1). Clearly, efforts are needed to decrease exposure to the sun and other carcinogenic factors associated with a concomitant decrease in skin tumors. The most common sites of metastases (which occur infrequently) are regional lymph nodes. Rarely, liver, lung, bone, and brain metastases are found. The primary treatment for skin tumors is local ablative therapy. This may consist of simple excisional procedures, excision and grafting or flap rotation, electrodesiccation and curettage, cryosurgery, Mohs' surgery, or radiation therapy. Each procedure is designed to ablate the tumor. Because local recurrence is the major risk—and the margin of excision needed to control these tumors may be less than for tumors like melanoma with discontinuous local extension—a variety of procedures have been developed to try to encompass the tumor while preserving normal skin, especially in cosmetically sensitive areas. One such technique, known after its originator as

Mohs' surgery, attempts to remove successive shells of tissue so as to take the minimal amount of tissue while completely excising the tumor. This is a time-consuming and costly procedure and has no place in the treatment of tumors like melanoma, where frozen sections are notoriously unreliable in assessing the presence of disease.

Radiation therapy is perhaps best used in older patients who may not tolerate the necessary surgery. Topical fluorouracil can be used to treat multiple basal cell carcinomas or actinic keratosis, in which the multiplicity of established or emerging new tumors in some patients makes surgical removal problematic [55,56]. β-carotene and isotretinoin have shown benefit in clinical trials and await definitive evaluation in this context. Patients with a history of xeroderma pigmentosum are at high risk because of UV associated mutations [57] and need to take special precautions against solar irradiation. Recently guidelines for care [58] have been published summarizing the local care of such lesions.

REFERENCES

1. Lotze MT, Dallal RM, Kirkwood JM, Flickinger JC: Cutaneous melanoma. In *Principles and Practice of Oncology*. Edited by DeVita V, Hellman S, Rosenberg S. Philadelphia: Lippincott-Raven; 2000.

2. Lipsker DM, Hedelin G, Heid E, *et al.*: Striking increase of thin melanomas contrasts with stable incidence of thick melanomas. *Arch Dermatol* 1999, 135:1451–1456.

3. Skolnick, MH, Cannon-Albright LA, Kamb A: Genetic predisposition to melanoma. *Eur J Cancer* 1994, 30A:1991–1995.

4. Whelan AJ, Bartsch D, Goodfellow PJ: A familial syndrome of pancreatic cancer and melanoma with a mutation in the CDKN2 tumor-suppressor gene. *N Engl J Med* 1995, 333:970–974.

5. Goldstein AM, Struewing JP, Chidambaram A, Fraser MC, Tucker MA: Genotype-phenotype relationships in U.S. melanoma-prone families with CDKN2A and CDK4 mutations. *J Natl Cancer Inst* 2000, 92:1006–1010.

6. Wang Y, Rao U, Mascari R, Richards TJ, *et al.*: Molecular analysis of melanoma precursor lesions. *Cell Growth Differ* 1996, 7:1733–1740.

7. Titus-Ernstoff L, Duray PH, Ernstoff MS, *et al.*: Dysplastic nevi in association with multiple primary melanoma. *Cancer Res* 1998, 48:1016–1018.

8. Ziegler A, Jonason AS, Leffel DJ, *et al.*: Sunburn and p53 in the onset of skin cancer. *Nature* 1994, 372:773–776.

9. Rhodes AR: Public education and cancer of the skin. *Cancer* 1995, 75:613–636.

10. Wang C, Brodland DG, Su WPD: Skin cancers associated with acquired immunodeficiency syndrome [abstract]. *Mayo Clin Proc* 1995, 70:766–772.

11. Cheson BD, Vena DA, Barrett J, Freidlin B: Second malignancies as a consequence of nucleoside analog therapy for chronic lymphoid leukemias. *J Clin Oncol* 1999, 17:2454–2460.

12. Maeurer MJ, Lotze MT: Immune responses to melanoma antigens. In *Cutaneous Melanoma*, edn 3. Edited by Balch CM, Houghton AN, Sober AJ, Soong S-J. St. Louis: Quality Medical Publishing, Inc.; 1998: 517–534.

13. Balch CM: A new AJCC staging system for cutaneous melanoma. *Cancer* 2000.

14. Poo-Hwu WJ, Ariyan S, Lamb L, *et al.*: Follow-up recommendations for patients with American Joint Committee on Cancer Stages I-III malignant melanoma. *Cancer* 1999, 86:2252–2258.

15. Essner R, Bostick PJ, Glass EC, *et al.*: Standardized probe-directed sentinel node dissection in melanoma. *Surgery* 2000, 127:26–31.

16. Balch CM, Seng-jaw S, Ross M, *et al.*: Long-term results of a multi-institutional randomized trial: Comparing prognostic factors and surgical results for intermediate thickness melanoma (1.0-4.0 mm). *Ann Surg Oncol* 2000, 7:87–97.

17. Karakousis CP, Velez A, Driscoll DL, Takita H: Metastasectomy in malignant melanoma. *Surgery* 1994, 115:295–302.

18. Manola J, Atkins M, Ibrahim J, Kirkwood J: Prognostic factors in metastatic melanoma: a pooled analysis of Eastern Cooperative Oncology Group trials. *J Clin Oncol* 2000, 18:3782–3793.

19. Kondziolka D, Patel A, Lunsford LD, *et al.*: Stereotactic radiosurgery plus whole brain radiotherapy versus radiotherapy alone for patients with multiple brain metastases. *Int J Radiat Oncol Biol Phys* 1999, 45:427–434.

20. Falkson CI, Falkson G, Falkson HC: Improved results with the addition of interferon alfa-2b to dacarbazine in the treatment of patients with metastatic malignant melanoma. *J Clin Oncol* 1991, 9:1403–1408.

21. Middleton MR, Grob JJ, Aaronson N, *et al.*: Randomized phase III study of temozolomide versus dacarbazine in the treatment of patients with advanced metastatic malignant melanoma. *J Clin Oncol* 2000, 18:158.

22. Rustoven JJ, Quirt IC, Iscoe NA, *et al.*: Randomized, double-blind, placebo-controlled trial comparing the response rates of carmustine, dacarbazine, and cisplatin with and without tamoxifen in patients with metastatic melanoma. *J Clin Oncol* 1996, 14:2083–2090.

23. Falkson CI, Ibrahim J, Kirkwood JM, *et al.*: Phase III trial of dacarbazine versus dacarbazine with interferon alfa-2b versus dacarbazine with tamoxifen versus dacarbazine with interferon alfa-2b and tamoxifen in patients with metastatic malignant melanoma: an Eastern Cooperative Oncology Group Study (E3690). *J Clin Oncol* 1998, 16:1743–1751.

24. Del Prete SA, Maurer LH, O'Donnell J, *et al.*: Combination chemotherapy with cisplatin, carmustine, dacarbazine and tamoxifen in malignant melanoma. *Cancer Treat Rep* 1984, 68:1403–1405.

25. Chapman PB, Einhorn LH, Meyers ML, *et al.*: Phase III multicenter randomized trial of the Dartmouth regimen versus dacarbazine in patients with metastatic melanoma. *J Clin Oncol* 1999, 17:2745–2751.

26. Kirkwood JM: Biologic therapy with interferon a and b: clinical applications: melanoma. In *Biologic Therapy of Cancer: Principles and Practice*. Edited by DeVita VT, Jr., Hellman S, Rosenberg SA. Philadelphia: JB Lippincott; 1995:388–411.

27. Lotze MT: The future role of interleukin-2 in cancer therapy. *Cancer J Sci Am* 2000, 6 (suppl 1):S58–S60.

28. Royal RE, Steinberg SM, Krouse RS, *et al.*: Correlates of response to IL-2 therapy in patients treated for metastatic renal cancer and melanoma. *Sci Am* 1996, 2:91–98.

29. Keilholz U, Scheibenbogen C, Tilgen W, *et al.*: Interferon-a and interleukin-2 in the treatment of metastatic melanoma: comparison of two phase II trials. *Cancer* 1993, 72:607–614.

30. Atkins MB, Lotze MT, Dutcher JP, *et al.*: High-dose recombinant interleukin-2 therapy for patients with metastatic melanoma: analysis of 270 patients treated from 1985–1993. *J Clin Oncol* 1999, 17:2105.

31. Hoon DS, Yuzuki D, Hayashida M, *et al.*: Melanoma patients immunized with melanoma cell vaccine induce antibody responses to recombinant MAGE-1 antigen. *J Immunol* 1995, 154:730–737.

32. Lotze MT, Shurin M, Esche C, *et al.*: Interleukin-2: developing additional cytokine gene therapies using fibroblasts or dendritic cells to enhance tumor immunity. *Cancer J Sci Am* 2000, 6 (suppl 1):S61–S66.

33. Lienard D, Ewalenko P, Delmotte JJ, *et al.*: High-dose recombinant tumor necrosis factor alpha in combination with interferon gamma and melphalan in isolation perfusion of the limbs for melanoma and sarcoma. *J Clin Oncol* 1992, 10:52–60.

34. Lienard D, Eggermont AM, Koops HS, *et al.*: Isolated limb perfusion with tumor necrosis factor-alpha and melphalan with or without interferon-gamma for the treatment of in-transit melanoma metastases: a multicenter randomized phase II study. *Melanoma Res* 1999, 9:491–502.

35. Barth A, Wanke LA, Morton DL: Analysis of prognostic factors in 1521 patients with metastatic melanoma [abstract]. *Proc ASCO* 1995, 14:410.

36. Flaherty LE, Robinson W, Redman BG, *et al.*: A phase II study of dacarbazine and cisplatin in combination with outpatient administered interleukin-2 in metastatic malignant melanoma. *Cancer* 1993, 71:3520–3525.

37. Sirott MN, Bajorin DF, Wong GY, *et al.*: Prognostic factors in patients with metastatic malignant melanoma: a multivariate analysis. *Cancer* 1993, 72:3091–3098.

38. Kirkwood JM, Wilson J, Whiteside TL, *et al.*: Phase IB trial of picibanil (OK-432) as an immunomodulator in patients with resected high-risk melanoma. *Cancer Immunol Immunother* 1997, 44:137–149.

39. Lear JT, Strange RC, Fryer AA: Relationship between sunlight exposure and a key genetic alteration in basal cell carcinoma. *J Natl Cancer Inst* 1997, 89:454–455.

40. Spitler LE: A randomized trial of levamisole versus placebo as adjuvant therapy in malignant melanoma. *J Clin Oncol* 1991, 9:736–740.

41. Kirkwood, JM, Strawderman MH, Ernstoff MS, *et al.*: Interferon alfa-2b adjuvant therapy of high-risk resected cutaneous melanoma: the Eastern Cooperative Oncology Group Trial EST1684. *J Clin Oncol* 1996, 14:7–17.

42. Cole BF, Gelber RD, Kirkwood JM, *et al.*: A quality-of-life-adjusted survival analysis of interferon alfa-2b adjuvant treatment for high-risk resected cutaneous melanoma: an Eastern Cooperative Oncology Group Study (E1684). *J Clin Oncol* 1996, 14:2666–2673.

43. Hillner BE, Kirkwood JM, Atkins MB, *et al.*: Economic analysis of adjuvant interferon alfa-2b in high-risk melanoma based on projections from ECOG 1684. *J Clin Oncol* 1997, 15:2351–2358.

44. Kirkwood JM, Ibrahim JG, Sondak VK, *et al.*: High- and low-dose interferon alfa-2b in high-risk melanoma: first analysis of intergroup trial E1690/S9111/C9190. *J Clin Oncol* 2000, 18:2444–2458.

45. Strom EA, Ross MI: Adjuvant radiation therapy after axillary lymphadenectomy for metastatic melanoma: toxicity and local control. *Ann Surg Oncol* 1995, 2:445–449.

46. Wallack MK, Sivanandham M, Balch CM, *et al.*: A phase III randomized, double-blind, multiinstitutional trial of vaccine melanoma oncolysate-active specific immunotherapy for patients with stage II melanoma. *Cancer* 1995, 75:34–42.

47. Mayordomo JI, Zorina T, Storkus WJ, *et al.*: Bone marrow-derived dendritic cells pulsed with synthetic tumor peptides elicit protective and therapeutic antitumor immunity. *Nature Medicine* 1995, 1:1297–1302.

48. Zitvogel L, Mayordomo JI, Tjandrawan T, *et al.*: Therapy of murine tumors with tumor peptide-pulsed dendritic cells: dependence on T cells, B7 costimulation, and T helper cell 1-associated cytokines. *J Exp Med* 1996, 183:87–97.

49. Luft T, Pang KC, Thomas E, *et al.*: Type I IFNs enhance the terminal differentiation of dendritic cells. *J Immunol* 1998, 161:1944–1953.

50. Nestle FO, Alijagic S, Gilliet M, *et al.*: Vaccination of melanoma patients with peptide- or tumor lysate-pulsed dendritic cells. *Nature Medicine* 1998, 4:328–332.

51. Favilla I, Favilla ML, Gosbell AD, *et al.*: Photodynamic therapy: a 5-year study of its effectiveness in the treatment of posterior uveal melanoma, and evaluation of haematoporphyrin uptake and photocytotoxicity of melanoma cells in tissue culture. *Melanoma Res* 1995, 5:355–364.

52. Coupland SE, Anastassiou G, Stang A, *et al.*: The prognostic value of cyclin D1, p53, and MDM2 protein expression in uveal melanoma. *J Pathol* 2000, 91:120–126.

53. Alexander HR, Libutti SK, Bartlett DL, *et al.*: A phase I-II study of isolated hepatic perfusion using melphalan with or without tumor necrosis factor for patients with ocular melanoma metastatic to liver. *Clin Cancer Res* 2000, 6:3062–70.

54. Preston DS, Stern RS: Nonmelanoma cancers of the skin. *N Engl J Med* 1992, 327:1649–1662.

55. Cullen SI: Topical fluorouracil therapy for precancer and cancers of the skin. *J Am Geriatr Soc* 1997, 27:529–535.

56. Ashton H, Beveridge GW, Stevenson CJ: Topical treatment of skin tumors with 5-flourouracil. *Br J Dermatol* 1970, 82:207–209.

57. Soufir N, Daya-Grosjean L, de La Salmoniere P, *et al.*: Association between INK4a-ARF and p53 mutation in skin carcinomas of xeroderma pigmentosum patients. *J Natl Cancer Inst* 2000, 92:1841–1847.

58. Miller SJ: The National Comprehensive Cancer Network (NCCN) guidelines of care for nonmelanoma skin cancers. *Dermatol Surg* 2000 26:289–292.

59. Kirkwood J, Ibrahim J, Lawson D, *et al.*: E2696: a trial of vaccination with or without IFNα2b in high-risk resected melanoma. *J Clin Oncol* 2001, in press.

INTERFERON α-2

Interferon α-2 has shown modest levels of antitumor activity as a single agent in patients with metastatic melanoma, ranging from 15% to 20% in multiple trials. The highest response rates with IFN α-2 were noted at the highest dosages in patients with the smallest bulk of disease. Immune mechanisms of antitumor response have their greatest impact in microscopic (or adjuvant) therapy rather than the advanced disease [30].

DOSAGE AND SCHEDULING

Arm A: high-dose IFN α-2b for 1 y
Induction therapy: 20 MU/m² QID IV for 5 d × 4 wk
Maintenance: 10 MU/m²/d 3 × weekly SC × 48 wk
Arm B: high-dose IFNα2b for 1 mo (induction as above, alone)

DOSAGE MODIFICATION: *Reduce dose if bilirubin is elevated (2.6–5 × ULN) or SGOT, alkaline phosphatase is elevated (2.6–5 × ULN).*

CANDIDATES FOR TREATMENT

High-risk patients with deep primary melanoma (> 4 mm Breslow depth) with or without lymph node involvement (T4, NO, MO)

TOXICITIES

Fever, chill, myalgia and arthralgia, fatigue, headache; neutropenia, anemia, thrombocytopenia (not dose limiting unless severe); hepatotoxicity (at high doses), hyperbilirubinemia, apparent hepatic necrosis (rare); proteinuria, elevated creatinine or BUN (at high doses)

ALTERNATIVE THERAPIES

Vaccination with cultured irradiated lines of tumor cells or partially purified proteins, whole tumor cells, partially purified proteins shed from cultured tumor cells, virus-modified tumor cell vaccine, defined gangliosides for immunization against melanoma, defined peptides and proteins for immunization against melanoma, antiidiotype antibodies as vaccine

ENTRY TO THE INTERGROUP STUDY

Patients may be formally entered into study by investigators in the Eastern Cooperative Oncology Group, Cancer and Leukemia Group B, and Southwest Oncology Group or at the MD Anderson and Memorial Sloan-Kettering Cancer Centers

DRUG INTERACTIONS

Aspirin, prostaglandin synthetase inhibitors, antihistamines, other immunomodulators, NSAIDs

CISPLATIN, VINBLASTINE, AND DACARBAZINE, ALONE OR IN COMBINATION WITH IL-2 AND IFN-α

The ECOG study group is conducting a phase III trial of cisplatin, vinblastine, and dacarbazine versus combined with interferon α-2, and IL-2 for surgically incurable metastatic melanoma. This trial is designed to confirm or refute initial reports that have suggested improved survival with IFN α-2 and IL-2.

Dacarbazine is the only single chemotherapy agent that is FDA approved for the indication of palliative therapy of metastatic melanoma. Combined chemotherapy for melanoma has not previously induced remissions significantly more frequently than dacarbazine nor prolonged survival. However, multiple single-center nonrandomized trials have suggested prolonged survival of patients with metastatic melanoma through combined-modality treatment with IL-2 given as an infusiant.

TRIAL DESIGN

Phase III comparison of cisplatin-vinblastine dacarbazine (CVD) combined with IL-2 and IFN α-2, versus CVD alone.

This trial design is now being participated in by the Southwest Cooperative Oncology Group, Cancer and Leukemia Group B, and the Eastern Cooperative Oncology Group, and will have a target accrual of 482 patients to adequately evaluate the potential for a 33% prolongation of survival by the chemo-biotherapy over chemotherapy alone.

CANDIDATES FOR TREATMENT

Histologically confirmed surgically incurable metastatic melanoma; measurable disease; performance status of 0–2; normal hematologic and biochemical values; SGOT < 3 times the upper limit of normal (unless deviation due to metastases); no prior chemotherapy; no prior radiotherapy to measurable disease; and no brain metastases
Exclusion criteria: ocular melanoma; angina pectoris, ventricular arrhythmias or myocardial infarction within 6 mo; prior malignancy; history of clinical depression

TOXICITIES

Flu-like syndrome (anorexia, fatigue and malaise, chills or rigors, myalgias and arthralgias); hematologic, renal, hepatic, CNS, and GI toxicities; weight gain (fluid retention) or loss (anorexia)

ALTERNATIVE THERAPIES

Three-drug regimen of cisplatin, vinblastine, decarbazine, with response rates of 50%, four-drug regimen of cisplatin, BCNU, tamoxifen, and dacarbazine with response rates of 50%; six-drug regimen with IFN α-2 and IL-2 added to the 4-day combination: response rates of up to 57%

HYPERTHERMIC PERFUSION WITH MELPHALAN

Locoregional spread of melanoma of the extremity is a problem for a subset of approximately 10% of patients. In spite of the lack of systemic spread, many patients develop local complications related to in-transit spread that are difficult to manage. Creech developed a method to apply locoregional perfusion using cytotoxic agents. The application of chemotherapy, heat, and/or immunotherapy using this method has been used by a variety of surgeons. One prospective randomized study showing benefit was carried out by Ghussen and colleagues from 1980 to 1983. In a control group ($n = 54$) the tumors were widely excised and the regional lymph nodes removed. The perfusion group received this treatment, as well as hyperthermic (42°C) perfusion with melphalan. After a median observation time of 5 years, 11 months, 26 recurrences were diagnosed in the control group and 6 noted in the perfusion group ($P < .001$). A survival advantage was also noted for the perfusion group ($P < .01$). Other studies have not shown a significant advantage, however. Recent variations that have used this approach have included coadministration of TNF and interferon γ [26,27].

Hyperthermic perfusion alone has been used with apparent antitumor effects. Subsequently, Stehlin reported that the antitumor effect could be increased by adding chemotherapy. Melphalan (L-phenylalanine mustard) is used most frequently in perfusates. Recently cisplatin has also been tested in some protocols. The maximally tolerated dose used in the randomized study was 1 mg/kg for the upper extremity and 1.5 mg/kg for the lower extremity. Morbidity and mortality for the isolation limb perfusion have been reported. A 6% to 39% morbidity, including requirement for major skin grafting and limb loss due to a compartment syndrome, has been reported in various series. Mortality is unusual but has been reported up to 3% in some series.

DOSAGE AND SCHEDULING

Upper extremity (UE): The axillary vein and artery are exposed through an incision from the clavicle to the anterior axillary line. The patient is heparinized systemically (100 U/kg), and the vessels are occluded and catheters inserted. The initial perfusate is whole blood using an extracorporeal heater/bubble oxygenator/low flow pump. Flow rates range from 250 to 400 mL/min.

Lower extremity (LE): The femoral vessels are exposed through an incision from a point medial to the anterosuperior iliac spine to the femoral triangle. The inferior epigastric and circumflex iliac vessels are temporarily occluded and catheters inserted into the external iliac vessels so that the catheters are lying in the proximal femoral vessels. An Esmarch is applied around the root of the limb to prevent circulation through cutaneous or subcutaneous blood vessels. Leakage is measured using dye dilution techniques.

The perfusate temperature is maintained at 42.5°C, monitored by thermistor probes between the muscles and in the subcutaneous tissues of the thigh and calf. Melphalan is given in the UE (1.0 mg/kg) and in the LE (1.5 mg/kg). The first half of the dose is administered when the limb has reached 40°C, and the balance is injected in 3 equal aliquots at 15, 30, and 45 minutes, the entire procedure taking place over 1 hour.

CANDIDATES FOR TREATMENT

Patients with deep primary melanoma of the extremity, or in transit, advanced locoregional melanoma; other advanced locoregional diseases confined to the extremity (squamous carcinomas, sarcomas)—currently under investigation

DRUG INTERACTIONS

TNFα and IFNγ (septic shock-like syndrome and death in some instances [5]) appear to enhance melphalan activity

TOXICITIES

Wound healing (5.7%), lymphatic fistulas (7.5%), low-grade fever, mild pain and erythema of the extremity, compartment syndrome (approximately 10%, amputation possibly required)

Give acetaminophen and/or indomethacin in the first 24–48 h to control fever and chills; observe perfusion of the extremities to assess circulation, swelling, and presence of pulse (using handheld Doppler device); monitor vital signs every 4 h during immediate postoperative period; refrain from movement of the extremity until drains are removed

PATIENT INFORMATION

Patient should be informed of benefits and side effects. Possible injury to the skin or other structures in the extremity may require additional operations and even amputation. The procedure is done under anesthesia and a hospital stay of approximately 1–2 wk is required

TOPICAL APPLICATIONS OF 5-FU

Patients with multiple actinic solar keratoses are at risk for development of nonmelanoma skin cancers. In addition, patients with established basal cell carcinomas or multiple basal cell carcinomas may be treated with a 5% fluorouracil cream.

Fluorouracil blocks the methylation reaction of deoxyuridylic acid to thymidylic acid. It inhibits the synthesis of DNA and, to a lesser extent, RNA. The primary effect of 5-FU is on rapidly growing cells, and topical application has been shown to lead to insignificant absorption and primarily local antitumor effects.

DOSAGE AND SCHEDULING

When Efudex is applied to a tumor, local inflammation occurs associated with erythema, blister formation, ulceration, local necrosis and ultimately reepitheliazation [43]. 5-FU cream or solution is applied twice daily in an amount sufficient to cover lesions [44]. The treatment is continued until inflammation resolves, usually for a period of 2 to 4 weeks. For treatment of basal cell carcinomas, applications for as long as 12 weeks may be required. A patient should be followed to determine the antitumor effects.

CANDIDATES FOR TREATMENT
Patients with Bowen's disease, actinic keratosis, or multiple basal cell carcinomas

SPECIAL PRECAUTIONS
Patients must not have a known hypersensitivity to any components of the drug

DRUG INTERACTIONS
None

TOXICITIES
Local reactions: pain, pyrites, hyperpigmentation, burning at the site of application; other reactions: contact dermatitis, scarring, tenderness, local infection, swelling

NURSING INTERVENTIONS
Instruct the patient in the expected side effects and to keep the area clean, dry, and potentially bandaged to prevent exposure to exogenous pathogens

PATIENT INFORMATION
This treatment is useful for patients thought to be at high risk for development of tumors of the skin or those who have had multiple previous tumors of the skin. In addition, some people with very early tumors, such as Bowen's disease or some basal cell carcinomas, will benefit from application of the cream. The cream should be applied in amounts sufficient to cover the lesions and the area lightly bandaged. Treatment may continue as long as 10 to 12 wk and will cause redness, swelling, some pain, and itching. The patient should be followed closely by the physician during the course of treatment and thereafter to insure that tumor eradication has occurred

Sarcomas are a histologically diverse group of tumors that arise most often from tissues of mesodermal origin. Despite the fact that approximately 75% of the body is derived from mesoderm, sarcomas are relatively rare, representing only 1% of all adult tumors and 15% of pediatric neoplasms. Approximately 6000 new cases of sarcoma are diagnosed each year, and half of these patients will eventually succumb to their disease. This chapter focuses on the current management of sarcomas arising in the soft tissue and bone in the adult population.

ADULT SOFT TISSUE SARCOMAS
Pathologic Classification, Grade, and Staging
Sarcomas are classified according to the differentiated tissue they most resemble histologically (Table 12-1). Although each subtype has distinct histologic features, tumor grade is the best predictor of the biologic aggressiveness for soft tissue sarcomas [1]. The major exceptions to this point are the pediatric sarcomas (rhabdomyosarcoma, Ewing's sarcoma, and peripheral neuroectodermal tumors) whose prognosis and treatment strategies differ based on the histologic subtype. Unfortunately, the criteria for grading soft tissue sarcomas is not standardized. Currently there exist three dominant systems for grading soft tissue sarcomas [2–4]: a four-grade system as proposed by Broders et al. [3], a three-grade system based on the American Joint Commission on Cancer (AJCC), and a binary system as used at Memorial Sloan-Kettering Cancer Center (MSKCC). Despite the lack of a standardized grading system, pathologists agree that cellularity, mitotic activity, nuclear atypia, and degree of necrosis are the most important histopathologic correlates of tumor grade.

Staging of soft tissue sarcomas is based on histologic grade, size of primary tumor, and presence or absence of distant metastases. Table 12-2 shows the current AJCC staging system [4]. Historically, staging has been predominantly based on histologic grade of the primary tumor. Low-grade lesions carry a low risk for developing distant metastases (< 15%) and an excellent survival rate, whereas high-grade lesions are associated with greater than 50% risk for developing distant metastases. The strong influence of tumor grade on prognosis, staging, and therapy of patients with soft tissue sarcomas combined with the lack of a uniform grading scheme underscores the importance of having all sarcoma specimens reviewed by a skilled pathologist experienced in sarcomas.

PRESENTATION AND DIAGNOSIS
Fifty percent of all soft tissue sarcomas arise in the extremities, with retroperitoneal (14%), visceral (15%), and truncal (10%) lesions accounting for the majority of other sites. These tumors typically present as a painless enlarging mass. Any enlarging or persistent (> 4 wk) soft tissue mass or any mass larger than 5 cm, should be biopsied. The choice of biopsy technique is critical and should provide maximal histopathologic information while not jeopardizing subsequent surgical procedures. Historically, incisional biopsy has been the preferred technique for lesions greater than 5 cm, but the complication rate and chance of spreading tumor cells through uncontaminated tissue planes is significant.

The accuracy of core needle biopsy in the diagnosis of soft tissue masses has been addressed by several investigators [5–7]. Barth et al. [5] at the National Cancer Institute (NCI) correlated the results of 27 core needle biopsies to the final resected specimen. Core needle biopsy correctly identified 16 of 16 malignant lesions and 10 of 11 benign lesions. In each of the malignant lesions, tumor grade was correctly identified by core needle biopsy. Heslin et al. [7] reviewed 60 core needle biopsies performed at MSKCC. In this series, results of core needle biopsy correlated with final pathology 95% of the time with respect to malignancy and 88% of the time with respect to tumor grade. The high specificity and sensitivity, coupled with the lower morbidity and cost of core needle biopsy, should make it the preferred technique when feasible. For lesions less than 5 cm, an excisional biopsy is adequate. Excisional biopsies should be performed with the intent to obtain negative margins. This will avoid an unsatisfactory re-resection of the surgical bed. Fine needle aspiration does not provide adequate sample to determine tumor grade and should not be routinely used in the initial diagnosis of soft tissue masses.

TREATMENT MODALITIES
Surgery
Surgery is the most effective modality in the treatment of localized soft tissue sarcomas. The goal of surgical excision should be complete removal of the tumor with a margin of normal tissue. In cases where the tumor abuts major neurovascular structures, every attempt at conservation should be made. Local control rates with limited wide local excision (limb-sparing surgery [LSS]) and adjuvant radiotherapy now approach those obtained historically with amputation [8]. Amputation, once the standard for surgical control of extremity soft tissue sarcomas, should only be applied in select cases of advanced or recurrent local regional disease. Currently, greater than 95% of all patients with extremity sarcomas are managed without amputation. For patients with stage I or II disease, surgery with adjuvant radiotherapy results in 5-year disease-free survival rates of 60% to 80%

Table 12-1. Common Histologic Subtypes of Soft Tissue Sarcomas

Histology	Cell Type	Frequency, %	Comments
Malignant fibrous histiocytoma	Fibroblast	22	Most common subtype; peak incidence 7th decade
Liposarcoma	Adipocyte	17	Occur commonly on thigh or retroperitoneum
Fibrosarcoma	Fibroblast	10	Peak incidence in 3rd to 5th decade
Synovial cell sarcoma	Synovial cells	7	Commonly occurs in young adults around knee
Leiomyosarcoma	Smooth muscle	19	Most common in viscera or retroperitoneum; surgery is primary treatment
Embryonal/rhabdomyosarcoma	Smooth muscle/mesoderm	4	Occur in young adults; treated primarily with chemoradiotherapy
Malignant peripheral nerve sheath (malignant schwannoma)	Schwann cell	5	Arise from nerve sheath; appearance in lower extremity or retroperitoneum common
Angiosarcoma	Mesoderm	1	Arise in chronic lymphedema, postirradiation, on scalp of elderly men, or in breast tissue

and overall survival rates of 80% to 98%. Small superficial lesions (< 5 cm) of the extremities regardless of histopathologic grade and depth may best be categorized into stage II lesions, because these patients have a greater than 90% chance of long-term event-free survival when treated with current standards [4,9].

Radiation

The role of radiation therapy is to treat local regional disease most often as an adjuvant to surgical resection, used prior to surgery as part of a combined modality approach to larger, initially inoperable primary lesions, and rarely for the definitive management of local recurrent disease.

Adjuvant radiotherapy combined with surgical resection results in improved local control over surgery alone for patients with soft tissue sarcoma of the extremities [8,10,11–14]. Postoperative adjuvant radiotherapy for high-grade lesions may be delivered in the form of external beam or brachytherapy. Brachytherapy delivers radiation to the tumor bed by way of interstitial catheters placed at the time of resection. This has several potential benefits over traditional external-beam radiotherapy, including shorter length of treatment, lower cost, and greater sparing of normal tissues [2,15]. In a prospective randomized trial of 164 patients from MSKCC, patients treated with surgery plus adjuvant brachytherapy had better local control

rates when compared with surgery alone (82% vs 69%; $P = 0.04$) [15]. Subset analysis revealed that patients with high-grade lesions benefited from adjuvant brachytherapy, whereas no improvement in local control rate was observed for patients with low-grade sarcomas.

The effectiveness of adjuvant external-beam radiotherapy in the treatment of soft tissue sarcomas of the extremities was addressed in a randomized trial [10,16]. At the National Cancer Institute (NCI), 91 patients with high-grade and 50 patients with low-grade soft tissue sarcomas of the extremity were randomly assigned to surgery alone or surgery plus adjuvant external-beam radiotherapy (6300 cGy). Patients with high-grade lesions all received adjuvant chemotherapy. Ninety-one patients with high-grade lesions were randomly assigned: 47 received radiotherapy and 44 did not receive radiotherapy. With a median follow-up of 9.6 years, a highly significant decrease ($P2 = 0.0028$) in the probability of local recurrence was seen with radiation, but no difference in survival. Of 50 patients with low-grade lesions randomly assigned 24 to resection alone and 26 to resection and postoperative, there was also a lower probability of local recurrence ($P2 = 0.016$) in patients receiving radiotherapy, again, without a difference in overall survival.

Several centers have reported on the use of preoperative adjuvant radiotherapy [17–21]. Local control rates for small (T1 and T2) lesions have been reported to be similar to those obtained with postoperative treatment. No randomized trial has addressed whether preoperative or postoperative radiotherapy is superior. Furthermore, given the excellent local control rates with small lesions, it is unlikely that a randomized trial could accrue enough patients to definitively answer this question. Studies are ongoing to explore the effectiveness of preoperative radiotherapy in the treatment of advanced local disease (large primary tumors >7 cm). Theoretically, the application of preoperative radiotherapy in this setting will allow for more limb-sparing resections.

In a clinical scenario in which surgical management is not feasible for medical reasons, definitive radiation to doses in the 7000 to 7500 cGy range result in local control and cure [22].

Chemotherapy

The role of chemotherapy is for the treatment of patients with metastatic disease, either postoperatively for those patients who are at risk of recurrence after primary management, or preoperatively for those patients who present with advanced localized disease.

Soft tissue sarcomas are among the most chemoresistant of all malignancies. Currently, there are only two agents that reproducibly demonstrate greater than 20% response rate in metastatic sarcoma: doxorubicin and ifosfamide. Doxorubicin is the single most effective agent against soft tissue sarcoma, with response rates reported from 9% to 70% [23–26]. Response to doxorubicin may well be dose related. Unfortunately, increasing the dose of doxorubicin is limited by severe myelosuppression, mucositis, and cardiotoxicity. Several anthracycline derivatives have been examined in an attempt to find agents with similar efficacy and less toxic profiles.

Epirubicin, an anthracycline derivative, was tested for activity in soft tissue sarcomas in a large randomized EORTC trial comparing doxorubicin with epirubicin. The two drugs showed similar overall response rates (18%) with no significant difference in toxicity profiles [27].

Ifosfamide, an analogue of the alkylating agent cyclophosphamide, also has activity as a single agent in the treatment of soft tissue sarcomas [28,29]. Ifosfamide has been shown to be superior to cyclophosphamide in a randomized trial conducted by the EORTC

Table 12-2. American Joint Committee on Cancer's Staging System for Soft Tissue Sarcomas

TNM Classification	Characteristics
Histologic Grade	
G1	Low grade, well differentiated
G2	Intermediate grade, moderately differentiated
G3	High grade, poorly differentiated
G4	High grade, undifferentiated
Primary Tumor	
T1	Tumor < 5 cm
a	Superficial tumor
b	Deep tumor
T2	Tumor > 5 cm
a	Superficial tumor
b	Deep tumor
Regional Nodes	
N0	No histologically verified lymph node metastases
N1	Histologically verified lymph node metastases
Distant Metastases	
M0	No distant metastases
M1	Distant metastases

Stage Group	5-y Survival, %
IA (G1–2,T1a–T1b,N0, M0)	98
IB (G1–2,T2a,N0,M0)	
IIA (G1–2,T2b,N0,M0)	81
IIB (G3–4,T1a–T1b,N0,M0)	
IIC (G3–4,T2a,N0,M0)	
III (G3–4,T2b,N0,M0)	51
IV (Any G,any T,N0,M0)	18

[30]. Ifosfamide is active in patients who have failed doxorubicin-based therapy [31]. The severe hemorrhagic cystitis associated with the use of ifosfamide has been greatly reduced by the introduction of the uroprotective agent mesna [32].

Dacarbazine (DTIC) is another agent frequently used in combination regimens for the treatment of soft tissue sarcomas. Using a single DTIC dose of 1.2 g/m^2, Durate et al. [33] reported limited effectiveness including patients who had progression after being treated with doxorubicin.

To improve on the response rates seen with single-agent therapies, several important randomized trials of combination chemotherapy have been conducted by the large cooperative groups (Table 12-3) [23,25,34–38]. The Eastern Cooperative Oncology Group (ECOG) conducted a series of randomized trails comparing single-agent doxorubicin to combination regimens. Higher response rates were observed for regimens combining doxorubicin with ifosfamide and doxorubicin with DTIC. However, the combination therapies offered no survival advantage and were associated with significantly higher toxicity [25,36]. The CyVADIC (cyclophosphamide, vincristine, doxorubicin, DTIC) regimen has been extensively studied by the Southwestern Oncology Group (SWOG). Several large randomized trials have demonstrated response rates ranging from 38% to 71% [37,39].

The EORTC showed no advantage to combination regimens over single-agent doxorubicin by comparing doxorubicin alone (75 mg/m^2 every 3 wk) or doxorubicin (50 mg/m^2) plus ifosfamide (5 g/m^2) to the CyVADIC regimen. Response rates were 23%, 28%, and 29%, respectively, with a median survival of 52, 51, and 55 weeks, respectively [38]. In a large randomized intergroup trial, the MAID (mesna, doxorubicin, ifosfamide, DTIC) regimen was shown to have DTIC (32% vs 17%) [34]. The overall survival advantage for the three-drug regimen was not significantly different (12 vs 13 mo). Moreover, toxicity was significantly greater in the MAID arm of this study, which resulted in significantly lower doses of doxorubicin delivered.

Testing the doxorubicin dose response, investigators have focused on dose intensification of doxorubicin with hematopoietic stem cell support, with no data to date to justify this approach outside of a clinical trial [40–43]. Another approach is to use hemopoietic growth factors. The SWOG reported that the addition of GM-CSF did not allow for significant dose intensification of doxorubicin [43]. The EORTC performed a phase III randomized trial comparing doxorubicin (50 mg/m^2) and ifosfamide (5 g/m^2) to doxorubicin (75 mg/m^2), a 50% increase in the doxorubicin dose, and ifosfamide (5 g/m^2) with granulocyte–macrophage colony-stimulating factor (GM-CSF) (250 μg/m^2) support. With more than 300 patients randomly assigned, there was no apparent difference in response rate or survival [44].

Another approach is to test the dose response for ifosfamide. For example, doses up to 24 g/m^2 have been reported with acceptable toxicity and the suggestion of higher response rates [45]. Several phase III trials are testing the ifosfamide dose response hypothesis or comparing that to doxorubicin as single agent.

Current research is focusing on the discovery of new agents. Newer agents with proven efficacy in other solid tumors have been evaluated in soft tissues sarcomas. The taxanes, both paclitaxel and docetaxel, have been evaluated and are marginally active as single agents [46–50]. Gemcitabine is another new agent, but based on phase II data is at best marginally effective [51,52] Similarly, topoi-

Table 12-3. Randomized Trials Comparing Efficacy of Combination Chemotherapy Regimens for Soft Tissue Sarcomas

Study	Agents	Patients, n	Response Rate, %	Improvement in response rate?*	Improvement in overall survival?*
ECOG [35]	Doxorubicin	200	27	—	—
	Doxorubicin/vincristine		19	No	No
	Cyclophosphamide, actinomycin-D, vincristine/cyclophosphamide		11	No	No
ECOG [36]	Doxorubicin (70 mg/m^2)	275	18	—	—
	Doxorubicin (45 mg/m^2)		16	No	No
	Doxorubicin/dacarbazine		30	Yes	No
ECOG [23]	Doxorubicin	298	17	—	—
	Doxorubicin/vindesine		18	No	No
ECOG [25]	Doxorubicin	262	20	—	—
	Doxorubicin/ifosfamide		34	Yes	No
	Mitomycin/doxorubicin, cisplatin		32	Yes	No
SWOG [37]	Doxorubicin/dacarbazine	276	33	—	—
	Doxorubicin/dacarbazine/cyclophosphamide		34	No	No
	Doxorubicin/dacarbazine/actinomycin-D		24	No	No
EORTC [38]	Doxorubicin	663	23	—	—
	Doxorubicin/ifosfamide		28	No	No
	Doxorubicin/vincristine/cyclophosphamide/actinomycin-D		28	No	No
ISSG [34]	Doxorubicin/dacarbazine	340	17	—	—
	Doxorubicin/ifosfamide/dacarbazine/mesna		32	Yes	No

*As compared with single-agent doxorubicin or control (indicated by a dash).
ECOG—Eastern Cooperative Oncology Group; EORTC—European Organization for Research in Cancer Therapy; ISSG—Intergroup Sarcoma Study Group; SWOG—Southwestern Oncology Group.

somerase I inhibitors are not effective [53]. Another approach is to develop new agents that target increasing known phenotypic characteristics of the transformed sarcoma cell. These agents are in early clinical development.

In summary, single-agent doxorubicin remains the standard for treatment of adult soft tissue sarcomas. Several studies provide evidence that combination regimens, including doxorubicin, and/or ifosfamide and/or DTIC can result in marginally higher response rates with no increase in survival at the cost of increased toxicity. The hope is that novel targeted agents and/or dose intensification may offer promise for better therapeutic results.

STAGE-SPECIFIC TREATMENT RECOMMENDATIONS

Figure 12-1 summarizes an algorithm for the approach to primary management of adult patients with soft tissue sarcoma.

Stage IA, IB, and IIA Adult Soft Tissue Sarcoma (Low grade)

Low-grade (1 or 2) soft tissue sarcomas have low metastatic potential. Surgical resection with negative tissue margins of at least 2 cm or more in all directions is the desired treatment, Small tumors generally have a favorable outcome with surgery alone [54]. Local recur-

rence is the greatest risk, so that if the surgical margins are compromised or for unresectable tumors, radiation therapy should be considered [10]. Adjuvant chemotherapy is usually not indicated.

Stage IIB, IIC, and III Adult Soft Tissue Sarcoma

The surgical management of high-grade localized soft tissue sarcoma is usually limb-sparing surgery that involves wide local excision in combination with preoperative or postoperative radiation therapy. For sarcomas of the extremities, local control comparable with that obtained with amputation and radiation may be achieved [10,21].

Patients with T1 primary extremity soft tissue sarcomas, even if they are high grade, have a greater than 90% long-term survival with only a 7% probability of distant recurrence and 11% local recurrence rate without adjuvant radiation and/or chemotherapy [4]. Conversely, for patients who have sarcomas larger than 5 cm that are high-grade have a more than 50% probability of eventually developing distant metastases.

The role of adjuvant chemotherapy is controversial. Chemotherapy is a treatment option for patients with resected high grade or larger than 5 cm tumors who have no evident disease, but are known to be at higher risk of recurrence, and for those patients with evident metastatic disease or local-regional disease that cannot be

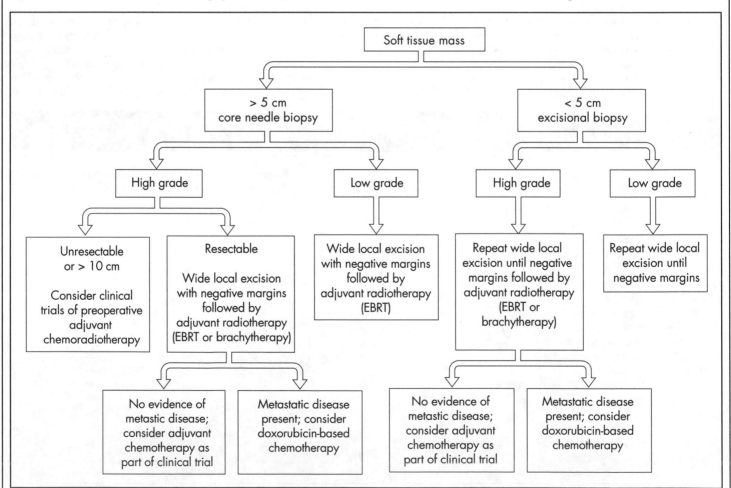

FIGURE 12-1.

Algorithm for management of primary soft tissue sarcoma. EBRT — external-beam radiotherapy.

controlled by surgery or radiation. Most authorities make the assumption that the best chemotherapy for patients with metastatic disease is the best chemotherapy for anterior or neoadjuvant therapy, and adjuvant therapy after surgical or radiation control of local-regional disease.

The goal of adjuvant chemotherapy is to improve survival by early elimination of microscopic hematogenous metastases. Successful adjuvant chemotherapy has been defined for a number of other cancers, including colon and breast cancer and osteosarcoma. However, adjuvant chemotherapy for patients with high-grade soft tissue sarcomas remains controversial. Table 12-4 summarizes several of the largest randomized trials examining adjuvant chemotherapy for this disease [55–68]. The two largest trials (European Organization for Research in Cancer Therapy [EORTC] and Scandinavian Sarcoma Group) do not support the use of adjuvant chemotherapy because neither showed a statistically significant improvement in overall survival [58,65]. Several smaller trials, including the update results from Italian Sarcoma Group, have shown a survival advantage for doxorubicin based adjuvant therapy; however, these studies have been extensively criticized for inadequate randomization, small size, and poor design [69].

To integrate the data from many of these trials, several meta-analyses have been performed [70–73]. The Sarcoma Meta-analysis Collaboration is the methodologically most rigorous analysis to date. Based on a meta-analysis of 1568 patients from 14 trials of doxorubicin-based adjuvant chemotherapy with a median follow-up 9.4 years, the statistical results demonstrated hazard ratios of 0.73 (95% CI, 0.56–0.94; P = 0.016) for local relapse free intervals, 0.70 (0.57–0.85; P = 0.0003) for distant relapse free survival, and 0.75 (0.64–0.87; P = 0.0001) for overall recurrence-free survival, correspond to absolute benefits from adjuvant chemotherapy of 6% (95% CI, 1–10), 10% (5–15), and 10% (5–15), respectively, at 10 years. For overall survival the hazard ratio of 0.89 (0.76–1.03) was not

significant (P = 0.12), but represents an absolute benefit of 4% (1–9) at 10 years. With further sub-set analyses, the best evidence of an effect of adjuvant chemotherapy for survival was seen in patients with high sarcomas of the extremities [70].

In summary, these data suggested a small advantage in recurrence of free survival and overall survival to doxorubicin-based adjuvant chemotherapy. However, these studies should be interpreted with caution. The low incidence of sarcoma and the diversity of this disease has made it difficult for many of these trials to accrue sufficient patients for meaningful randomization and statistical evaluation. Furthermore, the large heterogeneity in design, including patient selection bias, and methods of assessing outcome among the various trials makes synthesis of the data complex and potentially unreliable. Individual patient decisions must be based on specific prognostic factors, comorbidity, consideration of toxicity, and patient preference.

Another tactic is neoadjuvant chemotherapy, which has several theoretical advantages, including the early treatment of microscopic metastatic disease, ability to monitor the primary tumor to gauge responsiveness to particular agents, and shrinkage of advanced local tumors that may allow limb salvage. A retrospective analysis of 46 patients from the MD Anderson Cancer Center who received doxorubicin-based neoadjuvant chemotherapy found significantly improved disease free and overall survival in those patients whose primary tumors responded [74]. However, a prospective trial at MSKCC of 29 patients with large (> 10 cm) high-grade extremity sarcomas failed to demonstrate improved survival compared with historical controls [75]. Studies are ongoing to evaluate the efficacy of preoperative chemotherapy, especially in patients with large high-grade lesions [76].

Stage IV Adult Soft Tissue Sarcoma

Chemotherapy as outlined previously should be considered for those patients with metastatic disease. If possible, patients with limited

Table 12-4. Adjuvant Chemotherapy for Soft Tissue Sarcomas

Study	Regimen	Disease Sites	Patients, n	Improved Disease Free Survival?	Improved Overall Survival?
GOG [55]	Doxorubicin	Uterus	225	No	No
DFCI [56]	Doxorubicin	Extremities, trunk, head and neck, retroperitoneum	42	No	No
ECOG [57]	Doxorubicin	Extremities, trunk, head and neck, retroperitoneum	47	No	No
SSG [58]	Doxorubicin	Extremities, trunk, head and neck, breast, chest	240	No	No
Rizzoli [59]	Doxorubicin	Extremities	77	Yes	Yes
ISSG [60]	Doxorubicin	Extremities, trunk, head and neck, retroperitoneum	92	No	No
UCLA [62]	Doxorubicin	Extremities	119	No	No
MD Anderson [61]	Doxorubicin, cyclophosphamide, actinomycin-D, vincristine	Extremities, trunk	43	Yes	No
Mayo Clinic [63]	Doxorubicin, vincristine, dacarbazine, vincristine, actino-mycin-D, cyclophosphamide	Extremities, trunk	74	No	No
				No	No
NCI [64,67]	Doxorubicin, cyclophosphamide, methotrexate	Extremities	65	Yes	No
NCI [66]	Doxorubicin, cyclophosphamide, methotrexate	Trunk, breast, head and neck	57	No	No
EORTC [65]	Doxorubicin, cyclophosphamide, vincristine, dacarbazine	Extremities, trunk, head and neck	468	Yes*	No
Ravaud et al. [68]	Doxorubicin, cyclophosphamide, vincristine, dacarbazine	Extremities, trunk, head and neck, retroperitoneum	65	Yes	Yes

Limited to patients with head and neck or trunk lesions.
DFCI—Dana Farber Cancer Institute; ECOG—Eastern Cooperative Oncology Group; EORTC—European Organization for Research in Cancer Therapy; GOG—Gynecologic Oncology Group; ISSG—Intergroup Sarcoma Study Group; NCI—National Cancer Institute; SSG—Scandinavian Sarcoma Group; UCLA—University of California, Los Angeles.

pulmonary metastases should be considered for curative intent surgery by resection of the primary and/or pulmonary metastasectomy [77–79]. The role of adjuvant chemotherapy after metastasectomy is undergoing controlled clinical trial [80].

Unresectable and Recurrent Tumors

Despite adequate treatment of their primary tumors, 8% to 20% of patients with high-grade extremity sarcomas will recur locally. The link between local recurrence and the development of distant metastases is unclear and complex. Retrospective data correlates local recurrence with increased risk of developing distant metastases and decreased overall survival [77,78]. Yet in two prospective randomized trials, better local control rates did not translate into improved survival. In the NCI trial, local recurrence in the LSS arm was higher than with amputation, whereas overall survival did not differ between arms [10]. Similarly, in the adjuvant brachytherapy trial from MSKCC, improved local control in the adjuvant radiotherapy group did not result in improved overall survival [15]. It appears that survival is dictated by the biologic aggressiveness of the tumor and the presence of microscopic metastatic disease at the time of diagnosis. Local recurrence in patients with adequately treated primary tumors probably represents aggressive tumor biology, a harbinger for the development of distant disease.

The vast majority of these patients may be treated with re-resection and additional adjuvant radiotherapy [77,81]. A retrospective analysis suggested that if those patients whose tumors were previously resected and who were then referred for subsequent re-resection (two operations), the outcome was better correcting in a multivariant analysis of known prognostic factors [81]. In cases of multifocal recurrence or previous maximum radiotherapy, amputation may be necessary. In select patients with advanced unresectable or recurrent local disease, administration of chemotherapeutic drugs via direct arterial infusion or in the setting of isolated limb perfusion has been evaluated in an attempt to improve the rate of limb salvage. A review of 140 patients showed an 87% major response rate using a regimen of tumor necrosis factor and melphalan [82].

The management of pulmonary metastases is the metastatic site for almost all patients with extremity soft tissue sarcomas. In a retrospective study of more than 3000 patients, the important prognostic variables that were associated with a better outcome with metastasectomy were metastasis size, metastasis number, and primary tumor histologic grade [83].

Nonextremity and Atypical Soft Tissue Sarcomas

Retroperitoneal Sarcomas

Retroperitoneal sarcomas, although relatively rare, present additional treatment challenges. They account for approximately 15% of all sarcomas. Because of the large permissive nature of the retroperitoneal space, these patients will often present with large bulky tumors late in the course of their disease. The differential diagnosis of retroperitoneal masses should include lymphoma, sarcoma, and, in the male patient, metastatic testicular cancer. Complete surgical resection is often difficult because of the anatomic location, compromising the ability to achieve desired surgical margins. Unlike extremity tumors, for which the concern is pulmonary metastases, survival from retroperitoneal sarcomas is most dependent on locoregional control. Every attempt should be made to completely resect the tumor with negative margins at

initial exploration, because this is the only potentially curative therapy. Combined modality approaches are a standard of practice, but without evidence-based data to prove any disease-free or overall survival advantage [84,85].

Whenever necessary, adjacent viscera involved with the tumor should be removed en bloc with the specimen. Resectability of retroperitoneal sarcomas has been reported to be between 50% and 80% [84–86]. The 5-year actuarial survival for patients completely resected is 30% to 40% [85,86]. Despite complete resection, local recurrence will develop in 40% to 50 % of patients [84–86]. Local recurrences are managed by successive surgical resections that can go on for many years, increasing in frequency over time. Unfortunately, efforts to improve local control with adjuvant radiotherapy are limited by the radiosensitivity of overlying viscera. Attempts to minimize the dose of radiotherapy to normal tissue by means of intraoperative delivery of radiotherapy (IORT) have been successful in decreasing local failure rates but do not appear to improve survival [87]. Current studies are ongoing to evaluate methods to improve local control in these patients.

Sarcomas Arising in the Head and Neck or Trunk

Sarcomas arising in the head and neck region are uncommon, representing less than 5% of all sarcomas. The most common histologic subtypes in this region are fibrosarcoma, malignant schwannoma, and rhabdomyosarcoma. Treatment of these lesions is similar to sarcomas in other locations. Local failure is a significant problem for head and neck sarcomas. Surgical excision of the primary tumor with negative margins is more difficult, given the complex nature of this area. Adjuvant radiotherapy may play a role in preventing local recurrence. Successful treatment is predicted by the grade and size of the primary tumor, status of the surgical margins, and presence or absence of bony invasion [88]. Lymph node metastases, as with other sarcomas, are rare and routine; lymphadenectomy is not recommended. Five-year survival has been reported to vary from 20% to 68%. Sarcomas arising on the trunk or chest are managed primarily with surgery and adjuvant radiotherapy. As with other nonextremity sarcomas, local control is a significant problem with these lesions. Unlike extremity soft tissue sarcomas, survival correlates with the ability to locally control the primary tumor.

Rhabdomyosarcoma

Rhabdomyosarcoma is an uncommon histologic subtype of soft tissue sarcomas, occurring most commonly in childhood or adolescence. These tumors are more responsive to chemotherapy than other soft tissue sarcomas. The treatment of rhabdomyosarcomas is primarily nonsurgical, involving early and aggressive chemoradiation therapy.

Table 12-5. Common Histologic Types of Sarcomas Arising in Bone

Histologic Type	Comments
Osteosarcoma	Most common subtype; treated with adjuvant chemotherapy and surgery
Chondrosarcoma	Second most common sarcoma of bone; slow growing; low grade; treated primarily with surgery
Ewing's sarcoma	Small cell sarcoma; best treated with combination chemotherapy and radiation; surgery reserved for select cases

Kaposi's Sarcoma

Kaposi's sarcoma is an unusual vascular sarcoma that occurs in the skin of elderly men or in the setting of AIDS. The staging, prognosis, and therapy for Kaposi's sarcoma is completely different from that of other soft tissue sarcomas. Treatment strategies vary depending on the clinical scenario in which the tumor arises, but in general, systemic chemotherapy is the treatment of choice and excellent responses have been noted with single-agent vincristine, doxorubicin, vinblastine, taxanes, and/or etoposide.

SARCOMAS OF THE BONE
Pathologic Classification, Grading, and Staging

Sarcomas may arise form any of the four tissues that comprise mature bone: cartilage, bone, fibrous tissue, and marrow. As with soft tissue sarcomas, sarcomas of the bone are staged primarily on the grade. This is reflected in the staging system adopted by the Musculoskeletal Tumor Society (MSTS). Size of primary tumor and presence of distant metastases are also important prognostic factors.

Presentation and Diagnosis

The two most common histologic subtypes of bone sarcomas (osteosarcoma and Ewing's sarcoma) are most common in childhood or adolescence (Table 12-5). These tumors typically present as a painless mass firmly fixed to underlying bone. Radiographic evaluation is usually quite characteristic with a pattern of permeative cortical destruction, periosteal elevation, and soft tissue ossification. The biopsy of sarcomas arising in the bone must be performed with consideration for the definitive procedure. Poorly placed biopsies will often limit limb-sparing options later. In general, core needle biopsy is the preferred technique and will yield adequate specimen for diagnosis in the majority of cases [89].

Therapy

Surgery plus adjuvant chemotherapy is standard treatment of sarcomas arising from the bone. Prior to the 1980s, amputation of one joint above the lesion was the standard of care for all osteosarcomas [90]. Developments in reconstructive techniques and chemotherapy have made limb-sparing options more prevalent. As with soft tissue sarcoma, limited resections do not appear to affect survival. With current techniques, 50% to 80% of all osteosarcomas may be managed without amputation [90]. Contraindications to the use of limb-spar-

ing surgery include major neurovascular involvement, pathologic fractures, inappropriate biopsy site, infections, and skeletal immaturity.

Unlike soft tissue sarcomas, adjuvant chemotherapy effectively prolongs disease-free and overall survival in patients with osteosarcoma [91,92]. Currently, a majority of the regimens incorporate adriamycin and cisplatin with or without high dose methotrexate [90]. Other regimens used include bleomycin, cyclophosphamide, and dactinomycin [93]. Relapse-free survival rates between 40% and 60% have been reported using these regimens [93]. A major area of study in the treatment of osteosarcoma is the preoperative administration of adjuvant chemotherapy. Several early retrospective trials from MSKCC suggested that this approach may be better than traditional postsurgical adjuvant therapy [94–96]. However, preliminary results from a randomized trial by the Pediatric Oncology Group have failed to demonstrate a significant disease free survival advantage to preoperative chemotherapy versus traditional postsurgical adjuvant therapy [97]. Nevertheless, the response to preoperative chemotherapy remains the best predictor of future performance for patients with osteosarcoma.

It is known that patients whose primary tumors demonstrate significant histologic response are less likely to develop distant metastases and have better overall survival. This finding led to "custom tailoring" therapy, in which postsurgical adjuvant therapy is modified according to the response of the primary tumor to preoperative therapy. Early results from the T10 protocol conducted at MSKCC showed 70% to 90% long-term disease-free survival using this approach [98,99]. Subsequent multicenter trials have failed to reproduce these numbers [100,101]. It appears that poor responders will relapse and modifications of postsurgical chemotherapy do not significantly improve their survival. Current trials are evaluating dose intensification of preoperative chemotherapy in an attempt to increase the number of initial responders.

TREATMENT OF METASTATIC DISEASE

As with soft tissue sarcomas, the most common site of metastatic disease in osteosarcoma is the lung. The single most effective treatment for patients with isolated pulmonary metastases remains surgery. Long-term survival after pulmonary metastasectomy has been reported to vary from 15% to 30% [102–106]. Adjuvant therapy after metastasectomy has not been well studied, but some have suggested that it may be of use in select cases [93]. Despite the effectiveness of adjuvant chemotherapy for osteosarcoma, treatment of established metastatic disease is difficult and associated with poor response rates.

REFERENCES

1. Gaynor J, Tan C, Casper E, *et al.*: Refinement of clinicopathological staging for localized soft tissue sarcoma of the extremity: a study of 423 adults. *J Clin Oncol* 1992, 10:1317–1325.

2. Brennan MF, Casper ES, Harrison LB: Soft tissue sarcoma. In *Principles and Practice of Oncology*, edn 5. Edited by Rosenberg S, Devita V, Hellman S. Philadelphia: Lippincott-Raven; 1997:1738–1787.

3. Broders O, Hargrave R, Meyerding H: Pathological features of soft tissue fibrosarcomas with special reference to the grading of its malignancy. *Surg Gynecol Obstet* 1939, 69:237–241.

4. American Joint Committee on Cancer: *AJCC Cancer Staging Manual*, edn 5. Edited by Fleming I, Cooper J, Heuson D, *et al.* Philadelphia: Lippincott-Raven Publishers; 1997.

5. Barth R, Merino M, Solomon D, *et al.*: A prospective study of the value of core needle biopsy and fine needle aspiration in the diagnosis of soft tissue masses. Surgery 1992, 112:536–543.

6. Ball A, Fisher C, Pittan M, *et al.*: Diagnosis of soft tissues tumor by tru-cut biopsy. *Br J Surg* 1990, 77:756–760.

7. Heslin MJ, Lewis JJ, Woodruff JM, Brennan MF: Core needle biopsy for diagnosis of extremity soft tissue sarcoma. *Ann Surg Oncol* 1997, 4:425–431.

8. Spiro IJ, Rosenberg AE, Springfield D, Suit H: Combined surgery and radiation therapy for limb preservation in soft tissue sarcoma of the extremity: the Massachusetts General Hospital experience. *Cancer Investigation* 1995, 13:86–95.

9. Geer RJ, Woodruff J, Casper ES, Brennan MF: Management of small soft tissue sarcoma of the extremity in adults. *Arch Surg* 1992, 127:1285.

10. Yang JC, Chang AE, Baker AR, *et al.*: Randomized prospective study of the benefit of adjuvant radiation therapy in the treatment of soft tissue sarcomas of the extremity. *J Clin Oncol* 1998, 16:97–203.

11. Lindberg RD, Martin RG, Romsdahl MM, Barkley HT Jr.: Conservative surgery and postoperative radiotherapy in 300 adults with soft-tissue sarcomas. *Cancer* 1981, 47:2391–2397.

12. Abbatucci JS, Boulier N, de Ranieri J, *et al.*: Local control and survival in soft tissue sarcomas of the limbs, trunk walls and head and neck: a study of 113 cases. *Int J Radiat Oncol Biol Phys* 1986, 12:579–586.

13. Karakousis CP, Emrich LJ, Rao U, Krishnamsetty RM: Feasibility of limb salvage and survival in soft tissue sarcomas. *Cancer* 1986, 57:484–491.

14. Potter DA, Kinsella T, Glatstein E, *et al.*: High-grade soft tissue sarcomas of the extremities. *Cancer* 1986, 58:190–205.

15. Pisters PW, Harrison LB, Leung DH, *et al.*: Long-term results of a prospective randomized trial of adjuvant brachytherapy in soft tissue sarcoma. *J Clin Oncol* 1998, 14:859–868.

16. Yang J, Chang A, Baker A, *et al.*: A randomized prospective study of the benefit of adjuvant radiation therapy in the treatment of soft tissue sarcomas of the extremity. *J Clin Oncol* 1998, 16:197–203.

17. Spiro IJ, Gebhardt MC, Jennings LC, *et al.*: Prognostic factors for local control of sarcomas of the soft tissues managed by radiation and surgery. *Semin Oncol* 1997, 24:540–546.

18. Suit HD, Willett CG: Radiation therapy of sarcomas of the soft tissues. *Cancer Treat Res* 1991, 56:61–74.

19. Suit HD, Mankin HJ, Wood WC, Proppe KH: Preoperative, intraoperative, and postoperative radiation in the treatment of primary soft tissue sarcoma. *Cancer* 1985, 55:2659–2667.

20. Suit HD, Proppe KH, Mankin HJ, Wood WC: Preoperative radiation therapy for sarcoma of soft tissue. *Cancer* 1981, 47:2269–2274.

21. Temple WJ, Temple CL, Arthur K, *et al.*: Prospective cohort study of neoadjuvant treatment in conservative surgery of soft tissue sarcomas. *Ann Surg Oncol* 1997, 4:586–590.

22. Lindberg R, Martin R, Romsdahl M, *et al.*: Conservative surgery and radiation therapy for soft tissue sarcomas. In *Management of Primary Bone and Soft Tissue Tumors*. Chicago: Year Book Medical; 1977:289.

23. Borden EC, Amato DA, Edmonson JH, *et al.*: Randomized comparison of doxorubicin and vindesine to doxorubicin for patients with metastatic soft-tissue sarcomas. *Cancer* 1990, 66:862–867.

24. Casper ES, Gaynor JJ, Hajdu SI, *et al.*: A prospective randomized trial of adjuvant chemotherapy with bolus versus continuous infusion of doxorubicin in patients with high-grade extremity soft tissue sarcoma and an analysis of prognostic factors. *Cancer* 1991, 68:1221–1229.

25. Edmonson JH, Ryan LM, Blum RH, *et al.*: Randomized comparison of doxorubicin alone versus ifosfamide plus doxorubicin or mitomycin, doxorubicin and cisplatin against advanced soft tissue sarcomas. *J Clin Oncol* 1993, 11:1269–1275.

26. Verweij J, van Oosterom AT, Somers R, *et al.*: Chemotherapy in the multidisciplinary approach to soft tissue sarcomas: EORTC Soft Tissue and Bone Sarcoma Group studies in perspective. *Ann Oncol* 1992, 3 (suppl 2):S75–S80.

27. Mouridsen HT, Bastholt L, Somers R, *et al.*: Adriamycin versus epirubicin in advanced soft tissue sarcomas: a randomized phase II/phase III study of the EORTC Soft Tissue and Bone Sarcoma Group. *Eur J Cancer Clin Oncol* 1987, 23:1477–1483.

28. Stuart-Harris RC, Harper PG, Parsons CA, *et al.*: High-dose alkylation therapy using ifosfamide infusion with mesna in the treatment of adult advanced soft-tissue sarcoma. *Cancer Chemother Pharmacol* 1983, 11:69–72.

29. Stuart-Harris R, Harper PG, Kaye SB, Wiltshaw E: High-dose ifosfamide by infusion with mesna in advanced soft tissue sarcoma. *Cancer Treat Rev* 1983, 10 (suppl A):163–164.

30. Bramwell VH, Mouridsen HT, Santoro A, *et al.*: Cyclophosphamide versus ifosfamide: final report of a randomized phase II trial in adult soft tissue sarcomas. *Eur J Cancer Clin Oncol* 1987, 23:311–321.

31. Antman KH, Elias AD: Dana-Farber Cancer Institute studies in advanced sarcoma. *Semin Oncol* 1990, 17:7–15.

32. Elias AD, Eder JP, Shea T, *et al.*: High-dose ifosfamide with mesna uroprotection: a phase I study. *J Clin Oncol* 1990, 8:170–178.

33. Buesa JM, Mouridsen HT, van Oosterom AT, *et al.*: High-dose DTIC in advanced soft-tissue sarcomas in the adult: a phase II study of the EORTC Soft Tissue and Bone Sarcoma Group. *Ann Oncol* 1991, 2:307–309.

34. Antman KH, Crowley J, Balcerzak S, *et al.*: An Intergroup phase III randomized study of doxorubicin and dacarbazine with or without ifosfamide and mesna in advanced soft tissue and bone sarcomas. *J Clin Oncol* 1993, 11:1276–1285.

35. Schoenfeld DA, Rosenbaum C, Horton J, *et al.*: A comparison of adriamycin versus vincristine and adriamycin, and cyclophosphamide versus vincristine, actinomycin-D, and cyclophosphamide for advanced sarcoma. *Cancer* 1982, 50:2757–2762.

36. Borden EC, Amato DA, Rosenbaum C, *et al.*: Randomized comparison of three adriamycin regimens for metastatic soft tissue sarcomas. *J Clin Oncol* 1987, 5:840–850.

37. Baker LH, Frank J, Fine G, *et al.*: Combination chemotherapy using adriamycin, DTIC, cyclophosphamide, and actinomycin D for advanced soft tissue sarcomas: a randomized comparative trial: a phase III Southwest Oncology Group Study (7613). *J Clin Oncol* 1987, 5:851–861.

38. Santoro A, Tursz T, Mouridsen H, *et al.*: Doxorubicin versus CYVADIC versus doxorubicin plus ifosfamide in first-line treatment of advanced soft tissue sarcomas: a randomized study of the EORTC Soft Tissue and Bone Sarcoma Group. *J Clin Oncol* 1995, 13:1537–1545.

39. Pinedo HM, Bramwell VH, Mouridsen HT, *et al.*: Cyvadic in advanced soft tissue sarcoma: a randomized study comparing two schedules: a study of the EORTC Soft Tissue and Bone Sarcoma Group. *Cancer* 1984, 53:1825–1832.

40. Edmonson JH, Long HJ, Kvols LK, *et al.*: Can molgramostim enhance the antitumor effects of cytotoxic drugs in patients with advanced sarcomas? *Ann Oncol* 1997, 8:637–641.

41. Bokemeyer C, Franzke A, Hartmann JT, *et al.*: A phase I/II study of sequential, dose-escalated, high dose ifosfamide plus doxorubicin with peripheral blood stem cell support for the treatment of patients with advanced soft tissue sarcomas. *Cancer* 1997, 80:1221–1227.

42. Steward WP, Verweij J, Somers R, *et al.*: Doxorubicin plus ifosfamide with rhGM-CSF in the treatment of advanced adult soft-tissue sarcomas: preliminary results of a phase II study from the EORTC Soft-Tissue and Bone Sarcoma Group. *J Cancer Res Clin Oncol* 1991, 117(suppl 4):S193–S197.

43. Hicks LG, Balcerzak SP, Zalupski M: GM-CSF did not allow doxorubicin dose escalation in the MAID regimen: a phase I trial: a Southwest Oncology Group study. *Cancer Invest* 1996, 14:507–512.

44. Le Cesne A, Judson I, Crowther D, *et al.*: Randomized phase III study comparing conventional-dose doxorubicin plus ifosfamide versus high-dose doxorubicin plus ifosfamide plus recombinant human granulocyte-macrophage colony-stimulating factor in advanced soft tissue sarcomas: a trial of the European Organization for Research and Treatment of Cancer/Soft Tissue and Bone Sarcoma Group. *J Clin Oncol* 2000, 14:2676–2684.

45. Jaffar Z, Blum RH, Rosen G, *et al.*: Ifosfamide 14:24 GM/M^2: an outpatient study in sarcomas. *Proc Annu Meet Am Soc Clin Oncol* 1998, 17:1968.

46. Verweij J, Lee SM, Ruka W, et al.: Randomized phase II study of docetaxel versus doxorubicin in first- and second-line chemotherapy for locally advanced or metastatic soft tissue sarcomas in adults: a study of the European Organization for Research and Treatment of Cancer Soft Tissue and Bone Sarcoma Group. J Clin Oncol 2000, 18:2081–1086.

47. Amodio A, Carpano S, Paoletti G, et al.: Phase II study of docetaxel in patients with advanced stage soft tissue sarcoma. Clinical Trials 1998, 149:121–125.

48. Edmonson JH, Ebbert LP, Nascimento AG, et al.:Phase II study of docetaxel in advanced soft tissue sarcomas. Am J Clin Oncol 1996, 6:574–576.

49. Balcerzak SP, Benedetti J, Weiss GR, et al.: A phase II trial of paclitaxel in patients with advanced soft tissue sarcomas: a Southwest Oncology Group study. Cancer 1995, 76:2248–2252.

50. Casper ES, Waltzman RJ, Schwartz GK, et al.: Phase II trial of paclitaxel in patients with soft-tissue sarcoma. Cancer Invest 1998, 16:442–446.

51. Merimsky O, Meller I, Flusser G, et al.: Gemcitabine in soft tissue or bone sarcoma resistant to standard chemotherapy: a phase II study. Cancer Chemother Pharmacol 2000, 45:177–181.

52. Amodio A, Carpano S, Manfredi C, et al.: Gemcitabine in advanced stage soft tissue sarcoma: a phase II study. Clin Ter (Italy), 1999, 150:17–20.

53. Bramwell VH, Eisenhauer EA, Blackstein M, et al.: Phase II study of topotecan (NSC 609 699) in patients with recurrent or metastatic soft tissue sarcoma. Ann Oncol 1995, 6:847–849.

54. Geer RJ, Woodruff J, Casper ES, et al.: Management of small soft-tissue sarcoma of the extremity in adults. Arch Surg 1992, 127:1285–1289.

55. Omura A, Blessinf J, Major F, et al.: A randomized trial of adjuvant adriamycin in uterine sarcomas: a Gynecologic Oncology Group study. J Clin Oncol 1985, 3:1240–1245.

56. Antman K, Suit H, Amato D, et al.: Preliminary results of a randomized trial of adjuvant doxorubicin for sarcomas: lack of apparent difference between treatment groups. J Clin Oncol 1984, 2:601–608.

57. Lerner H, Amato D, Savlov E, et al.: Eastern Oncology Cooperative Group: a comparison of adjuvant doxorubicin and observation for patients with localized soft tissue sarcoma. J Clin Oncol 1987, 5:613–617.

58. Alvegard T, Sigurdsson H, Mouridsen H, et al.: Adjuvant chemotherapy with doxorubicin in high-grade soft tissue sarcoma: a randomized trial of the Scandinavian Sarcoma Group. J Clin Oncol 1989, 7:1504–1513.

59. Gherlinzoni F, Bacci G, Picci P, et al.: A randomized trial for the treatment of high-grade soft-tissue sarcomas of the extremities: preliminary observations. J Clin Oncol 1986, 4:552–558.

60. Antman KH, Ryan LM, Borden EC, et al.: Pooled results from three randomized adjuvant studies of doxorubicin versus observation in soft tissue sarcoma: 10-year results and review of the literature. In Adjuvant Therapy of Cancer VI. Edited by Salmon SE. Philadelphia: WB Saunders; 1990:529–543.

61. Benjamin RS, Terjanian TO, Fenoglio CJ, et al.: The importance of combination chemotherapy for adjuvant treatment of high risk patients with soft tissue sarcomas of the extremities. In Adjuvant Therapy of Cancer V. Edited by Salmon S. Orlando, FL: Grune and Stratton; 1987:735–744.

62. Eilber FR, Giuliano AE, Huth JF, Morton DL: Post operative adjuvant chemotherapy (adriamycin) in high grade extremity soft tissue sarcoma: a randomized prospective trial. In Adjuvant Therapy of Cancer V. Edited by Salmon S. Orlando, FL: Grune and Stratton; 1987:719–726.

63. Edmonson JH, Fleming TR, Ivins JC, et al.: Randomized study of systemic chemotherapy following complete excision of nonosseous sarcomas. J Clin Oncol 1984, 2:1390–1406.

64. Rosenberg SA, Tepper J, Glatstein E, et al.: Prospective randomized evaluation of adjuvant chemotherapy in adults with soft tissue sarcomas of the extremities. Cancer 1983, 52:424–434.

65. Bramwell VH, Rousse J, Steward WP, et al.: Adjuvant CYVADIC chemotherapy for adult soft tissue sarcoma-reduced local recurrence but no improvement in survival: a study of the European Organization for research and treatment of cancer, soft tissue and bone sarcoma group. J Clin Oncol 1994, 12:1137–1149.

66. Glenn J, Kinsella T, Glatstein E, et al.: A randomized, prospective trial of adjuvant chemotherapy in adults with soft tissue sarcomas of the head and neck, breast, and trunk. Cancer 1985, 55:1206–1214.

67. Chang AE, Kinsella T, Glatstein E, et al.: Adjuvant chemotherapy for patients with high-grade soft-tissue sarcomas of the extremity. J Clin Oncol 1988, 6:1491–1500.

68. Ravaud A, Bui NB, Coindre JM, et al.: Adjuvant chemotherapy with Cyvadic in high risk soft tissue sarcoma: a randomized prospective trial. In Adjuvant Therapy of Cancer. Edited by Salmon S. Philadelphia: WB Saunders; 1990:556–566.

69. Frustaci S, Gherlinzoni F, De Paoli A, et al.: Maintenance of Efficacy of Adjuvant Chemotherapy (CT) in Soft Tissue Sarcoma (STS) of the Extremities Up-Date of a Randomized Trial. Proc ASCO 1999:2108.

70. Sarcoma Meta-analysis Collaboration: Adjuvant chemotherapy for localised resectable soft-tissue sarcoma of adults: meta-analysis of individual data. Lancet 1997, 350:1647–1654.

71. Zalupski M, Ryan JR, Hussein ME, Baker LH: Systemic adjuvant chemotherapy for soft tissue sarcomas of the extremities. Surg Oncol Clin North Am 1993, 2:621–636.

72. Jones GW, Chouinard E, Patel M: Adjuvant adriamycin (doxorubicin) in adult patients with soft tissue sarcomas: a systematic overview and quantitative meta-analysis [abstract]. Clin Invest Med 1991, 14:A772.

73. Zalupski M, Ryan JR, Hussein ME: Defining the role of adjuvant chemotherapy for patients with soft tissue sarcoma of the extremities. In Adjuvant Therapy of Cancer VII. Edited by Salmon SE. Philadelphia: JB Lippincott; 1993:385–392.

74. Pezzi CM, Pollock RE, Evans HL, et al.: Preoperative chemotherapy for soft-tissue sarcomas of the extremities. Ann Surg 1990, 211:476–481.

75. Casper ES, Gaynor JJ, Panicek DM, Harrison LB: Preoperative and postoperative adjuvant chemotherapy for adults with high grade soft tissue sarcoma. Cancer 1994, 73:1644–1650.

76. Kraybill W, Spiro I, Harris J, et al.: RTOG 95-14: A phase II study of neoadjuvant chemotherapy and radiation therapy in the management of high risk, high grade, soft tissue sarcomas of the extremities and body wall: a preliminary report. Proc ASCO, in press.

77. van Geel AN, Pastorino U, Jauch KW, et al.: Surgical treatment of lung metastases: the European Organization for Research and Treatment of Cancer: Soft Tissue and Bone Sarcoma Group study of 255 patients. Cancer 1996, 77:675–682.

78. Casson AG, Putman JB, Natarajan G, et al.: Five-year survival after pulmonary metastasectomy for adult soft tissue sarcoma. Cancer 1992, 69:662–668.

79. Putnam JB Jr., Roth JA: Surgical treatment for pulmonary metastases from sarcoma. Hematology Oncology Clinics of North America 1995, 9:869–887.

80. Van Geel AN: EORTC Soft Tissue and Bone Sarcoma Group: phase III randomized study of neoadjuvant high-dose DOX/IFF with or without G-CSF followed by metastasectomy vs metastasectomy alone for lung metastases in patients with soft tissue sarcoma, EORTC-62933.

81. Singer S, Antman K, Corson J, Eberlein TJ: Long-term salvagability for patients with locally recurrent soft-tissue sarcomas. Arch Surg 1992, 127:548–554.

82. Eggermont AM, Schraffordt Koops H, Klausner JM, *et al.*: Isolation limb perfusion with tumor necrosis factor alpha and chemotherapy for advanced extremity soft tissue sarcomas. *Semin Oncol* 1997, 24:547–555.

83. Weiser MR, Downey RJ, Leung DH, *et al.*:. Repeat resection of pulmonary metastases in patients with soft-tissue sarcoma. *J Am Coll Surg* 2000, 191:184–190.

84. Jaques DP, Coit DG, Hajdu SI, Brennan MF: Management of primary and recurrent soft-tissue sarcoma of the retroperitoneum. *Ann Surg* 1990, 212:51–59.

85. Heslin MJ, Lewis JJ, Nadler E, *et al.*: Prognostic factors associated with long-term survival for retroperitoneal sarcoma: implications for management. *J Clin Oncol* 1997, 15:2832–2839.

86. Dalton RR, Donohue JH, Mucha P Jr, *et al.*: Management of retroperitoneal sarcomas. *Surgery* 1989, 106:725–732 (discussion 732–733).

87. Kinsella TJ, Sindelar WF, Lack E, *et al.*: Preliminary results of a randomized study of adjuvant radiation therapy in resectable adult retroperitoneal soft tissue sarcomas. *J Clin Oncol* 1988, 6:18–25.

88. Farhood A, Hajdu S, Shiu M, Strong E: Soft tissue sarcomas of the head and neck in adults. *Am J Surg* 1990, 160:365–369.

89. Mankin HJ, Lange TA, Spanier SS: The hazards of biopsy in patients with malignant primary bone and soft-tissue tumors. *J Bone Joint Surg Am* 1982, 64:1121–1127.

90. Malawer M, Link MP, Donaldson SS: Sarcomas of bone. In *Principles and Practice of Oncology*, edn 5. Edited by Rosenberg S, Devita V, Hellman S. Philadelphia: Lippincott-Raven; 1997:1789–1852.

91. Link MP, Goorin AM, Miser AW, *et al.*: The effect of adjuvant chemotherapy on relapse-free survival in patients with osteosarcoma of the extremity. *N Engl J Med* 1986, 314:1600–1606.

92. Elber F, Guiliano A, Eckardt J, *et al.*: Adjuvant chemotherapy for osteosarcoma: a randomized prospective trial. *J Clin Oncol* 1987, 5:21–26.

93. Mosende C, Gutierrez M, Caparros B, Rosen G: Combination chemotherapy with bleomycin, cyclophosphamide and dactinomycin for the treatment of osteogenic sarcoma. *Cancer* 1977, 40:2779–2786.

94. Rosen G, Marcove RC, Huvos AG, *et al.*: Primary osteogenic sarcoma: eight-year experience with adjuvant chemotherapy. *J Cancer Res Clin Oncol* 1983, 106(suppl):55–67.

95. Rosen G, Nirenberg A: Neoadjuvant chemotherapy for osteogenic sarcoma: a five year follow-up (T-10) and preliminary report of new studies (T-12). *Prog Clin Biol Res* 1985, 201:39–51.

96. Rosen G: Preoperative (neoadjuvant) chemotherapy for osteogenic sarcoma: a ten year experience. *Orthopedics* 1985, 8:659–664.

97. Goorin A, Baker A, Gieser P, Ayala A, *et al.*: No evidence for improved event free survival (EFS) with presurgical chemotherapy (PRE) for nonmetastatic extremity osteogenic sarcoma (OGS): preliminary results of randomized Pediatric Oncology Group (POG) trial [abstract]. *Proc Am Soc Clin Oncol* 1995, 14:444.

98. Meyers PA, Heller G, Healey J, *et al.*: Chemotherapy for nonmetastatic osteogenic sarcoma: the Memorial Sloan-Kettering experience. *J Clin Oncol* 1992, 10:5–15.

99. Glasser DB, Lane JM, Huvos AG, *et al.*: Survival, prognosis, and therapeutic response in osteogenic sarcoma: the Memorial Hospital experience. *Cancer* 1992, 69:698–708.

100. Provisor AJ, Ettinger LJ, Nachman JB, *et al.*: Treatment of nonmetastatic osteosarcoma of the extremity with preoperative and postoperative chemotherapy: a report from the Children's Cancer Group. *J Clin Oncol* 1997, 15:76–84.

101. Winkler K, Beron G, Delling G, *et al.*: Neoadjuvant chemotherapy of osteosarcoma: results of a randomized cooperative trial (COSS-82) with salvage chemotherapy based on histological tumor response. *J Clin Oncol* 1988, 6:329–337.

102. Beattie EJ, Harvey JC, Marcove R, Martini N: Results of multiple pulmonary resections for metastatic osteogenic sarcoma after two decades. *J Surg Oncol* 1991, 46:154–155.

103. Burk CD, Belasco JB, O'Neill JA, Jr., Lange B: Pulmonary metastases and bone sarcomas: surgical removal of lesions appearing after adjuvant chemotherapy. *Clin Orthop* 1991, 88–92.

104. Goorin AM, Delorey MJ, Lack EE, *et al.*: Prognostic significance of complete surgical resection of pulmonary metastases in patients with osteogenic sarcoma: analysis of 32 patients. *J Clin Oncol* 1984, 2:425–431.

105. Flye MW, Woltering G, Rosenberg SA: Aggressive pulmonary resection for metastatic osteogenic and soft tissue sarcomas. *Ann Thorac Surg* 1984, 37:123–127.

106. Putnam JB, Jr., Roth JA, Wesley MN, *et al.*: Survival following aggressive resection of pulmonary metastases from osteogenic sarcoma: analysis of prognostic factors. *Ann Thorac Surg* 1983, 36:516–523.

VMAID FOR THE TREATMENT OF ADVANCED SOFT TISSUE SARCOMA
Mesna, Doxorubicin, Ifosfamide, and Dacarbazine

Doxorubicin is the most effective single agent in the treatment of soft tissue sarcomas in the adult. Ifosfamide has been shown to also have good activity as a single agent. The combination regimen of doxorubicin and ifosfamide with or without dacarbazine (DTIC) has been shown to have higher response rates than treatment with single agents. Unfortunately, overall survival has not been shown to be improved by combination regimens. Moreover, toxicity is significantly greater. Efforts to limit myelosuppressive toxicity and increase the dose of doxorubicin in these regimens is currently being investigated.

RECENT EXPERIENCE AND RESPONSE RATES

Group	Regimen	Dose of A	Patients, n	RR, %	CR, %
DFCI [31]	MAID	60 mg/m² /course	108	47	10
SWOG [43]	MAID + GM-CSF	75 mg/m² /course	13	—	—
EORTC [44]	A + I + GM-CSF	60 mg/m² /course	145	45	10

A—doxorubicin; CR—complete response rate; DFCI—Dana-Farber Cancer Institute; EORTC—European Organization for Research in Cancer Therapy; GM-CSF—granulocyte–macrophage colony-stimulating factor; I—ifosfamide; MAID—mesna, doxorubicin, ifosfamide, and dacarbazine; RR—response rate; SWOG—Southwestern Oncology Group.

INDICATIONS

Doxorubicin is the only drug with labeled indication for the treatment of soft tissue sarcomas; combination regimens incorporating ifosfamide with mesna and/or dacarbazine have been shown in randomized trials to improve response rates in soft tissue sarcoma; currently little data exists to support the use of these drugs in the adjuvant setting outside of clinical trials; for patients with advanced disease, single-agent doxorubicin may provide palliative benefit; the greater response rates with combination regimens should be balanced against the increased toxicity

CANDIDATES FOR TREATMENT

Patients with advanced soft tissue sarcomas who have normal renal and cardiac function

TOXICITY

Enhanced myelosuppression with combination regimen: administration of hematopoietic growth factors may blunt severe neutropenia; severe nausea and emesis is common; alopecia is to be expected; **Doxorubicin:** cardiac toxicity is the single most important concern with doses exceeding 400 mg/m²; may also tinge urine red-orange; hyperpigmentation and creasing of nail beds may occur; should be administered through central venous line because local extravasation will result in severe cellulitis, vesication, and tissue necrosis; **Ifosfamide:** severe hemorrhaged cystitis; should only be administered with vigorous hydration in combination with uroprotective agent mesna; neurological manifestations (*eg*, somnolence, confusion, and hallucinations); **Dacarbazine:** severe nausea and vomiting are the most common toxicities

DRUG INTERACTIONS

Administration of live vaccines should be avoided in all patients receiving myelosuppressive chemotherapy; **Doxorubicin:** cyclosporine may induce coma and/or seizures; phenobarbitol increases elimination of doxorubicin; phenytoin levels may be decreased by concomitant administration of doxorubicin; **Ifosfamide and DTIC:** no specific interactions cited in literature; physician should be alert to possible combined drug interactions

NURSING INTERVENTIONS

Strict sterile technique when accessing central venous devices should be practiced; general supportive measures, including prophylactic antiemetics and mouth care to minimize symptoms from stomatitis; vigorous hydration with administration of ifosfamide; immediately report any symptoms of infection, bleeding, or shortness of breath

PATIENT INFORMATION

Common side effects from administration of these agents include nausea, vomiting, and stomatitis; in addition, doxorubicin may have direct cardiac toxicity manifested by acute left ventricular failure; immunosuppression is expected and occurs at a maximum of 10–14 d after therapy; patients should notify their physician immediately if they develop a fever, abnormal bleeding, or shortness of breath

ADMINISTRATION NOTES

Doxorubicin: (Rubex, Bristol-Meyers Squibb, Princeton, NJ) supplied as 10-mg, 50-mg, and 100-mg vials. Reconstitute with sterile sodium chloride (0.9%) to final concentration of 2 mg/mL. Reconstituted solution is stable up to 24 h at room temperature and 48 h under refrigeration (2°C–8°C)
Ifosfamide: (Ifex, Bristol-Meyers Squibb, Princeton, NJ) supplied as 1-g or 3-g single- or multiple-dose vials in combination packages with mesna. Should be reconstituted in sterile water to final concentration of 50 mg/mL. Should be refrigerated and used within 24 h of reconstitution
Dacarbazine: (multiple manufacturers) supplied as 100-mg or 200-mg vials. May be reconstituted and mixed with doxorubicin for injection.

MABCDP FOR TREATMENT OF OSTEOSARCOMA
Methotrexate, Doxorubicin, Bleomycin, Cyclophosphamide, Dactinomycin, and Cisplatin

Chemotherapy for osteosarcoma is most often given in the setting of adjuvant therapy. The development of effective regimens for these tumors has been largely empirical given the extremely poor response rates in macroscopic disease. Currently, the area under study is whether there is an advantage to early preoperative treatment versus traditional postoperative adjuvant therapy. Additionally, the value of modifying postoperative regimens in patients who respond poorly to preoperative therapy is being studied. The majority of randomized trials incorporate chemotherapy regimens based on doxorubicin and cisplatin. Other agents, such as high-dose methotrexate and the BCD (bleomycin, cyclophosphamide, dactinomycin) combination, are controversial.

INDICATIONS

FDA-approved: only doxorubicin has a labeled indication for the treatment of bone sarcomas; methotrexate, bleomycin, cyclophosphamide, dactinomycin, and cisplatin are all FDA-approved for the treatment of cancer and have shown effectiveness in various randomized trials against osteosarcoma

CANDIDATES FOR TREATMENT

Patients with osteosarcoma who have normal renal, cardiac, and pulmonary function

TOXICITIES AND ADVERSE REACTIONS

Enhanced myelosuppression with combination regimen: administration of hematopoietic growth factors may blunt severe neutropenia; severe nausea and emesis is common; alopecia is to be expected; **Doxorubicin:** cardiac toxicity is the single most important concern with doses exceeding 400 mg/m^2; may also tinge urine red-orange; hyperpigmentation and creasing of nail beds may occur; should be administered through central venous line because local extravasation will result in severe cellulitis, vesication, and tissue necrosis; **Methotrexate:** may result in renal failure or death if not given with appropriate support; cumulative toxicity includes hepatic fibrosis, osteoporosis, and pulmonary dysfunction; **Bleomycin:** severe idiosyncratic, anaphylactic reactions have been reported; pulmonary fibrosis that begins as pneumonitis is the most serious side effect, arising in 10% of patients treated; **Cyclophosphamide:** hemorrhagic cystitis; should be given with vigorous hydration; **Dactinomycin:** GI toxicity most predominate; locally irritating if extravasated

DRUG INTERACTIONS

Administration of live vaccines should be avoided in all patients receiving myelosuppressive chemotherapy; **Doxorubicin:** cyclosporine may induce coma and/or seizures; phenobarbitol increases elimination of doxorubicin; **Methotrexate:** nonsteroidal anti-inflammatories, ethanol, 5-fluorouracil, and salicylates. **Bleomycin:** granulocyte colony-stimulating factor may increase risk of pulmonary fibrosis

NURSING INTERVENTIONS

Strict sterile technique when accessing central venous devices should be practiced; general supportive measures, including prophylactic antiemetics and mouth care to minimize symptoms from stomatitis; vigorous hydration with administration of cyclophosphamide; immediately report any symptoms of infection, bleeding, pulmonary dysfunction, or symptoms of congestive heart failure

MABCDP FOR TREATMENT OF OSTEOSARCOMA (Continued)
Methotrexate, Doxorubicin, Bleomycin, Cyclophosphamide, Dactinomycin, and Cisplatin

RECENT EXPERIENCES AND RESPONSE RATES

Group	Preoperative regimen	Preoperative regimen	Patients, *n*	Disease-free survival, %	Overall survival, %
POG [97]	None or methotrexate, doxorubicin, and cisplatin	None or methotrexate, doxorubicin, and cisplatin	106	70.0 (preoperative) 72.8 (postoperative)	—
CCG [99]	Methotrexate and BCD	Methotrexate, doxorubicin, cisplatin, and BCD	231	53.0	60

BCD—bleomycin, cyclophosphamide, and dactinomycin; CCG—Children's Cancer Group; POG—Pediatric Oncology Group.

PATIENT INFORMATION

Common side effects from administration of these agents include nausea, vomiting, and stomatitis; in addition, doxorubicin may have direct cardiac toxicity manifested by acute left ventricular failure; bleomycin may result in severe pulmonary fibrosis; immunosuppression is expected and occurs at a maximum of 10–14 d after therapy; patients should notify their physician immediately if they develop a fever, abnormal bleeding or swelling, or shortness of breath

ADMINISTRATION NOTES

Doxorubicin: (Rubex, Bristol-Meyers Squibb, Princeton, NJ) supplied as 10-mg, 50-mg, and 100-mg vials. Reconstitute with sterile sodium chloride (0.9%) to final concentration of 2 mg/mL. Reconstituted solution is stable up to 24 h at room temperature and 48 h under refrigeration (2°C–8°C)

Cisplatin: (Bristol-Meyers Squibb) supplied as 10 mg or 50 mg of powder to be resuspended into solution at 50 mg/mL

Methotrexate: (multiple suppliers) supplied as 1-g vial lyophilized powder

Bleomycin: (Bristol-Meyers Squibb) supplied as 15-U vial

Cyclophosphamide: (Bristol-Meyers Squibb) supplied as 100-mg to 2-g vials

Dactinomycin: (Merck & Co., Whitehouse Park, NJ) supplied as 0.5-mg/mL vial

Leucovorin calcium: (multiple suppliers) 5–25-mg tablets; 3-mg/mL injection and 50–350-mg vial of powder for injection.

Tremendous strides have been made in the treatment of genitourinary malignancies in the past 10 to 15 years; the explosion of new findings in cell biology, physiology, biochemistry, pharmacology, immunology, and radiobiology continues to broaden and deepen our understanding of biology and treatment in the new century. This chapter summarizes present medical and surgical therapies employed for prostate, urinary bladder, testicular, and renal cancers. We highlight salient basic and clinical observations that have formed the foundation of our current therapeutic strategies in genitourinary cancers.

Testicular Cancer

Etiology and Risk Factors

Germ cell cancers arise from pleuripotent cells capable of differentiating along five different embryonic lines. These tumors are commonly classified as seminomatous and nonseminomatous. Seminoma tumors arise from the spermatocyte, the earliest cell with the greatest ability to differentiate into embryonic or placental tissue. Nonseminomatous tumors, often mixed, contain elements of embryonal cells, teratoma, yolk sac, and choriocarcinoma.

Germ cell tumors are rare, and if treatment for a suspicious testicular mass is approached promptly, clinical outcome for most patients is cure. It is of no surprise that screening for early-stage testicular malignancies has not proved to be beneficial [1]. Etiology and risk factors are described in Table 13-1.

Staging and Prognosis

Diagnosis and therapeutic approaches to germ cell tumor of the testis must consider the anatomy of lymphatic drainage and course of the neurovascular bundles, stage, histologic type, and the presence of vessel invasion (Table 13-2). In addition, relative sensitivity to chemotherapy or radiation therapy may dictate choice of treatment for these tumors. When testicular malignancy is suspected, a routine battery of laboratory and radiologic evaluations should be performed, including a complete blood count, lactate dehydrogenase, β-human chorionic gonadotropin (βhCG), α-fetoprotein, urine analysis, and computed tomography of the chest and abdomen. Magnetic resonance imaging and new modalities, such as positron-emission tomography (PET), may improve our ability to detect metastatic disease but have limited use in the present management of the disease. Preliminary reports of PET scanning suggest that this modality may help distinguish teratoma or scar from persistent tumor and may aid in evaluation of possible lymph node involvement for early stage disease. Other tests that may prove useful for the diagnosis and management of testicular tumors include testicular ultrasound and IV pyelography.

We are fortunate to have accurate tumor markers for assessment of germ cell cancers; these markers have become essential for the correct management of these malignancies (Table 13-3). Elevation of α-fetoprotein, βhCG, or both is found in 85% of nonseminomatous germ cell cancer, whereas only 10% of seminomas show mild elevation in βhCG. False elevations in serum markers are rare but should be recognized because treatment decisions are based, in part, on these measurements. Although lactate dehydrogenase is a nonspecific marker, it is helpful in suggesting bulky lymph node involvement.

For patients with metastatic disease, various prognostic factors have been used in devising staging systems [10–12]. Commonly used are the MD Anderson Classification, the Memorial Sloan-Kettering Cancer Institute Classification, and the Indiana Classification. These systems attempt to estimate the bulk of disease and do so relatively well. We use the Indiana system, which classifies patients with testicular cancer into three categories (Table 13-4).

Table 13-2. Staging of Testicular Cancers

Stage*	TNM Staging	Criteria
0	Tis N0 M0	Intratubular, preinvasive tumor
I (A)	T1 T2 N0 M0	Tumor limited to testes and/or rete testis Invasion beyond tunica albuginea or into epididymis
II (A)	T3 T4 N0 M0	Invasion of spermatic cord Invasion of scrotum Invasion of scrotum
III (B1)	Any T N1 M0	Metastasis to one lymph node ≤ 2 cm in dimension
IV (B2) (B3)	Any T N2 N3 M0	Metastasis to one lymph node 2–5 cm in size or multiple lymph nodes < 5 cm Metastasis to lymph node ≥ 5 cm in diameter
(C) or	Any T Any N M1	Distant metastases

*American Urological Association staging in parentheses.

Table 13-1. Risk Factors for Testicular Cancers

Genetic Factors
Association of Lewis antigen Le(a-b-) with germ cell tumors [2]
Association of HLABw41 with seminoma [3,4]

Acquired Factors
Cryptorchidism (relative risk of 7.4) [5]
Exposure to diethylstilbesterol in utero (relative risk 9.8) [6]
Decreased risk with birth order (for fourth or later child compared to first-born a relative risk of 0.3) [7]
Occupational exposure to extreme temperature (odds ratio 1.7) [8]

Table 13-3. Prognostic Factors for Patients with Stage I Testicular Cancers

Preoperative α-fetoprotein
Vascular invasion
Absence of teratoma

From Klepp et al. [9]; with permission.

Clinical outcome for minimal and moderate-stage metastatic germ cell cancer remains excellent, with 3-year survival rates of approximately 98% and 92%, respectively. A high percentage (≈ 90%) of advanced-stage metastatic cancers enters complete remission, with approximately 85% of patients free of disease at 2 years.

Primary Disease Therapy

There is no controversy about the appropriate initial diagnostic and therapeutic approach to suspected testicular malignancies (Table 13-5). An inguinal orchiectomy allows for control of blood and lymphatic vessels and en bloc removal of the affected testicle. Trans-scrotal biopsies or orchiectomy may lead to locoregional recurrences in as many as one quarter of patients and are therefore discouraged. Lymphatic pathways from the testicle pass first to the periaortic and preaortic lymph nodes on the left and interaortocaval, preaortic, and precaval lymph nodes on the right. Identifying the sympathetic nerves that supply the ejaculatory muscles and understanding which nodal groups are likely to be involved with tumor have allowed for an effective and more limited retroperitoneal lymph node dissection (RPLND), a procedure that preserves fertility. Laparoscopic technique for lymph node dissections has become available. As this technique becomes more popular, its role in evaluation of nodal status must be assessed.

Adjuvant Therapy for Regional Disease

The success of platinum-based multichemotherapy for the treatment of nonseminomatous testicular cancers has provided the foundation for the treatment of early-stage disease as well. The question in stage I nonseminomatous disease following inguinal orchiectomy and demonstration of no other metastases by serologic, radiologic, and physical examination is whether to do an elective RPLND or recommend surveillance. Studies of surveillance suggest that disease progression occurs in approximately 30% of patients and frequently presents with bulkier disease. Embryonal, yolk sac, and choriocarcinomatous histologic elements are highly prone to metastatic spread. Venous or lymphatic invasion and tumor outside the tunica albuginea or involving the epididymis (T2) suggest a tumor with the ability to metastasize. Vessel invasion was the single most important histologic risk factor in a report by the Testicular Cancer Intergroup Study. People with these findings are poor candidates for surveillance [12].

Approximately 25% of patients who undergo RPLND for clinical stage I disease have evidence of microscopic metastases. Approximately 10% to 15% of patients undergoing RPLND relapse with cancer, usually outside the operative field. Randomized studies have shown that two cycles of cisplatin, etoposide, and bleomycin (PEB) chemotherapy following RPLND for pathologic stage II disease yield a cure in approximately 98% of patients. Management of low-volume stage II disease (stage IIa, stage IIb, and patients with persistent marker elevation after orchiectomy) continued to generate considerable controversy. Lack of randomized, well-conducted studies and small sizes of prospective analyses have not clarified the controversies. One area of consensus is to reduce the type and number of therapies to minimize toxicity and cost.

Identification of factors that would predict benefit of combined RPLND and drug therapy could reduce the use of combined therapy by as much as 68% to 71% [13,14]. Baniel et al. [15] compared the direct costs, toxicity, and quality of life for nonseminomatous stage IIa/IIb cancers treated with primary RPLND plus adjuvant chemotherapy or cisplatin-based chemotherapy alone. They found that primary RPLND plus chemotherapy is equivalent to chemotherapy in producing 5-year disease-free status but is associated with lower overall rates of morbidity and mortality, lost weeks of work, and better fertility. If needed, postchemotherapy nerve-sparing RPLND is considerably more difficult and is associated with a decreased likelihood of preserving ejaculatory function.

Primary RPLND should be considered for patients with clinical stage IIa or IIb nonseminomatous germ cell tumors of the testes. Two cycles of cisplatin-based adjuvant chemotherapy following surgery are employed if tumor markers drop to normal levels.

The exception to this approach includes patients with large retroperitoneal masses (> 5 cm), high percentage of embryonal carcinoma, vascular invasion in primary tumor, or in multiple large lymph nodes where three cycles of PEB is curative therapy in more than 95% of patients.

Table 13-4. Indiana Staging System for Metastatic Testicular Malignancies

Minimal disease
Elevated βhCG and or α-fetoprotein
Palpable cervical nodes with or without nonpalpable retroperitoneal nodes
Unresectable, but nonpalpable, retroperitoneal nodes
Less than five metastatic lesions per lung field with none > 2 cm in largest diameter, with or without nonpalpable retroperitoneal nodes

Moderate disease
Palpable abdominal mass as only anatomical disease
Five to ten pulmonary metastases per lung field < 3 cm in largest diameter, or a mediastinal mass < 50% of the intrathoracic diameter, or a solitary pulmonary metastasis > 2 cm in largest diameter with or without nonpalpable retroperitoneal nodes

Advanced disease
Mediastinal mass > 50% of the intrathoracic diameter, or > 10 pulmonary nodules per lung field, or multiple pulmonary metastases > 3 cm with or without nonpalpable retroperitoneal nodes
A palpable abdominal mass with any pulmonary or intrathoracic metastases
Liver, bone, or CNS metastases

Other factors identified with poor outcome [12]
α-Fetoprotein > 500 IU/L
βhCG > 1000 IU/L
Age > 35 y

Factors associated with poor outcome in patients with low-volume disease (ie, minimal disease)
α-Fetoprotein > 1000 IU/L
βhCG > 10,000 IU/L

Adapted from Birch et al. [10] and Aass et al. [11]; with permission.

Table 13-5. Management of Early-Stage Primary Testicular Disease

Inguinal orchiectomy
Surveillance for good candidates
RPLND for nonseminomatous tumors to determine adjuvant chemotherapy
For seminoma, radiotherapy to nodal groups at risk

RPLND—retroperitoneal lymph node dissection.

Finally, patients with persistent elevation of tumor markers postorchicctomy in what otherwise appears to be stage I disease (so called "IIm") should be considered for primary chemotherapy because this may represent systemic rather than nodal metastases [16]. Newer markers and histopathologic factors may identify high-risk patients in this category, which allow for a more selective approach to adjuvant therapy.

Active Agents for Advanced Disease

Modern multiagent chemotherapy has had a significant impact on the treatment of testicular tumors. Whereas early trials demonstrated antitumor activity for actinomycin-D, vinblastine, and bleomycin, it was not until introduction of cisplatin in the mid-1970s that high reproducible cure rates were achieved. Cisplatin, velban, and bleomycin (PVB) came to comprise the most commonly used standard regimen. Toxicity of PVB chemotherapy was principally due to the high dose of vinblastine (0.4 mg/kg). Subsequent trials evaluated lower doses of vinblastine and led to a comparative randomized study of PVB chemotherapy versus PEB (cisplatin, etoposide, and bleomycin). This study demonstrated a significant reduction of toxicity for the PEB arm with equal or better response and survival rates (83% complete response [CR] for PEB vs 71% CR for PVB). Reduction in toxicity continues to be the focus of much clinical research. A multicenter, randomized trial compared the efficacy and toxicity of four cycles of carboplatin and etoposide versus cisplatin and etoposide in 270 patients with good-risk metastatic germ cell tumor [17]. Carboplatin doses ranged from 350 mg/m^2 to 500 mg/m^2. The carboplatin regimen was associated with greater hematologic toxicity, more relapses from CR, and lower event-free survival compared with the cisplatin-based therapy.

The feasibility of removing bleomycin from PEB chemotherapy was tested in a randomized study. The Eastern Cooperative Oncology Group (ECOG) study evaluating PEB versus cisplatin and etoposide (PE) in good-prognosis metastatic nonseminomatous cancers (minimal disease using Indiana staging) was discontinued after investigators noted that response rates were lower in the PE arm. A subsequent ECOG trial of three cycles of PEB (bleomycin 30 IU/wk for 9 weeks) versus four cycles of EP [18] again demonstrated superior relapse (23% vs 10%) and 3-year disease-free survival rates for the PEB arm. No cases of significant pulmonary toxicity were observed in either arm. The Australian Germ Cell Trial Group compared PVB with cisplatin and vinblastine (PV) in 222 patients with inoperable gonadal cancer. Patients were matched on prognostic risk factors. Minimum duration of follow-up was 4 years. Although relapse rates (7% for PV and 5% for PVB) and overall survival were not different for the two groups, tumor-related deaths occurred in 16 patients (15%) in the PV group and 6 patients (5%) in the PVB arm (P=0.02). Although toxicity was greater in the PVB arm, it was concluded that bleomycin significantly enhanced the therapeutic benefit of cisplatin and vinblastine [19]. Thus, the weight of the evidence at this time favors the continued inclusion of bleomycin in the treatment of good-risk metastatic germ cell tumors.

Response rates in metastatic seminoma to platinum-based combination chemotherapy regimens have proved to be as good as response rates in nonseminomatous cancers, with better than 80% cure rates. This has led to a rethinking of recommendations for radiotherapy, which was previously employed for the treatment of early-stage seminoma. Initial treatment of stage I and II disease has consisted of involved- and extended-field radiation therapy. Trials of radiation therapy for stage II disease reveal a 70% to 90% 5-year survival. In stage II disease, approximately 30% of patients have failures outside the radiation ports. Salvage of treatment failures with combination chemotherapy may be compromised by radiation damage to the bone marrow. We suggest treating stage II seminoma patients with evidence of residual cancer with initial chemotherapy followed by radiation therapy. Treatment strategies for stage I seminoma are more controversial. It appears that prophylactic radiation of the mediastinum does not provide survival advantage and adds to morbidity and late toxicity, as well as causing difficulty in administering chemotherapy at a later time if needed. Inguinal orchiectomy and postsurgery radiation therapy to abdominal lymph nodes are associated with 5-year survival of better than 98%. Chemotherapy is reserved for the few patients who have relapses.

With the use of platinum-based multiagent chemotherapy, extragonadal testicular tumors are treated with success that equals, stage for stage, that seen in primary gonadal tumors that have metastasized [20].

Options do exist for metastatic germ cell tumors of the testis that are refractory to or recur after cisplatin-based chemotherapy. Salvage chemotherapy (consisting of ifosfamide, cisplatin, and either vinblastine or etoposide) can cure up to 25% of these patients [21]. Use of high-dose carboplatin and paclitaxel (Taxol) with stem cell rescue in addition to cisplatin-based salvage chemotherapy in patients with refractory or recurrent disease [22] appears promising. Of 25 patients with a median follow-up, 56% were free from disease. High-dose chemotherapy with stem cell rescue is a viable option for refractory or recurrent malignancy but should be carried out in an experienced center.

Long-term follow-up for patients with testicular cancers should include evaluation for secondary leukemia in patients treated with chemotherapy, and solid organ malignancies, such as gastric carcinoma, in patients who received abdominal radiation therapy.

PROSTATE CANCER
Etiology and Risk Factors

Therapy for prostate cancer continues to generate controversy. A significant number of men are diagnosed with this cancer and die from their illness each year. In the United States, 180,400 men with prostate cancer will be diagnosed in 2000, and 39,200 deaths will be attributed to this disease. In autopsy studies, 30% of men between the ages of 50 and 70 years with no overt evidence of prostate cancer before death had evidence of prostate carcinoma. Prostate cancer risk factors (Table 13-6) include first-degree relatives with prostate

Table 13-6. Etiology and Risk Factors for Prostate Cancer

Age [23]

Race [23]

Family history [23]

Suspected but not yet fully accepted risk factors

Vasectomy (methodologic issues remain in the major studies evaluating vasectomy and prostate cancer) [24]

Dietary fat [25]

5-α reductase activity [26]

Socioeconomic status [27]

Cadmium [28]

cancer, race (in the United States), testosterone level, vasectomy, monounsaturated fat intake, and other dietary factors.

For the most part, prostate cancers are slow growing and metastasize late in their natural history. This presents to the treating clinician a therapeutic dilemma in patients with early-stage disease: which patients will have aggressive cancers needing treatment, and which will have indolent disease requiring no further therapy? Furthermore, if treatment is chosen, which treatment will provide the best outcome with the least morbidity? Although radical prostatectomy and radiotherapy have remained the keystones for initial therapy for early-stage prostate cancers (I and II), recent outcome analyses have questioned these approaches, raising more questions than answers [29,30]. These controversies over treatment for early-stage prostate cancer will continue; treatment for metastatic disease remains palliative, but the issue of when to begin therapy is unresolved.

Screening

Early diagnosis of prostate cancer is the focus of numerous screening modalities, including digital rectal examination, transrectal ultrasound, and serum prostate-specific antigen. No study has documented that screening affects overall survival from prostate cancer [31,32]. Furthermore, the controversy over treatment requirements for early-stage disease causes increasing difficulty in assessing the role of screening. Currently, the American Cancer Society, the National Cancer Institute, and the US Preventive Services Task Force recommends that information about prostate-specific antigen (PSA) and digital rectal examination (DRE) screening be made available to all men over the age of 50, or in high-risk individuals over the age of 40.

Assessment of PSA levels using 4 ng/mL as the upper limits of normal has been shown to improve prostate cancer detection [32]. Free PSA and other members of the human kallikrein gene family are also useful in the diagnosis of prostate cancer [33]. A survey of practicing urologists who are members of the American Urological Association (AUA) found that screening for prostate cancer was recommended for men between the ages of 50 and 80 years [34].

Staging and Prognosis

With early diagnosis comes the dilemma of identifying clinically aggressive cancer that causes significant morbidity by metastasizing or premature death. Except for invasion outside the capsule of the gland (T3, stage C) and histologic grade, which portend a bad prognosis, other factors have failed to delineate aggressive from indolent disease further, which causes considerable difficulty in interpreting screening results and confounding treatment decision (Tables 13-7 and 13-8).

Prostate cancer patients are evaluated with technetium pyrophosphate bone scan for patients with PSA above 10, chest radiography, computed tomography, or magnetic resonance imaging of the prostate and evaluation of blood work, including complete blood cell counts, coagulation profile measurement of tumor markers including prostate-specific antigen and lactate dehydrogenase. Usually, PSA alone, if elevated, is used in following patients with prostate cancer. Approximately 90% of nodal tissue can be examined using peritoneoscopy. The best clinical setting for the use of laparoscopic node dissection still needs to be determined. Another modality being tested for staging purposes is radiolabeled murine monoclonal antibodies. Small published series employing CYT-356 antibody (Prostascint; Cytogen, Princeton, NJ) suggest the use of this agent in detecting small microscopic foci. The U.S. Food and Drug Administration (FDA) has approved the use of Prostascint for detection of microscopic disease.

Table 13-7. Staging of Prostate Cancer

Stage*	TNM Staging	Criteria
0 (A1)	T1a	Tumor is incidental histologic finding in < 3 microscopic foci
(B1)	T2a	Tumor ≤ 1.5 cm with normal tissue on at least three sides in one lobe of the prostate gland
	N0	
	M0	
	G1	Well-differentiated cancer
I (A1)	T1a	
(B1)	or T2a	
	N0	
	M0	
	G2,G3–4	Moderately differentiated or poorly differentiated, respectively
II (A2)	T1b	Tumor is incidental histologic finding in > 3 microscopic foci
(B2)	or T2b	Tumor > 1.5 cm or in > 1 lobe
	N0	
	M0	
	Any G	
III (C1 or C2)	T3	Invasion of prostatic apex, or into or beyond prostatic capsule, bladder neck, or seminal vesicle, but not fixed
	N0	
	M0	
	Any G	
IV (C2)	T4	Tumor is fixed or invades adjacent structure other than those for T3
	N0	
	M0	
	Any G	
(D)	Any T	
	N1	Single lymph node, ≤ 2 cm involved with cancer
	N2	Metastasis in a single lymph node 2–5 cm in diameter or multiple lymph nodes < 5 cm
	N3	Metastasis to lymph node > 5 cm
	M0	
	Any G	
(D)	Any T	
	Any N	
	M1	Distant metastases
	Any G	

*American Urological Association staging in parentheses.

Table 13-8. Test for Evaluation of Prostate Cancer

Serum prostate-specific antigen

Chest radiograph

Bone scan

Computed tomography or magnetic resonance imaging of the pelvis and prostate

Coagulation profile

Lactate dehydrogenase

A new technique using reverse transcriptase-polymerase chain reaction (RT-PCR) allows the detection of circulating prostate cancer cells in the peripheral blood. RNA is extracted from 5 mL of circulating nucleated cells and, using primers for PSA, prostate cancer cells can be detected. This technique appears to be able to predict for capsular penetration with a sensitivity of approximately 67% and for detecting positive surgical margins with a sensitivity of approximately 87% [35]. A positive RT-PCR test result was found in 16 of 18 patients with metastatic disease. It is still too early to determine the ultimate utility of RT-PCR in the management of prostate cancer.

Patients with early-stage prostate cancers (A or B) and well- or moderately differentiated tumors have a 10-year survival of approximately 60% to 75%, whereas 20% to 40% of patients with poorly differentiated tumors may survive a decade. Fewer than half of patients with stage C disease may be expected to live 10 years or more. Gleason grade alone predicted for distant metastases in patients with D1 disease [36]. Gleason grades 8 to 10 correlated with rapid progression to distant metastases (85% at 5 years), whereas patients with a well- or moderately differentiated tumor had a 41% chance of distant metastases at 5 years.

Treatment of Early Stage Prostate Cancer

Initial treatment recommendations depend on clinical staging, radiographic findings, level of serum tumor markers, and histology. Assessment of clinical stage PSA level and histologic grade can be used to determine the likelihood of invasion outside the confines of the prostate gland or for metastatic spread. Survival of men with stage A1 (T1a) disease appears about the same as for age-matched controls and is followed with close observation and repeats biopsies of the prostate when clinically indicated. A mathematical model of patients with localized prostate cancer (A2, B1, B2, or T1b, T2a, T2b) suggests a benefit for therapeutic intervention (surgery or radiotherapy) only for men younger than 65 years. The model is provocative and suggests that a clinical trial should be performed to confirm to these predictions. The Prostate Intervention versus Observation Trial (PIVOT) for early-stage prostate cancer is being conducted as an intergroup study to address this question. The best initial treatment of stage A2 and B disease continues to be hotly debated between surgeons and radiotherapists. The only randomized study between radiation therapy and radical prostatectomy in patients with A2 and B disease was reported by Paulson *et al.* [37] in 1982, but it remains controversial owing to some methodologic concerns. Although the study suggests a survival advantage to surgery, the radiotherapy-treated patients appear to have a worse outcome than reported by other radiotherapy programs. The Veterans Administration Cooperative Urologic Research Group (VACURG) reported a small study of stage A and B patients randomly assigned to radical prostatectomy plus placebo versus placebo alone. Although there appeared to be a survival advantage for the patients treated in the placebo-alone arm, its small patient sample and high percentage of poorly differentiated tumors in the surgery arm flaw the study (there were none in the placebo arm). It is unlikely that an answer to this timeworn question is forthcoming in the foreseeable future.

Both surgical and radiation techniques continue to improve for the treatment of early-stage disease. One technique that most likely will yield a lower morbidity and higher dose of radiation is three-dimensional conformal radiotherapy, which allows specifically for more accurate delivery of the radiation dose. Recent attention has focused on the timing of adjuvant hormonal intervention.

Adjuvant Therapy for Regional Disease

Regional disease, defined as penetration through the capsule of the prostate gland (T3) with or without spread to neighboring organs (T4) or first-tier pelvic lymph nodes (N1), is incurable with surgical or radiotherapy techniques. Treatment choices must again reflect the natural history of the disease and development of symptoms. Several randomized studies have explored different schedules of adjuvant hormonal therapy with radiation treatment for patients with local advanced prostate cancer [38]. Goserelin 3.6 mg every 4 weeks for 3 years given in combination with 5 weeks of pelvic radiation (50 Gy with a 2-week boost of 20 Gy) and cyproterone acetate 150 mg for 1 month improved 5-year overall survival by 17% compared with radiation therapy alone. Even more striking was an 85% disease-free survival for the adjuvant hormone group compared with 48% in the radiotherapy group. The choice of adjuvant/hormonal therapy and the length of treatment have not yet been optimally defined. In a recent report, 98 men undergoing radical prostatectomy with positive nodes, were randomized to receive immediate antiandrogen therapy (gosorelin or orchiectomy) or observation. At a medium follow up of 7.1 years, 7 of 47 patients in the treatment group died compared with 18 of 51 deaths in the surgery only group. In this subset of men, adjuvant hormonal therapy improves overall survival and disease-free survival [39].

Active Single Agents for Advanced Disease

Hormone therapy using castration or estrogens has been considered standard therapy for D2 disease since the observations in the 1940s by Huggins and Hodges that hormonal intervention causes improvement in symptoms from bone metastases and decrease in alkaline phosphatase. With the advent of newer hormonal agents, the question of the optimal hormonal therapy must be addressed. Historically, the VACURG series of randomized studies provided the data supporting hormonal intervention as an effective therapy and determined the optimal dose of diethylstilbestrol. In addition, orchiectomy was found to be equivalent to diethylstilbestrol but without the cardiovascular complications associated with estrogen administration. These studies focused on surgical or medical castration. With the understanding that prostate cancer is under hormonal regulation, blockade of the adrenal source of testosterone with agents such as ketoconazole or cyproterone acetate was used as second-line therapy with only limited success. The concept of complete androgen blockade was introduced by Labrie *et al.* [40] and with the advent of both luteinizing hormone–releasing hormone (LHRH) agonists (or orchiectomy) and dihydrotestosterone receptor blockers, the question could be studied. A randomized, double-blind study evaluating the combination of flutamide and leuprolide versus leuprolide and placebo demonstrated a statistically significant superior progression-free and overall survival in favor of total androgen blockade, although the advantage was small. Because leuprolide and goserelin are LHRH agonists, initial stimulation of the pituitary-testis axis may cause a disease flare resulting in worsening symptoms, or in extremely rare isolated cases it may cause sudden death. We suggest the addition of flutamide or bicalutamide to begin concomitantly with LHRH agonists to prevent disease flare.

A meta-analysis performed by the Prostate Cancer Trialists' Collaborative Group analyzed 5710 patients from 22 randomized trials. They were unable to show any benefit of complete androgen blockade compared with surgical or medical castration [41]. A subsequent meta-analysis study by Caubet *et al.* [42] evaluated nine randomized studies demonstrating an improvement in overall survival and an increase in time-to-progression for maximum androgen blockade compared with monotherapy (orchiectomy vs LHRH). Furthermore, this study suggested an advantage for nonsteroidal antiandrogens over steroidal antiandrogens. These studies continue the ongoing controversy regarding the most appropriate hormonal therapy for metastatic prostate cancer.

There has been a suggestion of survival advantage with hormone therapy in the VACURG study, which compared placebo with three different doses of diethylstilbestrol in the treatment of advanced disease. A retrospective analysis of patients treated according to the ECOG prostate protocols suggested that continued androgen blockade despite progression of disease was associated with better survival.

The discovery of receptors for other growth factors, such as epidermal growth factor receptor (EGFr), provides a foundation for alternative treatment strategies. Suramin sodium is a polysulfonated naphthylurea used to treat African trypanosomiasis and onchocerciasis and has been found to bind the EGFr and block growth. Initial successes in clinical trials have not been completely fulfilled in larger randomized studies.

Finasteride, a 5-α-reductase, has been found to have moderate effects in patients with metastatic prostate carcinoma [43]. In a pilot study of 10 men with either stage C or D disease, the combination of finasteride and flutamide significantly decreased PSA. Eighty percent of the men remained potent, however, suggesting that this combination of hormone therapy may provide clinical benefit while allowing the patient to maintain potency [44].

Chemotherapy advances for metastatic prostate cancer patients have been encouraging, with high response rates and significant palliation of cancer-related symptoms. Mitoxantrone plus hydrocortisone has no survival benefit over hydrocortisone alone, but does improve time to treatment failure and improved cancer related pain [45]. The observation that estramustine inhibits mitosis through disrupting microtubules lead to a series of combination chemotherapies with excellent tolerance and activity in metastatic prostate cancer patients. Vinblastine (4 mg/m^2 IV weekly × 6 weeks) and estramustine (600 mg/m^2 PO daily × 6 weeks) gave a 30% response rate with improvement in symptoms [46]. Other combinations have included oral etoposide (50 mg/m^2/d) and estramustine (15 mg/kg/d) for 3 weeks. This combination produced a 53% response rate and was a well-tolerated regimen [47]. Most recently, paclitaxel (120 mg/m^2 over 96-hour continuous infusion) with estramustine (600 mg/m^2 daily) caused a 53% response rate but with greater than grade 2 toxicity in approximately one third of patients [48]. More recently, docetaxel has also been used either as a single agent or in combination with estramustine. Thus, it appears that estramustine-based combination therapies have a beneficial effect in patients with hormone-refractory prostate cancer. Much patient attention has been focused on the use of a Chinese herbal therapy, PC-SPES. This commercially available material contains extracts of eight herbs and has phytoestrogenetic effects. We have observed anecdotal PSA and objective responses in both hormone-sensitive and refractory patients. Although small series have reported PSA responses and improvement of quality of life [49], further study of this agent is warranted.

One of the most devastating complications for prostate cancer is the pain and dysfunction from bone metastases. External beam irradiation is useful in palliating isolated bone metastases. Unfortunately, patients with metastatic prostate cancer usually have multiple bone metastases. Two new approaches to the treatment of bone disease using radiation include hemibody irradiation and the use of bone-seeking compounds such as ^{89}Sr or ^{186}Re-hydroxyethylidene diphosphonate. Phase I and II studies of hemibody irradiation explored doses from 6 to 10 Gy and found the most effective dose for pain control to be 6 Gy for the upper body and 8 Gy for the middle and lower body. Delay in progression of bone metastases and a delay in the appearance of new disease within the field of hemibody irradiation have been seen in patients with breast and prostate cancer. Toxicities included hematologic effects, nausea, vomiting, diarrhea, anorexia, xerostomia, and loss of sense of taste.

^{89}Sr is a pure β-emitting radionuclide that follows the calcium metabolic pathways. The use of ^{89}Sr to treat malignant disease was first reported by Lawrence et al. in 1950 for multiple myeloma. Robinson et al. [50] reported palliative benefit in patients with osseous prostate cancer metastases. Porter and McEwan [51] confirmed the palliative nature of ^{89}Sr at 30 to 60 mCi/kg, a dose that does not result in toxicities.

Samarium-153 EDTMP (ethylene-diamine-tetramethylene-phosphonic acid) is a new radiopharmaceutical bone-seeking agent that has been reported to cause significant improvement in bone pain from metastasis [52].

TRANSITIONAL CELL CARCINOMA OF THE UROTHELIUM
Etiology and Risk Factors
Three major histologic types of cancers arise from the urothelium. Squamous cell and adenocarcinomas of the bladder present a different clinical and therapeutic problem and are not discussed here.

The major risk factor for transitional cell carcinoma remains tobacco use, particularly in association with a slow acetylator phenotype and exposure to β-naphthylamine (Table 13-9). Although dietary factors have been implicated in bladder cancer formation, there is no definitive evidence to date. Animal studies suggested that saccharin consumption is associated with the development of bladder tumors in the rat, but recent meta-analyses do not implicate this substance in bladder tumor formation in humans. Chlorine has been implicated in the carcinogenesis of bladder cancer. Meta-analysis has confirmed that the consumption of higher chlorinated water (chlorination by-products) is associated with a 1.21 relative risk for bladder cancer.

Screening tests for bladder cancer have not yet been developed fully. Preliminary results from the Drake Health Registry suggest that in high-risk people exposed to β-naphthylamine, screening with Papanicolaou cytology, fluorescence image analysis, measurement of urinary nuclear native proteins, urinary fibrin/fibrinogen degradation products, and urinalysis may be capable of identifying early changes, although the specificity of these changes is uncertain [53].

Staging and Prognosis
Transitional cell carcinoma of the bladder may be distinguished according to whether the tumor is superficial or invasive. Superficial tumors of the bladder represent local disease with little or no capability for metastasis and thus can be treated with local therapies. Histologic grading, tumor type (papillary or carcinoma in situ), muscle invasion, and differentiation are important clinicopathologic features that should be evaluated (Table 13-10).

Recurrence of superficial tumors (stage 0 or stage 1) and the need for intravesical therapy are determined by grade, tumor size, and whether multiple tumors are present [61]. True squamous differentiation in the tumor usually predicts for poor response to systemic chemotherapy.

Indices of proliferation and genetic markers are being studied as indicators for progression of superficial tumors (EGFr, p53, pRB, c-*erg*-2, nuclear matrix, metalloproteinases, and E-cadherin) [62,63]. Nuclear accumulation of p53 has been associated with tumor recurrences and tumor progression in transitional cell carcinoma of the bladder. A multivariable analysis of grade pathologic stage, lymph node status, and nuclear p53 status confirmed p53 overexpression as an independent predictor [62]. A study by Lacombe *et al.* [63] analyzed 196 tissue specimens from 98 patients (before and after treatment with intravesical bacille Calmette-Guérin [BCG]) for mutant nuclear p53 overexpression using immunohistochemistry and the relative risk of disease progression in patients with >20% expression of p53 in pretreatment samples. Although p53 expression could not predict response to BCG in patients who did not respond, it was strongly predictive of disease progression. Thus, patients with refractory tumors and mutant p53 overexpression should be considered candidates for cystectomy.

Primary Disease Therapy

Most uroepithelial tumors present with either gross or microscopic hematuria. Urinary cytology is an important part of the evaluation. Full assessment of the uroepithelium is indicated and is accomplished with cystoscopy and IV or retrograde pyelography. Transurethral resection of the bladder tumor (TURBT) is the initial treatment. Intravesical therapy is usually considered for high-grade tumors, carcinoma in situ, or recurrent low-grade tumors. Recent genetic evaluation of multiple simultaneous tumors arising in women suggests a clonal origin and the probability that tumors arose from a single cell that seeded other areas of uroepithelium. This process has been well established in experimental animal models.

Treatment for superficial bladder cancers is directed not only at tumor regression but also at reduction of the subsequent recurrence rate and prevention of tumor invasion. TURBT alone, for low-grade papillary transitional cell carcinoma, or in combination with intravesical chemotherapy and immunotherapy, can control local superficial tumor and prevent recurrences and invasion. Many therapeutic agents have been used in the treatment of superficial disease. BCG is considered the best of these agents, although its use is not without associated morbidity.

Herr *et al.* [64] performed a 10-year follow-up of a prospective randomized control trial comparing TURBT alone versus TURBT and intravesical BCG. The median time to progression had not been reached in the BCG-treated group, and 10-year progression-free survival was 61.9% versus 38% in the TURBT-alone group. It should be noted that all patients who received BCG experienced cystitis. A published 15-year update of this group found no significant differences with regard to overall progression rates and disease-specific survival [65]. In addition, there was a 31% incidence of upper tract tumors after a median of 7.3 years of follow-up. Although small (86 patients), this study demonstrates the necessity of close follow-up for extended periods, despite the initial advantage shown in the BCG-treated group.

Thiotepa, mitomycin C, and doxorubicin are the most common intravesical chemotherapies employed today and have been shown to be effective and safe agents. Burnand *et al.* [66] reported a randomized trial demonstrating that a single dose of thiotepa (90 mg over 30 minutes) can reduce recurrences by 40% at 1 year of follow-up compared with TURBT alone. Weekly thiotepa given for established superficial tumor can cause complete regression in approximately 30% of cases. The low molecular weight of thiotepa allows absorption across the bladder epithelium and may cause toxicity, specifically mild leukoneutropenia.

Mitomycin C appears to give the same clinical results as thiotepa, with less risk of leukoneutropenia but with increased risk for bladder irritation. Among intravesical chemotherapy agents, doxorubicin appears to give the best response rates in patients with established tumors, with a CR rate as high as 66%.

A randomized study of 262 patients with stage Ta and T1 papillary tumors or carcinoma in situ treated with either doxorubicin or

Table 13-9. Risk Factors for Transitional Cell Carcinoma

ß-Napthylamine
Tobacco [54]
Slow acetylator phenotype [55]
Chlorination by-products [56]
Diet (questionable) [57–60]
  High caloric intake from fat in those < 65 y
  Decrease risk with consumption of carotenoid in those < 65 y
  High sodium intake

Table 13-10. Staging of Transitional Cell Carcinoma of Urinary Badder

Stage*	TNM Staging	Criteria
0	Tis	Carcinoma in situ
	Ta	Noninvasive papillary cancer
	N0	
	M0	
I	T1	Invasion of subepithelial connective tissue
(A)	N0	
	M0	
II	T2	Invasion of muscle not extending beyond the inner half
(B1)	N0	
	M0	
III	T3a	Invasion of deep muscle—outer half of the bladder wall
(B2)	T3b	Invasion of perivesical fat
	N0	
	M0	
IV	T4	Invasion of neighboring anatomical structures: prostate, uterus, vagina, pelvic wall, abdominal wall
(C)		
	N0	
	M0	
	or	
(D)	Any T	
	N1	Metastasis to a single lymph node ≤ 2 cm
	N2	Metastasis to a single lymph node 2–5 cm in size or multiple lymph nodes < 5 cm in diameter
	N3	Metastasis in any lymph node > 5 cm in diameter
	M0	
	or	
	Any T	
	Any N	
	M1	Distant metastasis

*American Urological Association staging in parentheses.

BCG was reported by Lamm et al. [67]. Estimated 5-year disease-free survival was 17% for the doxorubicin-treated patients and 37% for BCG-treated patients with Ta or T1 lesions without carcinoma in situ (P=0.015). The median time to treatment failure in patients with carcinoma in situ was 5.1 months for doxorubicin and 39 months for BCG. Estimated 5-year disease-free survival in patients with carcinoma in situ was 18% for doxorubicin and 45% for BCG.

In a randomized prospective trial of 337 patients with high-risk superficial bladder tumors, Krege et al. [68] compared TURBT alone versus resection with BCG or resection with mitomycin-C. All patients underwent complete resection before starting intravesical therapy. Both groups treated with intravesical therapy had a lower relative risk of recurrence. Although there was no significant difference in the rates of progression between the two treatment groups, mitomycin-C demonstrated an initial modest advantage in patients with recurrent tumors. Side effects were more common with BCG. Thus, it seems reasonable to consider mitomycin-C intravesical therapy, especially in the context of recurrence. Other forms of intravesical immunotherapy, specifically interferon-alfa (IFN-α), appear to have benefits in superficial bladder cancer as well. We have conducted pilot studies of intravesical tumor necrosis factor. Although this agent can be given with a high degree of safety, clinical benefit has not yet been proven. Use of high dose intravesical IFN-α has also been explored in superficial bladder cancer. Little toxicity has been observed and although inferior to BCG or mitomycin C as first line therapy, its role as a single agent or in combination with other agents, is still being explored. Other agents and methods for intravesical therapies that are being explored include use of targeting antibodies, genetically modified BCG, and newer chemotherapy drugs.

Phototherapy for superficial bladder tumors is an alternative treatment but has not been tested against standard agents. Phototherapy employs laser treatments with photosensitizing agents, such as photofrin and polyporphyrin. This approach is under investigation in refractory superficial tumors.

Adjuvant Therapy for Regional Disease

The current standard therapy for locally invasive transitional cell carcinoma of the bladder remains cystectomy. The patient's risk of relapse depends on the depth of invasion into the wall of the bladder. Overall, there is a 40% to 60% chance of failure from cystectomy alone, raising the question of the need and effectiveness of adjuvant therapies. New pathologic techniques are becoming available to help distinguish metastatic potential of invasive bladder cancers, which include measurements of p53, NM23 RNA levels, DNA ploidy, and expression of the antigen T138 on the cell surface. Much recent work has been published regarding the use of concomitant chemotherapy with radiation and TURBT as a means of providing effective local and systemic therapy while preserving an intact bladder. Primary radiation therapy has a 5-year survival of 20% to 40% and results in dismal local control [69]. Based on in vitro data, the National Cancer Institute of Canada tested cisplatin plus radiation versus radiation alone in a randomized clinical trail [70]. Patients randomized to the chemotherapy group got three cycles of concomitant cisplatin at 100 mg/m² every 21 days with their radiation. There were no significant differences between the groups with regard to response, overall survival or progression-free survival, but there was significantly better local control with concomitant cisplatin and a trend toward better bladder preservation.

The role of radiotherapy combined with multiagent chemotherapy has been explored by Kaufman et al. [71]. A pilot study of 53 patients demonstrated a 77% survival rate at 54 months [72]. Pilot data from a protocol of complete transurethral resection, and outpatient multidrug chemotherapy followed by a short course of high-dose split-fraction radiotherapy, has shown similar excellent results with a 70% CR rate [73]. A phase I/II Southwestern Oncology Group (SWOG) study demonstrated that combination TURBT systemic therapy (methotrexate, vinblastine, cisplatin) and pelvic radiation (with concurrent cisplatin) could result in a combined CR of 56% (19 of 34 patients in this series). CR and improved survival with this protocol were associated with minimally invasive disease (T2 more than T3,4), lack of nodal involvement, complete resection at TURBT, and completion with as much planned chemotherapy as possible. However, local control was suboptimal in this trial with 11 of 19 complete responders experiencing local recurrence. Toxicity levels were acceptable.

The RTOG reported a phase II trial evaluation bladder preservation for invasive disease, using two cycles of methotrexate, cisplatin, and vinblastine (MCV) after incomplete resection followed by concomitant radiation and cisplatin in 91 patients [74]. Patients not entering a complete remission went to immediate cystectomy. If CR was achieved, the patient received a third cycle of cisplatin with consolidating radiation. The CR rate was 80% in this study, with an actuarial 4-year survival of 62% and an actuarial survival at 4 years of 44% with the bladder intact. Cystectomy ultimately was required in 40% (37 of 91). Toxicity was high, however, with 12% rate of leukopenia and 16 cases of severe delayed toxicity.

A group at MGH published a trial of 106 patients treated with as complete a TURBT as possible followed by the aforementioned RTOG regimen [75]. Only if the patients achieved T0 status, as in the RTOG trial, could they go on to cisplatin plus radiotherapy instead of cystectomy. The CR rate was 66%, and the 5-year actuarial survival was 52%, with 43% surviving with intact bladders. The 5-year freedom from invasive bladder recurrence was 79%. The survival figures were inversely proportional to stage with clinical T2 disease faring the best. In patients with T3 to T4 disease, the presence of hydronephrosis at study predicted poorer outcome. Toxicity, as in the RTOG trial, was substantial, with significant incidences of leukopenia and gastrointestinal toxicities.

Although large multicenter phase III trials have not definitively answered the questions regarding the ultimate utility of these combined-modality bladder-preserving approaches, it seems reasonable to offer this approach to patients unable or unwilling to undergo cystectomy. Common features of success from the above trials include resection of as much visible tumor as possible, completion of as much MCV as possible (given the toxicity), early stage (ie, T2), and lack of hydronephrosis. Should the patient not experience a CR, reconsideration of cystectomy is mandated. Although theoretical concerns regarding surgery after chemoradiation rationally exist, there are not current studies that demonstrate an increased complication rate, and none were reported in the above trials [74].

The role of adjuvant or neoadjuvant chemotherapy has not been definitively proven. Preliminary reports of randomized trials suggest that cisplatin-based multiagent chemotherapy may have a significant impact on the treatment of high-risk invasive bladder cancer. Stockle et al. [76] reported a study of 49 patients with pathologically staged T3b and T4a bladder cancer with or without lymph node involvement randomized to receive methotrexate, vinblastine (or epirubicin), doxorubicin, and cisplatin following cystectomy or cystectomy alone. Although time of follow-up is limited, only three of 18 patients treated with adjuvant chemotherapy have relapsed compared with 18 of 23 patients in the control arm. Freiha *et al.* [77] conducted a randomized control trial comparing radical cystectomy alone to radical cystectomy followed by four cycles of MCV-like chemotherapy in patients with pT3b or pT4 disease with or without nodal involvement. Twenty-five patients from each group were evaluable at 5 years. Of note, patients in the observation group received MCV therapy at first sign of recurrence. The recurrence rate in the adjuvant group was 48% (12 of 25 patients) versus 76% in the observation group. Although there was significant freedom from progression in the chemotherapy group, no difference was found in rates of overall survival. The authors contributed the latter finding to the crossover allowed in the design, indicating the benefit from chemotherapy could be seen with delayed treatment as well. Trials involving neoadjuvant multiagent cisplatin-based chemotherapy have been completed [78–80]. In a moderately size randomized clinical trial, the Radiation Therapy Oncology Group evaluated the role of two cycles of neoadjuvant MCV in muscle-invading bladder cancer treated with bladder preserving radiation. Patients received either MCV before radiation/cisplatin therapy or radiation/cisplatin therapy alone. Survival rates for the two arms were identical (5-year actuarial survival rates were 48% and 49%, respectively). A major criticism of the study is that overall only 74% of the patients completed the course of therapy: 67% in the neoadjuvant arm and 81% in the radiation/cisplatin alone arm [80].

In a study of 976 patients with T2, G3, T3, T4a N0-x or N0 who received either cystectomy or radiation for primary treatment ± 3 cycles of MCV neoadjuvant therapy, no improvement in 3-year survival rate was seen. Median follow-up in this study was 4 years [79].

These data suggest that the adjuvant or neoadjuvant therapy for invasive bladder cancer requires four or more cycles of multiagent chemotherapy with currently available agents. Newer agents, particularly gemcitabine and the taxanes, have encouraging activity in metastatic disease and will thus need to be tested in the adjuvant setting.

Chemotherapy for Advanced Disease

Advances in chemotherapy have been sought in the setting of metastatic transitional cell carcinoma of the urinary bladder. Phase II studies of single agents demonstrated significant activity (> 15%) for methotrexate, vinblastine, doxorubicin, cisplatin, and 5-fluorouracil. Until quite recently, cisplatin had been the single best agent and is currently the cornerstone of combination chemotherapy regimens. The most commonly used combinations today are M-VAC and MCV. M-VAC was found to be superior to cisplatin alone (objective response rates of 33% vs 15%, respectively; *P*=0.001) in a randomized ECOG trial evaluating the treatment of metastatic bladder cancer [81].

Concerns regarding the toxicity of cisplatin, especially in patients with baseline renal insufficiency, have led several investigators to explore the efficacy of carboplatin-based regimens. Based on phase II trials illustrating equivalent results with carboplatin and carboplatin-based therapies, Bellmunt [82] published a randomized control trial comparing standard MVAC with the carboplatin-based regimen M-CAVI (methotrexate, carboplatin at dose AUC of 5, and vinblastine). This study was stopped prematurely when it was clear that MVAC therapy had a clear survival advantage over that of M-CAVI. Response rates favored MVAC as well, but this was not significant (52% vs 39%, respectively, with three CRs in the MVAC arm). Toxicity, however, was clearly more frequent with MVAC. Given the favorable toxicity of M-CAVI, it is possible that an AUC of 5 was inadequate. The absence of doxorubicin could have also played a role in the observed differences. More trials are anticipated.

In an attempt to improve the toxicity profile on M-VAC, colony-stimulating factors have been employed. Although granulocyte colony-stimulating factor and granulocyte–macrophage colony-stimulating factor can reduce the length of leukoneutropenia and improve mucositis, response and survival rates have not differed significantly.

Nevertheless, the search for more active agents has proceeded. A phase II trial published by ECOG studied the activity of paclitaxel (a novel agent that blocks depolymerization of microtubules) in patients with previously untreated advanced transitional cell carcinoma of the bladder [83]. Twenty-six patients were treated with paclitaxel 250 mg/m^2 by 24-hour continuous infusion and granulocyte–macrophage colony-stimulating hormone support every 21 days until disease progression or intolerance. Forty-two percent of these patients demonstrated a response (11 of 26) with seven of 26 patients obtaining CR (27%), making paclitaxel the most active single agent against transitional cell carcinoma of the bladder studied thus far.

Several randomized studies have explored different multiagent chemotherapy regimens to improve response and to decrease toxicity in metastatic bladder cancer patients. In one study, a combination of methotrexate and vinblastine was clearly inferior to MCV [78]. Paclitaxel also has activity and has been used as a component of salvage therapy for metastatic disease [84]. In 405 patients, gemcitabine and cisplatin (GC) was found to be equivalent to MVAC therapy with regard to overall response, survival, and time to treatment failure [85]. GC was better tolerated.

RENAL CELL CARCINOMA

Etiology and Risk Factors

In 2000, approximately 31,200 people in the United States were diagnosed with renal cell carcinoma (RCC) and in about 50% of cases, the disease had not spread outside of the kidney at presentation. Although there are reports of long-term survivors with metastatic disease, the 5-year survival curves predict that virtually all patients will die from their disease by that time. Radical nephrectomy for local disease remains the only curative approach. Investigation of systemic therapies for RCC has provided insights into new treatment methods that may affect survival of a subset of patients.

Molecular genetic evaluation has provided greater insight into the nature of RCC. The most common chromosomal abnormality has been the loss of heterozygosity of 3p13-26, which is found in 66% to 98% of clear cell RCC tumors. Papillary tumors do not appear to have this abnormality. Patients with Hippel-Lindau disease have similar loss of heterozygosity of 3p. Further molecular genetic studies may uncover markers for metastatic behavior [88].

A causative relationship has been found between tobacco use and development of RCC. Beyond this major risk factor, obesity, analgesic abuse, and asbestos exposure have been linked with the development of RCC (Table 13-11). Use of Thorotrast as a contrast medium in the early part of the 20th century to visualize the kidney and liver has also been linked to the development of RCC. Other risk factors include acquired cystic disease of the kidney and end-stage renal failure.

Staging and Prognosis

Staging is presented in Table 13-12. Many prognostic schemes have been used to attempt to predict survival and outcome (Table 13-13). The sarcomatoid variant of RCC tends to have a worse prognosis, with median survival of less than 1 year. Performance status, disease-free survival more than 1 year (or in some schemes, 2 years), number of sites of metastases (one vs > one), and the presence of central nervous system metastases are common prognostic factors in most schemes.

Primary Disease Therapy

A radical nephrectomy may be performed with different approaches and includes complete resection of Gerota's fascia, kidney, and adrenal gland. The role of regional lymph node dissection remains unknown. Although no definitive proof exists that lymph node dissection prolongs survival, in the context of adjuvant therapy trials, it is imperative that staging is accurately assessed. In the usual lymph node dissection, the ipsilateral nodes from the diaphragm to the origin of the common iliac arteries and the renal hilar lymph nodes are removed. Available kidney-sparing operations include partial nephrectomy and excisional resection of the tumor. Although reports of these less radical procedures appear good, several pathologic series suggest that renal cell tumors may be multicentric. Partial nephrectomies should be considered in patients in whom preservation of renal function is an important goal of therapy, including patients with von Hippel-Lindau disease or unilateral kidney.

Radiation therapy for RCC has been directed at the palliation of metastatic sites, specifically, bone, spine, and brain. Stereotactic radiation or gamma knife therapy may be useful in conjunction with whole-brain radiation for palliation of single brain metastases of 2 cm or less. Initial reports on this modality suggest high sterilization rates. No clear evidence to date confirms that adjuvant radiotherapy to the bed of the kidney improves survival, and we do not routinely give adjuvant radiation therapy to patients who have had a nephrectomy.

Advanced Disease Therapy

Treatment of metastatic disease remains difficult. Biologic response modifiers have had the greatest impact on treatment of metastatic disease. High-dose interleukin (IL)-2 recently was approved by the FDA for the treatment of this condition.

Common toxic effects to IL-2 (>50%) in patients treated with high doses include chills, pruritus, nausea, vomiting, diarrhea, hyperbilirubinemia, oliguria with increased levels of blood urea nitrogen and creatinine, weight gain, edema, hypotension, and lymphopenia with eosinophilia. Respiratory distress with pulmonary edema secondary to leaky capillary syndrome, bronchospasm, pleural effusion, somnolence, disorientation, anemia, thrombocytopenia,

Table 13-11. Risk Factors for Renal Cell Carcinoma

Genetic [86,87]
   von Hippel-Lindau disease
   Familial RCC
Acquired traits
   Cystic kidney disease
   End-stage renal failure requiring dialysis
Environmental factors [88–90]•
   Tobacco use
   Asbestos exposure
   Analgesic abuse (phenactin)
   Obesity
   Thorotrast

Table 13-12. Staging of Renal Cell Carcinoma

Stage*	TNM Staging	Criteria
I (A)	T1	Limited to the kidney, ≤ 2.5 cm, surrounded by normal renal parenchyma
	N0	
	M0	
II (A)	T2	Tumor > 2.5 cm, limited to the kidney
	N0	
	M0	
III (C)	T1	Metastasis to a single lymph node ≤ 2 cm
	N1	
	M0	
or		
(C)	T2	Metastasis to a single lymph node 2–5 cm or multiple lymph nodes < 5 cm
	N2	
	M0	
or		
(B)	T3a	Tumor involving perinephric fat
	T3b	Tumor involving renal vein
	T3c	Involvement of infradiaphragmatic vena cava
	N0	
	M0	
or		
(C)	T3a	Tumor involving perinephric fat
	T3b	Tumor involving renal vein
	T3c	Involvement of infradiaphragmatic vena cava
	N1	
	M0	
or		
IV (D)	T4a	Tumor invasion beyond Gerota's fascia into surrounding organs
	T4b	Tumor involving supradiaphragmatic vena cava
	Any N	
	M0	
or		
	Any T	
	N2 or N3	Metastasis to a lymph node > 5 cm
	M0	
or		
	Any T	
	Any N	
	M1	Distant metastases

* Robson staging in parentheses.

Table 13-13. Prognostic Factors in Renal Cell Carcinoma

Histology (sarcomatoid variant)
Performance status
Disease-free survival
Central nervous system disease
Number of metastatic sites

From Palmer et al. [91]; with permission.

hypothyroidism, and arrhythmias is seen in 10% to 50% of patients. Rare toxic effects include myocardial infarction, central line sepsis, severe hypotension, renal failure, and death. In centers that have experience with high-dose IL-2, much of the toxicity can be managed with noninvasive monitoring and fluid replacement, antibiotics, H-2 blockers, antiemetics, and antihistamines. Awareness of early warning signals, such as slight change in mental status and skipping one or two doses, has improved the overall toxicity profile of high-dose IL-2. Blood pressure support is maintained with fluid replacement and adrenergic agonists, such as dopamine and norepinephrine. Rarely, intubation and mechanical ventilatory support are required. The IL-2 dose is held until the patient has cardiopulmonary stabilization. Usually this requires skipping a dose or two over the course of 1 week.

Although response rates to high-dose IL-2, alone or with adoptively transferred lymphokine-activated killer cells, vary from 4% to 35%, the duration of the response in those achieving a complete remission is significantly long. There was no difference in overall survival in patients with metastatic RCC treated in a randomized study of high-dose IL-2 with and without lymphokine-activated killer cells [92]. Objective clinical responses using high-dose IL-2 in the treatment of metastatic RCC have been reported to occur in 4% to 35% of cases. The summary of 255 patients treated with high-dose IL-2 reported to the FDA that established IL-2 as a treatment for metastatic RCC demonstrated an overall response rate of 14%. Approximately one third of responses are complete and patients usually maintain their response for about 2 years.

Although preliminary studies using lower doses of IL-2 were discouraging, a more recent randomized study of high-dose IL-2 versus a log lower dose of IV IL-2 (72,000 IU/kg) given on the same schedule found similar overall response rates: 7% CR, and 8% PR for low-dose IL-2 versus 3% CR and 17% PR for high-dose IL-2 [93].

Trials using IFN-α suggest a response rate from 10% to 20%. Initial studies employing Cantell preparations of human leukocyte IFN reported by Quesada *et al.* [94] and Kirkwood *et al.* [95] suggested a clinical role for IFN-α. These studies were limited by availability and specific activity of the material. Subsequent trials of recombinant DNA–produced IFN-α and lymphoblastoid IFN-α have confirmed activity of this cytokine in metastatic RCC, with response rates of 18%.

Flu-like symptoms are the most common acute toxicity to the IFNs and are seen in virtually 100% of patients. Flu-like symptoms begin about 1 to 2 hours following a dose of IFN-α and include fever, chill or rigor, myalgias, low backache, arthralgias, headache, and malaise. Gastrointestinal symptoms such as nausea, vomiting, and diarrhea are rare. Acetaminophen pretreatment usually blunts the flu-like symptoms of IFN-α. Tachyphylaxis of the flu-like symptoms occurs with repetitive doses. In the longer term, patients may have low-grade fever and with the decrease in appetite associated

with IFN-α develop subclinical dehydration, which contributes to the malaise. We recommend vigorous fluid intake by mouth to improve the tolerance to the agent. Occasionally, IV hydration on an outpatient basis may be warranted.

Central nervous system toxicity includes slight confusion, minimal paranoia, stupor, and coma and is associated with diffuse slowing on the electroencephalogram. These effects are reversible, but stupor and coma may take as long as 3 to 4 weeks to resolve. Peripheral neuropathy is also uncommon and is associated with the typical hand-glove paresthesias with slowing of nerve conduction.

Cardiovascular toxicity is usually characterized by supraventricular tachyarrhythmias, which may be controlled with β blockers or calcium channel blockers. Cardiac toxicity is usually seen at dosages of over 10 mU/d, in older patients (older than 70 years), and in patients with underlying heart disease.

Mild elevation in transaminases occurs in patients treated with IFN-α and clinical hepatitis rarely is seen. Elevation in bilirubin is unusual and should make the clinician search for another cause. Elevations in transaminases rarely are associated with liver pain.

Common hematologic abnormalities seen in patients treated with IFN-α are characterized by leukoneutropenia with a cellular marrow. Systemic infections are rare. Thrombocytopenia occasionally occurs.

Renal abnormalities include increase in protein excretion and the development of partially reversible nephrotic syndrome and renal failure. Metabolic abnormalities associated with high-dose IFN-α treatment are unusual and include hypocalcemia, hyperkalemia, and hypoalbuminemia. Prognostic features of responding patients have been identified, including tumor burden and performance status.

At present, IFN-α is a reasonable alternative for treatment in patients with metastatic renal cell carcinoma. We recommend subcutaneous treatment with 3 mU/m^2 three times weekly, and dose escalation to 10 mU/m^2 three times weekly as tolerated. We continue treatment for a minimum 2 to 3 months when possible. Patients with non–life-threatening minimal progression of disease, stable disease, or evidence of response during the first 2 to 3 months continue on treatment for up to 1 year.

Although preliminary studies of combination IFN-α and IL-2 have been encouraging, a randomized study of the combination versus high-dose IL-2 alone failed to demonstrate any benefit from the addition of IFN-α [96]. A confirmatory randomized study of high-dose IL-2 versus low-dose IL-2 plus IFN-α has recently been completed and is under evaluation by the Cytokine Working Group.

Newer immunotherapy approaches in the treatment of metastatic RCC have used tumor dendritic cell vaccines as well as miniallogeneic KLM transplants to advocate the appropriate T-cell compartment and induce antitumor cytolytic T lymphocytes [97–99]. These promising new approaches need to be tested in larger randomized studies before being adopted as standard therapies.

REFERENCES

1. Sladden M, Dickinson J: Testicular cancer: how effective is screening? *Aust Fam Physician* 1993, 22:1350–1356.

2. Dieckmann KP, Klan R, Bunte S: HLA antigens, Lewis antigens, and blood groups in patients with testicular germ-cell tumors. *Oncol J Clin Exp Cancer Res* 1993, 50:252–258.

3. Al-Jehani RM, Povey S, Delhanty JD, *et al.*: Loss of heterozygosity on chromosome arms 5q, 11p, 11q, 13q and 16p in human testicular germ cell tumors. *Genes Chromosomes Cancer* 1995, 13:249–256.

4. Reilly PA, Heerema NA, Sledge GW Jr., *et al.*: Unusual distribution of chromosome 12 in a testicular germ-cell tumor cell line (833K) and its cisplatin-resistant derivative (64CP9) *Cancer Genet Cytogenet* 1993, 68:114–121.

5. Pinczowski D, McLaughlin JK, Lackgren G, *et al.*: Occurrence of testicular cancer in patients operated on for cryptorchidism and inguinal hernia. *J Urol* 1991, 146:1291–1294.

6. Marselos M, Tomatis L: Diethylstilbestrol: I. Pharmacology, toxicology and carcinogenicity in humans. *Eur J Cancer* 1992, 28A:1182–1189.

7. Prener A, Hsieh CC, Engholm G, *et al.*: Birth order and risk of testicular cancer. *Cancer Causes Control* 1992, 3:265–272.

8. Zhang Z, Vena JER, Zielezny M, *et al.*: Occupational exposure to extreme temperature and risk of testicular cancer. *Arch Environ Health* 1995, 50:13–18.

9. Klepp O, Olsson AM, Henrikson H, *et al.*: Prognostic factors in clinical stage I nonseminomatous germ cell tumors of the testis: multivariate analysis of a prospective multicenter study. Swedish-Norwegian Testicular Cancer Group. *J Clin Oncol* 1990, 8:509–518.

10. Birch R, Williams S, Cone A, *et al.*: Southeastern Cancer Group: prognostic factors for favorable outcome in disseminated germ cell tumors. *J Clin Oncol* 1986, 4:400–407.

11. Aass N, Klepp O, Cavallin-Stahl E, *et al.*: Prognostic factors in unselected patients with nonseminomatous metastatic testicular cancer: a multicenter experience. *J Clin Oncol* 1991, 9:818–826.

12. Sesterhenn IA, Weiss BB, Mostofi FK, *et al.*: Prognosis and other clinical correlates of pathologic review in stage I and II testicular carcinoma: a report from the Testicular Cancer Intergroup Study. *J Clin Oncol* 1992, 10:69–78.

13. Lerner SE, Mann BS, Blute ML, *et al.*: Primary chemotherapy for clinical stage II nonseminomatous germ cell testicular tumors: selection criteria and long-term results. *Mayo Clin Proc* 1995, 70:821–828.

14. Horwich A, Norman A, Fisher C, *et al.*: Primary chemotherapy for clinical stage II nonseminomatous germ cell tumors of the testis. *J Urol* 1994, 151:72–77.

15. Baniel J, Roth BJ, Foster RS, *et al.*: Cost and risk benefit in the management of clinical stage II nonseminomatous testicular tumors. *Cancer* 1995, 75:2897–29903.

16. Culine S, Theodore C, Terrier-Lacombe MJ, *et al.*: Primary chemotherapy in patients with nonseminomatous germ cell tumors of the testis and biological disease only after orchiectomy. *J Urol* 1996, 155:1296–1298.

17. Bajorin DF, Sarosdy MF, Pfister DG, *et al.*: Randomized trial of etoposide and cisplatin versus etoposide and carboplatin in patients with good-risk germ cell tumors: multi-institutional study. *J Clin Oncol* 1993, 11:598–606.

18. Loehrer PJ Sr, Johnson D, Elson P, *et al.*: Importance of bleomycin in favorable-prognosis disseminated germ cell tumors: an ECOG trial. *J Clin Oncol* 1995, 13:470–476.

19. Levi JA, Raghavan D, Harvey V, *et al.*: The importance of bleomycin in combination chemotherapy for good-prognosis germ cell carcinoma. *J Clin Oncol* 1993, 11:1300–1305.

20. McAleer JJ, Nicholls J, Horwich A: Does extragonadal presentation impart a worse prognosis to abdominal germ-cell tumors? *Eur J Cancer* 1992, 28A:825–828.

21. Bosl GJ, Motzer RJ: Testicular germ cell cancer [review]. *N Engl J Med* 1997, 337:242–253.

22. Broun Erm Nichols CR, Gize G, *et al.*: Tandem high-dose chemotherapy with autologous bone marrow transplantation for initial relapse of testicular germ cell cancer. *Cancer* 1997, 79:1605–1610.

23. Pienta KJ, Esper PS: Risk factors for prostate cancer. *Ann Intern Med* 1993, 118:793–803.

24. DerSimonian R, Clemens J, Spirtas R, Perlman J: Vasectomy and prostate cancer risk: methodological review of the evidence. *J Clin Epidemiol* 1993, 46:163–172.

25. Hankin JH, Zhao LP, Wilkens LR, Kolonel LN: Attributable risk of breast, prostate and lung cancer in Hawaii due to standard fat. *Cancer Causes Control* 1992, 3:17–23.

26. Ross RK, Bernstein L, Lobo RA, *et al.*: 5-Alpha-reductase activity and risk of prostate cancer among Japanese and US white and black males. *Lancet* 1992, 339:887–889.

27. Bacquet CR, Horm JW, Gibbs T, *et al.*: Socioeconomic factors and cancer incidence among blacks and whites. *J Natl Cancer Inst* 1991, 83:551–557.

28. Elghany NA, Schumacher MC, Slattery ML, *et al.*: Occupation, cadmium exposure, and prostate cancer. *Epidemiology* 1990, 1:107–115.

29. Fleming C, Wasson JH, Albertsen PC, *et al.*: A decision analysis of alternative treatment strategies for clinically localized prostate cancer: Prostate Patient Outcome Research Team. *JAMA* 1993, 269:2650–2658.

30. Lu-Yao GL, McLerran D, Wasson J, *et al.*: An assessment of radical prostatectomy: time trends, geographic variation, and outcomes. The Prostate Patient Outcome Research Team. *JAMA* 1993, 269:2633–2636

31. Littrup PJ, Lee F, Mettlin C: Prostate cancer screening: current trends and future implications. *Cancer* 1992, 42:198–211.

32. Gerber GS, Thompson IM, Thisted R, *et al.*: Disease-specific survival following routine prostate cancer screening by digital rectal examination. *JAMA* 1993, 269:61–64.

33. McCormack RT, Rittenhouse HG, Finlay J, *et al.*: Molecular forms of prostate specific antigen and the human kallikrein gene family: a new era. *Urology* 1995, 45:729–744.

34. Thompson IM, Zeidman EJ: Current urological practice: routine urological examination and early detection of carcinoma of the prostate. *J Urol* 1992, 148:326–329.

35. Cama C, Olsson CA, Raffo AJ, *et al.*: Molecular staging of prostatic cancer: II. Comparison of application of enhanced reverse transcriptase polymerase chain reaction assay for PSA versus prostate specific membrane antigen. *J Urol* 1995, 153:1373–1378.

36. Sgrignoli AR, Walsh PC, Steinberg GD, *et al.*: Prognostic factors in men with stage D1 prostate cancer: identification of patients less likely to have prolonged survival after radical prostatectomy. *J Urol* 1994, 152:1077–1081.

37. Paulson DF, Lin GH, Hinshaw W: Radical surgery versus radiotherapy for adenocarcinoma of the prostate. *J Urol* 1982, 128:502–504.

38. Bolla M, Gonzalez D, Warde P, *et al.*: Improved survival in patients with locally advanced prostate cancer treated with radiotherapy and goserelin. *N Engl J Med* 1997, 337:295–300.

39. Messing EM, Manola J, Sarosdy M, *et al.*: Immediate hormonal therapy compared with observation after radical prostatectomy and pelvic lymphadenectomy in men with node-positive prostate cancer. *N Engl J Med* 1999, 341:1781–1788.

40. Labrie F, Luthy I, Veilleux R, *et al.*: New concepts on the androgen sensitivity of prostate cancer. *Prog Clin Biol Res* 1987, 243:145–172.

41. Prostate Cancer Trialists' Collaborative Group: Maximum androgen blockade in advanced prostate cancer: an overview of 22 randomized trials with 3283 deaths in 5710 patients. *Lancet* 1995, 346:265–269

42. Caubet JF, Tosteson TD, Dong EW, *et al.*: Maximum androgen blockade in advanced prostate cancer: a meta-analysis of published randomized controlled trails using nonsteroidal antiandrogens. *Urology* 1997, 49:71–78.

43. Presti JC Jr, Fair WR, Andriole G, *et al.*: Multicenter, randomized, double-blind, placebo controlled study to investigate the effect of finasteride (MK-906) on stage D prostate cancer. *J Urol* 1992, 148:1201–1204.

44. Fleshner NE, Trachtenberg J: Treatment of advanced prostate cancer with the combination of finasteride plus flutamide: early results. *Eur Urol* 1993, 24 (suppl):106–112.

45. Kantoff PW, Halabi S, Conaway M, *et al.*: Hydrocortisone with or without mitoxantrone in men with hormone-refractory prostate cancer: results of the cancer and leukemia group B 9182 study. *J Clin Oncol* 1999, 17:2506–2513.

46. Hudes GR, Greenberg R, Krigel RL, *et al.*: Phase II study of estramustine and vinblastine, two microtubule inhibitors, in hormone-refractory prostate cancer. *J Clin Oncol* 1992, 10:1754–1761.

47. Pienta LJ, Redman BG, Bandekar R, *et al.*: A phase II trial of oral estramustine and oral etoposide in hormone refractory prostate cancer. *Urology* 1997, 50:401–406.

48. Hudes GR, Nathan F, Khater C, *et al.*: Phase II trial of 96-hour paclitaxel plus oral estramustine phosphate in metastatic hormone-refractory prostate cancer. *J Clin Oncol* 1997, 15:3156–3163.

49. Pfeifer BL, Pirani JF, Hamann SR, *et al.*: A dietary supplement for the treatment of hormone-refractory prostate cancer. *Br J Urol Int* 2000, 85:481:208–485.

50. Robinson RG, Preston DF, Baxter KG, *et al.*: Clinical experience with strontium-89 in prostatic and breast cancer patients. *Semin Oncol* 1993, 20 (suppl):44–48.

51. Porter AT, McEwan AJ: Strontium-89 as an adjuvant to external beam radiation improves pain relief and delays disease progression in advanced prostate cancer: results of a randomized controlled trial. *Semin Oncol* 1993, 20 (suppl):38–43.

52. Serafini AN, Houston SJ, Resche I, *et al.*: Palliation of pain associated with metastatic bone cancer using samarium-153 lexidronam: a double-blind placebo-controlled clinical trial. *J Clin Oncol* 1998, 16:1574–1581.

53. Marsh GM, Callahan C, Pavlock D, *et al.*: A protocol for bladder cancer screening and medical surveillance among high-risk groups: the Drake Health Registry experience. *J Occup Med* 1990, 32:881–886.

54. Kadlubar FF, Butler MA, Kaderlik KR, *et al.*: Polymorphisms for aromatic amine metabolism in humans: relevance for human carcinogenesis. *Environ Health Perspect* 1992, 98:69–74.

55. Vineis P, Ronco G: Interindividual variation in carcinogen metabolism and bladder cancer risk. *Environ Health Perspect* 1992, 98:95–99.

56. Morris RD, Audet AM, Angelillo IF, *et al.*: Chlorination, chlorination byproducts, and cancer: a meta-analysis. *Am J Public Health* 1992, 82:955–963.

57. Vena JE, Graham S, Freudenheim J, *et al.*: Diet in the epidemiology of bladder cancer in western New York. *Nutr Cancer* 1992, 18:255–264.

58. Elcock M, Morgan RW: Update on artificial sweeteners and bladder cancer. *Regul Toxicol Pharmacol* 1993, 17:35–43.

59. Mills PK, Beeson WL, Phillips RL, Fraser GE: Bladder cancer in a low risk population: results from the Adventist Health Study. *Am J Epidemiol* 1991, 133:230–239.

60. Kiemeney LA, Witjes JA, Verbeek AL, *et al.*: The clinical epidemiology of superficial bladder cancer. Dutch South-East Cooperative Urological Group. *Br J Cancer* 1993, 67:806–812.

61. Tachibana M, Deguchi N, Baba S, *et al.*: Prognostic significance of bromodeoxyuridine high labeled bladder cancer measured by flow cytometry: does flow cytometric determination predict the prognosis of patients with transitional cell carcinoma of the bladder? *J Urol* 1993, 149:739–743.

62. Esrig D, Elmajian D, Groshen S, *et al.*: Accumulation of nuclear p53 and tumor progression in bladder cancer. *N Engl J Med* 1994, 331:1259–1264.

63. Lacombe L, Dalbagni G, Zhang Z, *et al.*: Overexpression of p53 in a high-risk population of patients with superficial bladder cancer before and after Bacillus Calmette-Guerin therapy: correlation to clinical outcome. *J Clin Oncol* 1996, 14:2646–2652.

64. Herr HW, Schwalb BM, Zhang Z, *et al.*: Intravesical Bacillus Calmette-Guerin therapy prevents tumor progression and death from superficial bladder cancer: ten-year follow-up of a prospective randomized trial. *J Clin Oncol* 1995, 13:1404–1408.

65. Cookson MS, Herr HW, Zhang Z, *et al.*: The treated natural history of high-risk superficial bladder cancer: 15-year outcome. *J Urol* 1997, 158:62–67.

66. Burnand KG, Boyd PJ, Mayo ME, *et al.*: Single dose intravesical thiotepa as an adjuvant to cystodiathermy in the treatment of transitional cell bladder carcinoma. *Br J Urol* 1976, 48:55–59.

67. Lamm DL, Crissmann J, Blumenstein B, *et al.*: Adriamycin versus BCG in superficial bladder cancer: a Southwest Oncology Group Study. *Prog Clin Biol Res* 1989, 310:263–270.

68. Krege S, Giani G, Meyer R, *et al.*: A randomized multicenter trial of adjuvant therapy in superficial bladder cancer: transurethral resection only versus transurethral resection plus mitomycin-C versus transurethral resection plus Bacillus Calmette-Guerin. *J Urol* 1996, 156:962–966.

69. Einstein AB Jr, Wolf M, Halliday KR, *et al.*: Combination transurethral resection, systemic chemotherapy, and pelvic radiotherapy for invasive (T2-T4) bladder cancer unsuitable for cystectomy: a phase I/II SWOG study. *Urology* 1996, 47:652–657.

70. Coppin CM Gospodarowica MK, James K, *et al.*: Improved local control of invasive bladder cancer by concurrent cisplatin and preoperative or definitive radiation: the NCI Canada Trials Group. *J Clin Oncol* 1996, 14:2901–2907.

71. Kaufman DS, Shipley WU, Griffin PP, *et al.*: Selective bladder preservation by combination treatment of invasive bladder cancer [see comments]. *N Engl J Med* 1993, 329:1377–1382.

72. Shipley WU, Kaufman DS, Heney NM, *et al.*: The integration of chemotherapy, radiotherapy and transurethral surgery in bladder-sparing approaches for patients with invasive tumors. *Prog Clin Biol Res* 1990, 353:85–94.

73. Zietman AL, Shipley WU, Kaufman DS: The combination of cisplatin based chemotherapy and radiation in the treatment of muscle-invading transitional cell cancer of the bladder. *Int J Radiat Oncol Biol Phys* 1993, 27:161–170.

74. Tester W, Caplan R, Heany J, *et al.*: Neoadjuvant combined modality program with selective organ preservation for invasive bladder cancer: results of RTOG phase II trial 8802. *J Clin Oncol* 1996, 14:119–126.

75. Kachnic LA, Kaufman DS, Heney NM, *et al.*: Bladder preservation by combined modality therapy for invasive bladder cancer. *J Clin Oncol* 1997, 15:1022–1029.

76. Stockle M, Meyenburg W, Wellek S, *et al.*: Advanced bladder cancer (stages pT3b, pT4a, pN1, pN2): improved survival after radical cystectomy and 3 adjuvant cycles of chemotherapy. Results of a controlled prospective study. *J Urol* 1992, 148:302–306.

77. Freiha F, Reese J, Torti FM: A randomized trial of radical cystectomy versus radical cystectomy plus cisplatin, vinblastine, and methotrexate chemotherapy for muscle invasive bladder cancer. *J Urol* 1996, 155:495–499.

78. Mead GM, Russel M, Clark P, *et al.*: A randomized trial comparing methotrexate and vinblastine (MV) with cisplatin, methotrexate and vinblastine (CMV) in advanced transitional cell carcinoma: results and a report on prognostic factors in a Medical Research Council study, MRC Advanced Bladder Cancer Working Party. *Br J Cancer* 1998, 78:1067–1075.

79. Neoadjuvant cisplatin, methotrexate, and vinblastine chemotherapy for muscle-invasive bladder cancer: a randomized controlled trial [international collaboration of trialists]. *Lancet* 1999, 354:526–527.

80. Shipley WU, Winter KA, Kaufman DS, *et al.*: Phase III trial of neoadjuvant chemotherapy in patients with invasive bladder cancer treated with selective bladder preservation by combined radiation therapy and chemotherapy: initial results of Radiation Therapy Oncology Group 89-03. *J Clin Oncol* 1999, 17:1327–1328.

81. Loehrer PJ Sr, Einhorn LH, Elson PJ, *et al.*: A randomized comparison of cisplatin alone or in combination with methotrexate, vinblastine, and doxorubicin in patients with metastatic urothelial carcinoma: a cooperative group study. *J Clin Oncol* 1992, 10:1066–1073.

82. Bellmunt J, Ribas A, Eres N, *et al.*: Carboplatin-based versus cisplatin alone or in combination with methotrexate, vinblastine, and doxorubicin in patients with metastatic urothelial carcinoma: a cooperative group study. *J Clin Oncol* 1992, 10:1066–1073.

83. Roth BJ, Dreicer R, Einhorn LH, *et al.*: Significant activity of paclitaxel in advanced transitional cell carcinoma of the urothelium: a phase II trial of the ECOG. *J Clin Oncol* 1994, 12:2264–2270.

84. Dreicer R, Gustin DM, See WA, *et al.*: Paclitaxel in advanced urothelial carcinoma: its role in patients with renal insufficiency and as salvage therapy. *J Urol* 1996, 156:1606–1608.

85. von der Maase H, Hansen SW, Roberts JT, *et al.*: Gemcitabine and cisplatin versus methotrexate, vinblastine, doxorubicin and cisplatin in advanced or metastatic bladder cancer: results of a large, randomized, multinational, multicenter, phase III study. *J Clin Oncol* 2000, 17:3068–3077.

86. McCredie M, Stewart JH: Risk factors for kidney cancer in New South Wales: IV. Occupation. *J Indust Med* 1993, 50:349–354.

87. van der Hout AH, van den Berg E, van der Vlies P, *et al.*: Loss of heterozygosity at the short arm of chromosome 3 in renal-cell cancer correlates with the cytological tumor type. *Int J Cancer* 1993, 53:353–357.

88. McCredie M, Stewart JH, Day NE: Different roles for phenacetin and paracetamol in cancer of the kidney and renal pelvis. *Int J Cancer* 1993, 53:245–249.

89. McCredie M, Stewart JH: Risk factors for kidney cancer in New South Wales: I. Cigarette smoking. *Eur J Cancer* 1992, 28A:2050–2054.

90. La Vecchia C, Negri E, D'Avanzo B, Franceschi S: Smoking and renal cell carcinoma. *Cancer Res* 1990, 50:5231–5233.

91. Palmer PA, Vinke J, Philip T, *et al.*: Prognostic factors for survival in patients with advanced renal cell carcinoma treated with recombinant interleukin-2. *Ann Oncol* 1992, 3:475–480.

92. Rosenberg SA, Lotze MT, Yang JC, *et al.*: Prospective randomized trial of high-dose interleukin-2 alone or in conjunction with lymphokine-activated killer cells for the treatment of patients with advanced cancer. *J Nat Cancer Inst* 1993, 85:622–632.

93. Yang JC, Topalian SL, Parkinson D, *et al.*: Randomized comparison of high-dose and low-dose intravenous interleukin-2 for the therapy of metastatic renal cell carcinoma: an interim report. *J Clin Oncol* 1994, 12:1572–1576.

94. Quesada JR, Swanson DA, Gutterman JU: Phase II study of interferon alpha in metastatic renal cell carcinoma: a progress report. *J Clin Oncol* 1985, 3:1086–1092.

95. Kirkwood JM, Harris JE, Vera R, *et al.*: A randomized study of low and high doses of leukocyte alpha-interferon in metastatic renal cell carcinoma: the American Cancer Society Collaborative Trial. *Cancer Res* 1985, 45:863–871.

96. Atkins MB, Sparano J, Fisher RI, *et al.*: Randomized phase II trial of high-dose interleukin-2 either alone or in combination with interferon alfa-2b in advanced renal cell carcinoma. *J Clin Oncol* 1993, 11:661–670.

97. Schwaab T, Heaney JA, Schned AR, *et al.*: A randomized phase II trial comparing two different sequence combinations of autologous vaccine and human recombinant interferon gamma and human recombinant interferon alpha2B therapy in patients with metastatic renal cell carcinoma: clinical outcome and analysis of immunological parameters. *J Urol* 2000, 163:1322–1327.

98. Kugler A, Stuhler G, Walden P *et al.*: Regression of human metastatic renal cell carcinoma after vaccination with tumor cell-dendritic cell hybrids. *Nat Med* 2000, 6:332–336.

99. Childs R, Chernoff A, Contentin N, *et al.*: Regression of metastatic renal cell carcinoma after nonmyeloablative allogeneic peripheral-blood stem cell transplantation. *N Engl J Med* 2000, 343:750–758.

100. Nichols CR, Catalano PJ, Crawford ED, *et al.*: Randomized comparison of cisplatin and etoposide and either bleomycin or ifosfamide in treatment of advanced disseminated germ cell tumors: an Eastern Cooperative Oncology Group, Southwest Oncology Group and CALGB study. *J Clin Oncol* 1998, 1287–1293.

101. deWit R, Stoter G, *et al.*: Four cycles of BEP vs four cycles of VIP in patients with intermediate-prognosis metastatic testicular non-seminoma: a randomized study of the EORTC Genitourinary Tract Cancer Cooperative Group. *Br J Cancer* 1998, 78:828–32.

PEB
(Cisplatin, etoposide, and bleomycin)

The success of platinum-based multichemotherapy for the treatment of nonsemi-nomatous testicular cancers has provided the foundation for the treatment of early-stage disease as well as metastatic testicular cancer. Randomized studies have demonstrated that three-drug combinations (PVB or PEB) are better than two-drug combinations (PV or PE).

Cisplatin's anticancer action is not exactly known but it is thought that its action is similar to that of a bifunctional alkylating agent. Cisplatin binds to plasma protein, and although serum half-life is calculated in hours, tissue levels have been detected as long as 4 mo after treatment. Cisplatin is excreted via the kidney.

Etoposide (VP16) is a podophyllotoxin from the mandrake plant. Although podophyllotoxins bind to tubulin, there is little discernible effect of etoposide on microtubular assembly. Etoposide blocks cell division at G_2. Stable ternary complexes are formed with DNA and topoisomerase II, causing single-strand DNA breaks. Elimination is principally renal although a significant amount of unchanged drug and metabolites can be found in the feces. Recent studies suggest that etoposide may be carcinogenic and lead to second malignancies.

Bleomycin is derived from the fungus *Streptomyces verticullus* and is classified as an antibiotic. The major isoform in the mixture is A_2. Bleomycin binds to DNA and ferrous ion. Ferrous ion oxidized, ultimately leading to oxygen radicals that cause DNA single- and double-strand breaks. The majority of the drug is excreted via the renal pathway.

DOSAGE AND SCHEDULING

	Day
Cisplatin 20 mg/m²/d x 5, q 3 wk	▬▬▬▬▬ (d 1–5)
Etoposide 100 mg/m²/d x 5, q 3 wk	▬▬▬▬▬ (d 1–5)
Bleomycin 30 U/wk	■ (d 2, 8, 15)
Chemistries, tumor markers with each cycle, d 1	□ (d 1)
CBC weekly and daily on subsequent doses if CBC counts are low, d 1,8	□ (d 1, 8)
CXR prior to therapy every 2 mo	
Day	1 2 3 4 5 6 7 8 9 10 11 12 13 14 15

DOSAGE MODIFICATIONS: *Maintain PEB schedule regardless of CBC counts; for granulopenic fever, reduce VP-16 dosage by 25%; for granulocytopenia on d 1 of 2nd, 3rd, or 4th cycle of therapy, do daily CBC counts and if WBC counts do not recover adequately, hold VP-16 on d 5; discontinue bleomycin if signs of pulmonary fibrosis develop*

CANDIDATES FOR TREATMENT
Patients with stage II nonseminomatous cancers (adjuvant) and those with metastatic seminoma and nonseminoma testicular malignancies

SPECIAL PRECAUTIONS
Dosage of PEB should be given on schedule regardless of CBC counts; for granulopenic fever, etoposide dosage is modified by a 25% reduction; for patients with granulocytopenia on d 1 of the second, third, or fourth cycle of therapy, daily blood cell counts are done and if leukocyte counts do not recover adequately, etoposide is held on d 5; bleomycin should be discontinued for signs of pulmonary fibrosis including respiratory lag, inspiratory rales, or radiographic changes; cisplatin can cause rash, magnesium wasting, Fanconi's syndrome, diabetes insipidus, peripheral neuropathy, hearing loss, and anaphylaxis

ALTERNATIVE THERAPIES
PVB (cisplatin, vinblastine, bleomycin); VAB-VI (vinblastine, dactinomycin, bleomycin, cyclophosphamide, cisplatin)

TOXICITIES
Cisplatin: leukopenia, thrombocytopenia, anemia, hemolytic anemia, nephrotoxicity, hyperuricemia, uric acid nephropathy, ototoxicity, anaphylaxis, neurotoxicity, optic neuritis, papilledema, stomatitis, syndrome of inappropriate diuretic hormone secretion, nausea, vomiting, diabetes insipidus, Fanconi's syndrome, magnesium wasting; **Bleomycin:** urticaria, Raynaud's phenomenon, pulmonary fibrosis, pneumonitis, burning at injection site, nail loss, fever, chills, anaphylaxis, stomatitis, confusion, wheezing, hepatotoxicity, pleuropericarditis, renal toxicity, cerebral arteritis, cerebral vascular accidents, myocardial infarction, thrombotic microangiopathy, rash, alopecia; **Etoposide:** anemia, leukopenia, thrombocytopenia, stomatitis, anaphylaxis, chemical phlebitis, neurotoxicity, anorexia, nausea, vomiting, lethargy, diarrhea, alopecia

DRUG INTERACTIONS
Cisplatin: allopurinol, colchicine, probenecid, sulfinpyrazone, antihistamines, buclizine, cyclizine, loxapine, meclizine, phenothiazines, thioxanthines, trimethobenzamid, bleomycin, radiation therapy, salicylates, vancomycin; **Etoposide:** radiation therapy, vaccines; **Bleomycin:** general anesthetics, concurrent radiation, cisplatin, vincristine

PEB (Continued)

RECENT EXPERIENCES AND RESPONSE RATES

Study	Evaluable Patients, *n*	Dosage and Schedule	Complete Response Rates
Williams *et al.*, *N Engl J Med* 1987, 316:1435–1440	121 nonseminoma	Cisplatin 20 mg/m²/d x 5 q3 wk Vinblastine 0.15 mg/kg d1 & 2 q3 wk Bleomycin 30 U/wk	61%
	123 nonseminoma	Cisplatin 20 mg/m²/d x 5 q3 wk VP-16 100 mg/m²/d x 5 q3 wk Bleomycin 30 U/wk	60%
Einhorn *et al.*, *J Clin Oncol* 1989, 7:387–391	88 nonseminoma	Cisplatin 20 mg/m²/d x 5 q3 wk VP-16 100 mg/m²/d x 5 q3 wk Bleomycin 30 U/wk 3 cycles	66 (75%)
	vs 96 nonseminoma	Cisplatin 20 mg/m²/d x 5 q3 wk VP-16 100 mg/m²/d x 5 q3 wk Bleomycin 30 U/wk 4 cycles	70 (73%)

NURSING INTERVENTIONS

Give antiemetics, maintain adequate IV fluid intake, monitor input and output closely, monitor weight; assess patient performance, mental and pulmonary status; use antidiarrheals as needed; monitor blood counts, liver function, and renal function; patients should be aware of delayed nausea and treated appropriately; instruct patient regarding the development of fever and urinary symptoms; advise the patient to stop smoking

PATIENT INFORMATION

Patient may experience nausea, vomiting, allergic reactions; patient should inform the physician if allergic types of reaction have occurred in the past; risk for pulmonary toxicity increased in smokers; watch for fever, chills, change in urinary habits, tarry stool, blood in the stool, change in hearing, pins and needles, rash, diarrhea, and sores in the mouth

ADMINISTRATION NOTES

Cisplatin: supplied as a powder and reconstituted in sterile water for injection, which should be stored at room temperature and should be protected from freezing and light; if solutions more dilute than 1 mg/mL are used, cisplatin should be diluted in 5% dextrose and saline; platinum will precipitate if it comes into contact with aluminum; reconstituted cisplatin is stable for 20 h at room temperature; **Etoposide:** supplied as a solution in a benzyl alcohol, polysorbate, and alcohol and should be stored below 40°C; may be diluted into either 0.9% saline or 5% dextrose solutions to a final dilution of 0.2–0.4 mg/mL; may precipitate at high concentrations; **Bleomycin:** supplied as sterile bleomycin sulfate and stored at room temperature; diluents containing benzyl alcohol are not recommended for neonates; reconstituted solutions with saline or dextrose are stable for 24 h at room temperature and for 2 wk at 4°C

VIP
(Vinblastine, ifosfamide, and cisplatin)

Cisplatin's anticancer action remains incompletely understood but it is thought that its action is similar to that of a bifunctional alkylating agent. Cisplatin binds to plasma protein, and although serum half-life is calculated in hours, tissue levels have been detected as long as 4 months after treatment. Cisplatin is excreted through the kidney.

Etoposide (VP16) is a podophyllotoxin from the mandrake plant. Although podophyllotoxins bind to tubulin, there is little discernible effect of etoposide on microtubular assembly. Etoposide blocks cell division at G2. Stable ternary complexes are formed with DNA and topoisomerase II, causing single-strand NDNA breaks. Elimination is principally renal although a significant amount of unchanged drug and metabolites can be found in feces. Recent studies suggest that etoposide may be carcinogenic and lead to second malignancies.

Vinblastine is an alkaloid from the plant *Vinca rosea*. Vinblastine binds to tubulin and inhibits microtubule formation. It disrupts cells during the M phase of mitosis. The drug is metabolized in the liver and excreted in the bile. Dose modifications are required for hyperbilirubinemia. One mechanism of resistance to vinblastine is through the adenosine triphosphate (ATP)-dependent efflux pump O-170 (MDR-1).

DOSAGE AND SCHEDULING

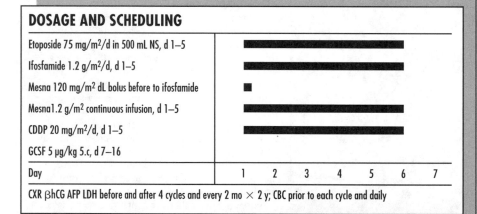

	Day	1	2	3	4	5	6	7
Etoposide 75 mg/m²/d in 500 mL NS, d 1–5								
Ifosfamide 1.2 g/m²/d, d 1–5								
Mesna 120 mg/m² dL bolus before to ifosfamide								
Mesna 1.2 g/m² continuous infusion, d 1–5								
CDDP 20 mg/m²/d, d 1–5								
GCSF 5 µg/kg 5.c, d 7–16								

CXR βhCG AFP LDH before and after 4 cycles and every 2 mo × 2 y; CBC prior to each cycle and daily

NURSING INTERVENTIONS

Give antiemetics, maintain adequate IV fluid intake, monitor input and output closely, monitor weight; assess patient performance, mental and pulmonary status; use antidiarrheals as needed; monitor blood counts, liver function, and renal function; patients should be aware of delayed nausea and treated appropriately; instruct patient regarding the development of fever and urinary symptoms; advise the patient to stop smoking

SPECIAL PRECAUTIONS

Dosage of VIP should be given on schedule regardless of CBC counts; for granulocytopenic fever dosage is modified by a 25% reduction, or GSF support can be given; Fanconi's syndrome, diabetes insipidus, peripheral neuropathy, hearing loss, and anaphylaxis

TOXICITIES

Cisplatin: leukopenia, thrombocytopenia, anemia, hemolytic anemia, nephrotoxicity, hyperuricemia, uric acid nephropathy, ototoxicity, anaphylaxis, neurotoxicity, optic neuritis, papilledema stomatitis, syndrome of inappropriate diuretic hormone secretion, nausea, vomiting, diabetes insipidus, Fanconi's syndrome, magnesium wasting; **Etoposide:** anemia, leukopenia, thrombocytopenia, stomatitis, anaphylaxis, chemical phlebitis, neurotoxicity, anorexia, nausea, vomiting, lethargy, diarrhea; **Ifosfamide:** gonadal depression, leukopenia, thrombocytopenia, hemorrhagic cystitis, nausea, vomiting, alopecia, anemia, ataxia, azotemic confusion, drowsiness, dysuria, hallucinations, seizures, psychosis and renal tubular necrosis; **Mesna:** diarrhea, dysgeusia, fatigue headaches, hematuria, hypotension, maculopapular rash, nausea, vomiting, pruritus, urticaria

DRUG INTERACTIONS

Cisplatin: allopurinol, colchicine, probenecid, sulfinpyrazone, antihistamines, buclizine, cyclizine, loxapine, meclizine, phenothiazines, thioxanthines, trimethobenzamide, bleomycin, radiation therapy, aminoglycosides, furosemide, vaccines, erythromycin, ethacrynic acid, salicylates, vancomycin; **Etoposide:** radiation therapy, vaccines; **Ifosfamide:** allopurinol, colchicine, probenecid, sulfinpyrazone, anticoagulants, radiation therapy, cocaine, hepatic enzyme inducers, lovastatin, succinylcholine, vaccines, aminoglycosides, amphotericin, anticoagulants, cimetidine

VIP (Continued)
(Vinblastine, Ifosfamide, and Cisplatin)

RECENT EXPERIENCES AND RESPONSE RATES

Study	Evaluable Patients, n	Dosage and Schedule	Complete Response Rate, %
Nichols et al., J Clin Oncol Oncol 1998, 4:1287–1293	145	VIP	37
	141	PEB	31
De Wit R et al., Br J Cancer 1998, 78:828–832.	84	VIP	74
	79	PEB	

NURSING INTERVENTIONS

Give antiemetics, maintain adequate IV fluid intake, monitor input and output closely, monitor weight; assess patient performance, mental and pulmonary status; use antidiarrheals as needed; monitor blood counts, liver function, and renal function; patients should be aware of delayed nausea and treated appropriately; instruct patient regarding the development of fever and urinary symptoms; advise the patient to stop smoking

INTERVENTIONS

Give antiemetics, maintain adequate IV fluid intake, monitor inputs and outputs closely, monitor weight; assess patient performance, mental and pulmonary status; use antidiarrheals as needed; monitor blood counts; check liver, pulmonary, and renal function; patients should be made aware of delayed nausea and treated appropriately; instruct patient regarding the development of fever and urinary symptoms; advise the patient to stop smoking; patient should be on adequate bowel regimen to prevent paralytic ileus, which may be caused by vinblastine

PATIENT INFORMATION

Patient may experience nausea, vomiting, allergic reactions; patient should inform the physician if allergic types of reactions have occurred in the past; risk for pulmonary toxicity increased in smokers; watch for fever, chills, change in urinary habits, tarry stool, blood in the stool, change in hearing, rash, diarrhea, and sores in the mouth; pins and needles may develop, as well as pain in the jaw; constipation may develop and should be treated aggressively but not from below because leukopenia may have developed

ADMINISTRATION NOTES

Cisplatin: supplied as a powder and reconstituted in sterile water for injection, which should be stored at room temperature and should be protected from freezing and light. If solutions more dilute than 1 mg/mL: are used, cisplatin should be diluted in 5% dextrose and saline; platinum will precipitate if it comes into contact with aluminum; reconstituted cisplatin is stable for 20 h at room temperature **Ifosfomide:** available in combination package with mesna, 1-g vial ifosfamide with 200-mg ampules of mesna; 3 gm vial of ifosfamide with 400 mg of mesna; 1 g vial of ifosfamide with 1 g ampule of mesna; **Etoposide:** supplied as a solution in a benzyl alcohol, polysorbate, and alcohol; should be stored below 40°C; may be diluted into either 0.9% saline or 5% dextrose solutions to a final dilution of 0.2 0.4 mg/mL; may precipitate at high concentrations; **Mesna:** mesna, or sodium 2-mercapto-ethanesulfonate is a chemoprotective agent against hemorrhagic cystitis. Mesna is a thiol that binds the urotoxic metabolites of ifosfamide. Although oral and continuous IV dosing of mesna has been used, the most common route of administration is by IV bolus before ifosfamide and after continuous infusion during ifosfamide treatment.

M-VAC
(Methotrexate, vinblastine, doxorubicin, and cisplatin)

The M-VAC regimen was found to be superior to cisplatin alone (objective response rates of 33% vs 15%, respectively; *P*=0.001) in a randomized trial evaluating the treatment of metastatic bladder cancer conducted by the Eastern Cooperative Oncology Group. Patients eligible for treatment with M-VAC include those with metastatic transitional cell carcinoma (TCC) of the uroepithelium who have adequate renal function. The role of M-VAC in the treatment of metastatic TCC is well documented. The use of M-VAC or other combination chemotherapy for adjuvant treatment of high-risk local TCCs has not yet been proven, and patients should be encouraged to participate in randomized trials evaluating these therapies.

Methotrexate is an antimetabolite that inhibits dihydrofolic acid reductase, thus interfering with DNA synthesis. Methotrexate is polyglutamated within cells, which allows the compound to remain in cells for prolonged periods of time. Renal excretion by glomerular filtration and active tubular secretion is the principal route of elimination, with as much as 90% of the drug excreted in the first 24 h.

Vinblastine is an alkaloid from the plant *Vinca rosea*. Vinblastine will bind to tubulin and inhibit microtubule formation. It disrupts cells during the M phase of mitosis. The drug is metabolized in the liver and excreted in the bile. Dose modifications are required for hyperbilirubinemia. One mechanism of resistance to vinblastine is through the ATP-dependent efflux pump P-170 (MDR-1).

Doxorubicin is a anthracycline antibiotic from *Streptomyces peucetius* (variety *caesius*). All of doxorubicin's mechanisms of action have not been elucidated, but it will enter the cell quickly and intercalate with DNA, thus inhibiting cellular division. Forty percent to 50% of the drug is excreted in the bile over a 7-d period. Patients with liver dysfunction require dose reduction.

Cisplatin's anticancer action is not exactly known but it is thought that its action is similar to that of a bifunctional alkylating agent. Cisplatin binds to plasma protein, and although serum half-life is calculated in hours, tissue levels have been detected as long as 4 mo after treatment. Cisplatin is excreted via the kidney.

DOSAGE AND SCHEDULING

		Day											
Methotrexate 30 mg/m² d 1, 15, 22	■							■	■		
Vinblastine 3 mg/m² d 2, 15, 22		■						■	■		
Doxorubicin 30 mg/m² d 2		■									
Cisplatin 70 mg/m² d 2		■									
Chemistries d 1	□										
BUN/creatinine d 1, 15, 22	□							□	□		
24-h CrCl d 1	□										
CBC d 1	□										
Day	1	2	3	4	5	6	7	10	15	20	22

Cycle repeated every 3 wk.

DOSAGE MODIFICATIONS: *Give full-dose methotrexate and vinblastine on d 15 and 22 if WBC count is 1999/mm³ and platelet count is > 74,999/mm³. If counts fall below, dose is held and restarted at 67% when counts return to normal. Omit d 15 and 22 if blood counts take more than 2 wk to recover. On d 15 and 22 methotrexate should be given on schedule regardless of CBC counts.*

CANDIDATES FOR TREATMENT

Patients with metastatic transitional cell carcinoma with renal, liver, cardiac, and adequate bone marrow function under some circumstances; patients at high-risk for relapse from local resected disease may be candidates

SPECIAL PRECAUTIONS

Dosage of M-VAC should be adjusted for toxicity; full-dose methotrexate and vinblastine should be given on d 15 and 22 for leukocyte count > 1999 cells/mm³ and platelet count > 74,999 mm³; for worse hematologic toxicity, chemotherapy dose should be held and restarted at 67% when the counts return to normal; omit d 15 and 22 if recovery of blood counts takes > 2 wk to recover; on d 15 and 22 should be given on schedule regardless of CBC counts; for granulocytic fever, dactinomycin and vinblastine dosage is modified by a 25% reduction; bleomycin should be discontinued for signs of pulmonary fibrosis including respiratory lag, inspiratory rales, or radiographic changes; can cause rash, magnesium wasting, Fanconi's syndrome, diabetes insipidus, peripheral neuropathy, hearing loss, and anaphylaxis

TOXICITIES

Methotrexate: nausea, vomiting, gingivitis, pharyngitis, stomatitis, diarrhea, enteritis, leukopenia, thrombocytopenia, hypogammaglobulinemia, erythematous rash, pruritus, urticaria, photosensitivity, depigmentation, alopecia, acne, hepatic atrophy and necrosis, cirrhosis, renal failure, cystitis, defective oogenesis or spermatogenesis, menstrual dysfunction, infertility, fetal defects, abortion, nephropathy, blurred vision, seizures, arachnoiditis, leukoencephalopathy, conjunctivitis; **Vinblastine:** leukoneutropenia, thrombocytopenia, cellulitis, stomatitis, jaw pain, loss of ankle jerk, peripheral neuropathy, nausea, vomiting, paralytic ileus, alopecia; **Doxorubicin:** leukoneutropenia, cardiotoxicity, arrhythmias, phlebosclerosis, facial flushing, alopecia, hyperpigmentation of the nail beds and dermal creases, recall reaction to radiation, erythematous streaking at IV site, tissue necrosis from extravasation, mucositis, conjunctivitis, nausea, vomiting, allergy including anaphylaxis; **Cisplatin:** leukopenia, thrombocytopenia, anemia, hemolytic anemia, nephrotoxicity, hyperuricemia, uric acid nephropathy, ototoxicity, anaphylaxis, neurotoxicity, optic neuritis, papilledema, stomatitis, syndrome of inappropriate diuretic hormone secretion, nausea, vomiting, diabetes insipidus, Fanconi's syndrome, magnesium wasting

DRUG INTERACTIONS

Methotrexate: alcohol, acetaminophen, amiodarone, estrogens, erythromycin, isoniazid, methyldopa, phenothiazines, phenytoin, piperacillin, rifampin, allopurinol, colchicine, sulfinpyrazones, nonsteroidal antiinflammatory agents, folic acid, oral neomycin, salicylates, sulfonamides, vaccines; **Vinblastine:** radiation therapy, vaccines, allopurinol, colchicine,

(Continued on next page)

M-VAC (Continued)

RECENT EXPERIENCES AND RESPONSE RATES

Study	Evaluable Patients, n	Dose and Schedule	Response Rates, % Complete/Partial
Sternberg et al., J Urol 1988, 139:461–69	92	Methotrexate 30 mg/m^2 d 1, 15, 22 Vinblastine 3 mg/m^2 d 2, 15, 22 Doxorubicin 30 mg/m^2 d 2 Cisplatin 70 mg/m^2 d 2	34/28
Sternberg et al., J Urol 1990, 144:396–397	121	Methotrexate 30 mg/m^2 d 1, 15, 22 Vinblastine 3 mg/m^2 d 2, 15, 22 Doxorubicin 30 mg/m^2 d 2 Cisplatin 70 mg/m^2	36/36
Connor et al., J Urol 1990, 144:397	14	Methotrexate 30 mg/m^2 d 1, 15, 22 Vinblastine 3 mg/m^2 d 2, 15, 22 Doxorubicin 30 mg/m^2 d 2 Cisplatin 70 mg/m^2	31/37
Scher et al., J Urol 1988, 139:470–477	41 neoadjuvant	Methotrexate 30 mg/m^2 d 1, 15, 22 Vinblastine 3 mg/m^2 d 2, 15, 22 Doxorubicin 30 mg/m^2 d 2 Cisplatin 70 mg/m^2	24/39
Scher et al., J Urol 1988, 139:478–487	5 extragonadal	Methotrexate 30 mg/m^2 d 1, 15, 22 Vinblastine 3 mg/m^2 d 2, 15, 22 Doxorubicin 30 mg/m^2 d 2 Cisplatin 70 mg/m^2	60/—

DRUG INTERACTIONS (Continued)

probenecid, sulfinpyrazone; **Doxorubicin:** allopurinol, colchicine, alcohol, amiodarone, estrogens, isoniazid, methyldopa, phenothiazines, phenytoin, piperacillin, rifampin, vaccines; **Cisplatin:** allopurinol, colchicine, probenecid, sulfinpyrazone, antihistamines, buclizine, cyclizine, loxapine, meclizine, phenothiazines, thioxanthines, trimethobenzamid, bleomycin, radiation therapy, aminoglycosides, furosemide, vaccines, erythromycin, ethacrynic acid, salicylates, vancomycin

NURSING INTERVENTIONS

Give antiemetics, maintain adequate IV fluid intact, monitor input and output closely, monitor weight. Assess patient performance, mental and pulmonary status. Use antidiarrheals as needed. Monitor blood counts and liver and renal function. Patients should be aware of delayed nausea and treated appropriately. Instruct patient regarding the development of fever and urinary symptoms. Patient should be on adequate bowel regimen to prevent paralytic ileus, which may be caused by vinblastine

PATIENT INFORMATION

Patient may experience nausea, vomiting, and allergic reactions. Patient should inform the physician if allergic types of reaction have occurred in the past. Watch for fever, chills, change in urinary habits, tarry stool, blood in the stool, change in hearing, pins and needles, rash, diarrhea, and sores in the mouth. Pins and needles may develop, as well as pain in the jaw. Constipation may develop and should be treated aggressively but not from below because leukopenia may have developed

ADMINISTRATION NOTES

Methotrexate: for IV use, provided as a preservative-free lyophilized powder, which is reconstituted in sterile 5% dextrose or 0.9% saline; concentration should not exceed 25 mg/mL; **Vinblastine:** provided in a lyophilized powder and is reconstituted in 0.9% sterile saline; final concentration of the drug is 1 mg/mL; once reconstituted, vinblastine sulfate has a shelf-life of 30 d at 2°C–8°C; **Doxorubicin:** provided as a sterile red-orange powder containing a 1:5 (w:w) ratio of lactose and a 1:0.1 ratio of methylparaben; powder may be stored at room temperature protected from light; doxorubicin is reconstituted with 0.9% sodium chloride injection to give a final concentration of 2 mg/mL; bacteriostatic diluents should be avoided; the reconstituted drug is stable for 15 d in the refrigerator and the dark; 5-fluorouracil and sodium heparin may cause doxorubicin to precipitate and should not be mixed with drug; the drug also may be obtained as a liquid with no preservatives; **Cisplatin:** supplied as a powder and reconstituted in sterile water for injection, which should be stored at room temperature and should be protected from freezing and light; if solutions more dilute than 1 mg/mL are used, cisplatin should be diluted in 5% dextrose and saline; platinum will precipitate if it comes into contact with aluminum; reconstituted cisplatin is stable for 20 h at room temperature.

Tumors of the female reproductive organs are heterogeneous with regard to histology, natural history, clinical behavior, and methods of treatment. Appropriate treatment requires careful diagnostic evaluation to distinguish them from other malignancies of the pelvis, including sigmoid, rectal, and bladder cancer, as well as from metastatic lesions, such as Krukenberg tumors. Accurate staging is critical because therapy is virtually always guided by extent of spread. Treatment of these malignancies requires a thorough understanding of their natural history and should not be attempted by those with little experience in this field. Optimal conditions for diagnosis, staging, and therapy require excellent communication between medical and radiation oncologists, the radiologist, and the surgeon. This is particularly true in those instances in which multimodality therapy is contemplated.

Tumor types discussed in this section include the common tumors of the ovary, uterine cervix, uterus, vulva, and gestational trophoblastic neoplasms (Table 14-1).

APPROACH TO THE THERAPY OF EPITHELIAL TUMORS OF THE OVARY

Etiology, risk factors, and screening

Tumors of this type comprise approximately 95% of all ovarian malignancies. The prevalence is 30 to 50 per 100,000 women with a lifetime incidence of one in 70 women. They occur most commonly in women in their sixth and seventh decades. Etiology and risk factors for ovarian cancer are shown in Table 14-2. Advanced age, nulliparity, prior history of cancer (endometrial, breast, or colon), Northern European or North American descent, or any history of familial syndromes increases the risk of developing ovarian cancer. Screening the general population is neither cost-effective nor practical; however, certain subpopulations of patients, defined by the risk factors described above, may be candidates. Three screening tests are currently employed: bimanual pelvic examination, cancer antigen (CA)-125, and transvaginal ultrasound. The pelvic examination is cost-effective and reliable when done by experienced hands, but it lacks adequate sensitivity and specificity as a screening test. It is estimated that physical examination detects only one in 10,000 ovarian carcinomas in asymptomatic women. The radioimmunoassay for CA-125, a tumor-specific antigen, is elevated in 80% of ovarian carcinomas, but only in 50% of women with cancer limited to the ovary. It may also be elevated in women with benign ovarian disease and in otherwise healthy women, which limits its specificity. In postmenopausal women with a pelvic mass, however, a serum CA-125 level above 65 U/mL is predictive for cancer in up to 75% of cases. Ultrasound techniques are not only expensive but also limited in their specificity and sensitivity. In one published study of 8500 asymptomatic women who underwent transvaginal ultrasound, 121 subsequently underwent surgery. Of those, 57 had serous cystadenomas, and eight had primary ovarian cancers (six, IA; one, IIC; one, IIIB); one had palpable ovarian enlargement and one had an elevated CA-125 level [1]. Therapy that combines CA-125 measurements and transvaginal ultrasound are promising in high-risk patients, but it should still be considered experimental.

Recommendations for screening

The 1994 National Institutes of Health Consensus Conference [2] concluded no effective method yet exists for screening and detecting early ovarian cancer. Nevertheless, some authorities consider it a reasonable strategy to screen such patients with a strong familial history or a familial cancer syndrome (see Table 14-2). Although an average woman has a lifetime risk of one in 70 of developing ovarian cancer, this increases to one in 20 in women with a first-degree relative with ovarian cancer, one in 14 to a woman with two first-degree relatives, and 40% for the hereditary ovarian cancer syndrome. Although no data demonstrate that screening reduces the mortality of the disease even in the higher risk groups, women who are at the highest risk ought to at least have an annual bimanual pelvic examination, assay for CA-125, and transvaginal ultrasound. Prophylactic oophorectomy is a consideration for women with a history of familial ovarian cancer syndrome.

The role of screening for genetic mutations (see next section) remains undefined. It would be inadvisable to offer genetic screening, although now commercially available, without adequate guidance from a clinical geneticist to interpret results and offer recommendations to patients.

Protective factors for women at risk for ovarian carcinoma include oral contraceptive use, full-term pregnancy, breast-feeding, and possibly tubal ligation. In women at high-risk who are undergoing abdominal surgery for other indications, prophylactic oophorectomy may be indicated. In this group, estrogen replacement should be discussed.

Role of genetic mutations

Approximately 10% of all epithelial ovarian cancers are associated with inheritance of an autosomal dominant genetic aberration, which confers cancer predisposition with a high penetrance. Perhaps the

Table 14-1. Common Tumors of the Female Genital Tract

Ovary
  Epithelial
  Stromal
  Germ cell
  Metastatic
Uterus
  Adenocarcinoma
  Sarcoma
    Leiomyosarcoma
    Mixed mesodermal tumors
    Endometrial stromal sarcoma
Cervix
  Squamous cell carcinoma
  Adenocarcinoma
  Adenosquamous carcinoma
Vulva
Gestational trophoblastic neoplasm
  Hydatidiform mole
  Invasive mole
  Choriocarcinoma

Table 14-2. Strategies for Early Diagnosis and Prevention of Ovarian Cancer

Identification of risk factors, including family history
Annual bimanual rectovaginal examination
Annual CA-125, transvaginal ultrasound in selected patients
Prophylactic oophorectomy in selected patients
Risk reduction strategies in selected patients

most important new dimension in understanding the etiology of some cancers of the ovary was the discovery of the role of mutations in *BRCA1*. The *BRCA1* gene, located on chromosome 17q12-21, is a tumor-suppressor gene. Mutations of *BRCA1* are associated with a higher incidence of breast cancer, especially but not exclusively, in women of Ashkenazi Jewish descent, and of ovarian cancer. Germline mutations of the gene are associated with a lifetime risk of breast cancer of up to 85% and of ovarian cancer in up to 45% for women with multiple family members who have ovarian and breast cancer over more than two generations. Incidence of germ-line mutations among women with ovarian cancer, however, is controversial and ranges from fewer than one in 47 to 5 in 115 [3,4]; it is in any case higher than that found in the general population (0.0006) [5]. One study detected probable germ-line mutations in *BRCA1* in 13 in 374 women with epithelial ovarian cancer younger than 70 years of age [6]. Women with mutations in *BRCA1* may have a greater likelihood of having breast cancer, and mutations are linked to the breast-ovary syndrome, which is linked to a lesser extent with mutations in *BRCA2* on chromosome 13q.

In addition to mutations in the *BRCA* genes, a higher incidence of ovarian cancer is observed in women who are members of families characterized by the Lynch II syndrome (hereditary nonpolyposis coli [HNPCC]). These families are characterized by a higher incidence of carcinomas of the ovary, breast, colon, and uterus, which occur more frequently than expected among a single generation and occur in multiple sequential generations, and which occur in a younger age population. The HNPCC syndrome is characterized by mutations in any of four known genes (*hMSH2, hMLH1, hPMS1,* and *hPMS2*), the human homologues of genes associated with mismatch repair, or more simplistically, genes that "proofread" errors in DNA replication, correcting errors in homopolymeric or dimeric repeats that occur frequently in human genes. In patients with mutations in these genes, mutations build up in the human genome, characterized by instability in microsatellites, portions of the genome with dimeric repeating sequences (*eg,* CACACACA . . .) or homopolymeric sequences (*eg,* AAAAAAA . . .). These patients are characterized by familial clustering of colon, breast, and endometrial carcinomas, as well as various other carcinomas that are less common. Thus, women with a well-defined familial history for these malignancies should be observed more carefully for the development of endometrial cancers.

For sporadic ovarian cancers, aberrations in various other protooncogenes, tumor-suppressor genes, and signal transduction pathways have been characterized. These include *ras, erbB2,* and *p53*. Mutations in *ki-ras2* occur at codon 12 most frequently, but also codon 13, and are found in between 30% and 50% of mucinous tumors, both borderline and invasive, and with a lower frequency in serous tumors. Mutations in *p53* occur rather late in the development of ovarian cancer, occurring in about 10% of early stage cancers and 40% of late stage tumors, but not borderline tumors. These mutations may correlate with worse overall outcome.

DIAGNOSIS AND MANAGEMENT OF EARLY STAGE DISEASE

Management of the adnexal mass

Detection of an adnexal mass either by physical or radiographic examination requires a management strategy. Although most are benign, between 13% and 21% of women undergoing surgery for a suspicious mass will have an ovarian malignancy. Recommendation for surgery depends on the degree of suspicion that this mass may be malignant; factors that should be considered include age, menopausal status, family history, size of the mass, type, duration, and characteristics of associated symptoms, CA-125, unilaterality versus bilaterality, and characteristics on ultrasound. Management may include observation with repeat examination, further radiographic tests, and laparoscopy, or laparotomy depending on the clinical circumstances.

Staging and management of early stage epithelial cancer
Overall goals
The natural history of ovarian cancer is dominated by locoregional spread, most commonly with peritoneal involvement. Precise histologic diagnosis and accurate staging are required before treatment. The International Federation of Gynecology and Obstetrics (FIGO) staging system of 1989 [7] is outlined in Table 14-3. Goals of therapy for early stage disease (FIGO I to III) include cure, and for later stage disease (suboptimal III to IV), palliation, particularly reduction of ascites, preservation of bowel function, adequate nutrition, and prevention of pain.

The cornerstone of treatment for epithelial ovarian tumors is surgery performed by an experienced gynecologic oncologist. Patients require a staging laparotomy with thorough inspection of the entire peritoneal cavity including the gutters, pelvis, and domes of the diaphragm, total abdominal hysterectomy and bilateral salpingo-oophorectomy, liver palpation, and biopsy, lymph node sampling, omentectomy, and peritoneal washings. All evidence of gross disease should be removed if possible. If surgical debulking is incomplete, the surgeon must estimate the size and extent of residual tumor. Patients who have had only a biopsy or incomplete debulking may be referred to an experienced gynecologic oncologist for consideration

Table 14-3. Staging and Prognosis of Ovarian Carcinoma

Stage	Characteristics
I	Disease confined to the ovaries
IA	One ovary, capsule intact, no ascites
IB	Both ovaries, capsule intact, no ascites
IC	IA or IB +: ascites, + washings, capsule ruptures, tumor on ovarian surface
II	Disease confined to the pelvis
III	Disease confined to the abdominal cavity, including surface of the liver, pelvic, inguinal or para-aortic lymph node, omentum, or bowel
IIIA	Negative nodes, + microscopic seeding of peritoneal surfaces
IIIB	Negative nodes, peritoneal implants ≤ 2 cm.
IIIC	Positive nodes and/or abdominal implants > 2 cm.
IV	Spread to liver parenchyma, lung (if effusion only, with positive cytology), or other extra-abdominal site

Prognosis

Stage	3-y Survival, %
IA, IB	90.4
IC, II	66.5
III	28.1
IV	10.4

Adapted from International Federation of Gynecology and Obstetrics [7].

for reoperation, because clinical outcome may be affected. Staging is performed per FIGO criteria.

OVARIAN CARCINOMA: SPECIFIC RECOMMENDATIONS FOR THE TREATMENT OF EARLY STAGE DISEASE

Approximately 25% of women with ovarian cancer have disease confined to one or both ovaries. Such women have a much more favorable prognosis. The primary therapy for patients with early stage ovarian cancer, either confined to the ovary (FIGO stage I) or confined to the pelvis (FIGO stage II), is surgery. Nevertheless, among selected subgroups, the failure rate is high enough to warrant adjuvant therapy with either radioisotopes, external beam irradiation, or chemotherapy. The Gynecologic Oncology Group has attempted to precisely define the subgroups that would benefit from adjuvant therapy and determine the optimal form of therapy for these patients. Two clinical trials were initiated in 1976 to accomplish these goals [9].

Stages Ia and Ib

The Gynecologic Oncology Group (GOG) 7601 included patients with stage Ia or Ib disease (growth limited to one or both ovaries with no ascites and negative peritoneal washings) and with well- or moderately-differentiated histologies. Patients were randomly assigned to observation or to receive oral melphalan, 0.2 mg/kg of body weight for 5 days every 4 to 6 weeks for 12 cycles. With a follow-up of 6 years, no difference was found between the two groups. Furthermore, the 5-year disease-free survival rate in the observation arm was 91% and the overall survival rate was 94%, thus suggesting that this subset of patients does well and should not receive adjuvant therapy [9].

Stages Iaii, Ibii, Ic–IIc and Ia or Ib with poorly differentiated histology

The GOG 7602 included patients with either a ruptured capsule or excrescences on the ovarian surface, high-grade histology, positive ascites, peritoneal washings, or spread to the uterus, fallopian tubes, or other pelvic tissues. Patients were randomly assigned to receive melphalan as already noted here or 15 mCi of intraperitoneal ^{32}P as chromic phosphate. The failure rate with a 6-year follow-up was 20% with failures distributed evenly between both groups. Toxicities were modest in both groups; however, those authors concluded that treatment with ^{32}P was preferable because of limited toxicity and no risk of developing leukemia, which has been observed with alkylating agents. In the replacement trial for the GOG, treatment with ^{32}P is compared with three cycles of cyclophosphamide/cisplatin [9]. Those investigators concluded that chemotherapy offered better progression-free survival and was well tolerated and thus the treatment of choice. The current recommendation from the Society of Gynecologic Oncologists indicates that most patients with epithelial tumors including early grade ovarian carcinomas receive adjuvant chemotherapy with the exception of grade 1, stage IA epithelial ovarian cancers [10].

OVARIAN CARCINOMA: RECOMMENDATIONS FOR TREATMENT OF OPTIMAL DISEASE

The largest single subgroup of women with ovarian carcinoma are those presenting with stage III disease [11]. Prognosis correlates well with extent of residual disease following primary debulking surgery. Patients with optimally debulked disease have been shown to have a favorable prognosis versus those in whom the tumor was too extensive to be debulked adequately. The cut-off for optimal disease is usually determined as either less than 1 or 2 cm, depending on the investigators' determination. It is likely that this is a continuum with those with the least tumor burden following surgery having the best prognosis and with prognosis worsening as the diameter of the smallest residual lesion increases, with about 40% of those with residual microscopic disease alive at 8 years versus 25% with residual disease less than 0.5 cm and 10% with residual disease between 0.5 and 2.0 cm.

The overall survival rate for women with optimally debulked disease is around 25%; thus, an appreciable cure rate is found in women treated with aggressive initial surgery followed by platinum-based chemotherapy. Following surgery, all women should receive at least six cycles of platinum-based therapy with either cisplatin or carboplatin in combination with paclitaxel. If cisplatin is employed, patients require careful monitoring of renal function and neurologic status. Dosage must be modified for either azotemia or for new onset of sensory neuropathy, because continued treatment at the same doses will likely lead to a worsening of both conditions. Systemic treatment with carboplatin is likely equivalent in this setting, although this remains to be proven definitively, because it does not result in permanent renal damage, ototoxicity, or neurologic deficits. Nevertheless, patients must be closely monitored for onset of neutropenic fevers and thrombocytopenia with attendant risk of hemorrhage.

For women receiving treatment with cisplatin, the major controversy concerns the route, intravenous (IV) or intraperitoneal (IP), by which the drug is to be optimally administered. A recent intergroup trial, led by the Southwest Oncology Group, which compared treatment with IV cyclophosphamide administered in combination with cisplatin administered either IP or IV, revealed a survival advantage for the group receiving IP cisplatin (49 vs 41 months; $P = 0.02$), and there was a significant reduction in sensory neuropathy with IP therapy [12].

Intraperitoneal therapy for patients with suboptimally debulked disease has not been widely accepted. Most such patients will still receive systemic therapy, which is considered next.

OVARIAN CARCINOMA: RECOMMENDATIONS FOR PATIENTS WITH SUBOPTIMALLY DEBULKED AND STAGE IV DISEASE

Women who have residual disease larger than 2 cm after initial debulking surgery have a substantially worse prognosis than those with optimally debulked disease. Nevertheless, a small proportion of these women will enjoy long-term disease-free survival. In contrast, women with disease outside the abdominal cavity or in the liver parenchyma, stage IV, have a worse prognosis and rarely enjoy long-term disease-free survival. In addition to residual tumor volume, other factors are associated with a poor prognosis, including gross residual tumor after first-line chemotherapy; grade 3 histology; aneuploidy; and increased S-phase or elevated Her 2/neu.

Evidence strongly suggests that chemotherapy can prolong survival in women with stage III disease, whether optimally or suboptimally debulked, and possibly in stage IV disease. Thus, women in these disease categories should be encouraged to receive chemotherapy as a treatment option following surgery. There are many active agents (Table 14-4). For patients with disease remaining after surgery, the usual treatment is combination therapy that includes paclitaxel [13] and a platinum compound.

Until recently, the standard of care for patients with advanced ovarian cancer was combination chemotherapy with paclitaxel plus cisplatin as administered in GOG 111 [14]. The superiority of this regimen over the older cyclophosphamide–cisplatin regimen was confirmed in a European Organization for Research and Treatment of Cancer (EORTC) study [15]. The major toxicities of this regimen are emesis and myelosuppression. Emesis may be controlled with newer antiemetics, such as ondansetron or granisetron. A hematopoietic growth factor, such as granulocyte-colony stimulating factor (G-CSF) or granulocyte-macrophage colony stimulating factor (GM-CSF), may decrease the duration of neutropenia and number of days of antibiotics but has not been shown to improve survival or response duration and should not be considered standard therapy. Use of a single alkylating agent, such as melphalan, is suboptimal therapy and should only be considered in those patients who cannot receive standard therapy. A recent study, GOG 132, compared treatment with cisplatin, 100 mg/m^2, as a single agent with paclitaxel, 200 mg/m^2, as a single agent, versus paclitaxel, 135 mg/m^2 plus cisplatin, 75 mg/m^2, administered concurrently, all regimens given every 3 weeks for six cycles, in women with suboptimally debulked disease [16]. Results of this trial failed to demonstrate the same median survival for women treated with the combination as in GOG 111. Furthermore, women who received cisplatin as a single agent or combination with paclitaxel had equivalent survival rates, whereas women receiving paclitaxel alone had an inferior result, demonstrating the superiority of platinum-based therapies. Given that the combination of cisplatin and paclitaxel was less toxic than cisplatin alone, the combination was considered the treatment of choice.

Recently, evidence has supported a new standard of care for patients with advanced ovarian cancer: combination therapy with carboplatin and paclitaxel. Paclitaxel is now administered most commonly in the outpatient setting as a 3-hour infusion, rather than a 24-hour infusion as was employed in GOG 111. Carboplatin

appears to preserve the efficacy of cisplatin, but is less toxic, as the toxicity profile of carboplatin differs from that of cisplatin with fewer irreversible ototoxicities, nephrotoxicities, and neurotoxicities. In addition, it is easier to administer carboplatin in the outpatient setting because of the absence of a requirement for pretreatment hydration. Indirect evidence supporting the carboplatin combination comes from a report from the Southwest Oncology Group demonstrating equal efficacy for the combination of cyclophosphamide plus carboplatin versus cyclophosphamide and cisplatin, but a lower incidence of irreversible toxicities associated with cisplatin treatment, including nephrotoxicity and neurotoxicity. Further evidence demonstrating the efficacy of carboplatin comes from a European trial comparing carboplatin alone with a combination of cyclophosphamide, doxorubicin, and cisplatin [17]. Adding carboplatin to a regimen containing cisplatin was equally effective, but more toxic, which discouraged use of this strategy [18].

Several early studies suggested that the combination of carboplatin and paclitaxel is equivalent in therapeutic outcome to cisplatin and paclitaxel. Two small studies from Nebraska and the Netherlands used 3-hour paclitaxel and carboplatin as a 30-minute infusion with acceptable toxicities and reasonable therapeutic outcome [19,20]. A small randomized study from the Netherlands confirmed that carboplatin-paclitaxel therapy had a better toxicity profile than the standard cisplatin-paclitaxel regimen, although the trial was underpowered to demonstrate therapeutic equivalence [21].

The Eastern Cooperative Oncology Group has tested the combination of short-infusion paclitaxel and carboplatin [23]. With objective response rates of 72% and overall survival for patients with measurable disease of 30.1 months, outcomes were essentially equivalent to those observed in women on GOG 132 receiving standard cisplatin-paclitaxel therapy [16], and in addition, an overall improvement in quality of life was observed. Thus, combinations of short-infusion paclitaxel over 3 hours and carboplatin administered in an outpatient setting would currently be considered an acceptable alternative to regimens such as that employed in GOG 111 [14] in women with suboptimally debulked and stage IV ovarian cancer.

Some controversy exists regarding the appropriate doses of carboplatin and paclitaxel to employ in this setting. The ECOG trial employed carboplatin at an area under the curve (AUC) of 5 and paclitaxel at 150 mg/m^2, which is somewhat lower than that employed in other studies. While some have argued that there is a dose response effect for carboplatin, the excellent results from the ECOG with minimal toxicity suggest that the dose employed in this trial may be acceptable.

DURATION OF THERAPY AND EVALUATION OF THE PATIENT ON THERAPY

Other considerations in the treatment of these patients must include the following findings. Before treatment, levels of the ovarian tumor marker CA-125 should be measured and used as adjunctive evidence of response to therapy. Levels should be measured routinely during the course of treatment. A consistent rise in CA-125 can be used as a measure of failure of treatment in the absence of radiographic and clinical changes. Likewise, a linear fall in serum levels of CA-125 can be used as a measure of treatment success in the absence of radiographic and clinical changes. Incorporation of CA-125 is a critical element in treatment. Levels of CEA and CA-19 may be elevated in women with mucinous carcinomas and may be potentially useful in following the course of the disease.

Table 14-4. Single-Agent Activity in Ovarian Cancer*

Drug	Patients, *n*	Response Rate, %
Cisplatin		
Low dose (30–60 mg/m^2)	71	45
Intermediate (60–90 mg/m^2)	31	55
High dose (100–120 mg/m^2)	21	52
Carboplatin	18	50
Cyclophosphamide		
Low dose	355	43
High dose	36	61
Melphalan	541	47
Thiotepa	337	48
Chlorambucil	40	23
Doxorubicin	58	34
Fluorouracil	92	20
Methotrexate	25	20
Hexamethylmelamine	59	34
Vinblastine	20	10
Taxol	124	24[†]
Ifosfamide	40	20[†]
Gemcitabine	38	13
Doxil	35	26
Topotecan	112	21

*Previously untreated patients except as noted.
†Most patients heavily pretreated.

Treatment should consist of four to eight cycles of therapy administered every 3 weeks or monthly. Residual disease should be measured before beginning therapy by visual inspection at the time of surgery, by CT scan if bulk disease remains, or by physical examination or chest radiograph when appropriate. Levels of CA-125 are followed as already described. If these levels rise or fail to decrease, resistance to treatment should be suspected. The role of positron-emission tomography (PET) scanning is currently being investigated and may add to the therapeutic investigation of these patients.

EVALUATION OF THE PATIENT AFTER INITIAL THERAPY

Following four to eight cycles of initial chemotherapy, patients who are clinically responding should be reevaluated using CA-125 levels and CT scan. Patients whose disease has clinically progressed through initial therapy have a poor prognosis [23]. Options for these patients include further treatment with a non–platinum-containing regimen or experimental therapy. Patients who initially responded to platinum-based therapy for longer than 6 months can be retreated with a platinum-based regimen.

Patients who have a clinical complete response on CT scan with either a normal or low CA-125 level may be candidates for second-look surgery. The role of second-look surgery is controversial. Second-look surgery clearly offers the most accurate assessment of response to chemotherapy and has important prognostic implications. The role of interval debulking, that is, a second debulking at the time of second look, has been advocated by some as having therapeutic utility, although improvement in survival has not been demonstrated [24]; however, one trial by the EORTC did demonstrate a survival advantage [25]. Furthermore, in the absence of effective second-line therapies, the entire therapeutic utility of second-look surgery remains unproven [26].

For patients enrolled in clinical trials requiring second-look surgery, such an approach is reasonable. If aggressive second-line treatment is contemplated, this may also be a reasonable approach.

TREATMENT OF RESIDUAL DISEASE

Patients who are found during second-look surgery to have small-volume residual disease may be candidates for various consolidation therapies. One reasonable approach is six additional cycles of platinum-based chemotherapy. A second approach, currently experimental, may be treatment with high-dose chemotherapy and peripheral stem-cell rescue. This was tested in the intergroup study GOG 164; however, this study unfortunately closed prematurely. Studies of conventional chemotherapy have failed to demonstrate a survival benefit for dose intensification of standard therapy. The use of higher doses with stem cell support requires further testing. Several recent editorials have recommended caution with such an approach [27].

A third option for patients with minimal residual disease after second debulking is intraperitoneal chemotherapy. This remains an experimental approach, although there are many preclinical and clinical data to suggest that it is of interest.

SALVAGE CHEMOTHERAPY

For patients in whom initial therapy with either frank progressive disease, positive disease on CT scan after 6 to 8 courses of treatment, or gross disease larger than 2 cm at time of second-look surgery, second-line chemotherapy may be an option. Currently, the topoiso-

merase I inhibitor, topotecan, is approved by the Food and Drug Administration for this use. In a European trial with 92 evaluable patients in which topotecan was administered in a daily × 5 schedule, the overall response rate was 16% with acceptable toxicities [28]. A second trial by the NY GOG employed topotecan as a 21-day infusion as second-line therapy with a 43% response rate and acceptable toxicities [29]. Furthermore, in another European trial, topotecan was slightly more effective than paclitaxel in the second-line setting, with response rates of 20% versus 13% [30].

Recently doxil, liposomally encapsulated doxorubicin, has been studied as salvage therapy in women with platinum- and paclitaxel-refractory ovarian carcinoma [31]. In this group of patients with an extremely poor prognosis, the response rate was 17% with acceptable toxicities, making this a worthwhile agent for second-line treatment. Other commercially available agents may also have modest activity in the second-line setting. These include gemcitabine, etoposide, hexamethylmelamine, 5-fluorouracil, leucovorin, and doxorubicin. Experimental agents are being tested by the GOG, NYGOG, and SWOG.

APPROACH TO THE TREATMENT OF THE PATIENT WITH CARCINOMA OF THE UTERINE CERVIX

General principles

Cervical cancer has a biphasic age distribution with peaks in the fourth and fifth decades and in the eighth and ninth decades. It affects nearly 14,000 women annually in the United States. Cervical cancer is more commonly found in poor women and in women who have been sexually active with multiple partners. It is more often found in women who have first intercourse early, have had multiple sexual partners, and have had multiple pregnancies. It is found less often in women who are nulliparous and those who are sexually inactive, such as nuns. A close association exists between infection with specific subtypes of human *Papillomavirus*, specifically types 16 and 18, and the development of cervical cancer and carcinoma in situ. The association with HIV infection is appreciable but has not been fully defined. Risk factors are listed in Table 14-5.

Screening, early detection, and diagnosis

The Papanicolaou (Pap) smear, or cytologic evaluation of cells obtained from the cervix, is one of the most sensitive, specific, and cost-effective screening tests for human cancers. International studies have demonstrated a significant reduction in the death rate from cervical cancer since introduction of this test. False-negative results are usually related to poor preparation of the smears or inadequate sampling. Combined with the relatively slow rate of development of invasive cervical cancer from the dysplastic lesions of the cervix, an annual Pap smear has a good probability of preventing the develop-

Table 14-5. Risk Factors for Cervix Cancer

Lower socioeconomic status, underdeveloped countries
First coitus at early age
Multiple sexual partners
Human papillomavirus types 16, 18, 31, 33, 35
AIDS–related malignancy
Carcinoma in situ

ment of invasive cancer. The technique for obtaining an adequate smear has been well described [32].

Management of patients with dysplastic lesions of the cervix is complex and beyond the scope of this chapter. Low-grade lesions require careful follow-up, although most regress spontaneously. Management of high-grade lesions is more controversial. Carcinoma in situ has an unacceptable rate of progression to invasive disease and requires either close follow-up or immediate surgical management. Entry of these patients into chemoprevention studies with novel agents may also be appropriate.

Diagnosis of invasive cervical cancer requires examination of tissue obtained from a cervical biopsy specimen. In the case of an abnormal Pap smear result, either a colposcopic biopsy or cone biopsy are adequate. For lesions that can be appreciated visually on speculum examination, a punch biopsy is adequate for diagnosis.

Approach to the patient with early stage disease

Goals of treatment in early stage disease are cure, and in late stage disease to prevent pain, preserve renal function, and prevent disease progression that can result in fistula formation, malodorous discharge, and thromboembolic events. Unlike carcinoma of the ovary, diagnosis is usually straightforward, because the cervix can be visually inspected and subjected to easy biopsy. Thus, 75% of cervical cancers are diagnosed at early stages, whereas only 25% of ovarian carcinomas are diagnosed before they have spread to the abdomen.

Unlike ovarian cancer, staging for cervical cancer is based on clinical findings (Table 14-6). Examination is optimally conducted with the patients under anesthesia. Other tests may be employed including cervical biopsy, cystoscopy, proctosigmoidoscopy, chest radiography, and intravenous pyelography (IVP) or CT scan of the abdomen. Thus, unlike ovarian cancer, surgical staging for cervical cancer is not warranted. However, surgical staging is acknowledged to be more accurate. The staging system is listed in Table 14-7.

As with ovarian cancers, precise staging is required as this correlates well with prognosis. Long-term survival rates are 76% for stage I (confined to the cervix), 55% for stage II (local spread to adnexa or upper vagina), 31% for stage III (spread to pelvic sidewalls or lower

vagina) and 7% for stage IV (spread beyond the pelvis). Furthermore, accurate staging is the foundation for further approaches to therapy. In addition to clinical staging, a chest roentgenogram is required to rule out pulmonary spread and a computed tomographic scan of the abdomen and pelvis is required to rule out lymph node and liver involvement. The role of nuclear magnetic resonance imaging remains unresolved.

For patients with disease confined to the pelvis, combination treatment with chemotherapy and radiation therapy has been recommended by a Consensus Panel from the National Institutes of Health in April, 1996 [34]. The basis for this statement was the publication of the results of four random assignment trials that all confirmed the benefit of cisplatin-based chemotherapy in combination with standard radiation therapy versus radiation therapy alone in patients with early-stage disease [35–38].

Radiation consists of external beam therapy at doses of 5000 to 6000 cGy, followed by brachytherapy with a cesium source to deliver 6500 to 7200 cGy to point A (ie, the bulkiest portion of the tumor). The optimal chemotherapeutic regimen remains to be determined. Concurrent chemotherapy appears to be superior to sequential chemotherapy and radiation therapy. Neoadjuvant therapy has consistently failed to demonstrate a clinical benefit.

Early stage cervical cancer (stage I or IIA) can be treated with radical hysterectomy with results equivalent to those in radiation therapy. Radical hysterectomy includes, in addition to total hysterectomy, en bloc resection of the parametrial connective tissues and the upper vagina, ureteral dissection, and total pelvic lymphadenectomy. The risks of surgical complications markedly increase compared with total hysterectomy.

Approach to the patient with metastatic or recurrent disease

For patients with positive findings in the para-aortic lymph nodes, therapy remains controversial. Treatment of microscopic disease in para-aortic nodes with extended field radiation therapy did prolong survival in one study [39]; however, this does not necessarily imply a clinical benefit for patients with macroscopic involvement. Such patients may be considered candidates for treatment of advanced disease; control of the primary lesion is indicated to prevent local complications.

Patients in whom local radiation therapy fails and who have no evidence of distant disease may be candidates for pelvic exenteration. This procedure, which is associated with high rates of morbidity, should only be attempted by clinicians with relevant expertise. Partial exenterative procedures (anterior or posterior) may be associated with lower rates of morbidity. Reconstructive procedures include construction of continent conduits, creation of a neovagina, and low rectal anastomosis.

Role of chemotherapy in patients with metastatic or recurrent disease

Patients in whom local therapy fails or who present de novo with disease at distant sites, such as liver, bone, or lung, are candidates for systemic therapy. Usefulness of single-agent therapy is limited; such activity is shown in Table 14-7.

The GOG conducted a randomized trial of three different doses and schedules of cisplatin [40]. The higher dose, 100 mg/m², produced higher response rates, but no improvement in duration of response or survival. Therefore, dose-intensive platinum therapy in patients with advanced cervical cancer is not indicated routinely. Other single agents, such as paclitaxel, may have modest clinical activity in women with advanced cervical cancer.

Table 14-6. Staging and Prognosis of Cervical Cancer

Stage	Characteristics
I	Microscopic or macroscopic disease confined to the cervix
II	Disease confined to the pelvis but not to the pelvic sidewall or to the lower one third of the vagina
III	Disease that has spread to the pelvic sidewall or the lower one third of the vagina or presents with hydronephrosis
IV	Disease that has involved the mucosa of the bladder or rectum or has spread outside the pelvis

Prognosis

Stage	Survival, %
I	76
II	55
III	31
IV	7

Adapted from Creasman [33].

The role of combination chemotherapy in cervical cancer is controversial. Although many clinicians prefer a cisplatin-based regimen, there is no standard therapy. Older combinations used cisplatin plus bleomycin with one or more additional agents, such as ifosfamide, often employed on an infusional schedule. More recently, combinations of paclitaxel and cisplatin or carboplatin have been studied. However, combination chemotherapy has not been shown to be more effective than single agent therapy and may accrue substantial toxicities.

Palliation of symptoms may be achieved with local radiotherapy. Surgical resection of late and isolated lung metastases may result in long-term survival in up to 25% of cases. Renal function may be preserved with a percutaneous renal stent; however, prolonged survival or palliation have not been demonstrated with this approach. Adequate pain control may be achieved with opiates, such as MS Contin or fentanyl patches. Patients with fistula formation often present with intractable problems including malodorous discharge, which may be partially controlled with charcoal-impregnated pads, or with infection requiring antibiotic therapy. Cachexia requires dietary counseling and nutritional supplementation.

APPROACH TO TREATMENT OF THE PATIENT WITH ENDOMETRIAL CARCINOMA

General principles

Cancer of the endometrium is the commonest tumor type of the female genital tract, accounting for approximately 33,000 cases of cancer annually in the United States. Because endometrial carcinoma is usually detected in early stages, this disease accounts for fewer deaths than carcinoma of the ovary. At time of diagnosis, 80% of cases fall into stage I disease, confined to the uterine corpus. This disease is usually easily diagnosed; however, well-differentiated tumors may be difficult to distinguish from endometrial hyperplasia.

Screening, early detection, and diagnosis

Risk factors are described in Table 14-9. Routine screening of asymptomatic, postmenopausal women is probably not warranted. Women older than 40 years of age with abnormal bleeding, with massive obesity, or history of endometrial hyperplasia may require routine screening, however, because they are at higher risk. The most provocative data on risk for endometrial carcinoma come from the recent NSABP trials in women with breast cancer receiving long-term tamoxifen therapy [41]. Incidence of endometrial

cancer increased among those women receiving tamoxifen, likely as a result of tamoxifen's estrogenic action on uterine tissue. The clinical, pathologic, and molecular characteristics of these tumors are now being analyzed and may offer some clues to the etiology of this disease. Women receiving long-term tamoxifen therapy require closer follow-up, which may indicate the development of a uterine carcinoma.

Among postmenopausal patients, use of hormone replacement therapy (HRT) is increasing because of salutary effects on bone density and cardiovascular disease. There is some controversy about whether HRT increases the risk of endometrial carcinoma, with most recent studies suggesting that it does not do so among the general population. There does appear to be an increased risk of breast cancer among women with a previous history of or family history of breast cancer. The possibility of an increased risk of cancer among women with a prior history of endometrial

Table 14-8. Risk Factors for Endometrial Carcinoma

Increased risk	Decreased risk
Obesity	Combination oral contraceptives
Nulliparity	
Late menopause	
Estrogen use	
Hypertension	
Diabetes	
Long-term tamoxifen use	
Familial cancer syndrome (Lynch II)	

Table 14-9. Staging and Prognosis of Endometrial Carcinoma

Stage	Characteristics
I	Disease confined to the corpus
IA	Confined to endometrium
IB	Invasion to less than half of the myometrium
IC	Invasion to more than half of the myometrium
II	Disease involves the corpus and cervix
IIA	Involves the endocervical gland
IIB	Invasion of the cervical stroma
III	Disease confined within the pelvis
IIIA	Invasion of serosa/adnexa or + peritoneal cytology
IIIB	Vaginal metastases
IIIC	+ Pelvic or para-aortic lymph nodes
IV	Advanced disease
IVA	+ Bladder or bowel mucosa
IVB	Distant metastases including abdominal or inguinal nodes

Prognosis

Stage	5-y Survival, %
I	72.3
II	56.4
III	31.5
IV	10.5

Adapted from International Federation of Gynecology and Obstetrics [42].

Table 14-7. Single-Agent Activity in Carcinoma of the Uterine Cervix

Drug	Patients, n	Response Rate, %
Cisplatin	52	40
Vincristine	44	23
Doxorubicin	78	10
Bleomycin	172	10
Cyclophosphamide	228	14
5-Fluorouracil	348	20
Methotrexate	77	16
Paclitaxel	52	17

cancer is currently being studied in an intergroup trial by the GOG and the ECOG.

There is also a familial risk factor for endometrial carcinoma. Endometrial carcinoma is part of the HNPCC or Lynch II familial cancer syndrome (see earlier description of this syndrome in this chapter in the section on ovarian carcinoma).

The peak age group for the development of endometrial carcinoma is in patients between 60 and 70 years old. The disease is associated with obesity and diabetes, which makes these patients somewhat older and less healthy than other patients with gynecologic malignancies. This accounts in part for the lesser role played by chemotherapy in the treatment of this disease.

The typical presentation of endometrial carcinoma is postmenopausal bleeding, which occurs in 80% of patients. Other symptoms include vaginal discharge and leukorrhea. Evaluation of postmenopausal bleeding includes fractional dilatation and curettage, with separation of cervical and endometrial specimens. Endometrial carcinoma must be distinguished from atypical hyperplasia. In addition to standard pathology, grading of the tumor is important in the subsequent management.

Staging and prognosis

Staging of endometrial carcinoma is described in Table 14-10. Factors that adversely affect survival include clear cell, papillary, or adenosquamous histologies; increased grade; increased uterine size; myometrial invasion; positive peritoneal cytology; positive pelvic or para-aortic lymph nodes; or adnexal spread. A high percentage of patients present with favorable factors; therefore, survival rates in endometrial carcinoma are higher than those of ovarian carcinoma.

Poor-risk subtypes of endometrial adenocarcinoma

Uterine papillary serous carcinoma (UPSC) is well-recognized as a more aggressive variant that clinically behaves more like an aggressive ovarian carcinoma than to the generally more indolent endometrial adenocarcinomas. Specifically, UPSC tends to metastasize earlier with involvement of the peritoneal cavity. Clear-cell, poorly differentiated adenocarcinomas, undifferentiated tumors and squamous cell carcinoma of the endometrium also have more aggressive clinical courses with a poorer outcome.

Uterine sarcomas

Sarcomas of the uterus include leiomyosarcoma, carcinosarcoma, and endometrial stromal sarcoma. These are uncommon, accounting for fewer than 5% of all endometrial tumors. These are aggressive tumors and survival beyond 2 years is uncommon. As with endometrial carcinomas, vaginal bleeding is the most frequently seen presenting symptom. Pain is also common and may be accompanied by prolapse of a uterine mass through the vagina. This may be accompanied by a foul-smelling discharge. Patients should undergo a biopsy before hysterectomy. Interpretation of the pathologic specimen is sometimes problematic in tumors with mixed histologies. These aggressive tumors require management in concert with an experienced surgeon and radiation therapist.

TREATMENT RECOMMENDATIONS FOR ENDOMETRIAL CARCINOMA

Treatment recommendations are summarized in Table 14-11. Specific recommendations are described here.

Treatment of stage I disease

For patients with disease confined to the uterine corpus, the treatment is total abdominal hysterectomy and bilateral salpingo-oophorectomy. The ovaries are removed because of occasional implants on ovaries or fallopian tubes. Suspicious pelvic nodes are also excised; if the frozen section is positive, para-aortic lymph node dissection is indicated. For patients at high risk of recurrence, adjuvant radiation therapy may be given. For patients who are not candidates for surgery, radiation therapy may provide equivalent results.

Treatment of stage II to III disease

For patients with gross involvement of the uterine cervix, either radical hysterectomy or preoperative radiation therapy is indicated followed by total abdominal hysterectomy and bilateral salpingo-oophorectomy (TAH-BSO). For patients with microscopic cervical spread, treatment includes TAH-BSO followed by postoperative radiation therapy. For patients with spread to other pelvic tissues, treatment includes TAH-BSO followed by pelvic irradiation.

Treatment of stage IV disease

For patients with disease that has spread beyond the pelvis, TAH-BSO plus pelvic irradiation may be required to prevent complications from hemorrhage. Systemic therapy would include either hormonal therapy or chemotherapy.

Hormonal therapy

Hormonal therapy is most successful in patients with a long disease-free interval (ie, 2 years or more), well-differentiated tumors, and progesterone–receptor rich tumors. There is a high degree of progesterone-receptor positivity in endometrial carcinomas, ranging from 33% to 64% in undifferentiated tumors to 81% to 95% in well-differentiated tumors and 70% to 72% overall [43]. The definition of the term receptor-rich is unclear. Overall, response to hormonal therapy with progestational agents is observed in 71% of patients with positive cytosolic progesterone receptors and 8% in patients without progesterone receptor protein [43]. One caution is that the assay for progesterone receptors must be performed properly on fresh tissue that has been rapidly frozen at - 70°C with appropriate controls.

The most commonly employed agent is the progestational agent megestrol acetate (Megace), which is administered at higher doses than those employed for breast cancer (320 mg/d). Progestational agents, such as 17-hydroxyprogesterone caproate (Delalutin) or 6-α-

Table 14-10. Treatment Recommendation by Stage for Endometrial Carcinoma

Stage	Treatment
I, II	TAH-BSO (en bloc)
	Para-aortic lymph node sampling (myometrial invasion only) with or without pelvic node sampling
	Peritoneal washings
	Postoperative radiation therapy for:
	High-risk: positive lymph nodes or adnexal spread
	?Intermediate risk: myometrial invasion >1/2, spread to cervix or vascular space, positive peritoneal washings, grade 3, incomplete surgical staging
	Adjuvant chemotherapy for papillary serous histology
III	Radiation alone or surgery plus radiation therapy
IV	Radiation therapy with or without hormonal therapy with or without chemotherapy

methyl-hydroxy progesterone acetate (Provera), are administered by injection. Toxicities with progestational agents are modest, with the commonest side effects fluid retention and weight gain. Response rates initially reported at 35% [44] have not been confirmed by later studies [45] with usual response rates in the 11% to 16% range, but with some responses still durable up to 29 months. The antiestrogenic agent, tamoxifen, and the synthetic 17-ethinyl testosterone derivative, danazol, also have activity in endometrial carcinoma, comparable with that of progestational agents. Combinations of hormonal agents have not proven superior to single-agent therapy.

New hormonal agents are currently being studied in clinical trials. Aromatase inhibitors, such as letrozole and anastrozole, which are active in women with breast cancer, are currently in clinical trials.

Chemotherapy

For patients in whom treatment with progestational agents has failed or who have life-threatening visceral involvement and are candidates for systemic chemotherapy, treatment with cytotoxic drugs is indicated. Single-agent activity is shown in Table 14-12.

Treatment with combination chemotherapy likely increases response rates over single-agent therapy with doxorubicin; however, the magnitude of the benefits are small and toxicities are increased. Two-drug therapy with doxorubicin–cisplatin has resulted in response rates of 33% [46]. In GOG 107, which compared doxorubicin alone to doxorubicin plus cisplatin, there was an advantage in response and to a lesser extent in progression-free survival, but not overall survival on preliminary analysis. Final analysis is pending.

Several studies have employed cyclophosphamide-doxorubicin-cisplatin (CAP) or cyclophosphamide-doxorubicin-vinblastine with response rates of 31% to 47%. In a randomized phase II study of cisplatin versus CAP conducted by the North Central Cancer Treatment Group, three of 14 responded to cisplatin and five of 16 to CAP. Only 7% and 12% of patients survived 2 years, respectively, and the authors concluded that treatment with experimental phase II agents was warranted [47]. These recommendations remain valid. Combinations of cytotoxic agents plus progestational agents have been tested and do not appear more active than single-agent chemotherapy.

Newer cytotoxic drugs appear to have activity in patients with advanced endometrial carcinoma. The ECOG trial E3E93 has demonstrated activity for topotecan, administered on a daily × 5 schedule, but with significant toxicities, mainly related to myelosup-

pression (unpublished data). Paclitaxel is also an active agent in the treatment of endometrial carcinoma. An NYGOG trial of paclitaxel and doxil demonstrated high response rates among women with uterine cancer [48].

Patients with advanced disease who are otherwise in good health may be candidates for clinical trials using experimental agents, after the risk and benefits of such an approach have been described to the patient.

TREATMENT OF UTERINE SARCOMAS

Treatment of these uncommon tumors is often complex. The foundation for the treatment of these tumors is surgery. The standard treatment is TAH-BSO. External radiation therapy is often employed as an adjunct to surgery, although few studies have documented the worth of radiation therapy. There is no standard approach to chemotherapeutic treatment in patients with advanced disease. In general, combinations of doxorubicin and cisplatin are employed. Recently, the New York Gynecologic Oncology Group has demonstrated significant clinical activity with the combination of doxil and paclitaxel [48].

APPROACH TO THE PATIENT WITH GESTATIONAL TROPHOBLASTIC NEOPLASM

General principles

Gestational trophoblastic neoplasms (GTN) comprise a family of related lesions that encompass molar pregnancy, placental site trophoblastic tumor and choriocarcinoma. Molar pregnancy may be classified as complete or partial based on histopathology and karyotype. Incidence of GTN varies widely among different parts of the world; it is five times more prevalent in Africa and Asia than Europe or North America. Although uncommon in North America, GTN is an important neoplasm to the medical oncologist because it is highly curable with chemotherapy. Even patients with high-risk disease enter remission in about 70% of cases with modern, aggressive combination chemotherapy regimens.

The etiology of GTN is not well established. Patients with a prior molar pregnancy have a higher risk for developing trophoblastic disease. Risk factors (Table 14-13) for development of a molar pregnancy include a uterus large for dates, although a molar pregnancy can occur in a normal-sized uterus. Time of evacuation may also increase the incidence of malignant sequelae with evacuations occurring earlier than 10 weeks being less likely to result in a malignancy.

Table 14-11. Single-Agent Activity in Carcinoma of the Endometrium

Agent	Response Rate, %
Cisplatin	42
Doxorubicin	37
Cyclophosphamide	21
5-Fluorouracil	23
Idarubicin	10
Mitoxantrone	5
Carboplatin	28
Megestrol acetate (high dose)	24
Hexamethylmelamine	9
Etoposide (oral)	0
Paclitaxel	36
Ifosfamide	24

Table 14-12. Risk Factors for Gestational Trophoblastic Neoplasms

Mole
  Asia greater risk than North America, Europe
  Age older than 50 y or younger than 16 y
  Prior hydatidiform mole
Postmolar gestational trophoblastic neoplasm
  Increased βhCG
  Increased maternal age
  Uterine enlargement
  Theca lutein cysts

Table 14-13. Prognostic Factors for Gestational Trophoblastic Neoplasm

Nonmetastatic GTN

Low risk

  Serum βhCG < 40,000 mIU/mL

  Duration < 4 mo

  No antecedent term pregnancy, prior chemotherapy, or brain or liver metastases

High risk

  Serum βhCG > 40,000 mIU/mL

  Duration > 4 mo

  Antecedent term pregnancy, failed prior chemotherapy, or brain or liver metastases

Screening and early diagnosis

Screening for GTN is not clinically indicated; however, it is important for the obstetrician and internist who are caring for the patient to be aware of this entity. In women who have had an evacuated molar pregnancy, indications for treatment include failure of human chorionic gonadotropin (hCG) to normalize following evacuation of a molar pregnancy, evidence of locally invasive disease, or evidence of metastatic disease. The commonest site of metastatic disease is in the lung; in later stages the liver, abdominal cavity, and brain may all become involved.

Treatment of women with gestational trophoblastic neoplasms

The clinical features have been reviewed previously [49]. Prognosis and approach to treatment are directly related to the clinical and histopathologic features of this disease (Table 14-14). Clinical features include degree of invasiveness (localized to uterine cavity, invasion into uterine myometrium, or metastatic to lungs or vagina [low risk], or to brain or liver [high risk]), disease-free interval and bulk of tumor [best assessed by levels of the tumor marker βhCG]). Important histopathologic features include the presence of complete or partial mole and the presence of choriocarcinoma.

Methotrexate was first reported to be curative in patients with metastatic choriocarcinoma in 1956 and has remained the mainstay of therapy for low-risk disease. The most commonly employed regimen is that developed at the New England Trophoblastic Disease Center, methotrexate (MTX) 1 mg/kg intramuscularly every other day for 8 days alternating with leucovorin rescue, 0.1 mg/kg intramuscularly every other day for 8 days. MTX has also been administered as a 12-hour intravenous infusion, orally and as weekly intramuscular therapy. Cure rates are high with all regimens; however, the accepted regimen is the alternating 8-day treatment. Actinomycin is also an active drug in the treatment of GTN, but is more toxic than the combination of MTX and leucovorin.

Patients with high-risk disease include patients with brain or liver metastases, large tumor burdens or high βhCG levels, prior failed chemotherapy, or long disease intervals. These patients require treatment with combination chemotherapy. Early regimens combined methotrexate and actinomycin with other agents (MAC [methotrexate, actinomycin D, cyclophosphamide]; CHAMOCA [cyclophosphamide, hydroxyurea, dactinomycin, methotrexate, vincristine, doxorubicin]). More recently, etoposide (VP-16) has been incorporated into GTN regimens with equivalent results to CHAMOCA, but less toxicity [50]. The two most important regimens are EMA/CO, which incorporates etoposide with methotrexate-leucovorin and actinomycin (EMA) and cyclophosphamide with vincristine (CO), and administers each on alternate weeks, as well as EMA and etoposide/cisplatin. Poor-risk patients had a survival rate of 84%; those in whom earlier therapy failed had a response rate of 74%. In a subsequent series, responses were observed in 76% of chemotherapy-naive, high-risk patients and in 57% of patients failed by prior treatment [50].

REFERENCES

1. Van Nagell JR, Gallion HH, DePriest PD: Ovarian cancer screening. *Cancer* 1995, 75:2642.

2. National Institutes of Health. Consensus Conference. *Gynecol Oncol* 1994; 55:S177.

3. Takahashi H, Behbakht K, McGovern PE, *et al.*: Mutation analysis of the BRCA1 gene in ovarian cancers. *Cancer Res* 1995, 55:2998–3002.

4. Merajver SD, Pham TM, Caduff RF, *et al.*: Somatic mutations in the BRCA1 gene in sporadic ovarian tumours. *Nat Genet* 1995, 9:439–443.

5. Ford D, Easton DF, Peto J: Estimates of the gene frequency of BRCA1 and its contribution to breast and ovarian cancer incidence. *Am J Hum Genet* 1995, 57:1457–1462.

6. Stratton JF, Gaythier SA, Russell P, *et al.*: Contribution of BRCA1 mutations to ovarian cancer. *N Engl J Med* 1997, 336:1125–1130.

7. International Federation of Gynecology and Obstetrics: Annual report on the results of treatment in gynecologic cancer. *Int J Gynecol Obstet* 1989, 28:189–190.

8. Society of Gynecologic Oncologists: Practice guidelines for gynecologic malignancies. *Oncology* 1997, 12:129–133.

9. Young RC, Walton LA, Ellenberg SS, *et al.*: Adjuvant therapy in stage I and stage II epithelial ovarian cancer: results of two prospective randomized trials. *N Engl J Med* 1990, 322:1021–1027.

10. Society of Gynecologic Oncology: Treatment recommendations. *Oncology* 1997, 12:129–133.

11. American College of Surgeons Commission on Cancer and the American Cancer Society: The National Cancer Data Base report on ovarian cancer treatment in United States hospitals. *Cancer* 1996, 78:2236–2246.

12. Alberts DS, Liu PY, Hannigan EV, *et al.*: Intraperitoneal cisplatin plus intravenous cyclophosphamide versus intravenous cisplatin plus intravenous cyclophosphamide for stage III ovarian cancer. *N Engl J Med* 1996, 335:1950–1955.

13. Rowinsky EK, Donehower RC: Paclitaxel (Taxol). *N Engl J Med* 1995, 332:1004–1007.

14. McGuire WP, Hoskins WJ, Brady MF, *et al.*: Cyclophosphamide and cisplatin compared with paclitaxel and cisplatin in patients with stage III and stage IV ovarian cancer. *N Engl J Med* 1996, 334:1–6.

15. Piccart MJ, Bertelsen K, James K, *et al.*: Randomized intergroup trial of cisplatin-paclitaxel versus cisplatin-cyclophosphamide in women with advanced epithelial ovarian cancer: three-year results. *J Natl Cancer Inst* 2000, 92:699–708.

16. Muggia FM, Braly PS, Brady MF, *et al.*: Phase III randomized study of cisplatin versus paclitaxel versus cisplatin and paclitaxel in patients with suboptimal stage III or IV ovarian cancer: a Gynecologic Oncology Group study. *J Clin Oncol* 2000, 18:106–115.

17. ICON Collaborators: ICON2: Randomised trial of single agent carboplatin against three-drug combination of CAP (cyclophosphamide, doxorubicin, and cisplatin) in women with ovarian cancer. *Lancet* 1998, 352:1571–1576.

18. Joly F, Heron JF, Kerbrat P, *et al.:* High-dose platinum versus standard dose in advanced ovarian carcinoma: a randomized trial from the Gynecologic Cooperative Group of the French Comprehensive Cancer Centers (FNCLCC). *Gynecol Oncol* 2000, 78:361–368.

19. Coleman RL, Bagnell KG, Townley PM: Carboplatin and short-infusion paclitaxel in high-risk and advanced-stage ovarian carcinoma. *Cancer J Sci Am* 1997, 3:246–253.

20. ten Bokkel Huinink WW, van Warmerdam LJC, *et al.:* Phase II study of the combination of carboplatin and paclitaxel in patients with ovarian cancer. *Ann Oncol* 1997, 8:351–354.

21. Neijt JP, Engelholm SA, Tuxen MK, *et al.:* Exploratory phase III study of paclitaxel and cisplatin versus paclitaxel and carboplatin in advanced ovarian cancer. *J Clin Oncol* 2000, 18:3084–3092.

22. Schink JC, Weller E, Harris LS, *et al.:*. Outpatient taxol and carboplatin chemotherapy for suboptimally debulked epithelial carcinoma of the ovary results in improved quality of life: an Eastern Cooperative Oncology Group phase II study (E2E93). *Ca J Sci Am* 2001, in press.

23. Eisenhauer EA, Vermorken JB, van Glabbeke M: Predictors of response to subsequent chemotherapy in platinum pretreated ovarian cancer: a multivariate analysis of 704 patients. *Ann Oncol* 1997, 8:963–968.

24. Tuxen MK, Straus G, Lund B, *et al.:* The role of second-look laparotomy in the long-term survival in ovarian cancer. *Ann Oncol* 1997, 8:643–648.

25. van der Burg MEL, van Lent, Kobierska A *et al.:* Intervention debulking surgery (IDS) does improve survival in advanced epithelial ovarian cancer (EOC): an EORTC Gynecologic Cancer Cooperative Group (GCCG) study. *Proc Am Soc Clin Oncol* 1993, 12:258.

26. van der Burg MEL. More than 20 years second-look surgery in advanced epithelial ovarian cancer: what did we learn. *Ann Oncol* 1997, 8:627–629.

27. Thigpen JT: Dose-intensity in ovarian carcinoma: hold, enough? *J Clin Oncol* 1997, 15:1291–1292.

28. Creemers GJ, Bolis G, Gore M, *et al.:* Topotecan, an active drug in the second-line treatment of epithelial ovarian cancer: results of a large European phase II study. *J Clin Oncol* 1996, 14:3056–3061.

29. Hochster H, Wadler S, Speyer J, *et al.:* Activity and pharmacodynamics of 21-day topotecan infusion in patients with ovarian cancer previously treated with platinum-based therapy. *J Clin Oncol* 1999, 17:2553–2561.

30. ten Bokkel Huinink WW, Gore M, Carmichael J, *et al.:* Topotecan versus paclitaxel for the treatment of recurrent epithelial ovarian cancer. *J Clin Oncol* 1997, 15:2183–2193.

31. Gordon AN, Granai CO, Rose PG, *et al.:* Phase II study of liposomal doxorubicin in platinum- and paclitaxel-refractory epithelial ovarian cancer. *J Clin Oncol* 2000, 18:3093–3100.

32. Wilkinson EJ: Pap smears and screening for cervical cancer. *Clin Obstet Gynecol* 1990, 33:817.

33. Creasman WT: New gynecologic cancer staging. *Gynecol Oncol* 1995, 55:157–158.

34. National Institutes of Health: Consensus statement. Cervical Cancer. 1996, 14:1–38.

35. Keys HM, Bundy BN, Stehman FB *et al.:* Cisplatin, radiation and adjuvant hysterectomy compared with radiation and adjuvant hysterectomy for bulky stage IB cervical carcinoma. *N Engl J Med* 1999, 340:1154–1161.

36. Rose PG, Bundy BN, Watkins EB, *et al.:* Concurrent cisplatin-based radiotherapy and chemotherapy for locally advanced cervical cancer. *N Engl J Med* 1999, 340:1144–1153.

37. Morris M, Eifel PH, Lu J, *et al.:* Pelvic radiation with concurrent chemotherapy compared with pelvic and para-aortic radiation for high-risk cervical cancer. *N Engl J Med* 1999, 340:1137–1143.

38. Peters WA, Liu PY, Barrett RJ, *et al.:* Concurrent chemotherapy and pelvic radiation therapy compared with pelvic radiation therapy alone as adjuvant therapy after radical surgery in high-risk early-stage cancer of the cervix. *Gynecol Oncol* 1999, 72:443.

39. Rotman M, Pajak TF, Choi K, *et al.:* Prophylactic extended-field irradiation of para-aortic lymph nodes in stages IIB and bulky IB and IIA cervical carcinomas. Ten-year treatment results of RTOG 79-20. *JAMA* 1995, 274:387–393.

40. Bonomi P, Blessing JA, Stehman FB, *et al.:* Randomized trial of three cisplatin dose schedules in squamous-cell carcinoma of the cervix: a Gynecologic Oncology Group study. *J Clin Oncol* 1985, 3:1079–1085.

41. Fisher B, Costantino JP, Redmond CK, *et al.:* Endometrial cancer in tamoxifen-treated breast cancer patients: findings from the National Surgical Adjuvant Breast and Bowel Project (NSABP) B-14. *J Natl Cancer Inst* 1994, 86:527–537.

42. International Federation of Gynecology and Obstetrics: Annual report on the results of treatment in gynecologic cancer. *Int J Gynecol Obstet* 1989, 28:189–190.

43. Richardson GS, MacLaughlin DT: The status of receptors in the management of endometrial cancer. *Clin Obstet Gynecol* 29:628-637, 1986

44. Reifenstein EC: The treatment of advanced endometrial cancer with hydroxyprogesterone caproate. *Gynecol Oncol* 1974, 2:377–414.

45. Podratz KC, O'Brien PC, Malkasian GD: Effects of progestational agents in the treatment of endometrial carcinoma. *Obstet Gynecol* 1985, 66:106–115.

46. Seltzer V, Vogl SE, Kaplan BH. Adriamycin and cis-diaminedichloroplatinum in the treatment of metastatic endometrial adenocarcinoma. Gynecol Oncol 19:308-313, 1984

47. Edmondson JH, Krook JE, Hilton JF, *et al.:* Randomized phase II studies of cisplatin and a combination of cyclophosphamide-doxorubicin-cisplatin (CAP) in patients with progestin-refractory advanced endometrial carcinoma. *Gynecol Oncol* 1987, 28:20–24.

48. Muggia FM, Hornreich G, Wadler S, *et al.:* Overview of toxicities from a combination of doxil-paclitaxel (Paclidox) in a New York Gynecologic Oncology Group (NYGOG) study on endometrial carcinomas and sarcomas. *Proc Am Soc Clin Oncol* 1999, 18:380a.

49. Berkowitz RS, Goldstein DP: Gestational trophoblastic diseases. *Semin Oncol* 1989, 16:410–416.

50. Newlands ES, Bagshawe KD, Begent RJH, *et al.:* Developments in chemotherapy for medium- and high-risk patients with gestational trophoblastic tumors (1979-1984). *Br J Obstet Gynecol* 93:63–69.

PACLITAXEL PLUS A PLATINUM COMPOUND FOR SUBOPTIMAL OVARIAN CARCINOMA

Chemotherapy for advanced suboptimally debulked (> 1 cm) or metastatic ovarian carcinoma is based on the combination of paclitaxel and a platinum compound. Cisplatin forms DNA adducts composed of intrastrand cross-links which act much in the same way as classic alkylating agents, preventing DNA transcription and synthesis and causing DNA strand breaks. Carboplatin is a cisplatin analogue with a different toxicity profile and different pharmacokinetic profile, but carboplatin also forms platinum adducts.

Paclitaxel is a natural product of the western yew which has a complex biochemical structure. Paclitaxel inhibits depolymerization of tubulin, a unique mechanism of action for a chemotherapeutic agent. Paclitaxel was introduced into front-line therapy based on excellent clinical activity in the second-line setting. In GOG 111, paclitaxel + cisplatin was compared with cyclophosphamide + cisplatin and the combination demonstrated a survival advantage.

A recent preliminary report by the GOG in which single agent cisplatin, single agent paclitaxel, and the combination were compared revealed that combination therapy and single-agent cisplatin, given at a higher dose than was administered in the combination, offered equivalent survival, and that both were better than single-agent paclitaxel.

Recent phase III trials have demonstrated compared survivals for combinations of paclitaxel and carboplatin versus paclitaxel and cisplatin. Thus, either combination would be accepted as a reasonable first-line therapy for women with advanced ovarian carcinoma. Because of the greater ease of administration of carboplatin and 3-hour paclitaxel, including the ability to administer treatment in the outpatient setting without aggressive hydration, this would be the preferred treatment of choice. The optimal regimen remains to be decided.

INDICATIONS

Advanced (stage III-IV) ovarian carcinoma; some patients with stage IC or II disease may be treated with this regimen

SPECIAL PRECAUTIONS

Patients must have adequate white blood cell and platelet counts and must not be dehydrated before initiating treatment. Myelosuppression was more profound when paclitaxel was administered with cisplatin. Ketoconazole may inhibit paclitaxel metabolism. Caution should be used when administering paclitaxel with these agents. Cisplatin should be discontinued with evidence of nephrotoxicity, ototoxicity, or neurotoxicity

DRUG INTERACTIONS

Paclitaxel: may accelerate neurotoxicity when used with other neurotoxic agents

TOXICITIES

Paclitaxel: Acute hypersensitivity reaction with wheezing, shortness of breath, urticaria, and hypotension occurred in 2% of patients receiving paclitaxel; alopecia, nausea, vomiting; profound granulocytopenia and myelosuppression; cardiac conduction abnormalities requiring a pacemaker, hypotension and bradycardia; peripheral neuropathy; arthralgias/myalgias; alopecia; diarrhea; and mucositis

Carboplatin: Granulocytopenia, thrombocytopenia, nausea, vomiting

RECENT EXPERIENCE AND RESPONSE RATES

Study	Regimen	Evaluable Patients, n	Response Rate, %	Median PFS, mo	Median OS, mo
McGuire et al.: N Engl J Med 1996, 334:1	Paclitaxel, 135 mg/m² (24-h infusion); cisplatin, 75 mg/m²	184	73	18	38
Muggia et al.: Proc Am Soc Clin Oncol 1997, 18:57	Cisplatin, 100 mg/m²	200	74	16.4	30.2
Muggia et al.: Proc Am Soc Clin Oncol 1997, 18:57	Paclitaxel, 200 mg/m²	213	46	11.4	26.0
Muggia et al.: Proc Am Soc Clin Oncol 1997, 18:57	Paclitaxel, 135 mg/m²; cisplatin, 75 mg/m²	202	72	14.1	26.6
Neijt et al.: Semin Oncol 1999, suppl 2:78–83	Paclitaxel, 175 mg/m²; carboplatin, AUC 5	213	NS	NS	NS
Du Bois	Paclitaxel, 185 mg/m²; carboplatin, AUC 6	800	70.5	69 wk	NS
Coleman et al.: Cancer J Sci Am 1997, 3:246–253	Paclitaxel, 175 mg/m²; carboplatin, AUC 7–7.5	22	84	NS	NS
Huinink et al.: Ann Oncol 1997, 8:351–534	Paclitaxel, 200 mg/m² (3-h infusion); carboplatin, 550 mg/m²	21	100	NS	NS
Schink et al.: Cancer J Sci Am 2000	Paclitaxel, 150 mg/m² (3-h infusion); carboplatin, AUC 5.0	48	72	11–17	25.7–30.1

AUC—area under the curve; NS—not significant; OS—overall survival; PFS—progression-free survival.

PACLITAXEL PLUS A PLATINUM COMPOUND FOR SUBOPTIMAL OVARIAN CARCINOMA (Continued)

DOSAGE AND SCHEDULING

Paclitaxel: 135–185 mg/m² can be administered as a 3-h infusion in the outpatient setting or as a 24-h inpatient infusion. Premedication to prevent allergic reaction should be administered including: cimetidine 300 mg IV, diphenhydramine (Benadryl; Werner-Lambert Co., Morris Plains, NJ) 50 mg IV, and decadron, 20 mg po 6- and 12-h before administering drug. Appropriate antiemesis should be instituted, because 50% of patients will develop nausea or vomiting. Patients should be monitored closely at the initiation of paclitaxel therapy, and the infusion should be discontinued for any sign of an allergic reaction (especially flushing or dyspnea).

Carboplatin: can be dosed at 5–7.5 AUC using the Calvert or other convenient formula to calculate the desired area under the curve. Unlike cisplatin, the drug does not require prehydration and can be given in the outpatient setting over 15 minutes. Treatment with the combination usually continues for 4–8 cycles. CBC, differential, platelet count, CA-125, BUN, creatinine should be monitored prior to each cycle. Failure of CA-125 to decrease suggests emerging resistance to drug treatment.

NURSING INTERVENTIONS

Combined blood count including platelets should be checked prior to administering drugs. Patients should be pretreated with adequate antiemetic therapy.

Renal function should be monitored. Patients should be monitored for signs of neurotoxicity.

Patients should be questioned regarding their fertility status, although it is unlikely patients with ovarian cancer are pregnant. Paclitaxel may be mutagenic and/or teratogenic. Patients should be cautioned regarding the development of fever 8–14 days after administration of paclitaxel

PATIENT INFORMATION

Patients should be informed about alopecia and cautioned regarding the hypersensitivity reactions thrombocytopenia and neutropenia

ADMINISTRATION NOTES

Paclitaxel is supplied in 30 mg/5 mL vials. Paclitaxel should be diluted in 0.9% sodium chloride for injection or 5% dextrose solution USP at 0.3-1.2 mg/mL. Because the vehicle reacts with polyvinyl chloride (PVC), administration of paclitaxel requires non-PVC bottles and polyethylene-lined tubing

COST

The cost to the pharmacist for each infusion of paclitaxel will probably exceed $1000. The cost to the pharmacist for an infusion of cisplatin is about $450

INTRAPERITONEAL THERAPY FOR OPTIMALLY DEBULKED OVARIAN CANCER

Therapy for optimally debulked (< 1 cm) ovarian cancer may differ from that of suboptimal disease. A recent intergroup study has demonstrated a survival benefit for women receiving intraperitoneal therapy compared with intravenous therapy. Whether the benefits of intensified therapy delivered in this manner will outweigh the inconvenience of placing an intraperitoneal port and the cumbersome administration with uncertain distribution of the drug remains to be demonstrated. Nevertheless, the impressive improvement in survival observed (49 mo vs 41 mo) is important.

DOSAGE AND SCHEDULING

Cyclophosphamide 600 mg/m^2 IV d 1
Cisplatin mg/m^2 in 2 L of normal saline administered rapidly intraperitoneally
Intraperitoneal therapy is warmed to body temperature prior to infusion and instilled rapidly through an intraperitoneal Tenckhoff or Drum catheter or Portacath; simultaneously, patients receive 1 L of normal saline with 3 g magnesium sulfate and 40 g mannitol IV.
Courses are repeated every 3 wk for 6 cycles; doses were held or modified for azotemia, neuropathy, or myelosuppression

INDICATIONS

Optimally debulked (< 1 cm) stage III ovarian carcinoma

SPECIAL PRECAUTIONS

Patients must have adequate white blood cell and platelet counts and must not be dehydrated prior to initiating treatment; patients must have adequate renal function; the catheter must be functioning properly with no evidence of bowel perforation; treatment should be stopped for refractory abdominal pain

DRUG INTERACTIONS

Cisplatin: may potentiate renal effects of nephrotoxic compounds such as aminoglycoside

TOXICITIES

Cisplatin: nephrotoxicity, ototoxicity, neurotoxicity, emesis, Coombs positive hemolytic anemia, electrolyte abnormalities; **Cyclophosphamide:** granulocytopenia, thrombocytopenia, nausea, vomiting, hemorrhagic cystitis, pneumonitis, alopecia

NURSING INTERVENTIONS

Combined blood count, including platelets, should be checked prior to administering drugs; patients should be pretreated with adequate antiemetic therapy; renal function should be monitored; patients should be monitored for signs of neurotoxicity

PATIENT ASSESSMENT

Patients should be questioned regarding their fertility status, although it is unlikely that patients with ovarian cancer will be pregnant; cyclophosphamide may be mutagenic and/or teratogenic

PATIENT INFORMATION

Patients should be cautioned regarding the development of fevers 8–14 d after administration of chemotherapy; patients should be informed about alopecia and cautioned regarding the potential for development of acute leukemia in patients treated with alkylating agents

ADMINISTRATION NOTES

The intraperitoneal solution should be prewarmed prior to administration; the bag should be checked to ensure that the solution is running into the peritoneal cavity freely; the fluid does not need to be drained

COST

The cost to the pharmacist for the cyclophosphamide is approximately $50; the cost to the pharmacist for an infusion of cisplatin is approximately $450

MEGACE FOR ADVANCED ENDOMETRIAL CARCINOMA

The mainstay of therapy for endometrial carcinomas are progestational agents. Megace (megestrol acetate) is available orally.

The precise mechanism of action is unknown. Progestins promote the differentiation and maintenance of endometrial tissues. In endometrial cancer, they probably act as negative growth regulators acting either directly or in concert with other growth factors, such as transforming growth factor β, which inhibits cell growth.

EXPERIENCES AND RESPONSE RATES

Study	Overall Response Rate ,%
Reifenstein *et al.*: *Gynecol Oncol* 1974, 2:377	35
Podratz *et al.*: *Obstet Gynecol* 1985, 66:106	11

DOSAGE AND SCHEDULING

Megace 40–80 mg/d PO
Liver function tests should be checked prior to treatment

INDICATIONS

Advanced endometrial and breast cancer

ELIGIBILITY AND EXCLUSIONS

Eligibility: advanced or refractory endometrial cancer;
Exclusions: none

SPECIAL PRECAUTIONS

Reduce dose in patients with preexisting liver disease; patients with congestive heart failure should be monitored carefully; liver function tests should be made before treatment

DRUG INTERACTIONS

None

TOXICITIES

Fluid retention, weight gain, liver function abnormalities (uncommon), thromboembolic phenomena (rare)

NURSING INTERVENTIONS

None

PATIENT INFORMATION

Patients should be warned about possible fluid retention; teratogenic

ADMINISTRATION

Available as 20-mg or 40-mg tablets

DOXIL AND PACLITAXEL FOR UTERINE SARCOMAS

DOXIL AND PACLITAXEL FOR UTERINE SARCOMAS

At present, no standard treatment exists for advanced high-risk endometrial carcinomas or sarcomas. For endometrial sarcomas, many physicians use a combination of doxorubicin, 50 mg/m^2, and cisplatin, 50 mg/m^2. For endometrial carcinomas, many physicians use either the same regimen (doxorubicin + cisplatin) or a combination of carboplatin and paclitaxel as already described elsewhere in this chapter. Recently, Muggia and coworkers described high response rates and acceptable toxicities in a preliminary report for the treatment of high-risk endometrial carcinomas and uterine sarcomas. The treatment incorporates doxil, which is a liposomally encapsulated form of doxorubicin, with paclitaxel, as previously described. Doxil has demonstrated a favorable pharmacologic profile and clinical activity in the treatment of refractory gastrointestinal malignancies. The report by Muggia and coworkers demonstrates that doxil and paclitaxel can be combined with high activity and acceptable toxicities.

RECENT EXPERIENCE AND RESULTS

Study	Sarcoma type	Doxorubicin dose, (mg/m^2)	CR + PR/evaluation
Sutton GP: *Am J Obstet Gyn* 1992, 166:556	LMSU	Dox, 60 q 3 wk, vs dox, 60 + DTIC q 3 wk	5 + 8/80 vs 7+9/66
Thigpen TJ: *Clin Oncol* 1991, 9:1962	LMSU	Cisplatin	7 PR/33
Sutton GP: *Proc ASCO* 1993, 12:271	LMSU	Dox 50 + Imesna	1 CR + 9 PR/27
Currie J: *Proc Soc Gyn Oncol* 1994	LMSU	Hydroxyurea, dox	2 CR + 5 PR/39
Sutton GP: *Gynecol Oncol* 1994, 53:24	MMT ovary	Ifos/Mesna	1 CR + 4 PR/28
Muss HB: *Am J Clin Oncol* 1990, 13:32	MMT, LMSU	Mitoxantrone	0/17 0/12
Slayton RE: *Invest New Drugs* 1991, 9:207	LMSU	Diaziquone	0/24
Asbury R, submitted	LMSU	Aminothiadazole	0/25 1 PR/22

Data from Muggia et al. (Personal communication).
LMSU — leiomyosarcoma uterus; MMT — mixed mesodermal tumor; MS — median survival.

DOSAGE AND SCHEDULING

Doxil is administered at 30 mg/m^2 on day 1, 21 and every 4 weeks. Paclitaxel is administered at 75 mg/m^2 weekly on days 1, 8, 15, 22, and so forth.

INDICATIONS

This is an experimental regimen that has not been tested in the phase III setting. Therefore, it should be used with caution. Nevertheless, clinical activity was observed in patients with high-risk endometrial carcinomas (uterine papillary serous carcinoma, poorly differentiated tumors, clear cell tumors) and uterine sarcomas (carcinomasarcoma and leiomyosarcoma) and in patients with carcinoma of the fallopian tubes

SPECIAL PRECAUTIONS

Patients should have normal white blood cell and platelet counts. Patients should have normal renal and hepatic function. Treatment should be administered through a functioning central line; the potential for extravasation should be considered. Patients should have normal cardiac ejection fraction; this should be tested before administration of doxil by echocardiogram or nuclear gated blood pool scan. Patients with pre-existing pulmonary obstructive disease may have severe exacerbation if there is an allergic reaction to paclitaxel. Patients should be pretreated with diphenhydramine (Benadryl), cimetidine, and decadron and be observed closely

DRUG INTERACTIONS

Paclitaxel may potentiate neurotoxicity in patients receiving other neurotoxic agents

TOXICITIES

Doxil: Skin toxicities predominate, primarily hand-foot syndrome and nail changes. Patients may develop troublesome cutaneous ulcerations on the vulva. Stomatitis and neutropenia are generally mild. Hypersensitivity reactions have been observed; the initial infusion should be slow with the first 25% administered over 1 hour and the remaining 75% over the second hour. Patients should be monitored for cardiac toxicity.
Paclitaxel: Acute hypersensitivity reaction with wheezing, shortness of breath, urticaria, and hypotension occurred in 2% of patients receiving paclitaxel; alopecia, nausea, vomiting; profound granulocytopenia and myelosuppression; cardiac conduction abnormalities requiring a pacemaker, hypotension and bradycardia; peripheral neuropathy; arthralgias/myalgias; alopecia; diarrhea, mucositis

NURSING INTERVENTIONS

Patients should be observed closely for extravasation reactions during administration of doxil, and for hypersensitivity reactions during administration of paclitaxel. Patients who develop shortness of breath, flushing, wheezing or other respiratory symptoms should have the infusion stopped. It can be restarted more slowly with careful observation. Patients should be cautioned about fevers during the period of granulocytopenia. Patients should be cautioned about alopecia, which is universal with paclitaxel

PATIENT INFORMATION

Patients should be cautioned about the development of fevers during the course of treatment; this may be a harbinger of severe infection, and they should be cautioned to have their blood counts checked. Patients should be warned that they will develop alopecia. They should be told of the high likelihood of cutaneous and nail toxicities including the possibility of vulvar ulcerations

ADMINISTRATION

Paclitaxel is supplied in 30-mg/5-mL vials. Paclitaxel should be diluted in 0.9% sodium chloride for injection or 5% dextrose solution USP at 0.3 to 1.2 mg/mL. Because the vehicle reacts with polyvinyl chloride (PVC), administration of paclitaxel requires non-PVC bottles and polyethylene-lined tubing. Doxil is mixed in D5W and is administered by IV infusion over 2 hours

COSTS

The cost to the pharmacist for each infusion of paclitaxel will probably exceed $1000. The cost to the pharmacist of each doxil treatment will be approximately $500

Primary central nervous system (CNS) tumors represent a diverse set of difficult-to-treat neoplasms. Affecting both children and adults, these tumors may either be indolent, slow-growing diseases cured with surgery alone, or rapidly proliferative lesions that can cause death within less than a year despite intensive treatment strategies. This chapter reviews the basic biology and current treatment strategies for primary CNS tumors. Although applicable for some types of childhood tumors, this discussion deals only with malignant glial lesions commonly found in adults.

EPIDEMIOLOGY

The overall annual incidence in the United States is 11 to 12 per 100,000 persons [1]. Primary brain tumors are the second most common cancer in childhood. Gliomas account for approximately 51% of CNS tumors; meningiomas, 25%; and a variety of other tumor types comprise the remainder. The Surveillance, Epidemiology, and End Results (SEER) Program trial conducted in 1994 for the leading causes of cancer deaths in the United States by sex and age reveal that in men between the ages of 15 and 34, CNS tumors are the leading cause of cancer death; for women in this same age group, such tumors are the fourth leading cause of cancer deaths [1]. Brain and other CNS tumors are the second leading cause of death after leukemia for children under age 15. The average age of onset for all primary brain tumors is 53 years, and is slightly higher in the more malignant phenotypes such as glioblastoma multiforme (GBM). Astrocytic tumors are more common in men, whereas meningeal tumors are more common in women, for reasons that are not clearly understood.

An increase in the incidence and mortality of brain tumors in the elderly has been noted during the past several decades—as high as 300% in developed countries [2,3]. For children, the incidence of primary malignant brain tumors has increased approximately 35% over the same period [4]. Some of these increases are certainly due to better diagnostic imaging and improved access to medical care. However, other causal factors may be important in this trend, and until specific risk factors are identified, the full explanation for these increases is still awaited.

Identification of risk factors has been problematic because of the heterogeneity of these tumors, the use of retrospective exposure analyses, and uncertain latency periods. One noninherited risk factor is ionizing radiation [5,6]. The low doses used to treat tinea capitis and skin hemangiomas in children have been associated with an increased risk of brain tumors, particularly nerve sheath tumors, meningioma, and glioma. In addition, an elevated risk of subsequent primary brain tumors has been observed after radiation treatment for childhood tumors (other than leukemia). In contrast, atomic bomb survivors in Japan have not shown an increased risk of CNS tumors [6]. However, prenatal radiation exposure does increase the risk. Electromagnetic fields may be associated with increased risk [7,8]. A recent meta-analysis suggests a nonsignificant increased risk of childhood brain tumors and leukemia in children living in homes with high electromagnetic field exposure, as well as an increased risk of brain cancer in electrical workers [9]. Despite these seemingly increased risks, however, a direct causal effect has not been proven. Several studies have been conducted evaluating the risk of certain occupations and industries with the development of brain tumors. Unfortunately, studies supporting or refuting the risk within the same industry have suggested that the inconsistencies may be due to, in part, a lack of an identified causal agent or cofactors. Certain industries do show increased risk, including pesticide and fertilization manufacturing, synthetic rubber processing, vinyl chloride industries, and petrochemical and oil refinery workers [5,6]. Some of the many difficulties encountered with this research include the fact that workers are only rarely exposed to a single suspected carcinogen, and only a small number of such workers ever are diagnosed with a brain tumor. Many chemical, biologic, or infectious agents may be considered potential causal agents, including *N*-nitroso compounds, organochlorides, nitrates and nitrites, formaldehyde, and vinyl chloride.

NEUROIMAGING

Magnetic resonance imaging (MRI) has been shown to be more sensitive than a CT scan for both detection and determining the extent of tumor. Hydrogen protons in water have low signal intensity on T_1-weighted images and high signal intensity on T_2-weighted images. Pathologic processes such as tumor, infections, and infarct all produce an increase in extracellular water. On T_1-weighted images, these pathologic regions show decreased signal on T_1-weighted images compared with normal brain tissue, and increased signal on T_2-weighted images. Tissue contrast is usually most apparent on T_2-weighted images on which high signal from pathologic processes is seen in contrast to the intermediate signal intensity of normal brain parenchyma. One of the major drawbacks of CT scanning is the insensitivity to lesions of the temporal lobes and posterior fossa due to the beam-hardening artifact from the adjacent skull. MRI, unaffected by bone artifact, is able to demonstrate temporal lobe and posterior fossa anatomy with superior detail. Another advantage of MRI is its ability to image directly in multiple planes. This usually permits the distinction of peripheral intra-axial masses from extra-axial lesions, *eg*, meningioma. Features favoring an extra-axial mass include broad attachment to the dura, white matter buckling, and a CSF cleft adjacent to the mass. Enhancement of the adjacent dura, the so-called "dural tail," can be seen with but is not pathognomonic of a meningioma. Despite the exquisite sensitivity of magnetic resonance for detection of cerebral neoplasms, multiple pathologic processes can demonstrate low signal intensity on T_1-weighted images and high signal intensity on T_2-weighted images. The magnetic resonance examination lacks specificity, and common processes can simulate intracranial neoplasms, *eg*, infarcts, inflammatory lesions, demyelination, and radiation necrosis. Diffusion-weighted imaging is helpful for confirming acute infarction within the first 7 to 10 days, demonstrating reduced diffusion typical of acute ischemic injury. If diffusion imaging is unavailable, a follow-up study in 10 days can be extremely helpful. With infarction, there is usually a rapid change in the enhancement pattern and mass effect as the infarct evolves from subacute to chronic stages. In general, most tumors will not exhibit much change over a 1- to 2-week period. Cerebral abscesses typically have a thin rim of enhancement compared with the thick and nodular enhancement seen in gliomas. Other features of cerebral abscesses include high intensity rim on precontrast T_1-weighted images and satellite images. However, enough imaging overlap exists between the two processes that usually the clinical history is vital in making the distinction. Occasionally, demyelinating disease such as multiple sclerosis may sometimes present in a tumefactive fashion. The acute plaque may demonstrate mass effect, enhancement, and vasogenic edema similar to primary brain tumors. Short-term follow-up magnetic resonance scans within 6 to 8 weeks usually demonstrate resolution of mass effect and enhancement.

Introduction of MRI contrast agents in 1988 had a tremendous impact on CNS tumor evaluation. The most commonly used MRI contrast agent is gadopentetate dimeglumine. Gadolinium is a rare earth metal with seven unpaired electrons. These unpaired electrons enable nearby protons to realign more quickly with the main magnetic field, thus shortening T_1 relaxation time. On a T_1-weighted image, molecules that realign rapidly with a magnetic field will have higher signal intensity than those that realign slowly. Thus, gadolinium enhancement results in an increase in the signal intensity on T_1-weighted images. Although gadolinium shortens both T_1 and T_2 relaxation times, the effect on T_1 is much greater, accounting for the exclusive use of T_1-weighted sequences after the administration of contrast material. Normal brain capillaries with an intact blood-brain barrier are impermeable to gadolinium complexes because of tight endothelial junctions. Regions of the brain normally lacking a blood-brain barrier, such as the pituitary gland, pineal gland, choroid plexus, and dura will enhance normally and should not be mistaken for pathology. Neoplasm-induced angiogenesis, especially in more malignant gliomas, results in capillaries with a discontinuous basic membrane that lacks a blood-brain barrier. These abnormal capillaries allow diffusion of gadolinium into adjacent brain parenchyma, which demonstrates enhancement on T_1-weighted images. These regions of enhancing tumor generally correspond to the areas of greatest concentration of the capillaries. Enhancement can help guide stereotactic biopsy and surgical resections; however, it does not necessarily reflect the most metabolically active portion of a tumor because necrosis may also occur within the region of contrast enhancement.

In general, higher grade gliomas generally enhance more frequently than lower grade gliomas. Nevertheless, benign or low-grade tumors, such as juvenile pilocystic astrocytoma, typically show intense enhancement reflecting their prominent vascularity. Likewise, higher-grade malignant tumors may occasionally demonstrate minimal, if any, enhancement.

Low-grade astrocytomas are diffusely infiltrating tumors composed of well-differentiated neoplastic astrocytes and account for approximately 25% of hemispheric gliomas. They typically occur in early adult life, with a peak incidence in the fourth and fifth decades. Microscopically, astrocytomas are ill-defined and tend to diffusely infiltrate the surrounding brain, resulting in enlargement and distortion of the structures involved. Calcification may be present in approximately 50% of cases, although this is rarely appreciated by magnetic resonance. The three major histopathologic variants are fibrillary, gemistocytic, and protoplasmic. On MRI, astrocytomas are typically well-defined, homogeneous masses that are hypointense on T_1-weighted images and hyperintense on T_2-weighted images. Mass effect and associated edema are usually minimal for the size of the tumor, although mass effect is always present to some degree. They are usually superficial in location and there may be involvement of the overlying gray matter. Enhancement is variable. Currently, it is not possible to predict with certainty the histologic grade of a glioma based on its MRI appearance [10].

Higher grade glial tumors can appear radiographically identical to lower grade gliomas.

Anaplastic astrocytomas occur later in life than astrocytomas, although they share a similar regional distribution. Anaplastic astrocytomas tend to be more heterogeneous on MR than astrocytomas. Characteristically, they have less well-defined borders and a greater degree of mass effect, vasogenic edema, and enhancement. Cysts and calcification can also be seen. Hemorrhage may be present, although it is more commonly seen in the higher grade GBM. On noncontrast T_1- and T_2-weighted images, heterogeneous signal intensity is usually present. The frequency of contrast enhancement is generally greater than in lower grade gliomas. It must be stressed, however, that these are general principles; variations from these observations are not uncommon.

Glioblastoma multiforme is the most common astrocytic tumor, representing 50% of astrocytic tumors and 15% to 20% of all intracranial tumors. The peak incidence is at 45 to 60 years of age. It occurs most commonly in the frontal lobes but can be seen in the cerebellum, brainstem, and spinal cord. A characteristic pattern of GBM is spread across the white matter tracts of the corpus callosum to involve the contralateral cerebral hemisphere (ie, the so-called "butterfly" appearance). Pathologically, GBM is often a heterogeneous tumor typically with areas of necrosis, hemorrhage, and endothelial proliferation. The magnetic resonance appearance of GBM reflects the heterogeneous pathologic features. Generally, GBMs exhibit heterogeneous signal intensity on both T_1- and T_2-weighted images, reflecting a combination of cysts, hemorrhage, and necrosis. Linear, serpiginous punctate regions of low signal on T_1- and T_2-weighted images may represent flow voids from tumor vascularity. The tumors are usually poorly defined with extensive mass effect and vasogenic edema. Contrast enhancement is more frequent in GBM than with other astrocytic tumors, occurring in up to 95% of all glioblastomas. The enhancement pattern is typically irregular or nodular with multiple foci extending throughout the lesion. It is not uncommon to see rests of contrast enhancement connected by nonenhancing regions of abnormal T_2 signal intensity.

Glioblastoma multiforme is almost always associated with a large region of high signal seen on T_2-weighted images. This region is composed of both vasogenic edema and microscopic tumor infiltration of the white and gray matter tracts and cannot be differentiated by magnetic resonance. In most cases, the extent of microscopic invasion is limited to a 2-cm margin surrounding the enhancing tumor, although malignant cells may extend several centimeters beyond the enhancing tumor margins. Tumor may be visualized on T_2 FLAIR (fluid attenuation inversion recovery) sequences coursing down white matter tracts such as the internal capsule and into the brainstem. Glioblastoma is the most common of the glial tumors to spread to the subarachnoid space. Contrast-enhanced magnetic resonance is far more sensitive than contrast CT in detecting leptomeningeal spread. An early indication of leptomeningeal spread is abnormal enhancement surrounding cranial nerves, most commonly seen along cranial nerves 5, 7, and 8.

Newer modalities of noninvasive tumor assessment are currently being evaluated. One of these is magnetic resonance spectroscopy (MRS). Available with routine MRI machines, areas of interest may be evaluated for intracellular metabolites, allowing differentiation of late radiation injury from that of tumor. Using proton MRS, three metabolites are of most interest: choline-containing compounds, creatine plus phosphocreatine, and N-acetyl aspartate. Tumors often show elevated levels of all three metabolites, whereas necrotic brain shows reduced levels [11,12]. Specific ratios of these compounds are used to express the relative changes to normal brain and determine tumor activity. Newer machines are now able to assess these regions with three-dimensional imaging techniques with simultaneous registration to the normal MRI data set, and with retrospective realignment with previous MRI and MRS data to allow sequential analysis over time. Continued research into these types of image analyses will greatly enhance our ability to assess response and toxicity to various modalities of therapies being used today.

TREATMENT

Treatment differs for GBM, anaplastic astrocytoma, and low-grade lesions. Surgery is critical to make an accurate diagnosis in each setting, however, with the goal to remove as much tumor as is safely possible, and to relieve symptoms. At least for malignant glioma, one prognostic factor that influences outcome is the extent of surgical resection [13–15]. Patients who undergo biopsy only will often survive a shorter period of time than a patient who has more extensive resection. Thus, whenever possible, surgical resection is preferred over biopsy procedures. Some investigators also believe that extent of surgical resection may alter outcome in low-grade tumors, although this is still controversial [16]. Numerous new technical modalities exist to assist the surgeon in this process, and in many cases complete resection of contrast-enhancing masses can be achieved with minimal risk of neurologic injury. There are occasions in which lesions in some areas of the brain cannot be safely removed, and will require biopsy only to establish the diagnosis. These procedures may be done under local anesthesia using stereotactic procedures, or via an open procedure. In general, the more tissue that is removed, the more accurate the pathologic diagnosis and the greater the likelihood of longer survival.

MALIGNANT GLIOMA

Malignant gliomas include GBM, anaplastic astrocytoma (AA), anaplastic oligodendroglioma (AO), and anaplastic mixed oligodendroglioma (AOA). Clinical studies conducted in the 1960s and 1970s included all of these various tumor types, making interpretation of outcome based on specific diagnosis difficult. Most clinical studies will now either restrict to one or the other type, or stratify based on histology. Survival expectations vary significantly with each of these lesions.

Patients with primary GBM are generally older, and will present with a large, contrast-enhancing necrotic lesion seen on MR imaging. As mentioned earlier, some cases of GBM are believed to arise from lower grade tumors and are called secondary GBM. Treatment remains the same for both types, and includes surgery and radiotherapy. The goal of surgery is to make a specific diagnosis, relieve symptoms, and reduce tumor bulk to the maximum extent possible. Radiation treatment is given following surgery, and treatment is directed to the local tumor volume plus a margin surrounding the tumor. Whole-brain radiation treatment is not used. When chemotherapy is used, it may be given in the neoadjuvant or adjuvant setting with radiotherapy. The chemotherapy most often used is single-agent BCNU (bis-chloroethyl-nitrosourea). The survival benefit of adjuvant chemotherapy is modest, at best, and frequently not used in the older patients [17]. With the combined approach of surgery, radiation, and adjuvant chemotherapy, median survival is approximately 50 weeks. Prognostic factors that will influence survival include younger age, a surgical resection greater than a simple biopsy, good performance status, and treatment with radiation therapy [15]. The precise extent of surgical resection that clearly confers a survival benefit has not been delineated beyond what is termed "subtotal resection." Some tumor locations may preclude a meaningful resection, such as in the motor cortex or brainstem, but most lesions are amenable to some degree of resection. If at all possible, an extensive resection should be considered. Radiotherapy has been proven in phase 3 studies to increase survival beyond best palliative care measures [17–24]. The use of single fractions, given daily until a dose of 60 Gy is reached, is considered the standard of care.

The target used to define the dose is the contrast-enhancing lesion and a margin of 2 to 3 cm beyond the edge of the lesion. Larger volumes or higher doses have not proven to be superior to focal radiation to 60 Gy. Numerous attempts to increase the therapeutic ratio of radiation have thus far been unsuccessful. These have included the use of radiation sensitizers and various dose-fractionation techniques such as hyperfractionation. Although still controversial, focal radiation using radiosurgery or interstitial brachytherapy may offer some chance at a longer survival, but comes at the risk of additional radiation injury [25–29]. The most common site of tumor relapse following surgery and focal radiation is in the original tumor site or within 2 to 4 cm of the margin. Although it is also known that tumor cells exist well beyond that margin, morbidity and mortality are generally consequences of more local than regional failure. Whole-brain irradiation has not been shown to increase survival over that seen with focal radiotherapy, and in fact can cause significant negative side effects, particularly in older patients, or in patients who survive beyond the median survival of 1 year. Currently, patients are treated with focal radiotherapy using three-dimensional conformal techniques to minimize dose to noninvolved brain. As mentioned, more intensive radiation is possible using interstitial brachytherapy or radiosurgery techniques. Some patients have been shown to have longer survival when additional radiation "boost" procedures are used. Patient selection factors (younger patients with small tumor volumes) may influence these survival expectations, and phase 3 studies have been inconclusive thus far, both favoring brachytherapy and showing no additional benefit. Further studies are ongoing, particularly with the use of radiosurgery. Adjuvant chemotherapy may improve survival in a small portion of patients [17]. Median survival remains unchanged with or without adjuvant BCNU, but younger patients with otherwise favorable prognostic factors do appear to have a slight 2-year survival advantage with adjuvant chemotherapy. Unfortunately, most patients will still die within 2 years, despite radiotherapy and adjuvant chemotherapy. The 5-year survival rate is less than 5%.

Patients with anaplastic tumors other than GBM have a different prognosis, with median survival expectations of 4 to 5 years [15,21,30–32]. Prognostic factors are similar to GBM, with younger patients having surgical resections, and a good performance status doing better than older, biopsy only, neurologically-impaired patients. In general, patients are treated with surgery, radiation therapy, and adjuvant chemotherapy. Retrospective review of large datasets of patients treated on various research protocols support the role of adjuvant chemotherapy in these tumor types. However, there has not yet been an adequately sized, prospective phase 3 trial assessing the role of chemotherapy. Because of the historical bias, it is unlikely that such a study will be conducted in this country. The current phase 3 study open within the Radiation Therapy Oncology Group (RTOG) for anaplastic gliomas other than GBM randomly assigns patients to irradiation and one of three adjuvant chemotherapy arms, with single-agent BCNU as the "control" arm. The experimental arms include the use of single-agent temozolomide, or BCNU plus temozolomide. A previous randomized phase 3 study compared the use of single-agent BCNU with PCV (procarbazine, CCNU [lomustine], and vincristine) in patients with GBM and anaplastic gliomas treated with radiation, and found a statistically significant survival advantage in patients with anaplastic gliomas treated with the three-drug combination [31]. No such advantage was seen for patients with GBM. The sample sizes were small, and only a partial cohort of patients with anaplastic gliomas was used in the subset analysis that suggested superior outcome. Other retrospective studies have been done showing no advantage with PCV over that seen with BCNU alone, and, thus, single-agent BCNU remains the control arm for the current phase 3 study described previously for this patient population [33]. Patients with pure AO or AOA also appear to have a more favorable response to treatment than patients with pure AA. Indeed, it has been shown that patients with a pure AO will frequently have a complete response to chemotherapy prior to radiotherapy, or when treated at the time of relapse [34,35]. The chemotherapy used in those studies was the combination of PCV. All of these lines of evidence strongly suggest that adjuvant chemotherapy is an appropriate modality for patients with anaplastic gliomas [17]. Disease-specific phase 3 studies may still need to be conducted to discover the benefit, or lack thereof, of chemotherapy for newly diagnosed patients with anaplastic gliomas.

TREATMENT AT RELAPSE

Treatment strategies used at the time of tumor recurrence for GBM include additional surgery, interstitial brachytherapy or radiosurgery, and chemotherapy. Patients are generally believed to be good candidates for surgery if a substantial resection is possible, they have good performance status, and additional therapy is available beyond that of surgery alone [14]. An additional reason for surgery is to treat with local therapies, eg, interstitial brachytherapy or with polymer-based drug delivery [36–39]. Again, these salvage therapies are most useful in very select patients, in whom there is a reasonable expectation that survival will be enhanced. Unfortunately, many patients are not candidates for additional surgery or radiotherapy because of a large tumor burden, or tumor location in areas of brain where surgery or focal radiation or chemotherapy would be dangerous. Systemic chemotherapy is often used in these patients, either as an adjuvant to additional surgery or radiotherapy, or alone as the single modality of therapy [35,40]. Survival expectations at the time of initial relapse are poor—often only 4 to 6 months.

As discussed for patients with recurrent GBM, patients with recurrent anaplastic gliomas should be considered for surgical re-resection, interstitial brachytherapy or radiosurgery, or other chemotherapy approaches. If patients have not received adjuvant chemotherapy, PCV or temozolomide chemotherapy is frequently used. Newer chemotherapy agents are often tested in this patient group. Patients in first relapse may be successfully retreated for 1 to 2 years, but will eventually become resistant to treatment and behave in a similar biologic fashion as recurrent GBM patients, with short survival expectation after successive relapses. With median survival expectations of 4 to 5 years, measured from the initial diagnosis, we have now seen more of the chronic effects of treatment, such as treatment-related second tumors, vascular abnormalities possibly secondary to radiotherapy, and chronic neurocognitive deficits.

LOW-GRADE GLIOMAS

Low-grade gliomas include grade 2 fibrillary or protoplasmic astrocytoma, oligodendroglioma, mixed oligoastrocytoma, juvenile pilocytic astrocytoma, ganglioglioma, gangliocytoma, pleomorphic xanthoastrocytoma, and dysembryoplastic neuroectodermal tumors. Obviously, with such a diverse spectrum of histologic subtypes, variations in clinical presentations and treatment approaches exist. In general, however, patients with these tumors are young adults or children, often diagnosed following a history of seizures, and may either have nonenhanc-

ing or enhancing tumors on MRI. Clinical and imaging characteristics may strongly suggest one tumor type over another, but most cases require at least a biopsy to confirm the specific pathology. Complete surgical resection may be all that is necessary for initial treatment for some of these tumors, and whenever possible should be considered. For instance, a completely resected pilocytic astrocytoma in the cerebellum would require no further therapy. Pilocytic astrocytomas in the hypothalamus or involving the optic nerves and chiasm, however, only rarely can be completely resected, and often these tumors will cause functional deficits, such as visual loss or endocrine abnormalities. Additional therapy is needed in this setting. In younger children, chemotherapy is frequently the first therapy used, and can successfully control tumor growth for many years, thus deferring the need for external beam radiotherapy [41–44]. Other tumors, such as the recently described dysembryoplastic neuroectodermal tumor (DNET), will have a favorable outcome, even with partial resection, and treatment beyond surgery is not recommended [45–47]. The same is true for most cases of pleomorphic xanthoastrocytoma, or ganglioglioma. Tumors may slowly grow over many years, before treatment would ever be considered. In these cases, re-resections should be considered.

Other tumors, particularly grade 2 infiltrating astrocytomas in young adults, have a different natural history than pilocytic astrocytomas. Treatment options for those tumors include the spectrum of no treatment, irradiation, chemotherapy, and, in some cases, the combination of irradiation plus chemotherapy [48,49]. Adults with these tumors can present in their early 20s or 30s following a seizure. In many cases, complete surgical resection is impossible because of the extent and location of the tumor. Surgical biopsy or partial resection is recommended, however, to confirm the diagnosis. Patients without symptoms may either be treated at the time of surgical or neuroimaging diagnosis, or followed with routine neurologic assessment and serial MRIs. If the lesion grows in size, or begins to produce symptoms, treatment can then be considered. It is not clear if either approach is superior to the other. Some studies strongly suggest that early intervention with radiotherapy is appropriate, whereas others take the approach that intervention later in the course of the disease will do no harm [50–54]. Again, prognostic factors will influence the outcome of these patients and should be considered when treatment decisions are made. Tumors in patients older than 50 tend to have a more aggressive biologic behavior than similar tumors in younger patients, and should be considered for immediate treatment, particularly if bulky residual disease is present [48]. Small surgical biopsies may underestimate the true malignant nature of some of these tumors, either because of sampling error or difficulty of accurate pathologic grading due to the small tissue specimen. Thus, older or younger patients with a short clinical history, have a large contrast-enhancing tumor, and who undergo a small biopsy procedure may actually have a higher grade tumor; these patients should be treated.

In addition to age, the extent of surgical resection may be an important predictor of survival. Several small retrospective studies of patients followed over long periods suggest an improvement in survival for patients who undergo a complete resection versus those who have partial removal or biopsy alone [16,52]. Patient selection factors, however, make it impossible to confirm these observations, and no controlled studies are available that randomly assign patients to biopsy alone versus intent to do a complete or subtotal resection, giving uniform treatment following surgery. It is unlikely that such a study would ever be conducted. However, one should at least consider an attempt at maximal surgical resection in these patients. Radiotherapy is given to the tumor area and a margin surrounding it, rather than to the whole brain. It is not clear what the optimal dose should be for treatment. In most cases, a dose of 54 Gy is used. Lower doses in some recent prospective studies appear to be similar in efficacy as 54 Gy, whereas other retrospective series suggest that higher doses are superior [50,51,54,55]. Further studies are needed to resolve this issue. Chemotherapy is generally reserved for tumor progression, and frequently PCV chemotherapy will be used. Patients with oligodendroglial tumors will often respond to this regimen with a reduction in tumor size, whereas pure astrocytomas more often stabilize or show no change for prolonged periods of time. Eventually, a series of relapses will occur, with shorter periods of progression-free survival at each relapse. Although it is true that many of these patients have a long natural history, most patients eventually die of tumor progression or transformation to a more malignant phenotype. Often, at the time of re-resection of what initially was called a grade 2 astrocytoma, pathologic features characteristic of glioblastoma multiforme will be found.

FUTURE STRATEGIES

As previously mentioned, the pace of laboratory research for CNS tumors has increased during the past 10 to 15 years, particularly in the area of molecular biology. A greater awareness of specific genetic abnormalities and their cellular consequences gives hope that this research will ultimately translate into novel, more specific treatment strategies for patients with these disorders. Specific areas of ongoing clinical research include the testing of new agents, modulation of mechanisms of resistance to standard chemotherapy agents, inhibitors of growth factors and their receptors, modification of angiogenesis and invasion, and gene therapy (Table 15-1).

Some of the newer drugs currently being tested in phase 2 or 3 trials include the agent temozolomide [56,57]. Temozolamide is an imidazotetrazine derivative with good oral bioavailability and minimal myelosuppression. Temozolomide has shown activity in recurrent malignant gliomas and was recently approved for this indication by the US Food and Drug Administration. It is being tested in many other settings, including newly diagnosed disease, and in combina-

tion with other chemotherapy and radiation treatment. Irinotecan, an inhibitor of topoisomerase-1, is also undergoing phase 2 testing using a variety of schedules [58]. Early results suggest modest activity in recurrent disease, and combination strategies are also underway, adding it to chemotherapy drugs such as temozolomide, and with radiation therapy. Inhibitors of angiogenesis have also completed several phase 1 and phase 2 trials. There are many new agents in this category, including TNP-470, SU-5416, and thalidomide. Antibodies to vasoactive endothelial growth factor have also now become available and, it is hoped, will soon begin phase 1 testing. Inhibitors of the matrix surrounding tumor cells also are a strategy being tested. Oral metalloproteinase inhibitors are currently in clinical trials, in phase 2 and 3 studies, alone and in combination with chemotherapy and radiation treatment, with the goal of reducing the invasive nature of these tumors. Inhibition of signal transduction through multiple pathways has become an area of intense research as well. Inhibition of protein kinase C is one such strategy, and the drugs bryostatin, UCN-01, and tamoxifen are being used in this regard. Inhibition of cell-cycle progression by regulation of the cyclin-dependent kinase family of genes by the use of flavoperidol is to begin testing in 2001. Other trials targeting platelet-derived growth factor receptor, epidermal growth factor receptor, and fibroblast growth factor as substrates for inhibitors of these growth factors have also begun phase 1 and 2 testing.

The herpes simplex thymidine kinase gene (*HSV-TK*) was the first gene to be used in humans with recurrent malignant brain tumors. New gene vectors have been developed with ongoing clinical trials to evaluate these newer constructs underway. In addition to retroviral delivery (such as with the *HSV-TK*), new phase 1 gene therapy trials have opened using the adenovirus as the vector-producing cell for the *HSV-TK* gene. In addition, a new study also recently opened to transfer the *p53* gene into tumor cells, again using an adenoviral vector. Other gene therapy studies are being planned as well.

Intratumor injection of toxins represents another line of research being developed [59–61]. In this strategy, various toxins are infused into the tumor-bearing area of brain using catheters and pump systems that can slowly cause diffusion of the agent over a period of time. To select for tumor cells, the toxin is conjugated to substrates that ideally will only be able to bind to tumor rather than normal brain. Various strategies are being developed, including the use of *Pseudomonas* exotoxin conjugated to interleukin-4 or interleukin-13 or to transforming growth factor-α [62–66]. Receptors to all of these factors are highly expressed on tumor cells and not in normal brain. Phase I studies with the interleukin-4 *Pseudomonas* exotoxin study have recently been completed, and new trials with the interleukin-13 and transforming growth factor-α *Pseudomonas* exotoxin study should open early in 2001.

CONCLUSIONS

Malignant glioma represents a unique challenge both within the laboratory and in the clinic. The biology of these tumors is being intensely investigated, and the information gathered supports a highly complicated, genetically heterogeneous lesion that currently confounds our ability to translate these data into successful treatments for patients. However, the pace of research and our general understanding of these tumors has increased tremendously in the last decade. New laboratory investigations using gene expression array and proteonomic arrays will hasten our knowledge of the biologic nature of the disease. New animal model systems, using transgenic

Table 15-1. Investigational New Agents in Current Clinical Research

Agent	Target
CCI-779	mTor (signal pathway)
Flavoperidol	Cyclin-dependent kinase inhibitor
STI-571	Platelet-derived growth factor
ZD-1839	Epidermal growth factor receptor
SU-5416	Vascular endothelial growth factor
06-BG	AGT (alkyl-guanine alkyltransferase)
CPT-11	Topoisomerase-2
IL-4/PE	IL-4 receptor
IL-13/PE	IL-13 receptor
TGF-α/PE	Epidermal growth factor receptor
Adeno-p53	p53 gene
R115777	Farnesly transferase/Ras
Fenretinide	Retinoid acid receptor

mice for instance, will support those investigations and help us model clinical strategies more efficiently. The empiricism of the past is now fortunately replaced by biologically driven models that will allow more specific clinical studies to emerge. Such studies are ongoing and the next decade should hopefully result in improved treatment responses and longer survival. Clearly, patients with malignant CNS tumors have many more options for participation in clinical research than was possible several years ago. Referral to specialized centers to discuss these options is highly recommended.

REFERENCES

1. Landis SH, Murray T, Bolden S, *et al.*: Cancer statistics 1998. *CA Cancer J Clin* 1988, 48:6–29. [Published errata appear in *CA Cancer J Clin* 1998, 48:192; and in *CA Cancer J Clin* 1998, 48:329.] *CA Cancer J Clin* 1998, 48:6–29.

2. Davis FG, Bruner JM, Surawicz TS: The rationale for standardized registration and reporting of brain and central nervous system tumors in population-based cancer registries. *Neuroepidemiology* 1997, 16:308–316.

3. Davis FG, Freels S, Grutsch J, *et al.*: Survival rates in patients with primary malignant brain tumors stratified by patient age and tumor histological type: an analysis based on Surveillance, Epidemiology, and End Results (SEER) data, 1973- 1991. J Neurosurg 88:1–10, 1998

4. Smith MA, Freidlin B, Ries LA, *et al.*: Trends in reported incidence of primary malignant brain tumors in children in the United States [see comments]. *J Natl Cancer Inst* 1998, 90:1269–1277.

5. Wrensch M, Bondy ML, Wiencke J, *et al.*: Environmental risk factors for primary malignant brain tumors: a review. *J Neurooncol* 1993, 17:47–64.

6. Preston Martin S: Epidemiology of primary CNS neoplasms. *Neurol Clin* 1996, 14:273–290.

7. Kaletsch U, Kaatsch P, Meinert R, *et al.*: Childhood cancer and residential radon exposure: results of a population-based case-control study in Lower Saxony (Germany). *Radiat Environ Biophys* 1999, 38:211–215.

8. Meinert R, Michaelis J: Meta-analyses of studies on the association between electromagnetic fields and childhood cancer. *Radiat Environ Biophys* 1996, 35:11–18.

9. Kheifets LI, Afifi AA, Buffler PA, *et al.*: Occupational electric and magnetic field exposure and brain cancer: a meta-analysis [see comments]. *J Occup Environ Med* 1995, 37:1327–1341.

10. Kondziolka D, Lunsford LD, Martinez AJ: Unreliability of contemporary neurodiagnostic imaging in evaluating suspected adult supratentorial (low-grade) astrocytoma [see comments]. *J Neurosurg* 1993, 79:533–536.

11. Wald LL, Nelson SJ, Day MR, *et al.*: Serial proton magnetic resonance spectroscopy imaging of glioblastoma multiforme after brachytherapy. *J Neurosurg* 1997, 87:525–534.

12. Nelson SJ, Huhn S, Vigneron DB, *et al.*: Volume MRI and MRSI techniques for the quantitation of treatment response in brain tumors: presentation of a detailed case study. *J Magn Reson Imaging* 1997, 7:1146–1152.

13. Ammirati M, Vick N, Liao YL, *et al.*: Effect of the extent of surgical resection on survival and quality of life in patients with supratentorial glioblastomas and anaplastic astrocytomas. *Neurosurgery* 1987, 21:201–206.

14. Barker FG II, Chang SM, Gutin PH, *et al.*: Survival and functional status after resection of recurrent glioblastoma multiforme. *Neurosurgery* 1998, 42:709–720.

15. Curran WJ, Jr., Scott CB, Horton J, *et al.*: Recursive partitioning analysis of prognostic factors in three Radiation Therapy Oncology Group malignant glioma trials [see comments]. *J Natl Cancer Inst* 1993, 85:704–710.

16. Berger MS, Deliganis AV, Dobbins J, *et al.*: The effect of extent of resection on recurrence in patients with low grade cerebral hemisphere gliomas [see comments]. *Cancer* 1994, 74:1784–1791.

17. Fine HA: The basis for current treatment recommendations for malignant gliomas. *J Neurooncol* 1994, 20:111–120.

18. Gaspar LE, Fisher BJ, Macdonald DR, *et al.*: Supratentorial malignant glioma: patterns of recurrence and implications for external beam local treatment. *Int J Radiat Oncol Biol Phys* 1992, 24:55–57.

19. Leibel SA, Scott CB, Loeffler JS: Contemporary approaches to the treatment of malignant gliomas with radiation therapy. *Semin Oncol* 1994, 21:198–219.

20. Papsdorf K, Wolf U, Hildebrandt G, *et al.*: Outcome and side effects in radiotherapy of glioblastoma: conventional fractionation versus accelerated hyperfractionation. *Front Radiat Ther Oncol* 1999, 33:158–165.

21. Prados MD, Larson DA, Lamborn K, *et al.*: Radiation therapy and hydroxyurea followed by the combination of 6-thioguanine and BCNU for the treatment of primary malignant brain tumors. *Int J Radiat Oncol Biol Phys* 1998, 40:57–63.

22. Prados MD, Berger MS, Wilson CB: Primary central nervous system tumors: advances in knowledge and treatment. *CA Cancer J Clin* 1998, 48:331–360.

23. Scott CB, Scarantino C, Urtasun R, *et al.*: Validation and predictive power of Radiation Therapy Oncology Group (RTOG) recursive partitioning analysis classes for malignant glioma patients: a report using RTOG 90-06. *Int J Radiat Oncol Biol Phys* 1998, 40:51–55.

24. Surawicz TS, Davis F, Freels S, *et al.*: Brain tumor survival: results from the National Cancer Data Base. *J Neurooncol* 1998, 40:151–160.

25. Larson DA, Gutin PH, McDermott M, *et al.*: Gamma knife for glioma: selection factors and survival [see comments]. *Int J Radiat Oncol Biol Phys* 1996, 36:1045–1053.

26. Prados MD, Gutin PH, Phillips TL, *et al.*: Interstitial brachytherapy for newly diagnosed patients with malignant gliomas: the UCSF experience. *Int J Radiat Oncol Biol Phys* 1992, 24:593–597.

27. Sneed PK, Gutin PH, Prados MD, *et al.*: Brachytherapy of brain tumors. *Stereotact Funct Neurosurg* 1992, 59:157–165.

28. Sneed PK, McDermott MW, Gutin PH: Interstitial brachytherapy procedures for brain tumors. *Semin Surg Oncol* 1997, 13:157–166.

29. Gutin PH, Prados MD, Phillips TL, *et al.*: External irradiation followed by an interstitial high activity iodine-125 implant "boost" in the initial treatment of malignant gliomas: NCOG study 6G-82-2. *Int J Radiat Oncol Biol Phys* 1991, 21:601–606.

30. Prados MD, Scott C, Sandler H, *et al.*: A phase 3 randomized study of radiotherapy plus procarbazine, CCNU, and vincristine (PCV) with or without BUdR for the treatment of anaplastic astrocytoma: a preliminary report of RTOG 9404 [see comments]. *Int J Radiat Oncol Biol Phys* 1999, 45:1109–1115.

31. Levin VA, Silver P, Hannigan J, *et al.*: Superiority of post-radiotherapy adjuvant chemotherapy with CCNU, procarbazine, and vincristine (PCV) over BCNU for anaplastic gliomas: NCOG 6G61 final report. *Int J Radiat Oncol Biol Phys* 1990, 18:321–324.

The information here is provided as guidance only. Prescribers should always consult the manufacturer's current prescribing information.

271

32. Levin VA, Prados MR, Wara WM, *et al.*: Radiation therapy and bromodeoxyuridine chemotherapy followed by procarbazine, lomustine, and vincristine for the treatment of anaplastic gliomas. *Int J Radiat Oncol Biol Phys* 1995, 32:75–83.

33. Prados MD, Scott C, Curran WJ, Jr., *et al.*: Procarbazine, lomustine, and vincristine (PCV) chemotherapy for anaplastic astrocytoma: a retrospective review of radiation therapy oncology group protocols comparing survival with carmustine or PCV adjuvant chemotherapy [In Process Citation]. *J Clin Oncol* 1999, 17:3389–3395.

34. Cairncross JG: Aggressive oligodendroglioma: a chemosensitive tumor. *Recent Results Cancer Res* 1994, 135:127–133.

35. Burton E, Prados M: New chemotherapy options for the treatment of malignant gliomas. *Curr Opin Oncol* 1999, 11:157–161.

36. Brem H, Tamargo R, Olivi A, *et al.*: Biodegradable polymers for controlled delivery of chemotherapy with and without radiotherapy in the monkey brain. *J Neurosurg* 1994, 80:283–290.

37. Brem H, Ewend M, Piantadosi S, *et al.*: The safety of interstitial chemotherapy with BCNU-loaded polymer followed by radiotherapy in the treatment of newly diagnosed malignant gliomas. *J Neurooncol* 1995, 26:111–123.

38. Scharfen CO, Sneed PK, Wara WM, *et al.*: High activity iodine-125 interstitial implant for gliomas. *Int J Radiat Oncol Biol Phys* 1992, 24:583–591.

39. Sneed PK, Stauffer PR, Gutin PH, *et al.*: Interstitial irradiation and hyperthermia for the treatment of recurrent malignant brain tumors. *Neurosurgery* 1991, 28:206–215.

40. Chang SM, Prados MD: Chemotherapy for gliomas. *Curr Opin Oncol* 1995, 7:207–213.

41. Packer RJ, Ater J, Allen J, *et al.*: Carboplatin and vincristine chemotherapy for children with newly diagnosed progressive low-grade gliomas. *J Neurosurg* 1997, 86:747–754.

42. Petronio J, Edwards MS, Prados M, *et al.*: Management of chiasmal and hypothalamic gliomas of infancy and childhood with chemotherapy. *J Neurosurg* 1991, 74:701–708.

43. Pollack IF: Pediatric brain tumors. *Semin Surg Oncol* 1999, 16:73–90.

44. Prados MD, Edwards MS, Rabbitt J, *et al.*: Treatment of pediatric low-grade gliomas with a nitrosourea-based multiagent chemotherapy regimen. *J Neurooncol* 1997, 32:235–241.

45. Daumas-Duport C, Varlet P, Bacha S, *et al.*: Dysembryoplastic neuroepithelial tumors: nonspecific histological forms. A study of 40 cases. *J Neurooncol* 1999, 41:267–280.

46. Cervera-Pierot P, Varlet P, Chodkiewicz JP, *et al.*: Dysembryoplastic neuroepithelial tumors located in the caudate nucleus area: report of four cases. *Neurosurgery* 1997, 40:1065–1069.

47. Daumas-Duport C: Dysembryoplastic neuroepithelial tumours. *Brain Pathol* 1993, 3:283–295.

48. Bauman G, Lote K, Larson D, *et al.*: Pretreatment factors predict overall survival for patients with low-grade glioma: a recursive partitioning analysis. *Int J Radiat Oncol Biol Phys* 1999, 45:923–929.

49. Cairncross JG, Laperriere NJ: Low-grade glioma. To treat or not to treat? *Arch Neurol* 1989, 46:1238–1239.

50. Karim AB, Maat B, Hatlevoll R, *et al.*: A randomized trial on dose-response in radiation therapy of low-grade cerebral glioma: European Organization for Research and Treatment of Cancer (EORTC) Study 22844. *Int J Radiat Oncol Biol Phys* 1996, 36:549–556.

51. Karim AB, Bleehen N, Afra D, *et al.*: Immediate postoperative radiotherapy in low-grade glioma improves progression-free survival but not overall survival: Preliminary results of an EORTC/MRC randomized trial [abstract]. *Proc of ASCO* 1998, 17:400.

52. Lote K, Egeland T, Hager B, *et al.*: Survival, prognostic factors, and therapeutic efficacy in low-grade glioma: a retrospective study in 379 patients. *J Clin Oncol* 1997, 15:3129–3140.

53. Shaw EG: The low-grade glioma debate: evidence defending the position of early radiation therapy. *Clin Neurosurg* 1995, 42:488–494.

54. Shaw EG AR, Scheithauer B, O'Fallon J, *et al.*: A prospective randomized trial of low-versus high-dose radiation therapy in adults with supratentorial low-grade glioma: initial report of a NCCTG-RTOG-ECOG study [abstract]. *Proceedings of ASCO* 1998, 17:401.

55. Shaw EG, Scheithauer BW, Gilbertson DT, *et al.*: Postoperative radiotherapy of supratentorial low-grade gliomas. *Int J Radiat Oncol Biol Phys* 1989, 16:663–668.

56. Yung WK, Prados MD, Yaya-Tur R, *et al.*: Multicenter phase II trial of temozolomide in patients with anaplastic astrocytoma or anaplastic oligoastrocytoma at first relapse: Temodal Brain Tumor Group. *J Clin Oncol* 1999, 17:2762–2771.

57. Newlands ES, O'Reilly SM, Glaser MG, *et al.*: The Charing Cross Hospital experience with temozolomide in patients with gliomas. *Eur J Cancer* 1996, 32:2236–2241.

58. Friedman HS, Petros WP, Friedman AH, *et al.*: Irinotecan therapy in adults with recurrent or progressive malignant glioma. *J Clin Oncol* 1999, 17:1516–1525.

59. Joshi BH, Plautz GE, Puri RK: Interleukin-13 receptor alpha chain: a novel tumor-associated transmembrane protein in primary explants of human malignant gliomas. *Cancer Res* 2000, 60:1168–1172.

60. Husain SR, Behari N, Kreitman RJ, *et al.*: Complete regression of established human glioblastoma tumor xenograft by interleukin-4 toxin therapy. *Cancer Res* 1998, 58:3649–3653.

61. Puri RK, Hoon DS, Leland P, *et al.*: Preclinical development of a recombinant toxin containing circularly permuted interleukin 4 and truncated Pseudomonas exotoxin for therapy of malignant astrocytoma. *Cancer Res* 1996, 56:5631–5637.

62. Debinski W, Gibo DM, Hulet SW, *et al.*: Receptor for interleukin 13 is a marker and therapeutic target for human high-grade gliomas. *Clin Cancer Res* 1999, 5:985–990.

63. Obiri NI, Husain SR, Debinski W, *et al.*: Interleukin 13 inhibits growth of human renal cell carcinoma cells independently of the p140 interleukin 4 receptor chain. *Clin Cancer Res* 1996, 2:1743–1749.

64. Debinski W, Obiri NI, Powers SK, *et al.*: Human glioma cells overexpress receptors for interleukin 13 and are extremely sensitive to a novel chimeric protein composed of interleukin 13 and pseudomonas exotoxin. *Clin Cancer Res* 1995, 1:1253–1258.

65. Husain SR, Obiri NI, Gill P, *et al.*: Receptor for interleukin 13 on AIDS-associated Kaposi's sarcoma cells serves as a new target for a potent *Pseudomonas* exotoxin-based chimeric toxin protein. *Clin Cancer Res* 1997, 3:151–156.

66. Phillips PC, Levow C, Catterall M, *et al.*: Transforming growth factor-alpha-Pseudomonas exotoxin fusion protein (TGF-alpha-PE38) treatment of subcutaneous and intracranial human glioma and medulloblastoma xenografts in athymic mice. *Cancer Res* 1994, 54:1008–1115.

PHASE-3 STUDY OF RT, BCNU, TEMOZOLOMIDE FOR NEWLY DIAGNOSED ANAPLASTIC ASTROCYTOMA

The RTOG 98-13 is a phase 3 randomized study of radiation therapy (RT) and temozolomide versus RT and BCNU versus RT and temozolomide and BCNU for anaplastic astrocytoma.

Objectives: This study is a three-arm phase 3 clinical trial for patients treated with RT, comparing single-agent BCNU (considered standard adjuvant chemotherapy treatment for anaplastic astrocytoma), to both single-agent temozolomide and the combination of temozolomide and BCNU. Objectives of this study include comparisons of overall survival, time to tumor progressions, relative toxicities of the drug regimens, and correlation of molecular analyses with survival rates and time to tumor progressions.

Rationale: Other than RT and BCNU, there is no clear standard of care for treatment of patients with anaplastic astrocytoma. Combined modality treatment will result in median survival between 3 and 5 years, depending on known prognostic factors such as patient age, performance status, and extent of resection. New approaches are needed to improve this outcome. One strategy is to test newer chemotherapy regimens. This study will primarily test the use of temozolomide in this setting. Temozolomide is a cytotoxic alkylating agent with modest toxicity and demonstrated clinical antitumor activity against malignant gliomas both at relapse and first diagnosis. It belongs to a group of compounds known as imidazotetrazinones. Temozolomide undergoes chemical degradation at physiologic pH to form MTIC (3-methyl-[triazen-1-y1]) imidazole-4-carboxamide, the active metabolite of dacarbazine, frequently used in the treatment of malignant melanoma. Dacarbazine differs, however, in that MTIC is formed only following drug metabolism in liver. The cytotoxicity of MTIC is thought to be primarily due to alkylation at the 06 position of guanine residues with additional alkylation occurring at the n7 position. Temozolomide has been found to penetrate the blood-brain barrier in both preclinical and phase I testing. There is one ongoing phase 2 clinical trial using the combination of temozolomide and BCNU for patients with recurrent malignant glioma. These phase 2 data are not yet available; however, in the prior phase 1 study, seven of 33 patients with malignant glioma had a partial response defined as a 50% reduction in tumor size; 12 of 33 had stable disease. Toxicity was predominantly hematologic. The rationale for the drug combination is clear, eg, two active drugs given together are more efficacious than single-agent therapy. Furthermore, it has been demonstrated that temozolomide can deplete 06-alkylguanine-DNA alkyltransferase (AT), the DNA repair enzyme, high levels of which are thought to contribute to glioma cell resistance to the nitrosoureas. However, because of the potential for increased toxicity with the combination of BCNU and temozolomide compared with either agent alone, it was felt that a third arm using temozolomide alone was appropriate, along with the control arm of BCNU alone.

CANDIDATES FOR TREATMENT

Histologically confirmed adult patients with anaplastic astrocytoma (central pathology review required). No prior treatment with irradiation or chemotherapy. KPS $\geq$ 60; hemoglobin $\geq$ 10; absolute neutrophils $\geq$ 1500; platelets $\geq$ 150,000. Therapy must begin within 5 weeks after tissue diagnosis. No spinal cord tumors or spinal cord metastases. DLCO $\geq$ 60% of predicted normal levels.

TOXICITIES

Expected radiation toxicities include hair loss, erythema or soreness of the scalp, nausea and vomiting, dry mouth, altered taste, fatigue, or temporary aggravation of brain tumor symptoms such as headaches, seizures, or weakness. Reactions in the ear canals and on the ear should be observed and treated symptomatically. Possible early delayed radiation effects include lethargy and transient worsening of existing neurologic deficits. Possible late delayed effects of RT include radiation necrosis, endocrine dysfunction, accelerated atherosclerosis, or radiation-induced neoplasms. Potential chemotherapy toxicity includes myelosuppression (platelets and neutrophils), which may be delayed with BCNU or the combination of BCNU and temozolomide. Cumulative myelosuppression may occur with BCNU treatment. Nausea or vomiting is possible. Reversible increases in hepatic enzymes may occur. Pulmonary toxicity is possible with single-agent BCNU and may potentially be increased with the combination of BCNU with temozolomide. Pulmonary fibrosis is especially prevalent with BCNU cumulative doses greater than 1200 mg/m^2

DOSING AND SCHEDULE

Arm 1 (RT + temozolomide): 59.4 Gy + temozolomide 200 mg/m^2 PO daily on days 1–5 of the first day of radiation, repeated every 28 d for 12 cycles

Arm 2 (RT + BCNU): 59.4 Gy + BCNU 80 mg/m^2 IV days 1, 2, 3 of the first week of radiation, repeated every 8 wk for 6 treatment cycles (maximum BCNU dose, 1440 mg/m^2)

Arm 3 (RT + BCNU and temozolomide): 59.4 Gy + BCNU 200 mg/m^2 IV on day 1 of radiation and temozolomide 150 mg/m^2 on days 1–5 of the first week of radiation, repeated every 6 wk for a total of 6 cycles

PHASE-3 STUDY OF RT ± PCV CHEMOTHERAPY FOR NEWLY DIAGNOSED LOW-GRADE GLIOMA

The RTOG 98-02 is a phase II study of observation in favorable low-grade glioma (LGG) and phase III study of RT with or without PCV(procarbazine, CCNU, vincristine) chemotherapy in unfavorable LGG.

Objectives: For low-risk patients, the goal is to identify the overall and relapse-free survival of low-risk (< 40 year old; gross total resection) adult patients with supratentorial LGG who are observed postoperatively without additional treatment. For the high-risk patients (all other patients with LGG), the goal is to compare the overall and relapse-free survival of these patients who are treated either with RT alone, or RT plus adjuvant chemotherapy using PCV.

Rationale: The most controversial issue in the management of the adult patient with a supratentorial LGG is whether or not to administer immediate versus delayed (*until the time of recurrence*) RT. Over a decade ago, when the Brain Tumor Study Group tried to randomize adults with supratentorial LGG to immediate versus delayed postoperative radiation, the study failed due to poor accrual, in part because some physicians did not want their good-prognosis patients to potentially be randomized to receive immediate postoperative radiation, whereas other physicians with poor-prognosis patients did not want the possibility that postoperative radiation might not be given.

Another controversial issue regarding RT is the appropriate dose. Despite the observation that doses of greater than 53 Gy were associated with significantly better survival than doses of less than 53 Gy, a recently published phase 3 prospective randomized trial from the European Organization for the Research and Treatment of Cancer (EORTC) failed to detect a significant difference in either overall or relapse-free survival between 45 Gy per 25 fractions and 59.4 Gy per 33 fractions in adults with supratentorial LGG (Karim *et al.*). A similar prospective study was completed in December 1994 by the North Central Cancer Treatment Group (NCCTG), Radiation Therapy Oncology Group (RTOG), and Eastern Cooperative Oncology Group (ECOG), randomizing between 50.4 Gy per 28 fractions and 64.8 per 36 fractions. No advantage in survival was noted comparing the higher dose with the lower dose radiation. Until results of this trial become available, the majority of radiation oncologists prefer to treat these patients with total doses in the mid–50 Gy range. The value of chemotherapy in patients with LGG has not been clearly demonstrated. Most studies have not reported response to treatment in relationship to tumor grade. There has been one randomized trial assessing the role of adjuvant chemotherapy in adult patients with supratentorial LGGs. The Southwest Oncology Group (SWOG) randomized 54 patients to either 55 Gy radiation alone (*n* = 19) or RT + CCNU (*n* = 35) in 1:2 randomization schema. Median survival was comparable between the two groups (2.8–3.1 years), but was considerably lower than in other series. More recently reported studies suggest a potentially beneficial role of chemotherapy. In a multi-institutional phase 2 trial, responses were seen in nine of 10 patients with recurrent oligodendroglioma who had presented initially with low-grade pure oligodendroglioma. Other studies reported responses in five of 15 (33%) patients with recurrent low-grade astrocytoma and two of five (40%) patients with recurrent low-grade oligoastrocytoma treated on a phase 2 North Central Cancer Treatment Group (NCCTG) trial with BCNU plus recombinant interferon-alfa. In a subsequent NCCTG phase 2 trial using nitrogen mustard, procarbazine, and vincristine, responses were seen in four of 20 (20%) patients with recurrent LGG. In both NCCTG trials, patients with recurrent LGG had higher response rates to the investigational regimen than those with any other histologic type, including anaplastic oligodendroglioma. As a group, these studies suggest modest chemosensitivity of recurrent LGGs. Less is known about the chemoresponsiveness of previously untreated LGG patients. In preliminary data from an ongoing NCCTG phase 2 trial of chemotherapy ("intensive" PCV for 6 cycles every 8 weeks) followed by radiation for patients with newly diagnosed LGG, responses have been noted in five of 15 patients who have completed the chemotherapy portion of the trial (unpublished data). Patients with astrocytoma, oligodendroglioma, and oligoastrocytoma have experienced tumor regression. Although there is evidence of antitumor activity of PCV in some untreated LGG patients, the frequency and duration of response are unclear. Nevertheless, preliminary data suggest that these patients are at least as responsive to chemotherapy as high-grade glioma patients in whom adjuvant chemotherapy confers modest but reproducible survival benefit, especially in younger patients and those with anaplastic astrocytoma. Given the uncertain frequency of tumor progression in patients receiving chemotherapy alone prior to radiation, we propose to administer RT first, followed by PCV chemotherapy.

CANDIDATES FOR TREATMENT

Adult patients (age ≥ 18 y) with histologic proof of a supratentorial LGG (WHO grade 2 astrocytoma, oligodendroglioma, oligoastrocytoma). Central neuropathology review mandatory prior to registration and treatment. KPS ≥ 60; absolute neutrophil count ≥ 1500, platelet count within institutional normal range, and serum creatinine, SGOT, and alkaline phosphatase < two times institutional normal range. Patients with other types of LGG are excluded, as are patients with tumors located in the optic chiasm, optic nerve, pons, medulla, cerebellum, or spinal cord

TOXICITIES

Expected radiation toxicities include hair loss, erythema or soreness of the scalp, nausea and vomiting, dry mouth, altered taste, fatigue, or temporary aggravation of brain tumor symptoms such as headaches, seizures, or weakness. Reactions in the ear canals and on the ear should be observed and treated symptomatically. Possible early delayed radiation effects include lethargy, transient worsening of existing neurologic deficits. Possible late delayed effects of radiotherapy include radiation necrosis, endocrine dysfunction, accelerated atherosclerosis, or radiation-induced neoplasms. Potential chemotherapy toxicity includes nausea and vomiting, fatigue, anorexia, weight loss, allergic reactions, and myelosuppression (platelets and neutrophils), which may be delayed with CCNU. Cumulative myelosuppression may occur with CCNU treatment. Reversible increases in hepatic enzymes may occur. Peripheral neuropathy, constipation, and fatigue is possible with vincristine, as is skin necrosis with extravasation. Foods rich in tyramine must be avoided while taking procarbazine

ADRENAL CORTICAL CARCINOMA

ETIOLOGY AND RISK FACTORS

Adrenal cortical carcinomas (ACC) are exceedingly rare tumors with an incidence of two cases per million population. There is a bimodal age distribution, with peak incidences in children under 5 years of age and in people in their fourth to sixth decades. Although no etiologic factors have been identified, ACC has been associated with certain hereditary syndromes (multiple endocrine neoplasia type I and a sarcoma, breast, and lung cancer syndrome).

Patients with ACC present with symptoms related to steroid hormone excess or an enlarging abdominal mass (Table 16-1). Women present more commonly with functioning ACC, whereas men are more likely to have nonfunctioning ACC. The most common hormone excess is hypercortisolism and associated Cushing's syndrome. Children most commonly present with virilization. Aldosterone-secreting ACC occurs but is exceedingly rare.

STAGING AND PROGNOSIS

The endocrinologic evaluation of functional ACC includes assessment of steroid hormone synthesis. The initial evaluation should include a single-dose overnight dexamethasone test. The etiology of the hypercortisolism can be further delineated by the clinical situation and the low- or high-dose dexamethasone suppression tests (or ovine corticotropin-releasing hormone test) as indicated. The presence of elevated, nonsuppressible steroid hormone levels can serve as a useful tumor marker for subsequent follow-up. Patients with clinically silent adrenal tumors should have a judicious clinical and biochemical evaluation [1].

Computed tomography (CT) of the adrenal glands is the technique most commonly used for radiologic evaluation of an adrenal mass. CT scan has 80% sensitivity for adrenal masses less than 1 cm and a sensitivity of 95% for tumors 3 to 4 cm in diameter. Abdominal CT scan can also identify local and distant metastases. However, adrenal CT scan is nonspecific in delineating a benign versus malignant mass. Magnetic resonance imaging (MRI) may be helpful in distinguishing benign adenomas from ACC, pheochromocytoma, or metastases to the adrenal gland based on relative brightness of the T2-weighted scan. MRI may aid in equivocal cases to improve the specificity of adrenal CT scan [2,3]. In some cases, iodocholesterol scanning can be useful to functionally localize the unilateral or bilateral nature of functional adrenal tumors [3]. The only definitive radiologic criteria for malignancy of a mass are evidence of local invasion or distant metastases.

Conversely, the frequent use of CT imaging of the abdomen has led to the discovery of adrenal "incidentalomas" in 0.6% of abdominal CT scans. The adrenal incidentaloma is usually benign but requires assessment by a clinician familiar with an efficient clinical and biochemical work-up of this issue. Although fewer than 1% of adrenal tumors that are less than 6 cm in size represent ACC, the risk of malignancy of lesions greater than 6 cm ranges from 35% to 98%. Therefore, it is recommended that all nonfunctioning tumors greater than 5 cm in diameter undergo surgical resection. Adrenalectomy is also warranted for all functional tumors, regardless of size. Biochemical screening for urinary catecholamines to exclude pheochromocytoma is obligatory before any needle biopsy or operation for an adrenal mass; such an intervention might precipitate a fatal hypertensive crisis if the patient has an unrecognized pheochromocytoma. Fine-needle biopsy of an adrenal mass does not aid in the differential between benign and malignant tumors. Therefore, fine-needle aspiration (FNA) is not routinely performed unless metastatic cancer or lymphoma are suspected.

The most important factors in the staging of ACC are tumor size and local invasion at presentation (Table 16-2). Prognosis in ACC depends on disease stage at presentation. Historically, approximately 70% of patients present with advanced (stage III or IV) disease; however, more recent series have nearly 50% lower-stage (I or II) patients [4]. Patients have an overall median survival of 2 years, with 5-year and 10-year survival rates of 22% to 30% and 10%, respectively. Patients with stage I or II disease have substantially better prognosis overall (~50% at 5 y); however, survival drops off quickly at stage III (median, 12 mo; only 20% alive at 5 y) and is very poor for patients with stage IV disease (median, 6 mo; 5% alive at 5 y) [4].

In addition to tumor size (>100 g), other factors associated with poor prognosis are vascular invasion, mitotic rate, necrosis, and nuclear ploidy. Factors of limited significance include capsular invasion, immunohistochemical staining, and functional status of the tumor.

PRIMARY DISEASE THERAPY

Complete surgical resection is the basis of effective treatment for ACC and offers the only curative therapy. The goal of the initial

Table 16-1. Presenting Clinical Features of Adrenal Cortical Carcinoma

Symptom	Rate, %
Cushing's syndrome	40–60
Virilization or feminization	10–20
Hypertension and hypokalemia	1
Abdominal symptoms only	30

Table 16-2. Staging Criteria for Adrenal Cortical Carcinoma

	Stage			
	I	II	III	IV
TNM Components	T1, N0, M0	T2, N0, M0	T1 or T2, N1, M0 or T3, N0, M0	Any T, any N, M1 or T3–T4, N1

Criteria
T1 — Tumor ≤ 5 cm, no invasion
T2 — Tumor > 5 cm, no invasion
T3 — Tumor outside adrenal in fat
T4 — Tumor invading adjacent viscera
N0 — No involved lymph nodes
N1 — Positive lymph nodes
M0 — No distant disease
M1 — Distant disease

operation is en bloc resection, which may involve adjacent viscera, vena cava, or diaphragm. The tumors tend to be quite locally invasive and require meticulous yet radical extirpation. Less than half of patients are resectable at time of presentation. Steroid hormone replacement is critical perioperatively and is continued postoperatively at replacement doses until complete recovery of the hypothalamic-pituitary axis. This may take up to 2 years after surgery [5]. Patients should be counseled regarding the dangers of Addisonian crisis during acute illnesses that require exogenous steroid replacement. Patients with stage I and II disease at surgical resection have a median survival of 5 years, whereas patients with invasion of contiguous structures have a mean survival of 2.3 years.

ADJUVANT THERAPY FOR REGIONAL DISEASE

Although surgical resection can be curative, a majority of patients have recurrence, with a median disease-free interval of 3 to 12 months for those cancers that do recur. Approximately one third recur locally, one third recur as distant metastases only, and one third demonstrate both local and distant disease at recurrence. There have been several studies recommending adjuvant mitotane after resection of localized disease. However, other studies have shown no increase in survival, and therefore, adjuvant therapy is not generally implemented. The disease-free interval was a significant prognostic factor in a report from the National Cancer Institute for select patients with recurrent or metastatic disease [6]. In this nonrandomized study, 15 patients treated with chemotherapy alone had a median survival from first recurrence of 11 months, whereas 18 patients whose recurrent disease was curatively re-resected in addition to chemotherapy had a median survival of 27 months. One third of the operated patients survived more than 5 years from initial re-resection. A more recent multicenter review of reoperative results demonstrated similar findings, ie, patients who presented with resectable recurrences and who were resected survived longer than those patients who recurred with unresectable disease or who elected to forgo re-resection [4]. These retrospective data would seem to support resection of local recurrences, or metastasectomy, when possible. Patients who have undergone curative resection should be followed for recurrences by urine steroid profiles and serial chest and abdominal CT scans. Of those who are unresectable at time of reoperation, palliative debulking of ACC has not been shown to have a survival benefit but significantly improves quality of life, especially in decreasing tumor bulk and functionality of the tumors.

THERAPY FOR ADVANCED DISEASE

Adrenal cortical carcinomas metastasize to lung (71%), liver (42%), and bone (26%). The pesticide analogue o,p-DDD (mitotane) has been used for treatment because of its adrenolytic properties. Chemotherapy for ACC has been largely ineffective, with most responses anecdotal and with no clear efficacy or documented benefit (Table 16-3) [7–10]. Mitotane is poorly tolerated and has not been studied in a randomized setting. Although there are isolated reports of long-term survivors, most of the 20% to 30% of patients who respond to mitotane have partial response of short duration. Pulmonary metastasectomy, isolated liver resection, and local-recurrence re-resection have been shown to induce remission in some patients [4,6]. External beam radiotherapy is ineffective except in the management of painful bony metastases.

Other agents under investigation include paclitaxel, but responses and experience have been limited. There is no information about immunotherapeutic strategies for metastatic ACC.

THYROID CANCER

ETIOLOGY AND RISK FACTORS

Thyroid cancer is the most common endocrine malignancy. Currently, there are 12,400 new cases of thyroid cancer diagnosed per year, with an estimated death toll of 1230. Thyroid cancer commonly presents as a thyroid nodule. Although 4% to 7% of the general population have thyroid nodules, only 10% of solid nodules are malignant. Important clinical factors that increase the likelihood of malignancy include patient age (< 20 y or > 50 y); growth on thyroid stimulating hormone (TSH) suppressive therapy; residence in an iodine-deficient geographic area; and a history of thyroiditis, goiter, or head and neck irradiation. Worrisome but nonspecific clinical features include neck pain, dysphagia, hoarseness, dyspnea, and cervical adenopathy. Although prior exposure to head and neck radiation is an etiologic factor in the development of papillary thyroid cancer, it is not a prognostic factor in its outcome. Patients with a history of childhood neck irradiation have a 33% to 37% chance of malignancy. Age of exposure and a radiation dose up to 2000 cGy have been shown to have a linear relation with the increased risk associated with ionizing radiation.

Papillary thyroid cancer has also been associated with several inherited tumor syndromes (Gardner's syndrome, Cowden's disease, and familial polyposis coli). A family history of thyroid cancer or other endocrine tumors should elicit the possibility of a multiple endocrine neoplasia syndrome (MEN). Direct DNA testing for mutation in *ret* proto-oncogene of individuals at risk for MEN type II is now routine. Subsequent prophylactic surgical management can be recommended in these patients.

Fine-needle aspiration biopsy has revolutionized the accuracy of diagnosing thyroid cancer. Thyroid scans are now largely unnecessary and the annual number of thyroidectomies has been substantially reduced with the advent of the FNA-cytology assessment. Between 70% and 94% of FNA biopsies give the correct cytologic diagnosis. FNA cytology is divided into categories of benign, suspicious or indeterminate, malignant, and insufficient sample. Patients with benign-appearing FNA cytology are placed on exogenous L-thyrox-

Table 16-3. Chemotherapy for Advanced Adrenal Cortical Cancer

Study	Agents	Response Rate
Decker *et al.* [7]	Mitotane, doxorubicin	19% = 3/16 PR
van Slooten *et al.*	Cisplatin, doxorubicin, cyclophosphamide	18% = 2/11 PR
Schlumberger *et al.* [8]	Cisplatin, doxorubicin, 5-FU	23% =1/13 CR, 2/13 PR
Bukowski *et al.* [9]	Mitotane, cisplatin	30% = 1/37 CR, 10/37 PR
Johnson *et al.*	Cisplatin, etoposide	2/2 PR
Hesketh *et al.*	Cisplatin, etoposide, bleomycin	1/4 CR, 2/4 PR
Berruti *et al.* [10]	Cisplatin, etoposide, doxorubicin	2/2 PR

CR—complete remission; 5-FU—5-fluorouracil; PR—partial remission.

ine therapy at a dose sufficient to suppress TSH to less than 0.4 mIU/mL. Approximately 20% to 40% of those who do not respond to this treatment will be diagnosed with thyroid cancer at time of subsequent operation. FNA cannot reliably distinguish between follicular adenoma and follicular thyroid cancer; patients with indeterminate follicular lesions require thyroidectomy to document the pathologic presence of vascular or capsular invasion by cancer. The rate of follicular cancer at surgery is 24% by this method of management. CT scan and MRI can be helpful in selected cases to evaluate the degree of tracheal deviation and compression, extension into the mediastinum, and carotid artery involvement by tumor.

STAGING AND PROGNOSIS

The most important factors in staging of thyroid cancer are patient age, tumor size, and cell type. The staging system is outlined in Table 16-4.

There are four primary cell types of thyroid cancer, with varying natural histories, treatments, and outcome. Well-differentiated thyroid cancer is the most common type, accounting for 90% of all thyroid cancers. This category is further subdivided into papillary (75%) and follicular (10%–15%) cancer. Mixed papillary follicular cancer has been reclassified as a follicular variant of papillary thyroid cancer due to the similar behavior and prognosis to usual papillary cancer. Follicular cancers are increasingly uncommon, except in iodine-deficient geographic areas. Follicular cancer with capsular invasion alone may have a better prognosis than more invasive lesions; follicular lesions without vascular or capsular invasion are benign follicular adenomas. Compared with papillary thyroid cancers, follicular cancer is less likely to metastasize to lymph nodes and more likely to pursue an aggressive course in older patients. The most important feature of a follicular cancer is the presence or absence of distant metastases at presentation in the elderly; when present, they portend a very poor, treatment-resistant course.

Prognosis for well-differentiated thyroid cancer is related primarily to risk group, although those of papillary histology have a slightly better prognosis than do the follicular cell types. Several widely used systems for determining risk have been developed based on multivariate analysis (AMES, AGES, MACIS). All systems have documented that a very important factor in predicting survival is patient age at presentation. Tumor invasion, size of primary tumor, and presence of distant metastases are also significant factors. Nuclear DNA content also has been cited as an important prognostic variable. Table 16-5 presents the most recent scoring system for papillary thyroid cancer [11]. The prognostic significance of cervical lymph node involvement is controversial; some studies have reported an univariant survival advantage with local nodal involvement. In general, the presence of cervical lymph node metastases is a predictor of local recurrence but does not influence survival (Table 16-6).

Hürthle cell cancers account for 2% to 4% of all well-differentiated cancers, and exhibit a poorer prognosis. Other less fortuitous histologies include tall cell, insular, and diffuse sclerosing papillary variants. Although the relatively uncommon Hürthle cell variant is staged with the other well-differentiated tumors, in some cases they metastasize early to lymph nodes, lung, and bone.

Medullary thyroid cancer (MTC) (5%–10% of patients) arises from the neuroendocrine parafollicular C cells, which secrete calcitonin. The serum levels of calcitonin can thus serve as a biochemical marker for this disease. MTC appears in four unique clinical settings: 1) sporadic (80% of cases), 2) inherited in association with MEN type IIa, 3) inherited in association with MEN type IIb, and 4) familial MTC. The three inherited forms arise from precursor C-cell hyperplasia and usually are multifocal. MTC can present either as a clinical thyroid nodule or as occult disease detected in a patient at risk for an inherited form. Direct DNA testing of the *ret* proto-oncogene has replaced provocative testing and has led to early thyroidectomy in those patients at risk [12,13].

Anaplastic thyroid cancer (2% of patients) is a highly malignant tumor arising from thyroid epithelium and, in some cases, from pre-existing well-differentiated thyroid cancer or long-standing goiter.

Table 16-4. Staging of Thyroid Cancers

Primary Tumor (T)	Nodal Involvement (N)	Metastases (M)
T1—T ≤ 1 cm within thyroid	N0—node negative	M0—No distant metastases
T2—1 cm < T ≤ 4 cm	N1a—ipsilateral node(s) involved	M1—Distant metastases
T3—T > 4 cm		
T4—Any size extending beyond capsule	N1b—contralateral, midline, or mediastinal node(s) involved	

Cancer Stage	Papillary or follicular, age < 45 y	Papillary or follicular, age ≥ 45 y	Medullary	Undifferentiated
I	Any T, any N, M0	T1, N0, M0	T1, N0, M0	—
II	Any T, any N, M1	T2, N0, M0	T2, N0, M0	—
		T3, N0, M0	T3, N0, M0	—
			T4, N0, M0	
III	—	T4, N0, M0	Any T, N1, M0	
		Any T, N1, M0		
IV	—	Any T, any N, M1	Any T, any N, M1	All stage IV

Adapted from Fleming et al. [27].

Table 16-5. MACIS Prognostic Index for Papillary Thyroid Cancer

Variable	Points Assigned
Age < 39	+ 3.1
Age > 40	+ 0.08 × age
Diameter of primary tumor	+0.3 × cm
Incomplete resection	+ 1
Extrathyroidal invasion	+ 1
Distant metastases	+ 3

MACIS Score	Metastasis at 10 y, %	Mortality at 20 y, %
< 6	3	1
6–6.9	18	13
7–7.9	40	45
8 +	60	76

Adapted from Hay et al. [11].

With earlier and more effective treatment of differentiated cancer, the incidence of anaplastic cancer has dropped dramatically over the past 50 years. Over half of the small cell variants of anaplastic thyroid cancer diagnosed in the past are now believed to be thyroid lymphomas. This important distinction is made today by immuno-histochemistry and flow cytometry, and is crucial to prognosis (Table 16-7) and management. One third to one half of cases of non-Hodgkin's lymphoma of the thyroid gland occur in the setting of pre-existing Hashimoto's thyroiditis.

PRIMARY DISEASE THERAPY

Primary treatment of thyroid cancer is based on histologic type. Surgical resection of well-differentiated cancers is the mainstay of treatment. Isolated papillary lesions smaller than 1 cm appear in 10% of thyroid glands at autopsy. After thyroid lobectomy is performed, these minimal thyroid cancers require no treatment other than expectant follow-up.

The extent of resection of papillary carcinomas remains controversial. At present there is a consensus that for low-risk, well-differentiated thyroid cancer, the minimal operation is a thyroid lobectomy and isthmectomy. Total or near-total thyroidectomy should be performed for lesions larger than 1.5 cm in angioinvasive follicular cancer, Hürthle cell cancer, or papillary cancer in association with prior neck irradiation or local invasion. A survival advantage for total thyroidectomy versus subtotal thyroidectomy or lobectomy has never been shown in a prospective randomized study but has been observed in retrospective series. Total thyroidectomy offers the significant advantage of simplifying postoperative surveillance and treatment of thyroid cancer. Major risks associated with total thyroidectomy include a 1% risk of permanent recurrent laryngeal nerve injury and a 1% to 3% chance of permanent hypoparathyroidism. These risks are demonstrably lower in the hands of expert surgeons. Neck dissection has no proven role in primary treatment of well-differentiated thyroid cancer, although some controversy does exist with the surgical management of lymph node involvement. Some advocate a formal dissection for clinically obvious lymph node metastases. Prognosis is noted in Table 16-6.

Surgical resection is the primary therapy for MTC. The operation of choice is total thyroidectomy and central node dissection. Modified or radical node dissection should be performed for palpable cervical disease. Patients with MEN type II should undergo total thyroidectomy on diagnosis of the syndrome because most patients will otherwise develop lethal MTC by their second decade. Prognosis is noted in Table 16-7.

Anaplastic cancer of the thyroid usually presents as a locally advanced tumor for which surgical intervention is not an curative option. Core or incisional biopsy may be required to definitely exclude lymphoma. An aggressive surgical debulking and tracheostomy may be warranted to forestall death from asphyxiation. Primary therapy for thyroid lymphoma is external radiation or combination chemotherapy, depending on stage.

ADJUVANT THERAPY FOR REGIONAL DISEASE

Postoperative management of patients with well-differentiated thyroid cancer includes hormonal therapy and radioactive iodine treatment (Table 16-8). Regardless of risk status, all patients with thyroid cancer should receive exogenous L-thyroxine suppressive therapy; considerable indirect evidence demonstrates that long-term TSH suppressive therapy favorably influences tumor recurrence, disease progression, and survival in well-differentiated thyroid cancer. Thyroglobulin is secreted by normal and cancerous thyroid cells and serves as a useful tumor marker for thyroid cancer persistence, recurrence, and progression. The sensitivity of this method is greatest when the patient is hypothyroid with high TSH levels. A poorly differentiated cancer may still secrete thyroglobulin after its iodine-concentrating ability has been lost.

Normal thyroid tissue concentrates radioiodine much more efficiently than thyroid cancer. Thus, any remaining thyroid tissue after

---

Table 16-6. Survival Rates for Papillary and Follicular Thyroid Cancer

	5 y, %	10 y, %	Distant Metastases at Presentation, %
Papillary	95	92	20
Follicular	82	70	18

Table 16-7. Prognosis for Medullary Thyroid Cancer, Anaplastic Thyroid Cancer, and Thyroid Lymphoma

Thyroid Cancer Subtype	Associated Endocrinopathies	16-y Survival, %
Medullary		
Sporadic	None	70–80
MEN-IIa	Pheochromocytoma, parathyroid hyperplasia	85–90
MEN-IIb	Pheochromocytoma, mucosal neuromas	< 40–50
FMTC	None	100%
Anaplastic	None	4–6 mo median survival
Thyroid lymphoma	None	50% at 5 y

FMTC—familial medullary thyroid cancer; MEN-IIa and MEN-IIb—multiple endocrine neoplasia, types IIa and IIb.

Table 16-8. Adjuvant Management of Well-differentiated Thyroid Cancer

1. Postoperative withdrawal of L-thyroxine for 4–6 wk.

2. When TSH is > 30 mIU/mL, obtain 131I scan and serum thyroglobulin level.

3. If, after total thyroidectomy, thyroid remnants or metastases are detected, or thyroglobulin level is > 10 mg/dL, administer calculated ablative/therapeutic dose of 131I, with post-therapy whole-body scan.

4. Begin/resume long-term L-thyroxine replacement to completely suppress TSH to < 0.1 mIU/mL.

5. Repeat hypothyroid 131I scan, thyroglobulin monitoring and radiotherapy every 6–12 mo until normal on 2 successive scans, then every 3–5 y (or until total 131I dose of 500–800 mCi). rTSH may be used for diagnostic scans but not treatment 131I doses.

thyroidectomy will decrease the efficacy of [131]I. Patients should have an ablative dose of ^{131}I while they are intentionally hypothyroid. [131]I is the treatment of choice for recurrent or metastatic differentiated thyroid cancer [14].

Radioiodine is not taken up by Hürthle cell, tall cell, medullary, or most anaplastic thyroid cancers and, thus, is not a therapeutic option. However, differentiated thyroid cancer that has lost affinity for radioiodine can still be treated successfully with large doses; 30% to 90% of patients with detectable thyroglobulin levels and a negative low-dose radioiodine scan who are treated with ^{131}I have uptake on their posttherapy scan. A treatment dose of 150 mCi delivers approximately 1000 cGy to the lesion. The risks of ^{131}I include temporary local pain, swelling, nausea and temporary myelotoxicity in up to a third of patients. Cases of leukemia and bladder cancer have been reported at high doses.

The most effective treatment for pulmonary metastases is ^{131}I, although it only offers palliation for bony metastases. External radiation therapy is reserved for palliation of bony metastases or for radioiodine-insensitive cases. Thyroid cancers that do not respond to radioiodine therapy are treated as advanced disease. Resection of recurrent regional disease offers no proven or theoretical advantage over [131]I. For locally advanced thyroid cancer, some have observed successful local control in a majority of patients treated with low-dose doxorubicin and hyperfractionated radiotherapy but no improvement in distant disease or in survival.

Treatment selection for regional MTC is based on the indolent growth of most of these tumors. Basal and stimulated calcitonin levels and serum carcinoembryonic antigen are followed postoperatively as indicators of recurrence and progression. With close surveillance and early reoperation, long-term survival rates as high as 86% have been reported. Most experts recommend resection of clinically or radiologically evident disease, but some advocate aggressive search for residual MTC, using invasive imaging techniques followed by comprehensive resection in an attempt to obtain a biochemical cure [15,16]. MTC is insensitive to ^{131}I and external radiation.

THERAPY FOR ADVANCED DISEASE

There has not been substantial recent progress in the treatment of relapsed and metastatic thyroid cancer. In 33% to 42% of patients, metastatic disease does not take up radioiodine, and these patients have significantly decreased survival rates (at 10 years, 83% for those who do take up ^{131}I vs < 1% for those who do not). The most active chemotherapeutic agent is doxorubicin; at a dose up to 75 mg/m^2, it produces a 17% to 33% response rate in metastatic non-MTC. Responses are partial and of a moderate duration (up to ~2 y); most patients die of pulmonary (80%) and cerebral (20%) metastases. The combination of doxorubicin with other agents, such as cisplatin or bleomycin, have not improved efficacy. Although there is much indirect evidence that autoimmune mechanisms may favorably influence the outcome of patients with metastatic thyroid cancer, no trials employing biologic response modifiers have been reported.

Chemotherapy in advanced MTC is generally not administered until the development of debilitating diarrhea (the main symptom of advanced disease), which occurs with calcitonin levels greater than 10,000 pg/mL. Doxorubicin alone or in combination has the highest response rate (15%–30%), with mean duration of response of 21 months. There is no documented survival benefit. Octreotide therapy has produced palliation of symptoms and objective biochem-

ical responses in several recent small studies; however, dose escalation usually was required to maintain the effect. Interferon α (IFN α) may provide similar palliative benefit as octreotide for advanced MTC.

Anaplastic thyroid cancer is stage IV by definition. Systemic chemotherapy has made no impact on the dismal prognosis. A protocol employing low-dose doxorubicin as a radiosensitizer for hyperfractionated external radiotherapy has been advocated. The multimodality therapy of radiotherapy, aggressive surgery, and combination chemotherapy may improve local control but offers no survival advantage.

CARCINOID TUMORS

ETIOLOGY AND RISK FACTORS

Carcinoid tumors arise from neuroendocrine enterochromaffin cells of neural crest origin and secrete the biogenic amine serotonin (5-hydroxytryptamine [5-HT]). Enterochromaffin cells are part of the amine precursor uptake and decarboxylation system, which is characterized by the potential for secretion of multiple amine and peptide hormones. Carcinoid tumors can also secrete adrenocorticotropic hormone (ACTH), somatostatin, α- and β-human chorionic gonadotropin, gastrin, and pancreatic polypeptide, which can disguise or complicate the clinical presentation of a carcinoid tumor. Precursor enterochromaffin cells are found submucosally throughout the gastrointestinal tract, bronchial tree, and genitourinary tract; carcinoid tumors arise from any of these sites.

Carcinoid tumors are clinically evident at a reported rate of 3.2 cases per 1 million, although this number underestimates their actual incidence according to autopsy studies. There are known associations of carcinoids with multiple endocrine neoplasia type I, of ampullary carcinoids with von Recklinghausen's disease, and of gastric carcinoids with hypergastrinemic states (eg, pernicious anemia, atrophic gastritis, and gastrinoma).

Carcinoid tumors have a characteristically indolent course that is heterogenous, depending on the histology and endocrine features of this diverse group of tumors. The median duration of symptoms prior to diagnosis is 21 months. Although one half of the symptomatic patients have unresectable disease at the time of diagnosis, over 50% of these patients will live 5 years or more after diagnosis. Median survival after onset of symptoms is 3.5 to 8.5 years.

The carcinoid syndrome is a spectrum of symptoms caused by the release of serotonin, histamine, and tachykinins into the systemic venous circulation. Symptoms include flushing, diarrhea, bronchospasm, and valvular heart disease (ie, tricuspid regurgitation, pulmonary stenosis). The severity of carcinoid syndrome is related directly to the bulk of tumor draining into the systemic circulation, which bypasses the first-pass effect of the portal circulation. The syndrome almost never occurs from midgut tumors unless they have metastasized to the liver. Rarely, carcinoid syndrome arises in patients with nonmetastatic gastrointestinal primary tumors, ovarian or testicular carcinoids, MTC, or pancreatic islet tumors. Precipitated by stress, FNA, alcohol, chemotherapy, or anesthesia, severe symptoms can present as carcinoid crisis associated with abdominal pain, hypotension, tachyarrhythmias, coma, and death. Carcinoid crisis is treated with parenteral (IV) octreotide in an emergent setting or administered prophylactically prior to FNA or surgery (100 μg SQ every 8 h).

In patients suspected to have a carcinoid tumor, the diagnosis is confirmed by measuring levels of 24-hour urine serotonin and 5-HIAA (serotonin metabolite). Measurement of platelet serotonin, serum chromogranin A, serotonin and substance P, and urinary 5-hydroxytryptophan (5-HTP, a serotonin precursor) can be helpful in ambiguous cases. Bronchial lavage for ACTH, and thymic vein sampling are of little value in the diagnosis of bronchial carcinoid. Tumor localization can be difficult, relying on endoscopy, colonoscopy, CT scan, and other studies, as appropriate. The use of radiolabeled somatostatin receptor scintigraphy (SRS) has greatly improved the sensitivity and specificity in the localization of carcinoid tumors and regional or distant metastases; SRS should be applied in any patient with foregut or midgut carcinoid, carcinoid syndrome, or evidence of metastasis [17,18].

STAGING AND PROGNOSIS

Carcinoid tumors are generally classified by their primary location, which helps explain their heterogeneity in biologic behavior and prognosis (Table 16-9). Foregut carcinoids usually appear in the bronchial tree as classic "coin lesions" on chest radiographs. Foregut tumors also include tumors of the thymus, stomach, duodenum, and pancreas. They typically have a low 5-HT content and often secrete other agents, such as 5-HTP, histamine, or ACTH. Gastric carcinoids are commonly multifocal in sporadic cases. Midgut carcinoids secrete 5-HT and can arise from the appendix, ileum, and rarely from the jejunum or right colon. Over half of appendiceal carcinoids are diagnosed at surgery for acute appendicitis (1:250 appendicitis cases), and 90% are less than 1 cm in size. Appendiceal carcinoids occur predominantly at the tip of the appendix. Jejunoileal carcinoids are usually multiple in 25% to 35% of patients (~15% are < 1 cm). Of jejunoileal tumors, 40% are found within 2 ft of the ileocecal valve. Hindgut carcinoid tumors rarely secrete 5-HT; they arise from the rectum and rarely from the bladder, ovary, testis, and left colon (80% are < 1 cm). During screening with endoscopy for adenomatous lesions, rectal carcinoids are recognized frequently, typically as a small yellow nodule protruding from the anterior or lateral rectal wall.

Important prognostic factors for carcinoid tumors are site of primary tumor (*see* Table 16-9), histologic subtype, size of primary tumor, and extent of tumor at presentation. Of the four histologic subtypes, the insular variant is considered to have the best prognosis, trabecular is intermediate, and glandular and undifferentiated have the worst prognoses. No histologic criteria can differentiate benign from malignant neoplasms. The size of the primary tumor is indicative of malignant potential, whereas race, age, gender, nuclear DNA content, and hormonal function have not proven to be significant prognostic factors. The most important predictor of survival is the presence of metastases (Table 16-10).

PRIMARY DISEASE THERAPY

The only curative therapy for carcinoid tumors is operative resection. The extent of surgery is determined by the size and extent of the primary tumor. Lesions less than 1 cm in size are generally amenable to simple full-thickness excision. The extent of surgery is still somewhat controversial for lesions 1 to 2 cm in size; other prognostic factors (*eg*, site and histology) are commonly taken into account. Results of this treatment strategy have been reportedly curative for appendiceal and rectal carcinoids [18]. For patients with appendiceal lesions greater than 2 cm in the appendix, a right hemicolectomy is recommended. Rectal tumors of 2 cm or greater in size require an abdominoperineal or low anterior resection. Perioperative octreotide blockade is recommended for patients with carcinoid syndrome.

THERAPY FOR REGIONAL DISEASE

This indolent group of tumors recurs in patients after a median disease-free interval of 16 years. Primary resection of involved regional lymph nodes is reportedly associated with improved survival (80% at 5 y). Resection of isolated hepatic metastases may also improve prognosis [18]. However, only 2% to 5% of patients with carcinoid syndrome are candidates for hepatic resection. Radiofrequency ablation of unresectable hepatic carcinoid metastases is now frequently employed for palliation and may contribute to control of disease progression as well.

As ileal carcinoids spread to the mesentery and lymph nodes, a marked fibrotic reaction can distort or infarct the bowel. Palliative resection is appropriate for bowel obstruction or bowel ischemia but has never been shown to prolong survival.

THERAPY FOR ADVANCED DISEASE

Carcinoid tumors metastasize to liver, bone, lymph nodes, and other less common sites (*eg*, the breast or heart). Resection of metastatic disease can be either curative or palliative. The benefit of palliative resection should not be overlooked. As these tumors are often indolent, resection can provide a long interval of relative stability in spite of known residual disease.

Table 16-9. Prognosis of Carcinoid Tumors

Site	Relative Frequency, %	Rate of Metastasis, %	5-y Survival, %	Incidence of Carcinoid Syndrome, %
Foregut				
Bronchi	12	20	87	13
Stomach	2	22	52	9.5
Midgut				
Appendix	40	2	99	< 1
Ileum	25	35	54	9
Hindgut				
Rectum	15	15	83	1

Adapted from Norton et al. [29].

Table 16-10. Prognosis for Carcinoid Tumors by Stage

	5-y Survival, %	10-y Survival, %
Localized disease	94	88
Regional lymph node metastasis	64	—
Distant metastases	18–30	0

Management of patients with the carcinoid tumor syndrome and unresectable disease should be separated into two distinct but related components. The syndrome should be managed by pharmacologic means, whereas the malignancy should be addressed by extirpative, embolic, radiofrequency ablation, or chemotherapeutic means. Management of the carcinoid syndrome can be helped by avoiding precipitating factors, such as caffeine or alcohol. In addition, there are a variety of pharmacologic agents that can be useful. Octreotide, in particular, can frequently provide outstanding palliation (Table 16-11). Octreotide LAR greatly simplifies management by allowing long-acting injection once every 3 to 4 weeks, compared with three times daily with octreotide.

Systemic treatment directed at the malignant component of the carcinoid tumor has been conventionally reserved until the tumor shows some evidence of progression. For metastatic disease mainly or completely confined to the liver, hepatic artery embolization (with or without concomitant chemotherapeutic agents) can have a substantial effect on the hormone production, although usually not on survival. Combination chemotherapeutic regimens of streptozotocin/5-fluorouracil or streptozotocin/adriamycin have similar, substantial partial response rates—particularly if hormone production is used as an endpoint—however, a survival advantage has not been evident (Table 16-12) [18]. Similarly, IFN α has been used extensively in some institutions with good results in managing patients over long periods of time; however, it is difficult to separate the effect of the therapy on survival from the indolent nature of the disease [19–21].

Immunotherapy of carcinoid metastases using leukocyte or recombinant IFN α has produced a good but variable biochemical response rate (29%–60%), with occasional complete remissions reported [22]. The median duration of response varies from 6 to 34 months. In addition, IFN α can offer excellent palliation of the carcinoid syndrome (30%–80% response rate). In a randomized study, therapy with IFN α had a significantly higher response rate and fewer side effects than did systemic 5-fluorouracil chemotherapy. Prior cytotoxic chemotherapy did not preclude effective treatment with IFN α [21]. The combination of IFN α and octreotide recently produced biochemical objective responses in 77% of patients, with median duration of remission of 12 months [22]. Therapy with IFN α has been less successful in reducing tumor size (15% response rate) [22].

PANCREATIC ENDOCRINE TUMORS

EPIDEMIOLOGY AND RISK FACTORS

Pancreatic endocrine tumors are rare malignancies that are similar to carcinoid tumors; they are derived from enterochromaffin cells. Although the incidence of clinically detected pancreatic islet cell tumors is approximately five cases per million population, autopsy series have revealed a prevalence of incidental pancreatic endocrine tumors up to 1.5%. Neoplasms of the endocrine pancreas are defined as functional when they secrete hormones that cause a clinical syndrome. A nonfunctional tumor is one not associated with a clinical syndrome despite the production of hormones. This latter category includes tumors secreting pancreatic peptide (PPoma) and neurotensin (neurotensinomas). Except for insulinomas, which are most commonly benign, pancreatic endocrine tumors have a high (60%–90%) malignant potential. Gastrinomas are the most common malignant pancreatic islet cell tumors and are well studied due to their association with Zollinger–Ellison syndrome and MEN type 1. The localization, surgical management, and therapies are similar for several of these rare tumors of the endocrine pancreas and are detailed together.

ZOLLINGER-ELLISON SYNDROME

In 1955, Zollinger and Ellison theorized a relationship between severe peptic ulcer disease and pancreatic tumors. At present, Zollinger–Ellison syndrome (ZES) is estimated to occur in 0.1% of patients with duodenal ulcer disease. Gastrinomas present commonly as sporadic cases but are associated with MEN type I syndrome in 25% of patients. The familial patients tend to present at younger ages and have multiple tumors.

The clinical presentation of ZES is a result of gastric acid hypersecretion secondary to hypergastrinemia. Patients typically present with abdominal pain, diarrhea, and peptic ulcer disease. The diagnosis of ZES is confirmed by a fasting hypergastrinemia and an elevated basal gastric acid secretion of at least 15 mEq/h. Other diagnoses that can mimic ZES (eg, retained gastric antrum syndrome, chronic gastric outlet obstruction, and antral G-cell hyperplasia) are excluded by history and provocative tests (eg, secretin stimulation test or standard meal test).

Gastrinomas occur in the head of the pancreas or duodenum up to 90% of the time in an area bounded by the sweep of the duodenum, the neck of the pancreas, and the junction of the cystic and common bile ducts (ie, the gastrinoma triangle) [23]. Histologically

Table 16-11. Pharmacotherapy for Carcinoid Syndrome

Agent	Flush	Diarrhea	Dose
Phenoxybenzamine	Better	No change	10–30 mg/d
Chlorpromazine	Better	No change	10–25 mg q 8 h
Methyldopa	Somewhat better	No change	4–6 g/d
Cyproheptadine	No change	Better	4–8 mg q 8 h
Ketanserin	Somewhat better	Better	40–160 mg/d
Methysergide	No change	Better	3–8 mg/d
Octreotide	Better (89%)	Better (74%)	50–150 μg SQ q 8 h
Octreotide LAR	Better	Better	30–100 mg SQ q 3–4 wk
rIFN α-2b	Better	Better	$9–30 \times 10_6$ U/m²/wk

Adapted from Norton et al. [29].

Table 16-12. Systemic Adjuvant Therapy for Carcinoid Tumors

Agent	Response Rate, %
Doxorubicin	21
Streptozocin	30
5-Fluorouracil	26
Streptozocin and 5-Fluorouracil	33
Streptozocin + doxorubicin	40
Interferon α	42–47 (median duration 36 mo)

indistinguishable, the malignant potential of pancreatic endocrine tumors is determined by the presence of metastases. Approximately 50% of patients with gastrinomas have metastasized to lymph nodes or liver at time of presentation.

Multiple modalities are used for the localization of pancreatic endocrine tumors. Abdominal CT scan locates primary tumors in approximately 50% of ZES cases, although this modality is dependent on tumor size and location. CT scan is more sensitive for pancreatic gastrinomas than it is for other typically smaller extrahepatic tumors. Visceral angiography can also be used to selectively focus on the arterial supply of the pancreas and peripancreatic area, with a variable success rate of 45% to 85%. Reports are limited regarding whether MRI is more sensitive than visceral angiography or CT scan for detecting metastases.

Somatostatin receptor scintigraphy is also a sensitive modality to localize primary gastrinomas (60%) and their metastases (90%). This technique is also useful for other pancreatic endocrine tumors except for insulinomas, which lack sufficient numbers of the type II somatostatin receptors [17,18]. In a small fraction of patients, the initial localization studies of CT scan, visceral angiography, and SRS will not identify the primary tumor. Portal venous hormone sampling and selective arterial secretin stimulation test may help localize the region of the functional tumor.

Other imaging modalities under ongoing evaluation are endoscopic and intraoperative ultrasonography (IOUS). A localization rate of 82% of primary gastrinomas using endoscopic ultrasonography has been reported in one institution; this modality has also been used for insulinoma [24–26]. Most authorities agree that IOUS is an important adjunct to the operative exploration for both gastrinoma and insulinoma [24,25]. A prospective study of the use of IOUS revealed a change in operative procedure in 10% of cases. Both of these techniques are sensitive for the detection of primary pancreatic neuroendocrine tumors but are highly user dependent. Intraoperative endoscopic duodenal transillumination may help in identification of small, duodenal gastrinomas, but duodenotomy and palpation of the lumen is standard now for most surgeons for gastrinoma [24].

TREATMENT OF ZOLLINGER-ELLISON SYNDROME
Medical Management
Treatment of ZES requires medical management of gastric acid hypersecretion and localization of primary tumor and metastatic disease. The peptic ulcer disease associated with ZES is successfully treated long-term with antisecretory medications: histamine H2 antagonists (cimetidine, famotidine), omeprazole, lansoprazole, or proton-pump inhibitors. These drugs should be adjusted to obtain a gastric pH > 5 during the hour prior to the next dose. These medications have been found to be efficacious and safe with long-term usage and have minimal side effects.

Surgical Management
With the success of antisecretory medications, the factor most responsible for the prognosis of gastrinomas is their malignant potential. Once gastric acid hypersecretion is controlled, the goal of surgical management is resection of gastrinoma in patients with ZES. The survival rate for ZES is more than 85% at 10 years. In patients who had undergone complete resection at the time of surgery, the rates improve to 94% at 10 years, respectively [29]. There is controversy as to the role of surgical management of gastrinomas in patients with MEN type I.

TREATMENT OF METASTATIC GASTRINOMA
Chemotherapy, hepatic artery embolization, cytoreductive surgery, hormonal therapy with somatostatin analog octreotide, immunotherapy with IFN, radiofrequency ablation of hepatic metastases, hepatic transplantation, or combinations of these have been studied in small numbers. These modalities have been examined for patients with pancreatic and neuroendocrine tumors, including carcinoids, with varying success. Although there has been a low response rate, the combination of streptozotocin and doxorubicin is commonly recommended as treatment for metastatic pancreatic endocrine tumors, including gastrinomas [19]. There have been small studies that show that hormonal treatment with octreotide and immunotherapy with IFN α can seem to stabilize progressive disease. Additional studies are needed to evaluate the efficacy of these therapies for gastrinomas and other malignant pancreatic endocrine tumors [19].

INSULINOMAS
The most common pancreatic endocrine tumor is insulinoma whose clinical syndrome was characterized by Whipple in 1935. Whipple's triad includes 1) symptoms of hypoglycemia during fasting, 2) a documented blood sugar below 50 mg/dL, and 3) relief of symptoms once glucose is administered. Insulinomas occur predominantly in women in their fourth decade with an overall incidence of 0.8 per million population. The symptoms of patients with insulinomas are classified into two categories: neuroglycopenic and adrenergic. These symptoms include confusion, seizure, personality change, coma or palpitations, trembling, diaphoresis and tachycardia. The diagnosis of an insulinoma is confirmed by a monitored 72-hour fast that documents symptoms associated with a blood sugar less than 50 mg/dL and a plasma insulin-to-glucose ratio above 0.4. To exclude other causes of hyperinsulinism (eg, reactive hypoglycemia and surreptitious administration of insulin or oral hypoglycemic agents) elevated plasma levels of C-peptide and proinsulin are documented [26].

Once the biochemical diagnosis of an insulinoma is confirmed, radiologic studies can be performed for preoperative tumor localization. Insulinomas are almost exclusively found in the pancreas; similar localization studies as outlined for gastrinomas can be undertaken. However, given the small nature of these pancreatic tumors, the rare incidence of malignancy, and the high likelihood of the presence of the tumor in the pancreas, IOUS is the most sensitive and most useful technique for localization of the primary tumor.

Unlike gastrinomas, only 10% of insulinomas are malignant. Management of these tumors focuses on surgical resection of primary lesion for control of symptoms. Medical therapy prior to surgery can include dietary control and the administration of octreotide and diazoxide, both of which have been shown to decrease hyperinsulinemia; however neither method provides adequate control of hypoglycemia for most patients. Tumor debulking can be performed for accessible metastases as well as combined chemotherapy and immunotherapy, as discussed previously for all pancreatic neuroendocrine tumors.

UNCOMMON PANCREATIC ENDOCRINE TUMORS
These rare tumors of the pancreatic endocrine cells are most frequently malignant; metastases are present in more than half of the patients at the time of diagnosis. The surgical management and treatment for metastatic disease is common to all pancreatic endocrine tumors as discussed previously.

VIPOMAS

The VIPoma syndrome (Verner–Morrison syndrome) is characterized by profuse watery diarrhea that leads to hypokalemia and dehydration. This syndrome is also referred to as the acronym WDHA (watery diarrhea, hypokalemia, and achlorhydria). Vipomas are diagnosed by elevated fasting levels of plasma VIP (vasoactive intestinal polypeptide) associated with severe secretory diarrhea. Management initially includes correction of electrolyte imbalances, acidosis, and dehydration. Octreotide has been found to decrease volume of diarrhea in a majority of patients. Surgical excision of these tumors, predominantly located in the pancreas, is the mainstay of palliative and potentially curative treatment.

GLUCAGONOMA

The syndrome associated with glucagonomas includes a dermatitis known as necrolytic migratory erythema, diarrhea, diabetes, anemia, and stomatitis. This rare tumor usually occurs as a large tumor that can be anywhere in the pancreas. The diagnosis is established by the documentation of elevated levels of plasma glucagon. Octreotide treatment eliminates the rash associated with glucagonomas, although it is not effective in treatment for the diabetes. Surgical excision is recommended, although the majority are metastatic on presentation.

SOMATOSTATINOMA

This is the most uncommon pancreatic endocrine tumor. Symptoms are attributed to the various hormonal functions of somatostatin and include diabetes, gallbladder disease, diarrhea, steatorrhea, and hypochlorhydria. Somatostatinomas are biochemically diagnosed by elevated plasma levels of somatostatin and are associated with von Recklinghausen's disease if located in the duodenum. Surgery, if technically feasible, is warranted.

REFERENCES

1. Ross NS, Aron DC: Hormonal evaluation of the patient with an incidentally discovered adrenal mass. *N Engl J Med* 1990, 323:1401–1405.

2. Doppman JL, Nieman LK, Travis WD, *et al.*: CT or MR imaging of massive macronodular adrenocortical disease: a rare cause of autonomous primary adrenal hypercortisolism. *J Comput Assist Tomogr* 1991, 15:773–779.

3. Yu KC, Alexander HR, Ziessman HA, *et al.*: Role of preoperative iodocholesterol scintiscanning in patients undergoing adrenalectomy for Cushing's syndrome. *Surgery* 1995, 118:981–987.

4. Bellantone R, Ferrante A, Boscherini M, *et al.*: Role of reoperation in recurrence of adrenal cortical carcinoma: results from 188 cases collected in the Italian national registry for adrenal cortical carcinoma. *Surgery* 1997, 122:1212–1218.

5. Doherty GM, Nieman LK, Cutler GB Jr, *et al.*: Time to recovery of the hypothalamic-pituitary-adrenal axis after curative resection of adrenal tumors in patients with Cushing's syndrome. *Surgery* 1990, 108:1085–1090.

6. Jensen JC, Pass HI, Sindelar WF, Norton JA: Aggressive resection of recurrent or metastatic disease in select patients with adrenocortical carcinoma. *Arch Surg* 1991, 126:457–461.

7. Decker RA, Elson P, Hogan TF, *et al.*: Eastern cooperative oncology group study 1989: mitotane and adriamycin in patients with advanced adrenocortical carcinoma. *Surgery* 1991, 110:1006–1013.

8. Schlumberger M, Brugieres L, Gicquel C, *et al.*: 5-Fluorouracil, doxorubicin, and cisplatin as treatment for adrenal cortical carcinoma. *Cancer* 1991, 67:2997–3000.

9. Bukowski RM, Wolfe M, Levine HS, *et al.*: Phase II trial of mitotane and cisplatin in patients with adrenal carcinoma: a Southwest Oncology Group study. *J Clin Oncol* 1993, 11:161–165.

10. Berruti A, Terzolo M, Paccotti P: Favorable response of metastatic ACC to etoposide, adriamycin and cisplatin. *Tumor* 1992, 78:345–348.

11. Hay ID, Bergstralh EL, Goellner JR, *et al.*: Predicting outcome in papillary thyroid carcinoma: development of a reliable prognostic scoring system in a cohort of 1779 patients surgically treated at one institution during 1940 through 1989. *Surgery* 1993, 114:1050–1057.

12. Chi DD, Toshima K, Donis-Keller H, Wells SA Jr: Predictive testing for multiple endocrine neoplasia type 2A based on the detection of mutations in the *ret* proto-oncogene. *Surgery* 1994, 116:124–132.

13. Wells SA Jr, Chi DD, Toshima K, *et al.*: Predictive DNA testing and prophylactive thyroidectomy in patients at risk for multiple endocrine neoplasia type 2A. *Ann Surg* 1994, 220:237–247.

14. Mazzaferri EL, Young RL: Papillary thyroid carcinoma: a 10-year follow-up report of the impact of therapy in 576 patients. *Am J Med* 1981, 70:511–518.

15. Moley JF, Wells SA Jr, Dilley WG, Tisell LE: Reoperation for recurrent or persistent medullary thyroid cancer. *Surgery* 1993, 114:1090–1096.

16. Moley JF, Dilley WG, DeBenedetti MK: Improved results of cervical reoperation for medullary thyroid carcinoma. *Ann Surg* 1997, 225:734–740.

17. Meko JB, Doherty GM, Siegel BA, Norton JA: Evaluation of somatostatin-receptor scintigraphy for detecting neuroendocrine tumors. *Surgery* 1996, 120:975–984.

18. Wiedenmann B, Jensen RT, Mignon M, *et al.*: Preoperative diagnosis and surgical management of neuroendocrine gastroenteropancreatic tumors: general recommendations by a consensus workshop. *World J Surg* 1998, 309–318 [review]

19. Arnold R, Frank M, Kajdan U: Management of gastroenteropancreatic endocrine tumors: the place of somatostatin analogues. *Digestion* 1994, 55:107–113.

20. Oberg K, Norheim I, Lundqvist G, Wide L: Cytotoxic treatment in patients with malignant carcinoid tumors: response to streptozocin alone or in combination with 5-FU. *Acta Oncol* 1987, 26:429–432.

21. Oberg K, Norheim I, Lind E, *et al.*: Treatment of malignant carcinoid tumors with human leukocyte interferon: long term results. *Cancer Treat Rev* 1986, 70:1297–1304.

22. Tiensuu-Janson EM, Ahlstrom H, Andersson T, Oberg KE: Octreotide and interferon alfa: a new combination for the treamtent of malignant carcinoid tumours. *Eur J Cancer* 1992, 28A:1647–1650.

23. Stabile BE, Morrow DJ, Passaro E: The gastrinoma triangle: operative implications. *Am J Surg* 1984, 147:25–31.

24. Doherty GM, Norton JA: Preoperative and intraoperative localization of gastrinomas. *Probl Gen Surg* 1990, 7:521–532.

25. Doherty GM, Doppman JL, Shawker TH, *et al.*: Results of a prospective strategy to diagnose, localize and resect insulinomas. *Surgery* 1991, 110:989–997.

26. Thompson NW, Czako PF, Fritts LL: Role of endoscopic ultrasonography in the localization of insulinomas and gastrinomas. *Surgery* 1994, 116:1131–1138.

27. Fleming ID, Cooper JS, Henson DE, *et al.* (eds): AJCC Cancer Staging Manual. Philadelphia: Lippincott–Raven; 1997.

28. Yu F, Venzon DJ, Serrano J, *et al.*: Prospective study of the clinical course, prognostic factors, causes of death and survival in patients with long-standing Zollinger-Ellison syndrome. *J Clin Oncol* 1999, 17:615–630.

29. Norton JA, Fraker DL, Alexander HR, *et al.*: Surgery to cure the Zollinger-Ellison syndrome. *N Engl J Med* 1999, 341:635–644.

MITOTANE AND CISPLATIN

Mitotane (o,p-DDD) is an isomer of the pesticide DDT that inhibits corticosteroid biosynthesis and, at high doses, causes selective adrenocortical atrophy and infarction. It is not effective in bulky retroperitoneal adrenal cortical cancer. Cisplatin is an alkylating agent that acts to cross-link DNA. In vitro, mitotane reverses the multidrug resistance mediated by MDR-1 expression that occurs in adrenal cortical cancer cells.

DOSAGE AND SCHEDULING

1. Prehydrate with saline 2 L IV and mannitol 12.5 g IV
2. Cisplatin 100 mg/m^2 IV, mannitol 25 g IV, and saline 1 L IV over 2 h, d 1
3. o,p-DDD 1 g PO four times daily, d 1 and daily while on regimen
4. Cortisone acetate and fludrocortisone acetate daily as needed

RECENT EXPERIENCE AND RESPONSE RATES

In a phase II clinical trial, these two agents in combination produced responses in 11 of 37 (30%) patients, with a median duration of response of 8 months and median time to response of 76 d [3]. Median survival from treatment was 11.8 mo. Although patients with complete surgical resection of tumor were not eligible for the study, a significant survival advantage was found for patients who had previously undergone surgical removal of primary tumor or bulky disease and for patients with a performance status of 0 or 1 [3]. Patients older than 65 y, those with extensive prior radiation, and those with poor tolerance to previous chemotherapy were considered high-risk and were given a lower dose of cisplatin.

CANDIDATES FOR TREATMENT

Patients with inoperable adrenal cortical cancer, regardless of tumor functionality

ALTERNATIVE THERAPIES

Dose escalation of mitotane to 8–16 g/d; possibly cisplatin and etoposide combination therapy, but currently insufficient data for recommendation [5–7]

SPECIAL PRECAUTIONS

Patients with significantly impaired renal function, myelosuppression, or hearing loss are ineligible

TOXICITIES

Drug combination: severe nausea and vomiting (22% of patients), mild mucositis, mild myalgias, weakness
Mitotane: dose-dependent anorexia, nausea, vomiting, diarrhea, confusion, somnolence, depression, dizziness, skin rash, cholestasis, male gynecomastia, visual disturbances
Cisplatin: nausea and vomiting, nephrotoxicity, irreversible paresthesias and neuropathies, cumulative ototoxicity, myelosuppression, anaphylaxis

DRUG INTERACTIONS

Anticonvulsants, aminoglycoside antibiotics, warfarin, exogenously administered steroids

NURSING INTERVENTIONS

Monitor renal function and obtain CBC, BUN, and creatine frequently throughout treatment; be prepared for anaphylactic reactions; provide proper antiemetics; hydrate well to prevent renal toxicity

PATIENT INFORMATION

Patient should be informed that mitotane may cause adrenal insufficiency

LOW-DOSE DOXORUBICIN AND RADIATION THERAPY

Most anaplastic thyroid cancers are metastatic at presentation and, uncontrolled, produce death from suffocation in 4–6 mo. Conventional radiotherapy often fails to induce significant regression of tumor around the airway. Doxorubicin is the single most active agent against thyroid carcinoma and, in addition, acts as a radiosensitizer of radioresistant hypoxic tumor cells, particularly at low doses. A hyperfractionated radiation therapy schedule may deliver more efficacious therapy to rapidly dividing tissues, while minimizing tissue morbidity.

DOSAGE AND SCHEDULING

Doxorubicin 10 mg/m^2 IV administered 1 × wk 1.5 h prior to radiation therapy and hyperfractionated radiation dose of 160 cGy per treatment, 2 × d for 3 d/wk; total tumor dose 5760 cGy delivered over 40 d

DOSAGE MODIFICATIONS: *70% of patients require a 1-wk respite during therapy due to toxicity*

LAB MONITORING: *clinical examination and subjective dyspnea, WBC*

RECENT EXPERIENCE AND RESPONSE RATES

Kim and Leeper reported that this regimen, which is under further investigation at the National Cancer Institute, resulted in complete tumor regression in eight of nine patients with anaplastic giant and spindle cell carcinoma of the thyroid gland [15]. Patients went on to die of distant metastatic disease (median survival from treatment 10 mo) without increased survival by comparison to historical controls. Findings were confirmed in a follow-up study published in 1987 (84% response rate) [12]. Median survival was 1 y from therapy.

CANDIDATES FOR TREATMENT

Patients with confirmed anaplastic thyroid cancer, patients with locally advanced well-differentiated thyroid cancer unresponsive to ^{131}I therapy

ALTERNATIVE THERAPIES

Systemic chemotherapy (with adriamycin-based regimens) or taxol-based therapy

SPECIAL PRECAUTIONS

Airway must be secured first

TOXICITIES

Therapy combination: increased toxicity to the myocardium, mucosae, skin, and liver with this combination;
Doxorubicin: minimal at this dose;
Radiation: mild-to-moderate pharyngoesophagitis and tracheitis; skin erythema, hyperpigmentation and late desquamation, laryngeal edema, cervical myelopathy

PATIENT INFORMATION

Patient should be informed that therapy may cause local pain and swelling

OCTREOTIDE AND INTERFERON α-2B

Octreotide, a long-acting analogue of the natural hormone somatostatin, suppresses the secretion of serotonin and gut peptides. It has been used effectively by many clinicians for the symptoms of carcinoid syndrome, but produces tumor regression at a low rate. Interferon α-2b (IFN α-2b) is believed to exert direct antiproliferative action against tumor cells as well as to modulate the host immune response to tumor. This protocol was designed to augment the response to octreotide by the addition of IFN α-2b, which itself has a 30%–60% response rate in malignant carcinoid tumors.

DOSAGE AND SCHEDULING

IFN α-2b 3×10^6 U SQ $3 \times$ wk and octreotide 100 μg SQ twice daily

DOSAGE MODIFICATIONS: *Weeks 8–16 — dose escalation of IFN α-2b to 5×10^6 U SQ $3 \times$ wk, as allowed by side effects and leukocyte count ($> 4 \times 10^9$/l); after week 16 — further escalation of IFN α-2b to 10×10^6 U SQ $3 \times$ wk, as allowed by side effects and leukocyte count*

LAB MONITORING: *Urine 5-HIAA, plasma serotonin, and other tumor markers q 4 wk; CBC, platelet count, glucose, renal function, response q 4 wk; thyroid function, gallbladder ultrasound q 8 wk*

RECENT EXPERIENCE AND RESPONSE RATES

In a recent phase II clinical trial, these two agents were administered together to 24 patients who, during initial treatment with octreotide (50–150 μg twice daily), had demonstrated progressive disease [23]. Administration of IFN α-2b together with octreotide produced an objective biochemical 77% response rate with median duration of response of 12 mo. Median survival from treatment was 58 mo. Symptoms of carcinoid syndrome were ameliorated in 10 of 18 patients (56%). No patient in this trial had significant objective tumor regression. No information is available concerning the efficacy of this regimen in patients not previously nonresponding to octreotide alone.

CANDIDATES FOR TREATMENT

Patients with inoperable metastatic carcinoid neoplasms, regardless of tumor functionality

SPECIAL PRECAUTIONS

Patients with significant preexisting cardiac disease or renal failure

ALTERNATIVE THERAPIES

Regimens with higher doses of octreotide (50–150 μg SQ TID) and IFN α-2b (10 mIUμ SQ daily); hepatic artery occlusion combined with chemotherapy or IFN α-2b (recently reported with comparable success rate)

TOXICITIES

Octreotide: changes in blood glucose mild and reversible, hypothyroidism, fat malabsorption, migratory thrombophlebitis; gallstones or sludge (15%–20% of patients) and acute cholecystitis (up to one third of patients with gallstones), prophylactic cholecystectomy may be appropriate;

IFN α-2b: flu-like syndrome and nausea and vomiting with first administration; may exacerbate pre-existing cardiac disease; anorexia, mild weight loss, bone marrow suppression, disturbed thyroid function including hypothyroidism and autoimmune thyroiditis, depression

DRUG INTERACTIONS

Octreotide: H_2-antagonists, antidiarrheal agents, insulin, sulfonureas, β-blockers, antihypertensives, thyroid replacement hormone; **Interferon α:** unknown

NURSING INTERVENTIONS

Monitor for development of gallstones and biliary colic; instruct patient in self-injection

PATIENT INFORMATION

Patients may self-administer injection after learning technique

ACUTE MYELOID LEUKEMIA

Acute myeloid leukemia (AML) is the most common type of acute leukemia that occurs in adults, accounting for over 80% of the leukemias diagnosed in patients over age 20. AML can affect all ages but is rare in childhood. The incidence increases with age, with a median age at the time of diagnosis of approximately 55 years. AML is rare compared with other malignancies, accounting for approximately three cases per 100,000. Whereas certain environmental exposures (chemicals such as petroleum solvents or radiation exposure) and occupations (*eg*, rubber workers) have been associated with an increased risk of AML, the etiology in the vast majority of cases remains unclear. The molecular events leading to AML are now only beginning to be elucidated.

Several inherited genetic disorders and immunodeficiency states are associated with an increased risk of AML. These include disorders with defects in DNA stability, leading to random chromosomal breakage, such as Bloom's syndrome and Fanconi's anemia. Li-Fraumeni kindreds have mutated p53 on chromosome 17, which may alter tumor suppressor gene functions. Down syndrome (trisomy 21) is associated with an 17-fold increase in the risk of AML [1]. Congenital immunodeficiency states, such as ataxia-telangiectasia and X-linked agammaglobulinemia, are also associated with increased rates of AML (Table 17-1).

AML that has arisen out of a prior myelodysplastic syndrome or other bone marrow failure syndrome is termed *secondary AML*. A prior exposure to particular chemotherapy agents or radiation therapy for other diseases is being increasingly recognized as a risk factor for secondary AML [2]. Exposure to alkylating agents in regimens such as MOPP (mechlorethamine, vincristine, procarbazine, and prednisone) chemotherapy for Hodgkin's disease is associated with a cumulative risk of AML at 10 years that can be as high as 10%. Exposure to epipodophyllotoxins is associated with the development of leukemia, often occurring within a few years of treatment and commonly having the specific chromosomal abnormality 11q23 [3,4]. Radiation therapy is also a risk factor for AML. The presence of prior myelodysplastic syndrome or other bone marrow failure syndrome is also associated with AML. An increasing incidence of myelodysplastic syndrome and associated secondary AML is being recognized following autologous bone marrow transplantation [5]. There is a 10% to 20% actuarial incidence of secondary AML/myelodysplasia after autologous bone marrow transplant when total body irradiation is part of the conditioning regimen for non-Hodgkin's lymphoma.

CLASSIFICATION AND PROGNOSIS

The diagnosis of AML is based on both the histologic and immunophenotypic evaluation of peripheral blood and bone marrow samples. Since 1976, the French-American-British (FAB) classification has been used to classify acute leukemia. Several modifications have been made since its creation, but the classification remains based on histologic appearance of the blasts and the use of histochemical stains. Eight subtypes of AML, designated M0 through M7, have been described. Currently, with the exception of the M3 (progranulocytic leukemia) subtype, initial therapy for remaining subtypes is similar. Various subtypes, however, may be associated with different prognoses.

Several prognostic factors have been identified in patients with AML (Table 17-2). These factors may be used to identify patients who have a high rate of cure with conventional chemotherapy alone. Conversely, patients with poor prognostic features may be considered for high-dose chemotherapy approaches (*eg*, bone marrow transplantation) early in the course of their disease, or they may be candidates for novel approaches to treat AML.

Older age has been demonstrated to be associated with inferior outcomes in numerous studies. Patients over 60 years of age have a lower rate of complete remission following induction chemotherapy compared with patients younger than 60 years of age. The higher death rate in this population is related to an increase in treatment-related toxicity (*eg*, death from infection) but also to an increased risk of death related to leukemia. The increased incidence of secondary AML, which is often more refractory to chemotherapy, may provide a partial explanation for the inferior outcome in this population. The benefits of high-dose postremission therapy in this population are also questionable.

Other adverse features of AML at the time of presentation include an elevated white blood cell count (WBC) of greater than 100,000. The reason for the impact of the high WBC on outcome is unclear but may suggest an increased proliferative capacity of the abnormal clone. Patients with high WBC are also at increased risk of leukostasis, which is an oncologic emergency created by the obstruction of the microvasculature by leukemic blasts. Patients with leukostasis may present with altered mental status or respiratory distress and have an increased early mortality.

Immunophenotypic analysis of leukemia cell surface antigens helps in the determination of myeloid or lymphoid lineage in cases in which histologic examination is not definitive. The prognostic significance of particular cell surface antigens has not yet been fully defined. Approximately 20% of myeloid leukemias may demonstrate

Table 17-1. Etiologic and Risk Factors in AML and ALL

AML	ALL
Chromosomal fragility syndromes	Chromosome fragility
Bloom's syndrome	
Fanconi's anemia	
Mutations of suppressor oncogenes (p53)	Down syndrome
Li-Fraumeni syndrome	
Age	Radiation exposure
Myelodysplasia	
Radiation or chemotherapy	

ALL—acute lymphoblastic leukemia; AML—acute myeloid leukemia.

Table 17-2. Prognostic Factors in Acute Myeloid Leukemia

Factor	Good Prognosis	Poor Prognosis
White blood count	< 100,000	> 100,000
Age	< 60	> 60
Cytogenetic findings	Translocations 8;21 and 15;17 and inversion 16	Deletions of 5 and 7; trisomy 8; multiple cytogenetic abnormalities

mixed-lineage antigens (both myeloid and lymphoid), and these leukemias are associated with a worse prognosis. AML with blasts expressing antigens that are associated with early hematopoietic development (eg, CD34) also have a poor outcome and may indicate the presence of a primitive malignant clone [6,7]. In one study, patients whose cells were CD14- or CD13-positive had a worse prognosis than those whose cells did not express these markers. The expression of combinations of cell-surface markers may be a more useful approach to defining a biologically meaningful phenotype. Patients whose cells expressed a "pan-myeloid" phenotype (myeloperoxidase, CD13, CD33, CDw65, and CD117) had superior DFS and OS compared to those with fewer myeloid markers [8]. The presence of certain cell surface markers in AML may serve as a target for emerging strategies using monoclonal antibodies as a part of treatment.

Specific cytogenetic abnormalities have been associated with clinical outcome. Translocations of 8;21, 15;17, and inversion 16 are associated with a good prognosis and an improved disease-free survival compared with patients with either normal chromosomes or other cytogenetic abnormalities [9]. Deletions of chromosomes 5 or 7 are associated with inferior outcomes, and these patients may be considered for early intensive therapy, such as bone marrow transplantation.

THERAPY

Chemotherapy

Treatment of AML has been divided into three stages: induction, postremission therapy, and therapy at the time of relapse [10]. The goal of induction therapy is to achieve a complete remission (CR) and then to proceed to the administration of postremission therapy in an attempt to achieve the maximal disease-free survival and cure. Induction for M3 AML should be considered distinct and is discussed below. Induction therapy for all types of AML includes the combination of cytosine arabinoside (cytarabine or Ara-C) with an anthracycline. Typically, patients receive cytarabine as a continuous infusion of 100 to 200 mg/m²/d for 7 days. This infusion is combined with an anthracycline (eg, daunorubicin, idarubicin [11,12]), or mitoxantrone for 3 days (Table 17-3). Two trials have compared daunorubicin/Ara-C and idarubicin/Ara-C in AML induction [11,12]. Idarubicin was associated with supe-

rior remission rates in patients under 60 years of age compared with daunorubicin. Of note, the daunorubicin arm of one study demonstrated a worse CR rate than that noted in larger comparative trials; therefore, the superiority of idarubicin has not been clearly demonstrated. Daunorubicin and idarubicin are both associated with cardiotoxicity at doses greater than 450 mg/m², whereas mitoxantrone is felt to be less cardiotoxic. Combination chemotherapy is associated with an induction CR rate of approximately 60% to 70% in patients younger than 60 years of age and 40% in patients older than 60 years of age.

Alternative induction regimens include high-dose cytarabine [13], high-dose cyclophosphamide and etoposide [14], or standard-dose cytarabine and etoposide [15]. In a single-institution trial, the addition of high-dose cytarabine following standard "7+3" improved the remission rate in patients with AML to 86% in patients under age 63 years of age [16]. This regimen has not been directly compared with the standard "7+3" regimen in a randomized study.

There is debate about whether older patients (> 70 y of age) and patients with secondary AML benefit from intensive induction approaches because in this population the CR rates remain low, and the treatment-related toxicity is significant [17]. Low-dose Ara-C (10–20 mg/m²/d) has been advocated by some in the treatment of older patients in an attempt to avoid the acute side effects associated with standard induction [18]. Although responses can be seen with low-dose Ara-C, many weeks of therapy may be required, and complications related to prolonged pancytopenia can be noted just as when following standard induction chemotherapy. In a recent large Southwestern Oncology Group trial, elderly patients (median age, 68 years) with favorable or normal cytogenetics had CR rates comparable with younger patients, suggesting that these patients may benefit from more aggressive induction regimens [19].

It is estimated that 1×10^9 leukemia cells may remain when patients are in complete remission. Postremission therapy is designed to further reduce and eliminate these cells. Postremission therapy may include reiterations of standard-dose cytarabine and anthracycline for two more courses or the use of other doses of cytarabine. In a prospective trial, Cancer and Leukemia Group B (CALGB) compared three different doses of cytarabine as postremission therapy [20]. Patients younger than 60 years of age received either 100 mg/m² for 5 days, 400 mg/m² for 5 days, or 3 g/m² every 12 hours for a total of six doses, each given four times over 4 to 6 months. This is followed by four more cycles of subcutaneous cytarabine at 100 mg/m² twice daily for 10 doses and daunorubicin 45 mg/m². Patients under 60 years of age receiving the high-dose cytarabine arm had a superior disease-free survival compared with the other groups, whereas there was no difference between arms in patients over 60 years of age.

Despite induction CR rates of greater than 60%, the long-term disease-free survival in patients with AML remains approximately 30% to 40%. Choice of chemotherapy at the time of relapse may be based on the duration of the first remission interval. Patients with a remission interval of greater than 1 year may respond to a similar regimen at the time of relapse, whereas patients with a shorter duration of remission should be considered for alternative regimens. Options for treatment of relapse include high-dose cytarabine, mitoxantrone and etoposide [21], carboplatin [20], or high-dose cyclophosphamide and etoposide [14] (Table 17-4). A second remission rate of approximately 40% to 50% is noted in these patients; however, these remissions are rarely durable, and long-term disease-free survival is unusual. A monoclonal antibody against CD33 conjugated to calicheamicin (Mylotarg) was recently approved for use in relapsed AML patients

---

Table 17-3. Initial Therapy for AML

1. Cytarabine via continuous infusion (100–200 mg/m² × 7 d)
   +
   Daunorubicin (45 mg/m² × 3 d)
   or
   idarubicin (12 mg/m²)
   or
   mitoxantrone (12 mg/m²)
2. High-dose cytarabine and anthracycline
3. Cytarabine via continuous infusion
   +
   Daunorubicin
   +
   High-dose cytarabine
4. Cyclophosphamide and etoposide

---

over 60 years of age [22]. This potent immunotoxin, given at 9 mg/m² body surface area 2 × 14 days apart, was capable of inducing complete remissions in patients with untreated first relapse. Although this immunotoxin does not produce some of the side effects associated with chemotherapy, it does produce significant myelosuppression, and there is a risk of hepatotoxicity.

Promyelocytic leukemia (APML) represents a distinct subgroup of AML. This subtype is characterized by promyelocytic blasts containing the 15;17 chromosomal translocation. This translocation leads to the generation of the fusion transcript comprised of the retinoic acid receptor (α-RAR) and a sequence called PML. Prior to the recognition of this molecular abnormality, the clinical observation had been made that retinoic acid induced differentiation of blasts in patients with APML, and investigators in France and China used retinoic acid to treat patients with APML [23]. All-*trans*-retinoic acid (ATRA) was found to be superior to *cis*-retinoic acid both in vitro and in vivo in APML and was capable of inducing complete remissions in patients with APML [24]. ATRA alone does not produce long-term CRs and should be used in combination with chemotherapy (Table 17-5). The combination of ATRA and chemotherapy at the time of induction leads to CR rates in greater than 85% of patients [25–27]. The exact timing of administration of ATRA and chemotherapy has yet to be fully determined [28]. Use of ATRA reduces the complications associated with induction chemotherapy in patients with APML, such as disseminated intravascular coagulation. Approximately 20% of patients treated with ATRA may develop the "retinoic acid syndrome" characterized by fever, pulmonary infiltrates, and hypoxemia with and without leukocytosis [29]. Therefore, it is important to distinguish APML from other subtypes of AML because ATRA should be used as part of the treatment regimen. In addition, studies suggest that high-dose cytarabine as consolidation therapy may not be associated with the same benefit in patients with APML as compared with other types of AML. For this reason, many groups have adopted a strategy of using subsequent courses of daunorubicin-based chemotherapy during the postremission period.

In an attempt to ameliorate the toxicity of induction chemotherapy related to prolonged pancytopenia, the use of human hematopoietic growth factors has been investigated. Granulocyte–macrophage colony-stimulating factor (GM-CSF) following induction chemotherapy for AML accelerates recovery of granulocytes and is not associated with an increased incidence of recurrent leukemia. Two large cooperative group trials have examined the effect of GM-CSF after induction chemotherapy [30,31]. An ECOG study demonstrated a higher remission rate and more rapid recovery of neutrophils associated with GM-CSF use, whereas a CALGB study did not demonstrate a benefit of GM-CSF compared with placebo. Both trials initiated GM-CSF on day 8; however, the ECOG trial employed the use of GM-CSF only if aplasia on day 8 was achieved. This may account for the benefit seen in the ECOG trial. A randomized trial that compared granulocyte colony-stimulating factor with placebo in patients with AML demonstrated a shortened duration of neutropenia and a need for antifungal therapy during induction and remission therapy [32]. Other recent studies, however, have demonstrated no benefit from the addition of growth factors during induction [33].

Bone Marrow Transplantation

Bone marrow transplantation (BMT) offers the best option for long-term disease-free survival in patients with AML in second and third remission. Both allogeneic and autologous transplantation lead to overall disease-free survival in 30% to 50% of patients. Conditioning regimens used for transplantation include high-dose cyclophosphamide and total-body irradiation [34], cyclophosphamide and busulfan [35,36], as well as regimens containing high-dose cytarabine or etoposide [37]. To date, the superiority of one regimen over another has not been demonstrated. Survival is less than 20% after allogeneic bone marrow transplant in patients with refractory disease.

Bone marrow transplantation at the time of first remission is associated with a higher disease-free survival than chemotherapy alone. Several randomized trials have been performed in AML in first CR comparing allogeneic BMT, autologous BMT, and chemotherapy at "standard" doses [38,39]. The variable design of these trials makes direct comparisons difficult. The major conclusion from these studies is that allogeneic BMT gives superior outcomes versus autologous BMT. Autologous BMT was superior to chemotherapy in all but one trial [39]. Current practice is to use peripheral blood progenitor cell transplantation in autologous transplants. No randomized trials comparing this approach with chemotherapy have been reported. The authors believe that patients without an HLA-matched donor or who are over 60 years of age and in CR1 should be offered autologous PBPC transplantation as consolidation therapy.

Allogeneic Bone Marrow Transplant

The best results of allogeneic BMT are reported in patients receiving transplants from HLA-identical siblings. Single-institution series suggest disease-free survival rates in patients with AML in first remission to be as high as 60% to 70%. Allogeneic BMT may be performed immediately after achieving a first CR without additional cytosine arabinoside–based consolidation therapy [40]. Transplantation in second and third remissions is associated with a much lower disease-free survival rate. Graft-versus-host disease (GVHD) remains the principle toxicity associated with BMT and

Table 17-4. Salvage Therapy for Leukemia

Acute Myeloid Leukemia	Acute Lymphocytic Leukemia
Etoposide and mitoxantrone	High-dose cytarabine and anthracycline
High-dose cytarabine and anthracycline	Teniposide and cytarabine
High-dose cyclophosphamide and etoposide	High-dose methotrexate
Mylotars	

Table 17-5. Treatment of Promyelocytic Leukemia

Induction
ATRA (45 mg/m²/d) until CR
followed by
Daunorubicin (60 mg/m² × 3 d)
+
Ara-C via continuous infusion (200 mg/m² ×7 d)

Consolidation
Ara-C
+
Daunorubicin

ARTA—all-trans-retinoic acid; CR—complete response.

reduces the overall effectiveness of this approach. The influence of the graft-versus-leukemia effect on disease-free survival does not appear to be as significant in AML as in chronic myelogenous leukemia (CML) [41]. Several groups have used T-cell depletion as a means to reduce the incidence of GVHD, an approach that does not appear to compromise disease-free survival [42,43]. Donor lymphocyte infusions may be used to treat patients who relapse after allogeneic BMT, but the complete response rate is only 20% [44].

For patients without a suitable sibling donor, the unrelated BMT registry may be used to identify a donor for up to 40% of patients [45]. The treatment-related mortality associated with an unrelated BMT remains significant, approaching 40% in registry series [46]. This approach may be considered for patients in second or subsequent remissions; however, its use in the first-remission setting remains controversial.

Autologous Bone Marrow Transplant

Autologous BMT is an option for patients without an HLA-matched sibling and for older patients. The treatment-related mortality associated with autologous transplantation is lower than allogeneic BMT, approaching 2% to 5%. Relapse after BMT remains the most significant complication of this approach. Both regimens containing chemotherapy only and those including total-body irradiation appear to be equally effective. Purging of the bone marrow to remove minimal residual disease can be performed by the use of either monoclonal antibodies, which are directed to antigens expressed on the surface of leukemia cells or by incubation of the marrow in cytotoxic drugs such as 4-hydroperoxycyclophosphamide [47,48]. To date, no clear benefit has been demonstrated by the purging of bone marrow by either technique. Long-term disease-free remission can be obtained in 30% to 50% of patients who receive autologous BMT in second or subsequent relapse.

ACUTE LYMPHOBLASTIC LEUKEMIA

ETIOLOGY AND RISK FACTORS

Acute lymphoblastic leukemia (ALL) is common in children but is rare in the adult population. Several factors, such as Down syndrome and radiation exposure, are associated with ALL, but the etiology is unknown in the majority of cases (see Table 17-1). Recent advances in the molecular genetics of ALL may allow for elucidation of the molecular events leading to ALL.

CLASSIFICATION AND PROGNOSIS

Acute lymphoblastic leukemia is a heterogeneous disease with distinct clinical features displayed by various subtypes. As with AML, the FAB classification is used to classify ALL. Three subtypes, L1 through L3, have been identified. Immunophenotyping identifies that the majority of cells are of B lineage and that most have characteristics consistent with a pre-B-cell phenotype. Approximately 25% of adult ALL are of T-cell lineage. Whereas earlier studies have suggested a worse prognosis associated with the T-cell phenotype, recent studies have not confirmed this finding [49–51].

Recurring cytogenetic abnormalities also have been demonstrated in ALL. The most common cytogenetic abnormality is the 9;22 translocation, which occurs in approximately 30% of adult ALL. Approximately one half of patients produce a fusion protein p190,

whereas the remaining patients demonstrate a p210 similar to patients with CML. The Philadelphia chromosome is a very poor prognostic finding, and these patients should be treated with allogeneic BMT if a donor is available [52–54]. Other translocations include translocation of 11q23 and translocation of chromosomes 1;9. Both of these abnormalities also appear to be associated with an inferior outcome. The recently identified 12;21 translocation, which is not detected on routine cytogenetic analysis, appears to associated with an improved prognosis in children with ALL [54–57]. The frequency of this translocation appears to be less in the adult ALL population compared with children. The prognostic importance of this translocation in adults has not been fully defined.

In addition to cytogenetic abnormalities, several clinical variables have also been associated with prognosis. These factors include age, sex, time to remission, and WBC at presentation [49] (Table 17-6). Extramedullary disease is common in these patients and treatment includes central nervous system (CNS) prophylaxis.

TREATMENT

Approximately one third to 40% of adults with ALL will be cured with modern chemotherapy. All induction regimens now include multiagent chemotherapy. The addition of anthracyclines to vincristine and prednisone alone or in combination with L-asparaginase has improved the induction CR rate in patients with adult ALL to over 70%. A CALGB study added cyclophosphamide to these four agents during induction, resulting in an 85% remission rate [45]. With intensive consolidation and CNS prophylaxis, the median survival in this study was 36 months. Prolonged maintenance therapy, which prevents relapse in children but has yet to be proven effective in adults, is standard in most ALL protocols and often includes methotrexate and 6-mercaptopurine in combination with "pulses" of vincristine and prednisone. A German multicenter study that used an induction phase containing eight drugs and an additional eight drugs during consolidation has been reported [50]. When combined with CNS prophylaxis, which includes both intrathecal methotrexate and cranial radiation, the remission rate was 74%. Treatment of the adult ALL L3 subtype using an intensive variation of this therapy over a short duration (six cycles) appears effective with a leukemia-free survival of 71% at 4 years [58].

Despite aggressive induction, the majority of adults with ALL relapse. A second remission may be obtained with chemotherapy in 10% to 70% of patients, depending on the regimen used. If relapse occurs after a prolonged remission, reinduction with similar agents used at the time of presentation may be used. The durability of second and subsequent remissions is poor, and these patients should be considered candidates for BMT.

Table 17-6. Prognostic Factors in ALL

Factor	Good Prognosis	Poor Prognosis
Age	< 35 y	> 35 y
Sex	Female	Male
Time to complete remission	< 4 wk	> 4 wk
Cytogenetic finding	T-cell phenotype Hyperdiploid cytogenetics	Philadelphia chromosome, t(9;22), t(4;11)
White blood count	< 30,000/µL	> 30,000/µL

BONE MARROW TRANSPLANTATION

Allogeneic Bone Marrow Transplantation

Allogeneic BMT for adults with ALL is associated with a 5-year disease-free survival of approximately 40% in patients undergoing BMT in first remission and 20% to 30% for patients undergoing BMT in second remission [59,60]. The role of allogeneic BMT in patients in first remission remains unclear. When results of allogeneic BMT in patients with ALL in first remission was compared with the results of chemotherapy alone, no clear benefit of early BMT was demonstrated [61]. The overall 5-year leukemia-free survival was 44% for patients who underwent BMT in first remission compared with 38% for patients receiving chemotherapy only. In this study, the treatment-related mortality in the patients undergoing BMT was high (39%); therefore, the benefits of transplantation may have been underestimated. In other series, allogeneic BMT in first remission in "high-risk" patients has been associated with a disease-free survival of over 60% [62]. Subgroups of patients with poor risk features may be considered for early consolidation with BMT.

Autologous Bone Marrow Transplantation

Autologous bone marrow transplantation provides an alternative source of stem cells for patients for whom no donor can be identified. Recent studies have shown that the residual leukemia cells infused at the time of marrow infusion can contribute to relapse [63]. A variety of approaches have been attempted to reduce the risk of marrow contamination by tumor cells, including immunologic purging using monoclonal antibodies, long-term culture strategies, and chemical purging in vitro. To date, no purging strategy has proved superior to the others, and some have been associated with prolonged time to engraftment [64].

Uncontrolled trials of autologous BMT in first and second remission have produced results superior to the disease-free survival often seen with chemotherapy alone. Prospective multicenter trials have not demonstrated a clear benefit in favor of autologous BMT in the treatment of adult patients in first remission. In one study, 96 patients were randomly assigned to autologous BMT, and 96 patients received chemotherapy alone. There was no significant difference in the incidence of treatment-related mortality, relapse, CR duration, or survival with a disease-free survival at 3 years of approximately 35% [65]. When autologous BMT is compared with allogeneic BMT, the treatment-related mortality associated with autologous BMT is much lower; however, the risk of relapse is significantly higher. Nonetheless, autologous BMT plays a significant role in the treatment of adult patients with ALL in second or subsequent remission in whom a donor is not available.

CHRONIC MYELOGENOUS LEUKEMIA

ETIOLOGY AND RISK FACTORS

Chronic myelogenous leukemia is a clonal myeloproliferative disorder of a pluripotent stem cell and is characterized by a specific chromosomal abnormality involving the translocation of chromosomes 9 and 22, creating the Philadelphia chromosome [66]. The median age of patients at the time of diagnosis is 55, but CML can be seen in both children and young adults. The causative factor in the majority of cases of CML is not known. Ionizing radiation is associated with the development of CML.

CLASSIFICATION AND PROGNOSIS

Patients with CML have an elevated WBC and are often asymptomatic at the time of presentation. The peripheral smear demonstrates mature leukocytes as well as other myeloid precursors (particularly basophils). The bone marrow is hypercellular and demonstrates a myeloid predominance. Chronic-phase CML is characterized by a WBC that is stable or easily controlled with chemotherapy and bone marrow without a significant number of blasts. The median survival for patients in stable phase is approximately 4 years. Patients eventually progress to an accelerated phase characterized by an increasingly difficult-to-control WBC. Finally, patients develop blast crisis, which is similar to acute leukemia. The majority of patients in blast crises have myeloid leukemia; however, approximately 20% to 30% of cases are lymphoid in derivation. The median survival after developing blast crises is only 3 months. Chemotherapy agents appropriate to the derivation of the leukemia (myeloid or lymphoid) are used to treat blast crisis. If remission is obtained, it is often of short duration.

THERAPY

Treatment options for patients in stable phase CML are initially directed at controlling the elevated WBC. Hydroxyurea is very effective in controlling the majority of patients. Busulfan is now rarely used because of the unpredictable effect on stem cells and occasional episodes of prolonged pancytopenia. After the WBC is stabilized on hydroxyurea, interferon alfa (IFN-α) may be initiated. A recent French study suggests both a survival benefit and an increased rate of major cytogenetic response (< 35% Ph+ cells in the bone marrow) from the combination of IFN-α and subcutaneous Ara-C compared with interferon alone [67]. It is important to appreciate that the time to maximal cytogenetic response after the initiation of IFN-α may be prolonged at least 6 to 9 months in some patients. The dose of IFN-α used is titrated according to the WBC, with a goal of approximately 2000 to 4000 cells/mm^3. The side effects of IFN-α can be significant and include fever, chills, malaise, headaches, anorexia, joint pains, and depression. Twenty percent to 30% of patients are not able to tolerate IFN-α secondary to these side effects.

Allogeneic BMT offers the only option for long-term disease-free survival in patients with CML. Transplants using HLA-identical siblings may be associated with an overall disease-free survival of 60% to 70% at 5 years. Transplants from unrelated donors have a high treatment-related mortality but are still associated with overall survival rates of 40% to 50% at 5 years [46]. The development of GVHD remains the principal obstacle to higher success rates. The graft-versus-leukemia effect is significant in CML, and T-cell–depleted transplants are associated with a higher incidence of relapse after transplant [41]. Donor lymphocyte infusions (DLI) have emerged as a powerful treatment for patients who have relapsed after allogeneic BMT. When administered at the time of cytogenetic relapse, DLI leads to complete cytogenetic response in over 70% of patients [44]. Strategies of combining T-cell–depleted BMT with delayed DLI are now being explored. Autologous transplantation in CML is associated with a high relapse rate and remains investigational.

The timing of transplant in patients with CML is important. Patients treated in early chronic phase (< 1 y after diagnosis) appear to have an improved disease-free survival compared with patients treated in late chronic phase [68]. Disease-free survival rates are much lower when patients undergo transplantation in the second chronic phase (accelerated or blastic phase) compared with the early chronic phase. Transplantation in blast crisis is successful in approximately 10% of cases. An investigational therapy targeting bcr-abl known as STI571 is showing promise in the treatment of CML [69]. This tyrosine-kinase inhibitor given in an oral formulation has been able to achieve hematologic and cytogenetic responses in a large proportion of patients with CML or CML in chronic phase refractory to interferon alfa therapy. A randomized trial comparing STI571 with interferon alfa and cytosine arabinoside is underway.

CHRONIC LYMPHOCYTIC LEUKEMIA

ETIOLOGY AND RISK FACTORS

Chronic lymphocytic leukemia (CLL) is the most common leukemia in the United States and occurs most often in patients older than 60 years of age. There are no known predisposing factors, although familial clustering has been reported.

CLASSIFICATION AND PROGNOSIS

A classification system developed by Rai (stages 0, I, II, III, and IV) has been used in the United States for many years. An alternative staging system (A, B, and C) has been proposed by Binet. Prognosis in CLL is linked to the stage of disease at presentation. Patients with lymphocytosis only (Rai stage 0 or Binet stage A) have a median survival of greater than 10 years from diagnosis. Patients presenting in more advanced stages have shorter survival expectancies (median survival: Rai stage I or II, 7 years; Rai stage III or IV, 4 years).

THERAPY

Treatment of chronic lymphocytic leukemia should be based on symptoms related to adenopathy or cytopenias. There is no benefit derived from treating patients solely to control the WBC. Patients may tolerate WBC > 300,000 without complications. Initial therapy can include the use of single alkylating agents. Chlorambucil may be administered chronically (often a daily dose of 6 to 8 mg) or by pulse dosing (0.4 to 0.8 mg/kg of body weight orally every 2 wk)

usually for no less than 8 to 12 months. There appears to be no benefit from the addition of prednisone to chlorambucil. Patients treated with combination chemotherapy regimens have a higher response rate, but survival is not improved. Other agents to treat CLL include the fluorinated analogue of adenine, fludarabine, possibly with cyclophosphamide [70] (Table 17-7). Recent data suggest that fludarabine is associated with a higher response rate, longer duration of response, and improved progression-free survival in a randomized trial of previously untreated patients compared with chlorambucil [71]. There is no benefit to the addition of prednisone to fludarabine, and it is actually associated with an increased risk of opportunistic infections [72]. Fludarabine leads to profound depression of T-cell subsets, particularly CD4+ cells. Patients receiving fludarabine should be considered candidates to receive prophylaxis for *Pneumocystis carinii* pneumonia. For young patients with advanced stage disease, both autologous and allogeneic BMT may be considered.

HAIRY CELL LEUKEMIA

Hairy cell leukemia is a chronic lymphoproliferative disease with a good prognosis. It is most commonly diagnosed in middle-aged men who present with pancytopenia and an enlarged spleen. A dry marrow aspiration in a patient with these symptoms is typical. Hairy cells have cytoplasmic projections that are fine or hair-like. Tartrate-resistant acid phosphatase (Trap stain) is present in the leukemic cells of most patients. Flow cytometry may be used to make the diagnosis because hairy cells express CD103.

Treatment options for patients with hairy cell leukemia have included splenectomy, chlorambucil, androgens, and interferons (Table 17-8). Formerly, treatment was often initiated when patients were symptomatic or had hematologic indications, such as anemia, thrombocytopenia, or neutropenia. With the recent availability of multiple systemic agents that are capable of inducing durable and complete hematologic remissions in a high percentage of patients, consideration should be given to treating patients early in the course of their disease. A single course of 2-chlorodeoxyadenosine appears to result in excellent long-term survival in more than 90% of patients with newly diagnosed hairy cell leukemia [73]. A second course of 2-chlorodeoxyadenosine, pentostatin, or interferon can be considered for patients who have evidence of recurrent disease [74].

Table 17-7. Therapy for Chronic Lymphocytic Leukemia

Agent	Overall Response Rate (CR), %
Chlorambucil	40–70 (rare)
Fludarabine (untreated)	80 (25–74)
Fludarabine (previously treated)	17–74 (0–20)

CR—complete response.

Table 17-8. Therapy for Hairy Cell Leukemia

Agent	Duration of Treatment	Overall Response Rate (CR), %
2-chlorodeoxyadenosine	1 wk	95 (80)
Pentostatin	3–6 mo	83 (57)
Interferon	12 mo	80 (9)

CR—complete response.

REFERENCES

1. Watson MS, Carroll AJ, Shuster JJ, *et al.*: Trisomy 21 in childhood acute lymphoblastic leukemia: a Pediatric Oncology Group study (8602). *Blood* 1993, 82:3098–3102.

2. Curtis RE, Boice JD Jr, Stovall M, *et al.*: Risk of leukemia after chemotherapy and radiation treatment for breast cancer [see comments]. *N Engl J Med* 1992, 326:1745–1751.

3. Pui CH, Ribeiro RC, Hancock ML, *et al.*: Acute myeloid leukemia in children treated with epipodophyllotoxins for acute lymphoblastic leukemia. *N Engl J Med* 1991, 325:1682–1687.

4. Hudson MM, Raimondi SC, Behm FG, Pui CH: Childhood acute leukemia with t(11;19)(q23;pl3). *Leukemia* 1991, 5:1064–1068.

5. Sobecks RM, Le Beau MM, Anastasi J, Williams SF: Myelodysplasia and acute leukemia following high-dose chemotherapy and autologous bone marrow or peripheral blood stem cell transplantation. *Bone Marrow Transplant* 1999, 23:1161–1165.

6. Borowitz MJ, Gockerman JP, Moore JO, *et al.*: Clinicopathologic and cytogenic features of CD34 (My 10)-positive acute nonlymphocytic leukemia. *Am J Clin Pathol* 1989, 91:265–270.

7. Campos L, Guyotat D, Archimbaud E, *et al.*: Surface marker expression in adult acute myeloid leukaemia: correlations with initial characteristics, morphology and response to therapy. *Br J Haematol* 1989, 72:161–166.

8. Legrand O, Perrot JY, Baudard M, *et al.*: The immunophenotype of 177 adults with acute myeloid leukemia: proposal of a prognostic score. *Blood* 2000, 96:870–877.

9. Mrozek K, Heinonen K, de la Chapelle A, Bloomfield CD: Clinical significance of cytogenetics in acute myeloid leukemia. *Semin Oncol* 1997, 24:17–31.

10. Bishop JF: The treatment of adult acute myeloid leukemia. *Semin Oncol* 1997, 24:57–69.

11. Wiemik PH, Banks PL, Case DC Jr, *et al.*: Cytarabine plus idarubicin or daunorubicin as induction and consolidation therapy for previously untreated adult patients with acute myeloid leukemia. *Blood* 1992, 79:313–319.

12. Berman E, Heller G, Santorsa L, *et al.*: Results of a randomized trial comparing idarubicin and cytosine arabinoside with daunorubicin and cytosine arabinoside in adult patients with newly diagnosed acute myelogenous leukemia. *Blood* 1991, 77:1666–1674.

13. Phillips GL, Reece DE, Shepherd JD, *et al.*: High-dose cytarabine and daunorubicin induction and postremission chemotherapy for the treatment of acute myelogenous leukemia in adults. *Blood* 1991, 77:1429–1435.

14. Brown RA, Herzig RH, Wolff SN, *et al.*: High-dose etoposide and cyclophosphamide without bone marrow transplantation for resistant hematologic malignancy. *Blood* 1990, 76:473–479.

15. Bishop JF, Lowenthal RM, Joshua D, *et al.*: Etoposide in acute nonlymphocytic leukemia: Australian Leukemia Study Group. *Blood* 1990, 75:27–32.

16. Mitus Aj, Nfiller KB, Schenkein DP, *et al.*: Improved survival for patients with acute myelogenous leukemia [see comments]. *J Clin Oncol* 1995, 13:560–569.

17. Estey EH: How I treat older patients with AML. *Blood* 2000, 96:1670–1673.

18. Tilly H, Castaigne S, Bordessoule D, *et al.*: Low-dose cytarabine versus intensive chemotherapy in the treatment of acute nonlymphocytic leukemia in the elderly. *J Clin Oncol* 1990, 8:272–279.

19. Estey E, Thall P, Beran M, *et al.*: Effect of diagnosis (refractory anemia with excess blasts, refractory anemia with excess blasts in transformation, or acute myeloid leukemia [AML]) on outcome of AML-type chemotherapy. *Blood* 1997, 90:2969–2977.

20. Mayer RJ, Davis RB, Schiffer CA, *et al.*: Intensive postremission chemotherapy in adults with acute myeloid leukemia: Cancer and Leukemia Group B [see comments]. *N Engl J Med* 1994, 331:896–903.

21. Lazzarino M, Morra E, Alessandrino EP, *et al.*: Mitoxantrone and etoposide: an effective regimen for refractory or relapsed acute myelogenous leukemia. *Eur J Haematol* 1989, 43:411–416.

22. Sievers EL, Appelbaum FR, Spielberger RT, *et al.*: Selective ablation of acute myeloid leukemia using antibody-targeted chemotherapy: a phase I study of an anti-CD33 calicheamicin immunoconjugate. *Blood* 1999, 93:3678–3684.

23. Degos L: [All-*trans*-retinoic acid in the treatment of acute promyelocytic leukemia]. *Presse Med* 1990, 19:1483–1484.

24. Warrell RP Jr, Frankel SR, Nhller WH Jr, *et al.*: Differentiation therapy of acute promyelocytic leukemia with tretinoin (all-*trans*-retinoic acid). *N Engl J Med* 1991, 324:1385–1393.

25. Fenaux P, Castaigne S, Dombret H, *et al.*: All-*trans*-retinoic acid followed by intensive chemotherapy gives a high complete remission rate and may prolong remissions in newly diagnosed acute promyelocytic leukemia: a pilot study on 26 cases. *Blood* 1992, 80:2176–2181.

26. Fenaux P, Le Deley MC, Castaigne S, *et al.*: Effect of all *trans*retinoic acid in newly diagnosed acute promyelocytic leukemia: results of a multicenter randomized trial: European APL 91 Group. *Blood* 1993, 82:3241–3249.

27. Tallman MS, Andersen JW, Schiffer CA, *et al.*: All-*trans*-retinoic acid in acute promyelocytic leukemia [see comments]. *N Engl J Med* 1997, 337:1021–1028.

28. Fenaux P, Chastang C, Sanz M, *et al.*: ATRA followed by chemotherapy (CT) vs ATRA plus CT and the role of maintenance therapy in newly diagnosed acute promyelocytic leukemia(APL): first interim results of APL 93 trial [abstract]. *Blood* 1997, 90:A533.

29. Frankel SR, Eardley A, Lauwers G, *et al.*: The "retinoic acid syndrome" in acute promyelocytic leukemia [see comments]. *Ann Intern Med* 1992, 117:292–296.

30. Rowe JM, Andersen JW, Mazza JJ, *et al.*: A randomized placebo-controlled phase III study of granulocyte-macrophage colony-stimulating factor in adult patients (>55 to 70 years of age) with acute myelogenous leukemia: a study of the Eastern Cooperative Oncology Group (El490). *Blood* 1995, 86:457–462.

31. Stone RM, Berg DT, George SL, *et al.*: Granulocyte-macrophage colony-stimulating factor after initial chemotherapy for elderly patients with primary acute myelogenous leukemia: Cancer and Leukemia Group B [see comments]. *N Engl J Med* 1995, 332:1671–1677.

32. Heil G, Hoelzer D, Sanz MA, *et al.*: A randomized, double-blind, placebo controlled, phase III study of filgrastim in remission induction and consolidation therapy for adults with de novo acute myeloid leukemia: the International Acute Myeloid Leukemia Study Group. *Blood* 1997, 90:4710–4718.

33. Lowenberg B, Boogaerts MA, Daenen SM, *et al.*: Value of different modalities of granulocyte-macrophage colony-stimulating factor applied during or after induction therapy of acute myeloid leukemia. *J Clin Oncol* 1997, 15:3496–506.

34. Clift RA, Buckner CD, Appelbaum FR, *et al.*: Allogeneic marrow transplantation in patients with acute myeloid leukemia in first remission: a randomized trial of two irradiation regimens [see comments]. *Blood* 1990, 76:1867–1871.

35. Copelan EA, Biggs JC, Thompson JM, *et al.*: Treatment for acute myelocytic leukemia with allogeneic bone marrow transplantation following preparation with BuCy2. *Blood* 1991, 78:838–843.

36. Copelan EA, Biggs JC, Szer J, et al.: Allogeneic bone marrow transplantation for acute myelogenous leukemia, acute lymphocytic leukemia, and multiple myeloma following preparation with busulfan and cyclophosphamide (BuCy2) [review]. *Semin Oncol* 1993, 20:33–38.

37. Blume KG, Long GD, Negrin RS, et al.: Role of etoposide (VP-16) in preparatory regimens for patients with leukemia or lymphoma undergoing allogeneic bone marrow transplantation. *Bone Marrow Transplant* 1994, 14(suppl 4):S9–S10.

38. Burnett AK, Goldstone AH, Stevens RM, et al.: Randomised comparison of addition of autologous bone-marrow transplantation to intensive chemotherapy for acute myeloid leukaemia in first remission: results of MRC AML 10 trial. UK Medical Research Council Adult and Children's Leukaemia Working Parties. *Lancet* 1998, 339:1649–1656.

39. Cassileth PA, Harrington DP, Appelbaum FR, et al.: Chemotherapy compared with autologous or allogeneic bone marrow transplantation in the management of acute myeloid leukemia in first remission [see comments]. *N Engl J Med* 1998, 339:1649–1656.

40. Tallman MS, Rowlings PA, Milone G, et al.: Effect of postremission chemotherapy before human leukocyte antigen-identical sibling transplantation for acute myelogenous leukemia in first complete remission. *Blood* 2000, 96:1254–1258.

41. Horowitz MM, Gale RP, Sondel PM, et al.: Graft-versus-leukemia reactions after bone marrow transplantation. *Blood* 1990, 75:555–562.

42. Papadopoulos EB, Carabasi MH, Castro-Malaspina H, et al.: T-cell-depleted allogeneic bone marrow transplantation as postremission therapy for acute myelogenous leukemia:freedom from relapse in the absence of graft-versus-host disease. *Blood* 1998, 91:1083–90.

43. Soiffer RJ, Fairclough D, Robertson M, et al.: CD6-depleted allogeneic bone marrow transplantation for acute leukemia in first complete remission. *Blood* 1997, 89:3039–3047.

44. Kolb HJ, Schattenberg A, Goldman JM, et al.: Graft-versus-leukemia effect of donor lymphocyte transfusions in marrow grafted patients: European Group for Blood and Marrow Transplantation Working Party Chronic Leukemia [see comments]. *Blood* 1995, 86:2041–2050.

45. Beatty PG. Hansen JA, Longton GM, et al.: Marrow transplantation from HLA matched unrelated donors for treatment of hematologic malignancies. *Transplantation* 1991, 51:443–447.

46. Szydlo R, Goldman JM, Klein JP, et al.: Results of allogeneic bone marrow transplants for leukemia using donors other than HLA-identical siblings. *J Clin Oncol* 1997, 15:1767–1777.

47. Selvaggi KJ, Wilson JW, Mills LE, et al.: Improved outcome for high-risk acute myeloid leukemia patients using autologous bone marrow transplantation and monoclonal antibody-purged bone marrow. *Blood* 1994, 83:1698–705.

48. Robertson MJ, Soiffer RJ, Freedman AS, et al.: Human bone marrow depleted of CD33-positive cells mediates delayed but durable reconstitution of hematopoiesis: clinical trial of MY9 monoclonal antibody-purged autografts for the treatment of acute myeloid leukemia. *Blood* 1992, 79:2229–2236.

49. Larson RA, Dodge RK, Burns CP, et al.: A five-drug remission induction regimen with intensive consolidation for adults with acute lymphoblastic leukemia: Cancer and Leukemia Group B study 8811. *Blood* 1995, 85:2025–2037.

50. Hoelzer D, Thiel E, Loffler H, et al.: Prognostic factors in a multicenter study for treatment of acute lymphoblastic leukemia in adults. *Blood* 1988, 71:123–131.

51. Linker CA, Levitt LJ, O'Donnell M, et al.: Treatment of adult acute-lymphoblastic leukemia with intensive cyclical chemotherapy: a follow-up report. *Blood* 1991, 78:2814–2822.

52. Barrett AJ, Horowitz MM, Ash RC, et al.: Bone marrow transplantation for Philadelphia chromosome-positive acute lymphoblastic leukemia. *Blood* 1992, 79:3067–3070.

53. Forman SJ, O'Donnell MR, Nademanee AP, et al.: Bone marrow transplantation for patients with Philadelphia chromosome-positive acute lymphoblastic leukemia. *Blood* 1987, 70:587–588.

54. Sierra J, Radich J, Hansen JA, et al.: Marrow transplants from unrelated donors for treatment of Philadelphia chromosome-positive acute lymphoblastic leukemia. *Blood* 1997, 90:1410–1414.

55. Golub TR, Barker GF, Bohlander SK, et al.: Fusion of the TEL gene on 12pl3 to the AML1 gene on 2lq22 in acute lymphoblastic leukemia. *Proc Natl Acad Sci U S A* 1995, 92:4917–4921.

56. Rubnitz JE, Shuster JJ, Land VJ, et al.: Case-control study suggests a favorable impact of TEL rearrangement in patients with B-lineage acute lymphoblastic leukemia treated with antimetabolite-based therapy: a Pediatric Oncology Group study. *Blood* 1997, 89:1143–1146.

57. McLean TW, Ringold S, Neuberg D, et al.: TEL/AML-1 dimerizes and is associated with a favorable outcome in childhood acute lymphoblastic leukemia. *Blood* 1996, 88:4252–4258.

58. Hoelzer D, Ludwig WD, Thiel E, et al.: Improved outcome in adult B-cell acute lymphoblastic leukemia. *Blood* 1996, 87:495–508.

59. Barrett AJ: Bone marrow transplantation for acute lymphoblastic leukaemia. *Baillieres Clin Haematol* 1994, 7:377–401.

60. Barrett AJ, Horowitz MM, Gale RP, et al.: Marrow transplantation for acute lymphoblastic leukemia: factors affecting relapse and survival. *Blood* 1989, 74:862–871.

61. Horowitz MM, Messerer D, Hoelzer D, et al.: Chemotherapy compared with bone marrow transplantation for adults with acute lymphoblastic leukemia in first remission. *Ann Intern Med* 1991, 115:13–18.

62. Snyder DS, Chao NJ, Amylon MD, et al.: Fractionated total body irradiation and high-dose etoposide as a preparatory regimen for bone marrow transplantation for 99 patients with acute leukemia in first complete remission. *Blood* 1993, 82:2920–2928.

63. Brenner MK, Rill DR, Moen RC, et al.: Gene-marking to trace origin of relapse after autologous bone-marrow transplantation. *Lancet* 1993, 341:85–86.

64. Gilmore MJ, Hamon MD, Prentice HG, et al.: Failure of purged autologous bone marrow transplantation in high risk acute lymphoblastic leukaemia in first complete remission. *Bone Marrow Transplant* 1991, 8:19–26.

65. Fiere D, Lepage E, Sebban C, et al.: Adult acute lymphoblastic leukemia: a multicentric randomized trial testing bone marrow transplantation as postremission therapy: the French Group on Therapy for Adult Acute Lymphoblastic Leukemia. *J Clin Oncol* 1993, 11:1990–2001.

66. Sawyers CL: Chronic myeloid leukemia [see comments]. *N Engl J Med* 1999, 340:1330–1340.

67. Guilhot F, Chastang C, Michallet M, et al.: Interferon alfa-2b combined with cytarabine versus interferon alone in chronic myelogenous leukemia: French Chronic Myeloid Leukemia Study Group [see comments]. *N Engl J Med* 1997, 337:223–229.

68. Goldman JM, Szydlo R, Horowitz NM, et al.: Choice of pretransplant treatment and timing of transplants for chronic myelogenous leukemia in chronic phase [see comments]. *Blood* 1993, 82:2235–2238.

69. Druker BJ, Talpaz M, Resta D, et al.: Clinical efficacy and safety of an abl specific tyrosine kinase inhibitor as targeted therapy for chronic myelogenous leukemia. *American Society of Hematology* 41st Annual Meeting, 1999.

70. Flinn IW, Byrd JC, Morrison C, et al.: Fludarabine and cyclophosphamide with filgrastim support in patients with previously untreated indolent lymphoid malignancies. *Blood* 2000, 96:71–75.

71. Rai K, Peterson B, Elias L, et al.: A randomized comparison of fludarabine and chlorambucil for patients with previously untreated chronic lymphocytic leukemia: a CALGB, SWOG, CTG /NCI-C and ECOG intergroup study [abstract]. *Blood* 1996, 88:A552.

72. Anaissie E, Kontoyiannis DP, Kantarjian H, *et al.*: Listeriosis in patients with chronic lymphocytic leukemia who were treated with fludarabine and prednisone. *Ann Intern Med* 1992, 117:466–469.

73. Piro LD, Carrera CJ, Carson DA, Beutler E: Lasting remissions in hairy-cell leukemia induced by a single infusion of 2-chlorodeoxyadenosine. *N Engl J Med* 1990, 322:1117–1121.

74. Saven A, Piro LD: Treatment of hairy cell leukemia. *Blood* 1992, 79:1111–1120.

CYTOSINE ARABINOSIDE AND ANTHRACYCLINE

The combination of cytosine arabinoside and one of the anthracycline antibiotics has become the standard induction regimen for acute myeloid leukemia around the world.

Cytosine arabinoside is an antimetabolite that interferes with DNA synthesis after conversion to ara-CTP, which is a potent inhibitor of DNA polymerase. In addition, metabolites of ara-CTP accumulate in DNA, causing a defect in ligation of newly synthesized fragments of DNA. Cytarabine may be inactivated by two intracellular enzymes: cytidine deaminase and deoxycytidine deaminase.

The anthracycline antibiotics are a class of drug that mediate their effects by binding to DNA and intercalation. The anthracyclines enter cells through a passive transport process and can be pumped out of cells through the multidrug resistance protein MDR1 or P glycoprotein. The natural substance daunorubicin has been used in the treatment of leukemia for over 20 years. More recently, a synthetic anthracycline, idarubicin, appears to have greater activity than daunorubicin, largely because of the persistence of an active metabolite. Another synthetic compound, mitoxantrone, has been used in the treatment of acute leukemia and has the advantage of possibly being less cardiotoxic.

DOSAGE AND SCHEDULING

STANDARD REGIMEN

Ara-c 100–200 mg/m²/d continuous infusion, d1–7	▬▬▬▬▬
Daunorubicin 45–50 mg/m²/d, IV bolus, d1–3	▬▬
Bone marrow	☐

SECOND COURSE (IF NEEDED BASED ON BONE MARROW)

Ara-c 100–200 mg/m²/d continuous infusion, d1–5	▬▬▬▬
Daunorubicin 45–50 mg/m²/d, IV bolus, d1–2	▬

Following achievement of complete remission: one or more courses of ara-C at high-dose (1.5–3 g/m² x 12 doses, lower for patients ≥ age 60 y) with daunorubicin daily for 3 d at completion of ara-C are recommended.

3 7 3 INDUCTION REGIMEN (ALTERNATIVE)

Cytarabine 100 mg/m² d 1–7	▬▬▬▬▬
Daunorubicin 45 mg/m² d 1–3	▬▬
Cytarabine 2 g/m² d 8, 9, 10	▬▬

CYCLE 1 AND 3

Cytarabine 200 mg/m² d 1–5	▬▬▬▬
Daunorubicin 60 mg/m² d 1, 2	▬

CYCLE 2

Cytarabine 2 g/m² d 1–3	▬▬
Etoposide 100 mg/m² d 4, 5	▬
Day	1 2 3 4 5 6 7 8 9 10 11 12 13 14

RECENT EXPERIENCE AND RESPONSE RATES

Most studies report complete remission rates of 60%–70% (lower in patients older than 60 y)

CANDIDATES FOR TREATMENT

Newly diagnosed patients with AML or relapsed AML (especially if first remission lasted 1 y)

SPECIAL PRECAUTIONS

Rapid cell turnover and hyperuricemia with possible renal damage (start patients on allopurinol 300 mg/d if necessary)

ALTERNATIVE THERAPIES

None is standard

TOXICITIES

Drug combination: extremely myelotoxic, resulting in marrow aplasia with attendant pancytopenia; neutropenia 2–4 wk following induction; overwhelming sepsis possible (institute antibiotics); platelet transfusions if platelet count < 20,000/mL; mucositis, alopecia; **ara-C:** hepatotoxicity, with transaminasemia and/or jaundice in some patients; **Anthracyclines:** cardiotoxicity (monitored with MUGA scans)

DRUG INTERACTIONS

None

NURSING INTERVENTIONS

Observe patients for any signs of infection; provide antiemetics, particularly during the daunorubicin phase of the protocol; monitor blood counts and liver function tests daily; wash hands carefully

PATIENT INFORMATION

Patients undergoing induction therapy for AML are often quite ill prior to therapy. Considerable counseling and reassurance are necessary at this phase of the patient's disease. The patient needs to be informed rapidly about the various treatment options available once remission is achieved (consolidation with chemotherapy, BMT)

INDUCTION AND CONSOLIDATION FOR PROMYELOCYTIC LEUKEMIA

All-*trans*-retinoic acid (ATRA) has emerged as an important component in the treatment of patients with promyelocytic leukemia (APML). ATRA reduces the acute complications associated with the administration of chemotherapy, such as disseminated intravascular coagulation. ATRA is combined with daunorubicin-based chemotherapy, and studies are currently being performed to optimize the time of administration of this agent. Administration of ATRA may be associated with the development of the retinoic acid syndrome. Fenaux *et al.* [28] reported a regimen that combines ATRA and chemotherapy and results in a complete response rate of 91% in patients with APML.

DOSAGE AND SCHEDULING

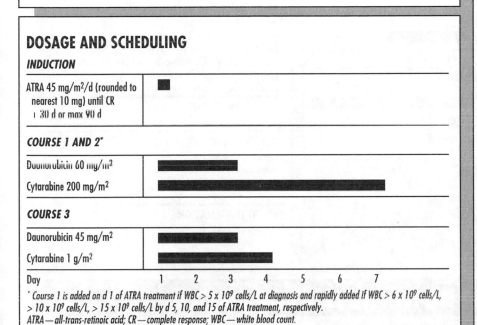

INDUCTION

ATRA 45 mg/m²/d (rounded to nearest 10 mg) until CR + 30 d or max 90 d	

COURSE 1 AND 2*

Daunorubicin 60 mg/m²	
Cytarabine 200 mg/m²	

COURSE 3

Daunorubicin 45 mg/m²	
Cytarabine 1 g/m²	

Day	1	2	3	4	5	6	7

*Course 1 is added on d 1 of ATRA treatment if WBC > 5 x 10⁹ cells/L at diagnosis and rapidly added if WBC > 6 x 10⁹ cells/L, > 10 x 10⁹ cells/L, > 15 x 10⁹ cells/L by d 5, 10, and 15 of ATRA treatment, respectively.

ATRA—all-trans-retinoic acid; CR—complete response; WBC—white blood count.

CANDIDATES FOR TREATMENT

Newly diagnosed patients with APML

SPECIAL PRECAUTIONS

Retinoic acid syndrome with rapidly increasing white blood count, hypoxia, and diffuse pulmonary infiltrates; coagulopathy may develop; treatment includes platelet transfusion; other considerations include heparin, tranexamic acid, and fresh frozen plasma; fibrinogen transfusions may be considered

ALTERNATIVE THERAPIES

Standard induction chemotherapy for acute myeloid leukemia

TOXICITIES

Drug combinations: extremely myelotoxic, resulting in marrow aplasia with attendant pancytopenia; neutropenia 2–4 wk following induction; sepsis possible; platelet transfusions in platelet count < 30,000/mL; mucositis; alopecia; **Ara-C:** hepatotoxicity with elevated transaminasemia and/or jaundice in some patients; **Anthracycline:** cardiotoxicity. **ATRA:** retinoic acid syndrome

DRUG INTERACTIONS

None

NURSING INTERVENTIONS

Same as for acute myeloid leukemia (*see* Cytosine Arabinoside and Anthracycline section)

PATIENT INFORMATION

Same as for acute myeloid leukemia (*see* Cytosine Arabinoside and Anthracycline section)

HIGH-DOSE CYTOSINE ARABINOSIDE

In an effort to increase the efficacy and durability of remissions, regimens containing cytosine arabinoside in high doses have been studied. High doses of ara-C give rise to higher levels of intracellular ara-C and increase the efficacy of the agent. As an induction regimen, high-dose ara-C is accompanied by an anthracycline antibiotic or L-asparaginase.

DOSAGE AND SCHEDULING

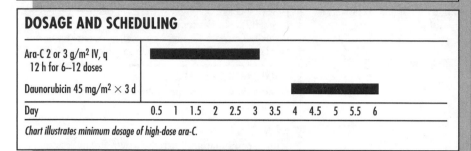

Ara-C 2 or 3 g/m² IV, q 12 h for 6–12 doses												
Daunorubicin 45 mg/m² × 3 d												
Day	0.5	1	1.5	2	2.5	3	3.5	4	4.5	5	5.5	6

Chart illustrates minimum dosage of high-dose ara-C.

RECENT EXPERIENCE AND RESPONSE RATES

Complete responses are seen in about 50% of patients tested in relapse

CANDIDATES FOR TREAMENT
AML in relapse

SPECIAL PRECAUTIONS
Tumor lysis syndrome with release of uric acid and phosphorus alkalinization of the urine should be induced and allopurinol, 300 mg/d, started immediately; NaCl or steroid eye drops for HD Ara-C

ALTERNATIVE THERAPIES
Standard-dose ara-C; Carboplatin

TOXICITIES
Drug combination: neutropenia and thrombocytopenia; nausea, vomiting, diarrhea; elevated liver function tests; **High-dose ara-C:** cerebellar toxicity (slurred speech, ataxia), ototoxicity, conjunctivitis; extreme myelotoxicity resulting in narrow aplasia and pancytopenia

DRUG INTERACTIONS
None

NURSING INTERVENTIONS
Observe patients for signs of infection; give antiemetic; monitor blood counts and liver function tests daily; wash hands carefully; watch for ataxia daily; manage conjunctivitis with glucocorticoid eyedrops every 6–8 h

PATIENT INFORMATION
Patients should be informed that this regimen is myelotoxic and that prolonged myelosuppresion is expected.

MITOXANTRONE AND ETOPOSIDE

Both mitoxantrone and etoposide have shown activity as single agents in acute myeloid leukemia (AML). A combination of the two agents is a relatively effective therapy for patients with relapsed disease. The regimen is relatively well tolerated.

DOSAGE AND SCHEDULING

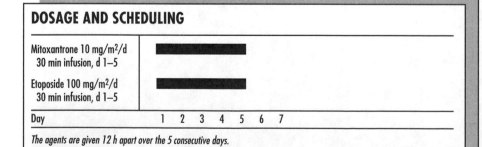

Mitoxantrone 10 mg/m²/d 30 min infusion, d 1–5							
Etoposide 100 mg/m²/d 30 min infusion, d 1–5							
Day	1	2	3	4	5	6	7

The agents are given 12 h apart over the 5 consecutive days.

RECENT EXPERIENCE AND RESPONSE RATES

Complete response rate of 45%–50%; as with most regimens used in relapse for AML, the duration of remission achieved is relatively brief. In a study by Lazzarino *et al.* [21], 61% of patients achieved complete remission including several patients with disease refractory to other therapy; the median CR duration was 5 mo with a range of 2 to 12 + mo.

CANDIDATES FOR TREATMENT
AML in relapse

SPECIAL PRECAUTIONS
Possibility of cardiotoxicity: obtain baseline MUGA scan

ALTERNATIVE THERAPIES
Ara-C and anthracycline, carboplatin, high-dose ara-C

TOXICITIES
Drug combination: myelosuppression; severe oral mucositis; reactivation of herpes virus (administer acyclovir); mild nausea and vomiting, diarrhea, transaminasemia, alopecia

DRUG INTERACTIONS
None

NURSING INTERVENTIONS
Parental hyperalimentation for grade 3 oral mucositis; monitor for myelosuppression

PATIENT INFORMATION
Patients undergoing induction therapy for AML are often quite ill prior to therapy. Considerable counseling and reassurance are necessary at this phase of the patient's disease. The patient needs to be informed rapidly about the various treatment options available once remission is achieved (consolidation with chemotherapy, BMT)

BFM INTENSIFIED INDUCTION AND CONSOLIDATION THERAPY

A significant advance in the treatment of acute lymphocytic leukemia (ALL) in adults has come from a series of German multicenter studies known as the BFM regimens (Berlin, Frankfurt, Munich). This intensive multiagent regimen has an induction phase with prednisone, vincristine, daunorubicin, and L-asparaginase followed by cyclophosphamide, cytarabine, 6-mercaptopurine, and methotrexate given over a period of 52 days. Following this, a reinduction phase is begun using dexamethasone, vincristine, doxorubicin, cyclophosphamide, ara-C, and thioguanine over the next 42 days. Then a maintenance phase with 6-mercaptopurine and methotrexate is started for up to 130 weeks. Central nervous system (CNS) prophylaxis consists of cranial irradiation with 24 Gy and intrathecal methotrexate (10 mg/m^2, maximum single dose 15 mg), once weekly for 4 wk during phase 2 when complete remission is achieved after phase 1. If complete remission is delayed until after completion of phase 2, CNS prophylaxis is given immediately thereafter.

Several important prognostic factors were uncovered during this study. Favorable outcome was seen in patients who achieved complete remission in less than 4 wk, who were younger than 35 years, whose initial leukocyte count was less than 30,000, and whose immunophenotype was T-ALL. The absence of these good prognostic factors resulted in an adverse outcome; that is, the presence of two or three adverse factors was associated with a median remission duration of 9.6 mo, whereas the absence of these factors resulted in a better outcome.

CANDIDATES FOR TREATMENT
Patients with ALL at diagnosis

SPECIAL PRECAUTIONS
Patients should have urine alkalinized (place on allpurinol 300 mg/dL)

ALTERNATIVE THERAPIES
Bone marrow transplantation after induction

TOXICITY
Myelosuppression with attendant problems

DRUG INTERACTIONS
None

NURSING INTERVENTIONS
Neutropenia is expected, therefore observe for any signs of infection; give antiemetics, particularly during daunorubicin phase of protocol; monitor blood counts and liver function tests daily; wash hands carefully

PATIENT INFORMATION
Patients undergoing induction therapy for ALL are often quite ill prior to therapy. Considerable counseling and reassurance are necessary at this phase of the patient's disease. The patient needs to be informed rapidly of the various treatment options available once remission is achieved (consolidation, BMT)

DOSAGE AND SCHEDULING

DRUG	DOSE AND DAYS
Induction	
Phase 1	
Prednisone	60 mg/m^2 d 1–21
Vincristine	1.5 mg/m^2 IV* d 1,8,15,22
Daunorubicin	25 mg/m^2 IV d 1,8,15,22
L-Asparaginase	5000 U/m^2 IV d 1–14
Phase 2	
Cyclophosphamide	650 mg/m^2 IV d 29,43,57
ara-C	75 mg/m^2 IV d 31–34,38–41,45–48,52–55
6-Mercaptopurine	60 mg/m^2 PO d 29–57
Methotrexate	10 mg/m^2 IT d 31,38,45,52
Consolidation	
Phase 1	
Dexamethasone	10 mg/m^2 PO d 1–28
Vincristine	1.5 mg/m^2 IV* d 1,8,15,22
Doxorubicin	25 mg/m^2 IV d 1,8,15,22
Phase 2	
Cyclophosphamide	650 mg/m^2 IV d 29
ara-C	75 mg/m^2 IV d 31–34,38–41
Thioguanine	60 mg/m^2 PO d 29–42
Maintenance	
6-Mercaptopurine	60 mg/m^2 PO/d, wk 10–18
Methotrexate	20 mg/m^2 PO/IV/wk and d 29–130

*Maximum dose of 2 mg.
CNS prophylaxis consisted of cranial irradiation with 24 Gy and intrathecal methotrexate, 10 mg/m^2 (maximum single dose, 15 mg/m^2), once weekly for 4 wk during phase II when complete remission was achieved.

RECENT EXPERIENCE AND RESPONSE RATES
Complete remission of 74%, with 34% of patients in continuous complete remission at 5 y; median survival is 28 mo.

ECOG INTENSIFIED INDUCTION AND CONSOLIDATION THERAPY

Modifications of the BFM protocol have been used by cooperative groups such as the Cancer and Leukemia Group. The Eastern Cooperative Oncology Group (ECOG) is joining with MRC of the UK to examine the role of bone marrow transplantation in the first remission of ALL. Patients receive the following induction regimen and are then randomized to autologous BMT (or assigned to allogenic BMT if a donor is available). Both groups receive intensification before either transplantation or conventional consolidation and maintenance.

DOSAGE AND SCHEDULING

DRUG	DOSE AND DAYS
Induction	
Phase 1	
Daunorubicin	60 mg/m² IV push d 1,8,15,21
Vincristine	1.4 mg/m² IV push* d 1,8,15,21
Prednisolone	60 mg/m² PO qd d 1–28
L-Asparaginase	10,000 U IM or IV in 100 ml D5W over 30 min qd d 17–28
Methotrexate	12.5 mg IT d 15 only

If CNS leukemia is present at diagnosis, methotrexate IT or via an Ommaya reservoir is given weekly until blasts are absent. 24 Gy cranial irradiation and 12 Gy to the spinal cord are administered concurrent with phase 2.

Phase 2 (weeks 5–8)	
Cyclophosphamide	650 mg/m² IV in 250 cc normal saline for 30 min, d 1,14,28
ara-C	75 mg/m² IV in 100 cc D5W for 30 min, d 1–4, 8–11, 15–18, 22–25
6-Mercaptopurine	60 mg/m² PO qd d 1–28
Methotrexate	12.5 mg IT d 1, 8, 15, 22

Postponed if total WBC count < 3 x 10⁹/L.

Intensification (weeks 13–16)	
HD Methotrexate	3 g/m² IV in NS 500 mL over 2 h, d 1,8,22
L-Asparaginase	10,000 Lu/m² IV in 100 mL D5W over 30 min, d 2,9,23
Leucovorin rescue	10 mg/m² IV D5W 50 mL q 6 h x 4 doses beginning 22–24 h after completion of methotrexate; then 10 mg/m² PO q 6 h x 72 h

Begin 4 wk from d 28 of induction, phase 2; postpone if WBC < 3 x 10⁹/L.
If randomized to autologous BMT or assigned to allogenic BMT, perform harvest (1–3 x 10⁸/kg nucleated cells) within 3–7 wk from start of intensification. Postpone harvest until marrow cellularity on biopsy ≥ 30%.

Day -6 to day -4: fractioned TBI total dose 1320 cGy; **For males only:** 400 cGy testicular boost; **Day -3:** etoposide 60 mg/kg IV; **Day 0:** allogeneic or autologous marrow infusion; **Day 0 — +27:** GM-CSF 250 µg/m²/day over 4–6 h IV

If randomized to chemotherapy, start conventional consolidation maintenance (beginning 1–2 mo after intensification).

Cycle I Consolidation	
ara-C	75 mg/m² IV in 500 mL D5W
Etoposide	100 mg/m² IV in 500 mL NS over 1 h, d 1–5
Vincristine	1.4 mg/m²,* d 1, 8, 15, 22
Dexamethasone	10 mg/m² PO, d 1–28

Cycles II, IV Consolidation	
ara-C	75 mg/m² IV in 500 mL D5W over 30 min, d 1–5
Etoposide	100 mg/m² IV in 500 mL normal saline x 60 min, d 1–5

Begin 4 wk from day 1 of each cycle or when WBC count > 3.0 x 10⁹/L, except cycle IV which begins 2 mo from day 1 following cycle III or when WBC count > 3.0 x 10⁹/L.

Cycle III Consolidation	
Daunorubicin	25 mg/m² IV push, d 1, 8, 15, 22
Cyclophosphamide	650 mg/m² IV in 250 mL normal saline over 30 min, d 29
ara-C	75 mg/m² IV 100 mL D5W over 30 min, d 31–34, 38–41
6-Thioguanine	60 mg/m² PO, d 29–42

Begin 4 weeks from day 1 of cycle II or when WBC count > 3.0 x 10⁹/L.

Maintenance Therapy	
Vincristine	1.4 mg/m² IV* every 3 mo
Prednisolone	60 mg/m² PO x 5 d every 3 mo
6-Mercaptopurine	75 mg/m² PO/d
Methotrexate	20 mg/m² PO or IV/wk for 2.5 y
Interferon alfa	3 MU SC 3 times/wk — Ph+ patients only

All drug doses are based on the lesser of the actual/corrected ideal body weight.
*Maximum dose of 2 mg.

CANDIDATES FOR TREATMENT
ALL at diagnosis

SPECIAL PRECAUTIONS
Patients should have their urine alkalinized (place on allopurinol 300 mg/d)

ALTERNATIVE THERAPIES
Bone marrow transplant after induction

RECENT EXPERIENCE AND RESPONSE RATES
60% complete response rate

TOXICITY
Myelosuppression with attendant problems

DRUG INTERACTIONS
None

NURSING INTERVENTIONS
Neutropenia is expected, therefore observe for any signs of infection; give antiemetics, particularly during daunorubicin phase of the protocol; monitor blood counts and liver function tests daily; wash hands carefully

PATIENT INFORMATION
Patients undergoing induction therapy for ALL are often quite ill prior to therapy. Considerable counseling and reassurance are necessary at this phase of the patient's disease. The patient needs to be informed rapidly about the various treatment options available once remission is achieved (consolidation with chemotherapy, BMT)

Hodgkin's disease is uncommon. The annual incidence is two per 100,000 people in the United States, accounting for about 14% of all newly diagnosed lymphomas. In developed countries, there is a bimodal age distribution with one peak in the late 20s and a second peak after age 45 years [1,2].

The etiology of Hodgkin's disease has not been definitively established. Immunologic and molecular evidence show that the Epstein–Barr virus is highly associated with histologic subtypes. However, a direct causal relationship has not yet been shown.

Pathologically, Hodgkin's disease is characterized by the presence of large abnormal cells with prominent nucleoli (Reed-Sternberg cells or mononuclear variants). However, most of the tumor is composed of a mixture of normal-appearing inflammatory cells. The recently proposed World Health Organization classification specifies two general categories: nodular lymphocyte-predominant Hodgkin's lymphoma and classical Hodgkin's lymphoma [3]. The classic category is further subdivided into four types: *nodular sclerosis, lymphocyte rich, mixed cellularity*, and *lymphocyte depletion*. Nodular sclerosis accounts for the vast majority of cases, whereas lymphocyte depletion is extremely rare. Lymphocyte rich is an uncommon new category that will require further clinical and pathologic correlation.

The diagnosis of Hodgkin's disease requires examination of a histologic sample by an experienced hematopathologist. Material from an excisional biopsy specimen usually is necessary to establish the initial diagnosis because fine needle aspiration often provides insufficient material or architectural information to render a definite diagnosis. Hodgkin's disease should be differentiated from non-Hodgkin's lymphomas, some of which may have a similar histologic appearance. Special immunohistochemical stains to test for cell surface markers may assist in establishing the diagnosis.

Most patients present with painless enlargement of the lymph nodes. The most common sites of involvement include the neck and the mediastinum. Other common sites are the axillae, spleen, and para-aortic lymph nodes. In most cases, the disease spreads in a nonrandom fashion to involve contiguous nodal sites. In advanced stages, the disease may spread to involve the liver, bone marrow, bone, or other extranodal sites. Constitutional symptoms, such as fevers, sweats, and weight loss, are also more common with advanced disease.

Accurate staging is crucial in planning the treatment of patients with Hodgkin's disease so that specific treatment can be tailored to the extent and location of disease. For example, radiotherapy alone can treat patients effectively with a limited extent of disease determined through careful and systemic staging. The widely accepted Ann Arbor Staging Classification System has been modestly revised. The Cotswold revision of the Ann Arbor Staging Classification System [4] is shown in Table 18-1. Staging evaluation requires a careful history to determine the duration and presence of fever, night sweats, and weight loss; a careful physical examination with special attention to sites of lymph nodes, liver, and spleen; laboratory evaluation including a complete blood count, erythrocyte sedimentation rate, alkaline phosphatase and lactate dehydrogenase levels, and tests for renal and hepatic function; and radiographic studies, including a chest radiograph and computed tomography (CT) scans of the chest, the abdomen, and the pelvis. A lower-extremity lymphangiogram may yield additional information about the architecture and size of retroperitoneal adenopathy beyond that provided by the CT scan. It also provides an inexpensive and simple way to monitor response to treatment. Bone marrow biopsies are indicated in patients with systemic symptoms and those with extensive or bulky clinical disease. Staging laparotomy (with splenectomy, liver biopsy, and retroperitoneal lymph node sampling) has been incorporated in staging when radiation therapy alone was being considered for primary therapy. Whereas staging provides critical information for determining therapy, several additional characteristics can provide further prognostic information. An international group of investigators identified seven factors that independently predict for outcome among patients with advanced disease [5]. These factors include serum albumin less than 4 g/dL, a hemoglobin level less than 10.5 g/dL, male sex, age of 45 years or older, stage IV disease, leukocytosis (a leukocyte count of $\geq 15,000/mm^3$), and lymphocytopenia (lymphocyte count < 600/mm^3 or a count < 8% of the total leukocyte count). The predicted outcome of patients ranged from a freedom from progression of 84% among patients with no risk factors to 42% among those with five or more. The internationally recognized prognostic score may aid in interpreting results of therapeutic trials, in the design of risk-adapted clinical studies, and in making individual therapeutic decisions.

TREATMENT MODALITIES
Radiation

Radiotherapy was the first modality demonstrated to be curative for Hodgkin's disease. There is a dose-response curve to therapy (greater rate of control with higher doses of radiation for a given tumor burden). Doses of 4000 to 4400 cGy are required for identifiable tumor masses, whereas subclinical disease in apparently uninvolved areas can be controlled with doses of 3000 to 3500 cGy [6]. Radiotherapy alone is curative in carefully staged patients with limited, asymptomatic disease and is a useful component of treatment in patients with bulky disease. The success of radiotherapy in favorable, limited disease is based on an understanding of the patterns of spread of disease and the inclusion of identifiable sites of disease as well as contiguous nodal sites in the radiation fields.

Table 18-1. Cotswold Revision of the Ann Arbor Stage in Classification of Hodgkin's Disease

Stage I: Involvement of a single lymph node region (*eg*, cervical, axillary, inguinal, mediastinal) or lymphoid structure, such as spleen, thymus, and Waldeyer's ring, or involvement of a single extralymphatic site (IE)

Stage II: Involvement of ≥ 2 lymph node regions or lymph node structures on the same side of the diaphragm; extralymphatic involvement on one side of the diaphragm by limited direct extension from an adjacent nodal site (IIE)

Stage III: Involvement of lymph node regions or lymphoid structures on both sides of the diaphragm, which may be accompanied by limited contiguous involvement of one extralymphatic site (IIIE)

Stage III$_1$: Spleen or splenic, hilar, celiac, or portal node involvement

Stage III$_2$: Paraaortic, iliac, or mesenteric node involvement

Stage IV: Extensive extranodal disease
A: Asymptomatic
B: Unexplained weight loss >10% of body weight in the previous 6 mo, or unexplained fever > 38°C during the previous month, or recurrent drenching night sweats during the previous month
X: Bulky disease

From Lister et al. [4].

Chemotherapy

The development of MOPP (mechlorethamine, vincristine, procarbazine, prednisone) chemotherapy in the 1960s represented a major advance in the treatment of patients with advanced-stage Hodgkin's disease, which to that time had been largely fatal. About 85% of patients achieved a complete response and over 50% were continuously free of disease at a median of 14 years' follow-up [7]. In the early 1970s, a second major advance came with the introduction of ABVD (doxorubicin, bleomycin, vinblastine, dacarbazine), a chemotherapy regimen containing drugs non–cross-resistant to those in MOPP. The activity of the ABVD regimen was demonstrated first in patients in whom MOPP failed and later as effective initial therapy [8].

A number of randomized, controlled trials have tested the efficacy of MOPP, ABVD, and various combinations of MOPP with ABVD (Table 18-2). The results from the Cancer and Leukemia Group B (CALGB) [9], Milan [10], and the European Organization for the Research and Treatment of Cancer [11] show that ABVD or an ABVD combination with MOPP yields superior response rates and freedom from progression compared with MOPP alone. However, the results with MOPP in these randomized studies are less favorable than those from the National Cancer Institute (NCI), possibly because of deviation from the dosing guidelines as specified by the original investigators. MOPP/ABV hybrid and MOPP-ABV alternating were equivalent in efficacy in studies from NCI Canada [12] and from Milan [13]. A superior response rate, relapse-free survival, and overall survival were seen with MOPP/ABV hybrid compared with a sequence of MOPP followed by ABVD in the Intergroup trial [14].

Table 18-2. Treatment of Advanced-Stage Hodgkin's Disease

Study	Evaluable Patients, *n*	Regimen	% (at 1y) CR	FFS	OS
Santoro et al. [8]	43	MOPP x 12	74	37 FPP	58 (10)
	45	MOPP/ABVD x 6/6	89	61* FFP	69
Somers et al. [9]	96	MOPP x 8	57	43	57 (6)
	96	MOPP/ABVD x 4/4	59	60*	65
Canellos et al. [7]	123	MOPP x 6–8	67	50	66 (5)
	115	ABVD x 6–8	82*	61*	73
	123	MOPP/ABVD x 6/6	83*	65*	75
Vivani [11]	204	MOPP/ABV x 6	89	69 FFP	72 (10)
	211	MOPP/ABVD x 3/3	91	67 FFP	74
Glick et al. [11a]	737	MOPP/ABV x 8	82*	77*	89* (2.5)
	total	MOPP x 6–8/ABVD x 3 (sequential)	73	65	82
Connors et al. [10]	146	MOPP/ABV x 8	85	75 FFP	84 (4)
	141	MOPP/ABVD x 4/4	83	70 FFP	84

*P<0.05
CR—complete response; FFP—freedom from progression; FFS—failure-free survival; OS—overall survival.

The results of the various randomized studies suggest that ABVD or a combination of ABVD and MOPP is superior to MOPP alone. An Intergroup trial has compared MOPP/ABV hybrid to ABVD alone. Preliminary results showed no difference in complete response rate, freedom from progression, or overall survival between treatments thus far. However, there was a significantly greater incidence of pulmonary, hematologic, and infectious toxicities with the hybrid treatment [15]. Longer follow-up is needed, however, before final conclusions can be made.

Several groups during the last 10 years have developed more intensive treatment regimens. Stanford University investigators developed a condensed 12-week chemotherapy program followed by radiation to sites of disease 5 cm or greater (Stanford V) [16]. Among 121 patients with advanced or bulky disease, overall survival was 95% at 5 years and failure-free survival (FFS) was 89%. Patients with 0 to 2 international prognostic factors had a FFS of 97%, whereas those patients with three or more factors had a FFS of 70%. An ongoing intergroup study is currently comparing the Stanford V regimen to ABVD among patients with 0 to 2 risk factors.

Investigators at the German Hodgkin's Lymphoma Study Group reported results of a time-condensed regimen, BEACOPP, in patients with advanced-stage disease. In this large, randomized, three-arm study, BEACOPP and intensified BEACOPP were compared to COPP/ABVD. Early analysis resulted in early closure of the COPP/ABVD arm because of superior complete remission rates, freedom from failure, and overall survival among the BEACOPP arms. A recent update showed that the intensified BEACOPP offered superior FFS (88% vs 79%) compared with standard BEACOPP [17]. The majority of patients in both arms also received consolidative radiotherapy. Overall survival, however, did not differ between groups. Seven of 403 patients in the intensified arm developed leukemia or myelodysplastic syndrome. Longer follow-up is needed to determine the late effects of therapy and the impact on survival.

TREATMENT STRATEGIES

Early-stage, Favorable Disease

One treatment option for patients with stage I or IIA nonbulky disease is radiotherapy alone. Clinical stage I or IIA patients with favorable features (nonbulky disease, absence of systemic symptoms, normal erythrocyte sedimentation rate, young age, < four nodal sites) may be treated with irradiation to the mantle and para-aortic fields. Recent results from the German Hodgkin's Study Group (HD7) suggests that brief chemotherapy (ABVD for two cycles) when combined with extended field radiotherapy offers improved freedom from treatment failure compared to extended field radiotherapy alone (96% vs 84% at 24 months). Survival rates among this favorable group of patients (stage I/II without clinical risk factors) was excellent in both arms (98% at 2 years) [18]. Less favorable stage I or IIA patients or those with constitutional symptoms are candidates for combined chemotherapy and radiotherapy. Results of radiotherapy in early stage disease are shown in Table 18-3. Most patients enter a sustained remission, and overall survival is very high in part because of effective treatments given at relapse.

Extended courses of treatment with chemotherapy alone, such as ABVD, have been tested in patients with early-stage disease. As expected, response rates and overall survival are excellent, although patients receive higher doses of potentially toxic agents [19].

Several groups are studying the use of less toxic or abbreviated chemotherapy and limited volume radiotherapy in early stage favorable disease. This strategy aims to avoid the complications associated with a staging laparotomy or extended field radiotherapy. Early results of this approach appear very promising. For example, the Stanford group reported a 3-year freedom from progression of 95% with an overall survival of 97% among 65 patients with stage I or II, nonbulky disease. Treatment consisted of 8 weeks of Stanford V chemotherapy followed by low dose radiotherapy (30 Gy) to sites of disease [20]. An ongoing study by the German Hodgkin's Study Group (HD10) will determine the optimum amount of chemotherapy and radiotherapy necessary for favorable early-stage disease. Patients are randomly assigned to either ABVD × 2 or × 4, and to either involved field radiotherapy to 20 Gy or to 30 Gy. Results of these and other randomized studies will help to determine the efficacy of abbreviated combined modality therapies. Long-term follow-up, however, will be needed to assess the effect on late side effects.

Bulky Mediastinal Disease

Patients with stage I or II disease with bulky mediastinal involvement (defined as the ratio of the maximum mediastinal diameter to the greatest internal transthoracic diameter greater than one third) should be treated with combination chemotherapy and radiation. Treatment of bulky disease with either radiation or combination chemotherapy alone is associated with a substantial relapse rate. In addition, using chemotherapy prior to radiotherapy will in most patients reduce the volume of required radiation and decrease the toxicity to adjacent organs.

Advanced-Stage Disease

Patients with stage III or IV should be treated with doxorubicin-containing combination chemotherapy such as ABVD. Although highly selected stage IIIA patients with upper abdominal disease and

no or only minimal splenic involvement may be treated with total lymphoid irradiation, this treatment is no longer in favor due to complications, primarily sterility. The selection of the particular regimen should be based on the potential toxicities expected, the tolerance of the individual patient, and the number of adverse prognostic factors. Consolidative radiotherapy is indicated in patients with bulky mediastinal involvement to decrease the chance of recurrence in that site. Patients with 0 to 2 prognostic factors may be eligible for the ongoing intergroup study comparing Stanford V plus radiotherapy to ABVD. Patients with more than two prognostic factors should be considered for the intergroup study comparing standard ABVD to ABVD for four cycles plus high-dose therapy with stem-cell support.

SECOND-LINE TREATMENT

The majority of patients with Hodgkin's disease are cured with initial therapy. However, a small portion of patients treated with radiotherapy alone for limited favorable disease, and a larger subset of patients treated with combination chemotherapy alone or with radiotherapy for advanced-stage or unfavorable disease, relapse after attaining an initial remission.

Patients relapsing after radiotherapy alone do as well with salvage combination chemotherapy as patients with advanced-stage disease who have never received radiation. Salvage treatment after relapse from combination chemotherapy is less successful. Retreatment with the initial chemotherapy regimen or employment of a non–cross-resistant regimen offers high response rates among patients with favorable characteristics at relapse, particularly those with a long duration of remission. Among this group, however, long-term disease-free survival is achieved in a minority of patients, and it is achieved in even fewer among those with early relapses or

Table 18-3. Treatment of Early-Stage Hodgkin's Disease

Study	Evaluable patients, n	Regimen	Stage	% (at 1 y)		
				CR	FFP	OS
Bates et al. [33]	30	VBM x 6-XRT	I-IIA	90	87	93 (2.5)
Hagemeister et al. [34]	79	NOVP x 3-XRT	I-II	95	87	98 (2.5)
Brusamolino et al. [35]	88	STNI	PS I-II (F)	94	69	96 (5)
	76	CT-XRT	I-II (U)	99	91	93
Noordijk et al. [36]	130	STNI	I-II (F)	94	81	99 (3)
	124	vs EBVP-IF XRT	I-II (F)	90	79	100
	156	MOPP/ABV x 6-IF XRT	I-II (U)	85	88*	92 (3)
	160	vs EBVP x 6-IF XRT	I-II (U)	82	72*	92
Horning et al. [37]	35	VBM x 6-IF XRT	I-II		87(5)	
	43	STNI			92	
Colonna et al. [38]	262	ABVD x 1–4-XRT	MMR < 1/3		94	93 (10)
			MMR > 1/3, < 0.45		87	87
			MMR > 0/45		63	78
Bonfante et al. [39]	37	ABVD x 4-STNI	I-II	100	100	100 (2)
	36	ABVD x 4-IF XRT		100	100	100
Tesch et al. [18]	571	EF-RT	I-II(F)	96	84(2)	98(2)
		ABVD + EF-RT		97	96(2)	98(2)

*P<0.01 CT:MOPP x 6 or ABVD x 3.
CR—complete response; EBVP—epirubicin, bleomycin, vinblastine, prednisone; F—favorable; FFP—freedom from progression; NOVP—novantrone, vincristine, vinblastine, prednisone; OS—overall survival; STNI—subtotal nodal irradiation; U—unfavorable; VBM—vinblastine, bleomycin, methotrxate, VF— very favorable.

other unfavorable characteristics. Wide-field radiotherapy as a salvage treatment can result in long remissions, but the number of optimal candidates for this treatment is limited.

High-dose therapy with autografting shows the greatest promise in the treatment of patients at relapse, with as many as half of patients event-free at several years follow-up. In addition, with greater experience, the morbidity and mortality associated with the procedure continue to decline. Predictors of improved outcome include less disease at time of transplant [21,22], fewer relapses [22,23], sensitive disease at time of transplant [22,24], better performance status [22], nodal disease, and absence of B symptoms at relapse [25]. The series by Reece *et al.* [25] consists only of patients in first relapse. With a median follow-up of 2.3 years, it is notable that 64% of the entire group is free from progression (FFP), with over 80% FFP among those patients with an initial remission greater than a year. Results such as these suggest that high-dose therapy and autografting should be used early after first relapse when more favorable characteristics are likely to be present. Despite the favorable results with high-dose therapy and autografting, few randomized studies have confirmed the apparent superiority of this approach. Some of the most compelling data come from a randomized study by the German Hodgkin's Study Group and the European Group for Blood and Marrow Transplantation [26]. A total of 161 patients with relapsed Hodgkin's disease received four courses of Dexa-BEAM or two courses of Dexa-BEAM followed by high-dose therapy (BEAM) with stem-cell support. Time to treatment failure among chemotherapy sensitive patients favored the high dose therapy arm, although overall survival did not differ. In spite of the favorable results with high-dose therapy and autografting, very few randomized studies have confirmed the apparent superiority of this approach. Yuen *et al.* [27] compared a group of patients treated with high-dose therapy who developed refractory disease or who were at first relapse with a matched group of patients who received conventional treatment. The group that received high-dose therapy had a better outcome overall and among patients who had refractory disease or an early relapse. However, there was no significant difference in outcome among patients who relapsed more than a year after initial therapy. Longer follow-up is needed to see if the apparent improvements will be sustained over time and also to better characterize long-term side effects associated with high-dose therapy and autografting.

SIDE EFFECTS OF TREATMENT

The satisfaction with success in the treatment of Hodgkin's disease over the last several decades must be tempered by increasing recognition of long-term side effects that limit the quality of life and survival of patients cured of their disease. Leukemias and second malignancies are among the most problematic of treatment-related side effects. Cardiac, pulmonary, and other organ toxicities also limit the quality of life of long-term survivors.

The risk of secondary leukemia is related to the extent of prior alkylator therapy. Recent estimates from Van Leeuwen *et al.* [28] show an eightfold risk of leukemia among patients treated with six or fewer cycles of nitrogen mustard plus procarbazine, with an increase to 40-fold among patients treated with more than six cycles. Whether or not the addition of radiotherapy to chemotherapy increases the leukemia risk is controversial [29,30], as is that of additional increased risk among patients who have had a splenectomy or splenic radiation [28,30,31]. Most patients in the series that reported an increased incidence of leukemia were treated with six or more cycles of MOPP chemotherapy, which is not currently favored. The incidence of leukemia among patients treated in the 1980s [28] or with ABVD [29] appears to be significantly less, though longer follow-up is needed to characterize the risk more completely.

The relative risks for non-Hodgkin's lymphoma, lung cancers, gastrointestinal cancers, urogenital cancers, melanoma, soft tissue sarcomas, and thyroid cancer [32] also are increased among Hodgkin's disease patients compared with the general population. Van Leeuwen *et al.* [33] found that the risk of lung cancer was related to the use of radiotherapy without additional risk from chemotherapy. Hancock *et al.* [34] found a sevenfold relative risk for breast cancer among patients younger than 30 years of age who had received radiation. The addition of MOPP increased the relative risk even further. Mauch *et al.* [35] confirmed the dramatically increased risk for breast cancer among younger women and showed that the risk of all second solid tumors continued to rise even after 15 years follow-up.

Hancock *et al.* [36] found about a threefold risk of cardiac death and acute myocardial infarction among patients who received more than 3000 cGy of mediastinal irradiation. The relative risk also increased for patients less than 20 years of age and for those with minimal cardiac blocking.

The risk of infertility is related to the chemotherapy regimen employed. MOPP chemotherapy is associated with a very high rate of azoospermia in males and amenorrhea in females. ABVD is associated with a much lower rate of infertility. MOPP/ABVD combinations have been associated with about 50% azoospermia even after prolonged follow-up [37].

Pulmonary toxicity associated with mantle radiation and chemotherapy has been found in up to 70% of patients by CT scanning shortly after starting radiotherapy [38]. Horning *et al.* [39] found a 20% decrease in pulmonary function tests at less than 15 months' follow-up among patients treated with mediastinal radiation.

In summary, the improvements in the treatment of Hodgkin's disease have come with a number of side effects that limit the quality and quantity of life after successful treatment of the disease. Increasing recognition of these effects should help to guide the development of safer and equally effective treatments.

REFERENCES

1. Medeiros L, Greiner T: Hodgkin's disease. *Cancer* 1995, 75:357–369.
2. MacMahon B: Epidemiological evidence of the nature of Hodgkin's disease. *Cancer* 1957, 10:1045–1054.
3. Harris N, Jaffe E, Diebold J, *et al.*: World Health Organization Classification of Neoplastic Diseases of the Hematopoietic and Lymphoid Tissues: report of the Clinical Advisory Committee Meeting, Airlie House, Virginia, November 1997. *J Clin Oncol* 1999, 17:3835–3849.
4. Lister TA, Crowther D, Sutcliffe SB, *et al.*: Report of a committee convened to discuss the evaluation and staging of patients with Hodgkin's disease: Cotswolds meeting. *J Clin Oncol* 1989, 7:1630–1636.
5. Hasenclever D, Diehl V: A prognostic score for advanced Hodgkin's disease. *N Engl J Med* 1998, 339:1506–1514.
6. Vijayakumar S, Myrianthopoulos L: An updated dose-response analysis in Hodgkin's disease. *Radiother Oncol* 1992, 24:1–13.

7. Longo DL, Young RC, Wesley M, *et al.*: Twenty years of MOPP therapy for Hodgkin's disease. *J Clin Oncol* 1986, 4:1295–1306.

8. Bonadonna G, Santoro A, Gianni AM, *et al.*: Primary and salvage chemotherapy in advanced Hodgkin's disease: the Milan Cancer Institute experience. *Ann Oncol* 1991, 1:9–16.

9. Canellos GP, Anderson JR, Propert KJ, *et al.*: Chemotherapy of advanced Hodgkin's disease with MOPP, ABVD, or MOPP alternating with ABVD. *N Engl J Med* 1992, 327:1478–1484.

10. Santoro A, Bonfante V, Viviani S, *et al.*: Decrease in mortality rate by Hodgkin's disease after ABVD vs MOPP: 10-year results. *Proc ASCO* 1991, 10:281.

11. Somers R, Carde P, Henry-Amar M, *et al.*: A randomized study in stage IIIB and IV Hodgkin's disease comparing eight courses of MOPP versus an alteration of MOPP with ABVD: a European Organization for Research and Treatment of Cancer Lymphoma Cooperative Group and Groupe Pierre-et-Marie-Curie controlled clinical trial. *J Clin Oncol* 1994, 12:279–287.

12. Connors JM, Klimo P, Adams G, *et al.*: Treatment of advanced Hodgkin's disease with chemotherapy comparison of MOPP/ABV hybrid regimen with alternating courses of MOPP and ABVD: a report from the National Cancer Institute of Canada Clinical Trials Group. *J Clin Oncol* 1997, 15:1638–1645.

13. Viviani S, Bonadonna G, Santoro A, *et al.*: Alternating versus hybrid MOPP and ABVD combinations in advanced Hodgkin's disease: ten year results. *J Clin Oncol* 1996, 14:1421–1430.

14. Glick J, Tsiatis A, Schilsky R, *et al.*: A randomized phase III trial of MOPP/ABV hybrid vs sequential MOPP/ABVD in advanced Hodgkin's disease: preliminary results of the Intergroup trial. *Proc ASCO* 1991, 10:271.

15. Duggan D, Petroni G, Johnson J, *et al.*: MOPP/ABV versus ABVD for advanced Hodgkin's disease: a preliminary report of CALGB 8952 (with SWOG, ECOG, NCIC). *Proc Am Soc Clin Oncol* 1997 16:5a.

16. Horning S, Hoppe R, Breslin S, *et al.*: Brief chemotherapy (Stanford V) and involved field radiotherapy are highly effective for advanced Hodgkin's disease. *Proc ASCO* 1998, 17:16.

17. Diehl V, Franklin J, Tesch H, *et al.*: Dose escalation of BEACOPP chemotherapy for advanced Hodgkin's disease in the HD9 trial of the German Hodgkin's Study Group (GHSG). *Proc ASCO* 2000, 19:4.

18. Tesch H, Sieber M, Ruffer J, *et al.*: Second interim analysis of the HD7 trial of the GHSG: 2 cycles ABVD plus extended field radiotherapy is more effective than radiotherapy alone in early stage HD. *Proc ASH* 1999, 94:268.

19. Rueda A, Alba E, Ribelles N, *et al.*: Six cycles of ABVD in the treatment of stage I and II Hodgkin's lymphoma: a pilot study. *J Clin Oncol* 1997, 15:1118–1122.

20. Horning S, Hoppe R, Breslin S, *et al.*: Very brief (8 week) chemotherapy and low dose (30 Gy) radiotherapy for limited stage Hodgkin's disease: preliminary results of the Stanford-Kaiser G4 study of Stanford V + RT. *Proc ASH* 1999, 94:387.

21. Rapoport AP, Rowe JM, Kouides PA, *et al.*: One hundred autotransplants for relapsed or refractory Hodgkin's disease and lymphoma: value of pretransplant disease status for predicting outcome. *J Clin Oncol* 1993, 11:2351–2361.

22. Anderson JE, Litzow MR, Appelbaum FR, *et al.*: Allogeneic, syngeneic, and autologous marrow transplantation for Hodgkin's disease: the 21-year Seattle experience. *J Clin Oncol* 1993, 11:2342–2350.

23. Armitage J: Early bone marrow transplantation in Hodgkin's disease. *Ann Oncol* 1994, 5:161–163.

24. Weaver CH, Petersen FB, Appelbaum FR, *et al.*: High-dose fractionated total-body irradiation, etoposide, and cylcophosphamide followed by autologous stem-cell support in patients with malignant lymphoma. *J Clin Oncol* 1994, 12:2559–2566.

25. Reece DE, Connors JM, Spinelli JJ, *et al.*: Intensive therapy with cyclophosphamide, carmustine, etoposide ± cisplatin, and autologous bone marrow transplantation for Hodgkin's disease in first relapse after combination chemotherapy. *Blood* 1994, 83:1193–1199.

26. Schmitz N, Sextro M, Pfistner B, *et al.*: High dose therapy followed by hematopoietic stem cell transplantation for relapsed chemosensitive Hodgkin's disease: final results of a randomized GHSG and EBMT trial (HD-R1). *Proc ASCO* 1999, 18:2.

27. Yuen AR, Rosenberg SA, Hoppe RT, *et al.*: Comparison between conventional salvage therapy and high-dose therapy with autografting for recurrent or refractory Hodgkin's disease. *Blood* 1997, 89:814–822.

28. van Leeuwen FE, Chorus AM, van den Belt-Dusebout AW, *et al.*: Leukemia risk following Hodgkin's disease: relation to cumulative dose of alkylating agents, treatment with teniposide combinations, number of episodes of chemotherapy, and bone marrow damage. *J Clin Oncol* 1994, 12:1063–1073.

29. Biti G, Cellai E, Magrini S, *et al.*: Second solid tumors and leukemia after treatment for Hodgkin's disease: an analysis of 1121 patients from a single institution. *Int J Radiation Oncol Biol Biophysics* 1994, 29:25–31.

30. Dietrich PY, Henry-Amar M, Cosset JM, *et al.*: Second primary cancers in patients continuously disease-free from Hodgkin's disease: a protective role for the spleen? *Blood* 1994, 84:1209–1215.

31. Hudson B, Hudson V, Linch D, Anderson L: Late mortality in young BNLI patients cured of Hodgkin's disease. *Ann Oncol* 1994, 5:65–66.

32. Sankila R, Garwicz S, Olsen JH, *et al.*: Risk of subsequent malignant neoplasms among 1641 Hodgkin's disease patients diagnosed in childhood and adolescence: a population-based cohort study in the five Nordic countries. *J Clin Oncol* 1996, 14:1442–1446.

33. van Leeuwen FE, Klokman WJ, Hagenbeek A, *et al.*: Second cancer risk following Hodgkin's disease: a 20-year follow-up study. *J Clin Oncol* 1994, 112:312–325.

34. Hancock SL, Tucker MA, Hoppe RT: Breast cancer after treatment of Hodgkin's disease. *J Natl Cancer Inst* 1993, 85:25–31.

35. Mauch PM, Kalish LA, Marcus KC, *et al.*: Second malignancies after treatment for laparotomy staged IA-IIIB Hodgkin's disease: long-term analysis of risk factors and outcome. *Blood* 1996, 87:3625–3632.

36. Hancock SL, Donaldson SS, Hoppe RT: Cardiac disease following treatment of Hodgkin's disease in children and adolescents. *J Clin Oncol* 1993, 11:1208–1215.

37. Viviani S, Ragni G, Santoro A, *et al.*: Testicular dysfunction in Hodgkin's disease before and after treatment. *Eur J Cancer* 1991, 27:1389–1392.

38. Mah K, Keane T, Van Dyk J, *et al.*: Quantitative effect of combined chemotherapy and fractionated radiotherapy on the incidence of radiation-induced lung damage: a prospective clinical study. *Int J Radiation Oncol Biol Biophysics* 1994, 28:563–574.

39. Horning SJ, Adhikari A, Rizk N, *et al.*: Effect of treatment for Hodgkin's disease on pulmonary function: results of a prospective study. *J Clin Oncol* 1994, 12:297–305.

ABVD
(Doxorubicin, Bleomycin, Vinblastine, Dacarbazine)

The ABVD regimen was developed to treat patients in whom MOPP chemotherapy had failed, and thus includes agents non–cross-resistant to the components of MOPP. The efficacy of ABVD was proven first as a second-line therapy in MOPP failures and later as superior to MOPP in randomized trials. The additional advantage of ABVD is in a lower incidence of sterility and very rare incidence of secondary leukemia. However, cardiac and pulmonary toxicities are associated with the use of doxorubicin and bleomycin components of the regimen.

CANDIDATES FOR TREATMENT
Patients with bulky disease or stage III or IV Hodgkin's disease

SPECIAL PRECAUTIONS
Patients with abnormal left ventricular function or history of coronary artery disease, significantly impaired respiratory function, or elevated bilirubin

ALTERNATIVE THERAPIES
MOPP/ABVD, MOPP/ABV, Stanford V

DOSAGE AND SCHEDULING

Doxorubicin 25 mg/m² IVP d 1, 15	■														■
Bleomycin 10 U/m² IVP d 1, 15	■														■
Vinblastine 6 mg/m² IVP d 1, 15	■														■
Dacarbazine 375 mg/m² IVP d 1, 15	■														■
CBC with diff. d 1,15	□														□
SMAC d 1	□														
Day	1	2	3	4	5	6	7	8	9	10	11	12	13	14	15

28-d cycle. Pulmonary function tests with DLCO approximately q 2–3 cycles or sooner if new, noninfectious pulmonary signs or symptoms develop; PA and lateral CXR q 2 cycles.

DOSAGE MODIFICATIONS

WBC	Platelets	Dose Adjustment [25]
>4000	>130,000	100% of all drugs
3000–3999	100,000–129,000	50% doxorubicin, vinblastine, & dacarbazine
2000–2999	80,000–99,000	50% dacarbazine & 25% doxorubicin & vinblastine
1500–1999	50,000–79,000	25% dacarbazine & NO doxorubicin or vinblastine
<1500	<50,000	NO doxorubicin, vinblastine or dacarbazine

RECENT EXPERIENCE AND RESPONSE RATES

Study	Evaluable Patients	CR, %	FFS, %	OS, %
Bonadonna et al. [6]	118	92*	81 (FFP)	77 (7 y)
Canellos et al. [7]	115	82	61	73 (5 y)

Includes use of radiotherapy.
CR—complete response; FFS—failure-free survival; FFP—freedom from progression; OS—overall survival.

MOPP AND ABVD

The proven activity of MOPP and ABVD as non–cross-resistant regimens led researchers to combine the two regimens in alternating fashion. The strategy was based on the Goldie-Coldman hypothesis that concludes that as many active drugs as possible should be administered as early in treatment as possible to prevent cells resistant to one drug from developing resistance to others. A superior response rate and failure-free survival of alternating MOPP and ABVD over MOPP alone has been observed in a number of studies, but a superior outcome of MOPP with ABVD over ABVD alone has not been observed.

CANDIDATES FOR TREATMENT
Patients with bulky disease or stage III or IV Hodgkin's disease

SPECIAL PRECAUTIONS
Patients with abnormal ventricular function or history of coronary artery disease, significantly impaired respiratory function, or elevated bilirubin; MAO inhibitor precautions with procarbazine

ALTERNATIVE THERAPIES
MOPP/ABV, ABVD, Stanford V

DOSAGE AND SCHEDULING

MOPP

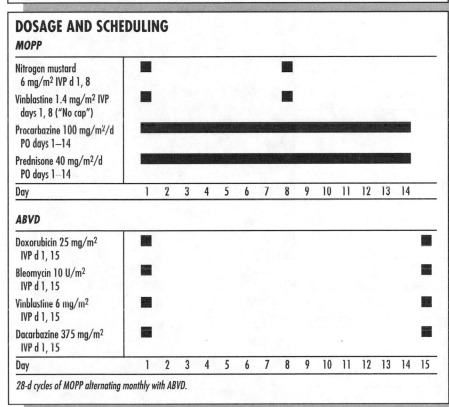

Nitrogen mustard
6 mg/m² IVP d 1, 8

Vinblastine 1.4 mg/m² IVP days 1, 8 ("No cap")

Procarbazine 100 mg/m²/d PO days 1–14

Prednisone 40 mg/m²/d PO days 1–14

Day   1 2 3 4 5 6 7 8 9 10 11 12 13 14

ABVD

Doxorubicin 25 mg/m² IVP d 1, 15

Bleomycin 10 U/m² IVP d 1, 15

Vinblastine 6 mg/m² IVP d 1, 15

Dacarbazine 375 mg/m² IVP d 1, 15

Day   1 2 3 4 5 6 7 8 9 10 11 12 13 14 15

28-d cycles of MOPP alternating monthly with ABVD.

RECENT EXPERIENCES AND RESPONSE RATES

Study	Evaluable Patients	CR, %	FFS, %	OS, %
Santoro et al. [8]	45	89	61 (FFP)	69 (10 y)
Connors et al. [10]	141	83	70 (FFP)	84 (4 y)
Canellos et al. [7]	123	83	65	75 (5 y)
Somers et al. [9]	96	59	60	65 (6 y)

CR—complete response; FFS—failure-free survival; FFP—freedom from progression; OS—overall survival.

MOPP/ABV HYBRID

The MOPP/ABV regimen was also developed according to the Goldie-Coldman theory. In this regimen, all agents are given by day 8 of the 28-d cycle, in contrast to MOPP alternating with ABVD, in which all agents are not introduced until the second month. The hybrid regimen was shown to be as effective as alternating MOPP-ABVD by Connors et al. [12] and superior to sequential MOPP-ABVD in regard to response and survival.

CANDIDATES FOR TREATMENT
Patients with bulky disease or stage III or IV Hodgkin's disease

ALTERNATIVE THERAPIES
MOPP/ABVD, ABVD, Stanford V

DOSAGE AND SCHEDULING

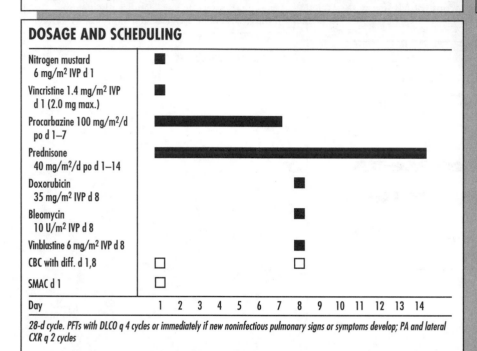

Nitrogen mustard
6 mg/m² IVP d 1

Vincristine 1.4 mg/m² IVP
d 1 (2.0 mg max.)

Procarbazine 100 mg/m²/d
po d 1–7

Prednisone
40 mg/m²/d po d 1–14

Doxorubicin
35 mg/m² IVP d 8

Bleomycin
10 U/m² IVP d 8

Vinblastine 6 mg/m² IVP d 8

CBC with diff. d 1,8

SMAC d 1

Day   1 2 3 4 5 6 7 8 9 10 11 12 13 14

28-d cycle. PFTs with DLCO q 4 cycles or immediately if new noninfectious pulmonary signs or symptoms develop; PA and lateral CXR q 2 cycles

RECENT EXPERIENCES AND RESPONSE RATES

Study	Evaluable Patients	CR, %	FFS, %	OS, %
Glick et al. [11]	370	82	77	89 (2.5 y)
Conners et al. [10]	146	85	77 (FFP)	84 (4 y)

CR—complete response; FFP—freedom from progression; FFS—failure-free survival; OS—overall survival.

STANFORD V

This novel chemotherapy regimen was designed to shorten the period of treatment, decrease the total doses of agents with the most significant long-term toxicities (alkylating agents, doxorubicin, and bleomycin), and maintain dose intensity. Adjuvant radiotherapy was administered to sites of bulky disease. The investigators at Stanford have reported excellent results in patients with bulky mediastinal involvement or with stage III or IV disease [16]. However, longer follow-up is needed, and the regimen should be tested in other centers and in a randomized comparison to confirm the very favorable results thus far.

CANDIDATES FOR TREATMENT
Patients with bulky disease or stage III or IV Hodgkin's disease

SPECIAL PRECAUTIONS
Patients with abnormal left ventricular function or history of coronary artery disease, significantly impaired respiratory function, or elevated bilirubin; elderly patients (constipation, obstipation)

ALTERNATIVE THERAPIES
MOPP/ABVD, MOPP/ABV, ABVD

TOXICITIES
Etoposide: moderately severe nausea and vomiting, hair loss

DRUG INTERACTIONS
As with ABVD regimen

NURSING INTERVENTIONS
As with ABVD regimen

PATIENT INFORMATION
As with ABVD regimen

DOSAGE AND SCHEDULING

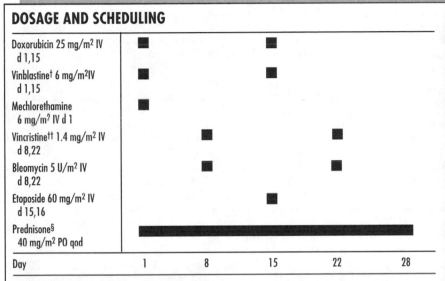

Doxorubicin 25 mg/m² IV
d 1,15

Vinblastine† 6 mg/m²IV
d 1,15

Mechlorethamine
6 mg/m² IV d 1

Vincristine†† 1.4 mg/m² IV
d 8,22

Bleomycin 5 U/m² IV
d 8,22

Etoposide 60 mg/m² IV
d 15,16

Prednisone§
40 mg/m² PO qod

Day   1   8   15   22   28

*Treatment repeated every 28 d for a total of 3 cycles.
†Vinblastine dose decreased to 4 mg/m², and vincristine dose decreased to 1 mg/m² during cycle 3 for patients ≥ 50 y of age.
§Tapered by 10 mg qod starting at week 10.
†Maximum dose, 2.0 mg

RECENT EXPERIENCES AND RESPONSE RATES

Study	Evaluable Patients	FFS, %	OS, %
Horning *et al.* [16]	121	89	95 (5 y)

CR—complete response; FFS—failure-free survival; OS—overall survival.

Non-Hodgkin's lymphomas (NHL) are a heterogeneous group of lymphoid malignancies defined by characteristic lymph node patterns and histology. Most NHL are B cell in origin, with fewer of the T-cell phenotype. Each histologic entity of NHL has a distinct clinical presentation, natural history, and survival pattern [1]. Several classification schema have previously been used to organize the different histologic entities of NHL. The International Working Formulation [2] recognizes three prognostic categories including those with low-, intermediate-, and high-grade histologies. Newer schemas like the REAL [3] and WHO classifications [4] use morphology, immunophenotyping, genetic and clinical features to characterize subtypes of NHL. The proposed WHO classification categorizes lymphoid neoplasms into B-cell and T-cell/NK cell neoplasms [4,5].

ETIOLOGY AND RISK FACTORS

Although the specific cause of NHL remains unknown, both genetic and environmental factors have been implicated. Established genetic factors include X-linked lymphoproliferative syndrome. Environmental exposures to viruses (eg, Epstein-Barr virus [EBV]), and to irradiation are also purported causative factors. Mucosa-associated lymphoid tissue (MALT) lymphomas are associated with *Helicobacter pylori* infection [6]. The human T-cell lymphotrophic virus (HTLV-1) retrovirus is associated with adult T-cell leukemia/lymphoma, a form of peripheral T-cell lymphoma. HIV-associated NHLs are related to retroviral infection as a result of virus-associated immunodeficiency rather than a direct tumor-promoting effect by the virus.

DIAGNOSIS

Diagnosis of NHL requires histopathology review in conjunction with immunophenotyping and molecular studies. The architectural pattern, either follicular or diffuse, is generally evaluated on lymph node rather than extranodal specimens. Immunohistochemical stains are used to characterize cell surface markers. Demonstration of B-cell clonality may be performed on fixed tissue using immunoperoxidase methods, by Southern blot analysis or by polymerase chain reaction (PCR) analysis. Identification of T-cell clonality is performed using molecular studies of fresh tissue for the T-cell receptor gene rearrangement. Specific immunophenotypic patterns may help distinguish histologic subtypes, which appear morphologically similar, such as mantle cell lymphoma and small lymphocytic lymphoma/chronic lymphocytic leukemia.

STAGING

After the diagnosis of NHL has been established by pathology review, a staging evaluation is performed to determine the extent of disease involvement. The Ann Arbor staging classification for Hodgkin's disease is often applied to NHL with some modifications. Standard staging studies for NHL are provided in Table 19-1. Diagnostic staging studies include a complete blood profile and lactate dehydrogenase (LDH), CT scans, and bone marrow biopsy. In patients with aggressive NHLs, a gallium scan is routinely performed at diagnosis to determine sites of disease and to follow response to treatment. The positron emission tomography (PET) scan is a newer dynamic imaging study being used in NHL. Although it appears to be a sensitive nuclear imaging tool, the role of PET scans in the management of NHL has not yet been clearly defined [7,8].

INDOLENT LYMPHOMAS

Follicular Lymphoma (Grades 1 and 2), Small Lymphocytic Lymphoma, and Marginal Zone Lymphoma

In the REAL and WHO classifications, several histologic subtypes correspond to the low-grade histologies defined in the Working Formulation. Small lymphocytic lymphoma is further subclassified into small lymphocytic lymphoma (chronic lymphocytic leukemia [CLL] type), lymphoplasmacytic lymphoma, and marginal zone lymphoma (nodal, splenic, or MALT types). It is now recognized that small lymphocytic lymphoma and CLL represent different clinical presentations of the same disease. Lymphoplasmacytic lymphoma is also considered a small lymphocytic lymphoma with plasmacytic differentiation and association with a IgM paraproteinemia [4].

Follicular lymphomas are subclassified into three histologic grades (grades 1, 2, and 3) according to the number of large cells present [4,9]. Follicular lymphomas—grades 1 and 2 are thought to be closely related to each other, and generally follow an indolent course of disease. Follicular lymphoma grade 3, while retaining a similar overall survival pattern as the lower grades, tends toward earlier relapses and is often treated like other large cell lymphomas (see section on Aggressive Lymphomas). The reciprocal t[14;18] translocation is identified in most cases of follicular lymphoma. This chromosomal aberration causes dysregulation and overexpression of *BCL-2*, an antiapoptosis oncogene.

Indolent lymphomas are generally considered incurable and follow a continual pattern of relapse despite good response to treatment [10]. They typically present in advanced stage with generalized adenopathy with or without bone marrow involvement. Hepatosplenomegaly or extranodal involvement (gastrointestinal [GI] tract, lung, skin, bone or epidural) may also occur. Gastrointestinal tract involvement is particularly common in MALT lymphomas, which is associated with *Helicobacter pylori* infection. Despite frequent bone marrow disease, meningeal involvement rarely occurs. Peripheral blood lymphocytosis is fairly common, as is the presence of a monoclonal gammopathy. Approximately 30% to 40% of patients with indolent lymphoma will eventually undergo histologic transformation to an aggressive non-Hodgkin's lymphoma [11,12].

Table 19-1. Diagnostic and Staging Evaluation for Non-Hodgkin's Lymphoma

Physical examination: examine peripheral lymph nodes, tonsils, spleen, and liver

Blood work: complete blood count and differential, peripheral blood smear, lactate dehydrogenase, renal function, liver function

Radiographic imaging

  CT scans of chest, abdomen, pelvis

  Gallium scan (for aggressive lymphomas); possibly PET scan

  Selected studies of the CNS, gastrointestinal tract, or bone depending on symptoms

Histopathology

  Lymph node biopsy

  Hematopathology review; classification according to REAL or WHO classification

  Immunophenotyping by immunohistochemistry or flow cytometry

  Bone marrow biopsy

  Cerebrospinal fluid cytology in aggressive lymphomas with documented bone, bone marrow, testicular, nasopharyngeal involvement, or multiple extranodal sites of disease

Few patients with indolent lymphomas present with limited stage disease, defined as clinical stage I or II. Patients with limited sites of disease in the periphery are candidates for regional radiation therapy alone. Treatment outcome is generally excellent with low morbidity [13] (Table 19-2).

Most affected patients present with advanced stage disease, defined as intra-abdominal stage II, III, or IV. Initial delay of chemotherapy does not decrease overall survival of patients with indolent NHL [14,15]. Rather, judicious use of chemotherapy may minimize potential adverse effects while preserving marrow function. Multiple studies have demonstrated that it is feasible to observe patients without directed therapy if there is no indication for treatment. Specific indications for treatment as defined by Groupe d'Etude Lymphomes Folliculaires (GELF) criteria for "high tumor burden" include a mass greater than 7 cm, three nodal sites each greater than 3 cm, systemic symptoms, splenomegaly, or end-organ compromise [16].

Many therapeutic options exist for patients with advanced stage disease. Criteria for selection among them remain controversial because curative treatment has not been established [17]. Standard chemotherapy programs for indolent lymphomas include single alkylating agents such as fludarabine or chlorambucil, or combination regimens like CVP or CHOP (eg, CVP [cyclophosphamide, vincristine, prednisone], or CHOP [cyclophosphamide, doxorubicin, vincristine, prednisone]). Combination chemotherapy with CVP and CHOP results in good clinical responses to treatment. Fludarabine has been shown to be superior to other single agents with response rates of 65% in follicular lymphomas but may cause significant bone marrow suppression [18,19].

Immunotherapy using monoclonal antibodies has also proven to be effective. Rituximab is an unlabeled monoclonal antibody targeting the CD20 antigen found on B lymphocytes. In a phase III trial evaluating rituximab as a single agent in low-grade or follicular lymphoma, the overall response rate was 48% [20]. Rituximab is at present approved for use in relapsed low-grade NHL. Combinations of chemotherapy with monoclonal antibody (eg, CHOP and rituximab) offer preliminary evidence of efficacy [21]. The GELA study group recently reported improvement in response rates with the addition of rituximab to CHOP compared with CHOP alone (CR, 76% vs 60%; P value 0.004). Although follow-up is short, there is preliminary evidence of improved survival with CHOP/rituximab [22]. Radioimmunotherapy agents are composed of radionuclides conjugated to monoclonal antibodies used to target radiation to tumor tissue. Radiolabeled monoclonal antibodies, such as ^{131}I tositumomab and ^{90}Y ibritumomab, are currently under investigation [23,24].

Autologous stem-cell transplantation (ASCT) has been evaluated in younger patients with follicular lymphoma in second or later remission [25,26]. Promising durable remissions have been reported after conventional allotransplantation of refractory indolent lymphoma [27]. Miniallogeneic bone marrow transplantation using nonmyeloablative doses of cytotoxic chemotherapy is under investigation, which appears promising with possibly less toxicity [28,29].

AGGRESSIVE LYMPHOMAS

Diffuse Large B-cell Lymphoma, Peripheral T-cell Lymphoma, Anaplastic Large Cell Lymphoma, and Follicular Lymphoma (Grade 3)

Aggressive NHLs are composed primarily of diffuse large B-cell lymphoma, but also include peripheral T-cell lymphomas, anaplastic large cell lymphomas, and follicular lymphoma (grade 3). Diffuse large B-cell lymphoma according to the WHO criteria includes diffuse large, diffuse mixed, and immunoblastic lymphomas previously described in the Working Formulation. Primary mediastinal large B-cell lymphoma is represented as a subcategory of diffuse large B-cell lymphoma in the present schema. Peripheral T-cell lymphomas have poor overall survival compared with diffuse large B-cell lymphomas, whereas anaplastic large cell lymphomas (T- or null-cell types) have overall survival similar to diffuse large B-cell lymphoma [1]. The t(2;5) translocation in T-cell anaplastic large cell lymphoma is an aberration of NPM-ALK.

Aggressive lymphomas share common clinical characteristics of male preponderance, presentation in middle age, rapidly enlarging adenopathy, and advanced stage. Masses are often bulky, particularly in the mediastinum or abdomen. Large masses in these sites may cause superior vena cava syndrome, tracheal compression, or ureteral compression. Extranodal sites often cause symptoms, such as ulcerated gastrointestinal lesions or lytic bone lesions. Lymphomatous meningitis may be detected in the presence of bone marrow, testicular or nasopharyngeal involvement.

The International Prognostic Index (IPI) for Non-Hodgkin's Lymphoma [30] describes five prognostic variables that predict outcome based on pretreatment clinical characteristics. Adverse prognostic variables include age over 60 years, elevated serum lactate dehydrogenase, poor performance status, advanced stage, and two or more extranodal sites of disease. Patients are stratified to low, low-intermediate, high-intermediate, or high-risk categories based on the number of poor prognostic features. Patients with IPI 4 are poor risk, and have significantly shortened survival (Table 19-3).

Table 19-2. Treatment Strategy for Indolent Lymphomas

Stages I and peripheral II: regional radiation therapy
Stages II (intra-abdominal), III, IV
  Consider observation
  Participation in a clinical trial of immune strategies
  Palliative chemotherapy (chlorambucil, fludarabine, or CVP)
  CHOP alone or with rituximab

Table 19-3. International Prognostic Index for Diffuse Large B-cell Lymphomas

Adverse Prognostic Features	Risk Group	Adverse Prognostic Factors	5-Year Survival, %
Age > 60 y	Low	0 or 1	73
Elevated serum LDH	Low–intermediate	2	51
Karnofsky Performance Score	High–intermediate	3	43
Advanced stage (III or IV)	High	4 or 5	26
Extranodal sites (> 1)			

Aggressive diffuse lymphomas are potentially curable. A curative outcome is obtained in approximately half of patients after first-line therapy. CHOP remains the standard first-line chemotherapy regimen. Several second-generation combination chemotherapy regimens have been evaluated; none has been proven superior to CHOP chemotherapy [31]. Patients with regional disease involvement (clinical stage I or II) may be treated with combination chemotherapy with or without regional irradiation. A randomized phase III study compared CHOP with CHOP plus involved field radiotherapy for early- stage disease with the finding of improved survival with combined modality therapy [32,33]. It is therefore feasible to give short-course chemotherapy followed by involved field radiotherapy for regional disease (Table 19-4).

Autologous stem cell transplantation (ASCT) in patients with high-risk IPI scores has been studied as upfront treatment in multiple clinical trials. Slow responders to CHOP, defined as incomplete responders to four cycles, were randomly assigned to receive four additional cycles of CHOP versus high-dose therapy followed by ASCT. No difference was found in the two treatment programs, but patients were not stratified into prognostic categories according to the IPI [34]. The various clinical data from multiple different trials in the upfront setting are currently under investigation.

ASCT has also been studied extensively for treatment of relapsed or refractory disease. Patients with chemosensitive disease in first or second relapse are candidates for ASCT. The PARMA trial evaluated patients with chemosensitive disease and demonstrated improved responses and overall survival for patients who received transplantation rather than additional chemotherapy [35,36]. The most significant predictor of a favorable outcome from ASCT is chemosensitivity at the time of transplantation. High-dose therapy has not proven to be useful for chemorefractory disease in first or subsequent relapse [37].

Cytoreductive regimens, such as DHAP [38] or ICE (ifosfamide, carboplatin, etoposide) [39], are given before the conditioning regimen and ASCT. Cytoreduction serves several purposes: to identify patients with chemosensitive disease, to allow a transplant to be performed with minimal disease burden, and to decrease potential contamination of the stem cell product. In addition, cytoreductive regimens together with cytokines are used to mobilize stem cells for collection.

Mantle Cell Lymphoma

Mantle cell lymphoma is a separately recognized histology incorporated into the REAL and WHO classifications, previously termed diffuse small cleaved cell lymphoma in the working formulation.

Table 19-4. Treatment Strategy for Aggressive Diffuse Lymphomas

Stages I and peripheral stage II: short-course CHOP or other doxorubicin-containing regimen with involved field radiation therapy

Stages II, III, and IV

  CHOP or other doxorubicin-containing regimen

    Central nervous system prophylaxis for patients with multiple extranodal sites, involvement of bone, bone marrow, testes, or paranasal region

    Tumor lysis precautions for bulky disease

    Localized GI tract involvement may be complicated by bleeding or perforation but rarely requires surgical resection

    Consider autologous stem cell transplantation for primary refractory or relapsed disease

Mantle cell lymphomas have aggressive disease features and often present in advanced stage with diffuse adenopathy, as well as bone marrow, peripheral blood, and splenic involvement. Extranodal disease sites are also common; diffuse GI tract involvement is referred to as lymphomatous polyposis. The typical cytogenetic aberration in mantle cell lymphoma is a reciprocal t(11;14) translocation causing dysregulation of *BCL-1* oncogene and overexpression of cyclin D1.

Mantle cell lymphomas have poor overall and failure-free survival rates [1]. No convincing evidence shows that conventional chemotherapy is curative, because there is no plateau in the overall survival curve. Investigational therapy with upfront transplantation appears promising, with durable remissions reported out to 4 years [40,41]. Single agent 2-CDA is a useful, well-tolerated palliative single drug [42].

Lymphoblastic Lymphoma

Lymphoblastic lymphoma shares similar features with acute lymphoblastic leukemia (ALL). This disease often presents with large mediastinal masses, and with leukemic as well as CNS involvement. Most lymphoblastic lymphomas are of immature T-cell origin, although some may have pre-B cell phenotypes. Lymphoblastic lymphoma is treated in the same manner as ALL with induction, intensive consolidation, and maintenance regimens.

Diffuse Small Noncleaved Cell Lymphomas (Burkitt's and Burkitt's-like)

Diffuse small noncleaved cell lymphomas (Burkitt's and non-Burkitt's) are identified as high-grade lymphomas in the International Working Formulation [2]. Small noncleaved cell lymphomas are characterized by young age, male preponderance, rapidly enlarging bulky adenopathy, and frequent bone marrow and meningeal involvement. The t[8;14] translocation identified in Burkitt's lymphoma causes dysregulation of the c-*myc* oncogene.

Small, noncleaved cell lymphomas have increased incidence within concurrent HIV infection. In this setting, sites of disease may be unusual, including the GI tract, brain, and soft tissue. Treatment of Burkitt's and Burkitt's-like lymphoma requires rapid initiation of high dose, short-course combination chemotherapy with central nervous system (CNS) prophylaxis [43,44]. When the patient is HIV positive, chemotherapy should be administered in conjunction with highly active antiretroviral therapy (HAART). Bulky disease may be associated with tumor lysis syndrome. Attention to hydration, alkalinization, prophylactic allopurinol, and monitoring of renal function, calcium, electrolytes, and phosphate balance during and after chemotherapy infusion are therefore necessary. With HIV infection, use of intensive chemotherapy may be significantly complicated by opportunistic infections. Use of HAART has decreased the incidence of opportunistic infections [45]. There have been anecdotal reports of HIV-infected patients who have achieved spontaneous regression of NHL after being treated with HAART [46].

HTLV-1 Associated Adult T-cell Leukemia/Lymphoma (Subtype of Peripheral T-cell Lymphoma)

HTLV-1–associated lymphomas are a subtype of mature peripheral T-cell neoplasm in the current WHO classification [4]. Many patients present clinically with the acute form, which is characterized by rapid onset, lytic bone lesions, subcutaneous nodules, hypercalcemia, and leukemic phase. The histologic subtype is typically a diffuse large cell or immunoblastic lymphoma. Prognosis for patients with aggressive presentations is poor, with only transient responses to intensive regimens. In southern Japan, where HTLV-1 incidence is endemic, a broader clinical spectrum is seen with both indolent and aggressive clinical and histologic subtypes.

REFERENCES

1. Armitage JO, DD Weisenburger: New approach to classifying non-Hodgkin's lymphomas: clinical features of the major histologic subtypes. *J Clin Oncol* 1998, 16:2780–2795.

2. National Cancer Institute: Summary and description of a working formulation for clinical usage: the Non-Hodgkin's Lymphoma Pathologic Classification Project. *Cancer* 1982, 49:2112–2135.

3. Harris NL, ES Jaffe, Stern H, *et al.*: A revised European-American classification of lymphoid neoplasms: a proposal from the International Lymphoma Study Group. *Blood* 1994, 84:1361–1392.

4. Jaffe ES, NL Harris, J Diebold, *et al.*: World Health Organization classification of neoplastic diseases of the hematopoietic and lymphoid tissues: report of the Clinical Advisory Committee Meeting. Airlie House, Virginia, November 1997. *J Clin Oncol* 1997, 17:3835–3849.

5. Harris NL, ES Jaffe, J Diebold, *et al.*: Lymphoma Classification: from controversy to consensus: the REAL and WHO classification of lymphoid neoplasms. *Ann Oncol* 2000, 11 (suppl 1):S3–S10.

6. Parsonnet J, Hansen S, Rodriguez L, *et al.*: Helicobacter pylori infection and gastric lymphoma. *N Engl J Med* 1997, 330:1267–1271.

7. Zinzani PL, Magagnoli M, Chierichetti F, *et al.*: The Role of Positron Emission Tomography [PET] in the Management of Lymphoma Patients. *Ann Oncol* 1999, 10:1181–1184.

8. Jerusalem G, Beguin Y, Fassotte MF, *et al.*: Whole-body positron emission tomography using 18F-fluorodeoxyglucose for post-treatment evaluation of Hodgkin's disease and non-Hodgkin's lymphoma has higher diagnostic and prognostic value than classical computed tomography scan imaging. *Blood* 1999, 94:429–433.

9. Mann R, Berard C: Criteria for the cytologic subclassification of follicular lymphomas: a proposed alternative method. *Hematology Oncology* 1982, 1:187–192.

10. Horning SJ, Rosenberg SA: The natural history of initially untreated low-grade non-Hodgkin's lymphomas. *N Engl J Med* 1994, 311:1471–1475.

11. Yuen AR, Kamel OW, Halpern J, Horning SJ: Long-term survival after histologic transformation of low-grade follicular lymphoma. *J Clin Oncol* 1995, 13:1726–1733.

12. Bastion Y, Sebban C, Berger F, *et al.*: Incidence, predictive factors, and outcome of lymphoma transformation in follicular lymphoma patients. *J Clin Oncol* 1997, 15:1587–1594.

13. McManus MP, Hoppe RT: Is radiotherapy curative for stage I and II low-grade follicular lymphoma? Results of a long-term follow-up study of patients treated at Stanford University. *J Clin Oncol* 1996, 14:1282–1290.

14. Portlock CS, Rosenberg SA: No initial therapy for stage III and IV non-Hodgkin's lymphomas of favorable histologic types. *Ann Intern Med* 1979, 90:10–13.

15. Young RC, Longo DL, Glatstein E, *et al.*: The treatment of indolent lymphomas: watchful waiting vs. aggressive combined modality treatment. *Semin Hematol* 1988, 25:11–16.

16. Brice P, Bastion Y, Lepage E, *et al.*: Comparison in low-tumor burden follicular lymphomas between an initial no-treatment policy, predmustine, or interferon alfa: a randomized study from the Groupe d'Etude des Lymphomes Folliculaires. *J Clin Oncol* 1997, 15:1110–1117.

17. Horning SJ: Treatment approaches to low-grade lymphomas. *N Engl J Med* 1988, 83:881–884.

18. Redman JR, Cabanillas F, Velasquez WS, *et al.*: Phase II trial of fludarabine phosphate in lymphoma: an effective new agent in low-grade lymphoma. *J Clin Oncol* 1992, 10:790–794.

19. Solal-Celigny P, Brice P, Brousse N, *et al.*: Phase II trial of fludarabine monophosphate as first-line treatment in patients with advanced follicular lymphoma: a multicenter study by the Groupe d'Etude des Lymphomes de l'Adulte. *J Clin Oncol* 1996, 14:514–519.

20. McLaughlin P, Grillo-Lopez AJ, Link BK, *et al.*: Rituximab chimeric Anti-CD20 monoclonal antibody therapy for relapsed indolent lymphoma: half of patients respond to a four dose treatment program. *J Clin Oncol* 1998, 16:2825–2833.

21. Maloney DG, Grillo-Lopez AJ, White CA, *et al.*: IDEC-C2B8 [Rituximab] anti-CD20 monoclonal antibody therapy in patients with relapsed low-grade non-Hodgkin's lymphoma. *Blood* 1997, 90:2188–2195.

22. Coiffer B, LePage R, Herbrecht R, *et al.*: Mabthera (Rituximab) plus CHOP is superior to CHOP alone in elderly patients with diffuse large B-cell lymphoma (DLCL): interim results of a randomized GELA trial. *Proc Am Soc Hematol* 2000:abstract 950.

23. Kaminski MS, Zasadny KR, Francis IR, *et al.*: Radioimmunotherapy of B-cell lymphoma with 131-I anti-B1 [anti-CD20] antibody. *N Engl J Med* 1993, 329: 459–465.

24. Witzig TE, White CA, Wiseman GA, *et al.*: Phase I/II of IDEC-Y2B8 radioimmunotherapy for treatment of relapsed or refractory CD20 positive B-cell non-Hodgkin's lymphoma. *J Clin Oncol* 1999, 17:3793–3803.

25. Rohatiner AZ, Johnson PW, Price CG, *et al.*: Myeloablative therapy with autologous bone marrow transplantation as consolidation therapy for recurrent follicular lymphoma. *J Clin Oncol* 1994, 12:1177–1184.

26. Bierman PJ, Vose JM, Anderson JR, *et al.*: High-dose therapy with autologous hematopoietic rescue for follicular low-grade non-Hodgkin's lymphoma. *J Clin Oncol* 1997, 15:445–450.

27. van Besien K, Khouri I, Champlin R, *et al.*: Allogeneic transplantation for low-grade lymphoma: long-term follow-up. *J Clin Oncol* 2000, 18:702–703.

28. Khouri IF, Keating M, Korbling M, *et al.*: Transplant-lite: induction of graft-versus malignancy using fludarabine based non-ablative chemotherapy and allogeneic blood progenitor cell transplantation as treatment for lymphoid malignancies. *J Clin Oncol* 1998, 16:2817–2824.

29. Shimomi A, Giralt S, Khouri I, *et al.*: Allogeneic hematopoietic transplantation for acute and chronic myeloid leukemia: non-myeloablative preparative regimens and induction of the graft-versus-leukemia effect. *Current Oncology Reports* 2000, 2:132–139.

30. Shipp M, Harrington D, Anderson J, *et al.*: A predictive model for aggressive non-Hodgkin's lymphoma: the International Non-Hodgkin's Lymphoma Prognostic Factors Project. *N Engl J Med* 1993, 329:987–994.

31. Fisher RI, Gaynor E, Dahlberg S, *et al.*: Comparison of a standard regimen CHOP with three intensive chemotherapy regimens for advanced non-Hodgkin's lymphoma. *N Engl J Med* 1993, 328:1002–1006.

32. Yahalom J, Varsos G, Fuks Z, *et al.*: Adjuvant cyclophosphamide, doxorubicin, vincristine, and prednisone chemotherapy after radiation therapy in stage I low-grade and intermediate grade non-Hodgkin's lymphoma. *Cancer* 1992, 71:2342–2350.

33. Miller TP, Dahlberg S, Cassady JR, *et al.*: Chemotherapy alone compared with chemotherapy plus radiotherapy for localized intermediate- and high-grade Non-Hodgkin's lymphoma. *N Engl J Med* 1998, 339:21–26.

34. Verdonck LF, van Putten WLJ, Hagenbeek A, *et al.*: Comparison of CHOP chemotherapy with autologous bone marrow transplantation for slowly responding patients with aggressive non-Hodgkin's lymphoma. *N Engl J Med* 1995, 332:1045–1051.

35. Philip T, Guglielmi C, Hagenbeek A, *et al.*: Autologous bone marrow transplantation as compared with salvage chemotherapy in relapses of chemotherapy-sensitive non-Hodgkin's lymphoma. *N Engl J Med* 1995, 333:1540–1545.

36. Philip T, Armitage JO, Spitzer G, *et al.*: High-dose chemotherapy and autologous bone marrow transplantation after failure of conventional chemotherapy in adults with intermediate grade or high grade non-Hodgkin's lymphoma. *N Engl J Med* 1987, 316:1493–1498.

37. Shipp MA, Abeloff MD, Antman KH, *et al.*: International consensus conference on high-dose therapy with hematopoietic stem cell transplantation in aggressive non-Hodgkin's lymphomas: report of the jury. *J Clin Oncol* 1999, 17: 423–429.

38. Velasquez WS, Cabanillas F, *et al.*: Effective salvage therapy for lymphoma with cisplatin in combination with high dose ara-C and dexamethasone [DHAP]. *Blood* 1998, 71:117–122.

39. Moskowitz CH, Bertino JR, Glassman JR, *et al.*: Ifosfamide, carboplatin, and etoposide: a highly effective cytoreduction and peripheral-blood progenitor-cell mobilization regimen for transplant eligible patients with non-Hodgkin's lymphoma. *J Clin Oncol* 1999, 17:3776–3785.

40. Khouri IF, Romajuera J, Kantarjian H, *et al.*: Hyper-CVAD and high-dose methotrexate/cytarabine followed by stem-cell transplantation: an active regimen for aggressive mantle cell lymphoma. *J Clin Oncol* 1988, 16:3803–3809.

41. Khouri I, Romajuera J, Kantarjian H, *et al.*: Update of the hyper-CVAD regimen followed by stem cell transplantation [SCT] in mantle cell lymphoma [abstract]. *1999 Proceedings of the American Society of Hematology.*

42. Inwards D, Brown D, Fonseca R, *et al.*: NCCTG phase II trial of 2-cholorodeoxyadenosine [2-CDA] as initial therapy for mantle cell lymphoma: a well-tolerated treatment with promising activity [abstract]. *1999 Proceedings of the American Society of Hematology.*

43. Magrath I, Adde M, Shad A, *et al.*: Adults and children with small non-cleaved cell lymphoma have a similar excellent outcome when treated with the same chemotherapy regimen. *J Clin Oncol* 1996, 14:925–934.

44. McMaster ML, Greer JP, Greco FA, *et al.*: Effective treatment of small-non-cleaved cell lymphoma with high intensity, brief-duration chemotherapy. *J Clin Oncol* 1996, 9:941–946.

45. Levine AM: Acquired immunodeficiency syndrome-related lymphoma: clinical aspects. *Semin Oncol* 2000, 27:442–453.

46. Fatkenheuer G, Hell K, Roers A, *et al.*: Spontaneous regression of HIV-associated T-cell non-Hodgkin's lymphoma with highly active antiretroviral therapy. *Eur J Med Res* 2000, 5:236–240.

CVP
(Cyclophosphamide, Vincristine, Prednisone)

CVP is a well-tolerated palliative regimen. Monthly cycles are repeated to maximum response plus two cycles. Randomized studies have demonstrated no response or survival advantage with the use CVP over continuous daily alkylating agent therapy. Responses are more rapid with CVP (within 3 mo), but not more durable.

Toxicity is primarily hematologic with drug-induced neutropenia. Hemorrhagic cystitis may occur and hydration reduces its frequency. Vinca-associated neurologic toxicity is mild with a capped 2-mg dose. Corticosteroid toxicities are infrequent with monthly cycles.

DOSAGE AND SCHEDULING

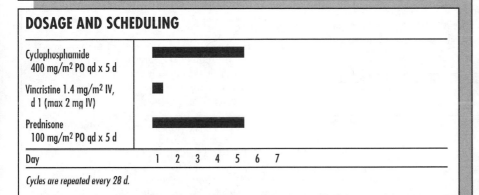

Cyclophosphamide 400 mg/m^2 PO qd x 5 d

Vincristine 1.4 mg/m^2 IV, d 1 (max 2 mg IV)

Prednisone 100 mg/m^2 PO qd x 5 d

Day: 1 2 3 4 5 6 7

Cycles are repeated every 28 d.

EXPERIENCES AND RESPONSE RATES

Study	Evaluable Patients, *n*	Complete Responses, %	Median Survival, *y*
Hoppe RT, *Blood* 1981, 58:592	40	85	7.5
Anderson T, *Cancer Treat Rep* 1977, 61:1057	49	67	7

CANDIDATES FOR TREATMENT
Patients with low-grade non-Hodgkin's lymphoma

ALTERNATIVE THERAPIES
Single-agent chlorambucil or cyclophosphamide; CHOP

TOXICITIES
Cyclophosphamide: myelosuppression with platelet sparing; nausea and vomiting, alopecia, darkening of skin and nails, mucositis (rare), hemorrhagic or sterile cystitis (5%–10% of patients, usually reversible, but can lead to fibrosis and bladder cancer), immunosuppression, SIADH; infertility; **Vincristine:** severe local inflammation possible if extravasated, alopecia, peripheral neuropathies, ileus; **Prednisone:** acne, thrush, thinning of the skin and striae; suppression of the adrenal–pituitary axis, hypokalemia, loss of muscle mass, increased appetite, myopathy, osteoporosis, cushingoid appearance, gastitis, peptic ulcer disease; euphoria, depression, psychosis, increased risk of infections and cataracts

DRUG INTERACTIONS
Cyclophosphamide: allopurinol, drugs that induce or block hepatic microsomal enzymes, sulfhydryl agents (*eg*, mesna); **Vincristine:** cisplatin, paclitaxel, and other drugs that affect peripheral nervous system

NURSING INTERVENTIONS
Give cyclophosphamide in the morning; administer vincristine as slow IV push to avoid extravasation; evaluate for neurologic deficit before each vincristine dose; maintain high fluid intake and encourage frequent voiding, stool softeners, and bulk diet

PATIENT INFORMATION
The most common side effects reported are leukopenia, hyperglycemia, weight gain, insomnia, alopecia, sensory neuropathy

CHOP
(Cyclophosphamide, Hydroxydaunorubicin, Vincristine, Prednisone)

CHOP is a potentially curative regimen for aggressive diffuse lymphomas. It may also be used in indolent lymphomas, particularly with evidence of histologic transformation. Responses are prompt (complete responses generally obtained in less than 4 months). CHOP chemotherapy is continued for two additional cycles beyond maximal response or for a minimum of 6 cycles. Complete remission is achieved in 60% to 75% of patients.

Prospective comparisons with more intensive second- and third- generation regimens have shown no significant difference in the response rates or survival outcomes of patients with aggressive diffuse lymphomas. CHOP remains the standard drug regimen in this setting.

Toxicity is moderate and reasonably well tolerated even in older patients. Adverse effects are similar to those outlined for CVP regimen. Potential cardiac toxicity from doxorubicin should be monitored closely; doses greater than 450 mg/m^2 should be avoided.

DOSAGE AND SCHEDULING

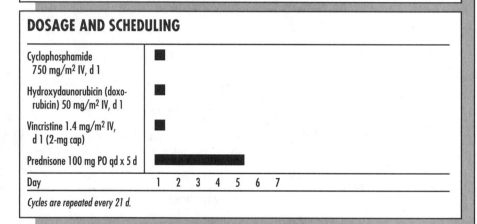

Cyclophosphamide 750 mg/m^2 IV, d 1

Hydroxydaunorubicin (doxo-rubicin) 50 mg/m^2 IV, d 1

Vincristine 1.4 mg/m^2 IV, d 1 (2-mg cap)

Prednisone 100 mg PO qd x 5 d

Day | 1 2 3 4 5 6 7

Cycles are repeated every 21 d.

EXPERIENCES AND RESPONSE RATES

Study	Evaluable Patients, *n*	Complete Responses, %	Median Survival
Armitage JD, *J Clin Oncol* 1984, 2:898	75	51	31% at 4–9 y
Gams RA, *J Clin Oncol* 1985, 3:1188	90	54	35% at 6 y
Dixon DO, *J Clin Oncol* 1986, 5:197	412	53	30% at 12 y

CANDIDATES FOR TREATMENT
Patients with indolent or aggressive diffuse non-Hodgkin's lymphoma

SPECIAL PRECAUTIONS
Patients with hepatic dysfunction; patients with impaired cardiac function (contraindicated)

ALTERNATIVE THERAPIES
ProMACE-CytaBOM, CEPP, C-MOPP, m-BACOD, MACOP-B

TOXICITIES
Prednisone: acne, thrush, thinning of the skin and striae, suppression of the adrenal–pituitary axis, hypokalemia, loss of muscle mass, increased appetite, myopathy, osteoporosis, cushingoid appearance, gastitis, peptic ulcer disease, euphoria, depression, psychosis, increased risk of infections and cataracts; **Cyclophosphamide:** myelosuppression with platelet sparing, nausea and vomiting, alopecia, darkening of skin and nails, mucositis (rare), hemorrhagic or sterile cystitis, immunosuppression, SIADH, infertility; **Vincristine:** severe local inflammation possible if extravasated, alopecia, peripheral neuropathies, ileus; **Doxorubicin:** myelosuppression (leukocytes and platelets), nausea and vomiting; mucositis, alopecia, radiation recall, local tissue damage progressing to necrosis if extravasated, hyperpigmentation, phlebitis, irreversible congestive heart failure (dose-dependent), acute arrhythmias

DRUG INTERACTIONS
Cyclophosphamide: allopurinol, drugs that induce or block hepatic microsomal enzymes, sulfhydryl agents (*eg*, mesna); **Vincristine:** cisplatin, taxol, and other drugs that affect peripheral nervous system; **Doxorubicin:** heparin, mediastinal radiation, interferon

NURSING INTERVENTIONS
Give cyclophosphamide in the morning; administer vincristine and hydroxydoxorubicin as slow IV push to avoid extravasation; evaluate for neurologic deficit before each vincristine dose; maintain high fluid intake and encourage frequent voiding, stool softeners, and bulk diet

PATIENT INFORMATION
The most common side effects reported are leukopenia, alopecia, nausea, vomiting, hyperglycemia, sensory neuropathy, insomnia

RITUXIMAB

Rituximab is an unlabeled chimeric monoclonal antibody targeting CD20 antigen on B lymphocytes. It is FDA-approved as single-agent therapy for the treatment of relapsed indolent non-Hodgkin's lymphomas. Studies are investigating the combination of rituximab with chemotherapy, and to evaluate its use in untreated patients.

DOSAGE AND SCHEDULING AS A SINGLE AGENT

375 mg/m^2 intravenous infusion over 3–4 h (titrated slowly as patient tolerates) on a weekly schedule for 4 weeks.

EXPERIENCE AND RESPONSE RATES

Study	Evaluable Patients, *n*	Overall Response Rate, %
McLaughlin *et al.*, J Clin Oncol 1988, 16:2825–2833.	166	48%

CANDIDATES FOR TREATMENT

Patients with relapsed low-grade or follicular B-cell non-Hodgkin's lymphoma.

SPECIAL PRECAUTIONS

Patients with peripheral blood lymphocytosis as in CLL or mantle cell lymphoma may develop a cytokine release syndrome; patients with underlying cardiovascular or pulmonary disease are at risk for developing infusion-related syndrome. Do not administer live vaccines during treatment.

ALTERNATIVE THERAPIES

CHOP, CVP, fludarabine

TOXICITIES

Symptoms related to the infusion: fevers, chills, headache, rigors, asthenia, throat irritation, abdominal pain. Neutropenia, leukopenia or thrombocytopenia; risk of infections due to decreased serum immunoglobulins or to leukopenia. Hypersensitivity reactions related to the infusion including hypotension, bronchospasm, or angioedema. Severe infusion-related reactions (usually with the first infusion) occur rarely and are characterized by hypoxia, pulmonary infiltrates, adult respiratory distress syndrome, ventricular fibrillation, or cardiogenic shock

DRUG INTERACTIONS

No specific drug–drug interactions. Contraindicated in patients with known type I hypersensitivity or anaphylactic reactions to murine proteins or to a component of rituximab

NURSING INTERVENTIONS

Careful monitoring is required during the first infusion with frequent blood pressure and heart rate monitoring within the first 2 hours of infusion. Supportive care measures include intravenous saline infusion and premedications with acetominophen, diphenhydramine and as needed to minimize infusion-related adverse effects. Keep meperidine on hand for infusion-related rigors. Rituximab infusion should be interrupted if significant side effects occur and resumed at a reduced rate only if side effects have resolved. Medications for treatment of hypersensitivity reactions such as epinephrine, antihistamines, and corticosteroids should be kept on hand in the event of a reaction

PATIENT INFORMATION

Most side effects are related to the infusion, such as fevers, chills and rigors. Patients do not experience alopecia

DHAP

DHAP is a second-line, salvage regimen for patients with intermediate grade or immunoblastic non-Hodgkin's lymphoma who have not attained a complete remission from up-front therapy or who have relapsed. Because only 45%–50% of patients are cured with their initial chemotherapy treatment program, many patients need to receive salvage chemotherapy. Depending on the patient's age, comorbidity, and performance status, the goals of second-line therapy vary. Transplant-eligible patients require only cytoreduction, whereas in transplant-ineligible patients a complete remission is desired.

DHAP is a treatment program that has the best reported efficacy in this setting. In the original report, 90 patients with progressive recurrent lymphoma were treated: 28 patients achieved a complete remission and 22 a partial remission for an overall response rate 56%.

Vigorous hydration with mannitol-induced diuresis was given in all patients. The acute tumor lysis syndrome was observed in 5 patients, emphasizing the need for frequent monitoring of electrolytes. Toxicity was severe with neutropenia, thrombocytopenia, renal, cerebellar, and gastroinstestinal dysfunction common.

DOSAGE AND SCHEDULING

Cisplatin: 100 mg/m² IV continuous infusion (CI) x 24 h, day 1 *or* 50 mg/m² as 1 h-infusion daily x 2
Ara-C: 2 g/m² x 2 IV: each infusion over 3 h q12 x 2 day 2
Dexamethazone: 40 mg IV or PO daily days 1–4

Patients are hospitalized to undergo treatment. Hydration with normal saline at 150–250 mL/h is administered for a 36-h period and after the first 6 hours of hydration cisplatin can be administered. Therapy is repeated every 3–4 weeks for a maximum of 4 cycles after maximal tumor response. Patients aged older than 70 years received ara-C are treated with a dose of 1 g/m².

TOXICITIES

Profound myelosuppression with marked neutropenia and thrombocytopenia, especially in patients with lymphomatous involvement of the bone marrow or previous pelvic irradiation. Documented infections were seen in 30% of patients with a mortality of 33% in these patients. Tumor lysis syndrome occurred in 5% of patients. Renal insufficiency is seen in 20% and can be irreversible. Acute cerebellar dysfunction and tinnitus has been reported.

Neutropenia can be shortened by growth factor support (G-CSF or GM-CSF).

CANDIDATES FOR TREATMENT

Patients with refractory or relapsed intermediate grade or immunoblastic non-Hodgkin's lymphoma

SPECIAL PRECAUTIONS

Patients who are elderly; patients with renal or neurological dysfunction; patients with compromised bone marrow reserve

ALTERNATIVE THERAPIES

Ifosamide and etoposide alone or with cisplatin or carboplatin C-MOPP

DRUG INTERACTIONS

Aminoglycoside antibiotics should be avoided; any drugs that have renal or ototoxicity must be used with caution

NURSING INTERVENTIONS

Monitor renal function and obtain BUN, creatinine and 12-h urine collection for creatinine clearance; provide proper antiemetics, hydrate well; observe for signs of infection; neutropenia is expected; severe thrombocytopenia occurs, and signs for bleeding should be monitored

PATIENT INFORMATION

The most common side effect include fever when the blood counts are low, nausea, vomiting, and alopecia

ICE (IFOSFAMIDE, CARBOPLATIN, ETOPOSIDE)

This salvage combination chemotherapy regimen for aggressive large cell non-Hodgkin's lymphomas is often used for cytoreduction and for stem-cell mobilization in transplant-eligible patients with relapsed or refractory non-Hodgkin's lymphoma. This regimen causes less renal toxicity than DHAP, and is fairly well tolerated except for significant myelosuppression.

DOSING AND SCHEDULING: ICE REGIMEN*

Agent	Day of Cycle													
	1	2	3	4	5	6	7	8	9	10	11	12	13	14
Etoposide	X	X	X											
Ifosfamide		X												
Carboplatin		X												
Mesna		X												
Filgastrim						X	X	X	X	X	X			

Ifosfamide, 5 g/m^2 IV on day 2; carboplatin (AUC 5), IV on day 2; etoposide, 100 mg/m^2 on days 1, 2, and 3. Mesna 5 g/m^2 IVCI over 24 h on day 2 with ifosfamide. Filgastrim is given midcycle.

EXPERIENCES AND RESPONSE RATES

Study	Evaluable Patients, n	Overall Response, %
Moskowitz et al., J Clin Oncol 1999, 17:3776–3785.	163	66.3%

CANDIDATES FOR TREATMENT

Relapsed or refractory aggressive diffuse lymphomas as salvage therapy or as cytoreduction prior to autologous stem cell transplantation.

SPECIAL PRECAUTIONS

Patients who are older or with marginal performance status; patients with renal or neurologic dysfunction; and patients with poor bone marrow reserve. Ifosfamide should be given with MESNA at similar dosages to prevent hemorrhagic cystitis.

ALTERNATIVE THERAPIES

DHAP, ESHAP, ifosfamide and etoposide without carboplatin, C-MOPP, or CEPP

TOXICITIES

Ifosfamide: myelosuppression, nausea and vomiting, alopecia, hemorrhagic cystitis, CNS toxicity, infertility, renal impairment; **Carboplatin:** myelosuppression, nausea and vomiting, renal dysfunction, liver function abnormalities, electrolyte disturbances, peripheral neuropathy; **Etoposide:** myelosuppression, nausea, vomiting, alopecia, mucositis

DRUG INTERACTIONS

Ifosfamide: coumadin; **Carboplatin:** aminoglycoside antibiotics, phenytoin; **Etoposide:** ara-C, methotrexate, cisplatin, calcium channel blockers, coumadin, cyclosporine, tamoxifen

NURSING INTERVENTIONS

Supportive care during infusion includes adequate intravenous hydration, and pretreatment antiemetics. Renal function, electrolytes, blood counts, and signs of bleeding should all be monitored

PATIENT INFORMATION

Common side effects include fevers when blood counts are low; alopecia, nausea and vomiting. Low platelet counts as a consequence of treatment will increase the risk of bleeding, which may require platelet transfusions depending on severity

VANDERBILT REGIMEN
(Cyclophosphamide, Etoposide, Vincristine, Bleomycin, Methotrexate, Leucovorin, Prednisone)

Small noncleaved cell lymphomas—Burkitt's and non-Burkitt's types—are rare high-grade lymphomas. When associated with HIV infection, this phenotype is one of the most common histologies. HIV-negative small, noncleaved cell lymphoma is a highly curable disease with high-dose, short-course therapy [24]. CNS prophylaxis is essential. As with lymphoblastic lymphoma, tumor lysis is a serious complication of effective initial therapy and must be anticipated with initiation of hydration, alkalinization, and allopurinol, and frequent monitoring of electrolytes, renal function, and calcium and phosphate balance.

Severe myelosuppression is to be expected with this drug protocol. Even with growth factor support, nadir fever should be anticipated as well as the need for platelet support. Mucositis may occur in up to half of all patients. Nevertheless, maintaining treatment schedule is important whenever possible to combat this rapidly growing neoplasm.

DOSAGE AND SCHEDULING

Agent	Cycle 1						Cycle 2					
	Day 1	Day 2	Day 3	Day 8	Day 15	Day 22	Day 29	Day 30	Day 31	Day 36	Day 43	Day 50
CTX	X	X					X					
ETOP	X	X	X				X	X	X			
ADR							X	X				
VCR				X		X				X		X
BLEO				X		X				X		X
MTX					X						X	
LV			X		X						X	
PRED	X	X		X			X	X	X	X		

REGIMEN

In cycle 1, CTX—cyclophosamide 1500 mg/m²; ETOP—etoposide 400 mg/m²; VCR—vincristine 1.4 mg/m² (2 mg max), BLEO—bleomycin 10 U/m²; MTX—methotrexate 200 mg/m²; LV—leucovorin 15 mg/m² (q 6 h x 6); PRED—prednisone 60 mg/m². In cycle 2, etoposide dose is reduced to 100 mg/m² and ADR (doxorubicin) is added at 45 mg/m². Allopurinol is routinely given. Patients with meningeal involvement at diagnosis receive methotrexate 12 mg/m² IT weekly x 5 and whole-brain radiation 2000 cGy in 10 fractions. Prophylactic intrathecal therapy is recommended.

DOSAGE MODIFICATIONS: Cycle 2 can be delayed if ANC < 1000. Reduce bleomycin, if renal failure develops; withhold methotrexate if creatinine clearance ≤ 60 mL/min.

EXPERIENCE AND RESPONSE RATES

Study	Evaluable Patients, n	Complete Responses, %	Disease-Free Survival
McMaster et al., J Clin Oncol 1991; 9:941–946	20	85	65% at 29 mo

CANDIDATES FOR TREATMENT
Patients with high-grade non-Hodgkin's lymphoma

SPECIAL PRECAUTIONS
Patients with renal dysfunction

ALTERNATIVE THERAPIES
Stanford regimen using combined modality

TOXICITIES
Cyclophosphamide, prednisone, vincristine: see CVP protocol for list of toxicities; **Bleomycin:** alopecia, stomatitis, nail bed thickening, hyperpigmentation and skin desquamation (common), acute anaphylaxis with ARDS, dose-related pneumonitis progressing to pulmonary fibrosis (max cumulative dose of 200 U/m²); frequently severe fever; **Methotrexate:** myelosuppression, nausea and vomiting, severe mucositis with ulceration and bloody diarrhea, irreversible cirrhosis (rare), pneumonitis, alopecia, renal tubular necrosis, **Etoposide:** myelosuppression (leukopenia and thrombocytopenia), nausea and vomiting, alopecia, mucositis

DRUG INTERACTIONS
Cyclophosphamide, prednisone, vincristine: see CVP protocol for list of interactions; **Bleomycin:** radiation therapy, nephrotoxic drugs; **Etoposide:** ara-C, methotrexate, cisplatin, calcium antagonists, coumadin; **Methotrexate:** aspirin, NSAIDs, alcohol, 5-FU, L-asparaginase

NURSING INTERVENTIONS
See CVP protocol for list of interventions; test dose of bleomycin (1 U IM) prior to first dose; use glass containers for infusion of bleomycin; administer etoposide over 1 h to avoid hypotension and extravasation; mix intrathecal methotrexate with buffered nonbacteriostatic solution; monitor methotrexate levels if renal dysfunction develops and maintain leucovorin every 6 h until methotrexate levels are nontherapeutic

PATIENT INFORMATION
These most common side effects reported are pancytopenia, infections, alopecia, bleeding, mucositis, peripheral neuropathy

CODOX-M AND IVAC
(Cyclophosphamide, Doxorubicin, Vincristine, Methotrexate, Cytarabine, Ifosfamide, Etoposide)

Diffuse small noncleaved cell lymphomas, both Burkitt's and non-Burkitt's, are considered high-grade lymphomas. These subtypes are commonly detected in the setting of HIV infection. Small noncleaved cell lymphomas not related to HIV infection are curable with high-dose, short-course chemotherapy. CNS prophylaxis is an essential component of the treatment regimens. Because tumor lysis syndrome may occur after the initiation of therapy, it is important to include intravenous hydration, alkalinization of the urine, and administration of allopurinol. Frequent monitoring of electrolytes, renal function, serum calcium, and phosphate is also necessary. Although adverse effects such as myelosuppression and neutropenic fevers are common, the treatment schedule should be maintained because these are rapidly growing tumors.

Patients with favorable small noncleaved cell lymphoma defined as nonbulky stage I or II disease may be treated with three cycles of CODOX-M regimen [37]. Patients with unfavorable small noncleaved cell lymphoma may be treated with CODOX-M alternating with IVAC regimen for a total of four treatment cycles. The Vanderbilt Regimen is also an effective regimen for small noncleaved cell lymphomas.

DRUG INTERACTIONS

Cyclophosphamide: allopurinol, drugs that induce or inhibit hepatic microsomal enzymes, sulfhydryl agents (*ie*, mesna); **Doxorubicin:** heparin, mediastinal irradiation, interferon; **Vincristine:** cisplatin, paclitaxel, other drugs that affect the peripheral nervous system. **Cytarabine:** possibly flucytosine; **Ifosfamide:** coumadin; **Etoposide:** ara-C, methotrexate, cisplatin, calcium channel antagonists, coumadin, cyclosporine, tamoxifen. **Methotrexate:** aspirin, NSAIDs, alcohol, fluorouracil, L-aspariginase; penicillin.

NURSING INTERVENTIONS

Mix intrathecal methotrexate with buffered nonbacteriostatic solution; monitor methotrexate levels if renal dysfunction develops; administer leucovorin every 6 hours until methotrexate levels are nontherapeutic.

PATIENT INFORMATION

The most common side effects are pancytopenia, predisposition to infections, alopecia, bleeding, mucositis, and peripheral neuropathy.

DOSAGE AND SCHEDULING: CODOX-M REGIMEN

Agent	Day of Cycle																	
	1	2	3	4	5	6	7	8	9	10	11	12	13	14	15	16	17	18
CTX	X	X	X	X	X													
DOXO	X																	
VCR	X							X							(X)			
MTX										X								
LEUCO											X	X	X	X				
IT CYTAR	X		X															
IT MTX															X			

Cyclophosphamide (CTX) 800 mg/m² IV on day 1, then 200 mg/m² IV on days 2 to 5; doxorubicin (DOXO) 40 mg/m² IV on day 1; vincristine (VCR) 1.5 mg/m² IV on days 1 and 8 of cycle one, and on days 1, 8, and 15 on cycle 3. High-dose methotrexate (MTX) is administered as a 24-hour infusion starting on day 10: 1200 mg/m² IV over 1 hour, then 240 mg/m²/h × 23 h. IV each hour for 23 hours. Leucovorin (LEUCO) begins about 36 hours after starting high-dose methotrexate and continues until serum methotrexate level decreases to nontoxic levels. Intrathecal cytarabine (IT CYTAR) on days 1 and 3; intrathecal methotrexate (IT MTX) on day 15.

DOSAGE AND SCHEDULING: IVAC REGIMEN*

Agent	Day of Cycle																	
	1	2	3	4	5	6	7	8	9	10	11	12	13	14	15	16	17	18
Cytarabine	X	X																
Ifosfamide	X	X	X	X	X													
Etoposide	X	X	X	X	X													
Mesna	X	X	X	X	X													
IT MTX					X													

*High-dose cytarabine 2 g/m² IV every 12 hours on days 1 and 2 (total, four doses). Ifosfamide 1500 mg/m² IV on days 1 through 5 with Mesna. Etoposide 60 mg/m² IV on days 1 through 5. Intrathecal methotrexate (IT MTX) on day 5.

(Continued on next page)

CODOX-M AND IVAC (Continued)
(Cyclophosphamide, Doxorubicin, Vincristine, Methotrexate, Cytarabine, Ifosfamide, Etoposide)

RECENT EXPERIENCES AND RESPONSE RATES

Study	Patients, n	Event-free Survival at 2 y, %
Magrath et al., J Clin Oncol 1996, 14:925–934	72 (39 adults)	56% (CODOX-M) 92% (IVAC)

CANDIDATES FOR TREATMENT
Patients with diffuse small noncleaved cell non-Hodgkin's lymphoma

SPECIAL PRECAUTIONS
Patients with renal dysfunction

ALTERNATIVE THERAPIES
Vanderbilt regimen

TOXICITIES
Cyclophosphamide: myelosuppression, nausea and vomiting, alopecia, mucositis (rare), hemorrhagic or sterile cystitis, SIADH (syndrome of inappropriate antidiuretic hormone), infertility; **Doxorubicin:** myelosuppression, nausea and vomiting, mucositis, alopecia, radiation recall, local tissue damage if extravasated; phlebitis, congestive heart failure, arrhythmias; **Vincristine:** local inflammation if extravasated, alopecia, peripheral neuropathy, ileus; **Methotrexate:** myelosuppression, nausea and vomiting, severe mucositis with ulceration and bloody diarrhea, cirrhosis (rare), pneumonitis, alopecia, renal tubular necrosis; **Cytarabine:** nausea, vomiting, neuropathy, neurotoxicity, rash myelosuppression; ocular toxicity; **Ifosfamide:** myelosuppression, nausea and vomiting, alopecia, hemorrhagic cystitis, CNS toxicity, infertility, renal impairment; **Etoposide:** myelosuppression, nausea, vomiting, alopecia, mucositis

INCIDENCE AND ETIOLOGY

The incidence for multiple myeloma in the United States exceeds 3 people per 100,000 and appears to be increasing. Myeloma accounts for 1% of malignant disease and over 10% of hematologic malignancies. The occurrence of myeloma is more common in men than in women and more common in African Americans than in whites (Table 20-1). It most commonly presents in the seventh decade, with fewer than 2% of patients younger than age 40 years.

The cause of multiple myeloma remains unknown. Monoclonal gammopathy of undetermined significance (MGUS) may offer a clue to its pathogenesis [1]. More than 33% of patients with apparent benign monoclonal gammopathy will develop myeloma, another lymphoplasmacellular malignancy, or progression of their monoclonal gammopathy. The incidence of myeloma in patients with MGUS is 25% after 20 to 35 years of follow-up. These observations implicate MGUS as a premalignant clonal disorder that, on further transforming damage to the clone, can give rise to multiple myeloma.

Table 20-1. Risk Factors for the Development of Multiple Myeloma

African-American race
Male gender
Advanced age
Monoclonal gammopathy of undetermined significance (MGUS)
Chronic immune stimulation
Exposure to ionizing radiation
Occupational exposure to pesticides, paints, and solvents
Genetic predisposition

Table 20-2. Clinical Staging System for Myeloma

Stage	Criteria	Myeloma Cell Mass, cells/m²
I	All of the following:	$< 0.6 \times 10^{12}$ (low)
	1. Hemoglobin > 10 g/dL	
	2. Serum calcium value normal ($\leq$ 12 mg/100 mL)	
	3. On x-ray, normal bone structure or solitary bone plasmacytoma only	
	4. Low M-component production rates	
	a. IgG value < 5 g/100 mL	
	b. IgA value < 3 g/100 mL	
	c. Urine light chain M-component on electrophoresis < 4 g/24 h	
II	Fitting neither stage I nor III	$0.6–1.2 \times 10^{12}$ (intermediate)
III	One or more of the following:	1.2×10^{12} (high)
	1. Hemoglobin < 8.5 g/100 mL	
	2. Serum calcium value > 12 mg/100 mL	
	3. Advanced lytic bone lesions	
	4. High M-component production rates	
	a. IgG value > 7 g/100 mL	
	b. IgA value > 5 g/100 mL	
	c. Urine light chain M-component on electrophoresis > 12 g/24 h	
Subclass		
A	Serum creatine < 2 mg/100 mL	
B	Serum creatine $\geq$ 2 mg/100 mL	

Adapted from Durie and Salmon [4].

Genetic predisposition, radiation exposure, chronic antigenic stimulation, and various environmental or occupational conditions have been observed as factors but account for only a small percentage of all myeloma. Recent reports demonstrate the importance of autocrine stimulation of the malignant clone by IL-6 and the apparent role of oncogene activation at various stages of the disease. The recent identification of the human herpesvirus 8 in the bone marrow of myeloma patients provides a possible new etiologic factor in this disease [2,3]. Interestingly, these studies showed this virus to be present in nonmalignant dendritic cells, suggesting a novel mechanism by which viruses in general may stimulate malignant transformation and growth. If this virus proves etiologic, it may also become a new target for therapeutic approaches in the future. These and other recently appreciated factors provide insight into the pathogenesis of myeloma, but their relationship to the original malignant event is not yet spelled out.

DIAGNOSIS AND STAGING

Diagnosis of myeloma is made by the presence of malignant plasma cells in the bone marrow (usually > 10%) or by biopsy proof of a plasmacytoma plus either protein evidence of myeloma with a monoclonal serum or urine protein or characteristic osteolytic lesions. For the past 20 years, the most commonly used staging system has been that proposed by Durie and Salmon (Table 20-2). It correlates tumor burden with the presence or absence of severe anemia, hypercalcemia, advanced skeletal disease, and the amount of monoclonal protein detected in serum or urine [4].

Clinical stage has proved to be predictive of survival in many series. Stage I patients generally survive over 5 years, whereas the median survival for Stage II patients is 3 to 4 years and for Stage III rarely more than 2 years. The presence of renal failure has an important negative prognostic significance in myeloma. More recent studies have demonstrated that elevated plasma ß-2 microglobulin and elevated plasma cell labeling index are also important adverse prognostic signs that may at times override the significance of clinical stage [5]. Although renal dysfunction will result in elevated serum β-2 microglobulin levels, this protein is an independent prognostic factor in myeloma [6]. The presence of both low plasma ß-2 microglobulin and elevated plasma cell labeling index appears to be a strong predictor of long survival in patients with myeloma.

Several other factors have been found to have prognostic importance in myeloma (Table 20-3). They relate to patient factors, tumor burden, and tumor biology. Recently, specific chromosomal abnor-

Table 20-3. Prognostic Factors

Patient factors	Tumor biology
Age	Plasma cell labeling index (PCLI)
Performance status	C reactive protein (CRP)
Concomitant illness	Circulating soluble IL-6 receptor (sIL-6R)
Renal function	Lactic dehydrogenase
Serum albumin	ras Gene mutations
	p53 and p16 abnormalities
Factors reflecting tumor burden	Plasmablastic subtype
Clinical stage (see Table 20-2), including component factors Hb, M-component concentration, serum calcium, osteolytic lesions	Chromosomal abnormalities
β 2-microglobulin	Circulating tumor cells
Bone marrow plasma cell percent	

malities (especially those involving chromosomes 11 and 13) have portended poor outcome in these patients [7]. In one study [3], multivariate analysis identified serum creatinine, B2M, plasma cell percent (by immunofluorescent technique) along with 3 biologic factors, PCLI, CRP, and sIL-6R as the independent prognostic variables. The presence of abnormalities on magnetic resonance imaging in early-stage disease may also suggest an adverse outcome [9].

PRIMARY DISEASE THERAPY

Although high-dose therapy followed by hematopoietic support may result in long-term survival in a few cases, the goals of treatment in

most cases are to extend survival several years, to produce objective disease regression with its attendant relief from pain and other disease symptoms, and to protect the patient's ability to lead an active life for as long as possible. For the past three decades the standard treatment for multiple myeloma has been widely considered to be use of the single alkylating agent, melphalan, or a combination of melphalan and prednisone (MP), which is usually given in a high-dose, intermittent, outpatient regimen (Fig. 20-1) [10]. When this treatment is used, objective responses, documented by a 50% or greater decrease in serum M-protein levels and control of other major manifestations of disease, are seen in 50% of patients. Unfortunately, response duration is generally less than 2 years and

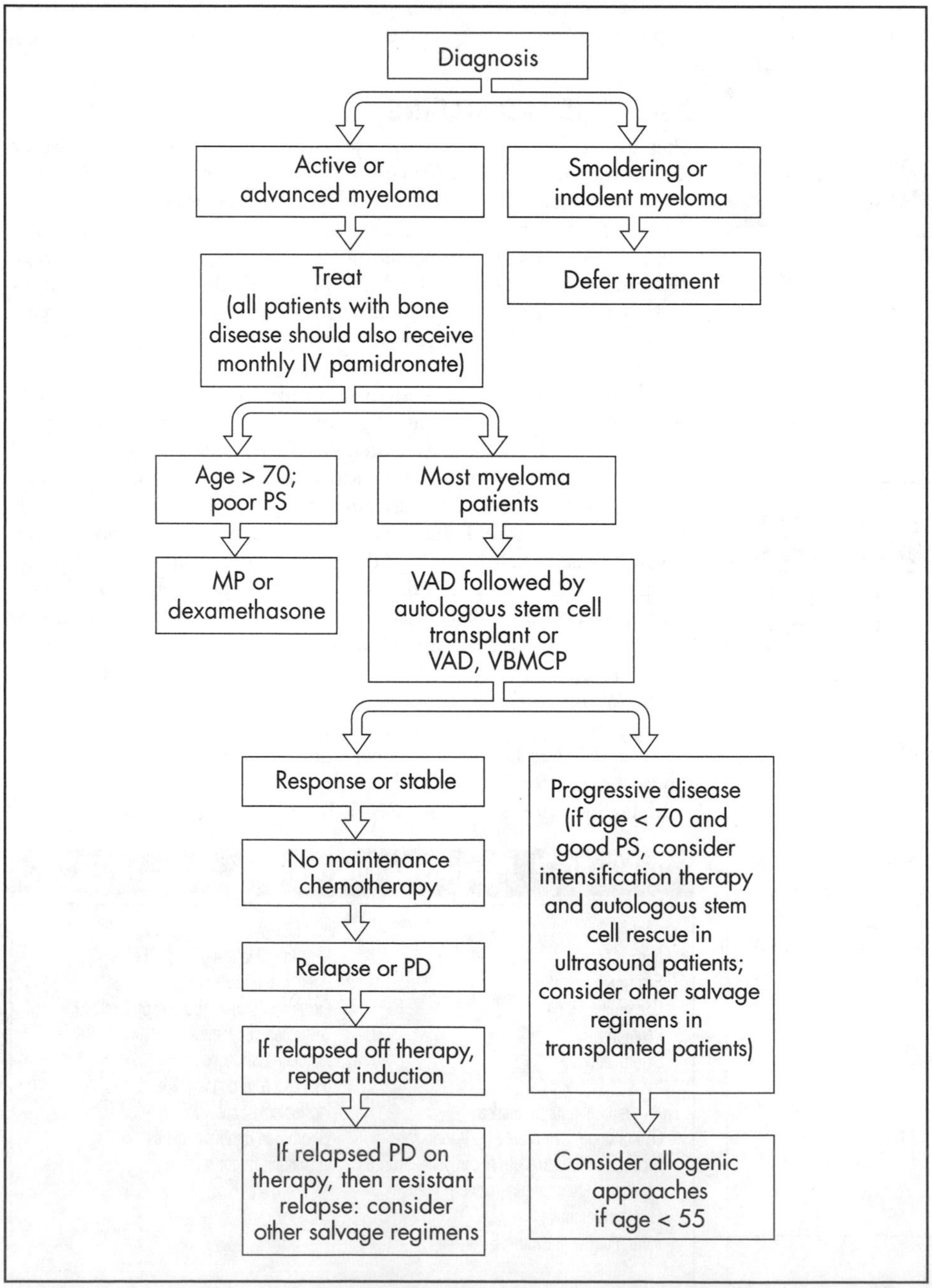

FIGURE 20-1.

Treatment strategy for myeloma. MP—melphalan and prednisone; PD—progressive disease; PS—performance status; VAD—vincristine, doxorubicin, and dexamethasone; VBMCP—vincristine, carmustine (BCNU), melphalan, cyclophosphamide, and prednisone.

The information here is provided as guidance only. Prescribers should always consult the manufacturer's current prescribing information.

324

the median duration of survival is 30 months. Survival durations exceeding 5 years are achieved in fewer than 20% of patients.

Numerous combination chemotherapy regimens have been developed in an attempt to improve on the results obtained from use of the MP regimen (Table 22-4). Most resemble either the vincristine, carmustine (BCNU), melphalan, cyclophosphamide, and prednisone (VBMCP) regimen or the VMCP/VBAP regimen, consisting of alternating cycles of vincristine plus prednisone combined with either melphalan plus cyclophosphamide or with BCNU plus doxorubicin. Because of promising preliminary results, several randomized clinical trials have been conducted to compare MP with more aggressive multidrug regimens. However, most randomized trials and meta-analyses have suggested that these more aggressive combination chemotherapy regimens with their added toxicity may slightly improve response rates, but these therapies have made no significant impact on overall survival. Results of the recent Eastern Cooperative Oncology Group (ECOG) trial comparing VBMCP (vincristine, carmustine [BCNU], melphalan, cyclophosphamide, and prednisone) with MP (melphalan and prednisone) showed response rates of 72% and 51%, respectively; but more importantly, no difference was found in overall survival between patients receiving these two regimens [10].

Other commonly used combination chemotherapy regimens include VMCP (vincristine, melphalan, cyclophosphamide, and prednisone) alternating with VBAP (vincristine, BCNU, doxorubicin, and prednisone) [11], ABCM (doxorubicin, BCNU, cyclophosphamide, and melphalan) [12], and VMCPP alternating with VBAPP [13]. Recent studies show the efficacy of high-dose oral glucocorticosteroids alone in these patients without the bone marrow toxicity produced by use of alkylating agents. A recent promising, newer steroid-containing combination without alkylator therapy from MD Anderson Cancer Center that consists of VAD (infusional vincristine and adriamycin with oral dexamethasone) results in both rapid and high response rates [14]. Although an historical comparison of this combination to oral dexamethasone alone showed an improvement in response rate, it did not produce an improvement in overall survival [15].

In determining what type of therapy to initiate in the newly diagnosed patient, it is important to consider the extent of disease, other clinical conditions, and whether the patient is a candidate for high-dose therapy regimens. For example, several small randomized trials have demonstrated no benefit to treating asymptomatic early-stage patients with chemotherapy. A "wait and watch" approach is warranted in this group of patients until more effective therapies become available. In patients who are candidates for high-dose therapy followed by autologous hematopoietic support, regimens without alkylating agents are preferable because of the difficulty in collecting adequate stem cells in patients exposed to these agents prior to stem cell mobilization. Thus, VAD is ideally suited for initial therapy in these patients. In elderly patients or in those persons unable to tolerate more aggressive chemotherapy, oral dexamethasone alone or MP is the preferred form of treatment.

Initial chemotherapy is generally given for 6 to 12 months and rarely results in complete responses. Responding patients demonstrate a reduction in tumor mass as reflected in decreases in paraprotein levels, and enter a plateau phase, at which point the monoclonal protein level remains constant despite continued chemotherapy.

MAINTENANCE THERAPY

The use of continued chemotherapy during plateau phase does not improve overall survival as demonstrated in several large randomized trials. In fact, continuation of therapy leads to a permanent reduction in bone marrow reserve and increases the risk of secondary leukemia. Recent attempts to prolong survival with maintenance therapy have largely involved the use of interferon α-2 (IFN α-2). Used alone as initial therapy, this agent has little demonstrated antimyeloma activity, which may in fact reflect its ability to reduce immunoglobulin production by plasma cells without actually reducing tumor cell growth [16]. Although some single-arm trials have suggested a benefit with the addition of this agent to other chemotherapy, several large randomized trials have not shown an improvement in overall survival with the addition of IFN α-2 to other initial chemotherapeutic regimens. However, an early large randomized Italian study suggested that this drug may have a role in maintenance therapy as demonstrated by its ability to prolong plateau and possibly prolong overall survival in certain subgroups [17]. Patients with stable disease during induction chemotherapy did not appear to benefit from treatment. Unfortunately, most subsequent trials with the exception of the Canadian study have shown little impact on overall survival with maintenance IFN α-2 therapy [13,18–21]. A recent unpublished meta-analysis of randomized trials suggests a slight but significant benefit in both progression-free and overall survival with use of maintenance IFN α-2 therapy; but included in the analysis, were several positive studies that have not been published in peer-reviewed publications. As a result, one must weigh the considerable toxicity and expense against the minimal possible benefit of this agent before using it in patients responding to initial chemotherapy. A recently published Southwest Oncology Group (SWOG) trial comparing maintenance therapy of IFN plus prednisone versus IFN alone showed a survival advantage for patients receiving the combination treatment [22]. However, it was unclear from this study whether the combination was necessary or glucocorticosteroids alone could be used as effective maintenance therapy. The results of the recently completed SWOG 9210 study provide clear evidence for the benefit of alternate-day prednisone 50 mg as maintenance therapy for patients responding to induction VAD chemotherapy [23].

HIGH-DOSE THERAPY

Based on the higher response rates achieved with more aggressive combinations of alkylating agents, high-dose chemotherapy with or without hematopoietic support has been studied. Initial trials involved patients with resistant multiple myeloma who were treated with melphalan in doses of 70 to 140 mg/m^2. Although dramatic responses were noted, these responses were short-lived and associated with significant morbidity related to protracted myelosuppression. Hematopoietic support using autologous bone marrow was added to shorten the duration of granulocytopenia, allowing for more intensive preparative conditioning with higher doses of melphalan (200 mg/m^2) alone or lower doses (140 mg/m^2) combined with total body irradiation (TBI) or busulfan and cyclophosphamide. In these early studies, despite treatment eligibility based on resistance to conventional chemotherapy, impressive cytoreduction was achieved, but progression-free survival was brief. Several favorable prognostic factors for sustained response were identified and included chemotherapy-sensitive myeloma and a shorter duration of primary treatment. Based on these results, autologous bone marrow transplantation was used on recently diagnosed patients with chemotherapy-responsive disease. These studies showed very high response rates with a high frequency of complete remissions, and suggested improved long-term myeloma-free survival compared with patients treated with conventional chemotherapy alone.

In a randomized French study of 200 untreated patients with intermediate- to high-stage multiple myeloma, patients assigned to high-dose chemotherapy and autologous bone marrow transplantation achieved higher overall response rates and better progression-free and overall survival than that achieved by patients continued on conventional chemotherapy [24]. A recent update of this study continues to show similar benefits in patients on the high-dose arm. However, data have recently been presented showing no benefit to high-dose therapy among patients with advanced myeloma [26]. In that French trial, 191 patients with advanced multiple myeloma underwent several courses of VAD and then were randomized to receive either high-dose therapy followed by autologous support or another form of conventional therapy (VMCP). There was no difference in event-free or overall survival between the arms. Several other similar, large randomized trials comparing patients receiving high-dose therapy with those patients obtaining conventional treatment are also currently in progress. A potential problem unresolved by the use of autologous bone marrow support is the presence of clonogenic plasma cells in the autologous bone marrow product. One approach to overcome this problem has been to change the source of hematopoietic support from bone marrow to autologous peripheral blood progenitor cells obtained by leukaphereses. This latter product contains much less tumor contamination than what is found in bone marrow harvests. A further possible way to reduce the risk of tumor cell contamination in the autograft is through purification of the leukapheresis material by negatively purging with a battery of anti–B-cell antibodies or by positive selection for hematopoietic progenitor cells.

The lack of uniform expression of B-cell antigens on malignant plasma cells reduces the efficacy of the former technique. On the other hand, in a recent single-arm study of positive hematopoietic progenitor cells selected by their expression of the early hematopoietic CD34 antigen, residual tumor cell contamination of the autograft was markedly reduced by this procedure, and yet these CD34-selected progenitor cells produced rapid hematologic recovery of neutrophils and platelets [27]. A recently completed randomized trial using this selection technique in 134 patients confirmed these results, and showed most patients receiving CD34-enriched autografts contained tumor-free products to the sensitivity of the assay [28]. Despite the reduction in tumor burden, there was no difference in progression-free or overall survival between the arms [29]. Analysis of the tumor burden in bone marrow and peripheral blood from these patients suggests that there is only a modest reduction of tumor burden (1–2 logs) from the high-dose therapy procedure [30]. Thus, reduction of the small amount of tumor in the autograft is unlikely to significantly benefit patients undergoing myeloablative chemotherapy until more effective treatment strategies are developed.

Given the high response rate and likelihood of prolonged progression-free survival with relatively low treatment-related mortality (< 2%) in patients undergoing high-dose chemotherapy with autologous progenitor cell support, this treatment modality should be considered for patients aged 70 years or less with intermediate- to advanced-stage multiple myeloma responsive or stable following conventional chemotherapy.

Because of the encouraging results from the French Intergroup trial, several groups have conducted trials involving multiple courses of high-dose therapy. Although a nonrandomized trial from the University of Arkansas suggested a survival benefit in patients undergoing two courses of high-dose therapy [31], early results from the randomized French Intergroup trial show no survival difference between patients undergoing two courses versus one course of high-dose therapy [32].

Allogeneic bone marrow transplantation has also been used in myeloma. Its potential advantage includes the complete absence of malignant cells in the infused product as well as a possible therapeutic form of adoptive immunotherapy or graft-versus-tumor effect mediated by the allogeneic bone marrow. Occasionally, patients relapsing after autologous transplantation have been treated with this procedure, but the outcome has been generally poor. Due to age restrictions and lack of available donors, very few studies have been published, and most contain small numbers of patients. The results have been disappointing, with a high risk of treatment-related mortality attributable to early transplant-related organ toxicity and graft-versus-host disease. Although early results from the largest study of allogeneic transplants from the European Bone Marrow Transplant Registry were encouraging [33], a recently published update showed that many patients have relapsed, with very few patients alive and free of disease. Thus, there has been no demonstrated clinical advantage of allogeneic transplantation as hematopoietic support following myeloablative chemotherapy in multiple myeloma.

A new possible approach has been the use of donor leukocyte infusions (DLIs) with a possible graft-versus-myeloma effect observed in several patients undergoing this procedure [34]. However, many of these patients died from opportunistic infections soon after DLI. In addition, many of these patients also were receiving glucocorticosteroids as immunosuppressive therapy, so some of the responses may have resulted from these agents rather than the DLIs. Recent results from a European trial were encouraging using this approach in a group of 27 myeloma patients who either relapsed or were refractory to conventional allogeneic transplantation [35]. Recently, the MD Anderson group developed an allogeneic transplantation procedure involving lower doses of conditioning chemotherapy, which may allow the graft-versus-myeloma effect to occur without the high treatment-related mortality [36].

THERAPY FOR REFRACTORY OR RELAPSED DISEASE

Thirty percent to 50% of multiple-myeloma patients will have progressive disease despite conventional therapy and have a particularly poor prognosis. Even in patients who do achieve an initial response, nearly all will ultimately relapse and develop disease unresponsive to initial therapy. When these patients relapse, repeat use of the original induction regimen may achieve remissions (usually lasting < 1 y) especially in patients with a long duration of their initial remission. Numerous studies of standard-dose alkylating agents, anthracyclines, spindle toxins, and other drugs have failed to produce results in refractory patients. Likewise, nucleoside antagonists, taxanes, and nitrosoureas have been tried without therapeutic effect. A recent SWOG study suggests topotecan may have some activity in previously treated patients [37]. High-dose glucocorticosteroids (eg, prednisone 200 mg every other day [or pulse 60 mg/m^2 daily for 5 d every 8 d] or dexamethasone 40 mg daily for 4 d repeated every 8–14 d) may produce excellent responses even in refractory patients. However, the duration of response is usually less than 1 year. Toxicities include insomnia, hyperglycemia, mental status changes, and increased risk of infections. VAD may be used in patients who initially failed MP, but its efficacy in patients who previously failed high-dose dexamethasone therapy alone is less impressive. This salvage regimen remains one of the most active treatments even in patients relapsing after high-dose therapy and is very well tolerated by most patients.

Recently, use of another anthracycline (idarubicin) with dexamethasone (both given orally) has produced encouraging results in preliminary studies. Etoposide with cyclophosphamide or in other regimens, such as EDAP (etoposide, dexamethasone, cytarabine, and cisplatin) or ICE (etoposide, cyclophosphamide and idarubicin), have also demonstrated some activity in refractory myeloma. Other idarubicin-containing regimens have also shown efficacy in patients with relapsing or refractory disease [38]. Intravenous cyclophosphamide alone may also produce responses in patients with resistant myeloma [39].

Because patients relapsing frequently develop expression of a protein involved in multidrug resistance, P-glycoprotein approaches to block the expression of this protein have been developed [40]. Early approaches involved the addition of cardiotoxic drugs (eg, quinine and verapamil or the nephrotoxic agent cyclosporine) to patients receiving VAD-type regimens after failing a similar type of chemotherapy initially. With the newer multidrug resistance inhibitor PSC 833, encouraging results have been observed in small single-arm trials, but significant neurotoxicity was also found in some patients [41]. This agent is now being investigated in several large randomized trials.

Intensive treatment with high-dose alkylating agents and radiation may produce dramatic response in patients with refractory disease. However, these responses are short-lived and cannot be considered a standard form of salvage treatment. A recent French study suggests that high-dose therapy may be equally effective when done at the time of first relapse as when done as part of the patient's initial treatment. Thus, this certainly is an option in patients who have relapsed following conventional therapy. However, induction of disease stabilization or response with conventional chemotherapy should be achieved prior to attempting a high-dose program, otherwise the outcome is extremely poor. In patients relapsing following high-dose therapy, another high-dose treatment regimen may be used if the initial therapy resulted in a relatively long remission following the first transplant. Alternatively, in patients who previously underwent autologous transplantation, allogeneic support may be tried, but the high risk of treatment-related mortality must be considered in any decision regarding this form of treatment.

BONE DISEASE

Bone disease is the major cause of morbidity in multiple myeloma, resulting from stimulation of osteoclasts by bone-resorbing cytokines (tumor necrosis factor, interleukin-1-β and interleukin-6), which are overabundant in the myeloma bone marrow. Osteolytic lesions and generalized osteoporosis may lead to severe pain, pathologic fractures, and spinal cord compression and collapse. These complications often require radiation therapy to relieve pain or to treat actual or impending pathologic fractures or spinal cord compression. Plasma cell tumors are relatively responsive to radiation treatment. Responses typically occur rapidly, with most lesions treated with approximately 3000 cGy. However, it is important to avoid unnecessary radiotherapy because its myelosuppressive effect may limit the ability to deliver cytotoxic doses of systemic chemotherapy. Often the latter treatment alone will be effective for relieving skeletal pain. High doses of analgesics may be necessary until pain control is achieved with radiation treatment or chemotherapy. Surgery may be necessary to treat actual fractures or prevent large lytic lesions from developing fractures. The placement of intramedullary rods is usually the surgical procedure of choice. Spinal disease may require surgical decompression or stabilization of the spine. Previous attempts to reduce the development of these skeletal complications with calcium, sodium fluoride, androgenic steroids, or combinations of the three have been unsuccessful.

Bisphosphonates inhibit osteoclastic activity and are effective in the treatment of hypercalcemia associated with myeloma. Previous attempts to use relatively weak first-generation bisphosphonates (etidronate or clodronate) orally as an adjunct to chemotherapy had no significant effect on the development of skeletal complications in myeloma patients. A recent large randomized trial compared the effect of the more potent second-generation agent pamidronate (given as a 90-mg 4-h infusion every 4 wk for 21 cycles) with placebo on the development of bony complications in patients on chemotherapy [42,43]. At study entry, patients were stratified according to whether they were receiving first-line chemotherapy or had already failed initial chemotherapy. In both strata, pamidronate was successful in both reducing the percentage of patients developing at least one skeletal event as well as reducing the number of events experienced by the patient. In addition, patients experienced less pain after beginning pamidronate therapy, their requirement for analgesic usage was less than that of placebo-treated patients, and individuals treated with the bisphosphonate showed a better ECOG performance status. Interestingly, pamidronate also led to a significant improvement (50%) in overall survival in the stratum of patients who entered the trial having failed initial chemotherapy. Several recent in vitro studies suggest that these agents may have both a direct and indirect antitumor effect on myeloma. Although the clinical trial involved patients with Durie-Salmon stage III myeloma, it is likely that this drug will also be efficacious in reducing these complications in patients at earlier stages of the disease. Newer, more potent bisphosphonates are in clinical development. Although results were disappointing among 199 patients randomized to receive either intravenous monthly ibandronate or placebo [44], several recent studies suggest the potential for intravenous zoledronic acid to improve upon the results achieved with monthly intravenous pamidronate. Specifically, in a randomized Phase III trial, zoledronic acid (4 or 8 mg) was superior to pamidronate (90 mg) in achieving normocalcemia among patients with tumor-induced hypercalcemia [45], and early Phase I and II studies [46,47] demonstrated that monthly doses ≥ 2 mg led to sustained and marked suppression of bone resorption markers and a reduction in skeletal complication among breast cancer and myeloma patients with osteolytic bone disease.

NEW THERAPY APPROACHES

A number of new therapeutic strategies for myeloma are now in clinical development. Previous studies have shown a high degree of angiogenesis in multiple myeloma and its association with a poor outcome among these patients [48]. The most exciting therapeutic development has been the demonstrated anti-myeloma effect of thalidomide in a group of patients, most of whom had failed high-dose therapy [49]. However, the dose used in the first trial is poorly tolerated by most patients, and more recent trials have suggested similar activity with lower doses of this drug especially in combination with glucocorticosteroids [50]. Although an initial study suggested the efficacy of oral clarithromycin in relapsing myeloma [51], other studies have failed to show any benefit with single-agent therapy [52,53]. However, a high response rate has recently been observed when this macrolide antibiotic was combined with low-dose thalidomide and dexamethasone [54]. Whether the clarithromycin adds to the benefit of the thalidomide-dexamethasone is still not clear but deserves further study. In addition, several other new drugs including a proteosome inhibitor, PS-341 [55], and arsenic trioxide [56] have shown responses in relapsing myeloma patients in early trials, and are now entering larger Phase II studies. Use of antagonists to interleukin-6 have been evaluated in early phase I trials. In one myeloma patient, vaccination of an allogeneic donor with purified paraprotein induced an immune response to the monoclonal protein by the donor, and these donor cells were used clinically in the patient [57]. Whether this approach will prove generally useful awaits larger clinical trials, which have been initiated. Use of ex vivo–generated dendritic cells specifically armed with part of the monoclonal protein is another new immunologic approach that is being explored. However, the presence of a possible etiologic agent (human herpesvirus-8) for myeloma in these types of immune cells must be considered in these therapeutic strategies. Because of the encouraging results on overall survival from the recent pamidronate trial, higher doses of bisphosphonates alone are being used to treat previously treated patients in clinical trials.

In summary, many regimens will produce responses in patients with myeloma, but long-term disease control is uncommon. High-dose therapy with peripheral blood stem cell support seems to offer both longer progression-free and overall survival than conventional treatment but is not curative in the vast majority of patients. Use of intravenous pamidronate reduces the bony complications while improving the quality of life of these patients; it may even improve overall survival in some patients. Newer immunologic or other novel approaches will be required to improve these patients' outcomes.

REFERENCES

1. Kyle RA: "Benign" monoclonal gammopathy after 23 years of follow-up. *Mayo Clinic Proc* 1993, 68:26–36.

2. Rettig MB, Ma HJ, Vescio RA, *et al.*: Kaposi's sarcoma-associated herpesvirus infection of bone marrow dendritic cells from multiple myeloma patients. *Science* 1997, 276:1851–1854.

3. Said JW, Rettig MR, Heppner K, *et al.*: Localization of kaposi's sarcoma-associated herpesvirus in bone marrow biopsy samples from patients with multiple myeloma. *Blood* 1997, 90:4278–4282.

4. Durie BGM, Salmon SE: A clinical staging system for multiple myeloma. *Cancer* 1975, 36:842–854.

5. Greipp PR, Lust JA, O'Fallon M, *et al.*: Plasma cell labeling index and beta2-microglobulin predict survival independent of thymidine kinase and c-reactive protein in multiple myeloma. *Blood* 1993, 91:3382–3387.

6. Durie B, Stock-Novack D, Salmon S, *et al.*: Prognostic value of pretreatment serum beta2 microglobulin in myeloma: a Southwest Oncology Group Study. *Blood* 1990, 75:823–830.

7. Tricot G, Barlogie B, Jagannath S, *et al.*: Poor prognosis in multiple myeloma is associated only with partial or complete deletions of chromosome 13 or abnormalities involving 11q and not with other karyotype abnormalities. *Blood* 1995, 86:4250–4256.

8. Greipp PR, Gaillard JP, Klein B, *et al.*: Independent prognostic value for plasma cell labeling index, immunofluorescence microscopy plasma cell percent, beta 2-microglobulin, soluble interleukin-6 receptor and C-reactive protein in myeloma trial E9487. *Blood* 1994, 84:385.

9. Kusumoto S, Jinnai I, Itoh K, *et al.*: Magnetic resonance imaging patterns in patients with multiple myeloma. *Br J Haematol* 1997, 99:649–655.

10. Oken MM, Harrington DP, Abramson N, *et al.*: Comparison of melphalan and prednisone with vincristine, carmustine, melphalan, cyclophosphamide, and prednisone in the treatment of multiple myeloma. *Cancer* 1997, 79:1561–1567.

11. Salmon SE, Tesh D, Crowley J, *et al.*: Chemotherapy is superior to sequential hemibody irradiation for remission consolidation in multiple myeloma: a Southwest Oncology Group Study. *J Clin Oncol* 1990, 8:1575–1584.

12. MacLennan ICM, Chapman C, Dunn J, *et al.*: Combined chemotherapy with ABCM vs melphalan for treatment of myelomatosis. *Lancet* 1993, 339:200–205.

13. Salmon SE, Crowley JJ, Grogan TM, *et al.*: Combination chemotherapy, glucocorticoids, and interferon alpha in the treatment of multiple myeloma: a Southwest Oncology Group study. *J Clin Oncol* 1994, 12:2405–2414.

14. Barlogie B, Smith L, Alexanian R: Effective treatment of advanced multiple myeloma refractory to alkylating agents. *N Engl J Med* 1984, 3:1353–1356.

15. Alexanian R, Dimopoulos MA, Delasalle K, *et al.*: Primary dexamethasone treatment in multiple myeloma. *Blood* 1992, 80:887–890.

16. Palumbo A, Battaglio S, Napoli P, *et al.*: Recombinant interferon-gamma inhibits the in vitro proliferation of human myeloma cells. *Br J Haematol* 1994, 86:726–732.

17. Mandelli F, Avvisati G, Amadori S, *et al.*: Maintenance treatment with recombinant interferon alfa-2b in patients with multiple myeloma responding to conventional induction chemotherapy. *N Engl J Med* 1990, 322:1430–1434.

18. Powles R, Raje N, Cunningham D, *et al.*: Maintenance therapy for remission in myeloma with intron A following high-dose melphalan and either an autologous bone marrow transplantation or peripheral stem cell rescue. *Stem Cells Daytona* 1995, 13:114–117.

19. Browman GP, Rubin S, Walker I, *et al.*: Interferon alpha-2b maintenance therapy prolongs progression-free and overall survival in plasma cell myeloma: results of a randomized trial. *Proc Am Soc Clin Oncol* 1994, 13:408.

20. Peest D, Deicher H, Coldewey R, *et al.*: A comparison of polychemotherapy and melphalan/prednisone for primary remission induction, and interferon-alpha for maintenance treatment, in multiple myeloma: a prospective trial of the German Myeloma Treatment Group. *Eur J Cancer* 1995, 31A:146–151.

21. The Nordic Myeloma Study Group: Interferon alpha-2b added to melphalan-prednisone for initial and maintenance therapy in multiple myeloma: a randomized, controlled trial. *Ann Intern Med* 1996, 124:212–222.

22. Salmon S, Crowley J: Alpha interferon plus alternate day prednisone (IFN/P) improves remission maintenance duration in multiple myeloma (MM) compared to IFN alone. *Proc Am Soc Clin Oncol* 1997, 16:46.

23. Berenson J, Crowley J, Barlogie B, Salmon S: Alternate day oral prednisone maintenance therapy improves progression-free and overall survival in multiple myeloma patients. *Blood* 1998, (Suppl 1):318a.

24. Attal M, Harousseau J-L, Stoppa A-M, *et al.*: A prospective, randomized trial of autologous bone marrow transplantation and chemotherapy in multiple myeloma. *N Engl J Med* 1996, 335:91–97.

25. Attal M, Harousseau JL, Stoppa AM, *et al.*: Autologous transplantation-clinical results in multiple myeloma. *Blood* 1997, 90:1858.

26. Fermand JP, Ravaud P, Katsahian S, *et al.*: High-dose therapy (HDT) and autologous blood stem cell (ABSC) transplantation versus conventional treatment in multiple myeloma (MM): Results of a randomized trial in 190 patients 55 to 65 years of age. *Blood* 1999, 94:368a.

27. Schiller G, Vescio R, Freytes C, *et al.*: Transplantation of CD34+ peripheral blood progenitor cells after high-dose chemotherapy for patients with advanced multiple myeloma. *Blood* 1995, 86:390–397.

28. Vescio R, Stewart A, Ballester O, *et al.*: Myeloma cell tumor reduction in PBPC autografts following CD34 selection: the results of a phase III trial using the CEPRATE device. *Blood* 1997, 90:1872.

29. Stewart KA, Vescio R, Schiller G, *et al.*: Purging of autologous peripheral blood stem cells in multiple myeloma by CD34+ selection does not improve overall or progression free survival following high dose chemotherapy: results of a multi-center randomized controlled trial. *J Clin Oncol.* In press.

30. Vescio RA, Schiller HJ, Stewart AK, *et al.*: Quantitative assessment of myleoma peripheral blood and bone marrow tumor burden in patients undergoing autologous transplantation. *Blood* 1996, 88:641a.

31. Barlogie B, Jagannath S, Vesole DH, *et al.*: Superiority of tandem autologous transplantation over standard therapy for previously untreated multiple myeloma. *Blood* 1997, 89:789–793.

32. Attal M, Payen C, Facon T, *et al.*: Single versus double transplant in myeloma: a randomized trial of the Inter Groupe Francais du Myelome (IFM). *Blood* 1997, 90:1859.

33. Gahrton G, Tura S, Ljungman P, *et al.*: European Group for bone marrow transplantation: allogeneic bone marrow transplantation in multiple myeloma. *N Eng J Med* 1991, 325:1267.

34. Tricot G, Vesole DH, Jagannath S, *et al.*: Graft-versus-myeloma effect: proof of principle. *Blood* 1996, 87:1196–1198.

35. Lokhorst HM, Schattenberg A, Cornelissen JJ, *et al.*: Donor lymphocyte infusions for relapsed multiple myeloma after allogenic stem-cell transplantation: predictive factors for response and long-term outcome. *J Clin Oncol* 2000, 18(16):3031–3037.

36. Giralt S, Estey E, van Besien K, *et al.*: Induction of graft-versus-leukemia without myeloablative therapy using allogeneic PBSC after purine analog containing regimens. *Blood* 1996, 88:2444.

37. Kraut EH, Crowley JJ, Wade JL, *et al.*: Evaluation of topotecan in resistant and relapsing multiple myeloma: a Southwest Oncology Group Study. *J Clin Oncol* 1998, 16:589–592.

38. Parameswaran R, Giles C, Boots M, *et al.*: CCNU (lomustine), idarubicin and dexamethasone (CIDEX): an effective oral regimen for the treatment of refractory or relapsed myeloma. *Br J Haematol* 2000, 109(3):571–575.

39. Lenhard RE Jr, Oken MM, Barnes JM, *et al.*: High-dose cyclophosphamide: an effective treatment for advanced refractory multiple myeloma. *Cancer* 1984, 53:1456–1460.

40. Grogan TM, Spier CM, Salmon SE, *et al.*: P-glycoprotein expression in human plasma cell myeloma: correlation with prior chemotherapy. *Blood* 1993, 81:490–495.

41. Sonneveld P, Marie J-P, Huisman C, *et al.*: Reversal of multidrug resistance by SDZ PSC 833, combined with VAD (vincristine, doxorubicin, dexamethasone) in refractory multiple myeloma: a phase I study. *Leukemia* 1996, 10:1741–1750.

42. Berenson J, Lichtenstein A, Porter L, *et al.*: Long-term pamidronate treatment of advanced multiple myeloma patients reduces skeletal events. *J Clin Oncol* 1998, 16: 593–602.

43. Berenson J, Lichtenstein A, Porter L, *et al.*: Efficacy of pamidronate in reducing skeletal events in patients with advanced multiple myeloma. *N Eng J Med* 1996, 334:488–493.

44. Fontana A, Hermann Z, Menssen HD, *et al.*: Effects of intravenous ibandronate therapy on skeletal related events (SRE) and survival in patients with advanced multiple myeloma. *Blood* 1998, 92:106a.

45. Major P, Lortholary A, Hon J, *et al.*: Zoledronic acid is superior in the treatment of hypercalcemia of malignancy: A pooled analysis of two randomized, controlled clinical trials. *J Clin Oncol* 2001, 19:558–5671

46. Berenson J, Vescio R, Rosen L, *et al.*: A Phase I dose-ranging trial of monthly infusions of zoledronic acid for the treatment of osteolytic bone metastases. *Clin Cancer Res.* In press.

47. Berenson J, Rosen LS, Howell A, *et al.*: Zoledronic acid reduces skeletal related events in patients with osteolytic metastases: A double-blind, randomized dose-response study. *Cancer.* In press.

48. Munshi N, Wilson CS, Penn J, *et al.*: Angiogenesis in newly diagnosed multiple myeloma: Poor prognosis with increased microvessel density (MVD) in bone marrow biopsies. *Blood* 1998, 92 (Suppl 1):98a.

49. Singhal S, Mehta J, Desikan R, *et al.*: Antitumor activity of thalidomide in refractory multiple myeloma. *N Engl J Med* 1999, 18:1565–1571.

50. Rajkumar SV, Hayman S, Fonseca R, *et al.*: Thalidomide plus dexamethazone (THAL/DEX) and thalidomide alone (THAL) first line therapy for newly diagnosed myeloma (MM). *Blood* 2000, 96:722.

51. Weber DM, Rankin K, Gavino M, *et al.*: Thalidomide with dexamethasone for resistant multiple myeloma. *Blood* 2000, 96:719.

52. Durie BGM, Villarette L, Farvard M, *et al.*: Clarithromycin (Biaxin®) as primary treatment for myeloma. *Blood* 1997, 90:2578–2579a.

53. Stewart AK, Trudel S, Al Berouti BM, *et al.*: Lack of response to short-term use of clarithromycin (BIAXIN) in multiple myeloma. *Blood* 1999, 93(12):4441.

54. Moreau P, Huynh A, Facon T, *et al.*: Lack of efficacy of clarithromycin in advanced multiple myeloma. *Leukemia* 1999, 13(3):490–491.

55. Coleman M, Leonard J, Nahum H, *et al.*: Non-myelosuppressive therapy with BLT-D (Biaxin®, low-dose thalidomide and dexamethasone) is highly active in Waldenstrom's macroglobulinemia and myeloma. *Blood* 2000, 96:167a.

56. Stinchcombe TE, Mitchell BS, Depcik-Smith N, *et al.*: PS-431 is active in multiple myeloma: Preliminary report of a phase I trial of the proteasome inhibitor PS-341 in patients with hematologic malignancies. *Blood* 2000, 96:2219.

57. Desikan M, Zangari A, Badros S, *et al.*: Marked antitumor effect of arsenic trioxide (AS_2O_3) in high-risk refractory multiple myeloma. *Blood* 1999, 94:123a.

58. Kwak LW, Taub DD, Duffey PL, *et al.*: Transfer of myeloma idiotype-specific immunity from an actively immunised marrow donor. *Lancet* 1995, 345:1016–1020.

MP
(Melphalan and Prednisone)

Melphalan and prednisone is the prototype regimen in the single-alkylating-agent therapy for multiple myeloma. The high-dose intermittent schedule has proved a simple, relatively safe way to administer melphalan. A 1972 study reported that prednisone doubled the response rate to melphalan and that it produced modest improvement in survival. MP became, and for some, remains, the standard chemotherapy for multiple myeloma. Treatment is generally administered in cycles of 3–6 wk duration and is continued for 1–2 y, although it sometimes has been continued until disease progression.

An important problem with this protocol is the erratic absorption of oral melphalan, which sometimes leads to inadequate bioavailability in some patients who take apparently adequate oral doses.

DOSAGE AND SCHEDULING

	Day 1 2 3 4 5 6 7 8 9 10 11 12 13 14
Melphalan 8 mg/m² PO d 1–4	████████
Prednisone 60 mg/m² PO d 1–4	████████
CBC, serum creatinine; cycle 1, 4, 7, etc. d 1, 14 (cycle 1 only)	☐ ☐

Cycle duration, 4 wk; treatment duration, 1 to 2 y.

DOSAGE MODIFICATIONS: After first cycle, modify melphalan dose for depressed blood counts as follows: ANC 1000–2000/μL—give 75%; ANC 750–1000 or platelets 50,000–100,000/μL—give 50%; delay treatment for ANC < 750/μL or platelets < 50,000/μL.

EXPERIENCES AND RESPONSE RATES

Study	Evaluable Patients, n	Dosage and Scheduling	Objective Response (%)	Median Survival (mo)
Alexanian et al., Cancer 1972, 30:382–389	77	Melphalan 0.25 mg/kg PO d 1–4 Prednisone 2 mg/kg PO d 1–4 Cycle duration, 6 wk	47*	24
Abramson et al., Cancer Treat Rep 1982, 66:1273–1277	72	Melphalan 8 mg/m² PO d 1–4 Prednisone 75 mg PO d 1–7 Cycle duration, 4 wk	43‡	25
Oken et al., Proc ASCO 1987, 6:203	217	Melphalan 8 mg/m² PO d 1–4 Prednisone 60 mg/m² PO d 1–4	51†	30
Bergsagel et al., N Engl J Med 1979, 301:743–748	125	Melphalan 9 mg/m² PO d 1–4 Prednisone 100 mg PO d 1–4 Cycle duration, 4 wk	40*	28

*Response requires ≥ 75% decrease in M-protein production.
†Response requires ≥ 50% decrease in M-protein value.
‡Response evaluated at 6 mo only.

CANDIDATES FOR TREATMENT
Patients with active or advanced myeloma, particularly those who are elderly and frail

SPECIAL PRECAUTIONS
Risk for infection greater during early cycles (use allopurinol to prevent hyperuricemia during early months); treatment-associated myelodysplastic syndrome and acute leukemia occur in some

ALTERNATIVE THERAPIES
Melphalan alone, VMCP/VBAP, ABCM

TOXICITIES
Melphalan: bone marrow suppression leading to neutropenia with increased risk for infection, thrombocytopenia with risk for bleeding, erythroid hypoplasia with risk for symptomatic anemia; long-term toxicity: testicular atrophy, amenorrhea, risk for treatment-induced acute leukemia; **Prednisone:** immunosuppression, infection, edema, exacerbation of diabetes, weight gain, menstrual abnormalities, mental status dysfunction (especially in elderly)

DRUG INTERACTIONS
None

NURSING INTERVENTIONS
Instruct patient to seek medical attention if fever or other specific or subjective symptoms develop that could represent infection; monitor blood glucose if diabetic; antacid therapy may be used

PATIENT INFORMATION
Patient should take melphalan on empty stomach, prednisone after meals; anticipate possibility of mood and appetite changes or fluid retention; be alert to early signs of bleeding or infection

VBMCP
(Vincristine, BCNU, Melphalan, Cyclophosphamide, Prednisone)

VBMCP is a prototype combination chemotherapy regimen that is more intensive than standard MP. Initial reports of a markedly increased response rate in comparison with MP were confirmed in a large randomized trial. The regimen is one of multiple alkylating agents plus the vinca alkyloid vincristine and prednisone. Full-dose melphalan plus prednisone is part of the regimen but is administered at 5-wk rather than 4-wk intervals. Part of the increase in response rate may be attributed to the addition of three intravenous drugs to the sometimes erratically absorbed, orally administered melphalan.

BCNU, or carmustine, is a nitrosourea that is primarily an alkylating agent, as are both cyclophosphamide and melphalan. Vincristine is a vinca alkyloid and is cell cycle–specific for the M phase, interfering with the mitotic spindle formation.

DOSAGE AND SCHEDULING

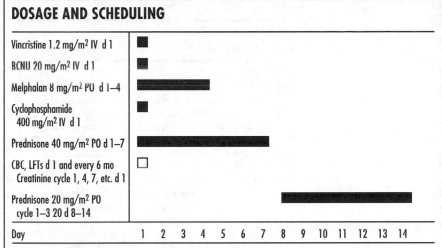

Vincristine 1.2 mg/m² IV d 1

BCNU 20 mg/m² IV d 1

Melphalan 8 mg/m² PO d 1–4

Cyclophosphamide 400 mg/m² IV d 1

Prednisone 40 mg/m² PO d 1–7

CBC, LFTs d 1 and every 6 mo
Creatinine cycle 1, 4, 7, etc. d 1

Prednisone 20 mg/m² PO
cycle 1–3 20 d 8–14

Day 1 2 3 4 5 6 7 8 9 10 11 12 13 14

Cycle duration, 5 wk; treatment duration, 1 to 2 y.

DOSAGE MODIFICATIONS: *After first cycle, modify melphalan, BCNU, cyclophosphamide for depressed blood counts as follows: ANC 1000–2000/µL—give 75%; ANC 750–1000 or platelets 50,000–100,000/µL—give 50%; delay treatment for ANC < 750/µL or platelets < 50,000/µL vincristine dose reduction required for hepatic insufficiency.*

EXPERIENCES AND RESPONSE RATES

Study	Evaluable Patients, *n*	Dosage and Scheduling	Response, %	Median Survival, *mo*	5-Y Survival, %
Case *et al., Am J Med* 1977, 63:897–903 Lee *et al.,* In Wiernik (ed.) *Controversies in Oncology* 1982, pp 61–79	81	Vincristine 0.03 mg/kg IV d 1 BCNU 0.5 mg/kg IV d 1 Melphalan 0.25 mg/kg PO d 1–4 Cyclophosphamide 10 mg/kg IV d 1 Prednisone 1 mg/kg PO d 1–7, then 0.5 mg/kg d 8–14, then taper	78*	38	—
Oken *et al., Proc ASCO* 1987, 6:203	214	Vincristine 1.2 mg/m² IV d 1 BCNU 20 mg/m² IV d 1 Melphalan 8 mg/m² PO d 1–4 Cyclophosphamide 400 mg/m² IV d 1 Prednisone 60 mg/m² PO d 1–7; (20 mg/m² PO d 8–14 cycle 1–3)	72*	31	26

*Response requires ≥ 50% decrease in M-protein value.

CANDIDATES FOR TREATMENT
Patients with active myeloma unless they are elderly (> 70 years) and frail

SPECIAL PRECAUTIONS
Risk for infection greater during early cycles (use allopurinol to prevent hyperuricemia during early months); treatment-associated myelodysplastic syndrome and acute leukemia occur in some; VBMCP poorly tolerated by patients > 70 years of age and frail—MP is better choice

ALTERNATIVE THERAPIES
MP, VMCP/VBAP, ABCM, melphalan alone, VBMCP and interferon

TOXICITIES
Drug combination: long-term toxicity: testicular atrophy, amenorrhea, risk for treatment-induced acute leukemia; **Melphalan:** bone marrow suppression leading to neutropenia with increased risk for infection, thrombocytopenia with increased risk for bleeding, erythroid hypoplasia with risk for symptomatic anemia; **Prednisone:** immunosuppression, infection, exacerbation of diabetes, weight gain, edema, mental status dysfunction—especially in elderly; **BCNU:** bone marrow suppression possibly longer than that with melphalan or cyclophosphamide, pain in injected extremity or at IV site, nausea, vomiting, liver or renal dysfunction; pulmonary fibrosis (rare); **Cyclophosphamide:** bone marrow suppression but relatively platelet sparing, nausea, vomiting, hemorrhagic cystitis, alopecia; rarely, pulmonary fibrosis, liver dysfunction; **Vincristine:** peripheral neuropathy, cranial nerve neuropathy, constipation, alopecia, vesicant if extravasated; SIADH (rare)

DRUG INTERACTIONS
Cyclophosphamide: barbiturates, phenytoin, chloral hydrate

NURSING INTERVENTIONS
Push fluids for 24 hours after cyclophosphamide to reduce risk for hemorrhagic cystitis; give antiemetic before administration; monitor blood glucose if diabetic; antacid therapy may be used

PATIENT INFORMATION
Maintain good fluid intake; take melphalan on empty stomach, prednisone after meals; anticipate possibility of mood and appetite changes or fluid retention; be alert to early signs of bleeding or infection; call physician for blood in urine; vincristine may cause severe constipation: monitor bowel pattern carefully, use mild laxatives, seek medical attention if persistent or severe

VMCP/VBAP AND ABCM

(Vincristine, Melphalan, Cyclophosphamide, Prednisone/Vincristine, BCNU, Doxorubicin, Prednisone; and Doxorubicin, BCNU, Cyclophosphamide, Melphalan)

This regimen consists of alternating cycles of vincristine plus prednisone combined with either melphalan plus cyclophosphamide or with BCNU plus doxorubicin. The strategy of rapid alternating cycles provides maximum early exposure to active combinations and theoretically could prevent or delay the emergence of resistant clones. An alternative strategy of giving three cycles of VMCP followed by three cycles of VBAP yielded essentially identical results in a SWOG study. Therefore, these results are pooled. A third variation on VMCP/VBAP, the ABCM regimen, eliminates vincristine and prednisone and yields similar results.

DOSAGE AND SCHEDULING

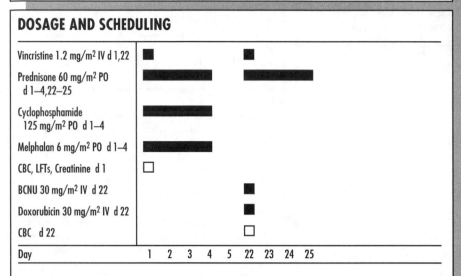

	Day	1	2	3	4	5	22	23	24	25

Vincristine 1.2 mg/m² IV d 1,22
Prednisone 60 mg/m² PO d 1–4,22–25
Cyclophosphamide 125 mg/m² PO d 1–4
Melphalan 6 mg/m² PO d 1–4
CBC, LFTs, Creatinine d 1
BCNU 30 mg/m² IV d 22
Doxorubicin 30 mg/m² IV d 22
CBC d 22

DOSAGE MODIFICATIONS: *Reduce dose of vincristine and doxorubicin for impaired liver function or significant treatment-induced cytopenias*

EXPERIENCES AND RESPONSE RATES

Study	Evaluable Patients, *n*	Dosage and Scheduling	Response, %	Median Survival, *mo*	5-Y Survival, %
VMCP/VBAP Durie *et al.*, *J Clin Oncol* 1986, 4:1227–1237, Salmon *et al.*, *J Clin Oncol* 1990, 8:1575–1584	614	Vincristine 1.0 mg IV d 1, 22 Prednisone 60 mg/m² PO d 1–4, 22–25 Melphalan 6 mg/m² d 1–4 Cyclophosphamide 125 mg/m² PO d 1–4 BCNU 30 mg/m² IV d 22 Doxorubicin 30 mg/m² IV d 22	38*	30	27
ABCM Maclennan *et al.*, *Lancet* 1992, 339:200–205	314	Doxorubicin 30 mg/m² IV d 1 BCNU 30 mg/m² IV d 1 Cyclophosphamide 100 mg/m² PO d 22–25 Melphalan 6 mg/m² PO d 22–25	61†	32	25

*Response requires ≥ 75% decrease in M-protein production.
†Response—achievement of plateau phase.

CANDIDATES FOR TREATMENT

Patients with active myeloma who are elderly and frail (partially or totally bedridden)

SPECIAL PRECAUTIONS

Risk for infection greater during early cycles (use allopurinol to prevent hyperuricemia during early months); treatment-associated myelodysplastic syndrome and acute leukemia occur in some; do not use doxorubicin in patients with significant cardiac decompensation (ejection fraction < 45%, signs of congestive heart failure [CHF], recent myocardial infarction [MI], or unstable angina); do not exceed cumulative doxorubicin dose of 450 mg/m²

ALTERNATIVE THERAPIES

MP, melphalan alone, VMCP/VBAP, ABCM

TOXICITIES

Melphalan: bone marrow suppression leading to neutropenia with increased risk for infection, thrombocytopenia with increased risk for bleeding, erythroid hypoplasia with risk for symptomatic anemia; **Prednisone:** immunosuppression, infection, Cushing's syndrome, exacerbation of diabetes, weight gain, edema, mental status dysfunction—especially in elderly; **BCNU:** bone marrow suppression possibly longer than that with melphalan or cyclophosphamide, pain in injected extremity or at IV site, nausea, vomiting, liver or renal dysfunction; pulmonary fibrosis rare at this dose range; **Cyclophosphamide:** bone marrow suppression but relatively platelet sparing, nausea, vomiting, alopecia, hemorrhagic cystitis, pulmonary fibrosis (rare), liver dysfunction (rare); **Vincristine:** peripheral neuropathy, cranial nerve neuropathy, constipation, alopecia, vesicant if extravasated; SIADH (rare); **Doxorubicin:** myelotoxicity, nausea, vomiting, alopecia, cardiotoxicity—generally at higher doses, vesicant if extravasated; **long-term toxicity:** testicular atrophy, amenorrhea, risk for treatment-induced acute leukemia

DRUG INTERACTIONS

Cyclophosphamide: barbiturates, phenytoin, chloral hydrate

NURSING INTERVENTIONS

Push fluids for 24 h after cyclophosphamide to reduce risk for hemorrhagic cystitis; give antiemetic before administration; monitor blood glucose if diabetic; antacid therapy may be used

PATIENT INFORMATION

Patient should maintain good fluid intake; take melphalan on empty stomach, prednisone after meals; anticipate possibility of mood and appetite changes or fluid retention; be alert to early signs of bleeding or infection; seek medical attention for blood in urine; vincristine may cause severe constipation: monitor bowel pattern carefully, use mild laxatives, seek medical attention if persistent or severe

VAD
(Vincristine, Doxorubicin, Dexamethasone)

The VAD regimen combines vincristine and adriamycin by 4-d infusion with high-dose oral dexamethasone. It is primarily a salvage regimen in patients who have relapses but has gained an additional application as a treatment to be used prior to autologous bone marrow transplant harvest when alkylating agents are to be avoided. Responses to this regimen usually occur within 2 mo, making VAD more rapid than MP or VMCP/VBAP and, possibly, VBMCP. The repeated cycles of high-dose corticosteroids are an important component in this regimen's effectiveness and may generate most of the activity in patients with refractory disease.

DOSAGE AND SCHEDULING

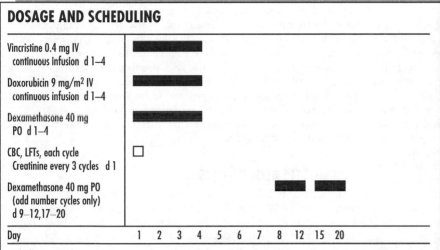

| | Day | 1 | 2 | 3 | 4 | 5 | 6 | 7 | 8 | 12 | 15 | 20 |

Vincristine 0.4 mg IV continuous infusion d 1–4

Doxorubicin 9 mg/m² IV continuous infusion d 1–4

Dexamethasone 40 mg PO d 1–4

CBC, LFTs, each cycle Creatinine every 3 cycles d 1

Dexamethasone 40 mg PO (odd number cycles only) d 9–12, 17–20

Cycle duration, 4 wk.
Trimethoprim/sulfamethoxazole 1 DS PO daily and clortrimazole troches, 10 mg 3×d as prophylaxis while receiving therapy. During dexamethasone, patients should receive an H₂-receptor antagonist, such as ranitidine, at full dose.

DOSAGE MODIFICATIONS: *Reduce dose of vincristine and doxorubicin for impaired liver function; reduce dexamethasone for severe dyspepsia, edema refractory to diuretics, myopathy, severe hypertension, severe corticosteroid withdrawal symptoms or cushingoid changes, steroid psychosis or hallucinations; after first cycle, reduce doxorubicin for myelotoxicity: 75% if ANC is 1500–1000/mm³, 50% if ANC is 750–1000 or platelets are 50,000–100,000/μL.*

EXPERIENCES AND RESPONSE RATES

Study	Evaluable Patients, n	Dosage and Scheduling	Cycle Duration, wk	Objective Response, %
Alexanian et al., Ann Intern Med 1986, 105:8–11	39	Vincristine 0.4 mg IV d 1–4 Doxorubicin 9 mg/m² IV d 1–4; both by continuous infusion Dexamethasone 40 mg PO d 1–4, 9–12, 17–20, 25–28	6	46†
Lokhorst et al., Br J Haemotol 1989, 71:25–30	31	Vincristine 0.4 mg IV d 1–4 Doxorubicin 9 mg/m² IV d 1–4; both by continuous infusion Dexamethasone 40 mg PO d 1–4, 9–12, 17–20 (odd # cycles) Dexamethasone 40 mg PO d 1–4 (even # cycles)	4	60‡

*In previously treated patients
†Response requires ≥ 75% decrease in M-protein production.
‡Response requires ≥ 50% decrease in serum M-protein level.

CANDIDATES FOR TREATMENT

Alternative primary regimen for patients under consideration for stem cell harvest. Most often used in patients with relapsed myeloma.

SPECIAL PRECAUTIONS

Regimen is contraindicated in patients with poor liver function; prophylactic trimethoprim/sulfamethoxazole and clotrimazole troches advised during therapy; use allopurinol to prevent hyperuricemia during early months; doxorubicin is contraindicated in patients with significant cardiac decompensation (ejection fraction < 45%, signs of CHF, recent MI, or unstable angina); do not exceed cumulative doxorubicin dose of 450 mg/m²; to prevent dyspepsia or ulcer, administer an H₂-receptor agonist at full dosage during dexamethasone

TOXICITIES

Vincristine: peripheral neuropathy, cranial nerve neuropathy, constipation, alopecia, vesicant if extravasated; SIADH (rare); **Doxorubicin:** myelotoxicity, nausea, vomiting, alopecia, flare, cardiotoxicity (generally at higher doses), vesicant if extravasated; **Dexamethasone:** immunosuppression, infection, Cushing's syndrome, osteoporosis, exacerbation of diabetes, weight gain, hypertension, edema, mental status dysfunction—especially in elderly

DRUG INTERACTIONS

Doxorubicin and vincristine are compatible

NURSING INTERVENTIONS

Carefully place venous access catheter before initiating VAD; do not use a peripheral IV site—would expose patient to excessive risk for doxorubicin or vincristine extravasation injury; if right atrial catheter or central venous port is in place, administer doxorubicin and vincristine in an ambulatory outpatient setting with portable infusion pump; doxorubicin and vincristine may be mixed together; monitor regularly for hypertension, CHF, severe fluid retention, behavioral changes, symptoms of ulcer or dyspepsia, infections—including local Candida infections

PATIENT INFORMATION

Patient should anticipate possibility of mood and appetite changes or fluid retention; be alert to early signs of infection; vincristine may cause severe constipation: monitor bowel pattern carefully, use mild laxatives, seek medical attention if persistent or severe

The accumulation of fluid in the pleural or pericardial space, as a result of either cancer or its treatment, leads to a progressive reduction in the ability of the patient to oxygenate. This inability to oxygenate, first manifested as dyspnea on exertion, is a result of reduced cardiac output or compromised pulmonary reserve. Although the end result of progressive respiratory failure is the same, the presenting signs and symptoms of malignant pleural or pericardial effusions differ (Table 21-1) [1,2].

PATHOPHYSIOLOGY

The causes of both effusions are essentially identical, reflecting a profound imbalance in the production and clearance of normal fluid through the respective space. In both instances, the presence of active malignancy in either space leads to the production of an exudative effusion that exceeds the capacity of normal lymphatic channels to clear it. The presence of significant amounts of tumor in the mediastinal lymph nodes, or the obstruction of mediastinal lymphatics by radiation-induced fibrosis, greatly exacerbates the clinical problem. Although reduced oncotic pressure due to hypoproteinemia or concurrent infection can exacerbate a malignant effusion, the direct presence of malignancy and the obstruction of mediastinal lymphatic flow are the primary contributing factors to the development of clinically significant, malignant pleural, and pericardial effusions.

In the case of the pericardium, the development of symptoms is a function of the rapidity with which the fluid accumulates, the amount of fluid produced, and the premorbid condition of the underlying myocardium [1]. Slowly accumulating fluid can produce no symptoms until a relatively massive amount of fluid has developed because the pericardium has time to stretch. Eventually, the combination of volume of fluid and speed of onset results in resistance to ventricular filling during diastole and a progressive compromise of cardiac output [6].

In the pleural space, the pathway is similar, but the speed of onset is of less importance in determining the onset of symptoms. However, the development of dyspnea is a function of the amount of fluid produced and the condition of the lungs prior to the onset of the effusion. At a point that varies among patients, the increase in accumulated fluid and the degree of prior pulmonary compromise intercept to produce a sense of dyspnea.

CLINICAL PRESENTATION

The interplay between volume and underlying organ function leads to a wide spectrum of presenting symptoms and signs. Radio-

graphically obvious but clinically silent pleural and pericardial effusions are common. In both instances, the initial presentation is usually shortness of breath on exertion. It is important to remember that patients with malignant pericardial effusions present with dyspnea on exertion, but the critical diagnostic test—the echocardiogram—usually is done at rest. This can result in a delay in therapy when the echo shows no evidence of tamponade. As outlined in Table 21-1, the two syndromes go on to manifest different signs and symptoms, reflecting the primarily cardiac or pulmonary organ systems being stressed. In malignant pleural effusions the progression of symptoms usually is linear and relatively predictable. On the other hand, pericardial effusions can lead to a rapid change in clinical status as critical pressures are exceeded [3]. Consequently, the presence of the classical findings of a positive Kussmaul's sign and pulsus paradoxus are actually very late findings indicative of the potential for rapid clinical deterioration in patients with malignant pericardial effusions. The use of potent diuretics, therefore, can impact rapidly on ventricular filling pressures and exacerbate the symptoms of pericardial tamponade.

DIAGNOSTIC ALGORITHMS

Figures 21-1 and 21-2 outline recommended diagnostic and treatment algorithms for malignant pleural and pericardial effusions. These are predicated on the assumption that the patient in question either has or is highly suspected to have a malignancy known to cause malignant effusions. These algorithms do *not* apply to the general medical patient who presents with a wider spectrum of possible diagnoses.

The approach to the patient with a suspected malignant pleural effusion is outlined in Figure 21-1 [4]. Most cases are detected during a routine chest radiograph or during computed tomography (CT) done to assess disease response or stability. The presence of new or worsening dyspnea often leads to the radiograph study. Obvious infection, heart failure, or an immunologic disorder usually can be excluded by the history and physical examination. The diagnostic thoracentesis can then complete the initial evaluation. Although literally hundreds of pleural fluid markers have been described, the diagnosis can be made by the simple use of cytologic examination and a comparison of serum and pleural fluid levels of lactate dehydrogenase and protein (Table 21-2). In my practice, the use of blind, transcutaneous needle biopsies as a next step has been virtually abandoned. If a transudate is present, there is no evidence of a malignant effusion. A cytologically negative exudate can present diagnostic dilemmas for the physician, but if a second diagnostic thoracentesis is negative I usually move directly to thoracoscopy, which allows direct visualization of the pleural space and biopsy of any suspicious area directly.

The approach to the patient with a suspected malignant pericardial effusion is outlined in Figure 21-2. Many cases are detected by changes on the chest radiograph. The "water bottle" cardiac silhouette is the most common change, although any significant change in cardiac width is important. At least 1- to 1.5-cm differences in cardiac width between films must be allowed for cardiac-cycle–related variation, but beyond 2 cm there is rarely any question about the diagnosis. Patients often have chest CT scans done for purposes of measuring tumor response, and this, too, can be an effective means of diagnosing a malignant pericardial effusion, especially one with an associated thick layer of tumor "cake." The history and physical examination rule out most instances of heart failure,

Table 21-1. Signs and Symptoms of Malignant Effusions in the Chest		
	Pleural	**Pericardial**
Common	Dyspnea (exertion)	Dyspnea (exertion)
	Dyspnea (rest)	Dyspnea (rest)
	Cough	Jugular venous distension
	Dullness to percussion	Distant heart sounds
	Egophony	
Uncommon	Cyanosis	Cyanosis
	Anorexia	Peripheral vasoconstriction
	Chest pain	Pulsus paradoxus
		Narrow pulse pressure (Kussmaul's sign)
		Electrical alternans

infection, and recent myocardial infarction. The optimal diagnostic test is the echocardiogram, which can both establish the presence of fluid and determine if diastolic filling is impaired. Pericardiocentesis to ascertain the cytologic nature of the fluid is usually less important because the diagnosis can be made rapidly during therapy. In unusual settings, the pericardiocentesis is the preferred procedure (*eg*, when the patient has such a poor prognosis from their systemic cancer that an operative procedure is believed to be relatively or absolutely contraindicated).

THERAPY OF MALIGNANT EFFUSIONS IN THE THORAX

Figures 21-1 and 21-2 also outline the recommended therapeutic approach to patients with malignant intrathoracic effusions. The decision to treat or not to treat must be individualized for each patient. Only in the moribund or rapidly progressive end-stage patient do I proceed with either no treatment or needle aspiration only. In both the pleural and pericardial spaces, it is associated with a relatively rapid recurrence of fluid and little prolonged palliative benefit. On the

other hand, I take a relatively aggressive approach to the patient who is asymptomatic but who has a significant effusion. For the patient with a pericardial effusion, the prolonged presence of an exudative effusion can increase the risk of a more constrictive presentation, requiring a more extensive surgical procedure later. The patient who will live more than 3 to 4 months following their systemic disease is a good candidate for early intervention to prolong the palliative effect.

The therapy of malignant pleural effusions depends on the responsiveness of the underlying cancer to systemic chemotherapy. Newly diagnosed responsive tumors such as lymphomas or small cell lung cancer can be treated directly with systemic therapy unless the volume of the effusion is life-threatening. During relapse, these cancers often migrate to the occasionally or rarely responsive subgroups. Patients with breast cancer typify a group of patients that are often responsive to systemic therapy. They can be treated by simple drainage followed by a trial of systemic therapy. During failure, they too often migrate to the refractory group. For patients whose effusion is caused by a tumor that is generally refractory to therapy, the treatment of choice is tube thoracostomy followed by

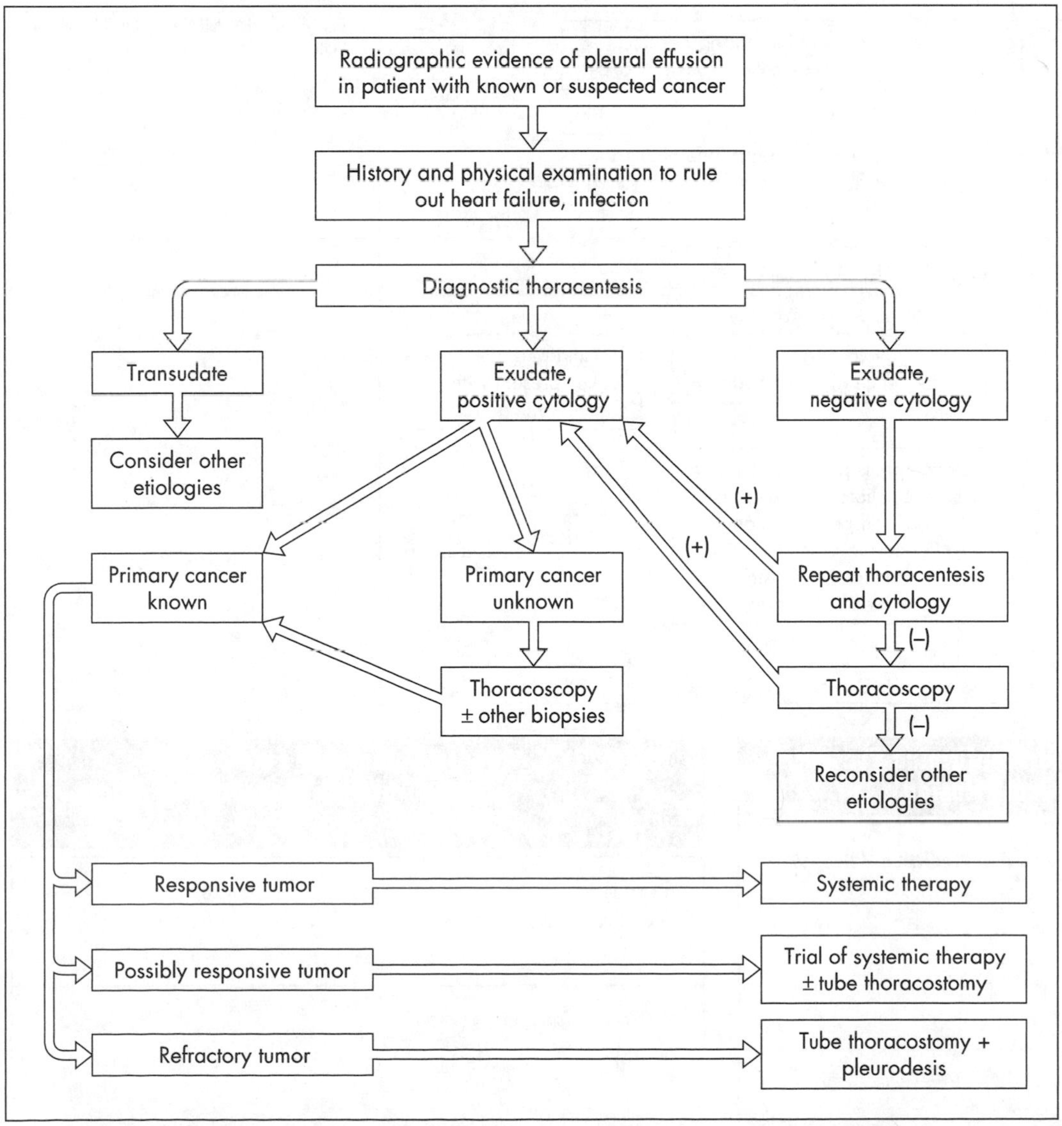

FIGURE 21-1.

Approach to the diagnosis and therapy of malignant pleural effusion. (*Adapted from* Ruckdeschel [4].)

pleurodesis. Several of the more commonly employed agents for pleurodesis are listed in Table 21-3 [1,7,8].

There are, however, some general points to be made about intrapleural therapy. The effusion should not be tapped to total dryness during the diagnostic thoracentesis because this may lead to an increased risk of lung puncture and the possibility of adhesions that prevent full reexpansion of the lung. The lung must fully reexpand for therapy to be effective. A conventional chest tube or smaller bore tubes can be used, although good trials have not been done comparing them. Drainage by suction is required. Recently, several trials have been conducted comparing outcome with comparatively small catheter drainage and sclerosis. The results have been encouraging, and for straightforward, nonloculated, free-flowing effusions, small-bore pigtail catheter drainage followed by sclerosis is effective and recommended [9,10]. These smaller catheters are less painful and better tolerated overall. Disadvantages include inability to drain more viscous, malignant effusions effectively and poor delivery of talc if used as a sclerosant. Typically, whether a standard-bore (28-F)

chest tube or a smaller (12- to 16-F) pigtail is used, patients require hospitalization for several days.

Several groups have reported the efficacy of simple pigtail catheter drainage attached to a closed, portable drainage system that the patient can monitor and empty. This allows outpatient management. In the vast majority of patients treated (> 80%), Putnam *et al.* [11] report excellent effusion control and increased patient mobility. Most importantly, patients can be discharged immediately and can simply monitor the drainage amount daily. Typically within 2 to 3 weeks, drainage subsides, sclerosis has been achieved without sclerosant, and the tube can be removed. In several trials, excellent results were obtained with greater than 85% effusion control with drainage for 30 days or less without additional sclerosant [11,12]. Potential drawbacks of this approach include patient discomfort from prolonged catheter placement (> 2 to 3 weeks), inconvenience of bulb drainage, and a small chance of infection.

This approach can be especially helpful in patients with trapped lung in whom any form of sclerotherapy is ineffective.

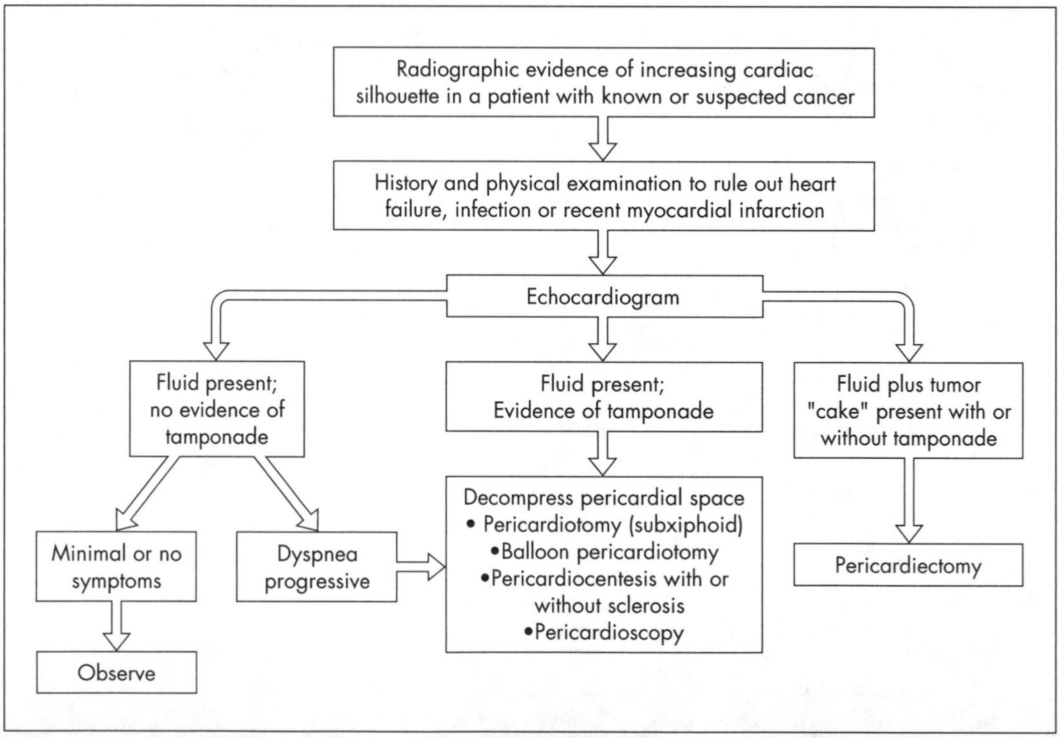

FIGURE 21-2.

Approach to the diagnosis and therapy of malignant pericardial effusion.

Table 21-2. Diagnostic Test for Confirming Presence of Malignant Pleural Effusion	
Test	**Positive Predictive Value, %**
Cytology	100
Fluid LDH > 200 U	100
Fluid/blood LDH ratio > 0.6	99
Fluid/protein ratio > 3 g	95
Fluid/blood protein ratio > 0.5	99

Adapted from Health and Public Policy Committee, American College of Physicians [5].

Table 21-3. Agents Commonly Employed as Intrapleural Therapy for Malignant Effusions	
Bleomycin	60 U*
Doxycycline	1–1.5 g
Talc	4–5 g

*Also used for malignant pericardial effusions.

For patients who have significant hydrothorax and a sense of "chest tightness," chronic catheter drainage is effective. Alternatives include pleuroperitoneal shunt placement or pleurectomy and decortication. A pleuroperitoneal shunt can palliate symptoms in a patient with advanced disease but has a high failure rate and is rarely used. Problems with longstanding drainage include significant fluid and protein loss in typically already nutritionally depleted patients [13]. There is some controversy about how much control of the drainage is needed. Most reports suggest getting the daily drainage down to 100 to 250 mL per 24 hours before introducing the sclerosing agent, but hard data have been elusive. There are studies of shorter drainage periods with little attention paid to the volume of drainage. In reality, a strict cutoff of the volume of daily effusion drainage prior to sclerosant is not needed. Once the majority of the effusion is drained (usually within the first 24 to 36 hours of chest tube placement) and especially if the lung re-expands fully, then the pleural space should be sclerosed promptly. Waiting for daily drainage volumes to decrease below 200 to 300 cc is usually not warranted. This can actually lead to less ineffective pleurodesis due to the chest tube becoming "walled off" within the pleural cavity.

Historically, a wide array of agents have been employed for intrapleural therapy. Tetracycline in its parenteral form was the most common agent employed until it was taken off the market by its manufacturer [14–16]. Several tetracycline derivatives (doxycycline, minocycline) have been proposed as alternatives, but it is not clear that they work as well as tetracycline did; several reports describe the need for multiple injections before control is achieved [17–19]. Bleomycin, an anticancer drug, was shown to be superior to tetracycline in one of the few randomized trials in this area, but concerns have been raised about its cost [20,21]. Many surgeons prefer the use of talc as an intrapleural agent, but it requires an operative procedure for insufflation or the use of a slurry of sterile talc that can be difficult to obtain [22–24]. Several large clinical trials are addressing this issue. Several smaller trials have compared the efficacy of chest tube (pigtail or conventional tube thoracostomy) drainage and talc slurry sclerosis versus intraoperative, minimally invasive thoracoscopic drainage and talc poudrage (direct insufflation). In these trials for otherwise uncomplicated malignant effusions, drainage and talc slurry was equally effective and obviated the need for a general anesthetic and operative procedure [25,26].

The study attempting to answer this question definitely has been performed by the Cancer and Leukemia Group B (CALGB) intergroup. This trial had to be extended initially due to insufficient patients for analysis despite large numbers of patients enrolled (< 400 patients). The trial has recently closed. Preliminary analysis suggests no significant advantage in either arm, with 30-day control ranging from 80% (slurry) to 85% to 90% (poudrage).

Many agents are effective as primary sclerosants, including mechanical abrasion, chemical sclerosant (antibiotics, chemotherapeutics (eg, bleomycin [27], cisplatin), recombinant cytokines (eg, interleukin-2 [28], tumor necrosis factor [29]), talc remains the most cost-effective and least painful way to achieve sclerosis and effusion control.

Route of talc administration either via slurry or direct insufflation has to be tailored to the individual patient's situation. In patients who have loculated effusions or an element of trapped lung, we prefer thoracoscopy. With a short 30- to 60-minute anesthetic, the pleural space can be inspected, the complete effusion drained, loculations broken down, and talc insufflated.

In patients with uncomplicated effusions, especially those that are recently diagnosed without evidence of bulky tumor, loculations or lung entrapment, either pigtail or tube thoracostomy drainage with talc slurry is highly effective and usually definitive.

The predominant therapy for malignant pericardial effusions should be subxiphoid pericardiotomy [28,29], although many centers persist in using needle pericardiocentesis with insertion of a drainage catheter and sclerosing agent [30,31]. I reserve needle pericardiocentesis for the urgent clinical situation when a surgeon or operating room is not available and for the patient with an extremely limited prognosis. The increasing availability of video-assisted thoracoscopic equipment has led to an increased use of pericardioscopy to drain the pericardial space and make a more certain diagnosis when the etiology is in question [32]. As in the pleural space, the thoracoscopic approach allows better visibility of lesions for direct biopsy. Despite this, a limited subxiphod incision (3 to 4 cm) is highly effective and allows excellent exposure to the pericardium for malignant effusion decompression and tissue diagnosis. Thoracoscopy does not offer any significant advantage unless concomitant pleural disease is present. A new procedure has been described, percutaneous balloon pericardiotomy, that allows for the nonsurgical creation of a pericardial window [33]. Although its potential is exciting, the role of this procedure in managing pericardial effusions has yet to be fully assessed. Several series have demonstrated good pericardial effusion control with pigtail drainage and sclerosis, similar to the approach and results in malignant pleural effusions. In these patients, usually with advanced stage disease, this approach is attractive. Furthermore, in patients with large pericardial effusions, induction of general anesthesia can be problematic due to underlying tamponade and right ventricular dysfunction. In the hands of experienced clinicians, pericardial catheter placement and drainage is safe and effective. Severe right ventricular failure after relief of tamponade has been described and is one more reason to treat as early as possible [34]. When malignant effusions are drained operatively, caution must be taken to decompress the pericardial tamponade gradually (over several minutes) to avoid the rare but often fatal complication of acute right ventricular distention and failure.

OUTCOME

Therapy for malignant pleural effusions controls the effusion in nearly 70% of cases treated with bleomycin or tetracycline derivatives. Talc controls the effusion in about 90% of cases, but the issues of patient selection have not been addressed, and results of clinical trials that address this are pending. Pericardiotomy by the traditional surgical approach controls nearly all effusions except those with a significant tumor cake, for which a pericardiectomy is required. (Whether to escalate to a full thoracic operation in this setting is unclear, and the risks must be balanced against the potential benefits for each patient.) Pigtail drainage with sclerosis is an effective alternative to balloon pericardotomy. Balloon pericardotomy has not proven to be a significant advance.

Whatever the therapy for malignant effusions involving either the pleural or pericardial spaces, it must be stressed that the purpose of the therapy is strictly palliative. Survival is short for both groups, particularly for those with pericardial effusions. Consequently, the therapy of this disorder must be sensitive to the balance of risk and benefit.

REFERENCES

1. Mills SA, Graeber GM, Nelson MG: Therapy of malignant tumors involving the pericardium. In *Thoracic Oncology*, edn 2. Edited by Roth J, Ruckdeschel JC, Weisenburger T. Philadelphia: WB Saunders, 1995:492–513.

2. Moores DWO, Ruckdeschel JC: Pleural effusions in patients with malignancy. In *Thoracic Oncology*, edn 2. Edited by Roth J, Ruckdeschel JC, Weisenburger T. Philadelphia: WB Saunders, 1995:556–566.

3. Hankins JR, Satterfield JR, Aisner J, *et al.*: Pericardial window for malignant pericardial effusion. *Ann Thorac Surg* 1980, 30:465.

4. Ruckdeschel JC: Management of malignant pleural effusion: an overview. *Semin Oncol* 1988, 15(suppl 3):24–28.

5. Health and Public Policy Committee, American College of Physicians: Diagnostic thoracentesis and pleural biopsy in pleural effusions. *Ann Intern Med* 1985, 103:799–802.

6. Hancock EW: Neoplastic pericardial disease. *Card Clin* 1990, 8:673.

7. Anderson CB, Philpott GW, Ferguson TB: The treatment of malignant pleural effusions. *Cancer* 1974, 33:916–922.

8. Tattersall MHN, Boyer MJ: Management of malignant pleural effusions. *Thorax* 1980, 45:81–82.

9. Saffran L, Ost DE, Fein AM, Schiff MJ: Outpatient pleurodesis of malignant pleural effusions using small-bore pigtail catheter. *Chest* 2000 118:417–421.

10. Bloom AI, Wilson MW, Kerlan RK, Jr., *et al.*: Talc pleurodesis through small-bore percutaneous tubes. *Cardiovasc Intervent Radiol* 1999, 22:433–436.

11. Putnam JB, Jr., Walsh GL, Swisher SG, *et al.*: Outpatient management of malignant pleural effusion by a chronic indwelling pleural catheter. *Ann Thorac Surg* 2000, 69:369–375.

12. Putnam JB, Jr., Light RW, Rodriguez RM, *et al.*: A randomized comparison of indwelling pleural catheter and doxycycline pleurodesis in the management of malignant pleural effusions. *Cancer* 1999, 86:1992–1999.

13. Genc O, Petrou M, Ladas G, Goldstraw P: The long-term morbidity of pleuroperitoneal shunts in the management of recurrent malignant effusions. *Eur J Cardiothorac Surg* 2000, 18:143–146.

14. Wallach HW: Intrapleural therapy with tetracycline and lidocaine for malignant pleural effusions (letter). *Chest* 1975, 73:246.

15. Gupta M, Opfell RW, Padova J, *et al.*: Intrapleural bleomycin versus tetracycline for control of malignant pleural effusion: a randomized study. *Proc Am Assoc Cancer Res Am Soc Clin Oncol* 1980, 21 (abstract):189.

16. Johnson CE, Curzon PGD: Comparison of intrapleural bleomycin and tetracycline in the treatment of malignant pleural effusion. *Proc Br Thorac Soc Thorax* 1985, 40:210.

17. Robinson LA, Fleming WH, Gailbraith TA: Intrapleural doxycycline control of malignant pleural effusions. *Ann Thorac Surg* 1993, 55:1115–1121.

18. Vaughn LM, Walker PB, Sahn SA: Alternatives to tetracycline pleurodesis. *Ann Pharmacol* 1992, 26:562.

19. Manson T: Treatment of malignant pleural effusion with doxycycline. *Scand J Infect Dis* 1988, 53(suppl):29–34.

20. Ruckdeschel JC, Moores D, Lee JY, *et al.*: Intrapleural therapy for malignant pleural effusions: a randomized comparison of bleomycin and tetracycline. *Chest* 1991, 100:1528–1535.

21. Ostrowski MJ: An assessment of the long-term results of controlling the reaccumulation of malignant effusions using intracavitary bleomycin. *Cancer* 1986, 57:721–727.

22. Jones GR: Treatment of recurrent malignant pleural effusion by iodized talc pleurodesis. *Thorac* 1969, 24:69–73.

23. Adler RH, Sayek I: Treatment of malignant pleural effusion: a method using tube thoracostomy and talc. *Ann Thorac Surg* 1976, 22:8–15.

24. Fentiman IS, Rubens RD, Hayward JL: A comparison of intracavitary talc and tetracycline for the control of pleural effusions secondary to breast cancer. *Eur J Cancer Clin Oncol* 1986, 22:1079–1081.

25. Yim AP, Chan AT, Lee TW, *et al.*: Thoracoscopic talc insufflation versus talc slurry for symptomatic malignant pleural effusion. *Ann Thorac Surg* 1996, 62:1655–1688.

26. Monjanel-Mouterde S, Frenay C, Catalin J, *et al.*: Pharmacokinetics of intrapleural cisplatin for the treatment of malignant pleural effusions. *Oncol Rep* 2000, 7:171–175.

27. Liu G, Crump M, Goss PE, *et al.*: Prospective comparison of the sclerosing agents doxycycline and bleomycin for the primary management of malignant pericardial effusion and cardiac tamponade. *J Clin Oncol* 1996, 14:3141–3147.

28. Little AG, Kremser PC, Wade JI, *et al.*: Operation for diagnosis and treatment of pericardial effusions. *Surgery* 1984, 96:738.

29. Appelqvist P, Maamies T, Grohn P: Emergency pericardiotomy as primary diagnostic and therapeutic procedure in malignant pericardial tamponade: report of three cases and review of the literature. *J Surg Oncol* 1982, 21:18.

30. Wong B, Murphy J, Chang CJ, *et al.*: The risk of pericardiocentesis. *Am J Cardiol* 1979, 44:1110.

31. Gatenby RA, Hertz WH, Kessler HB: Percutaneous catheter drainage for malignant pericardial effusion. *J Vasc Interv Radiol* 1991, 2:151.

32. Millaire A, Wurtz A, deGroote P, *et al.*: Malignant pericardial effusions: usefulness of pericardioscopy. *Am Heart J* 1992, 124:1030.

33. Ziskind AA, Pearce AC, Lemon CC, *et al.*: Percutaneous balloon pericardiotomy for the treatment of cardiac tamponade and large pericardial effusions: description of the technique and report of the first 50 cases. *J Am Coll Cardiol* 1993, 21:1–5.

34. Anguera I, Pare C, Perez-Villa F: Severe right ventricular dysfunction following pericardiocentesis for cardiac tamponade. *Int J Cardiol* 1997, 59:212–214.

MALIGNANT PLEURAL EFFUSIONS

Malignant pleural effusions are a common consequence of advanced solid tumors that lead to significant morbidity and mortality. They can be diagnosed and treated readily. Treatment depends on the condition of the patient and the potential responsiveness of the underlying cancer to systemic chemotherapy.

MANAGEMENT OR INTERVENTION

1. If responsive tumor, treat systemically.
2. If an unresponsive tumor, drain through tube thoracostomy, then ensure complete lung expansion, instill bleomycin 60 U, or talc 4–5 g, or tetracycline substitute 1–1.5 g. Consider drainage with a small-bore catheter in patients with good performance status.

CAUSATIVE AGENTS

Tumor in the pleural space or tumor extensively involving mediastinal lymph drainage

PATHOLOGIC PROCESS

Excessive production of exudative fluid with reduced clearance due to blocked mediastinal lymphatics; radiation fibrosis may exacerbate

DIFFERENTIAL DIAGNOSIS

Infection, including tuberculosis, mesothelioma, congestive heart failure, parapneumonic effusion, lymphatic obstruction, and rheumatologic disorders

PATIENT ASSESSMENT

History and physical examination thoracentesis: cytology; LDH and protein

MALIGNANT PERICARDIAL EFFUSIONS

Malignant pericardial effusions are less common and cause symptoms by reducing cardiac output. They are much more sensitive to speed of onset. Treatment depends on adequate drainage of pericardial space.

MANAGEMENT OR INTERVENTION

Drain pericardial space
Pericardiocentesis with sclerosis (bleomycin) if poorer prognosis
Subxiphoid pericardiotomy
Video-assisted pericardioscopy
Balloon pericardiotomy
Pericardiectomy if large tumor cake and otherwise better prognosis

CAUSATIVE FACTORS

Tumor in the pericardial space or tumor obstructing mediastinal lymph nodes

PATHOLOGIC PROCESS

Excessive fluid production in pericardial space with reduced clearance due to blocked mediastinal lymphatics; radiation fibrosis may exacerbate

DIFFERENTIAL DIAGNOSIS

Infection (especially viral), cardiomyopathy, recent myocardial infarction, rheumatologic disorders, and congestive heart failure

PATIENT ASSESSMENT

History and physical examination: pulsus paradoxus, Kussmaul's sign, echocardiogram

Despite the sophisticated diagnostic tools available to establish the diagnosis of human neoplasia, oncologists frequently are asked to evaluate and treat a subset of patients with metastatic cancer in whom detailed investigations fail to identify a primary anatomic site. The reported prevalence of unknown primary carcinoma (UPC) varies with the practice setting and the definition used from 0.5% to 9% of all patients who are diagnosed with cancer [1,2]. Because identification of the primary has formed the basis for predicting the expected behavior and assigning appropriate therapy of malignant diseases, the absence of a primary poses a major challenge. The inability to identify a primary generates anxiety for the patient, who may believe that the physician's evaluation has been inadequate or that the prognosis would be improved if a primary could be established.

As suggested by the aforementioned prevalence statistics, the definition of UPC has not been standardized, varying in published reports primarily with regard to the extent of evaluation required to accept this diagnosis. A recent definition includes patients with UPC as those who have a biopsy-proven malignancy for which the anatomic origin remains unidentified after history and physical examination, including breast palpation and pelvic examination in women and testicular and prostate examination in men; laboratory studies, including liver and renal function tests; hemogram; chest radiograph; computed tomography of abdomen and pelvis; and mammography in women. Only positive findings on this initial evaluation are then investigated in detail [3,4]. Depending on the clinical situation, additional studies might include sputum cytology, computed tomography of the chest, breast ultrasonography, or gastrointestinal endoscopy.

In practice, however, considerable controversy surrounds the evaluation of patients with UPC. It is clear that despite understanding their limitations, unnecessary studies are often carried out because treatment planning is based on both the anatomic origin and the histologic type of the malignancy. The arguments for an exhaustive versus directed evaluation of patients with UPC have been outlined by many authors [5–15]. The most effective strategy takes into account the projected natural history and duration of survival and provides a reasonable probability of locating the primary anatomic site without compromising quality of life with difficult and time-consuming diagnostic studies. The overall goal is to identify the treatable patient subsets or occult primaries through a rapid, rational, calculated approach.

Several recent studies have evaluated whether 2[^{18}Fl] fluoro-2-deoxy-D-glucose (FDG) positron emission tomography (PET) contributes to the diagnostic evaluation of UPC. The question is whether PET scanning would result in a more efficient, less costly, and potentially less invasive work-up that would increase the likelihood of identifying the primary tumor or tumors in a timely manner. The series were small (15 to 53 patients) and focused primarily on patients with cervical or supraclavicular lymphadenopathy. Because patients with metastatic lymph nodes in these regions often are treated empirically with extensive radiotherapy for a primary head and neck tumor, or conversely may be eligible for radical neck resection, this subset in particular may benefit from additional testing to identify the primary.

In general, PET was able to consistently visualize known metastatic lesions, and demonstrated true positive primary tumor identification rates of 45% [16], 37.8% [17], and 47% [18]. False-positive rates were as high as 20%. Another study of 13 patients showed no improved rate of identification of squamous carcinomas of the neck compared with panendoscopy [19]. There is great variability in tissue-specific tracer uptake rates as well as interpatient glucose metabolism, which may contribute to test variability. Further, although PET is a promising diagnostic modality, it is not clear whether identification of the primary and, thus, potentially more directed therapy, will lead to improved survival in patients with UPC.

BIOLOGIC ASPECTS

Patients with UPC are heterogeneous and composed of numerous underlying primary cancers that remain occult during observation of the patient. Many different primary cancers can remain occult during observation of the patient. This concept is supported by studies showing that a detailed postmortem anatomic investigation frequently establishes a primary in patients [5,20]. Detailed clinical and biochemical study of UPC cells, although heterogeneous in their origins, may represent a valuable resource for understanding fundamental aspects of the metastatic phenotype [21–24]. As is the case for the specific well-defined primary neoplasms discussed elsewhere in this book, it is the phenomenon of metastasis, as purely exemplified by the patient with UPC, that causes the majority of cancer deaths.

The fact that numerous occult anatomic sites can give rise to carcinomas that present with only metastatic disease supports the possibility that specific interactions of genetic and environmental insults could give rise to genomic and biochemical changes that lead to the early development of the metastatic phenotype without the associated changes supporting local growth in the organ of origin [25]. Although this concept must be considered highly speculative, it is an hypothesis that can be tested through analysis of available biomarkers, such as oncogenes and tumor suppressor genes, which have been characterized for cancers with known anatomic origins, such as lung, pancreatic breast, and colorectal carcinomas. Either the absence of genetic changes typical for malignancies with established primaries or the presence of unusual variants of known genetic alterations support this hypothesis.

Whether the biology of UPC is fundamentally different from known primary carcinoma with systemic metastases remains controversial. Nystrom et al. [26] have argued that the distribution of metastatic sites in patients with UPC in which the primary subsequently is found is sufficiently different from known primary carcinoma to support the hypothesis that UPC is biologically unique. A preliminary analysis of a consecutive series of UPC patients shows that there are no significant differences in the patterns of metastases [27], although overall survival for UPC patients was inferior to patients in whom the primary was found [4]. Continued study of UPC patients is necessary to resolve this controversy.

The reason the primary organ site cannot be diagnosed remains unknown. Previous investigators have speculated that the tumor may remain below the limits of clinical or radiographic detection or that it spontaneously regressed [25]. Another possibility is that a clinically detectable primary never develops because of the development of specific genetic changes that support metastatic over local growth.

PATHOLOGY

An early, accurate pathologic assessment of biopsy material is essential in the initial evaluation of the patient with suspected UPC. In this context, the pathologist usually is able to confirm that the lesion is neoplastic and may be able to judge if the lesion is primary or metastatic. In some situations, however, it may be impossible to determine if the tumor has arisen from the biopsied organ site. This problem often complicates the cytologic evaluation of fine-needle aspirate specimens and emphasizes the need for close communication between the clinician and the pathologist.

The initial pathologic assessment of the biopsied material usually is initiated by light microscopic examination of paraffin sections stained with hematoxylin and eosin. Based on established cytologic criteria [28], the pathologist usually can place the tumor into broad groups, such as carcinoma, sarcoma, or lymphoma. Additionally, many carcinomas are immediately recognized as manifesting at least some glandular differentiation (adenocarcinoma). When glandular differentiation is absent, patients with UPC frequently are diagnosed with poorly differentiated carcinoma or undifferentiated carcinoma. Other specimens lack any cytologically distinguishing features, in which case a diagnosis of an undifferentiated malignancy is reported. In these groups with poorly differentiated carcinoma, undifferentiated carcinoma, or undifferentiated malignancy, additional pathologic studies, including histochemistry, immunohistochemistry, and electron microscopy, are employed most frequently and productively. A vast array of tissue markers is available; however, in practice, regular use is limited to a few [29]. Emphasis should be placed on the identification of patients with lymphoma because these neoplasms are curable with therapy. Increasingly, pathologists are using cytokeratin immunohistochemical stains to distinguish between neoplasms of epithelial origin as discussed in detail by Lagendijk *et al.* [30].

Because special studies usually are not performed routinely unless there is a reasonable suspicion that they will be contributory, direct discussions between the pathologist and clinician are critical to ensure the most focused pathologic characterization possible. Random use of large numbers of tissue markers are rarely helpful for establishing a diagnosis or planning therapy.

CLINICAL CHARACTERISTICS AND NATURAL HISTORY

The clinical presentations of UPC are extremely varied. Historically, patients have been characterized as to whether they have disease above or below the diaphragm [31]. Given the heterogeneity and widespread metastases that characterize this disease, however, this arbitrary division is of doubtful value. Other investigators have begun to subclassify patients based largely on clinicopathologic criteria of histology, involved organ sites, and responsiveness to therapy. This approach has led to the definition of well-characterized patient subsets, which are discussed subsequently. Despite these efforts at subclassification, the majority of patients present with solitary or multiple areas of involvement in a variety of visceral sites. In most cases, the presenting symptoms and physical signs simply reflect the neoplastic involvement of these organ sites.

The demographics of the UPC patient population mirror those of the general population of patients referred to a large cancer center,

Table 22-1. Major Sites of Tumor Involvement and Histologic Diagnoses Identified in 1196 Patients With Unknown Primary Carcinoma

	Patients, *n*	%
Histologic diagnosis		
Adenocarcinoma	706	59.0
Carcinoma	335	28.0
Squamous carcinoma	75	6.3
Neuroendrocrine carcinoma	54	4.5
Unknown/other*	26	2.2
Major metastatic sites		
Lymph nodes	519	43.4
Liver	404	33.8
Bone	334	27.9
Lung	315	26.3
Pleura and pleural space	129	10.8
Peritoneum	118	9.9
Brain	84	7.0
Adrenal	71	5.9
Skin	41	3.4

*Includes malignant neoplasm, 5; and unknown, 21.
Adapted from Abbruzzese et al. [2].

Table 22-2. Univariate and Multivariate Survival Analyses

Univariate Survival Analysis

Variable	Grouping	*P**	Effect on Survival
Age, y	20–39, 40–49, 50–59, 60–69, 70+	0.43	None
Sex	Male, female	0.0018	Decreased survival for men
Race	White, other	0.86	None
Organ sites, *n*	1, 2, 3+	0.0018	Decreased survival with more organ sites
Involved organ sites			
Lung	—	0.0014	Deleterious
Bone	—	0.0005	Deleterious
Liver	—	0.0050	Deleterious
Pleura	—	0.0019	Deleterious
Brain	—	0.014	Deleterious
Lymph nodes	—	<0.0001	Advantageous
Axillary	—	0.0003	Advantageous
Supraclavicular	—	0.44	None
Peritoneum	—	0.59	None
Skin	—	0.69	None
Histology			
Adenocarcinoma	—	<0.0001	Deleterious
Carcinoma	—	0.0058	Advantageous
Squamous carcinoma	—	0.058	Advantageous
Neuroendocrine	—	0.0009	Advantageous

Multivariate Survival Analysis

Variable	Relative Risk†	*P**	Effect on Survival
Male sex	1.39	0.0007	Deleterious
Increasing no. of organ sites	1.23	<0.0001	Deleterious
Involved organ sites			
Liver	1.33	0.0064	Deleterious
Lymph nodes	0.46	<0.0001	Advantageous
Supraclavicular	1.56	0.013	Deleterious
Peritoneum	0.59	0.0099	Advantageous
Histology			
Adenocarcinoma	1.46	0.0001	Deleterious
Neuroendocrine carcinoma	0.30	0.0005	Advantageous

*Log-rank test.
†Calculated from the Cox proportional hazards regression.
Adapted from Abbruzzese et al. [2].

except for an excess of men among the UPC patients [2]. The median age is approximately 60 years. The family history frequently identifies additional cancers with established origins in other family members; however, no clearly familial instances of UPC have been reported. Table 22-1 shows the distribution of metastatic sites and histologic classification of 1196 UPC patients from one series. These data have remained unchanged as compared with the original series reported in 1994 [2].

The clinical features outlined have been analyzed to determine their effect on survival. There are considerable differences in survival for the four most frequently encountered pathologic subtypes of UPC. The median survival for patients with squamous carcinoma (exclusive of patients with mid-high cervical adenopathy) was 13 months; adenocarcinoma, 6 months; carcinoma 11 months; and neuroendocrine carcinoma, 27 months. The state of differentiation or mucin production does not significantly influence the poor survival of patients with adenocarcinoma. The influence of other clinicopathologic features of UPC on survival has been assessed using univariate and multivariate analyses. These data are summarized in Table 22-2. Other studies have documented similar results [32].

THERAPEUTIC APPROACH AND RESPONSE TO THERAPY

Unknown primary carcinomas are a heterogeneous group of tumors with widely varying natural histories; therefore, in discussing treatment and survival, it is imperative to understand the patient population studied. When all patients are considered, UPC is a highly aggressive neoplasm with an overall median survival of 3 to 4 months in older series [6,26]. Most recent studies have documented median survivals of 9 to 12 months [33–35]. In a series of 657 consecutive patients, the median survival was 11 months [2], and this number has remained consistent in the expanded series of 1196 patients.

The treatment of UPC continues to evolve. Although the majority of patients are treated with systemic chemotherapy, the careful integration of surgery, radiation therapy, and even periods of observation is important in the overall management of these patients [12]. Observation is particularly important for patients with single sites of disease that have received adequate local therapy.

The most common problem is treatment of the patient with progressive metastatic carcinoma or adenocarcinoma involving two or more organ sites [36–60]. Table 22-3 outlines the results from five trials. Recently, Hainsworth et al. [61] reported that a combination of carboplatin, paclitaxel, and etoposide was effective for some patients with UPC. Use of a chemosensitivity assay may help guide the selection of the optimal combination [62]. Treatment of these patients remains suboptimal and awaits discovery of novel strategies applicable to other highly resistant adenocarcinomas, such as those originating in the lung or gastrointestinal tract. This situation is contrasted with the management of the favorable subsets described. These patients have been grouped together primarily on the basis of their responsiveness to therapy or favorable natural histories. The number of patients who fall into these groups is small; however, they are important to recognize because specific treatment may significantly extend survival.

Table 22-3. Selected Chemotherapeutic Trials in Unknown Primary Carcinoma

Author	Histology	Regimen	Patients, n	Response, %	Median Survival, mo
Pasterz et al. [32]	Adenocarcinoma and undifferentiated carcinoma	5-FU/adria/cytoxan/cisplatin	44	28	NS
Greco et al. [33]	Poorly differentiated carcinoma and adenocarcinoma	CDDP/vinblastine bleo ± doxorubicin	68	56 (22% CR)	18*
Moertel et al. [36]	Adenocarcinoma	5-FU	88	16	NS
Woods et al. [39]	Adenocarcinoma and undifferentiated carcinoma	Adria/mito-C	25	36	4.5
Raber et al. [46]	Adenocarcinoma and undifferentiated carcinoma	CDDP/VP-16/5-FU	36	22	NS
Lenzi et al. [48]	Adenocarcinoma and poorly differentiated carcinoma	CDDP/5-FU/folinic acid	31	30	18
Hainsworth et al. [49]	Poorly differentiated carcinoma	CDDP/etoposide	32	60 (32% CR)	NS
Hainsworth et al. [61]	Adenocarcinoma and poorly differentiated carcinoma and adenocarcinoma	Paclitaxel/carboplatin/etoposide	55	47	13.4
Greco et al. [92]	PDA, PDC neuroend SSC	Docetaxel + cisplatin or carboplatin	26 / 47	26 / 22	8 / 12
Culine et al. [93]	WDA, PDC, PDA, Pdneu	HD AC, EP PBSC support	60	42 / 39	11
Briasoulis et al. [94]	PDC, PDA, well/mod DA	Carbo, EP Epirubicin	62	37%	8 [visceral] † 10 [nodal]
Briasoulis et al. [95]	PDA, PDC	Carbo Paclitaxel	77	47.8 / 68.4 / 15.1	13 / 15 / 10

*Calculated from data presented.
†This study provided response rates and survival data for two patient groups: those with 1) predominantly nodal disease or midline involvement, and 2) predominantly splanchnic involvement.
NS—not stated; PDA—poorly differentiated adenocarcinoma; PDC—poorly differentiated carcinoma; Pdneu—poorly differentiated neuroendocrine carcinoma; SSC—small cell carcinoma; WDA—well-differentiated adenocarcinoma.

REFERENCES

1. Greco FA, Hainsworth JD: Cancer of unknown primary site. In *Cancer: Principles and Practice of Oncology*, edn 4. Edited by De Vita VT Jr, Hellman S, Rosenberg SA. Philadelphia: JB Lippincott, 1993:2072–2092.

2. Abbruzzese JL, Abbruzzese MC, Hess KR, *et al.*: Unknown primary carcinoma: natural history and prognostic factors in 657 consecutive patients. *J Clin Oncol* 1994, 12:1272–1280.

3. Abbruzzese JL: An effective strategy for the evaluation of unknown primary tumors. *Cancer Bull* 1989, 41:157.

4. Abbruzzese JL, Abbruzzese MC, Lenzi R, *et al.*: Analysis of a diagnostic strategy for patients with suspected tumors of unknown origin. *J Clin Oncol* 1995, 13:2094–2103.

5. Nystrom JB, Weiner JM, Wolf RM, *et al.*: Identifying the primary site in metastatic cancer of unknown origin: inadequacy of roentgenographic procedures. *JAMA* 1979, 241:381.

6. Newman KH, Nystrom JS: Metastatic cancer of unknown origin: non-squamous cell type. *Semin Oncol* 1982, 9:427.

7. Stewart JF, Tattersall MHN, Woods RL, *et al.*: Unknown primary adenocarcinoma: incidence of over investigation and natural history. *Br Med J* 1979, 1:1530.

8. Karsell PR, Sheedy PF II, O'Connell MJ: Computed tomography in search of cancer of unknown origin. *JAMA* 1982, 248:340–343.

9. Didolkar MS, Fanous N, Elias EG, *et al.*: Metastatic carcinoma from occult primary tumors: a study of 254 patients. *Ann Surg* 1977, 186:625.

10. McMillan JH, Levine E, Stephens RH: Computed tomography in the evaluation of metastatic adenocarcinoma from an unknown primary site. *Radiology* 1982, 143:143–146.

11. Walsh JW, Rosenfield AT, Jaffe CC, *et al.*: Prospective comparison of ultrasound and computed tomography in the evaluation of gynecologic pelvic masses. *AJR Am J Roentgenol* 1978, 131:955–960.

12. Raber MN, Abbruzzese JL, Frost P: Unknown primary tumors. *Curr Opin Oncol* 1992, 4:3.

13. Shahangian S, Fritsche HA: Serum tumor markers as diagnostic aids in patients with unknown primary tumors. *Cancer Bull* 1989, 41:152.

14. Koch M, McPherson TA: Carcinoembryonic antigen levels as an indicator of the primary site in metastatic disease of unknown origin. *Cancer* 1981, 48:1242.

15. Abbruzzese J, Raber M, Frost P: The role of CA-125 in patients with unknown primary tumors. *Proc Am Soc Clin Oncol* 1990, 9:118.

16. Lassen U, *et al.*:18F-FDG whole body positron emission tomography (PET) in patients with unknown primary tumors (UPT). *Eur J Cancer* 1999, 35:1076—1082.

17. Bohuslavizki KH, Klutmann S, Kroger S, *et al.*: FDG PET detection of unknown primary tumors. *J Nucl Med* 2000, 41:816–822.

18. Os AA, *et al.*: Metastatic head and neck cancer: role and usefulness of FDG PET in locating occult primary tumors. *Radiology* 1999, 210:177–181.

19. Greven KM, Keyes JW, Jr, Williams DW III, *et al.*: Occult primary tumors of the head and neck: lack of benefit from positron emission tomography imaging with 2-[F-18]fluoro-2-deoxy-D-glucose. *Cancer* 1999, 86:114–118.

20. Le Cesne A, Le Chevalier T, Caille P, *et al.*: Metastases from cancers of unknown primary site: data from 302 autopsies. *Pesse Med* 1991, 20:1369–1373.

21. Motzer RJ, Rodriguez E, Reuter VE, *et al.*: Genetic analysis of an aid in diagnostic for patients with midline carcinomas of uncertain histologies. *J Natl Cancer Inst* 1991, 83:341.

22. Ilson DH, Motzer RJ, Rodriguez F, *et al.*: Genetic analysis in the diagnosis of neoplasms of unknown primary site. *Semin Oncol* 1992, 20:229–237.

23. Motzer RJ, Rodriguez E, Reuter VE, *et al.*: Molecular and cytogenetic studies in the diagnosis of patients with poorly differentiated carcinomas of unknown primary site. *J Clin Oncol* 1995, 13:274–182.

24. Bar-Eli M, Abbruzzese JL, Lee-Jackson D, *et al.*: p53 Mutation spectrum in human unknown primary tumors. *Anticancer Res* 1993, 13:1619–1624.

25. Frost P, Raber M, Abbruzzese J: Unknown primary tumors—are they a unique subgroup of neoplastic disease? *Cancer Bull* 1987, 39:216.

26. Nystrom JS, Weiner JM, Heffelfinger-Juttner J, Irwin LE: Metastatic and histologic presentations in unknown primary cancer. *Semin Oncol* 1977, 4:53.

27. Abbruzzese JL, Raber MN: Unknown primary carcinoma. In *Clinical Oncology*. Edited by Abeloff MD, Armitage JO, Lichter AS, Niederhuber JE. New York: Churchill Livingstone; 1995, 1822–1845.

28. Mackay B, Ordoñez NG: The role of the pathologist in the evaluation of poorly differentiated tumors and metastatic tumors of unknown origin. In *Poorly Differentiated Neoplasms and Tumors of Unknown Origin*. Edited by Fer MF, Greco AF, Oldham RK. Orlando; Grune & Stratton, 1986:3.

29. Hainsworth JD, Wright EP, Johnson DH, Davis BW, Greco FA: Poorly differentiated carcinoma of unknown primary site: clinical usefulness of immunoperoxidase staining. *J Clin Oncol* 1991, 9:1931–1938.

30. Lagendijk JH, Mullink H, Van Diest PJ, *et al.*:Tracing the origin of adenocarcinomas with unknown primary using immunohistochemistry: differential diagnosis between colonic and ovarian carcinomas as primary sites. *Hum Pathol* 1998, 29:491–497.

31. Ultmann JE, Phillips TL: Cancer of unknown primary site. In *Cancer: Principles and Practice of Oncology*. Edited by DeVita VT Jr, Hellman S, Rosenberg SA. Philadelphia: JB Lippincott, 1989: 1941–1950.

32. Pasterz R, Savaraj N, Burgess M: Prognostic factors in metastatic carcinoma of unknown primary. *J Clin Oncol* 1986, 4:1652.

33. Greco FA, Vaughn WK, Hainsworth JD: Advanced poorly differentiated carcinoma of unknown primary site: recognition of a treatable syndrome. *Ann Intern Med* 1986, 104:547.

34. Sporn JR, Greenberg BR: Empiric chemotherapy in patients with carcinoma of unknown primary site. *Am J Med* 1990, 88:49.

35. Kambhu SA, Kelsen D, Fiore J, Niedzwiecki D, *et al.*: Metastatic adenocarcinomas of unknown primary site. *Am J Clin Oncol* 1990, 13:55.

36. Moertel CG, Reitmeier RJ, Schutt AJ, *et al.*: Treatment of patient with adenocarcinomas of unknown origin. *Cancer* 1972, 30:1469.

37. McKeen E, Smith F, *et al.*: Fluorouracil (F), Adriamycin (A), and mitomycin (M), FAM for adenocarcinoma of unknown origin. *Proc AACR ASCO* 1980, 21:358.

38. Rodnick S, Tremont S, *et al.*: Evaluation and therapy for adenocarcinoma of unknown primary (ACUP), *Proc AACR ASCO* 1981, 22:379.

39. Woods RL, Fox RM, *et al.*: Metastatic adenocarcinomas of unknown primary site. *N Engl J Med* 1980, 303:87–89.

40. Valentine J, Rosenthal S, *et al.*: Combination chemotherapy for adenocarcinoma of unknown primary origin. *Cancer Clin Trials* 1979, 2:265–268.

41. Bedikian AY, Bodley GP, *et al.*: Sequential chemotherapy for adenocarcinoma of unknown primary. *Am J Clin Oncol* 1983, 6:219–224.

42. Goldberg R, Smith F, Veno W, Ahlgren J, Schein P: Treatment of adenocarcinoma of unknown primary with fluorouracil, adriamycin, and mitomycin-C (FAM). *Am Soc Clin Oncol* 1986, 5:129.

43. Walach N: Treatment of adenocarcinoma of unknown origin with cyclophoshamide (C), Oncogin (O), Methotrexte (M), and 5-fluorouracil (F), (COMF). *Proc Am Soc Clin Oncol* 1986, 5:125.

44. Shildt RA, Kennedy PS, Chen TT, *et al.*: Management of patients with metastatic adenocarcinoma of unknown origin: a Southwest Oncology Group study. *Cancer Treat Rep* 1983, 67:77–79.

45. Anderson H, Thatcher N, Rankin E, *et al.*: VAC (Vincristine, Adriamycin, Cyclophosphamide) chemotherapy for metastatic carcinoma from an unknown site. *Eur J Cancer Clin Oncol* 1983, 19:49–52.

46. Raber MN, Faintuch J, Abbruzzese JL, *et al.*: Continuous infusion 5-fluorouracil, etoposide and cis-diamminedichloroplatinum in patients with metastatic carcinoma of unknown primary origin. *Ann Oncol* 1991, 2:519.

47. LeChevalier T, Tremblay J, Rouesse J; *et al.*: Phase II trial of methotrexate-FAM in adenocarcinoma of unknown primary. *Proc ASCO* 1987, 6:130.

48. Lenzi R, Raber MN, Frost P, Schmidt S, Abbruzzese JL: Phase II study of cisplatin, 5FU, and folinic acid in patients with tumors of unknown primary origin. *Eur J Cancer* 1993, 29A:1634.

49. Hainsworth JD, Johnson DH, Greco FA: The role of etoposide in the treatment of poorly differentiated carcinoma of unknown primary site. *Cancer* 1991, 67:310.

50. Lenzi R, Raber MN, Gravel D, Frost P, Abbruzzese JL: Phase I and II trials of a laboratory derived synergistic combination of cisplatin and 2'-deoxy-5-azacytidine. *Int J Oncol* 1995, 6:447–450.

51. Kelsen D, Martin DS, Coloriore J, *et al.*: A Phase II trial of biochemical modulation using *N*-phosphonacetyl-L-aspartate, high-dose methotrexate, high-dose 5-flourouracil, and leucovorin in patients with adenocarcinoma of unknown primary site. *Cancer* 1992, 70:1988.

52. Gill I, Guaglianone P, Gruneberg SM, *et al.*: High dose intensity of cisplatin and etoposide in adenocarcinoma of unknown primary. *Anticancer Res* 1991, 11:1231–1235.

53. Porta C, Moroni M, Nastasi G, *et al.*: COMF combination chemotherapy for the treatment of adenocarcinoma of unknown primary origin. *Ann Oncol* 1992, 3(suppl):48.

54. Trudeau M, Thirlwell MP, Boos G, *et al.*: Cancer of unknown primary syndrome (CUPS): Predictive value of CA-125 in patients treated with 5-fluorouracil, doxorubicin and cisplatin (FAP) [abstract]. *Proc Am Soc Clin Oncol* 1993, 12:399.

55. Ahlgren JD, Bern M, Booth B, *et al.*: Protracted infusional 5FU (PIF): An active, well-tolerated regimen in metastatic adenocarcinoma of undetermined primary (AUP): a mid-Atlantic oncology program (MOAP) study [abstract]. *Proc Am Soc Clin Oncol* 1993, 12:401.

56. Colleoni M, Buzzoni R, Bajetta E: Fluorouracil plus folinic acid in metastatic adenocarcinoma of unknown primary site suggestive or a gastrointestinal primary. *Tumori* 1993, 79:116–118.

57. van der Gaast A, Henzen-Logmans SC, Planting AS, *et al.*: Phase II study of oral administration of etoposide for patients with well- and moderately-differentiated adenocarcinomas of unknown primary site. *Ann Oncol* 1993, 4:789–790.

58. de Campos ES, Menasce LP, Radford J, *et al.*: Metastatic carcinoma of uncertain primary site: a retrospective review of 57 patients treated with vincristine, doxorubicin, cyclophosphamide (VAC) or VAC alternating with cisplatin and etoposide (VAC/PE). *Cancer* 1994, 73:470–475.

59. Akerley W, Thomas A, Miller M, *et al.*: Phase II trial of oral etoposide for carcinoma of unknown primary (CUP) [abstract]. *Proc Am Soc Clin Oncol* 1994, 13:406.

60. Merrouche Y, Lasset C, Trillet-Lenoir V, *et al.*: Phase II study of cisplatin and etoposide in a subgroup of patients with carcinoma of unknown primary [abstract]. *Proc Am Soc Clin Oncol* 1994, 13:401.

61. Hainsworth JD, Erland JB, Kalman LA, *et al.*: Carcinoma of unknown primary site: treatment with 1-hour paclitaxel, carboplatin, and extended-schedule etoposide. *J Clin Oncol* 1997, 15:2385–2393.

62. Hanauske AR, Clark GM, Von Hoff DD: Adenocarcinoma of unknown primary: retrospective analysis of chemosensitivity of 313 freshly explanted tumors in a tumor cloning system. *Invest New Drugs* 1995, 13:43–49.

63. Jesse RH, Perez CA, Fletcher GH: Cervical lymph node metastases: unknown primary cancer. *Cancer* 1973, 31:854.

64. Wang RC, Geopfert H, Barber AE, Wolf P: Unknown primary squamous cell carcinoma metastatic to the neck. *Arch Otolaryngol Head Neck Surg* 1990, 116:1388.

65. Weir L, Keane T, Cummings B, *et al.*: Radiation treatment of cervical lymph node metastases from an unknown primary: an analysis of outcome by treatment volume and other prognostic factors. *Radiother Oncol* 1995, 35:206–211.

66. Marcial-Vega VA, Cardenes H, Perez CA, *et al.*: Cervical metastases from unknown primaries: radiotherapeutic management and appearance of subsequent primaries. *Int J Radiat Oncol Biol Phys* 1990, 19:919.

67. Carlson LS, Fletcher GH, Oswald MJ: Guidelines for the radiotherapeutic techniques for cervical metastases from an unknown primary. *Int J Radiat Oncol Biol Phys* 1986, 12:2101.

68. Talmi YP, Wolf GT, Hazuka M, *et al.*: Unknown primary of the head and neck. *J Laryngol Otol* 1996, 110:353–356.

69. De Braud F, Heilbrun LK, Ahmed K, *et al.*: Metastatic squamous cell carcinoma of an unknown primary localized to the neck: advantages of an aggressive treatment. *Cancer* 1989, 64:510.

70. Lee NK, Byers RM, Abbruzzese JL, Wolf P: Metastatic adenocarcinoma to the neck from an unknown primary. *Am J Surg* 1991, 162:306.

71. Patel J, Nemoto T, Rosner D, *et al.*: Axillary lymph node metastasis from an occult breast cancer. *Cancer* 1981, 47:2923.

72. Ashikari R, Rosen PP, Urban JA, Senoo T: Breast cancer presenting as an axillary mass. *Ann Surg* 1976, 183:415.

73. Henry-Tillman RS, Harms SE, Westbrook KC, *et al.*: Role of breast magnetic resonance imaging in determining breast as a source of unknown metastatic lymphadenopathy. *Am J Surg* 1999, 178:496–500.

74. Ellerbrook N, Holmes F, Singletary E, Evans H, *et al.*: Treatment of patients with isolated axillary nodal metastases from an occult primary carcinoma consistent with breast origin. *Cancer* 1990, 66:1461.

75. Jackson B, Scott-Conner C, Moulder J: Axillary metastasis from occult breast carcinoma: diagnosis and management. *Am Surg* 1995, 61:431–434.

76. Rosen PP: Axillary lymph node metastases in patients with occult noninvasive breast carcinoma. *Cancer* 1980, 46:1298.

77. August CA, Murad TM, Newton M: Multiple focal extraovarian serous carcinoma. *Int J Gynaecol Pathol* 1985, 4:11.

78. Dalrymple JC, Bannatyne P, Russell P, *et al.*: Extraovarian peritoneal serous papillary carcinoma: a clinicopathologic study of 31 cases. *Cancer* 1989, 64:110.

79. Strnad CM, Grosh WN, Baxter J, *et al.*: Peritoneal carcinomatosis of unknown primary site in women. *Ann Intern Med* 1989, 111:213.

80. Ransom DT, Patel SR, Keeney GL, *et al.*: Papillary serous carcinoma of the peritoneum: a review of 33 cases treated with platin-based chemotherapy. *Cancer* 1990, 66:1091.

81. Lenzi R, Hess KR, Abbruzzese MC, *et al.*: Poorly differentiated carcinoma and poorly differentiated adenocarcinoma of unknown origin: favorable subsets of patients with unknown primary carcinoma? *J Clin Oncol* 1997, 15:2056–2066.

82. Farrugia DC, Norman AR, Nicolson MC, *et al.*: Unknown primary carcinoma: randomised studies are needed to identify optimal treatments and their benefits. *Eur J Cancer* 1996, 32A:2256–2261.

83. van der Gaast A, Verweij J, Henzen-Logmans SC, Rodenburg CJ, *et al.*: Carcinoma of unknown primary: identification of a treatable subset? *Ann Oncol* 1990, 1:119.

84. Jones A, Farrow G, Richardson FL: The extragonadal germ cell cancer syndrome: the Mayo Clinic experience. *Poorly Differentiated Neoplasms and Tumors of Unknown Origin.* Edited by Fer MF, Greco FA, Oldham RK. Orlando: Grune & Stratton, 1986:203.

85. Richardson RL, Shoumacher RA, Fer MF, *et al.*: The unrecognized extragonadal germ cell cancer syndrome. *Ann Intern Med* 1981, 94:181.

86. Fox RM, Woods RL, Tattersall MHN: Undifferentiated carcinoma in young men: the atypical teratoma syndrome. *Lancet* 1979, 1:1316.

81. Currow DC, Findlay M, Cox K, *et al.*: Elevated germ cell markers in carcinoma of uncertain primary site do not predict response to platinum based chemotherapy. *Eur J Cancer* 1996, 32A:2357–2359.

88. Hainsworth JD, Johnson DH, Greco FA: Cisplatin-based combination chemotherapy in the treatment of poorly differentiated carcinoma and poorly differentiated adenocarcinoma of unknown primary site: results of a 12-year experience. *J Clin Oncol* 1992, 10:912–922.

89. Hainsworth JD, Johnson DH, Greco FA: Poorly differentiated neuroendocrine carcinoma of unknown primary site. A newly recognized clinicopathologic entity. *Ann Intern Med* 1988, 109:364–371.

90. Moertel CG, Kvols LK, O'Connell MJ, Rubin J: Treatment of neuroendocrine carcinomas with combined etoposide and cisplatin: evidence of major therapeutic acitivty in the anaplastic variants of these neoplasms. *Cancer* 1991, 68:227.

91. Hess K, Abbruzzese MC, Lenzi R, *et al.*: Classification and regression tree analysis of 1000 consecutive patients with unknown primary carcinoma [abstract]. *Proc Am Soc Clin Oncol* 1996, 15:452.

92. Greco FA, *et al.*: Carcinoma of unknown primary site: phase II trials with docetaxel plus cisplatin or carboplatin. *Ann Oncol* 2000, 11:211–215.

93. Culine S, Fabbro M, Ychou M, *et al.*: Chemotherapy in carcinomas of unknown primary site: a high-dose intensity policy. *Ann Oncol* 1999, 10:569–575.

94. Briasoulis E, Tsavaris N, Fountzilas G, *et al.*: Combination regimen with carboplatin, epirubicin and etoposide in metastatic carcinomas of unknown primary site: A Hellenic Co-Operative Oncology Group Phase II study. *Oncology* 1998, 55:426–430.

95. Briasoulis E, Kalofonos H, Bafaloukos D, *et al.*: Carboplatin plus paclitaxel in unknown primary carcinoma: a phase II Hellenic Cooperative Oncology Group Study. *J Clin Oncol* 2000, 18:3101–3107.

SQUAMOUS CARCINOMA INVOLVING MID-HIGH CERVICAL LYMPH NODES

High cervical adenopathy with squamous carcinoma is an important clinical subset because of its well-defined natural history and responsiveness to therapy [63–66]. With appropriate evaluation, including direct visualization of the hypopharynx, nasopharynx, larynx, and upper esophagus, an occult primary lesion will be frequently identified. When no primary is found, aggressive local therapy is applied to the involved neck [65–67]. Thirty percent to 50% of 5-year survivals have been reported with radical neck surgery, high-dose radiotherapy, or a combination of both modalities. A potential advantage of radiation therapy is that the suspected primary anatomic sites (nasopharynx, oropharynx, and hypophar-ynx) can be included in the radiation port [65,66]. Recent studies suggest that the eventual emergence of the primary site adversely affects the prognosis [68]. The role of chemotherapy in these patients is unclear. One randomized study, however, suggested that chemotherapy with cisplatin and 5-fluorouracil improved the response rate and median survival relative to radiation alone [69].

Patients with adenocarcinoma involving mid-high cervical nodes and patients with lower cervical or supraclavicular adenopathy of all histologies have a much poorer prognosis [70]. These patients are managed with local measures (usually radiation therapy) or may be candidates for systemic chemotherapy protocols.

RECOMMENDED THERAPY

Low N-stage (NX, N1, or N2A): surgery followed by radiation therapy (> 50 Gy) or radiation therapy alone (minimum 50 Gy) to ipsilateral neck with or without nasooropharynx.
High N-stage (N2B, N3A, N3B) or poorly differentiated tumors: cisplatin 100 mg/m^2 d 1, 22, and 43 with concurrent radiation therapy **or** cisplatin 100 mg/m^2 d 1 plus 5-FU 1000 mg/m^2/d by continuous infusion d 1–5. Repeat courses of cisplatin and 5-FU every 3–4 wk for three courses followed by radiation therapy.

WOMEN WITH ISOLATED AXILLARY ADENOPATHY

Isolated axillary adenopathy secondary to metastatic adenocarcinoma usually occurs in women and has unique clinical features. Many of these women have occult breast primaries, which can be identified in 40% to 70% of these patients who undergo mastectomy [71,72]. In this setting, rebiopsy of involved axillary nodes for estrogen and progesterone levels should be considered in view of the influence of this information on diagnosis and management. Breast magnetic resonance imaging has been shown to provide significant diagnostic accuracy in identifying occult breast carcinoma in women with axillary lymphadenopathy [73]. This may aid substantially in treatment planning for those patients considering surgery versus whole breast irradiation; however, it would not change the need for systemic chemotherapy in these women. Management is based on the treatment of stage II breast cancer, and this should include both local and systemic therapies. Prognosis following treatment is comparable to women with stage II breast cancer [73,74]. Older series have advocated modified radical mastectomy and axillary dissection for primary treatment [71,72,75]. A series of 42 patients suggested that survival was superior in patients receiving systemic chemotherapy, and local control was improved by irradiating the breast and the axilla [74]. The actuarial disease-free survival in this study was 71% at 5 years and 65% at 10 years.

Patients with axillary adenopathy and involvement of additional sites (usually liver or bone) or with nonadenocarcinoma histology constitute a much more heterogeneous group composed of equal numbers of men and women as well as a broader histologic spectrum with poorly differentiated carcinoma and neuroendocrine carcinomas represented in addition to adenocarcinoma. The survival of patients with axillary adenopathy and other involved organ sites is intermediate between that of the overall UPC population and women with isolated axillary adenopathy [27].

The management of patients with involvement of the axilla as well as other sites or nonadenocarcinoma histology is less certain. These patients generally are approached using a combination of local and systemic modalities and again may be good candidates for novel systemic chemotherapy protocols.

RECOMMENDED THERAPY

General principles are based on the management of women with stage II breast cancer. Tamoxifen is added to the systemic therapy of patients with estrogen receptor–positive neoplasms.

Modified radical mastectomy with axillary nodal dissection followed by systemic chemotherapy with 5-FU, doxorubicin, FAC or similar regimen for six courses **or** chemotherapy with FAC, or similar regimen for six to eight courses followed by radiation therapy to the ipsilateral breast and axillary nodes. (Axillary dissection can be considered before chemotherapy to assess receptor status and complete nodal staging but increases the risk of arm edema following radiation therapy.)

PERITONEAL CARCINOMATOSIS

Women with diffuse peritoneal carcinomatosis with adenocarcinoma constitute another recently recognized subset. These patients form a distinctive subset because of their clinical similarities to typical ovarian carcinoma. Often, papillary histology and elevations in CA-125 are found, but exploratory laparotomy fails to document a primary [77,78]. Other workers have also recognized this patient subset, terming this syndrome peritoneal papillary serous carcinoma or multifocal extraovarian serous carcinoma. These patients frequently respond to platinum-based chemotherapy [78–80]. Many patients in these series also underwent exploratory laparotomy with surgical debulking followed by chemotherapy. Median survivals are reported to be 16 months to 2 years.

The natural histories of men with isolated peritoneal carcinomatosis or patients with histologies inconsistent with ovarian carcinoma (*eg*, mucin-positive adenocarcinoma) or additional metastatic sites are much more poorly characterized, but overall survival, even with therapy, is poor.

RECOMMENDED THERAPY

Papillary serous carcinoma of the peritoneum: surgical debulking followed by systemic chemotherapy with carboplatin AUC-6 d 1 plus paclitaxel 175 mg/m^2 both IV d 1, repeat every 3–4 wk.
Adenocarcinoma of the peritoneum: systemic chemotherapy using cisplatin 75 mg/m^2 IV d 1; folinic acid 500 mg/m^2 in 200 mL normal saline IV over 2 h d 1–5; 5-FU 375 mg/m^2 IV after 1 h of folinic acid d 1–5; carboplatin AUC-6 d 1 plus paclitaxel 175 mg/m^2 both IV d 1, repeat every 3–4 wk; or a similar regimen.

POORLY DIFFERENTIATED AND UNDIFFERENTIATED CARCINOMA

Approximately one third of patients with UPC are defined as having this histologic picture. In this subset, detailed histochemical or immunohistochemical studies are most likely to identify highly treatment-responsive patients with lymphoma (leukocyte common antigen), germ cell (β-HCG, AFP), or neuroendocrine (neuron-specific enolase, chromogranin) neoplasms [29]. Additionally, Greco *et al.* [33] have identified a group of patients with poorly differentiated carcinoma or poorly differentiated adenocarcinoma that are responsive to platinum-based chemotherapy. Other investigators, however, conclude that these highly responsive patients are infrequently encountered in a consecutive series of UPC patients [81,82]. Most of these patients had clinical features (young age, mediastinal and retroperitoneal involvement, and rapid growth) of the extragonadal germ cell syndrome [83–86]. Many of these patients are male and have elevated β-HCG or AFP, although the usefulness of these serum tumor markers in predicting response is in question [81,87]. Motzer *et al.* [21] identified abnormalities in chromosome 12 specific for germ cell neoplasms in a group of male patients with poorly differentiated carcinoma involving midline structures confirming the germ cell origin of these tumors.

Combination chemotherapy regimens specific for germ cell carcinoma of testicular origin have usually been employed in the treatment of these patients [33,88]. These regimens have produced documented complete responses and an actual 10-year disease-free survival of 16% [88].

RECOMMENDED TREATMENT

Cisplatin 20 mg/m^2 d for 5 d plus etoposide 100 mg/m^2 d for 3–5 d with or without bleomycin 30 U/wk. Assess response after two courses of therapy; total of four to six courses for responding patients. Alternative approaches include carboplatin AUC-6 plus paclitaxel 200 mg/m^2 by 1-h infusion plus oral etoposide 50 mg/m^2 in 200 mL normal saline IV over 2 h d 1–5, 5-FU 375 mg/m^2 IV after 1 h of folinic acid d 1–5.

POORLY DIFFERENTIATED NEUROENDOCRINE CARCINOMA

Poorly differentiated (anaplastic) neuroendocrine carcinoma is an emerging clinicopathologic entity recognized primarily for its responsiveness to therapy. There is probably considerable overlap with extrapulmonary small cell carcinomas, anaplastic carcinoid, anaplastic islet cell tumors, Merkel's cell tumors, and paragangliomas. Histologically, these tumors are poorly differentiated, but histo-chemical stains are positive for chromogranin or neuron-specific enolase. These patients often present with diffuse hepatic or bone metastases but do not have the indolent histologic or clinical features of typical carcinoid tumors, islet cell tumors, or paragangliomas, and thus observation may not be appropriate. These tumors are also highly responsive to cisplatin-based chemotherapy [89,90].

RECOMMENDED THERAPY

Etoposide 130 mg/m^2 daily for 3 d plus cisplatin 45 mg/m^2 on d 2 and 3; courses repeated every 4 wk.

PATIENTS WITH ADENOCARCINOMA OR CARCINOMA OF UNKNOWN ORIGIN

The optimistic results for the favorable patients described previously do not apply to the vast majority of patients with UPC. Two thirds of UPC patients have metastatic adenocarcinoma with involvement of two or more visceral sites, usually some combination of liver, lung, lymph nodes, or bone. In addition, many men and women with poorly differentiated carcinoma or poorly differentiated adenocarcinoma have none of the clinical features outlined and respond poorly to chemotherapy [81]. Even in series showing optimistic results for selected patients with poorly differentiated carcinoma or poorly differentiated adenocarcinoma, the overall median survival remains poor at 12 months [88].

For unselected patients, numerous empiric chemotherapy combinations have been reported. Many have been based on doxorubicin, 5-fluorouracil, or cisplatin. A recent report using carboplatin, paclitaxel, and etoposide reported that 47% (25 of 53 patients) had objective responses [61]. In this series, seven patients (13%) experienced complete responses. The actuarial median survival for the entire group, however, was 13.4 months. The disappointing aspect of this survival statistic is that it is not substantially different from the 11-month median survival reported in large consecutive series of UCP patients [2,91]. There is little information on the use of biologic agents alone or with chemotherapy. Response rates generally range from 20% to 30%; however, most responses are partial and brief, resulting in little or no impact on median survival. Newer regimens continue to be tested; however, there has been no substantial progress in the treatment of these patients to date (*see* Table 23–3).

RECOMMENDED THERAPY

Cisplatin 20 mg/m^2 for 5 d plus etoposide 100 mg/m^2 for 3–5 days **or** cisplatin 100 mg/m^2 plus etoposide 100 mg/m^2 for 3 d (repeat courses administered every 3–4 wk); **or** paclitaxel 200 mg/m^2 by 1 h IV infusion d 1, carboplatin calculated AUC=6 IV d 1, etoposide 50 mg alternated with 100 mg/m^2 PO d 1–10 (repeat courses administered every 21 d); **or** cisplatin 75 mg/m^2 IV d 1, folinic acid 500 mg/m^2 in 200 mL normal saline IV over 2 h d 1–5, 5-FU 375 mg/m^2 IV after 1 h of folinic acid 1–5, or similar regimen (repeat courses administered every 28 d).

CHAPTER 23: AIDS-RELATED MALIGNANCIES

Afshin Dowlati, Scot C. Remick

With the close of the second decade of the AIDS epidemic, it is apparent that the spectrum of neoplasia in the background of underlying HIV infection and acquired immune deficiency remains dynamic. The evolution of primary antiretroviral therapy during this period, especially in more industrially developed portions of the world, has had a great impact on this aspect of the epidemic. Thus, we must reconcile the natural history and therapeutic interventions reported for various AIDS-related malignancies in the context of the evolution of current primary antiretroviral therapy. The highly active antiretroviral therapy (HAART) era dates back to 1996 with the general availability of the protease inhibitors (saquinavir was the first agent of this class to be approved for use in the United States by the Food and Drug Administration in 1995). It is now possible with the emergence of HAART therapies to achieve more sustained elevations in CD4 lymphocyte counts (immunologic response) and near complete suppression of HIV viral load (virologic response). Of these outcome measures, complete response (immunologic and virologic) and immunologic response seem important in achieving at least partial immune restoration, reduction in short-term opportunistic infectious complications, and prolongation of overall survival [1]. Throughout this chapter, in which references to the pre- and post-, or current HAART therapy era are made, the impact of this therapeutic era on malignant complications of HIV disease is elucidated.

AIDS-defining neoplasms include Kaposi's sarcoma, CNS lymphoma, non-Hodgkin's lymphoma, and invasive cervical cancer. In general, these neoplasms are characterized by aggressive clinical behavior with higher-grade lesions, more advanced stage, and shortened survival compared with similar neoplasms in HIV-seronegative or HIV-indeterminate individuals [2]. Reports from follow-up of the Multicenter AIDS Cohort Study (MACS), and other epidemiologic studies in the United States, Europe, Africa, and Australia have identified several neoplasms that increase in incidence in patients with underlying HIV infection [3–7]. These neoplasms include pediatric leiomyosarcoma and other soft tissue sarcomas, intraepithelial anogenital neoplasia and invasive anal cancer, Hodgkin's disease, squamous cell carcinoma of the conjunctiva (in Africa), brain tumors, lip cancer, seminoma, and plasma cell neoplasms including multiple myeloma and perhaps also plasmacytoma. In addition, other neoplasms are encountered in this particular patient population that are well characterized and include squamous cell carcinoma of the skin; nonseminomatous germ cell tumors; carcinoma of the oral mucosa, head, and neck; lung cancer; and malignant melanoma [8–10]. Although some cancers are clearly seen in increased incidence in patients with AIDS, some of these tumor types may not necessarily be related to immune deficiency. For instance, although rates of invasive cervical cancer and anal cancer are excessive among persons with AIDS, most of this excess can be attributed to the confounding occurrence from sexually transmitted human papillomavirus (HPV) infection rather than from immune deficiency [6,7]. Reports have been made of other tumors that are encountered in this setting, including hepatocellular carcinoma, penile cancer, and vaginal and vulvar cancer but estimated relative risk in comparison with the general US population for these tumors remains undefined [6]. At the dawn of the third decade of the epidemic, the spectrum of malignancy in HIV-infected patients is expanding (Table 23-1). Clearly, KS and NHL remain the dominant neoplasms encountered in this setting. This chapter briefly comments on putative pathogenetic mechanisms of neoplasia in HIV infection. The major focus is on the evolving therapeutic approach to patients with AIDS-related KS, NHL, and the diagnostic approach in patients with AIDS-related primary lymphoma of the central nervous system (CNS). A limited discussion about salient clinical aspects and treatment of other neoplasms that are encountered in the AIDS setting is also included.

PATHOGENESIS

The clinical paradigm for analyzing these observations on HIV-associated malignancy includes development of neoplastic complications in patients who have undergone solid organ transplantation. It is known that KS and NHL are seen in increased incidence in patients with other immunodeficient states, whether congenital or acquired. What is less well recognized is that other tumors, especially squamous cell carcinoma of the skin and lips, cervical carcinoma, and other anogenital tract neoplasms, are also seen in increased incidence in patients who have undergone organ transplantation. Gastric carcinoma has been described in increased incidence in other immunodeficient states as well. It may not be surprising, therefore, to see increased numbers of HIV-infected patients develop solid tumors other than those that have been so characteristic since the epidemic began.

Progressive immunologic deterioration is the hallmark of HIV infection, and malignancy evolves in this context in most HIV-infected patients. The pathogenesis of AIDS-defining and HIV-associated neoplasia is no doubt complex and multifactorial, and much remains to be elucidated. The HIV virus is generally not thought oncogenic. However, one report suggests a more direct pathogenetic role for HIV infection because HIV viral genome has been found incorporated into the fur gene complex on chromosome 15 in non–B cell malignant lymphoma cells [11]. This suggestion warrants further study. What is known is that the HIV tat gene protein product is a potent growth factor for KS and NHL [12]. These observations lend further support to the existence of a more direct link between HIV infection and malignancy. Other concurrent viral infections in HIV-infected patients such as those resulting from Epstein-Barr virus (EBV), human papillomavirus (HPV), HBV, and HCV are likely involved in the development of malignancy as well. There are well recognized epidemiologic links to malignancy and/or capacity for oncogenic transformation for each of these viruses. Another study has identified EBV viral genome in smooth-muscle cells in leiomyosarcomas in pediatric patients and another young man, all of whom were HIV-infected [13]. In another study of HIV infection and Hodgkin's disease, 78% of cases were EBV associated [14]. Sequences of an apparently new herpes-like virus (HHV-8) have also been identified in patients with AIDS-related KS, body cavity–based NHL (primary effusion lymphoma), and multicentric Castleman's disease [15–18]. In addition, this virus has also been demonstrated to infect bone marrow cells in HIV-seronegative patients with multiple myeloma [19]. Other reports have suggested that patients receiving prolonged antiretroviral (ie, zidovudine) therapy with progressive and severe underlying immunosuppression (CD4 lymphocyte count < 50/μL) may have an increased probability of developing malignant lymphoma. It is paradoxical that as HIV-infected patients live longer because of improvements in antiretroviral therapy and the recognition, management, and prophylaxis of opportunistic infections, they will be at increased risk for the development of neoplastic disease. The spectrum of malignancy in HIV infection is complex and heterogeneous. Improved understanding of the pathogenesis of HIV infection will likely lead to better insight of malignant transformation.

KAPOSI'S SARCOMA

Epidemiology

At the outset of the HIV epidemic up to 40% to 50% of patients presented with KS as their index AIDS-defining illness. Nearly half of these patients presented with disseminated disease, they died soon thereafter, and therapy complicated by the underlying immunosuppression of HIV infection [20,21]. Many of these clinical features of AIDS-related KS were akin to those initially described in the African endemic form in children in the 1960s. It is recognized that HIV-infected gay men have a 100,000-fold increased risk of developing Kaposi's sarcoma compared with the US general population and that this risk is approximately seven times greater than that for other HIV risk-behavior groups. At present, incidence of AIDS-associated KS is declining, which to a great extent may be attributable to the use of HAART as employed in the clinic [6,22]. Other contributing factors may be a manifestation of the changing risk-behavior profile of HIV-infected patients, new surveillance case definition (with CD4 lymphocyte count < 200/μL meeting clinical criteria for AIDS), and the development of wasting or other illnesses that may precede a diagnosis of KS. The annual risk of developing KS remains fairly constant over the duration of HIV infection, and as patients live longer it is more likely that they will develop the disease. It is projected that 15% to 20% of patients with HIV infection will develop KS. Given the global implications of the AIDS epidemic, KS is now recognized as the leading cancer in males (48% of registered cases) and the second commonest cancer in females (18%) in Kampala, Uganda, which parallels the evolution of the epidemic [23]. There appears to be an early peak of KS in African children as well. Incidence of childhood disease has risen more than 40-fold in the era of AIDS, and 78% of patients tested were HIV-seropositive [23].

Virology of Kaposi's Sarcoma and Human Herpes Virus-8

By the end of 1994, Chang *et al.* [15] were the first to report a unique DNA sequence associated with KS in patients with AIDS using representational difference analysis. These sequences were of nonhuman origin and were closely homologous to minor capsid and tegument protein genes of the Gammaherpesvirinae (*Rhadinovirus* subgroup), herpesvirus samiri, and EBV. It was soon recognized that this new virus was also present in KS patients without HIV infection. With the discovery of KS-associated KSHV/HHV-8, it is now known that KSHV is found in essentially all forms of KS (95% of patients) regardless of HIV serostatus; the virus is localized to KS lesions in spindle cells and not in normal skin; the virus also infects peripheral blood mononuclear cells (PBMCs) and is found in semen; KSHV-antibody seroprevalence matches KS risk groups and geographic distribution with higher rates in the Mediterranean, eastern Europe, and Africa; background seroprevalence in areas with a lower incidence of KS such as the United Kingdom and United States are 2% to 3%; and approximately 50% of AIDS-associated KS patients seroconvert within 10 years before developing the disease [22,24–29]. All of these epidemiologic and biologic features of KSHV link this virus to the disease and are suggestive of a more direct pathogenetic role. This virus has also been implicated in the pathogenesis of the emerging and distinct clinicopathologic entity of body cavity–based or primary effusion lymphoma and multicentric Castleman's disease in HIV-infected patients [17,18].

Pathogenesis

It has been well established that the HIV *tat* gene protein product is a potent growth factor for KS [12]. This protein increases bFGF [RL2]and promotes migration and adhesion of vascular endothelial cells, which are deemed to be important in the development of the spindle tumors characteristic of KS [30,31]. Additional pathogenetic mechanisms that are involved include HIV-associated immune activation and dysregulation of cytokine modulatory pathways (with inflammatory cytokines interleukin [IL]-1β, IL-6, tumor necrosis factor-α [TNF-α], and interferon gamma [IFN-γ]); and angiogenic cytokines (bFGF and vascular endothelial growth factor [VEGF] having pivotal roles) and coexisting viral infection [32,33]. The KSHV/HHV-8 virus is no doubt implicated in the development of KS, but at present no direct proof confirms that the virus is oncogenic or capable of immortalizing infected B cell or endothelial cell lines (ie, a transforming virus). This is substantiated by the lack of any animal or in vitro models and it is noteworthy that the KS Y-1 cell line, an immortal neoplastic KS cell line, is without evidence of HHV-8 infection [34]. Nonetheless, the virus does contain numerous homologous genes that stimulate cellular proliferation (v-cyclin, v-G

Table 23-1. Spectrum of Neoplastic Disease in HIV Infection

Tumor Type	Relationship to Immune Deficiency
US Centers for Disease Control AIDS-defining neoplasms	
Kaposi's sarcoma	Strong
Primary central nervous system lymphoma	Strong
Non-Hodgkin's lymphoma	Strong (especially high-grade)
Cervical carcinoma	Weak
Neoplasms with an increased incidence	
Hodgkin's disease	Strong
Pediatric leiomyosarcoma	Strong
Anogenital neoplasia and invasive anal cancer	Possible
Brain	Possible
Squamous cell carcinoma conjunctiva (in Africa)	Possible
Lip cancer	Possible
Seminoma	Possible
Plasmacytoma and multiple myeloma (likely)	Possible
Nonmelanoma skin cancer	Insufficient data

protein-coupled receptor [vGCR]/vIL-8R,and v-IFN regulatory factor [vIRF]); inhibit apoptosis (vbcl-2, vFLIP, and vIL-6); and play a role in recruitment of inflammatory cells and angiogenesis (vIL-6 and v-macrophage inflammatory protein [vMIP-1]) [32,35,36]. The virus is potentially equipped to maintain a latent state in B-cells or KS-associated endothelial cells but does not contain the necessary genes as seen in other rhadinoviruses (Stp, Tip), which can result in malignant transformation. In addition, there are no corresponding EBV nuclear antigens (EBNAs) and latent membrane proteins (LMPs), which are crucial for maintenance of viral latency and for growth transformation of the host cell. In summary, likely infection of normal mesenchymal progenitor cells by KSHV/HHV-8 results in activation/transformation to a "pre-KS" cell. Unlike normal mesenchymal progenitors, these cells acquire responsiveness to HIV tat and various cellular cytokines such as bFGF, IL-1, IL-6, onco-statin-M, and TNF-α [32,33]. The resultant cytokine dysregulation, secondary to the underlying HIV infection, promotes proliferation and differentiation of the KS tumor by various endogenous and exogenous (autocrine and paracrine) growth factors. Proliferation is further stimulated by progressive immunosuppression, cytokine perturbations associated with HIV infection, and modulation by HIV tat. Ultimately, these cells grow in an uncontrolled manner, which may be clonal in nature and recognized clinically as KS. Androgen receptor fragment analysis and recent detection of terminal repeat sequences of HHV-8 viral genome suggest that in some instances the transformation process may proceed to clonal proliferation [37,38]. An improved understanding of the pathogenesis of KS will no doubt lead to pathogenesis or mechanistically based therapeutic interventions, some of which are currently being investigated in the clinic.

Emerging Therapeutic Targets and Novel Agents

Advances in understanding the pathogenesis of KS have provided a framework with which to rationally approach the development of more effective treatment strategies. Several cytokines, both proinflammatory (IL-1, IL-6, TNF-α, and IFN-γ) and angiogenic (bFGF, VEGF, and IL-8), have been identified as autocrine growth factors for KS as already discussed. Accordingly, modulation of the expression of these cytokines and the vascular endothelium are emerging therapeutic targets. Several novel anti-angiogenic compounds (ie, angiogenesis inhibitors) are in fact in the midst of evaluation in the clinic. Two of the first antiangiogenic compounds evaluated were pentosan polysulfate [38,39] and tecogalan sodium [41,42]. Little or no antitumor activity was seen with either of these agents. Another antiangiogenic agent studied in AIDS-KS was fumagallin analogue, TNP-470 [43]. An 18% partial remission rate was observed in patients receiving this agent as a weekly intravenous infusion. Other angiogenesis inhibitors are currently in the midst of early phase and phase III clinical trial evaluation in the US National Cancer Institute (NCI)–sponsored AIDS Malignancy Consortium (AMC). A phase III study (AMC protocol #013) of IM862, a dipeptide (L-glutamic acid plus L-tryptophan) that demonstrates potent cell activating properties and marked antiangiogenic activity both in vitro and in xenograft models, is near completion. A recently reported randomized trial of this agent given intranasally demonstrated a 36% complete response rate with an additional 11% partial response [44]. SU5416 is a competitive inhibitor of the VEGF receptor, Flk1/KDR. Initial reports of a phase I dose-escalating trial of SU5416 in AIDS-KS showed several complete and partial responses [45]. IL-12 has been shown to inhibit angiogenic activity potently through induction of IFN-κ, which in turn upregulates

inducible protein 10 (IP-10). A dose finding trial of IL-12 in AIDS-KS demonstrated several clinical responses [46]. Similarly, in a phase II trial of thalidomide in AIDS-associated KS, eight of 17 patients obtained partial remission [47]. The potential for angiogenesis inhibition as a target and therapeutic implication of these agents remains to be borne out by current clinical trials. Given these preliminary observations, it is fair to say at this juncture that the clinical investigation of this strategy is warranted.

Therapeutic Approach

A prospective follow-up and validation of the AIDS Clinical Trials Group (ACTG) clinical TIS staging system [T: tumor, ulceration, edema, nodular oral disease, or visceral involvement; I: immune status, CD4 lymphocyte count of 200/μL or more; and S: systemic illness, KPS more than 70%, B symptoms: including fever, weight loss, night sweats or diarrhea, and prior AIDS-defining opportunistic infection) has recently confirmed its prognostic value [48]. This TIS system gives a score of 0 (good risk) or 1 (poor risk) for each of these factors. Tumor (T) stage and CD4 lymphocyte count (I), especially less than 150/μL, provide the most predictive information. AIDS-related KS is much more aggressive, associated with shortened duration of response, and generally pursues a relentless progressive course, the tempo of which may be variable at the outset when compared with de novo disease. For this reason, it is often not desirable to "watch and wait" or delay treatment. In addition, there are clearly acceptable cosmetic indications to pursue some form of therapy, including liquid nitrogen cryotherapy, intralesional chemotherapy, or interferon. In patients with AIDS-related KS, radiation is usually reserved as a last resort for palliative intervention, given that it often precludes administration of effective doses of systemic therapy into the tumor bed. Nonetheless, radiation can provide effective palliation [49].

Many chemotherapeutic agents have documented efficacy in KS; these primarily include bleomycin, doxorubicin, etoposide, and the vinca alkaloids (eg, vinblastine and vincristine) [50,51]. Single-agent chemotherapy is clearly better tolerated with a broad range of response rates ranging between 10% and 75% [50]. Newer agents such as the liposomal anthracyclines (doxorubicin and daunorubicin as first-line therapy) and paclitaxel (as salvage therapy) are also efficacious [52–56]. Vinorelbine is a new vinca alkaloid, which is currently undergoing evaluation in KS as well. Combination chemotherapy regimens, historically bleomycin and vincristine (BV and ABV), are known to yield higher response rates (40%–85%) with greater toxicity levels [50]. Results from randomized clinical trials suggest that single-agent liposomal anthracyclines have an improved therapeutic index over ABV [52,54]. For many patients, liposomal anthracyclines constitute appropriate first-line therapy. The AMC and Eastern Cooperative Oncology Group (ECOG) are currently conducting a randomized phase III intergroup trial comparing liposomal doxorubicin with paclitaxel as first-line therapy in advanced KS (AMC protocol #009). In patients with severe pulmonary disease, it may be prudent to administer ABV, because this regimen has been demonstrated to be helpful in this setting. Perhaps more important, with the improved understanding of the pathogenesis of KS, therapeutic interventions are evolving that are mechanistically based [57]. It will be of interest to define the impact of current protease inhibitor and HAART regimens on the natural history of the disease [58]; to explore the impact of antiviral therapy on the underlying viral disease and whether this may result in prophylaxis of KS in high-risk patient populations [59] and begin to tailor treatment strategies that modulate the various cytokine perturbations that have been demonstrated to promote tumor growth (*eg*, angiogenesis inhibitors [49,39–46]; thalidomide → ↓TNF-α [47]; IL-4 → ↓IL-6; metalloprotease inhibitors → ↓bFGF; neutralizing Ab → IL-1; topical retinoids; βHCG [60]; and antiviral therapy → HHV-8 [58,59]).

NON-HODGKIN'S LYMPHOMA

Epidemiology

Shortly after the onset of the AIDS epidemic, systemic B-cell NHL was seen in increased incidence in HIV-infected patients and added to the case definition list. Approximately 5% to 10% of HIV-infected patients are destined to develop lymphoma [61]. NHL is the AIDS-defining illness in approximately 3% of HIV-infected patients. As experience with nucleoside analogue antiretroviral monotherapy (zidovudine) was gained, some initial concern was raised about long-term administration and risk of developing NHL [62,63]. Clearly, the risk of developing lymphoma steadily increases with duration of HIV infection and advancing immunosuppression. Prospects for significantly increased short- and long-term survival are enhanced with the emergence of HAART therapy as already mentioned. The significance of this remains to be sorted out but it is conceivable that long-term survivors of HIV infection will likely remain at increased risk for NHL. This would be reminiscent of the experience with patients undergoing solid organ transplantation and the lifelong increased risk of lymphoma, among other tumors, because of attendant iatrogenic immunosuppression. Nonetheless, albeit early observations of lymphoma incidence as the HAART era evolves reveals negligible impact on systemic lymphoma (in some instances perhaps a small nonsignificant decline is seen), but an apparent substantial decline in primary CNS lymphoma [64]. This could in part be explained by short-term improvement in immune function. Longer follow-up periods and epidemiologic studies of larger cohorts are clearly needed to help sort the risk of lymphoma.

Pathogenesis

The pathogenesis of lymphoma in the setting of HIV infection is no doubt complex and much about it remains to be elucidated. What is known is that progressive immune suppression, chronic antigen stimulation and B-cell proliferation, associated immune activation and dysregulation of cytokine modulatory pathways (IL-6 and IL-10 in particular), altered *bcl-6*, *p53*, and *c-myc* protooncogene expression, and coexisting viral infection(s) are all implicated [2,65–68]. Several developments have further unveiled the potential role of viral oncogenesis in the pathogenesis of AIDS-related lymphoma and perhaps other B-cell neoplasms: 1) EBV's long-standing association with systemic and CNS NHL; 2) HIV viral genome has been found incorporated into the fur gene complex on chromosome 15 in non-B-cell lymphoma cells upstream to *c-fes*, a protooncogene [11,69]; 3) KSHV/HHV-8 has recently been identified in HIV-infected patients with body-cavity-based NHL or primary effusion lymphoma, multicentric Castleman's disease, and in bone marrow dendritic cells of HIV-seronegative multiple myeloma patients [17–19,70].

Therapeutic Approach

In general, AIDS-related NHL is characterized by higher grade (40% to 60%), greater predilection for extranodal disease (80%), more advanced clinical stage (60% to 70% stage III/IV) and shortened survival (median 7 to 8 months) when compared with lymphomas in HIV-seronegative patients [61,71,72]. At time of presentation, the

median CD4 lymphocyte count is 100/μL [73]. It was recognized early on that the clinical course was much more aggressive. This in fact led to the evaluation of more aggressive and dose-intense combination chemotherapy regimens in this disease at the outset. Early results were dismal, regimens were poorly tolerated, and there was a trend for shortened survival. More traditional NHL combination chemotherapy regimens were then evaluated in conjunction with antiretroviral therapy; incorporation of colony-stimulating factors (CSFs), of which granulocyte-macrophage CSF (GM-CSF) is known to upregulate HIV viral replication; and use of various CNS prophylaxis strategies because of the proclivity of AIDS-related lymphoma to disseminate or relapse in this site. Complete responses ranged between 20% and 60% with median survival duration of between 4 and 7 months [71,72].

In June 1997, the ACTG reported the largest randomized clinical trial in AIDS-related NHL. The ACTG 142 study compared standard dose (SD) m-BACOD with GM-CSF with a dose-modified (low dose [LD]) m-BACOD regimen [73]. All patients received intrathecal cytosine arabinoside for meningeal prophylaxis during the first cycle of chemotherapy. The results of this study confirm that hematologic toxicity was significantly lower and overall the dose-modified regimen better tolerated with equivalent efficacy: complete response (CR) 41% LD and CR 52% SD ($P = 0.56$); with median survival duration of 35 weeks. LD and 31-week SD ($P = 0.25$), respectively. Poor prognostic factors were identified inclusive of age older than 35 years, history of injecting drug use, stage III/IV disease, and (most important) a CD4 lymphocyte count of less than 100/(L [73,74]. In the ACTG study, patients with no or one adverse prognostic factors had a median survival of 46 weeks; those with two had 44 weeks; and those with three or four, 18 weeks [74]. This resulted in 3-year survival rates of 30% for no or one adverse prognostic factors, 17% for two, and 0% for three or four [74]. A 3% CNS relapse rate was observed.

The longest median survival reported for AIDS-related NHL in the preprotease inhibitor era is 18 months in a single institutional study of 46 patients [75–77]. These patients were treated with a 96-hour continuous infusion of cyclophosphamide-doxorubicin-etoposide (CDE). The overall CR rate is 57% with this regimen [75–77]. Confirmatory evaluation is ongoing in both HIV-seropositive/negative patients with NHL in the cooperative group (*eg*, ECOG) setting. Preliminary results were presented at both the 1999 annual American Society of Clinical Oncologists' and Third National AIDS Malignancy meetings [78,79]. In all, 48 patients with AIDS-related NHL were treated in this confirmatory multi-institutional phase II study of infusional-CDE. A 46% complete response rate was observed with a median survival of 8.2 months, 1-year survival rate of 48%, and 2-year survival rate of 35% [78,79]. The regimen is myelotoxic, with 75% and 52% of patients experiencing grade 4 neutropenia and thrombocytopenia, respectively, and a 10% (five patients) treatment-related mortality rate [78,79].

An oral combination chemotherapy regimen has been developed inclusive of CCNU, etoposide, cyclophosphamide and procarbazine (also a single-institution study) [80,81]). The rationale for his regimen is straightforward and takes advantage of oral administration, in vitro synergy, known first-line efficacy of the drugs in NHL, and inclusion of two agents (CCNU and procarbazine) that cross the blood-brain barrier. This regimen precludes the potential cardiotoxicity of doxorubicin-based regimens and avoids the additional immunosuppressive effects of corticosteroids. The addition of G-CSF to the regimen decreased the frequency of hospitalization for febrile neutropenia and decreased the discontinuation of chemotherapy because of leukopenia [81]. Thrombocytopenia, however, was more severe. The overall objective response rate with this regimen is 66% (CR 34%) with a 5% CNS relapse rate, and median survival duration of 7.0 months [80,81]. In addition, one third of patients survived 1-year, 11% 2 years, and half of patients survived free from progression of their lymphoma. None of the patients treated with the oral chemotherapy regimen received protease inhibitor–based antiviral therapy.

At the Third National AIDS Malignancy Conference in 1999, preliminary results of CHOP (cyclophosphamide, hydroxydaunomycin, vincristine sulfate [Oncovin], and prednisone) chemotherapy regimen in combination with HAART (AMC clinical trial #005) were presented [82]. In this study, patients were randomized to receive either a modified-dose or full-dose CHOP regimen with HAART (stavudine [d4T], lamivudine [3TC], and indinavir). In total, 65 patients were treated (63 patients remain currently evaluable). The CR rate was comparable in each study arm, 30% modified-dose (40 patients) and 32% full-dose (25 patients) [82]. Grade 3 or 4 neutropenia occurred in 55% and 32% of patients on the dose-modified and standard dose arms, respectively [82]. Encouraging follow-up results were also presented at this meeting with EPOCH infusional chemotherapy, in which a 79% (19 of 24 patients) CR rate and 72% overall 2-year survival rate were observed [83]. This single institution study did treat a very favorable group of patients, in that 67% of patients had a CD4 lymphocyte count of 100/µL or more [83]. In this study, HIV viral burden was monitored closely in eight patients on days 1 and 6 of each cycle and at 3 and 6 weeks' postchemotherapy. Antiretroviral therapy was withheld during chemotherapy because of the potential of overlapping toxicity, pharmacokinetic interactions between HAART therapy and cyclophosphamide in particular, and to ensure that dose schedule of chemotherapy would be maintained. There was no apparent worsening of viral burden during chemotherapy administration and in fact there was a trend for lower viral burden between days 1 and 6; median day 1, 17,000 RNA copies per µL plasma versus median day 6, 8150 RNA copies per µL of plasma ($P < 0.01$) [84]. These observations suggest that cytotoxic chemotherapy may not adversely effect underlying HIV viral burden and clearly need to be extended to larger numbers of patients with AIDS-related NHL. Most recently, at the Fourth International AIDS Malignancy Conference in March 2000, updated information on infusional CDE and EPOCH regimens was reported [85,86]. In the ECOG trial of CDE, the confirmed 42% CR rate (data analysis incomplete), 17.8 month median survival duration, and 55% 1-year survival rate were reported for infusional-CDE in the post-HAART era versus 46% CR, 8.2 months median survival time, and 48% 1-year survival, respectively, in the pre-HAART era [85]. Further follow-up from the EPOCH trial did not identify further risk of progressive HIV infection with the temporary suspension of antiretroviral therapy during chemotherapy administration [86]. Results from recent AIDS lymphoma trials are summarized in Table 23-2.

Observations of recent clinical trials show that approximately 10% to 20% of patients may be cured or, more appropriately, survive free from progression of their lymphoma. In patients with good prognostic factors at presentation, up to 30% may survive 3 years and some patients may be appropriate candidates for more traditional or aggressive cytotoxic therapy [74]. As a result, salvage therapy may become increasingly important, which to date has been discouraging. Nonetheless, preliminary results with mitoguazone (MGBG) have been promising [87]. The AMC is currently evaluating the role of ifosfamide-etoposide combination chemotherapy as salvage therapy followed by the addition of IL-12 in responding patients (AMC protocol #008).

Treatment recommendations can be summarized as follows. The results of ACTG 142 (conducted in the pre-HAART era) imply that a dose-modified chemotherapeutic approach is appropriate for most patients with AIDS-related non-Hodgkin's lymphoma. In the HAART therapy era, however, it is important to individualize systemic therapy options as the natural history of the underlying HIV disease is so drastically changing and patients are in fact better able to tolerate standard-dose systemic therapy. It is by no means standard practice to withhold antiviral therapy during chemotherapy, although preliminary results with this strategy employing EPOCH chemotherapy are encouraging. Furthermore, it remains to be established which is the optimal therapeutic regimen. Given this backdrop, participation on clinical trials addressing these issues is to be encouraged at all times. All patients should receive prophylaxis for *Pneumocystis carinii* pneumonia. It is likely preferable to continue effective antiretroviral regimens with chemotherapy, although this is under investigation. CSF support is likely warranted in most patients. The role of routine CNS prophylaxis has yet to be defined and should be discouraged. Exceptions may include patients with high-grade histologies, bone marrow involvement, and bulky lesions, particularly those affecting the head and neck/paranasal sinus and epidural areas that may invade the CNS. Patients with no adverse prognostic factors may be candidates for standard treatment approaches to improve the overall survival; dose-intense strategies are being revisited. The next-generation chemotherapy trial for AIDS-related NHL in the AMC is the addition of CD20-monoclonal antibody (rituximab) to CHOP combination chemotherapy (AMC protocol #010).

PRIMARY CENTRAL NERVOUS SYSTEM LYMPHOMA

Epidemiology and Pathogenesis

Since the AIDS epidemic began, primary CNS lymphoma (PCL) has been regarded as an AIDS-defining neoplasm. Approximately 1% to 2% of HIV-infected patients develop primary CNS lymphoma [61]. Overall incidence of this neoplasm in the general population is increasing independent of the AIDS epidemic; the incidence in the HAART therapy era in the HIV setting is declining [6,64,65]. Invariably, this tumor is encountered in patients with profound immunodeficiency (ie, CD4 lymphocyte counts below 50/µL) and there is the nearly constant association of this tumor with EBV infection. This latter observation may in fact be of considerable diagnostic importance.

Diagnostic Evaluation

Diagnosis of AIDS-related primary CNS lymphoma is challenging because of its protean manifestations. The lack of focal findings and the broad differential diagnosis in HIV-infected patients who present with nonconfirmatory neurologic findings often contributes to a delayed or missed diagnosis [88]. In one series of AIDS patients with primary CNS lymphoma, an antemortem diagnosis was established in only half of these patients. The initial evaluation of an HIV-infected patient with suspected CNS lymphoma should establish whether the disease is systemic or primary. This can often be established by a complete physical examination, routine blood work, and chest radiography. If these limited clinical staging procedures reveal no obvious pathology, then further systemic evaluation such as body CT-MRI scanning, gallium scan, and bone marrow aspiration and biopsy, are of low yield and can be avoided.

Single and multiple contrast-enhancing lesions, in most cases, may be seen on head CT and MRI scan. In AIDS-related CNS lymphoma, lesions are usually hypodense in the absence of contrast; involve the basal ganglia, cerebellum, brain stem, and cerebral hemispheres; classic ring enhancement may be demonstrated in up to 40%of cases; and up to 10% may show no contrast enhancement. MRI is thought to be more sensitive than CT in identifying primary CNS lymphoma. These radiographic findings are too inconsistent to be the only method of diagnosis. The differential diagnosis of a space occupying CNS mass lesion in an HIV-infected patient is broad and primarily includes toxoplasmosis, which may decline with HAART. Progressive multifocal leukoencephalopathy (PML), fungal and bacterial abscesses, tuberculosis, gummatous lesions, infarct, hemorrhage, and glioma can also present as focal lesions. Because serologic techniques for diagnosis of toxoplasmosis are unreliable in a significant number of AIDS patients and ring enhancement is often an accompanying radiographic sign, biopsy is necessary to establish a diagnosis. Tissue can be obtained by various methods including of brain parenchyma with stereotactic brain biopsy; lumbar puncture for CSF cytology (between 20% and 25% of AIDS patients have positive findings on cytology); or orbit through aqueous tumor cytology. A careful ophthalmologic and slit-lamp examination may prove helpful to establish vitreal involvement. The preferable approach depends on the available expertise at any treatment center.

It is often appropriate to embark on a course of empiric treatment for toxoplasmosis for many patients in whom their clinical status is stable and their CNS lymphoma is not their AIDS-defining illness. In this instance, antitoxoplasma therapy is administered for 7 to 14 days and head CT-MRI is repeated to document resolution of CNS mass lesions, thus establishing a diagnosis of toxoplasmosis. If the lesions persist, it is appropriate to proceed to biopsy. For patients in whom their CNS mass lesion is their AIDS-defining event alone, or also in those with clinically significant intracranial disease (eg, mass effect) it is generally advisable to attempt biopsy to offer diagnosis-specific therapy. Current investigational modalities, which may greatly facilitate diagnostic evaluation in this setting, include detection of EBV DNA in CSF and thallium single-photon emission computed tomography (SPECT) scanning [89]. Initial studies suggest that the presence of EBV DNA in CSF as detected by polymerase chain reaction (PCR) has a specificity of 100% and a sensitivity of between 80% and 98.5% [90,91]. In a large series of 61 patients, investigators at the University of Miami reported that 95.2% of AIDS-related CNS lymphoma patients have positive SPECT scans [92]. In another smaller study, thallium-brain SPECT scanning had a sensitivity of 100% and a specificity of 90% [93]. These modalities may prove valuable in establishing a diagnosis of primary CNS lymphoma and complement or replace current diagnostic methods. The diagnostic approach for HIV-infected patients with a CNS mass lesion is summarized in Figure 23-1.

Therapeutic Approach

Overall median survival for AIDS-related primary CNS lymphoma ranges between 2 to 3 months [88]. Survival is likely to be improved in patients without prior AIDS-defining opportunistic infections and good performance status (Karnofsky performance status rating above 70%) [88,94,95]. This aspect of the natural history of the disease is important to consider in clinical decision-making, given that up to 20% of patients may survive 1 year following a course of radiotherapy [94,95]. For patients suspected of CNS lymphoma with profound immunosuppression, advanced stage AIDS, and poor clinical status, it may be moot to establish a diagnosis or offer therapy because survival is so poor [61].

Radiotherapy historically has been the primary treatment modality for CNS lymphoma. It appears that combined modality chemotherapy and radiation in HIV-seronegative/indeterminate primary CNS lymphoma improves median survival (≈ 3 years) and is the preferred approach [108]. This clearly must be regarded an investigational approach in the HIV setting, and trials are currently under way to

Table 23-2. Summary of Results with Combination Chemotherapy Regimens from Reported Trials in AIDS-related non-Hodgkin's Lymphoma

Regimen	Route of Administration	Patients, n	CR Rate, %	MST	Long-term Survival	CSF Prophylaxis	HAART era[†]	Study
m-BACOD					30% / 17% / 0% 3-y by adverse factors*			
SD	IV bolus	94	52	31 wk		Yes	Pre	Kaplan et al. [87],
LD		98	41	35 wk				Straus et al. [93]
CDE						Yes (high grade; bone marrow +)	Pre	Sparano et al. [104]
Pre	96-h CI	48	46	8.2 mo	48% 1-y		Post	
Post		60	42	17.8 mo	55% 1-y			
CHOP								
SD	IV bolus	25	32	Not available	Not available	No	Post	Ratner et al. [101]
LD		40	30					
EPOCH	96-h CI	33	77	Not reached	72% 2-y	Yes	Post	Little et al. [105]
Oral therapy	PO	38	34	7.0 mo	32% 2-y 13% 2-y	No	Pre	Remick et al. [99,100]

*Three-year survival rates were reported for the AIDS Clinical Trials Group for all patients (not by arm of study) by number of adverse prognostic factors: 0 or 1, 30%; 2, 17%; 3 or 4, 0%; see Straus et al. [93] for details.
†Pre and post highly active antiretroviral (HAART) therapy.
m-BACOD—???; CDE—cyclophosphamide, doxorubicin, and etoposide; CHOP—cyclophosphamide, doxorubicin, vincristine, and prednisone; CI—continuous infusion; CR—complete response rate; EPOCH—etoposide, prednisone, vincristine, cyclophosphamide, and doxorubicin; MST—median survival time; PO—by mouth; SD/LD—standard dose/low dose.

define feasibility, toxicity, and efficacy. The AMC is currently investigating induction antiviral therapy with zidovudine, ganciclovir, and IL-2 in a pilot study (AMC protocol #019). In the absence of a clinical trial, we generally offer definitive radiation therapy, add concurrent chemotherapy in select patients for one cycle, and attempt to wean such patients from any corticosteroids as rapidly as possible.

OTHER TUMORS

Hodgkin's disease, testicular cancer, lung cancer, and anogenital (including invasive anal and cervical carcinoma) neoplasms are increasingly diagnosed in HIV-infected patients. A more detailed discussion about the therapeutic approach to these neoplasms is beyond the scope of this chapter's discussion. Key points regarding the natural history and therapeutic approach are, however, briefly summarized.

Hodgkin's Disease

It has been established that Hodgkin's disease is clearly seen in increased incidence in HIV-infected patients [2–4,6]. This tumor

has been well characterized, especially in injecting drug users in Europe [14]. Several features of the natural history of this disease in this setting are worthy of comment. Most patients present with stage III and IV disease, often with extranodal disease, and as a result systemic chemotherapy is the mainstay of treatment [14,95,96]. There is little mediastinal involvement, which can be explained by the predominance of mixed cellularity and lymphocyte depletion histologies and lack of nodular sclerosis subtype. The frequency of EBV genome expression appears to be higher in HIV-related Hodgkin's disease compared with de novo disease. Current treatment approaches have generally focused on traditional chemotherapy for Hodgkin's disease with the greatest experience reported for the ABVD regimen. The CR rate is approximately 50% and median survival is approximately 18 months [95,96]. The optimal chemotherapy regimen remains to be established and various regimens are currently under investigation; it is not yet known whether a dose-modified approach akin to that for non-Hodgkin's disease is appropriate; and prospects for progression-free and long-term survival need to be identified.

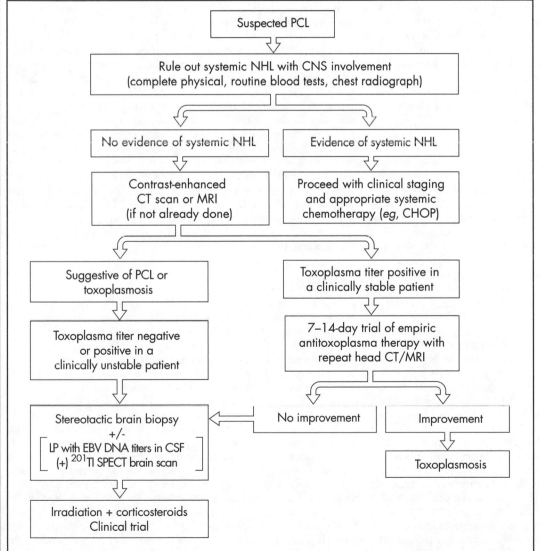

FIGURE 23-1.

Diagnostic algorithm in HIV-infected patients with central nervous system (CNS) mass lesion(s) and suspected primary CNS lymphoma (PCL). CHOP—cyclophosphamide, doxorubicin, vincristine, prednisone; CSF—colony-stimulating factor; CT—computed tomography; EBV—Epstein–Barr virus; MRI—magnetic resonance imaging; LP—lumbar puncture; NHL—non-Hodgkin's lymphoma; SPECT—single-photon emission computed tomography.

TESTICULAR NEOPLASMS

Seminoma has been described in increased incidence in HIV infection [3,4]. NSGCTs are less commonly encountered. It appears on review of reported cases of testicular neoplasms in the HIV-infected patient population. The histopathologic subtype and clinical stage are no different than in the general population (50% seminoma versus 50% nonseminomatous germ cell tumor; and 40% stage I, 40% for II, and 20% for III) [8,9]. One must recognize that HIV-infected testicular cancer patients may be inappropriately downstaged, that is, from stage I to II, because of benign retroperitoneal lymphadenopathy, which is secondary to their underlying HIV infection and not metastasis [8,9]. This has obvious prognostic and therapeutic implications that are difficult to sort out in otherwise healthy asymptomatic HIV-infected patients with relatively high CD4 lymphocyte counts. There is no correlation of CD4 count and clinical stage of testis cancer in these patients. Sound clinical judgment regarding the staging of these patients is imperative. What is interesting is that most HIV-infected testicular cancer patients as reported in the literature tolerate standard systemic combination chemotherapy alone or in combination with radiotherapy very well [8,9]. This contrasts with the toxicity encountered in most HIV-infected patients with other neoplasms who generally present with advanced underlying immunodeficiency. A 95% CR rate was observed in 20 patients, approximately half of whom received chemotherapy, and the other half radiation [118]. Fewer than 50% of these patients experienced severe grade III and IV hematologic toxicity. Median survival approaches 40 months for patients with CD4 counts more than 200/μL and 26 months for patients with CD4 counts less than 200/μL [8,9].

Lung Cancer

As the HIV epidemic advances, lung cancer is more commonly recognized. Review of AIDS surveillance and cancer registry databases has not yet identified a true increased incidence of this neoplasm in HIV infection. Nonetheless, there are several features of lung cancer that develop in this setting that suggest an altered natural history of the disease. There is a clear correlation of cigarette smoking and risk of lung cancer in HIV-infected patients; a significantly younger age at time of diagnosis (median 45 years); a predominance of adenocarcinoma histology (> 50%) and paucity of small-cell carcinoma (< 10%); approximately 85% of patients, mostly male, present with stage III and IV disease versus 20% stage I disease in HIV-seronegative or indeterminate patients; and the clinical course is more aggressive with shortened survival [8–10]. Median CD4 lymphocyte count is 233/μL, which suggests that profound immunosuppression and symptomatic HIV infection may not be significant cofactors in the pathogenesis of lung cancer in these patients [10]). The most important clinical implication of these observations is that lung cancer must be included in the differential diagnosis of an abnormal chest radiograph in HIV-infected patients, especially a solitary mass lesion. Patients with good medical or operative risk and stage I disease are best managed with surgical resection. HIV seropositivity alone is not a contraindication to resection. There are, however, limited published data on the follow-up of HIV-infected lung cancer patients with stage I disease. For patients with regionally advanced disease and good clinical status it would be prudent to offer sequential rather than concurrent chemotherapy and irradiation because of the enhanced toxicity. Patients with metastatic disease are managed similarly to HIV-seronegative or indeterminate patients, and clinical performance status may be of particular prognostic value

as well. It will be interesting to identify the activity of the novel topoisomerase I inhibitors (topotecan, 9-aminocamptothecin), which are known to have antiretroviral activity and are currently being evaluated in AIDS-related KS [98]. Overall median survival for HIV-infected lung cancer patients is 3 months, no 5-year survival rates have been published, and unfortunately treatment and survival results are inconsistently reported [8–10].

Anogenital Tumors: Invasive Anal and Cervical Carcinoma

These neoplasms are clearly encountered in increased incidence in HIV-infected individuals. Because immunodeficiency advances in HIV infection while patients live longer, there appears to be increased risk for the development of high-grade intraepithelial lesions both of the anus, especially in homosexual men who practice anoreceptive intercourse, and of the cervix. Consequently, appropriate anogenital tract surveillance that includes gynecologic examination with Papanicolaou smear and colposcopy in women, anal examination and colposcopy in high-risk HIV-seropositive men, and provision of local modalities for treatment of high-risk lesions is warranted and must be incorporated into primary care. The precise strategy of surveillance for anal intraepithelial neoplasia is currently being identified. The therapeutic approach to HIV-infected patients with invasive cervical carcinoma is identical to that for HIV-seronegative women. Surgery and radiation remain the cornerstones of therapy. There are few published chemotherapy data for patients with systemic disease and overall the clinical course in much more aggressive [99]. HIV-infected patients with anal squamous cell carcinoma are similarly managed as HIV-seronegative patients with combined modality therapy. Chemotherapy with mitomycin, 10 to15 mg/m^2 intravenously on day 1, and 5-fluorouracil (5-FU), 1000 mg/m^2 as a 24-hour continuous infusion on days 1 to 4, with radiotherapy (3000 cGy over 3 weeks) has been administered concomitantly to patients who are not HIV infected. Up to 80% of patients have a complete remission and abdominoperineal resection can be avoided. In the HIV setting, toxicity is much more pronounced and it may be advisable to do sequential therapy [100]. There are as yet no AIDS-specific or dose-modified therapeutic approaches for HIV-infected patients with invasive cervical or anal cancer.

CONCLUSIONS

As the HIV epidemic advances and patients live longer owing to improvements in antiretroviral therapy and recognition, management, and prophylaxis of opportunistic infections, it is apparent that various neoplasms, both AIDS defining and non-AIDS defining, will likely be of increasing clinical concern. Clinicians must continue to define the spectrum and biology of malignant disease in this setting with attention to the underlying HIV infection, quality of life, and prospects for improved survival. General supportive care recommendations for most patients with AIDS-related neoplasms include 1) optimize protease inhibitor–based combination antiretroviral therapy to achieve complete or near complete HIV viral load suppression; 2) provide adequate prophylaxis for opportunistic infection (usually all patients receiving cytotoxic chemotherapy should receive prophylaxis for *P. carinii* (pneumonia); and 3) closely monitor for myelosuppression, with a low threshold to add cytokine/growth factor support. At present, a dose-modified chemotherapy approach has only been confirmed to be efficacious in AIDS-related NHL, and in the current HAART therapy era, usefulness of this approach may be limited. In many instances, patients with AIDS-related malignancies are more susceptible to the toxicity of antineoplastic therapy or are too ill to withstand such therapy for which a dose-modified approach may be warranted. More important, patients with AIDS-related malignancies should at all times be considered appropriate candidates for participation on clinical trials to help resolve and improve the therapeutic approach for these diseases.

REFERENCES

1. Grabar S, Le Moing V, Goujard C, *et al.:* Clinical outcome of patients with HIV-1 infection according to immunologic and virologic response after 6 months of highly active antiretroviral therapy. *Ann Intern Med* 2000, 133:401–410.

2. Levine AM: AIDS-related malignancies: the emerging epidemic. *J Natl Cancer Inst* 1993, 85:1382–1397.

3. Lyter DW, Bryant J, Thackeray R, *et al.:* Incidence of human immunodeficiency virus-related and nonrelated malignancies in a large cohort of homosexual men. *J Clin Oncol* 1995, 13:2540–2546.

4. Rabkin CS: Epidemiology of malignancies other than Kaposi's sarcoma and non-Hodgkin's lymphoma in HIV infection. *J Acquir Immune Defic Syndr Hum Retrovirol* 1997, 14:A12.

5. Grulich A, Wan X, Law M, *et al.:* Rates of non-AIDS defining cancers in people with AIDS. *J Acquir Immune Defic Syndr* 1997, 14:A18.

6. Goedert JJ: The epidemiology of acquired immunodeficiency syndrome malignancies. *Semin Oncol* 2000, 27:390–401.

7. Goedert JJ, Cote TR, Virgo P, *et al.:* Spectrum of AIDS-associated malignant disorders. *Lancet* 1998, 351:1833–1839.

8. Remick SC: The spectrum of Non-AIDS-defining neoplastic disease in HIV infection. *J Invest Med* 1996, 44:205–215.

9. Remick SC: Non-AIDS-defining cancers. *Hematol Oncol Clin North Am* 1996, 10:1203–1213.

10. Vyzula R, Remick SC: Lung cancer in patients with HIV infection. *Lung Cancer* 1996, 15:325–339.

11. Shiramizu B, Herndier BG, McGrath MS Identification of a common clonal human immunodeficiency virus integration site in human immunodeficiency virus associated lymphoma. *Cancer Res* 1994, 54:2069–2072.

12. Prakash O, Z-Y Tang, He Y, *et al.:* Human Kaposi's sarcoma cell-mediated tumorigenesis in human immunodeficiency type 1 Tat-expressing transgenic mice. *J Natl Cancer Inst* 2000, 92:721–728.

13. McClain KL, Leach CT, Jenson HB, *et al.:* Association of Epstein-Barr virus with leiomyosarcomas in young people with AIDS. *N Engl J Med* 1995, 332:12–18.

14. Tirelli U, Errante D, Dolcetti R, *et al.:* Hodgkin's disease and human immunodeficiency virus infection: clinicopathologic and virologic features of 114 patients from the Italian Cooperative Group on AIDS and Tumors. *J Clin Oncol* 1995, 13:1758–1767.

15. Chang Y, Cesarman E, Pessin MS, *et al.:* Identification of herpesvirus-like DNA sequences in AIDS-associated Kaposi's sarcoma. *Science* 1994, 266:1865–1869.

16. Moore PS, Chang Y: Detection of herpesvirus-like DNA sequences in Kaposi's sarcoma in patients with and those without HIV infection. *N Engl J Med* 1995, 332:1181–1185.

17. Cesarman E, Chang Y, Moore PS, *et al.:* Kaposi's sarcoma-associated herpesvirus-like DNA sequences in AIDS-related body cavity-based lymphomas. *N Engl J Med* 1995, 332:1186–1191.

18. Cesarman E, Knowles D:. Herpes-like DNA sequences, AIDS-related tumors, and Castleman's disease. *N Engl J Med* 1995, 333:798–799.

19. Rettig MB, Ma HJ, Vescio RA, *et al.:* Kaposi's sarcoma-associated herpesvirus infection of bone marrow dendritic cells from multiple myeloma patients. *Science* 1997, 276:1851–1854.

20. Dezube BJ: Clinical presentation and natural history of AIDS-related Kaposi's sarcoma. *Hematol Oncol Clin North Am* 1996, 10:1023–1029.

21. Dezube BJ: Acquired immunodeficiency syndrome-related Kaposi's sarcoma: clinical features, staging, and treatment. *Semin Oncol* 2000, 27:424–430.

22. U.S. Centers for Disease Control and Prevention: Surveillance for AIDS-defining opportunistic illnesses 1992–1997. *MMWR Morb Mortal Wkly Rep* 1999, 48:1–24.

23. Wabinga HR, Parkin DM, Wabwire-Mangen F, *et al.:* Cancer incidence in Kampala, Uganda, in 1989-91: changes in incidence in the era of AIDS. *Int J Cancer* 1993, 54:26–36.

24. Gao S-J, Kingsley L, Hoover DR, *et al.:* Seroconversion to antibodies against Kaposi's sarcoma-associated herpesvirus-related latent nuclear antigens before development of Kaposi's sarcoma. *N Engl J Med* 1996, 335:233–241.

25. Huang YO, Li JJ, Kaplan MH, *et al.:* Human herpesvirus-like nucleic acid in various forms of Kaposi's sarcoma. *Lancet* 1995, 345:759–761.

26. Miller G, Rigsby MO, Heston L, *et al.:* Antibodies to butyrate-inducible antigens of Kaposi's sarcoma-associated herpesvirus in patients with HIV-1 infection. *N Engl J Med* 1996, 334:1292–1297.

27. Purvis SF, Katongole-Mbidde E, Johnson J, *et al.:* High incidence of Kaposi's sarcoma-associated herpesvirus and Epstein-Barr virus in tumor lesions and peripheral blood mononuclear cells from patients with Kaposi's sarcoma in Uganda. *J Infect Dis* 1997, 175:947–950.

28. Whitby D, Howard MR, Tenant-Flowers M, *et al.:* Detection of Kaposi's sarcoma associated herpes virus in peripheral blood of HIV-infected individuals and progression to Kaposi's sarcoma. *Lancet* 1995, 346:799–802.

29. Martin JN, Ganem DE, Osmond DH, *et al.:* Sexual transmission and the natural history of human herpesvirus 8 infection. *N Engl J Med* 1998, 338:948–954.

30. Ensoli B, Gendelman R, Markham P, *et al.:* Synergy between basic fibroblast growth factor and HIV-1 tat protein in induction of Kaposi's sarcoma. *Nature* 1994, 371:674–680.

31. Ensoli B, Markham P, Kao V, *et al.:* Block of AIDS-Kaposi's sarcoma (KS) cell growth, angiogenesis, and lesion formation in nude mice by antisense oligonucleotide targeting basic fibroblast growth factor: a novel strategy for the therapy of KS. *J Clin Invest* 1994, 94:1736–1746.

32. Dezube BJ: The role of human immunodeficiency virus-1 in the pathogenesis of acquired immunodeficiency syndrome-related Kaposi's sarcoma: the importance of an inflammatory and angiogenic milieu. *Semin Oncol* 2000, 27:420–423.

33. Miles SA: Pathogenesis of AIDS-related Kaposi's sarcoma: evidence of a viral etiology. *Hematol Oncol Clin North Am* 1996, 10:1011–1021.

34. Lunardi-Iskandar Y, Gill PS, Lam VH, *et al.:* Isolation and characterization of an immortal neoplastic cell line (KS Y-1) from AIDS-associated Kaposi's sarcoma. *J Natl Cancer Inst* 1995, 87:974–981.

35. Neipel F, Albrecht J-C, Fleckenstein B: Cell-homologous genes in the Kaposi's sarcoma-associated rhadinovirus human herpesvirus-8: determinants of its pathogenicity. *J Virol* 1997, 71:4187–4192.

36. Russo JJ, Bohenzky RA, Chen MC, *et al.:* Nucleotide sequence of the Kaposi's sarcoma-associated herpesvirus (HHV-8). *Proc Natl Acad Sci U S A* 1996, 93:14862–14867.

37. Rabkin CS, Janz S, Lash A, *et al.:* Monoclonal origin of multicentric Kaposi's sarcoma lesions. *N Engl J Med* 1997, 336:988–993.

38. Jean-Gabriel J, Lacoste V, Briere J, *et al.:* Monoclonality and oligoclonality of human herpesvirus 8 terminal repeat sequences in Kaposi's sarcoma and other diseases. *J Natl Cancer Inst* 2000, 92:729–736.

39. Pluda JM, Shay LE, Foli A, et al.: Administration of pentosan polysulfate to patients with human immunodeficiency virus-associated Kaposi's sarcoma. *AIDS* 1999, 13(suppl A):S215–S225.

40. Schawartzmann G, Sprinz E, Kalakun L, et al.: Phase II study of pentosanpolysulfate (PPS) in patients with human immunodeficiency virus-associated Kaposi's sarcoma. *Tumori* 1996, 82:360–3636.

41. Eckhardt SG, Burris HA, Eckhardt JR, et al.: A phase I clinical and pharmacokinetic study of the angiogenesis inhibitor, tecogalan sodium. *Ann Oncol* 1996, 7:491–496.

42. Tulpule A, Snyder JC, Espina BM, et al.: A phase I study of tecogalan, a novel angiogenesis inhibitor in the treatment of AIDS-related Kaposi's sarcoma and solid tumors. *Blood* 1994, 84(suppl 1):248a.

43. Dezube BJ, VonRoenn JH, Holden-Wiltse J, et al.: Fumagilin analog in the treatment of Kaposi's sarcoma: a phase I AIDS Clinical Trials Group Study. *J Clin Oncol* 1997, 16:584–589.

44. Tulpule A, Scadden DT, Espina BM, et al.: Results of a randomized study of IM862 nasal solution in the treatment of AIDS-related Kaposi's sarcoma. *J Clin Oncol* 2000, 18:716–723.

45. Miles S, Arasteh K, Gill P, et al.: A multicenter dose-escalating study of SU5416 in AIDS-related Kaposi's sarcoma. *Proc Am Soc Clin Oncol* 2000, 19:176a.

46. Pluda JM, Wyvill K, Little R, et al.: A pilot/dose finding study of interleukin 12 (IL-12) administered to patients (pts) with AIDS-associated Kaposi's sarcoma (KS). *Proc Am Soc Clin Oncol* 1999, 18:547a.

47. Little RF, Wyvill KM, Pluda JM, et al.: Activity of thalidomide in AIDS-related Kaposi's sarcoma. *J Clin Oncol* 2000, 18:2593–2602.

48. Krown SE, Testa MA, Huang J, et al.: AIDS-related Kaposi's sarcoma: prospective validation of the AIDS Clinical Trials Group staging classification. *J Clin Oncol* 1997, 15:3085–3092.

49. Swift PS: The role of radiation therapy in the management of HIV-related Kaposi's sarcoma. *Hematol Oncol Clin North Am* 1996, 10:1069–1080.

50. Lee F-C, Mitsuyasu RT: Chemotherapy of AIDS-related Kaposi's sarcoma. *Hematol Oncol Clin North Am* 1996, 10:1051–1068.

51. Remick SC, Reddy M, Herman D, et al.: Continuous infusion bleomycin in AIDS-related Kaposi's sarcoma. *J Clin Oncol* 1994, 12:1130–1136.

52. Northfelt DW, Dezube B, Miller B, et al.: Randomized comparative trial of Doxil vs Adriamycin, bleomycin, and vincristine (ABV) in the treatment of severe AIDS-related Kaposi's sarcoma (AIDS-KS). *Blood* 1995, 86:382A.

53. Northfelt DW, Dezube BJ, Thommes JA, et al.: Efficacy of pegylated-liposomal doxorubicin in the treatment of AIDS-related Kaposi's sarcoma after failure of standard chemotherapy. *J Clin Oncol* 1996, 15:653–659.

54. Gill PS, Wernz J, Scadden D, et al.: Randomized phase III trial of liposomal daunorubicin versus doxorubicin, bleomycin, and vincristine in AIDS-related Kaposi's sarcoma. *J Clin Oncol* 1996, 14:2353–2364.

55. Saville MW, Lietzau J, Pluda JM, et al.: Treatment of HIV-associated Kaposi's sarcoma with paclitaxel. *Lancet* 1995, 346:26–28.

56. Gill PS, Tulpule A, Reynolds T, et al.: Paclitaxel (Taxol) in the treatment of relapsed or refractory advanced AIDS-related Kaposi's sarcoma. *Proc Am Soc Clin Oncol* 1996, 15:306.

57. Karp JE, Pluda JM, Yarchoan R: AIDS-related Kaposi's sarcoma: a template for the translation of molecular pathogenesis into targeted therapeutic approaches. *Hematol Oncol Clin North Am* 1996, 10:1031–1049.

58. Routy J-P, Urbanek A, MacLeod J, et al.: Significant regression of Kaposi's sarcoma following initiation of an effective antiretroviral combination treatment. *J Acquir Immune Defic Syndr* 1997, 14:22a.

59. Mocroft A, Youle M, Gazzard B, et al.: Anti-herpesvirus treatment and risk of Kaposi's sarcoma in HIV infection. *AIDS* 1996, 10:1101–1105.

60. Gill PS, Lunardi-Iskandar Y, Louie S, et al.: The effects of preparations of human chorionic gonadotropin on AIDS-related Kaposi's sarcoma. *N Engl J Med* 1996, 335:1261–1269.

61. Remick SC: Acquired immunodeficiency syndrome-related non-Hodgkin's lymphoma. *Cancer Control* 1995, 2:97–103.

62. Levine AM, Bernstein L, Sullivan-Halley J, et al.: Role of zidovudine antiretroviral therapy in the pathogenesis of acquired immunodeficiency syndrome-related lymphoma. *Blood* 1995, 86:4612–4616.

63. Pluda JM, Venzon DJ, Tosaro G, et al.: Parameters affecting the development of non-Hodgkin's lymphoma in patients with severe human immunodeficiency virus infection receiving antiretroviral therapy. *J Clin Oncol* 1995, 11:1099–1107.

64. Klein C, Miccikren G, Dolan J, et al.: Impact of highly active antiretroviral therapy (HAART) on HIV-associated primary central nervous system lymphoma (PCNSL). *J Acquir Immune Defic Syndr* 2000, 23:A26.

65. Tirelli U, Spina M, Gaidano G, et al.: Epidemiological, biological and clinical features of HIV-related lymphomas in the era of highly active antiretroviral therapy. *AIDS* 2000, 4:1675–1688.

66. Ballerini P, Gaidano G, Gong J, et al.: Molecular pathogenesis of HIV-associated lymphomas. *AIDS Res Hum Retroviruses* 1992, 8:731–735.

67. Herndier BG, Kaplan LD, McGrath MS: Pathogenesis of AIDS lymphoma. *AIDS* 1994, 8:1025–1049.

68. Gaidano G, LoCoco F, Ye BH, et al.: Rearrangements of the *bcl-6* gene in AIDS-associated non-Hodgkin's lymphoma: association with diffuse large-cell subtype. *Blood* 1994, 84:397–402.

69. Mack KD, Wei R, Herndier B, et al.: HIV insertional cis-activation of the proto-oncogene *c-fes* in AIDS associated lymphomagenesis. *J Acquir Immune Defic Syndr* 1997, 14:A44.

70. Nador RG, Cesarman E, Chadburn A, et al.: Primary effusion lymphoma: a distinct clinicopathological entity associated with the Kaposi's sarcoma associated virus. *Blood* 1996, 88:646–656.

71. Levine AM. Acquired immunodeficiency syndrome-related lymphoma. *Blood* 1992, 80:8–20.

72. Levine AM. Acquired immunodeficiency syndrome-related lymphomas: clinical aspects. *Semin Oncol* 2000, 27:442–453.

73. Kaplan LD, Straus DJ, Testa M, et al.: Low-dose compared with standard-dose m-BACOD chemotherapy for non-Hodgkin's lymphoma associated with human immunodeficiency virus infection. *N Engl J Med* 1997, 336:1641–1648.

74. Straus DJ, Huang J, Testa MA, et al.: Prognostic factors in the treatment of human immunodeficiency virus-associated non-Hodgkin's lymphoma: analysis of ACTG 142 (low-dose vs. standard-dose m-BACOD plus granulocyte-macrophage colony-stimulating factor). *J Clin Oncol* 1998, 16:3601–3606.

75. Sparano JA, Wiernik PH, Strack M, et al.: Infusional cyclophosphamide, doxorubicin, and etoposide in HIV- and HTLV-1 related non-Hodgkin's lymphoma: a highly active regimen. *Leuk Lymphoma* 1994, 14:263–271.

76. Sparano JA, Wiernik PH, Hu X, et al.: Pilot trial of infusional cyclophosphamide, doxorubicin, and etoposide plus didanosine and filgrastim in patients with human immunodeficiency virus-associated non-Hodgkin's lymphoma. *J Clin Oncol* 1996, 14:3026–3035.

77. Sparano JA, Wiernik PH, Strack M, et al.: Infusional cyclophosphamide, doxorubicin, and etoposide in human immunodeficiency virus type 1-related non-Hodgkin's lymphoma: a highly active regimen. *Blood* 1993, 81:2810–2815.

78. Sparano JA, Lee S, Chen M, et al.: Phase II trial of infusional cyclophosphamide, doxorubicin, and etoposide (CDE) in HIV-associated non-Hodgkin's lymphoma: an Eastern Cooperative Oncology Group Trial (E1494). *Proc Am Soc Clin Oncol* 1999, 18:12a.

79. Sparano JA, Lee S, Chen M, *et al.:* Phase II trial of infusional cyclophosphamide, doxorubicin, and etoposide (CDE) in HIV-associated non-Hodgkin's lymphoma (NHL): an Eastern Cooperative Oncology Group Trial (E1494). *JAIDS J Acquir Immune Defic Syndr* 1999, 21:A39.

80. Remick SC, McSharry JS, Wolf BC, *et al.:* Novel oral combination chemotherapy in the treatment of intermediate-grade and high-grade AIDS-related non-Hodgkin's lymphoma. *J Clin Oncol* 1993, 11:1691–1702.

81. Remick SC, Sedransk N, Haase RF, *et al.:* Oral combination chemotherapy in conjunction with filgrastim (G-CSF) in the treatment of AIDS-related non-Hodgkin's lymphoma: evaluation of the role of G-CSF; quality of life analysis; and long-term follow-up. *Am J Hematol* 2001 (in press).

82. Ratner L, Redden D, Hamzeh A, *et al.:* Chemotherapy for HIV-associated non-Hodgkin lymphoma (HIV-NHL) in combination with highly active antiretroviral therapy (HAART) is not associated with excessive toxicity. *JAIDS J Acquir Immune Defic Syndr* 1999, 21:A32.

83. Little RF, Pearson D, Franchini G, *et al.:* Dose-adjusted EPOCH chemotherapy (CT) in previously untreated HIV-associated non-Hodgkin's lymphoma (HIV-NHL): preliminary report of efficacy, immune reconstitution, and HIV control following therapy. *J Acquir Immune Defic Syndr* 1999, 21:A33.

84. Little R, Franchini G, Pearson D, *et al.:* HIV viral burden (VB) during EPOCH chemotherapy (CT) for HIV-related lymphomas. *J Acquir Immune Defic Syndr* 1997, 14:A42.

85. Sparano JA, Lee S, Henry DH, *et al.:* U. Infusional cyclophosphamide, doxorubicin, etoposide in HIV-associated Non-Hodgkin's lymphoma: a review of the Einstein, Aviano, and ECOG experience in 182 patients. *J Acquir Immune Defic Syndr* 2000, 23:A11.

86. Little RF, Pearson D, Gutierrez M, *et al.:* Dose-adjusted EPOCH chemotherapy (CT) with suspension of antiretroviral therapy (ART) for HIV-associated Non-Hodgkin's lymphoma (HIV-NHL). *JAIDS J Acquir Immune Defic Syndr* 2000, 23:A11.

87. Levine AM, Tulpule A, Tessman D, *et al.:* Mitoguazone therapy in patients with refractory or relapsed AIDS-related lymphoma: results from a multicenter phase II trial. *J Clin Oncol* 1997, 15:1094–1103.

88. Fine HA, Mayer RV: Primary central nervous system lymphoma. *Ann Intern Med* 1993, 119:1093–1104.

89. Ruiz A, Post MJ, Bundschu C, *et al.:* Primary central nervous system lymphoma in patients with AIDS. *Neuroimaging Clin North Am* 1997, 7:281–296.

90. Cinque P, Brytting M, Vago L, *et al.:* Epstein-Barr virus DNA in cerebrospinal fluid from patients with AIDS-related primary CNS lymphoma of the central nervous system. *Lancet* 1993, 42:398–401.

91. Cingolani A, De Luca A, Larocca LM, *et al.:* Minimally invasive diagnosis of acquired immunodeficiency syndrome-related primary central nervous system lymphoma. *J Natl Cancer Inst* 1998, 90:364–369.

92. Patel P, Raez LE. Primary central nervous system lymphomas in patients with acquired immunodeficiency syndrome (AIDS). *J Acquir Immune Defic Syndr* 1997, 14:A40.

93. Lorberboym M, Estok L, Machac J, *et al.:* Rapid differential diagnosis of cerebral toxoplasmosis and primary central nervous system lymphoma by thallium-201 SPECT. *J Nucl Med* 1996, 37:1150–1154.

94. Baumgartner JE, Rachlin JR, Beckstead JH, *et al.:* Primary central nervous system lymphoma: natural history and response to radiation therapy in 55 patients with acquired immunodeficiency syndrome. *J Neurosurg* 2000, 73:206–211.

95. Levine AM: HIV-associated Hodgkin's disease: biologic and clinical aspects. *Hematol Oncol Clin North Am* 1996, 10:1135–1148.

96. Spina M, Vaccher E, Nasti G, *et al.:* Human immunodeficiency virus-associated Hodgkin's disease. *Semin Oncol* 2000, 27:480–488.

97. Bernardi D, Salvioni R, Vaccher E, *et al.:* Testicular germ cell tumors and human immunodeficiency virus infection: a report of 26 cases. *J Clin Oncol* 1995, 13:2705–2711.

98. Li CJ, Zhang LJ, Dezube BJ, *et al.:* Three inhibitors of type 1 human immunodeficiency virus long terminal repeat-directed gene expression and virus replication. *Proc Natl Acad Sci U S A* 1993, 90:1839–1842.

99. Klevins PM, Fleming PL, Mays MA, *et al.:* Characteristics of women with AIDS and invasive cervical cancer. *Obstet Gynecol* 1996, 88:269–273,.

100. Chadha M, Rosenblatt EA, Malamud S, *et al.:* Squamous-cell carcinoma of the anus in HIV-positive patients. *Dis Colon Rectum* 1994, 37:861–865.

ABV THERAPY FOR KAPOSI'S SARCOMA
Single-Agent and Combination Doxorubicin, Bleomycin, and Vincristine

Single-agent chemotherapy in the management of AIDS-related Kaposi's sarcoma (AIDS-KS) is clearly easier to administer and less toxic than combination chemotherapy. In the absence of a requirement for immediate cytoreduction, single-agent chemotherapy is an attractive initial therapeutic intervention for many patients. Early studies of vinca alkaloids, bleomycin, podophyllotoxins, and anthracyclines established the activity of these agents in classical KS disease. It is important to mention that early studies of AIDS-KS used traditional solid-tumor and often disease-specific response criteria to varying degrees, which makes it difficult to analyze and compare clinical trial data. Clinical trial reporting will be streamlined with the adoption of the AIDS Clinical Trials Group (ACTG) clinical staging and response criteria across current generation and future studies.

Vinblastine, which has very high response rates in classical KS (90%), has a response rate of 30%–50% in AIDS-KS when administered at a dose of 4–8 mg/wk. Vincristine at a dose of 2 mg/wk as a single agent has been reported to have a response rate of 20%–60%. Doxorubicin (Adriamycin) alone in low weekly to biweekly doses (10–20 mg/m^2) has been associated with response rates of 10%–50%. Single-agent bleomycin administered on various dose schedules, including 72-h continuous infusion (20 mg/m^2/d), yielded response rates ranging between 40%–70%. Paclitaxel has substantial activity in AIDS-KS. At doses up to 100–175 mg/m^2 IV 3-h infusion every 2–3 wk, paclitaxel induces partial and complete responses in more than 50% of previously treated patients. Its effect appears to be qualitatively different from those of other agents, with a rapid, substantial reduction in tumor-associated edema. Moderate neutropenia requiring granulocyte–macrophage colony-stimulating factor (GM-CSF) is common. The various single and combination chemotherapy regimens that have been reported have response rates ranging between 30%–84%. Randomized controlled studies stratified by tumor stage have not been conducted with any of these regimens to date, and impact on survival has not been clearly demonstrated. There is, however, clear documentation of effective palliation with systemic cytotoxic chemotherapy and likely improved survival in many settings.

It is important to briefly touch on the supportive care issues in managing patients with AIDS-KS. These therapeutic principles are apropos for all HIV-infected patients with neoplastic complications of their disease. For a variety of AIDS-related neoplasms, clinical trials are addressing the issue of concurrent antiretroviral therapy with cytotoxic chemotherapy regimens. Published reports from the ACTG trial 075 defined 10 mg/m^2 of doxorubicin as the maximum tolerated dose (MTD) when used in combination with zidovudine (600 mg/d), vincristine (2 mg), and bleomycin (10 U/m^2) every other week. Hematologic and immunologic toxicity were the primary side effects. A later study adding GM-CSF to this regimen (ACTG 094) showed an overall better response rate, but it was the same MTD for doxorubicin. The ACTG 163 study administered ABV as follows: 20 mg/m^2 doxorubicin, 10 mm^2 bleomycin, 1 mg vincristine IV every 2 wk with dideoxyinosine (200 mg twice daily if $\geq$ 60 kg or 125 mg twice daily if < 60 kg) or with dideoxycytidine (0.75 mg three times daily if $\geq$ 50 kg or 0.375 mg three times daily if < 50 kg) with comparable and acceptable toxicity and response rates of 58% and 60%, respectively.

In the protease-inhibitor era, it is clearly preferable to maximize antiretroviral therapy prior to embarking on systemic cytotoxic chemotherapy because significant objective tumor regression may be encountered. It may be important to continue effective antiretroviral therapy with maximal viral suppression in conjunction with chemotherapy until further clinical studies address this issue. Because many patients are likely to have very complicated medical regimens, it is imperative to closely monitor for potential drug interactions and be alert for myelosuppression, immunologic side effects with emergence of opportunistic infectious complications, and other side effects commonly seen with cytotoxic chemotherapy. As a result, all patients should receive *Pneumocystics carinii* pneumonia prophylaxis when receiving cytotoxic chemotherapy irrespective of CD4 lymphocyte count. Other prophylactic strategies and interventions need to be made on an individual patient basis. In many instances of myelosuppression, it may be prudent to administer cytokine CSFs (*eg*, G-CSF, GM-CSF [generally given in conjunction with antiretroviral therapy to offset HIV upregulation], and erythropoietin). Thrombopoietin and other platelet factors are currently under investigation.

RECENT EXPERIENCES AND RESPONSE RATES

Study	Regimen	Evaluable Patients, *n*	Response Rate	Median Duration of Response, *mo*
Gill *et al.* (ACTG 075). *AIDS* 1994, 8:1695.	ABV + ZDV	24	71%	Not specified
Mitsuyasu *et al.* (ACTG 163). *Proc ASCO* 1995, 14:289.	ABV (ddI/ddC)	81	58% (ddI) 60% (ddC)	20 wk (ddI) 19 wk (ddC)
Saville *et al. Lancet* 1995, 346:26.	Paclitaxel	20	65%	34 wk
Gill *et al. Proc ASCO* 1996, 15:306.	Paclitaxel	30	53%	Not specified

ABV—doxorubicin, bleomycin, and vincristine; ddC—dideoxycytodine; ddI—dideoxyinosine; ZDV—zidovudine.

ABV THERAPY FOR KAPOSI'S SARCOMA (Continued)

DOSAGE AND SCHEDULING

Chemotherapy	Dose	Interval
Single agents		
Doxorubicin	10–15 mg/m2 IV	Every wk
	20.0 mg/m^2 IV	Every 2 wk
Bleomycin	20.0 mg/m^2/d as 72-h continuous infusion	Every 3 wk
Vincristine	1.4 mg/m^2 IV (maximum 2.0 mg)	Every 2 wk
	1.0 mg IV	Every wk
Paclitaxel	100.0 mg/m^2 IV (3 h)	Every 2 wk
	135.0 mg/m^2 IV (3 h)	Every 3 wk
ABV regimen		
Doxorubicin	10.0–20.0 mg/m^2 IV, d 1	Every 2 wk
Bleomycin	10.0 mg/m^2 IV, d 1	
Vincristine	1.0–2.0 mg IV, d 1	
BV regimen		
Bleomycin	10.0 mg/m^2 IV, d 1	Every 2 wk
Vincristine	2.0 mg (total) IV, d 1	

CANDIDATES FOR TREATMENT

Management of patients with AIDS-KS should take into consideration not only prospects for symptomatic palliation and tumor regression but also the potential for myelotoxicity and immunosuppressive side effects of the therapeutic regimen; for patients with symptomatic disease or life-threatening organ involvement, prompt and effective cytoreductive treatment is required; patients with moderate disease (> 25 cutaneous lesions and no tumor edema or pulmonary involvement) can be treated with single agents; patients may also have fewer lesions but in cosmetically strategic locations, for which systemic therapy may also be appropriate; vinblastine, vincristine, doxorubicin, or bleomycin are appropriate in these situations; recent published data on liposomal anthracycline formulations (see Liposomal Anthracyclines section) for AIDS-KS suggest these agents may be suitable first-line alternatives; patients with rapidly progressing disease and/or significant visceral disease, especially symptomatic pulmonary involvement, should be treated with higher doses of liposomal anthracyclines or preferably the ABV combination regimen; paclitaxel is currently approved as second-line therapy

SPECIAL PRECAUTIONS AND NURSING INTERVENTIONS

Anthracyclines (including the liposomal formulations): patients with underlying cardiac disease (eg, HIV-related cardiomyopathy); **Bleomycin** chronic lung disease; **Vinca alkaloids and paclitaxel:** HIV-related peripheral neuropathy and constipation; in many of these circumstances it may be appropriate to avoid the offending cytotoxic agent altogether or closely monitor the functional status of the patient (eg, left ventricular ejection fraction by radionuclide scanning, diffusion capacity for carbon monoxide, and careful neurologic examination)

TOXICITIES

HIV-infected patients may be more susceptible and/or have more pronounced mucosal toxicity; for the majority of patients, the ABV regimen is not particularly troublesome in terms of nausea and vomiting; an occasional patient may require aggressive antiemetic support; myelosuppression remains the most important side effect for any cytotoxic agent and is generally more severe with combination regimens; bone marrow function and reserve is certainly compromised for the majority of HIV-infected patients with late-stage disease secondary to underlying disease, opportunistic infection, and myelotoxic antiretroviral therapy; complete blood counts (including platelets) need to be monitored and neutropenia, in particular, closely followed; it is advisable to have a low threshold to add G-CSF (usually 5 µg/kg administered subcutaneously) to the cytotoxic regimen between periods of chemotherapy administration and to maintain appropriate neutrophil counts, ideally > 1500/µL). Alternatively, GM-CSF (usually in conjunction with concurrent antiretroviral therapy) and erythropoietin can also be administered. Myelosuppression, neuropathy, and alopecia are all problematic with paclitaxel; myalgias are also commonly encountered; the optimal dose and schedule of this agent are to be determined; lower doses of this agent may lessen the toxicity and improve therapeutic index

PATIENT INFORMATION

General instructions for all HIV-infected patients receiving chemotherapy for AIDS-KS and other related neoplasms include the following: patients should at all times maintain adequate fluid intake and maximize good nutrition as feasible; patients should maintain excellent oral hygiene throughout therapy; it is appropriate to aggressively screen patients prior to embarking on systemic cytotoxic therapy for poor oral hygiene, dentition, and periodontal disease; patients need to be alerted for the prospects of mucosal and gastrointestinal side effects from the various regimens; blood counts need to be monitored closely and patients instructed to report and monitor signs and symptoms suggestive of infection (eg, fever, chills, cough, dyspnea, and sore throat); patients also need to be alerted for potential exacerbation of symptoms secondary to peripheral neuropathy while receiving vinca alkaloids and constipation, especially if receiving concurrent analgesic drugs; most regimens will likely lead to alopecia, and it is important to educate patients about this; myalgias may also be troublesome for patients receiving paclitaxel; finally, because many patients are bound to be taking multiple medications, there are no clear contraindications or specific drug-interactions that preclude the coadminstration of the various antineoplastic agents and the currently available antiretroviral agents inclusive of the protease inhibitors; pharmacokinetic studies are underway to help identify some of these issues

LIPOSOMAL ANTHRACYCLINES

Liposomal formulations (microscopic phospholipid spheres) of some anthracyclines [doxorubicin (Doxil; Sequus Pharmaceuticals, Menlo Park, CA) and daunorubicin (DaunoXome; Nexstar, San Dimas, CA)] have been shown in animal models and early clinical trials in human patients to improve the therapeutic index when compared with the native anthracycline preparation, with less toxicity and comparable and/or improved efficacy in patients with AIDS-KS. Pharmacokinetic advantages of these formulations include a several-fold increase in plasma half-life with resultant prolonged circulation time, reduced clearance, a small volume of distribution, and markedly increased area under the curve. A putative advantage of the pegylated liposomal formulation (*eg*, liposomal doxorubicin) over the simple liposomal formulations is that the pegylated liposome reduces liposome opsonization and inhibits uptake by the reticuloendothelial system. The clinical significance of this remains to be sorted out, and to date, there are no comparative data of the two newly approved liposomal formulations of doxorubicin and daunorubicin. It is advisable for the clinician to become familiar and knowledgeable with one of the two agents. It is noteworthy in the trial data outlined below that both liposomal formulations were compared with an ABV (doxorubicin, bleomycin, and vincristine) combination regimen; however, for liposomal daunorubicin, the ABV regimen was dose-modified when compared with the traditional regimen.

Liposomal doxorubicin was investigated in an early phase II setting in patients with advanced KS. All 34 patients had poor prognostic disease as judged by AIDS Clinical Trials Group criteria. Patients were treated with 20 mg/m^2 of liposomal doxorubicin IV every 3 wk on an outpatient basis. Nineteen of 34 patients had received prior chemotherapy for KS, although no patient had received prior anthracyclines. An overall response rate of 73.5 % was observed with a complete response rate of 5.8%. In patients who had received previous chemotherapy, the response rate was 68.4%. Median duration of response was 9 wk. The major toxicity was neutropenia. Liposomal doxorubicin has also been investigated in patients with advanced KS who have failed standard chemotherapy. While receiving standard ABV or BV (bleomycin and vincristine) chemotherapy, fifty-three patients who experienced disease progression or intolerable toxicity received liposomal doxorubicin at a dose of 20 mg/m^2 IV every 3 wk. Nineteen patients (36%) had a partial response and one patient had a clinical complete response. The most common adverse effect was leukopenia, which occurred in 40% of patients.

Preliminary results of the largest randomized phase III clinical trial of liposomal doxorubicin versus ABV in 258 AIDS-KS patients have been reported [36]. In this study, the liposomal doxorubicin yielded a superior response rate of 43.0% versus 24.5% (*a much lower response rate than previously reported for the ABV regimen*). The toxicity profile also favored the liposomal formulation with 1) less alopecia, nausea/vomiting, and peripheral neuropathy; 2) comparable leukopenia; and 3) more stomatitis/mucositis. Liposomal daunorubicin has also been investigated in a prospective randomized phase III trial. In this study, 232 patients were randomized to receive liposomal daunorubicin (40 mg/m^2) or an ABV regimen (10 mg/m^2, 15 mg, and 1 mg, respectively, which is reduced vs standard ABV) both given IV every 2 wk. The overall response rate for liposomal daunorubicin was 25%, similar to the 28% in the ABV group. There was significantly less alopecia and peripheral neuropathy but significantly more grade 4 neutropenia in patients treated on the liposomal daunorubicin arm.

RECENT EXPERIENCES AND RESPONSE RATES

Study	Drug	Evaluable Patients, *n*	Dosage Schedule	Complete and Partial Response Rate, %
Harrison *et al. J Clin Oncol* 1995, 13:914.	Liposomal doxorubicin	34	20 mg/m^2 every 3 wk	73.5
Gill *et al. J Clin Oncol* 1996, 14:2353.	Liposomal daunorubicin	116	40 mg/m^2 every 2 wk	25.0
Northfelt *et al. J Clin Oncol* 1996, 15:653.	Liposomal doxorubicin	53	20 mg/m^2 every 3 wk	38.0

DOSAGE AND SCHEDULING

Chemotherapy	Dose	Interval
Liposomal doxorubicin	20 mg/m^2 IV (30 min)	Every 2–3 wk
Liposomal daunorubicin	40 mg/m^2 IV (1 h)	Every 2 wk

LIPOSOMAL ANTHRACYCLINES (Continued)

CANDIDATES FOR TREATMENT

Patients with rapidly progressive disease, extensive disease with edema, or pulmonary involvement, should be treated aggressively; liposomal anthracyclines may be used in this setting; clinicians should be alert to opportunistic infections; all patients should receive prophylaxis for *P. carinii* pneumonia

ALTERNATIVE THERAPIES

ABV combination chemotherapy regimen

SPECIAL PRECAUTIONS AND NURSING INTERVENTIONS

Experience with liposomal anthracyclines is limited in patients with cardiac disease or risk factors; until further experience is recorded with these agents, the recommended total cumulative dose of liposomal doxorubicin is identical to that reported for doxorubicin; liposomal daunorubicin is perhaps less cardiotoxic; the drug with appropriate monitoring of left ventricular function (at 320 mg/m^2, 480 mg/m^2, and then 240 mg/m^2 increments thereafter) can be escalated. The pharmacokinetics of the liposomal anthracyclines have not been studied in patients with hepatic impairment and renal insufficiency, and dose modifications are recommended in these settings; both agents are not as likely as either native drug to cause severe extravasation; caution is advised, however, in both the administration and monitoring of infusion to avoid extravasation

TOXICITIES

In summary, liposomal formulations, when compared with ABV regimens, appear to be characterized by 1) significantly less alopecia, neurotoxicity, and gastrointestinal toxicity; 2) more stomatitis/mucositis; and 3) comparable myelosuppression, especially neutropenia; principal clinical toxicities include myelosuppression (60% risk of leukopenia) and an approximate 10% chance of thrombocytopenia and cardiotoxicity; infusion reactions occurring with the first cycle of therapy are not uncommon with liposomal doxorubicin (6.8% incidence); these are characterized by flushing, shortness of breath, facial swelling, headache, chest tightness, and back pain; the reactions generally do not recur with later cycles; palmar-plantar erythrodysesthesia occurs in 3.4% of patients receiving liposomal doxorubicin and is characterized by swelling, pain, erythema, and (in some circumstances) desquamation of the skin of the hands and feet; the incidence may be increased with higher dosage or more frequent administration; similarly, a triad of back pain, flushing, and chest tightness has been reported in 13.8% of patients receiving liposomal daunorubicin; this usually occurs during the first 5 minutes of the infusion and subsides with interruption of the infusion; in both situations, reduction of the infusion rate may be helpful, and these reactions do not preclude further therapy

DRUG INTERACTIONS

No formal drug-interaction studies have been conducted with liposomal anthracyclines; until specific compatibility data are available, it is not recommended that liposomal anthracyclines be mixed with other drugs; liposomal anthracyclines may interact with drugs known to interact with the conventional formulation of doxorubicin or daunorubicin

PATIENT INFORMATION

The liposomal anthracycline formulations compared with ABV regimens in controlled clinical trials cause significantly less alopecia; this is likely an important consideration for many patients.

DOSE-MODIFIED M-BACOD THERAPY FOR NHL
Methotrexate, Bleomycin, Doxorubicin, Cyclophosphamide, Vincristine, and Dexamethazone

In an attempt to ascertain if "less is better," the AIDS Clinical Trials Group (ACTG) recently completed the largest randomized trial in AIDS-related non-Hodgkin's lymphoma, comparing a standard dose of m-BACOD and a low dose (less cyclophosphamide, doxorubicin, and dexamethasone) of the same regimen. Patients treated with low-dose m-BACOD had significantly fewer hematologic toxic effects and spent fewer days in the hospital than patients treated with conventional doses of m-BACOD. These results justify the treatment of most patients who have AIDS-related lymphoma with reduced doses of cytotoxic chemotherapy. This study also demonstrated that CD4 lymphocyte count is a more important predictor of survival than dose intensity of chemotherapy. Febrile neutropenia was an infrequent complication in this trial, perhaps because granulocyte–macrophage colony-stimulating factor (GM-CSF), which was administered concurrently, shortened the duration of severe neutropenia. Opportunistic infections occurred in 20% of patients. Intrathecal cytosine arabinoside (ara-C) was used to prevent CNS relapse and resulted in a CNS relapse rate of 3.4%. The ACTG also explored the use of GM-CSF with escalating doses of m-BACOD, noting that full dose m-BACOD could be given safely without clinical progression of HIV disease.

RECENT EXPERIENCES AND RESPONSE RATES

Study	Regimen	Evaluable Patients, n	CR, %	Median Survival, mo
Levine et al. JAMA 1991, 266:84	Low-dose m-BACOD	35	46	6.50
Kaplan et al. N Engl J Med 1997, 336:1641.	Low-dose m-BACOD + GM-CSF	94	41	8.75
	Standard-dose m-BACOD + GM-CSF	81	52	7.75

CR—complete response rate; GM-CSF—granulocyte–macrophage colony-stimulating factor.

DOSAGE AND SCHEDULING

Chemotherapy*	Dose
Methotrexate	200 mg/m^2 IV d 15
Bleomycin	4 U/m^2 IV d 1
Doxorubicin	25 mg/m^2 IV d 1 (45 mg/m^2 standard dose)
Cyclophosphamide	300 mg/m^2 IV d 1 (600 mg/m^2 standard dose)
Vincristine	1.4 mg/m^2 IV d 1 (maximum 2 mg)
Dexamethasone	3 mg/m^2 PO d 1–5 (6 mg/m^2 standard dose)
GM-CSF	5 mug/kg SC d 4–13 as needed
CNS prophylaxis (ara-C)	50 mg IT d 1,8,15,22

* Cycle length every 21 d (minimum of 4 cycles; 2 after complete response).
Ara-C—cytarabine; CNS—central nervous system; GM-CSF—granulocyte–macrophage colony-stimulating factor; IT—intrathecally.

CANDIDATES FOR TREATMENT

The optimal therapy for AIDS-lymphoma remains to be defined; therapy must be tailored to the individual patient; for the majority of patients, a dose-modified approach may be appropriate, and the greatest experience has been reported for low-dose m-BACOD; individuals with favorable prognostic factors (none or one of the following: age > 35 y, history of injecting drug use, stage III/IV disease, and CD4 lymphocyte count < 100/µL) may be candidates for full-dose/standard chemotherapy in the hope of improving the complete response rate and prospect for long-term survival; a stratified therapeutic approach based on risk factors has yet to be applied in the management of AIDS-related lymphoma; furthermore, there are no data on the substitution of liposomal formulations in anthracycline-based combination chemotherapy regimens; finally, the role of routine central nervous system prophylaxis has not been definitively addressed in well-controlled clinical trials and may not be warranted in all patients (*see* text for details); in any event, most patients with AIDS-lymphoma should be offered a trial of chemotherapy; although not curative of the lymphoma in most individuals, chemotherapy may result in significant palliation of symptoms and improve quality of life; if there is no response after 2 cycles of therapy or if there is a decline in performance status, discontinuation of chemotherapy is appropriate

ALTERNATIVE THERAPIES

Infusional CDE (cyclophosphamide, doxorubicin, and etoposide), oral combination chemotherapy, EPOCH, or CHOP (cyclophosphamide, doxorubicin, vincristine, and prednisone); a suggested dose-modified CHOP regimen is as follows—**Cyclophosphamide:** 375 mg/m^2 IV d 1; **Doxorubicin:** 25 mg/m^2 IV d 1; **Vincristine:** 1.4 mg/m^2 (maximum 2.0 mg) IV d 1; **Prednisone:** 100 mg PO d 1–5 (cycle length every 21 d)

SPECIAL PRECAUTIONS AND NURSING INTERVENTIONS

Special precautions are needed for patients with underlying cardiac disease (*eg*, HIV-related cardiomyopathy) for the anthracyclines, chronic lung disease for bleomycin, and HIV-related peripheral neuropathy and constipation for the vinca alkaloids; in many of these circumstances, it may be appropriate to avoid the offending cytotoxic agent altogether or to closely monitor the functional status of the patient (*eg*, left ventricular ejection fraction by radionuclide scanning, diffusion capacity for carbon monoxide, and careful neurologic examination); given the immunosuppressive effects of chemotherapy regimens for lymphoma, the majority of which include corticosteroids, all patients should receive *P. carinii* pneumonia prophylaxis regardless of CD4 lymphocyte count

TOXICITIES

Fifty-one percent of the patients receiving dose-modified m-BACOD will experience grade 3 or higher toxic effects; 50% will develop grade 4 neutropenia; episodes of febrile neutropenia will complicate approximately 6% of the cycles administered; 11% will develop grade 3 or higher thrombocytopenia; grade 3 or higher anemia will occur in 32% of patients; opportunistic infection will complicate the course of treatment in ~20% of patients

PATIENT INFORMATION

Traditional cytotoxic chemotherapy regimen dose-modified for AIDS patients with lymphoma.

INFUSIONAL CDE
Cyclophosphamide, Doxorubicin, Etoposide

Investigators at Albert Einstein initially reported this regimen in a pilot study with 12 patients. The regimen consists of a continuous 96-h infusion of cyclophosphamide, doxorubicin, and etoposide. Patients with small noncleaved-cell lymphoma and those with bone marrow involvement received central nervous system (CNS) prophylaxis consisting of intrathecal chemotherapy and whole-brain radiotherapy. This study and their subsequent reports demonstrated a response rate of 58%–93%. Their initial study had a long median survival of 17.4 mo. Therapy was generally well tolerated and was given on an outpatient basis using a portable infusion pump. The Eastern Cooperative Oncology Group is currently conducting a phase II pilot study of infusional CDE, coupled with dideoxyinosine (ddI) and granulocyte–macrophage colony-stimulating factor (protocol E1494-NHL). Updated clinical trial data with this regimen has been presented in abstract form (see text for discussion and Table 24-2 for details). Regardless of CD4 count, all patients should receive prophylaxis for *P. carinii* pneumonia during treatment.

RECENT EXPERIENCES AND RESPONSE RATES

Study	Evaluable Patients, n	Response Rate, %	Median CD4 Count	Median Survival, mo
Sparano *et al. Blood* 1993, 81:2810	14	93	Not specified	17.4
Sparano *et al. Leuk Lymphoma* 1994, 14:263	21	86	84	18.0
Sparano *et al. J Clin Oncol* 1996, 14:3026	25	58	85	18.0

DOSAGE AND SCHEDULING

Chemotherapy*	Dose	Interval
Cyclophosphamide	150 mg/m^2 as 96-h CIV	Every 4 wk
Doxorubicin	50 mg/m^2 as 96-h CIV	Every 4 wk
Etoposide	240 mg/m^2 as 96-h CIV	Every 4 wk
G-CSF	5 μg/kg SC d 6 until ANC > 10,000/μL	
CNS prophylaxis (in select patients; *see above*)		
Cytarabine	45 mg/m^2 IT d 1, cycle 1	
Methotrexate	12 mg IT d 3 & 5, cycles 1 & 2	

* Maximum of 6 cycles (2 cycles after complete response).
ANC—absolute neutrophil count; CIV—continuous infusion; CNS—central nervous system; G-CSF—granulocyte colony-stimulating factor; IT—intrathecal.

ALTERNATIVE THERAPIES
Low dose m-BACOD, oral combination chemotherapy, EPOCH or CHOP (cyclophosphamide, doxorubicin, vincristine, and prednisone)

TOXICITIES
Opportunistic infection is of primary concern, especially if CD4 lymphocyte counts are < 25/μL; concomitant use of steroids increases this risk; the combination of this regimen and ddI is associated with significantly less neutropenia and thrombocytopenia and fewer erythrocyte and platelet transfusions; CDE results in a significant decrease in CD4 and CD8 lymphocytes, an effect not abrogated by coadministration with ddI; nonhematologic toxicity consists of nausea and vomiting (72%) and stomatitis (56%); one patient developed heart failure due to this regimen

PATIENT INFORMATION
This regimen requires placement of a central venous access device and patients will likely have to be hospitalized for 4 d in the absence of appropriate home-care support or if clinician is not familiar with the regimen; nonetheless, this regimen has resulted in the longest survival reported for patients with AIDS-related lymphoma; confirmatory multi-institutional trials are underway.

ORAL-COMBINATION CHEMOTHERAPY

Recent studies have been investigating novel methods of drug scheduling and delivery, including protracted infusion and oral administration of chemotherapy in the treatment of AIDS-related lymphoma. An oral-combination chemotherapy regimen has been reported in 38 patients; it achieved complete remission in 13 of 38 patients (34%), an overall objective response rate of 66%, and an overall median survival of 7 mo. The 1-y, 18-mo, and 2-y survival rates are 34%, 21%, and 11%, respectively. Two of 38 patients (5%) developed CNS relapse or progression without prescribed CNS prophylaxis, which raises the possibility of CNS activity of lomustine and procarbazine. Although significant myelotoxicity was observed, the protocol was convenient and less costly to administer than standard intravenous chemotherapy. Interestingly, the incidence of clinically significant ($\geq$ grade 2) nausea, vomiting, diarrhea, and stomatitis seen with other intravenous chemotherapy is low with this regimen. Treatment is self-administered, and consequently, patient compliance is a very important consideration. A dose-modified oral regimen is being developed.

RECENT EXPERIENCES AND RESPONSE RATES

Study	Regimen	Evaluable Patients, n	CR, n	Median Survival, mo
Remick *et al. J Clin Oncol* 1993, 11:191	Oral chemotherapy	18	39	7
Remick *et al. Am J Hematology* 2001 (in press)	Oral chemotherapy + G-CSF	20	30	7

CR — complete response rate; G-CSF — granulocyte colony-stimulating factor.

DOSAGE AND SCHEDULING

Chemotherapy*	Dosage
Lomustine	100 mg/m^2 (cycles 1 & 3) d 1
Etoposide	200 mg/m^2 d 1–3
Cyclophosphamide	100 mg/m^2 d 22–31
Procarbazine	100 mg/m^2 d 22–31
G-CSF	5 µg/kg SC d 5–21, 33–42
CNS prophylaxis	Not given

* Cycles administered every 6 wk for a total of 3 cycles; all chemotherapy drugs given orally.
CNS — central nervous system; G-CSF — granulocyte colony-stimulating factor.

ALTERNATIVE THERAPIES

Low dose m-BACOD, infusional CDE (cyclophosphamide, doxorubicin, and etoposide), EPOCH, and CHOP (cyclophosphamide, doxorubicin, vincristine, and prednisone)

TOXICITIES

The overall toxicity of this regimen compares favorably with that of others; myelosuppression is the most frequent and severe toxicity encountered, with leukopenia being more pronounced than thrombocytopenia; there is a 57% incidence of $\geq$ grade 3 neutropenia and 49% incidence of $\geq$ grade 3 thrombocytopenia with the oral chemotherapy regimen; a total of 21 episodes of febrile neutropenia (21% of treatment cycles) have occurred; The coadministration of granulocyte colony-stimulating factor significantly reduced both the number of hospitalizations for febrile neutropenia and the incidence of discontinuation of chemotherapy because of neutropenia; thrombocytopenia was, however, more severe with the administration of granulocyte colony-stimulating factor; interestingly, the incidence of clinically significant ($\geq$ grade 2) nausea, vomiting, diarrhea, and stomatitis seen with other regimens is low with this regimen

PATIENT INFORMATION

Administration of oral chemotherapy may be attractive to patients for a variety of reasons; some patients are often receiving complicated antiretroviral regimens and many other medications, a situation that may be cumbersome; if a patient's compliance cannot be assured, perhaps it is best to offer IV chemotherapy for their lymphoma; this regimen does not require CNS prophylaxis; the CNS relapse rate observed with this regimen is clinically acceptable.

Palliative care is comprehensive care focused on alleviating suffering and maximizing quality of life for patients with life-threatening illness, including cancer. Achieving these goals requires careful pain and symptom management, psychosocial and spiritual support of patients and families, and understanding of patient and family preferences and goals. Palliative care was once viewed as relevant mainly for patients very near death; however, newer models of palliative care (Fig. 24-1) highlight its role along the continuum of care from diagnosis until death. Oncologists must develop skills in providing excellent palliative care from the time of diagnosis through all phases of a patient's illness. Specific times to address the goals of palliation include when bad news is conveyed (*eg*, when disease progresses, when therapeutic options are limited or when cure is not possible); times of increased symptomatology (*eg*, when chemotherapy is given or when disease progression leads to further symptoms); and times of increased family stress (*eg*, when decisions regarding end-of-life care must be made). Oncologists need to recognize and respond to these transition points in a patient's care. One of the most difficult transitions is when the focus of care shifts from disease-oriented, anticancer therapy to symptom-oriented palliative care. Helping patients and families recognize this transition point requires the accurate assessment of their understanding of the diagnosis and prognosis; effectively communicating details of the illness including likely disease course and outcomes, and potential benefits and burdens of available treatment options (including palliative care). A multidisciplinary team including physicians, nurses, social workers, chaplains, and psychologists can most effectively meet the diverse physical, psychosocial, spiritual, financial, and practical needs of patients and families facing a life-threatening illness.

PALLIATIVE CARE ASSESSMENT

Specific elements of a comprehensive palliative care assessment include a thorough review of the patient's symptoms; advanced care planning including determination of the patient and family's understanding of the diagnosis and prognosis as well as clarification of the patient's goals and preferences for care; evaluation of the patient's social supports including practical and financial concerns; and identification of spiritual or existential concerns.

A successful palliative care assessment relies on effective communication between patients and clinicians. Physicians can elicit a patient's concerns, goals, and values by asking open-ended questions and following up on a patient's response before discussing specific clinical decisions. Physicians can acknowledge patients' emotions, explore the meaning of these emotions, and encourage patients to say more about difficult topics. Examples of open-ended questions that may lead to further discussion include "What concerns you most about your illness?" "How is treatment going for you?" "What are your hopes and expectations for the future?" [1]. The minimal time invested in these discussions will often foster a more effective doctor-patient relationship as well as minimizing misunderstandings and unaddressed concerns.

Validated screening instruments may also help identify otherwise unrecognized issues. Examples include the Edmonton Symptom Assessment Scale [2] and the Memorial Symptom Assessment Scale [3] as well as tools for assessing quality of life (see chapter 30). In addition, educational materials are available to better inform patients and families about their options for end-of-life care [4,5].

Symptom Management

Many patients fear pain and physical suffering as death approaches [6,7]. Unfortunately, unrelieved symptoms remain common in patients with advanced cancer [8,9] despite better management options. A study of patients admitted to a palliative care unit revealed that patients were experiencing an average of 13 different symptoms and that symptom burden correlated with their perceived quality of life [10]. Unrelieved physical suffering precludes any possibility of relieving associated psychologic, social, and spiritual suffering.

The general approach to managing symptoms in advanced illness is identical to the standard approach to managing any illness. A thorough history and physical examination, and laboratory and radiologic investigations are used to understand the underlying etiology and pathophysiology of the symptom and guide treatment decisions. If further investigative studies are not consistent with an individual patient's goals, a therapeutic trial aimed at the most likely etiology based on history and physical examination alone is appropriate. Similarly, if the underlying etiology is known but not amenable to specific therapy, treatment strategies aimed at symptom relief alone may be needed. Frequent reassessment is critical because patients' conditions may change rapidly.

Education and involvement of the patient and family are key to successful management. Patients may make assumptions about disease status or progression based on the development of new or worsening symptoms. Assessing the meaning a patient attaches to a symptom enables clinicians to treat the patient's worry as well as the symptom.

Pain

Pain in patients with cancer is common and often undertreated [11]. At the time of diagnosis, 30% to 45% of cancer patients experience moderate to severe pain. As the disease progresses, more than 75% of cancer patients report pain [12]. Cancer pain can be controlled by relatively simple means using the principles described later in approximately 90% of patients [12]. Oncologists play a crucial role in the optimal assessment and management of cancer pain.

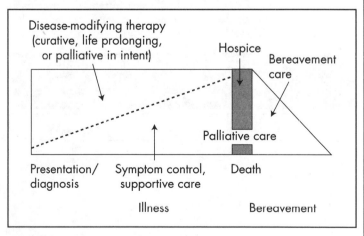

FIGURE 24-1.

Continuum of care. Disease-modifying therapy with curative, life-prolonging, or palliative intent wanes as the illness progresses toward the end of a person's life, tapering to nonexistence as active dying begins in the last hours of life. Comfort-oriented symptom control and supportive care increases over time, maximizing as dying culminates in death. Often people receive this care through a hospice program. Anticipatory grief over many different losses begins before death. Bereavement continues for some time after death. Palliative care provides for all three phases, for the family as well as the patient. (*Adapted from* the American Medical Association's Education for Physicians on End-of-Life Care (EPEC) Curriculum.)

Assessment

Prompt, careful assessment of the patient's pain is essential to the timely design and implementation of a rational treatment plan. Assessment should be carried out at the time of the initial report of pain, at regular intervals thereafter, and with any treatment changes. Cancer patients often experience more than one type of pain and each pain complaint should be individually assessed and prioritized. Pain is a subjective phenomenon and the patient's report must be believed.

A careful pain history includes the intensity, duration, location, and quality of the pain as well as aggravating and alleviating factors and associated symptoms. A numeric rating scale should be used to quantify pain intensity and follow it over time. The impact of the pain on the patient's psychosocial functioning and activities of daily living should be determined. The Brief Pain Inventory [13] contains a validated subscale that assesses pain-related interference with function, mood, and enjoyment of life. Appropriate physical examination elements and diagnostic studies should be performed to determine the underlying cause of the pain when possible. Specific pains respond to specific therapies. Identification of the underlying cause of pain will guide management.

Management

After a thorough assessment has been completed and the cause of the pain identified, if possible, an appropriate treatment regimen can be instituted. Pharmacologic and nonpharmacologic modalities are often combined to maximally manage the pain.

Pharmacologic Measures

The World Health Organization analgesic ladder provides a standard initial approach to drug selection for cancer pain based on pain severity and previous analgesic use. The ladder begins with the use of acetaminophen, aspirin, or nonsteroidal anti-inflammatory drugs (NSAIDs) for mild to moderate pain. When pain persists or increases, an opioid is added. Pain that is moderate or severe at presentation or more persistent should be treated with opioids at higher dosages or with a stronger opioid preparation. The simplest route and dosage schedule and the least invasive pain management

measures are preferred for initial use. Chronic cancer pain requires around-the-clock dosing, supplemented by as-needed ("rescue") doses for breakthrough pain.

Acetaminophen and NSAIDs have analgesic and antipyretic effects, with NSAIDs having additional anti-inflammatory effects. These drugs do not produce tolerance or dependence, but there is a ceiling to their analgesic effects beyond which no further analgesia is obtained. Adding NSAIDs or acetaminophen to an oral opioid regimen can boost the analgesia obtained, which may allow lower dosing of opioids and possibly limiting side effects. NSAIDs have significant risk of serious side effects, especially in elderly patients and patients with renal or hepatic insufficiency. Newer COX-2 inhibitors provide similar analgesia without platelet inhibition but at increased cost [14].

Opioids are highly effective, easily titrated, and generally well tolerated. Dosage requirements vary greatly among patients and with time; therefore, careful and ongoing titration is necessary to achieve and maintain adequate analgesia. Dose titration for acute pain is best achieved by using a short-acting opioid and rapidly increasing the dose until pain resolves. The dose can be increased at the end of each dosing interval, by 25% to 50% for mild to moderate pain and by 50% to 100% for more severe pain. Once the acute pain is controlled or at the initial assessment for chronic pain, a long-acting opioid preparation can be dosed twice daily. Short-acting opioids should remain available for episodes of breakthrough pain. Breakthrough doses should be approximately 10% to 20% of the total 24-hour dose of the long-acting preparation and should be used every 2 to 4 hours as needed.

An equianalgesic table (Table 24-1) facilitates conversions between different opioids and different routes of administration. Codeine is the least potent opioid. Doses of 15 to 30 mg provide pain control comparable with that achieved with full analgesic doses of aspirin, acetaminophen, or NSAIDs. The related compounds oxycodone and hydrocodone are more potent than codeine and are

Table 24-1. Oral and Parenteral Opioid Analgesic Equivalences and Relative Potency of Opioids as Compared with Morphine*†

Opioid Agonist	Parenteral, mg‡	Oral, mg§
Morphine	30	3–4
Oxycodone	20–30	3–4
Hydromorphone	7.5	3–4
Meperidine¶	300	3
Fentanyl	—	1–2
Codeine	200	3–4
Hydrocodone	25–30	—

*When converting from one opioid to another, allow for incomplete cross-tolerance between different opioids by using 50%–75% of the equivalent dose (may need to titrate up rapidly and use as-needed dose to ensure effective analgesia for the first 24 h).
†Avoid intramuscular injections because of inconsistent absorption and patient discomfort.
‡Parenteral opiate onset of action, 15–30 min; peak, 15 min.
§Oral opiate onset of action, 15–30 min; peak, 45–60 min.
¶Should not be used longer than 48 h or > 600 mg/d; contraindicated with monoamine oxidase inhibitors.

Table 24-2. Single Opioid Formulations and Strengths

Drug	Short Acting, mg	Long Acting
Morphine	Tablets: 10, 15, 30 Capsules: 15, 30 Oral solution: 10/5 mL, 20/mL Suppository: 5, 10, 20, 30	MS Contin* (q 12 h): 15, 30, 60, 100, 200 mg Kadian† (q 24 h): 20, 50, 100 mg
Oxycodone	Tablets and capsules: 5, 15, 30 Oral solution: 5/5 mL; Oxyfast, 20/mL	Oxycontin‡ (q 12 h): 10, 20, 40, 80, 160 mg
Hydromorphone (Dilaudid§)	Tablets: 1, 2, 3, 4, 8 (brand scored) Oral solution: 1/mL Suppository: 3	—
Codeine	Tablets: 15, 30, 60	—
Fentanyl	—	Transdermal patch: 25, 50, 75, 100 μg/h Q 3 d

*Purdue Frederick Company, Norwalk, CT.
†Zeneca Pharmaceuticals, Wilmington, DE.
‡Purdue Pharma LP, Norwalk, CT.
§Knoll Pharmaceutical Company, Mount Olive, NJ.

similar in potency to morphine. These opioids are available in combination with aspirin and acetaminophen (Tables 24-2 and 24-3). The toxicities of the nonopioids in these formulations limit the overall dose that can be administered daily (maximum, 4 g of acetaminophen or aspirin in 24 hours). Morphine and oxycodone are available in sustained-release preparations, allowing 12-hour dosing (Table 24-2). These long-acting formulations cannot be crushed or chewed. Hydromorphone (Dilaudid; Knoll Pharmaceutical Company, Mount Olive, NJ) is more potent than morphine and currently is available in short-acting formulations only. Fentanyl, a potent opioid, is available as a transdermal preparation that provides 3 days of analgesia. Its slow onset and prolonged effect require careful titration (not more often than every 24 hours) to avoid excessive sedation. Methadone can be used effectively and inexpensively for chronic cancer pain and is usually dosed every 6 to 8 hours when used for pain. Careful dose titration is essential to prevent excess sedation with repeated dosing given its prolonged half life. Meperidine (Demerol; Sanofi-Synthelabo, New York, NY) is not recommended for chronic cancer pain because of its short duration of action, rapid inactivation of oral dosing, and toxicity of its active metabolite, normeperidine, which causes central nervous system irritability including seizures, especially in patients with renal dysfunction.

Common opioid side effects include constipation and sedation, with nausea, pruritus, dry mouth, and myoclonus occurring less frequently. Tolerance occurs to all of the side effects of opioids except constipation. A bowel regimen (Fig. 24-2), including a stimulant laxative and stool softener, should be prescribed for all patients taking opioids more than intermittently to prevent problematic constipation. Sedation related to opioids typically improves within several days but if persistent can be managed by rotating to a different opioid or by adding a psychostimulant such as methylphenidate (Ritalin; Novartis Pharmaceuticals, Summit, NJ). A commonly feared side effect, respiratory depression, is extremely rare and not a concern in carefully conducted management of chronic pain.

Table 24-3. Combination Opioid Formulations and Strengths

Drug	Formulation Strength
Hydrocodone/acetaminophen* (Lorcet†)	Tablets: 5/500. 7.5/650, 10/650 mg
Hydrocodone/acetaminophen§ (Lortab**)	Tablets: 2.5/500, 5/500 (brand scored), 7.5/500, 10/500 mg
	Elixir: 2.5/167 mg/5 mL
Oxycodone/acetaminophen§ (Percocet††)	Tablets: 5/325 mg
Oxycodone/ASA (Percodan‡‡)	Tablets: 5/325, 2.5/325 mg
Oxycodone/acetaminophen§ (Roxicet)	Tablets: 5/325 mg
	Caplets: 5/500 mg
	Oral solution: 5/325 mg/5 mL
Acetaminophen/codeine§ (Tylenol with codeine)	Tablets: 15/300 (#4)
	Elixir: 12 mg/120 mg/5 mL
Hydrocodone/acetaminophen§ (Vicodin)	Tablets: 5/500, 7.5/750, 10/660 mg

*Maximum daily dose, 4 g.
†Forest Pharmaceuticals, Inc., St. Louis, MO.
‡UCB Pharma, Inc., Smyrna, GA.
§Endo Pharmaceuticals Inc., Wilmington, DE.
¶Roxane Laboratories, Inc., Columbus, OH
**Ortho-McNeil Pharmaceuticals, Raritan, NJ.
††Knoll Pharmaceutical Company, Mount Olive, NJ.

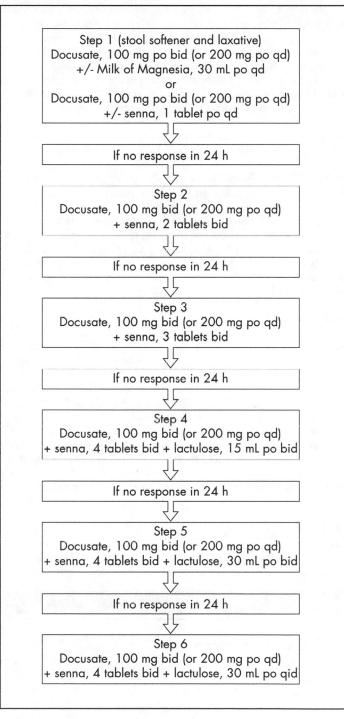

FIGURE 24-2.

Example bowel regimen. With few exceptions, all patients on opioid therapy need an individualized bowel regimen. If the patient has not been on a bowel regimen, the step 1 regimen should be started. At any given time, if there has been no bowel movement in 4 days or more, a sodium phosphate or mineral oil enema should be administered. If this is not effective, a high colonic tap water enema should be administered. Be aware of the possibility of bowel obstruction or fecal impaction. A digital rectal examination should be performed prior to starting a bowel regimen and if no bowel movement for 4 days.

When an effective regimen is found, it should be continued for the duration of the opioid therapy.

Adjuvant analgesics (Table 24-4) can be used for specific pain syndromes to enhance the effectiveness of the previously discussed analgesics. Tricyclic antidepressants and anticonvulsants represent important adjuvants for neuropathic pain. Newer anticonvulsants, particularly gabapentin, have proved particularly effective for neuropathic pain and have a better side effect profile than earlier agents. Psychostimulants can be used to combat opioid-induced sedation [15]. Glucocorticoids may lessen the pain associated with tumor-associated inflammation or infiltration while enhancing appetite and sense of well-being. Patients with pain caused by bone metastases may benefit from therapy with bisphosphanates, which inhibit osteoclast activity and reduce bone pain.

Nonpharmacologic Measures

Physical modalities such as heat, cold, massage, vibration, acupuncture, and transcutaneous electrical nerve stimulation may help to manage pain when used in conjunction with appropriate analgesics. Relaxation techniques, guided imagery, hypnosis, and biofeedback can be helpful, especially for episodic pain and pain associated with specific activities. These modalities are easy to use and relatively inexpensive with minimal morbidity, and they can give patients a sense of control over the pain.

Invasive Modalities

Patients in whom adequate pain control is not achieved with well-designed pharmacologic therapy or who experience intolerable side effects may be candidates for invasive anesthetic procedures. Epidural or intrathecal injection of opioids and local anesthetics can be used for control of intractable pain in the lower part of the body. Operator expertise is essential to ensure proper catheter placement and to manage potential complications, including respiratory depression, hypotension, and infection. Nerve blocks utilize the application of a local anesthetic, corticosteroid, or neurolytic to control intractable pain related to an identifiable nerve structure. Again, precise technique is required for the successful implementation of a nerve block and to prevent damage to surrounding tissue and other nerves.

DYSPNEA

Dyspnea is one of the most frightening and distressing symptoms for patients, families, and caregivers, occurring in 12% to 74 % of patients with advanced malignancies [16]. Various underlying cancer-related etiologies cause dyspnea, including pulmonary embolism, airway obstruction, pulmonary edema, cardiac tamponade, anemia, pleural effusion, and pneumonia. The specific underlying cause of dyspnea should be treated when possible and when compatible with the overall patient goals. If maximal treatment of the underlying cause is inadequate or not possible, palliative measures to control the symptom take precedence. Symptomatic relief of dyspnea includes oxygen, opioids, and anxiolytics.

Measurements of hypoxemia (pulse oximetry, blood gas determination) do not reliably correlate with a patient's self-report of dyspnea. Therefore, a trial of supplemental oxygen therapy is reasonable for most dyspneic patients regardless of objective measures. However, there may be a significant placebo effect; for example, air from a room fan moving across a patient may be equally effective.

Opioids have been demonstrated to relieve the sensation of dyspnea in many patients, although the exact mechanism remains unclear. The principles for opioid prescribing for pain outlined previously also apply for dyspnea, although in opioid-naive patients, smaller doses may be effective for managing dyspnea. Respiratory depression has not been demonstrated at the doses used to relieve breathlessness. Respiratory depression can occur when an opioid-naïve patient is started on long-acting or continuous opioids.

Dyspnea is frequently associated with anxiety. Benzodiazepines and opioids can be combined safely and effectively in managing dyspnea. Behavioral interventions, including relaxation techniques, distraction, and hypnosis can play an important role in managing dyspnea. Simple measures such as fresh air from an open window and repositioning the patient in bed can be quite helpful.

FATIGUE

Multiple studies confirm fatigue (asthenia) as the most frequent distressing symptom of advanced cancer [17,18]. Patients and families often focus on the symptom itself rather than the underlying disease, feeling that the patient is "giving up" because of this lack of energy. Patient and family education and simple nonpharmacologic measures represent important management elements. Patients can be encouraged to conserve energy by adapting activities of daily living. Physical and occupational therapy can teach energy conservation measures and provide assistive devices as needed.

Limited pharmacologic therapy exists for managing fatigue, with corticosteroids and psychostimulants having some role. Dexamethasone in doses of 2 to 20 mg/d (dosed in the morning) may result in increased energy and feeling of well-being; however, the effect may wane after 4 to 6 weeks. Psychostimulants such as methylphenidate (Ritalin) may also increase energy as well as combating opioid-induced sedation. Starting doses of methylphenidate are 2.5 to 5 mg dosed in the early morning and midday to prevent insomnia with dose titration until maximal effect is observed. Methylphenidate can be used safely even in debilitated or elderly patients, although patients should be monitored for adverse effects, including insomnia, anxiety, and tremulousness. Finally, recent data suggest that erythropoeitin relieves fatigue and improves the sense of well-being in patients undergoing chemotherapy [19,20]. Some have postulated that a similar effect may occur in terminally ill patients, although empirical data are lacking.

DEPRESSION

Depression can cause significant mental and emotional suffering in patients facing the end of life and is often underdiagnosed and under-

Table 24-4. Adjuvant Analgesics

Drug	Usual Adult Dose Range, *mg*
Antidepressants	
Amitriptyline	10–150 q HS
Nortriptyline	10–150 q HS
Anticonvulsants	
Gabapentin	100–800 tid
Carbamazepine	100–800 tid
Phenytoin	300–500 qd
Psychostimulants	
Dextroamphetamine	5–10 qd–bid
Methylphenidate	2.5–20 qd–bid
Glucocorticoids	
Dexamethasone	4–96 qd–qid
Prednisone	10–100 qd–bid

treated in this patient population. As many as 25% to 77 % of cancer patients experience major depression [21]. Although initial intense sadness is commonly experienced when facing a diagnosis of a serious illness, persistent symptoms of depression are not normal or inevitable for patients at the end of life. Diagnosis of depression in patients with serious physical illness must rely more on psychologic and cognitive symptoms (feelings of helplessness, hopelessness, worthlessness; loss of self-esteem, pervasive despair) rather than somatic symptoms (changes in appetite, energy level, sleep), which may simply be related to the underlying disease. One study found that asking "have you felt down, depressed, or hopeless most of the time for the last 2 weeks?" or "have you been able to do things that you enjoy?" are both sensitive and specific for depression [22]. Combined psychotherapeutic and pharmacologic interventions are most effective in managing depression. Pharmacologic management is guided by the time available for treatment to take effect. Selective serotonin reuptake inhibitors represent the typical choice for patients in whom a 2- to 4-week or longer response time is acceptable. Patients in whom a more rapid response is required (limited life expectancy, more severe symptoms) may benefit from psychostimulants. Dosing is similar to that described for fatigue above. A newer antidepressant, mirtazapine (Remeron; Organon Inc., West Orange, NJ), may have a role in depression in advanced illness given its appetite-stimulating effects, but data in terminally ill patients are meager.

GASTROINTESTINAL SYMPTOMS

Nausea and vomiting, constipation, diarrhea, and anorexia are covered in chapter 26. The treatment modalities discussed when these symptoms result from chemotherapy also apply in patients near the end of life, but with the general principles described here guiding management in this setting.

TERMINAL SYMPTOMS

The final days of a progressive illness may be very significant, providing a last opportunity for patients and loved ones to say goodbye, find peace, and attain life closure. Health care professionals can play a crucial role in managing these final days to relieve physical, emotional, and psychologic suffering of patients and families and provide smooth passage for the dying person.

Education of families and caregivers about expected changes as death approaches is essential because many laypersons have not witnessed the dying process. Changes such as increasing weakness, decreasing oral intake, decreasing perfusion and urine output, and changes in respiratory pattern may be alarming if not described and discussed in advance.

General symptom management as death approaches requires eliminating unnecessary interventions and medications while converting medications needed to maintain comfort to routes that can be continued as the patient becomes unable to take medications orally. Many medications, including opioids, benzodiazepines, and neuroleptics are available as concentrated oral elixirs that can be administered against the buccal mucosa in patients who can no longer swallow.

Agitated terminal delirium and excessive oral secretions may require specific pharmacologic management if symptoms remain distressing to patients or families after careful explanation and discussion. Build-up of oropharyngeal secretions as death approaches may lead to gurgling, crackling, or rattling with each breath.

Caregivers at the bedside may fear that the patient is choking or suffocating. The first intervention involves explaining these changes as an expected part of the dying process that are not usually distressing to the patient. If the symptom remains bothersome, anticholinergic agents can be used to diminish production of secretions. Scopolamine can be administered transdermally (1.5 mg per patch every 72 hours), subcutaneously (SC) or intravenously either intermittently (0.2–0.4 mg SC every 4 hours) or by continuous infusion (0.1–1.0 mg/h). Other options include glycopyrrolate SC or intravenously intermittently (0.2 mg every 4–6 h) or continuously (0.4–1.2 mg/d) or hyoscyamine elixir, 0.125 to 0.25 sublingually every 6 to 8 hours. Suctioning provides only very short-term relief and can be uncomfortable for patients and unpleasant for caregivers to witness; thus it should generally be avoided.

Agitated terminal delirium fortunately occurs in the minority of dying patients but can be very distressing to families and caregivers who may interpret the agitation and associated moaning and groaning as uncontrolled pain. Whereas identifying and treating underlying causes of delirium is appropriate earlier in the disease process, efforts to manage symptoms are primary in the imminently dying patient.

Benzodiazepines are often used to manage terminal delirium given their anxiolytic, muscle relaxant, and antiseizure effects. Lorazepam elixir, 1 to 2 mg, can be administered against the buccal mucosa as often as hourly until the patient settles, and then on a scheduled basis to maintain symptom control. Neuroleptics can also be used to manage terminal delirium, especially in patients who have had paradoxic responses to benzodiazepines. Haloperidol (starting doses, 0.5–2.0 mg) or a more sedating neuroleptic such as chlorpromazine (starting doses, 10–25 mg) can be administered every 6 hours sublingually, rectally, or intravenously with dose titrated to the desired effect.

ADVANCED CARE PLANNING

Advanced care planning should be a routine part of medical care especially for cancer patients. The process of determining a terminally ill patient's goals, as well as whom they would like to make decisions for them if they are unable to themselves, ideally should begin at the initial visit and continue throughout the disease course. The purposes of these conversations range from building a therapeutic relationship by ensuring that the patient understands your interest in their values, to determining goals for patients for whom life-prolonging therapies are not an option, to discussing specific therapeutic options. Physicians can also encourage patients to discuss these issues with their families because surrogates are likely to be involved in end-of-life decision-making. It is important in these conversations to develop an understanding of each patient's goals and values related to their illness. This can be done in various ways such as asking about past experiences with serious illness in the patient or others known to him or her, or describing likely scenarios and trying to discern the values that underlie the patient's decision-making. Conversations should focus both on the treatments that will not be used (because they are inconsistent with the patient's goals) and the palliative treatments that will be used to promote the patient's goals. An example of the steps involved in advanced care planning is described in Table 24-5. Validated worksheets exist to facilitate the process of determining patient preferences [4]. Once preferences are established, they can be discussed with the patient's proxy and health care providers and entered into the medical record. The patient's advanced directive should be reviewed and updated on a periodic basis in response to changes in the patient's medical and life circumstances.

PSYCHOSOCIAL NEEDS

A careful assessment of the psychosocial needs of the patient and family is essential. Ideally, a comprehensive assessment by a qualified mental health professional (*ie*, psychologist, psychiatrist, or social worker) will be a routine part of the patient's medical care, but this assessment can also be initiated by other members of the healthcare team. Areas to address include availability of community support through the patient and family's workplace, school, church, or neighborhood organizations; and financial impact of the illness on the family. Practical assessment of the presence of caregivers to assist with daily chores such as cooking, cleaning, shopping, paying bills, and providing transportation is essential to providing optimal care.

SPIRITUAL AND EXISTENTIAL ISSUES

Spiritual and existential issues (including how people find meaning, purpose, and value in life) become especially important as a patient approaches death. Physicians should screen for unaddressed spiritual or existential concerns [1]. Unresolved issues in personal matters and relationships may be a prominent focus of the experience of patients facing the end of life. Such issues can be elicited by asking "Given all that is happening, what concerns you the most? When you look at the future, what are your major concerns?" Physicians and other members of the healthcare team can facilitate the process of life review with questions such as "As you look back, what has given your life the most meaning? What are the things that matter most to you?" Other helpful questions to explore existential concerns include "What are some of the things that give you a sense of hope? How have you tried to make sense of what is happening to you?" [1]. Physicians can explore these issues fully depending on their interest, comfort, and skill, or involve other members of a multidisciplinary team including social workers and chaplains to fully address these concerns.

Important elements of a spiritual assessment include how spiritual the person has tended to be in the past, how inclined toward spiritual life the person is now, whether the patient would like to visit with a pastoral care provider, and whether there are religious rituals that are important. Screening questions might include "Are you a spiritual person? What role does religion play in your life? Is faith or spirituality important to you in this illness?" [1]. Community clergy and hospital chaplains may be important resources to provide spiritual support and guidance to patients and families.

HOSPICE CARE

Hospice programs provide comprehensive, multidisciplinary care for dying patients and their families. Unfortunately, hospice care continues to be greatly underutilized due to lack of referrals or very late referrals. The average length of stay in a hospice program is less than 2 months, with more than 15% of patients dying within 2 weeks [23]. Late referrals compromise good end-of-life care. Optimal palliative care requires time for the hospice team to assess the patient's needs and to develop a trusting relationship with the patient and family.

Eligibility for hospice services (as defined under the Medicare Hospice Benefit) include a physician-certified prognosis of less than 6 months if the disease runs its normal course, and treatment goals that are palliative rather than curative. Individual hospice agencies may impose additional criteria, including a "do not resuscitate" order and no plans for total parenteral nutrition, artificial hydration, chemotherapy or blood products, although these are often negotiable depending on specific patient circumstances.

Hospice services include nursing visits to optimize symptom control; home health aide services to help with bathing, dressing, and other physical care; social services for psychologic and financial counseling for patients and families as well as preparation for death including completion of advanced directives, wills and funeral planning; chaplain services for spiritual and existential support; volunteers for relief of family members; and bereavement care for the family after the patient's death. In addition, all medications related to the terminal illness, durable medical equipment, and ancillary services (*eg*, physical therapy, dietary counseling) are fully covered under the hospice benefit. Patients and families must understand that hospice does not provide 24-hour custodial care. Family or privately hired caregivers are generally needed to provide the bulk of daily care, especially as the disease progresses. Hospice care is predominately provided in the home, but limited coverage exists for inpatient care for symptom management, terminal distress, or family respite.

Table 24-5. Components of Advanced Care Planning*

Introduction

  Make sure the setting is appropriate and that other significant people are present.

  Explain why this is being brought up now (*eg*, may relate to prognosis of illness, recent hospitalization, fact that you always do this)

  Explain that the purpose is to respect patient's wishes.

  Reassure that death is not believed to be imminent (if true) — but avoid false reassurance.

Information

  Make sure patient understands course of illness and prognosis — achieve shared understanding.

  Explain any treatments that are discussed in terms of patient's experience and outcome.

Elicit preferences

  Gain an understanding of patient's goals regarding treatment (*eg*, persistent vegetative state) and what risks they would take to avoid these states.

  Discuss probabilities and ask how patient would manage uncertainty.

  Ask about artificial nutrition and hydration specifically if patient indicates that he or she would not want treatment in any given situation.

  Give positive options — discuss what you *will* do to meet the patient's goals. Emphasize that you will be there and remain actively involved regardless of what goals you and the patient choose.

Proxies

  Identify who is to be proxy (one person or a larger group?).

  Stress need for patient to communicate with proxy.

  Ask how much leeway proxy should have in decision-making.

Documents

  Provide an opportunity for documentation (*eg*, chart note, living will).

Communication

  Attend to affect, and provide opportunities for patient to talk.

  Avoid vague terms — or define them.

  Ask for questions.

  Remind patients that they do not need to make an immediate decision and can always change their mind.

  Ensure shared understanding of conversation.

Courtesy of James Tulsky (Duke University Medical Center, Durham, NC), Bob Arnold, and Gary Fischer (University of Pittsburgh Medical Center, Pittsburgh, PA).

GRIEF AND BEREAVEMENT

Physicians can play an important role in providing bereavement support for families after a patient's death. A call, note of condolence, or attendance at funeral services by the physician or other members of the medical team shows clearly that the patient was an important and valued individual while offering a crucial opportunity for lingering unanswered questions, regrets, or concerns to be addressed. Physicians should be able to recognize signs of complicated grief (*eg*, absence of sadness, prolonged grieving, self-destruc- tive behaviors, deterioration in other relationships, extreme guilt and self-reproach) and make appropriate referrals for counseling as needed. Recently, growing research has focused on unresolved grief [24]. Investigators have termed this *traumatic grief* because the syndrome has features in common with posttraumatic stress disorder. The syndrome is distinct from depression and seems to have serious implications for the individual's function and quality of life. Further research is needed to better characterize the syndrome and determine effective treatment.

REFERENCES

1. Lo B, Quill T, Tulsky J: Discussing palliative care with patients. *Ann Intern Med* 1999, 130:744–749.

2. Bruera E, Kuehn N, Miller M, *et al.*: The Edmonton Symptom Assessment System (ESAS): a simple method for the assessment of palliative care patients. *J Palliat Care* 1991, 7:6–9.

3. Portenoy R, Thaler H, Kornblith A, *et al.*: The Memorial Symptom Assessment Scale: an instrument for the evaluation of symptom preva- lence, characteristics and distress. *Eur J Cancer* 1994, 30:1326–1336.

4. Martin D, Emanuel L, Singer P: Planning for the end of life. *Lancet* 2000, 356:1672–1676.

5. Lynn J, Harrold J: *Handbook for Mortals: Guidance for People Facing Serious Illness*. New York: Oxford University Press; 1999.

6. Singer P, Martin D, Kelner M: Quality end-of-life care: patients' perspectives. *JAMA* 1999, 281:163–168.

7. Steinhauser K, Christakis N, Clipp E, *et al.*: Factors considered impor- tant at the end of life by patients, family, physicians, and other care providers. *JAMA* 2000, 284:2476–2482.

8. The SUPPORT Principal Investigators: A controlled trial to improve care for seriously ill hospitalized patients: the study to understand prognoses and preferences for outcomes and risks of treatments (SUPPORT). *JAMA* 1995, 274:1591–1598.

9. Field M, Cassel C, eds.: *Approaching Death, Improving Care at the End of Life: Committee on Care at the End of Life*. Washington, DC: Institute of Medicine; National Academy Press: 1997.

10. Fainsinger R, Miller M, Bruera E: Symptom prevalence during the last week of life on a palliative care unit. *J Palliat Care* 1991, 7:5–11.

11. Cleeland C, Gonin R, Hatfield A, *et al.*: Pain and its treatment in outpatients with metastatic cancer. *N Engl J Med* 1994, 330:592–596.

12. Jacox A, Carr D, Payne R, *et al.*: *Management of Cancer Pain: Clinical Practice Guideline No. 9*. Rockville, MD: Agency for Health Care Policy and Research; US Department of Health and Human Services: AHCPR Publication No. 94-0592; March 1994.

13. Dalal S, Melzack R: Potentiation of opioid analgesia by psychostimu- lant drugs: a review. *J Pain Symptom Manage* 1998, 16:245–253.

14. Daut R, Cleeland C, Flanery R: Development of the Wisconsin Brief Pain Inventory to assess pain in cancer and other diseases. *Pain* 1983, 17:197–210.

15. Emery P, Zeidler H, Kvien T: Celecoxib versus diclofenac in long- term management of rheumatoid arthritis: randomised double-blind comparison. *Lancet* 1999, 354:2106–2111.

16. Billings JA: *The Management of Common Symptoms: Outpatient Management of Advanced Cancer*. Philadelphia, PA: JB Lippincott; 1985.

17. Conill C, Verger E, Henriquez I, *et al.*: Symptom prevalence in the last week of life. *J Pain Symptom Manage* 1997, 14:328–331.

18. Ng K, von Gunten: Symptoms and attitudes of 100 consecutive patients admitted to an acute hospice/palliative care unit. *J Pain Symptom Manage* 1998, 16:307–316.

19. Demetri G, Kris M, Wade J, *et al.*: Quality-of-life benefit in chemotherapy patients treated with epoetin alfa is independent of disease response or tumor type: results from a prospective community oncology study. *J Clin Oncol* 1998, 16:3412–3425.

20. Soignet S: Management of cancer-related anemia: epoetin alfa and quality of life. *Semin Hematol* 2000, 37:9–13.

21. Block S: Assessing and managing depression in the terminally ill patient. *Ann Intern Med* 2000, 132:209–218.

22. Chochinov H, Wilson K, Enn M, Lander S. "Are you depressed?" Screening for depression in the terminally ill. *Am J Psychiatry* 1997, 154:674–676.

23. American Society of Clinical Oncology: Cancer care during the last phase of life. *J Clin Oncol* 1998, 16:1986–1996.

24. Prigerson H, Shear M, Jacobs S, *et al.*: Consensus criteria for traumatic grief: a preliminary empirical test. *Br J Psychiatry* 1999, 174:67–73.

Patients receiving chemotherapy or radiation therapy experience certain side effects. Some (*eg*, acute nausea and vomiting) occur acutely and are managed with medications or intravenous fluids designed to counteract these effects. Other side-effects (*eg*, alopecia), although uncomfortable and perhaps damaging in terms of patient self-image, are not dangerous and do resolve at the conclusion of therapy. Among all side effects seen, those associated with the effects of anticancer therapy on the bone marrow (BM) represent a potentially dangerous and even life-threatening circumstance [1]. Because most anticancer treatments affect rapidly dividing cells preferentially, BM is an ideal target for these effects. This is the primary reason that myelosuppression is among the complications most frequently seen.

Temporary damage to BM can result in decreases in all three major strains of peripheral blood, although effects on leukocytes and especially the myeloid series tend to dominate, given that they have the shortest survival of all BM-derived cells (Table 25-1). This results in a drop in the infection-fighting neutrophil series, with an associated increased risk of infection. Although these patients are at increased risk for both bacterial and fungal forms of infection, the former tends to be more commonly seen. Generally, only patients with long-term severely low (absolute neutrophil count < 250 cells/μL) for lengthy periods experience mycotic infections. Bodey *et al.* [2] reviewed the experience at the National Institutes of Health leukemia service, which defined that both the depth and duration of neutropenia play roles in the risk of developing systemic infectious complications. Because in most cases, neutropenia is of a short duration, the average risk of infection with standard chemotherapy is relatively low. Among the remaining lineages, anemia is most often cumulative in nature. A current controversy disputes which level of anemia represents a sufficiently significant drop to warrant intervention with medical therapy even though transfusion therapy continues to be a mainstay of management of this side effect. This complication most often lowers patients' quality of life by fatiguing them. Finally, a small percentage of patients develops clinically significant thrombocytopenia from cancer therapy. The risk of clinically severe bleeding in patients with thrombocytopenia is low and occurs primarily when the platelet count falls to dangerously low levels. Overall, development of myelosuppression as a complication of cancer therapy can be related to a range of variables (Table 25-2); the development of other complications such as disseminated intravascular coagulopathy or other underlying illness can complicate this issue.

PATHOPHYSIOLOGY

Production of blood cells by BM is an orderly process controlled by both positive and negative regulators termed hematopoietic growth factors (HGFs) and cytokines (Table 25-3) [2]. These include both early-acting stem cell factors (primarily interleukins 1, 3, 6, as well as stem cell factors) and the lineage-specific colony-stimulating factors (*eg*, granulocyte colony-stimulating factors [G-CSF], granulocyte-macrophage colony-stimulating factors [GM-CSF], and erythropoietin). These biologic agents control the proliferation, differentiation, and maturation of multipotential precursor cells that can be directed to various lineages based on the relative expression of specific factors in a BM microenvironment. Hematologic lineages are regulated by a series of feedback loops such as that of the renal tubules that control erythropoietin expression in response to hematocrit.

Blood cell production begins with the multipotential stem cell, which has the ability to self replicate and thereby ensure that adequate precursor cells are always available. The exhaustion of this stem cell supply, although theoretical, could lead to severe BM aplasia and hypoproduction of all blood cells. Although BM aplasia as a result of cancer therapy is rare, it generally only happens with the most intensive chemotherapy regimens.

In general, the environment in which the stem cells exist needs to be conducive to their growth and development. Severe fibrosis from diseases, such as the myeloproliferative disorders or chronic changes as a result of radiation therapy, tends to make BM space inhospitable to blood cell production. This therefore can contribute significantly to the development of myelosuppression.

Kinetically, the myelosuppressive effects of cancer therapy tend to be related to what stage of development is damaged by the agent in question. Neutrophils, which usually survive 7 hours in circulation, are most sensitive to treatment effects. Similarly, platelets that last 7 to 10 days are more commonly affected than erythrocytes, which last 120 days in circulation. The progression of hematopoietic development is similar for all lineages taking approximately 7 days to progress from stem cell to committed progenitor and another 7 to 10 days to progress from committed progenitor to mature cell, ready for release into the circulation. It is this latter 7- to 10-day period that can be compressed by the available CSFs to accelerate blood cell production rapidly.

CAUSES

The principal forms of cancer therapy that cause myelosuppression are chemotherapy and radiation therapy. In the case of radiation, the damaging effect is not limited to the hematopoietic compartment, but to the marrow microenvironment itself. Not uncommonly, it can take up to several years for recovery of a previously irradiated area. In

Table 25-1. Categories of Cytopenias

Lineage	Approximate Survival (in Circulation)	Deficiency
Myeloid	7 h	Neutropenia
Erythroid	120 d	Anemia
Megakaryocyte	7–10 d	Thrombocytopenia

Table 25-2. Factors Associated With Myelosuppression

Therapy
    Choice of chemotherapy agents and dose-intensity
    Radiation therapy including total dose and volume radiated
Bone marrow reserve
    Patient's age and nutritional status
    Prior therapy
    Bone marrow involvement with malignancy or other process
    Bone marrow involvement with cancer or other process
    Comorbid conditions such as autoimmune processes
    Drug-related effects (nonchemotherapy)
    Infection-related complications (*ie*, disseminated intravascular coagulation)

contrast to these two therapies, biologic therapy (*eg*, immunotherapy) may cause myelosuppression by inducing a peripheral consumptive state related to hypersplenism or some similar mechanism. This former effect most commonly resolves quickly following discontinuation of these agents. In some cases of antibody-directed irradiation (using a monoclonal antibody to target radiation particles), the impact can be more significant.

Chemotherapy

Chemotherapy affects hematologic cells in much the same way it does cancer cells. Chemotherapy drugs can be classified into categories based on mechanism of action. Alkylating agents typically bind to nucleotide bases of DNA and thereby inhibit protein synthesis and replication. This effect is similar to that of the antitumor antibiotics such as doxorubicin or daunorubicin that intercalate into DNA strands, thus preventing DNA synthesis. Vinca alkaloids (vincristine or vinblastine) and the taxanes (paclitaxel and docetaxel) inhibit microtubular synthesis that inhibits spindle formation preventing cells from actively undergoing mitosis. Finally, antimetabolites frequently substitute themselves for purine or pyrimidine nucleotides, thereby blocking DNA or RNA synthesis. These latter agents may also block specific enzymes required for nucleotide synthesis. BM cells take up these chemotherapy drugs in much the same way as cancer cells. Hence, BM, because of its rapidly proliferating state, often tends to be more sensitive to the effects of chemotherapy because unlike cancer cells, these progenitors often lack mechanisms of resistance to the chemotherapy. An outline of cancer chemotherapeutic agents and their relative effects on different lines is shown in Table 25-4. Several agents such as vincristine, low-dose methotrexate, L-asparaginase, and oral cyclophosphamide generally do not cause significant myelosuppression. Conversely, agents such as the nitrosureas and mitomycin-C frequently induce delayed and prolonged myelosuppression because of their relative effects on the stem cell population.

Immunotherapy

Biologic agents can be divided into two specific groups with regard to their effects on the hematologic system. The first group, which includes the interferons (alfa, beta, and gamma), can exert a direct suppressive effect on BM and although not specifically myelotoxic,

certainly is not myelosuppressive. This impact on blood counts is typically relatively rapidly reversible after the drug has been discontinued. In contrast, lymphopenia and neutropenia associated with interleukin-2 (IL-2) appear to be predominantly related to peripheral consumption by immunostimulated cells or by vascular margination of pools of cells. Both these side effects are rapidly reversible, appear to be dose related, and generally are not associated with infectious complications. In addition to the IL-2–mediated neutropenia, this agent has the ability to induce neutrophil dysfunction, which lasts longer than quantitative neutropenia and may be associated with increased infectious risk.

Radiation Therapy

Radiation therapy induces cell death by causing lethal double-stranded DNA breaks. These DNA breaks result in cell death and apoptosis when the cell enters the cell cycle. For this reason, it is cells in G_0 that tend to be more sensitive to DNA damage than those in G_1 or S-phase, which tend to be more resistant due to their ability to correct damage enzymatically. Hence, myelosuppression associated with radiation therapy is often related to the volume of BM irradiated, the total radiation dose, and the patient's overall BM reserve (which may be compromised by either prior therapy or BM involvement with cancer).

DIAGNOSIS

The first evidence of myelosuppression is often a defined drop in the number of peripherally circulating blood cells. Because of the kinetics and life span of blood cells as previously noted, leukopenia and neutropenia are typically the first deficiencies noted. This drop, which may be mild, is frequently found 7 to 10 days following the completion of therapy, although more intensive treatments may accelerate the process. In the case of moderately to severely intensive regimens, thrombocytopenia may be noted at or around the same time. Anemia, as a side-effect of therapy, is more commonly cumulative and develops over time or a series of cycles.

In typical situations, response to the development of cytopenias is an increase in BM production of blood cells. This generally corrects mild leukopenia or thrombocytopenia in a short time (7 to 14 days). In some cases, in which more severe or prolonged myelosuppression occurs, further investigation may be necessary.

Table 25-3. Hematopoietic Growth Factors and Cytokines

	Name	Lineage	Approval Status
Colony-stimulating factors	G-CSF	m	Approved
	GM-CSF	m, mo	Approved
	EPO	e	Approved
	TPO	p	Investigational
	M-CSF	mo	No longer under study
Interleukins	Interleukin-11	p	Approved
	Interleukin-3	m, e, p	No longer under study
	Interleukin-6	p	No longer under study
	Interleukin-1	m, e, p	No longer under study

e—erythroid; G-CSF—granulocyte colony-stimulating factor; GM-CSF—granulocyte–macrophage colony-stimulating factor; EPO—erythropoietin; m—myeloid; mo—monocytic; M-CSF—macrophage colony-stimulating factor; p—platelet; TPO—thrombopoietin.

Peripheral Blood

Evaluation of a peripheral blood (PB) smear is the easiest form of "tissue biopsy" available. Comprehensive review of a PB smear can provide significant insight both before and after chemotherapy as to the risk and complications of chemotherapy administration. In addition to being able to evaluate leukocytes, erythrocytes, and platelets quantitatively, a PB smear allows qualitative evaluation. Prechemotherapy evaluation may demonstrate important findings such as that of a leukoerythroblastic picture (elevated numbers of early leukocytes and nucleated erythrocytes) consistent with BM involvement with tumor or fibrosis. Both these situations may increase the risk of more severe myelosuppression.

After therapy has been administered, a review of the PB smear will allow a differential count to be performed on the PN leukocytes and a calculation of the absolute neutrophil count (ANC), which is the total number of leukocytes multiplied by the percentage of

Table 25-4. Drug-Induced Myelosuppression

	Route of administration	Degree of suppression*	Time to nadir (wk)*	Time to recovery (wk)*	Affected cell type
Alkylating agents					
Busulfan	PO	Moderate–marked	2–4	6–8	L,P
Chlorambucil	PO	Moderate	2–3	4–8	L
Cyclophosphamide	IV,PO	Mild–moderate	1–2	2–4	L
Ifosfamide	IV	Moderate	1–2	2–4	L,P
Melphalan	PO	Moderate	2–3	4–7	L,P
Thiotepa	IV	Moderate–marked	2–3	4–6	P,L
Antibiotics					
Bleomycin	IV	0–mild	1–2	2–3	P,L
Daunorubicin	IV	Marked	2	3–4	L,P
Doxorubicin	IV	Marked	2	3–4	L,P
Epirubicin	IV	Moderate–marked	1–2	2–3	L,E
Idarubicin	IV	Marked	2	3–4	L,P
Mitoxantrone	IV	Marked	1–2	3	L,P
Mitomycin	IV	Moderate	Up to 8	Up to 10	L,P
Antimetabolites					
2-Chlorodeoxyadenosine	IV	Moderate	1–2	3–4	L,P
Cytosine arabinoside	IV	Moderate–marked	2	3	L,P
Fludarabine	IV	Mild–moderate	2–3	3–5	L,P
Fluorouracil	IV	Mild–moderate	1–2	2–3	L,P
Gemcitabine	IV	Moderate-marked	1–2	2–3	L,E,P
Mercaptopurine	IV	Moderate	1–2	3–4	L,P
Methotrexate	PO	Moderate–marked	1–2	2–3	L,P
Vinca alkaloids/ Epipodophyllotoxins					
Etoposide	IV,PO	Mild–moderate	1–2	3	P
Teniposide	IV	Moderate–marked	1	2–3	L,P
Vinblastine	IV	Moderate	1–2	2–3	L
Vincristine	IV	Mild	1–2	2	L
Vinorelbine	IV	Moderate–marked	1–2	3–4	L
Miscellaneous					
L-asparaginase	IV	0–mild	1–2	—	L
Cisplatin	IV	Moderate	2–3	4–6	G,P,E
Carboplatin	IV	Moderate	2–3	4–6	G,P,E
Dacarbazine	IV	Mild	2–3	4–5	G,P
Docetaxel	IV	Moderate — marked	1–2	2–3	L,E
Hydroxurea	PO	Moderate — marked	1	2–3	G,P
Paclitaxel	IV	Moderate — marked	1–2	2–3	L,P
Procarbazine	PO	Moderate	3–4	4–6	P,G

*Dependent on dose, administration, and scheduling.
E—erythrocytes; L—leukocytes; P—platelets.

segmented neutrophils plus band forms. The ANC is a critical calculation on which treatment of patients with fever during leukopenia is based. Early BM recovery is typically heralded by a PB monocytosis. Monocytes, a more primitive type of anti-infectious cell, tend to increase in number transiently before granulocytosis.

In addition to quantitative evaluation of blood cells, qualitative analysis of the PB smear is critical. Complications such as infection with disseminated intravascular coagulation (DIC) may be identified on the smear based on the features of fragmented erythrocytes and deficient platelets. Furthermore, patients with prolonged leukopenia, who are at risk for secondary malignancies following chemotherapy with or without radiation, may demonstrate signs of an underlying myelodysplastic syndrome. Evidence in support of this diagnosis may include pseudo Pelger-Huet neutrophils (unilobed or bilobed segmented neutrophils), hypogranularity of the myeloid series, or long-standing PB monocytosis with erythrocyte macrocytosis.

Bone Marrow

In some settings, BM evaluation may be necessary to explore etiologies for relative or absolute cytopenias. Examples of such diagnoses include the superimposed autoimmune cytopenias. This is conducted through BM aspiration and biopsy, typically on the posterior iliac spine unless the pelvis has been previously irradiated. In that case, a sternal BM aspirate alone is appropriate. A sternal BM aspirate is performed in the region approximately 2 to 3 cm below the sternomanubrial joint in the midline. The key feature of a successful BM aspirate is the presence of spicules, which represent small bony particles around which hematopoietic precursors develop. Occasionally, it may be impossible to attain an adequate aspirate due to the lack of spicules (as may be the case in severely aplastic marrows) or because of a "dry tap," which may occur due to scarring or fibrosis in the BM space. In these situations, a BM biopsy is critical to adequately evaluate the BM pathophysiology. Magnetic resonance imaging (MRI) to investigate BM cellularity using the difference in water content between hypocellular BM (high fat content) and hypercellular BM is being investigated. Abnormal signal in the BM may also be seen on MRI, which may indicate involvement of the BM space with malignant tumor.

HEMATOLOGIC TOXICITY
Neutropenia

As noted previously, neutropenia is one of the first findings consistent with myelosuppression. It is of potential value in terms of monitoring the effect of orally administered chemotherapy in which variable absorption may play a role in activity of the drug. Such is the case for oral melphalan in the setting of multiple myeloma in which serial blood counts demonstrating development of mild-to-moderate neutropenia is indicative of adequate drug absorption.

Neutropenia is a deficiency of the number of circulating neutrophilic granulocytes. As the primary bacterial infection-fighting cell of the body, it is responsible for preventing overwhelming pyogenic infections. A pool of neutrophils exists in a marginated state and some patients, particularly those of African descent, have a relative neutropenia that responds to the administration of low doses of epinephrine, which redistributes the marginated pool. This is more of a pseudoneutropenia and is not associated with an increased risk of infection.

Absolute neutrophil count (ANC) levels below 1000 cells/μL are associated with increased risk of infection. This is common in instances in which patients are receiving combination chemotherapy.

Incidence of infection is directly related to the depth of the neutropenia as well as its absolute duration (how low and for how long) [3]. As has been noted previously, recovery of ANC to normal levels may take approximately 2 weeks following administration of standard dose chemotherapy. During the period when patients are effectively neutropenic, close monitoring for signs or symptoms of infection must take place. Any clinically significant fever must be met with a thorough investigation of potential sources of infection including risk of infection related to indwelling central venous catheters.

After a patient with neutropenia has been determined to have a fever (temperature at or above 38.5°C), appropriate antibiotic coverage with a third-generation cephalosporin is indicated. This monotherapy is appropriate for all patients with culture-negative febrile neutropenia with an adjustment of the antibiotic coverage for positive blood cultures. Patients with indwelling central venous catheters are candidates for the addition of vancomycin either at the initiation of antibiotic coverage or within 48 to 72 hours if fever continues (if a source is not found). Antibiotics should be continued until the ANC exceeds 500 cells/μL and the patient is afebrile. Patients with positive blood cultures and an indwelling central catheter require treatment based on culture and symptom. It is rare in the setting of short-lasting neutropenia for patients to develop fungal infections. In a case in which systemic fungal infection develops, intravenous therapy with amphotericin B is appropriate; duration of this therapy is defined by the severity of the infection and the fungal isolate.

The two hematopoietic colony-stimulating factors (G-CSF, GM-CSF) entered into clinical use in the early 1980s. Approved several years later, G-CSF has demonstrated the ability to reduce the depth and duration of chemotherapy-induced neutropenia associated with combination chemotherapy [4]. As a result of this effect, it also significantly decreases incidence of febrile neutropenia. Although GM-CSF has similar biologic activities, its benefits are seen in the setting of BM transplantation in which it accelerates recovery of neutrophils and hastens the ability to discharge the patient from the hospital [5]. Anecdotal use of these agents in the setting of drug-induced neutropenia also suggests a benefit. The value of CSF use for the treatment of radiation-induced neutropenia remains unclear; at least one study in non–small cell lung cancer demonstrates that concomitant GM-CSF and radiation therapy results in poorer survival compared with radiation alone. Of significance, no study has demonstrated a survival advantage to the use of CSFs in conjunction with cancer therapy. Hence they remain as supportive care and their use is based on a physician's perception of the individual risk-benefit ratio.

Anemia

The past several years have seen more and more attention focused on the impact of anemia on patient tolerance of chemotherapy and their overall quality of life. Anemia is defined as a drop in the hemoglobin or hematocrit to a level below the lower limit of normal. In most institutions, this is represented by a fall below 12 g/dL or a hematocrit of 36%. Although most patients at this level are minimally symptomatic in terms of fatigue, new studies suggest that mild anemia may contribute to slowing of the mental processes with decision making. This so-called "executive function" is a critical new endpoint in anemia research. Evaluation for contributing factors such as nutritional deficiencies (folic acid or vitamin B_{12}) or a destructive process must be completed.

Declines in hematocrit levels tend to be cumulative in that patients progressively develop more symptoms, which include fatigue, exercise intolerance, tachycardia, dyspnea on exertion and, in extreme cases, exacerbation of preexisting cardiopulmonary disease. Most of these symptoms can be alleviated by the transfusion of packed erythrocytes, although transfusions are expensive and not without risks (eg, viral infections). As an alternative to transfusions, use of recombinant human erythropoietin has been explored [6,7]. Proven as beneficial to decrease the need to erythrocyte transfusions, it is widely perceived as a therapy that also improves quality of life for patients receiving chemotherapy, although this has not been widely confirmed in a randomized trial. Optimal timing of the initiation of erythropoietin use is before patients require transfusions. Current initial dose is a once weekly, subcutaneously administered, treatment at a dose of 40,000 units per week.

Thrombocytopenia

Thrombocytopenia represents a deficiency in the number of circulating platelets, which normally circulate at levels between 150 and $400,000/\mu L$. Levels of $50,000/\mu L$ and higher are generally adequate for hemostasis to allow minor or major surgical procedures. The degree to which patients develop thrombocytopenia is directly related to the incidence of bleeding complications. Spontaneous minor bleeding episodes increase in frequency when the platelet count falls below 20,000/(L. Major bleeding complications occur in the setting of more severe thrombocytopenia (platelet counts below 10,000/L). With the use of more intensive regimens, newer drugs, and patients' receiving overall more chemotherapy, thrombocytopenia is becoming more common.

Increased risk of bleeding can be seen in patients with coagulation disorders contributing to their thrombocytopenia. In these cases, processes such as DIC, which can be associated with metastatic cancer as well as infection, can increase risk of bleeding. In addition, this risk can also be affected by drugs that either affect platelet function (eg, aspirin or other nonsteroidal anti-inflammatory agents) or coagulation function (eg, heparins or coumadin).

Recent studies have validated an acceptable threshold of $10,000/\mu L$ for transfusion of platelets and have recognized single donor or pooled random donor platelets as reasonable options for transfusion. This lower threshold has the potential not only to limit viral infection exposure and potentially reduce the development of alloimmunization, but also to reduce costs related to transfusion support.

Advances in the field of hematopoietic growth factors have resulted in the approval of interleukin-11 (Neumega [oprelvekin; Genetics Institute, Cambridge, MA]) for prevention of severe chemotherapy-induced thrombocytopenia [8]. These data support its use in settings in which the risk of severe thrombocytopenia and the likelihood of the need for transfusion are high.

OTHER INTERVENTIONS: PROGENITOR CELL INFUSIONS

Use of PB progenitor or stem cells (PBPC or PBSC) has become increasingly widespread although the overall value of such high-dose chemotherapy that typically necessitates its use remains controversial in many settings. The addition of PBPC to dose-intensive regimens appears to be able to shorten the duration of myelosuppression and has allowed implementation of outpatient administration of this type of therapy [9].

Although autologous PBPC has become a relatively commonly used procedure for many different diseases, its use in the allogeneic setting or most recently in the setting of minitransplants is the largest new use. It is anticipated that although HGFs may be used to enhance the mobilization of these progenitors into the PB, that they alone may be adequate to reconstitute hematologic recovery without additional therapy involving cerebrospinal fluid.

REFERENCES

1. De Vita V, Jr: Principles of cancer management: chemotherapy. In *Cancer: Principles and Practice of Oncology*. Edited by De Vita V, Jr, Hellman, Rosenberg. Philadelphia: Lippincott-Raven; 1997:333–348.

2. Bodey G, Buckley M, Sathe Y, *et al.*: Quantitative relationships between circulating leukocytes and infection in patients with acute leukemia. *Ann Intern Med* 1966, 64:328–340.

3. Bagby G, Jr, Segal G: Growth factors and the control of hematopoiesis. In *Hematology: Basic Principles and Practice*. Edited by Hoffman B, Jr, Shattil *et al*. New York: Churchill Livingstone; 1995:207–241.

4. Crawford J, Ozer H, Stoller R, *et al.*: Reduction by granulocyte colony-stimulating factor of fever and neutropenia by chemotherapy in patients with small-cell lung cancer. *N Engl J Med* 1991, 325:164–170.

5. Nemunaitis J, Rabinowe S, Singer J, *et al.*: Recombinant granulocyte-macrophage colony-stimulating factor after autologous bone marrow transplantation for lymphoid cancer. *N Engl J Med* 1991, 324:1773–1778.

6. Glaspy J, Bukowski R, Steinberg D, *et al.*: Impact of therapy with epoetin alfa on clinical outcomes in patients with nonmyeloid malignancies during cancer chemotherapy in community oncology practice: Procrit Study Group. *J Clin Oncol* 1997, 15:1218–1234.

7. Demetri G, Kris M, Wade J, *et al.*: Quality-of-life benefit in chemotherapy patients treated with epoetin alfa is independent of disease response or tumor type: results from a prospective community oncology study. Procrit Study Group. *J Clin Oncol* 1998, 16:3412–3425.

8. Tepler I, Elias L, Smith JI, *et al.*: A randomized, placebo-controlled, trial of recombinant human interleukin-11 in cancer patients with severe thrombocytopenia due to chemotherapy. *Blood* 1996, 87:3607.

9. Glaspy J: Economic considerations in the use of peripheral blood progenitor cells to support high-dose chemotherapy. *Bone Marrow Transpl* 1999, 23 (suppl 2):S21–S27.

The information here is provided as guidance only. Prescribers should always consult the manufacturer's current prescribing information

378

NEUTROPENIA

Neutropenia is defined as a deficiency in the number of functional neutrophil granulocytes. The criterion for neutropenia is an absolute neutrophil count less than 1000/µL. Patients with neutropenia are at greater risk of developing infections, particularly if they are undergoing dose-intensified or prolonged chemotherapy.

INTERVENTIONS

1. Prevention
   a. Avoid concurrent myelosuppressive agents and radiation therapy
   b. Chemotherapy dose reduction, if appropriate, maintaining schedule
   c. Delay interval between treatment cycles until neutrophil recovery
   d. Interrupt radiation therapy until neutrophil recovery
   e. Hematopoietic growth factor support (G-CSF, GM-CSF)
   f. Nutritional support
2. Prevention and treatment of sequelae
   a. Avoid exposure to infection and reverse isolation
   b. Meticulous personal hygiene
   c. Early antimicrobial treatment for associated fevers (broad-spectrum antibiotics, with staphylococcal and gram-negative coverage; biliary tree–enteric anaerobe; bowel-enteric anaerobe)
   d. Transfusion of neutrophils
   e. Prophylactic antibiotics

GRANULOCYTE–COLONY-STIMULATING FACTOR (G-CSF) OR FILGRASTIM

1. **Indications:** Patients with malignancies receiving myelosuppressive chemotherapy associated with a significant (minimal 40%) incidence of severe neutropenia and fever (contraindicated in patients with known hypersensitivity to *E. coli*–derived proteins)
2. **Dosage and administration:** 5 µg/kg/d SC or IV to begin ≥ 24 h after chemotherapy
3. **Lab monitoring:** Baseline CBC and platelet counts, biweekly thereafter
4. **Adverse reactions:** medullary bone pain, increased uric acid, alkaline phosphatase, LDH, transient decreased blood pressure (rare)

GRANULOCYTE-MACROPHAGE–COLONY-STIMULATING FACTOR (GM-CSF) OR SARGRAMOSTIM

1. **Indications:** Patients with non-Hodgkin's lymphoma, acute lymphocyte leukemia, and Hodgkin's disease undergoing high-dose chemotherapy with progenitor cell support and elderly patients with acute myeloid leukemia receiving chemotherapy (contraindicated in patients with known hypersensitivity to GM-CSF, yeast-derived products or any component of the product)
2. **Dosage and administration:** 250 µg/m^2/d for 21 d by 2-h IV infusion beginning 2–4 h after ABMT; discontinue therapy when neutrophil count is > 20,000/mm^3
3. **Lab monitoring:** If blast cells appear, discontinue therapy; biweekly monitoring of renal and hepatic function and CBC with differential
4. **Adverse reactions:** > 5% incidence over placebo; diarrhea, exacerbation of preexisting asthma, renal or hepatic dysfunction, rash, exacerbation of arrhythmia, malaise, fever, headache, bone pain, hives, myalgia, dyspnea, peripheral edema

CAUSATIVE FACTORS

Primary: benign; chronic—severe, congenital, cyclic, idiopathic; **secondary:** neoplastic—hematologic malignancy, metastatic tumor; nonneoplastic—autoimmune, drug-related (chemotherapy, antibiotics, anticonvulsants, antidepressants); infection (bacterial, viral, mycobacterial); radiation; hematologic disease (aplastic anemia, myelofibrosis, paroxysmal nocturnal hemoglobinuria, T-gamma syndrome), organomegaly, nutritional deficiency

PATHOLOGIC PROCESS

Many unknown, possibly overproduction of cytokine suppressors or loss of growth factor receptors on progenitors, inhibition of nucleic acid and protein syntheses, maturation arrest, overproduction of hematopoietic inhibitors, antibody-induced destruction, drug-induced destruction, replacement of bone marrow by tumor or fibrosis, defective folate metabolism

DIFFERENTIAL DIAGNOSES

See Causative Factors

PATIENT ASSESSMENT

Leukocyte count and differential, review of smear for morphology, bone marrow aspiration and biopsy, karyotype, culture bone marrow, special bone marrow stains, including reticulin and acid-fast bacilli; serum B$_{12}$ and folate levels, analysis for T-cell receptor gene rearrangement; review of medication

TOXICITY GRADING

	0	1	2	3	4
WBC x 10^3	> 4.5	3.0– < 4.5	2.0– < 3.0	1.0– < 2.0	< 1.0
Neutrophil x 10^3	> 1.9	1.5– < 1.9	1.0– < 1.5	0.5– < 1.0	< 0.5

THROMBOCYTOPENIA

Thrombocytopenia is a shortage of functional platelets due to decreased production, increased consumption, defective function, or splenic pooling. The condition is often exacerbated by cancer therapy and can place the patient at risk of hemorrhage.

INTERVENTIONS

1. Prevention
    a. Avoid antiplatelet agents (*eg*, ASA)
    b. Chemotherapy dose adjustment, maintaining schedule
2. Prevention and treatment of sequelae
    a. Avoid invasive procedures (IM injections, rectal supp)
    b. Use progesterones to prevent menses
    c. GI tract prophylaxis (*ie*, antacids, stool softeners)
    d. Platelet transfusion (see below)

PLATELET TRANSFUSION

1. **Indications:** Prophylaxis for patients with platelet counts < 10,000–20,000/mm^3, prophylaxis for surgery if counts < 50,000/mm^3, treatment of hemorrhage if < 50,000–100,000/mm^3; signs and symptoms indicating need for transfusion: easy bruisability, petechiae, mucous membrane bleeding
2. **Preparations:** All are ABO compatible and may be leukocyte-depleted at the bedside; from whole blood (random donor), $\geq 5.5 \times 10^{10}$/bag; apheresis (single donor), $> 3 \times 10^{11}$/bag; leukocyte-poor and single donor delay development of alloimmunization; HLA matched—for patients already alloimmunized
3. **Dose and administration:** 6 U (random donor) or 1 bag (single donor) IV infusion. Count should increase 5,000–10,000/μl/random donor bag. A poor response in platelet increment may be due to splenomegaly, fever, sepsis, disseminated intravascular coagulation (DIC), alloimmunization (1-h increment < 50% of expected suggests alloimmunization)
4. **Risks and adverse reactions:** *immune*—fever, allergic reaction, graft-versus-host reaction; *nonimmune*—volume overload, transmission of infection

INTERLEUKIN-11 (IL-11)

1. **Indications:** Patients with nonmyeloid malignancies receiving dose-intensive chemotherapy and at a high risk for the development of severe chemotherapy-induced thrombocytopenia (contraindicated in patients with known hypersensitivity to *E. coli*–derived products)
2. **Dosage and administration:** 50 μg/kg/d SC to begin following chemotherapy (no sooner than 6 h after chemotherapy) and continued until a postnadir platelet count of 50,000/μL is achieved or for a maximum of 21 d (do not round to vial size)
3. **Lab monitoring:** Twice weekly complete blood and platelet counts
4. **Adverse reactions:** Asthenia, edema, dyspnea, rare incidence of atrial arrhythmias

CAUSATIVE FACTORS

Quantitative: *decreased production*—congenital, acquired: alcoholism, drug-related (chemotherapy and radiation, diuretics, H2 blockers), infections (viral), nutritional deficiency, tumor involvement of bone marrow, myelofibrosis, primary hematologic disorder; *increased consumption*—autoimmune (ITP, TTP, hematologic malignancy), DIC, drug-related (heparin, antibiotics, infection); **qualitative:** *drug-related*—nonsteroidal antiinflammatory agents, antimicrobials, psychiatric drugs, alcohol; *concomitant illness*—uremia, chronic liver disease, myeloproliferative disorders

PATHOLOGIC PROCESS

Clot formation, antibody-induced destruction, inhibition of nucleic acid synthesis, bone marrow replacement with tumor or fibrosis, sequestration in enlarged spleen, defective maturation, drug-induced acetylation of platelet cyclooxygenase

DIFFERENTIAL DIAGNOSES

See Causative factors

PATIENT ASSESSMENT

CBC, peripheral blood smear, mean platelet volume, bone marrow aspiration or biopsy, karyotype, platelet aggregation studies, bleeding time (if platelet count adequate).

TOXICITY GRADING

	0	1	2	3	4
Platelet					
x 10^3	>130	90– < 130	50– < 90	25– < 50	< 25

ANEMIA

The patient with anemia has an abnormally low concentration of erythrocytes and hemoglobin. The potential risks of anemia are less serious than those of neutropenia and thrombocytopenia; however, with the trend toward intensified therapy doses and BMT, the incidence and severity of anemia are increasing. Transfusion continues to be the conventional method of support.

INTERVENTIONS

1. Prevention—erythropoietin support
2. Prevention and treatment of sequelae; transfusion of erythrocytes; management of fatigue

TRANSFUSION OF ERYTHROCYTES

1. **Indications:** Patients with symptomatic anemia requiring increased red cell mass and improved oxygen-carrying capacity. Symptoms may include tachycardia, dyspnea, angina, decreased mentation, transient ischemic attacks, syncope, postural hypotension, inability to maintain reasonable level of daily activity (contraindicated in asymptomatic patients with vitamin-responsive anemia, Fe-responsive anemia, erythropoietin-responsive anemias)
2. **Preparations:** *All ABO-compatible and cross-matched*—PRBC is blood component of choice, majority of plasma removed, 50–75 mL remain in each unit; preservative solution added; Hct = 70%–80%; 1 U increases Hb in 70 kg adult by 1–1.5 g/dL; *leukocyte-poor erythrocytes*—used to prevent febrile transfusion reactions and alloimmunization to leukocyte, antigen and platelet transfusion; *washed erythrocytes*—for patients with history of transfusion-related allergic reactions (usually due to plasma proteins), Hct = 50%–70%
3. **Dosage and administration:** Dose based on severity. In otherwise healthy patients, transfuse to Hb ≥ 8 g/dL. In patients with cardiac disease, frequently transfuse to Hb ≥ 10 g/dL. Infuse over 4 h via IV catheter with normal saline for flushing
4. **Risks and adverse reactions:** *Nonimmune*—volume overload, Fe overload, transmission of infections: hepatitis (1–2:100 transfusions), cytomegalovirus, HIV, HTLV-1, Epstein–Barr virus, bacterial infections (rare), Lyme disease, babesiosis, Chagas' disease, brucella, malaria, possibly TB; *immune*—acute or delayed hemolysis, fever (most common reaction with transfusion), allergic (urticaria, wheezing, angioedema), graft-versus-host (prevented by radiation therapy of blood product with 1500–3000 cGy)

ERYTHROPOIETIN (EPO)

1. **Indications:** Patients with chronic renal failure (CRF), patients with anemia due to chemotherapy (contraindicated in patients with uncontrolled hypertension or with hypersensitivity to mammalian cell–derived products of human albumin)
2. **Dose and administration:** CRF—50–100 U/kg IV three times pre week, reduce dose if target Hct is reached or if Hct increases > 4% in 2 wk; increase dose if target not reached or no increase of 5%–6% in 8 wk; maintenance dose is individualized; chemotherapy— 150 U/kg IV/SC three times per week with an increase to 300 U/kg three times per week if no response after 8 weeks. *Alternatively, weekly dosing can be used with 40,000 U SC/week.*
3. **Lab monitoring:** blood pressure, Hct 1–2 × wk during dose adjustment, Fe and Fe-binding capacity
4. **Adverse reactions:** *CRF patients*—hypertension, thrombotic events, headache, shortness of breath, tachycardia, hypercalcemia, nausea and vomiting, diarrhea (most frequent); flu-like symptoms, rash, urticaria, and seizures (rare); *patients receiving chemotherapy*: diarrhea, edema; fever, shortness of breath, paresthesia, URI (less frequent)

CAUSATIVE FACTORS

Blood loss, chemotherapy and radiation, chronic disease: tumor, infection, drug-related (zidovidine), hemolysis: autoimmune—tumor (CLL, lymphoma), drug-related; mechanical—chemotherapy (mitomycin C), DIC (tumor- or infection-related); nutritional deficiency: poor nutrition, postsurgery of gastrointestinal tract; bone marrow involvement: hematologic malignancy, metastatic tumor, myelofibrosis; concomitant illness: renal insufficiency, endocrine deficiencies

PATHOLOGIC PROCESS

Defective hemoglobin production, defective glucolysis, defective DNA synthesis, defective iron and B_{12} absorption, defective purine and pyrimidine synthesis, blockade in folate metabolism, erythrocyte parasites, bacterial toxins, antibody-induced destruction, erythropoietin deficiency, production of cytokines that inhibit hematopoiesis, replacement of bone marrow by tumor or fibrosis

DIFFERENTIAL DIAGNOSES

See Causative Factors

PATIENT ASSESSMENT

Erythrocyte count, hemoglobin concentration, hematocrit, mean corpuscular hemoglobin, mean corpuscular volume, mean corpuscular hemoglobin concentration, reticulocyte count, erythrocyte morphology, additional tests based on clinical evaluation: total and fractionated bilirubin, serum iron, total iron binding capacity, stool hematocrit, serum vitamin B_{12}, red cell folate, hemoglobin electrophoresis, direct and indirect Coombs' test, bone marrow aspiration and biopsy, thyroid function tests

TOXICITY GRADING

	0	1	2	3
Hbg g%,	> 11,	9.5–10.9,	< 9.5,	Transfusion required
Hct%	> 32	28–31.9	< 28	Transfusion required

NAUSEA AND VOMITING

Nausea and vomiting are among the most frequent and noticeably unpleasant side effects of anticancer therapy. Consequences of uncontrolled nausea and vomiting include dehydration, electrolyte disturbance, weight loss, and patient discomfort that may result in avoidance of further anticancer therapy, anticipatory emesis, or both. Additional side effects may include gastrointestinal bleeding, esophagogastric tears, and aspiration pneumonia.

PATHOPHYSIOLOGY

The chemoreceptor trigger zone and the vomiting center are involved in chemotherapy-induced nausea and vomiting. The chemoreceptor trigger zone is located in the area postrema of the fourth ventricle. This area is outside the blood-brain barrier and has a rich vascular supply, making it susceptible to irritation by anticancer agents and their metabolites. The vomiting center is located in the medulla oblongata and is responsible for mediating the physiologic events of the emetic response, including contraction of the abdominal muscle and diaphragm, tachycardia, vasoconstriction, salivation, diaphoresis, and intestinal retroperistalsis. Stimulation of the vomiting center through the afferent nerves may originate in the chemoreceptor trigger zone, gastrointestinal tract, vestibular system, higher cortical centers, or the limbic system.

SYMPTOMS AND ASSESSMENTS

Patient risk factors for experiencing nausea and vomiting include poor control during earlier chemotherapy, female gender, history of low alcohol intake (< 100 g/d), and younger age. Patients with high alcohol intake for several years may experience less nausea and vomiting with emetogenic anticancer therapy.

The emetic effect of an anticancer agent can be reliably measured by counting the number of episodes of nausea or vomiting that occur in a 24-hour period. This measure has been shown to correlate well with a patient's satisfaction with their emetic control [1]. The National Cancer Institute (NCI) Common Toxicity Criteria grades for vomiting, which are based on the number of episodes in 24 hours, are a useful means of comparing the severity of emetic events, both within the same patient and across therapies.

Anticancer agents can be categorized as having high (occurring in at least 30% of patients), intermediate (10% to 30% frequency), or low (< 10% frequency) emetogenic potential.

Agents that typically induce nausea and vomiting in 90% or more of patients include [2] cisplatin ($\geq$ 50 mg/m^2), mechlorethamine, streptozocin, cyclophosphamide (> 1500 mg/m^2), carmustine (> 250 mg/m^2), and dacarbazine.

MANAGEMENT

Although multiple mechanisms are likely to exist, serotonin receptors appear to play a significant role in acute nausea and vomiting. Pretreatment with 5-hydroxytryptamine$_3$ (5-HT$_3$) antagonists, especially when used with corticosteroids, has resulted in virtually complete control of acute emesis during the first 24 hours after chemotherapy in most patients [3]. The mechanism behind delayed nausea and vomiting is less clear-cut. Corticosteroids are the mainstay of treatment for delayed nausea and vomiting. Anxiety appears to play a role in anticipatory nausea and vomiting for which antianxiolytics, behavioral modification, and appropriate antiemetic therapy can be beneficial.

Chemotherapy-induced nausea and vomiting is classified as acute (occurring during or up to 24 hours after chemotherapy), delayed (occurring > 24 hours after chemotherapy), or anticipatory (occurring before administration of chemotherapy).

Tables 26-1 to 26-3 provide guidelines for appropriate antiemetic therapy. The contents of these tables are based on guidelines developed by the American Society of Clinical Oncologists [3], the Multinational Association of Supportive Care in Cancer [2], and the American Society of Health-System Pharmacists [4].

General principles for administering antiemetic therapy [3] are as follows: antiemetic therapy for combination chemotherapy should be based on the most highly emetogenic agent; oral agents are as effective as intravenous agents at biologically equivalent doses; single doses can often be used instead of multiple doses with equivalent effectiveness; only doses with proven efficacy are recommended.

Table 26-1. Prevention of Nausea and Vomiting Induced by Chemotherapy of High Emetogenic Potential*

Chemotherapeutic Agent	Acute (0–24 h)	Delayed (> 24 h)
Actinomycin-D	5-HT$_3$ antagonist plus corticosteroid†	Corticosteroid plus either metoclopramide or 5-HT$_3$ antagonist†
Carboplatin		
Carmustine		
Cisplatin		
Cyclophosphamide		
Cytarabine		
Dacarbazine		
Daunorubicin		
Doxorubicin		
Epirubicin		
Hexamethylmelamine		
Idarubicin		
Ifosfamide		
Lomustine		
Mechlorethamine		
Streptozocin		

*Occurs in at least 30% of patients.
†See Tables 26-4 and 26-5.

Table 26-2. Prevention of Nausea and Vomiting Induced by Chemotherapy of Intermediate Emetogenic Potential*

Chemotherapeutic Agent	Acute (0–24 h)	Delayed (> 24 h)
Docetaxel	Pretreatment with corticosteroid (see Table 26-5)	No routine use of preventive antiemetics.
Etoposide		
Gemcitabine		
Irinotecan		
Mitomycin		
Mitoxantrone		
Paclitaxel		
Teniposide		

*Occurs in 10% to 30% of patients.

STOMATITIS AND MUCOSITIS

Those cells comprising the mucous lining of the mouth and esophagus provide a protective lining against bacteria, fungus, chemicals, and irritants. The balanced environment of the oral cavity requires a functioning mucous lining, oral flora, proper occlusion, care of gingiva and dentition, and production of saliva. Anticancer therapies can disrupt this protective barrier in various ways, leading to toxicity that can vary from annoying to serious morbidity and occasionally hospitalization and mortality.

Table 26-3. Prevention of Nausea and Vomiting Induced by Chemotherapy of Low Emetogenic Potential*

Chemotherapeutic Agent	Acute (0–24 h)	Delayed (> 24 h)
2-Chlodeoxyadenosine	No routine use of preventive emetics	No routine use of preventive antiemetics
Bleomycin		
Busulphan		
Chlorambucil		
Fludarabine		
Fluorouracil		
Hydoxyurea		
L-asparaginase		
Melphalan		
Mercaptopurine		
Methotrexate		
Tamoxifen		
Thioguanine		
Vinblastine		
Vincristine		
Vindesine		
Vinorelbine		

Occurs in fewer than 10% of patients.

Pathophysiology

Chemotherapies that are most likely to produce mucositis are cytotoxics with mechanisms of action that affect actively dividing cells. These classes of drugs include anthracyclines, alkylating agents, antimetabolites, fluoropyrimidines, antifolates, vinca alkaloids, topoisomerase I and II inhibitors, nucleoside analogues, epipodophyllotoxins, and nitrosoureas. It is estimated that between 40% and 70% of patients receiving chemotherapy experience mucositis during active treatment, the higher rates being seen in patients undergoing bone marrow transplantation.

Risk factors for developing therapy-related mucositis include hematologic malignancies, patient age less than 20 years, poor oral health (baseline periodontal disease), class of drug and intensity of regimen administered, and radiation therapy to the head and neck [5]. Despite being used at standard dosage, cytotoxic chemotherapy can destroy cells lining the upper gastrointestinal tract, thus allowing bacteria volume to increase, invade, and inflame normal tissues resulting in tissue necrosis.

Symptoms and Assessments

The classic symptoms of pain, ulceration, bleeding dysphagia, and infection are related to tissue damage. The NCI grading system uses these symptoms to assign a level of severity to mucositis. Assignment of grading can be a useful guideline for patient management and subsequent chemotherapy dose reduction. These symptoms can lead to decreased nutritional status, hospitalization for management of infection, pain, or nutrition and, at times, cause patients to withdraw from therapy. Some patients have described severe mucositis as "having a mouthful of broken glass" or "it's like having a thousand open ulcers and someone pours acid on them."

Radiation-induced mucositis is a known adverse event that occurs in 100% of patients receiving treatment for head and neck cancer. The oral effects of radiation therapy go beyond mucositis and include osteonecrosis (long-term sequelae) and significant decrease in saliva production that can produce loss of appetite. The NCI toxicity criteria have a separate scale for radiation-induced mucositis.

Treatment regimens for mucositis can be divided into prevention (Table 26-7) and primary treatment (Tables 26-8 and 26-9).

Table 26-4. Doses and Schedules of Antiemetics with High Activity

Antiemetic Agent	Dose and Schedule per Published Guidelines*	Dose and Schedule per Package Insert
5-HT$_3$ antagonists		
Dolasetron	PO: 100 mg prior to chemotherapy	PO: 100 mg prior to chemotherapy
	IV:100 mg or 1.8 mg/kg prior to chemotherapy	IV:100 mg or 1.8 mg/kg prior to chemotherapy
Granisetron	PO: 2 mg prior to chemotherapy	PO: 2 mg prior to chemotherapy, or 1 mg bid
	IV: 1 mg or 10 µg/kg prior to chemotherapy	IV: 10 µg/kg prior to chemotherapy
Ondansetron	PO: 12–24 mg prior to chemotherapy	PO: 0.15 mg/kg prior to chemotherapy and repeated 4 and 8 h later, or 32 mg IV prior to chemotherapy
	IV: 8 mg or 0.15 mg/kg prior to chemotherapy	PO prior to chemotherapy, then tid for up to 1–2 d after chemotherapy completed
		10–20 mg IV prior to chemotherapy; 8 mg IV followed by 4 mg PO every 6 h × 4 doses
Corticosteroids		
Dexamethasone	IV: 20 mg prior to chemotherapy	None recommended
	For delayed emesis, PO 8 mg bid for 2–3 d (3–4 d for high-dose cisplatin)	
Methylprednisolone	IV: 40–125 mg prior to chemotherapy (may use equivalent doses of methylprednisolone in place of dexamethasone if desired)	

Adapted from Gralla et al. [1] and the Antiemetic Subcommittee of the Multinational Association of Supportive Care in Cancer [2].
IV—intravenously; PO—orally.

Management

Management of therapy-induced mucositis begins before therapy period with a complete history and physical examination, awareness of the planned therapies, and a patient-education program. Combination therapy standards for local treatment of mucositis are numerous and can be based on institution preference.

Interleukin-11 increases mucosal cell proliferation in animal models of chemotherapy or radiotherapy-induced mucositis. Results from recent phase I trials support assessment for efficacy in randomized trials.

A promising, although currently unapproved, agent in clinical trials is keratinocyte growth factor (KGF). This is a recombinant form of a naturally occurring epithelial tissue growth factor that stimulates the growth and development of cells that comprise the surface lining of the gastrointestinal tract. KGF is in phase 2 clinical trials to determine whether it can reduce the severity and duration of oral mucositis when administered to cancer patients receiving some forms of chemotherapy and radiation therapy.

Preventive treatment of patients undergoing mucositis-producing therapy, particularly radiation therapy to the head and neck, starts with a pretherapy comprehensive dental examination. Patients benefit by physicians' using an interdisciplinary approach to management as outlined in the NIH consensus statement (1989) [16], which recommends including a preventative dental oncology service during the treatment planning stage.

Dental disease is a potential source of infection and, when possible, ought to be corrected before beginning therapy. Examples of this include poorly fitted dentures, plaque formation, periactical or periodontal disease, third molars, and dental caries.

Topical fluorides provide most effective protection from radiation-induced injury and can be applied using various formulations: rinses, gels, or drips [17]. When patients develop xerostomia (dryness of the mouth because of thickened, reduced, or absent salivary flow), they can no longer distinguish between sweet and sour tastes. This leads to poor nutrition, weight loss, and confounding illnesses.

Treatment includes monitoring medications, nutritional status, and plaque development as well as periodontal disease. Mechanical débridement of the tongue with a soft toothbrush and spraying formulations allow the taste buds to function properly during food intake. Therapy-induced decrease in the quantity and quality of saliva can benefit by preventive addition of sialagogues. These saliva substitutes, such as Xerolube (RP Scherer, Inc., Basking Ridge, NJ) or Salivart (Gebauer Company, Cleveland, OH) can be applied four to six times per day in rinse form. Pilocarpine can stimulate saliva flow from the parotid glands.

CHEMOTHERAPY-INDUCED DIARRHEA

Diarrhea is a common side-effect of a number of chemotherapeutic regimens, especially those including 5-fluorouracil (5-FU) and irinotecan. From published clinical trials, the incidence of "any" diarrhea ranged from 26% to 56% and the incidence of "severe" diarrhea was 5% to 23% in patients with advanced colorectal cancer receiving 5-FU–based chemotherapy [19]. The addition of leucovorin or other biochemical modulators of 5-FU has been shown to increase the frequency and severity of diarrhea in several randomized trials. Other chemotherapy agents that can produce diarrhea include capecitabine, UFT, methotrexate, topotecan, and cytosine arabinoside. If not promptly evaluated and treated, chemotherapy-induced diarrhea (CID) can lead to hospitalization and death.

Pathophysiology

The pathophysiologic factors of CID are not completely understood in relation to most chemotherapeutic agents; however, it is thought to be a multifactorial process affecting the small bowel. The mechanisms for CID depend on the causative agent. Fluoropyrimidines have been shown to cause mitotic arrest of the intestinal epithelial crypt cells that results in a relative increase of immature secretory cells to mature absorptive cells. This imbalance leads to abnormal absorption and secretion of fluid and electrolytes. Unlike 5-FU, irinotecan-induced

Table 26-5. Doses and Schedules of Antiemetics with Intermediate Activity

Antiemetic Agent	Dose and Schedule per Published Guidelines*	Dose and Schedule per Package Insert
Dopamine Receptor Antagonists		
Metoclopramide	IV:2–3 mg/kg prior to chemotherapy, and repeated 2 h after chemotherapy × 1. For delayed emesis: 30–40 mg PO bid to qid for 2–3 d (2–4 d for high-dose cisplatin)	IV: 1–2 mg/kg prior to chemotherapy, then q 2–3 h × 3–5 doses. IV or PO: 10–20 mg q 4–6 h PRN
Prochlorpherazine	PO, IV, IM: 5–20 mg q 6 h PR: 25 mg q 12 h SR: 15–30 mg q 12 h	PO, IV, IM: 5–10 mg q 6–8 h PR: 25 mg q 12 h PO: SR 10–15 mg q 12 h

IV—intravenously; IM—intramuscularly; PO—orally; PR—rectally; prn—as required; SR—?.
*Adapted from Gralla et al. [1] and the Antiemetic Subcommittee of the Multinational Association of Supportive Care in Cancer [2].

Table 26-6. Doses and Schedules of Antiemetics with Low Activity

Antiemetic Agent	Dose and Schedule per Published Guidelines*	Dose and Schedule per Package Insert
Benzodiazepines		
Diazepam	PO, IV: 5 mg q 6 h	PO: 2–10 mg bid to qid IV:2–10 mg bid 2–10 mg bid
Lorazepam	PO, SL, IM: 1–2 mg q 6 h	IV: 0.025 mg/kg or 1.5 mg/m² (max dose, 3 mg) prior to chemotherapy PO: 0.5–2 mg bid to tid prn for anxiety
Butyrophenones		
Haloperidol	PO, IV, IM: 1–4 mg q 6 h	IM: 2–5 mg prior to chemotherapy, then q 4–6 h
Phenothiazines		
Chlorpromazine	PO: 25–50 mg q 4–6 h PR: 50–100 mg q 6 h	PO: 10–25 mg PO q 4–6 h IM: 12.5–50 mg q 3–4 h PR: 50–100 mg q 6–8 h
Perphenazine	IV: 2–4 mg q 6 h	PO, IM:2–4 mg q 6 h
Thiethylperazine	PO, IM, IV: 10 mg q 4–6 h	PO, IM, PR:10 mg qid–tid

IM—intramuscularly; IV—intravenously; PO—orally; PR—rectally; prn—as required; SL—sublingually.
*Adapted from Gralla et al. [1] and the Antiemetic Subcommittee of the Multinational Association of Supportive Care in Cancer [2].

diarrhea is related to the direct toxic effects of its active metabolite, SN-38, which is formed by intestinal bacteria [19].

When a patient with cancer presents with diarrhea, the initial step is to assess the onset and duration of the diarrhea, as well as its volume. A complete evaluation may rule out other contributing factors such as infection (eg, *Clostridium difficile*, parasites), malabsorption syndromes (eg, partial small-bowel obstruction, short bowel, bowel-wall edema), dietary causes (dairy products), endocrine factors (eg, hyperthyroidism, vasoactive intestinal peptide–secreting tumor, gastrinoma), and inter-current medications (eg, antibiotics, laxatives, metoclopramide).

Management

Management of CID depends on the severity of diarrhea and its complications. In all cases, chemotherapy should be stopped immediately as well as ingestion of all lactose-containing products and laxatives. Fluid and electrolyte replacement can be given orally but an intravenous route is recommended for patients with severe watery or bloody diarrhea, overt dehydration, and cramping abdominal pain. Two opioids, diphenoxylate and loperamide, are the drugs most commonly used to treat CID. Aggressive antidiarrheal therapy with loperamide is effective in reducing the incidence of irinotecan-induced diarrhea, which typically occurs 2 to 14 days after therapy and is part of standard treatment with irinotecan. One dosage regimen for loperamide used in phase II trials of irinotecan consisted of the following: 4 mg orally at the first onset of diarrhea and then 2 mg every 2 hours (4 mg every 4 hours at night) until diarrhea-free for at least 12 hours [20]. Octreotide, a synthetic somatostatin analogue, has been shown to be effective in the control of severe diarrhea induced by 5-FU–based chemotherapy regimens [21]. Octreotide, 100 to 150 µg subcutaneously every 8 hours, is generally used in treating patients who continue to experience low-grade diarrhea after 24 hours of loperamide therapy as well as those with more severe diarrhea; however, because the optimal dose of octreotide has not been determined, the dose may need to be increased to 500 to 1500 µg as subcutaneous or intravenous bolus every 8 hours [22]. Octreotide LAR, a depot preparation of the long-acting SMS analogue octreotide, is under clinical investigation for the prophylaxis of CID due to irinote-can-containing regimens. A proposed algorithm for the treatment of CID is presented in Figure 26-1 [19].

CONSTIPATION

Pathophysiology

Constipation may occur in patients due to change in physiologic factors, habits, the progression of disease, or administered therapy [23]. Factors that can predispose a patient to constipation include advancing age, inactivity, change in diet, depression, or physical obstruction. Of course, many of these factors are not unique to the patient with cancer. During the course of therapy or disease progression, metabolic disturbances, such as dehydration, nausea and vomiting, hypercalcemia, and hypokalemia can lead to constipation as well. Additionally, damage to nerves central to bowel function will lead to constipation; among these are damage to the sacral plexus, cauda equina, or spinal cord. Drug-induced constipation is common in cancer patients, although it is more often attributed to concomitant medications than the primary anticancer therapy. For example, vinca alkaloids are known to produce a neurotoxicity of which constipation is one sequela. Other constipation-inducing medications commonly prescribed to patients with cancer include opioids, drugs with anti-cholinergic actions, antacids, diuretics, iron, or 5-HT$_3$ antagonists.

Symptoms and Assessments

Various clinical signs and symptoms are associated with constipation including nausea, vomiting, anorexia, abdominal distension and

---

Table 26-8. General Treatment Measures

Analgesics, topical, oral, or systemic for pain control
    This includes narcotics for significant pain
Maalox (Novartis Consumer Health, Inc., Summit, NJ) and Mylanta (Johnson & Johnson–Merck Consumer Pharmaceuticals, Ft. Washington, PA)
    30 mL; frequently used in combination therapy
Diphenhydramine
    30 mL; frequently used in combination therapy
Nystatin
    30 mL; frequently used in combination therapy
Imidazoles (ketoconazole or fluconazole)
    Useful for patients with *Candida*; may have limited use in patients who are not eating
Sucralfate
    Topical application may confer benefit with one placebo-controlled, randomized study
        showing that a decrease in mucositis, pain, and dysphagia is seen in the sucralfate group
Acyclovir
    Particularly useful for those patients undergoing bone marrow transplant and test positive for
        Herpes simplex virus antibody (50%–90% of patients) [10]
Allopurinol
    A negative trial was reported in patients treated with 5-FU [11]
Vitamin E
    One small study was positive for reduced mucositis [12]
β-carotene, MGI 209 (Oratect Gel)
    One small study has been positive for mucositis reduction
Antibiotics
    Nonabsorbable antibiotic lozenge may not substantially alter radiation-induced mucositis [13]
Granulocyte colony-stimulating factor (G-CSF)
    Oral ulcerations may frequently appear during periods of neutropenia and begin healing on
        recovery of blood counts. Studies have suggested that a reduction in mucositis is seen with
        G-CSF administration in patients with chemotherapy-induced mucositis [14], but not head
        and neck patients receiving radiochemotherapy [15].

Table 26-7. Preventive Measures

Cryotherapy
    Placement and retention of an ice chip in the patient's mouth during chemotherapy administration. Ice chips in mouth 5 minutes prior to 5-FU, continuously swished in the mouth and replenished for a total of 30 min [6]. Cryotherapy may be effective for doxorubicin-induced mucositis [7].
Saline rinses
    As effective as glycerine-based rinses and povidine iodine rinse 0.5%. Rinse 2–4 times/d; do not swallow. When combined with prophylaxis of nystatin, dexpanthenol, rutoside, and immunoglobin, incidence of radiotherapy-induced mucositis was reduced [8].
Chlorhexidine gluconate (Peridex; Zila Inc., Phoenix, AZ)
    This reduces levels of microflora and symptoms of chemotherapy-induced (but probably not radiation-induced) mucositis in most studies. Of the three large randomized trials, no clear reduction of symptoms was seen [9].
Sodium bicarbonate and peroxide rinses
    May slow mucosal regeneration.
Improve and maintain good oral hygiene
    Patients should be instructed to attend to their oral hygiene, use soft bristled brushes, floss, and use mouthwashes. If severe mucositis is present, then use of chlorhexidine-soaked foam brushes are recommended.

---

pain, and even diarrhea, the latter being related to liquefaction of impacted stool.

An approach to a patient at risk for constipation or with evidence of constipation begins with a detailed history and physical examination that would include review of the differential diagnosis and consideration of serious events (spinal cord involvement or bowel obstruction). A rectal examination is an important part of the total physical examination in such patients but is not performed in 59% of patients [24]. An abdominal radiograph can assist in determining the presence of fecal masses. Advice to all patients includes increasing fluid intake and dietary fiber and ensuring that impaction is not present.

Management

Therapy for constipation includes adding a daily stool-softening agent and occasional use of an osmotic laxative or contact cathartic (most frequently used for opioid-related constipation). In refractory cases, use of suppositories, intermittent enemas, colonic lavage, or naloxone for opioid-induced diarrhea needs to be considered. If a dose of naloxone exceeds about 5 mg, a reversal of opioid-induced analgesia may occur. If these therapies are not effective, prokinetic agents may be employed. Bethanecol, metoclopramide, and domperidone are among this class of agents whereas cisapride has been withdrawn from the US market. Of note, the current toxicity scale ranks constipation intensity by the type of therapy administered, not symptoms or signs.

GASTROINTESTINAL BLEEDING

Pathophysiology

Patients undergoing treatment for cancer occasionally experience gastrointestinal bleeding. Common causes of upper gastrointestinal bleeding, such as peptic ulceration, erosive gastritis, varices, and esophagogastric tears, need to be considered. Cytotoxic chemotherapy, corticosteroids, and anti-inflammatory drugs may induce or exacerbate gastritis or esophagitis. Intractable nausea and vomiting can lead to an

---

Table 26-9. Examples of Combination Treatments of Mucositis

Treatment of Mucositis and Pain

Dephenhydramine (Benadryl; Pfizer Warner-Lambert Consumer Group; Morris Plains, NJ; 12.5 mg/5 mL)
   30 mL
Viscous lidocaine, 2%
   30 mL
Diphenhydramine, 12.5 mg/5 mL
   30 mL
Tetracycline or penicillin, 125 mg/5 mL suspension
   60 mL
Nystatin oral suspension, 100,000 U/mL
   45 mL
Viscous xylocaine 2%
   30 mL
Hydrocortisone suspension, 10 mg/5 mL
   30 mL
Sterile water
   45 mL

Adapted from Sonis [5].

---

esophagogastric tear (Mallory-Weiss syndrome). Inasmuch as gastric erosions frequently develop in patients with increased intracranial pressure, patients with brain tumors or brain metastases are at risk. Primary tumors of the esophagus and stomach generally cause chronic blood loss but rarely produce massive bleeding. Lower gastrointestinal bleeding is commonly associated with colorectal and anal cancers. Among nongastrointestinal cancers, melanoma that has metastasized to the bowel is one of the most frequent causes of bleeding. However, common causes of this finding include hemorrhoids, anal fissures, and fistulas, as well as infections. Upper and lower gastrointestinal bleeding can be complicated by chemotherapy-induced thrombocytopenia and coagulation defects.

Symptoms and Assessments

A patient who is bleeding requires rapid evaluation to assess the site, extent, and rate of bleeding. Maintaining adequate intravascular volume and hemodynamic stability is a primary concern. Before performing a history and physical examination, vital signs should be obtained, blood sent for typing and cross-matching, and a large-bore intravenous line placed. The history and physical examination should determine the choice of invasive diagnostic procedures. Hematemesis almost always indicates proximal bleeding. Melena usually indicates bleeding from the esophagus, stomach, or duodenum, but lower lesions can produce melena if gastrointestinal transit time is prolonged. If an upper gastrointestinal source for the bleeding is suggested, nasogastric aspiration should be performed to confirm whether the bleeding is proximal to the ligament of Treitz. After a nasogastric tube is in place, saline irrigation may be initiated to assess the rate of bleeding and clear the stomach of old blood in preparation for possible endoscopy. Hematochezia generally indicates bleeding distal to the ligament of Treitz and is evaluated by digital examination, anoscopy, or sigmoidoscopy. Endoscopy is the most accurate diagnostic procedure for both upper and lower bleeding. Two additional procedures may be useful if endoscopy is nondiagnostic: radiolabeled erythrocyte scans and arteriography. Radiolabeled erythrocyte scans are more sensitive than arteriography in detecting blood loss of 0.1 mL/min.

Management

Management often depends on the source of the bleeding. The use of blood products is determined by the clinical and laboratory parameters. Diffuse upper bleeds associated with chemotherapy are generally managed conservatively with intravenous H_2 blockers. The American College of Gastroenterology recommends octreotide, 50µg IV bolus followed by 50 µg/h X 5 days, for acute management of bleeding esophageal varices [25]. Intravenous vasopressin is usually reserved for persistent bleeding because of potentially serious side effects. Endoscopic coagulation with a yttrium-aluminum-garnet laser, heater probe, or electrocautery can control single or multiple bleeding sites. External beam radiation to primary tumors may also be an effective alternative to these procedures. If upper gastrointestinal lesions are associated with arterial blood loss at 0.5 mL/min, radiographic embolization may be helpful in controlling bleeding. Endoscopic sclerosis and banding of varices can be effective in treating bleeding esophageal varices. Depending on the patient, surgery is an option when nonoperative measures have failed and the source of bleeding can be excised.

ANOREXIA

Pathophysiology

Anorexia is a loss of appetite that becomes problematic when it leads to undesired weight loss. Cancer-related causes are multiple, includ-

---

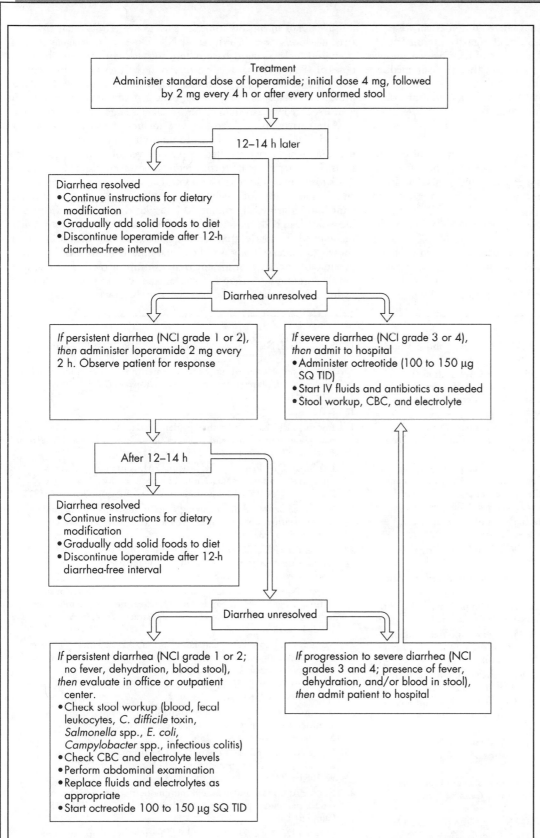

Treatment
Administer standard dose of loperamide; initial dose 4 mg, followed by 2 mg every 4 h or after every unformed stool

12–14 h later

Diarrhea resolved
• Continue instructions for dietary modification
• Gradually add solid foods to diet
• Discontinue loperamide after 12-h diarrhea-free interval

Diarrhea unresolved

If persistent diarrhea (NCI grade 1 or 2), then administer loperamide 2 mg every 2 h. Observe patient for response

If severe diarrhea (NCI grade 3 or 4), then admit to hospital
• Administer octreotide (100 to 150 μg SQ TID)
• Start IV fluids and antibiotics as needed
• Stool workup, CBC, and electrolyte

After 12–14 h

Diarrhea resolved
• Continue instructions for dietary modification
• Gradually add solid foods to diet
• Discontinue loperamide after 12-h diarrhea-free interval

Diarrhea unresolved

If persistent diarrhea (NCI grade 1 or 2; no fever, dehydration, blood stool), then evaluate in office or outpatient center.
• Check stool workup (blood, fecal leukocytes, C. difficile toxin, Salmonella spp., E. coli, Campylobacter spp., infectious colitis)
• Check CBC and electrolyte levels
• Perform abdominal examination
• Replace fluids and electrolytes as appropriate
• Start octreotide 100 to 150 μg SQ TID

If progression to severe diarrhea (NCI grades 3 and 4; presence of fever, dehydration, and/or blood in stool), then admit patient to hospital

FIGURE 26-1

Recommended treatment algorithm for chemotherapy-induced diarrhea. *C. difficile*—*Clostridium difficile*; *E. coli*—*Escherichia coli*; CBC—complete blood count; NCI—National Cancer Institute; SQ—subcutaneous; TID—three times daily. (*Adapted from* Wadler *et al.* [19].)

ing metabolic or cytokine abnormalities related to underlying disease, malabsorption syndromes, obstruction of the gastrointestinal tract, and diagnosis-related depression. Side effects of therapies commonly administered to cancer patients (*eg*, anticancer therapy, pain medication) can also result in anorexia.

Side effects that may be related to anorexia include mucositis, nausea, vomiting, constipation, and diarrhea.

Symptoms and Assessment

Patient interview, physical examination, and a review of current medications are necessary components for discerning the cause(s) of anorexia in individual patients. Although preferences vary, therapeutic intervention should be considered when patients lose of 5% of their weight over a 6-month period [26].

Management

Appropriate management of side effects of therapy assists in the treatment or prevention of anorexia. Previous sections of this chapter review guidelines for management of these side effects. If needed, additional intervention may include a nutritional assessment and diet plan, and possible use of an appetite stimulant such as megestrol acetate (Megace; Bristol-Meyers Squibb, Princeton, NJ). Doses of that agent ranging from 160 to 1600 mg/d have been associated with benefit; however, doses of 480 to 800 mg/d have achieved the best results with acceptable levels if side effects [27]. An oral suspension form is available that provides convenient dosing for the patient. Unfortunately, the weight gain associated with use of megestrol acetate is largely in adipose tissue.

Alternatives to megestrol acetate include therapy with corticosteroids such as dexamethasone, methylprednisolone, and prednisolone, which have resulted in patient weight gain during clinical trials. Long-term use of corticosteroids, however, requires increasing doses to maintain effect and can exacerbate progressive muscle wasting and weakness [26]. Although not reported in cancer patients, recombinant human growth hormone (0.1 mg/kg/d) has been effective in increasing lean body mass in HIV-positive patients so long as dosing is maintained. Similarly, thalidomide, 100 mg four times/d, has been shown to increase body weight in patients who are HIV positive, presumably because of an antitransforming growth factor effect. However, antitumor necrosis factor agents such as pentoxifylline and hydrazine sulfate have not been effective in therapy for anorexia.

REFERENCES

1. Gralla RJ, Clark RA, Kris MG, *et al.*: Methodology in anti-emetic trials. *Eur J Cancer* 1991, 27:S5–S8.

2. Antiemetic Subcommittee of the Multinational Association of Supportive Care in Cancer (MASCC): Prevention of chemotherapy- and radiotherapy-induced emesis: results of the Perugia Consensus Conference. *Ann Oncol* 1998, 9:811–819.

3. Gralla RJ, Osoba D, Kris MG, *et al.*: Recommendations for the use of antiemetics: evidence-based, clinical practice guidelines. *J Clin Oncol* 1999, 17:2971–2994.

4. ASHP Commission on Therapeutics: ASHP therapeutic guidelines on the pharmacologic management of nausea and vomiting in adult and pediatric patients receiving chemotherapy or radiation therapy or undergoing surgery. *Am J Health-Syst Pharm* 1999, 56:729–764.

5. Sonis S, Clark J: Prevention and management of oral mucositis induced by antineoplastic therapy. *Oncology* 1991, 5:11–22.

6. Loprinzi CL: Alleviation of cytotoxic therapy-induced normal tissue damage. *Semin Oncol* 1995, 22:95–97.

7. Twelves C: Mouth cooling to prevent doxorubicin-induced stomatitis. *Ann Oncol* 1991, 9:695.

8. Rahn R: Povidone-iodine to prevent mucositis in patients during antineoplastic radiochemotherapy. *Dermatology* 1997, 2:57–61.

9. Karthaus M, Rosentahl C, Ganser A: Prophylaxis and treatment of chemo- and radiotherapy induced oral mucositis: are there new strategies. *Bone Marrow Transpl* 1999, 24:1095–1108.

10. Redding SW: Role of herpes simplex virus reactivation in chemotherapy-induced oral mucositis. *NCI Monogr* 1990, 9:103–105.

11. Loprinzi CL: A controlled evaluation of an allopurinol mouthwash as prophylaxis against 5-FU-induced stomatitis. *Cancer* 1990, 65:1879–1882.

12. Wadleigh R, Redman R, Graham M, *et al.*: Vitamin E in the treatment of chemotherapy -induced oral mucositis. *Am J Med* 1992, 92:481–484.

13. Okuno SH: A randomized trial of a nonabsorbable antibiotic lozenge given to alleviate radiation-induced mucositis. *Cancer* 1997, 17:2193–2199.

14. Crawford J: Reduction of oral mucositis by filgrastim (r-metHuG-CSF) in patients receiving chemotherapy. *Cytokines Cell Mol Ther* 1999, 5:187–193.

15. Schneider S, Nishimura RD, Zimmerman RP, *et al.*: Filgrastim (r-metHuG-C-CSR) and its potential use in reduction of radiation-induced oropharyngeal mucositis: an interim look at a randomized, double-blind, placebo-controlled trial. *Cytokines Cell Mol Ther* 1999, 5:175–180.

16. NIH.

17. Lockhart PB, Clark J: Pretherapy dental status of patients with malignant conditions of the head and neck. *Oral Surg Oral Med Oral Pathol Oral Radiol Endodontics* 1994, 77:236–241.

18. Leichman CG, Fleming TR, Muggia FM, *et al.*: Phase II study of fluorouracil and its modulation in advanced colorectal cancer: a Southwest Oncology Group study. *J Clin Oncol* 1995, 13:1303–1311.

19. Wadler S, Benson AB, Engelking C, *et al.*: Recommended guidelines for the treatment of chemotherapy-induced diarrhea. *J Clin Oncol* 1998, 16:3169–3178.

20. Rothenberg ML, Eckardt JR, Kuhn JG, *et al.*: Phase II trial of irinotecan in patients with progressive or rapidly recurrent colorectal cancer. *J Clin Oncol* 1996, 14:1128–1135.

21. Petrelli N, Rodriquez-Bigas M, Creaven P, *et al.*: Efficacy of somatostatin analogue (SMS), Sandostatin, for treatment of chemotherapy induced diarrhea in colorectal cancer [abstract]. *Proc Am Soc Clin Oncol* 1992, 11:170.

22. Kornblau S, Benson AB, Catalano R, *et al.*: Management of cancer treatment-related diarrhea: issue and therapeutic strategies. *J Pain Symptom Manage* 2000, 19:118–129.

23. Bruera E: Constipation in advanced cancer patients. *Support Care Cancer* 1998, 6:356–364.

24. Bruera E: The assessment of constipation in terminal cancer patients admitted to a palliative care unit: a retrospective review. *J Pain Symptom Manage* 1994, 9:515–519.

25. Grace N: Diagnosis and treatment of gastrointestinal bleeding secondary to portal hypertension. *Am J Gastroenterol* 1997, 92:1081–1091.

26. Bunn PA: Cancer and acquired immunodeficiency syndrome wasting syndromes: current and future therapies. *Semin Oncol* 1998, 25 (suppl 6):1–3.

27. Ottery FD, Walsh D, Strawford A: Pharmacologic management of anorexia/cachexia. *Semin Oncol* 1998, 25(suppl 6):35–44.

MUCOSITIS

Mucositis is a common side effect of chemotherapy and radiation therapy and may result in significant pain, dehydration, malnutrition, poor quality of life, limitation in cancer therapy, and secondary systemic infection. Radiation and certain chemotherapeutic agents cause direct damage to the oral mucosa, the severity of which depends on dose intensity, schedule, and concomitant treatment. In addition, chemotherapy-induced myelosuppression increases the risk for serious intra-oral infections. Effective management requires thorough pretreatment assessment, correction of preexisting oral pathology, a comprehensive preventative oral hygiene program, treatment of infection, and attention to pain control.

PREVENTION AND MANAGEMENT

1. Pretreatment measures
   a. Complete oral and dental evaluation
   b. Correction of underlying pathology
2. Routine oral hygiene
   a. Daily brushing with soft brush and fluoride toothpaste
   b. Daily flossing unless severely thrombocytopenic
   c. Mouthwash four times daily
   d. Lip lubrication
3. Prophylactic measures
   a. Chlorhexidine gluconate 0.12% mouth rinse bid for intensive chemotherapy
   b. Severely myelosuppressed or HSV antibody positive patients should receive oral acyclovir, 200 mg five times per day
   c. Oral cryotherapy with ice chips for 30 min immediately before and after 5-FU
4. Mild to severe mucositis
   a. Complete examination and culture of oral cavity if indicated
   b. Patients should be on bland diet and instructed to pay strict attention to adequate fluid intake
   c. Administer topical anesthetics
   d. Administer topical or systemic antibiotics based on findings
   e. Administer systemic analgesics as needed

CAUSATIVE AGENTS

Antimetabolites: methotrexate, fluorouracil, cytosine arabinoside, mercaptopurine, hydroxyurea; **Alkylating agents:** nitrogen mustard, cyclophosphamide, ifosfamide, procarbazine; **Antibiotics:** bleomycin, doxorubicin, daunorubicin, plicamycin, mitomycin; **Vinca alkaloids:** vincristine, vinblastine; **Biologics:** IL-2, IFN-α

PATHOLOGIC PROCESS

Direct stomatotoxicity of chemotherapeutic agents due to high proliferative rate of mucosal cells of the upper digestive tract, resulting in mucosal atrophy that may lead to frank ulceration, and indirect stomatotoxicity due to chemotherapy or biologic-induced myelosuppression and oral infections from bacterial, fungal, and viral colonizing pathogens

DIFFERENTIAL DIAGNOSES

Bacterial: *Pseudomonas, Klebsiella, Escherichia coli, Serratia, Enterobacter, Proteus, Staphylococcus, Streptococcus;* **Fungal:** *Candida;* **Viral:** herpes simplex, varicella zoster

PATIENT ASSESSMENT

Baseline assessment: clinical evaluation of oral health, identify risk factors (performance status, age, agents given), education of family and other care providers; **Overt symptoms:** complete oral examination and grading of toxicity, CBC, culture of lesions if appropriate, attention to fluid status

TOXICITY GRADING

1	2	3	4
Painless erythema	Painful erythema	Painful erythema	Requires parenteral or enteral support
Ulcers	Edema	Edema	
Mild soreness	Ulcers	Ulcers	
	Can eat	Cannot eat	

NAUSEA AND VOMITING

Nausea and vomiting are among the most distressing and feared side effects of cancer treatment. Elucidation of the pathophysiology of chemotherapy-induced nausea and vomiting and the role of a variety of neurotransmitters have greatly enhanced prevention and treatment. Chemotherapeutic agents differ markedly in their emetic potential, and symptoms depend on dose, schedule, and concomitant medications. There is also considerable interpatient variability. Effective management requires patient and family education and early prophylactic treatment. Combinations of antiemetics with differing mechanisms of actions and side effects are more effective than single agents alone.

PREVENTION AND MANAGEMENT

1. Prophylactic administration of antiemetic therapy based on emetogenic potential of the chemotherapy (*see* Table 26-4)
2. Provide patient support and guidelines for psychological and behavioral adjustments

TOXICITY GRADING

1	2	3	4
Vomiting	2–5 episodes in 24 h	6–10 episodes in 24 h	> 10 episodes in 24 h or requiring parenteral support
1 episode in 24 h			
Nausea			
Able to eat, reasonable intake	Intake significantly reduced	No significant intake	

CAUSATIVE AGENTS

Highly emetogenic: cisplatin, dacarbazine, nitrogen mustard, streptozocin; **Moderately emetogenic:** cyclophosphamide, ifosfamide, cytosine arabinoside, hexamethylmelamine, carboplatin, doxorubicin, mitomycin C, procarbazine, etoposide, paclitaxel; **Minimally emetogenic:** fluorouracil, bleomycin, methotrexate, vincristine, vinblastine

PATHOLOGIC PROCESS

Neuronal reflex arch mediated by the chemoreceptor trigger zone rich in serotoninergic and dopaminergic receptors. After further coordination in the vomiting center in the central nervous system, efferent neuronal pathways mediate autonomic and somatic responses that result in nausea and vomiting.

DIFFERENTIAL DIAGNOSES

Chemotherapy; narcotics; radiation to brain, abdomen, chest, spine; brain metastasis; gastrointestinal or biliary tract obstruction; hypercalcemia; hyponatremia; uremia

PATIENT ASSESSMENT

Increased risk of severe symptoms if history of "nervous stomach," motion sickness, poor emetic control with previous chemotherapy; patients with a history of heavy alcohol tolerate chemotherapy with less nausea and vomiting; young patients experience more anticipatory nausea and vomiting and are more susceptible to the extrapyramidal side effects of many antiemetics

DIARRHEA

Diarrhea results from a direct toxic effect on the gastrointestinal mucosa. It is most frequently seen with antimetabolites and is related to dose and intensity of drug administration. There is considerable interpatient variability. Symptoms may range from mild to severe. All chemotherapy should be stopped at the first signs of significant diarrhea. Appropriate management requires strict attention to hydration and the institution of antidiarrheals and antibiotics if the diarrhea is severe or bloody or there is concomitant fever or neutropenia. For patients experiencing severe diarrhea, all subsequent chemotherapy should be given with great caution and at reduced dose intensity.

PATIENT ASSESSMENT

For moderate or severe diarrhea: evaluation of volume status; CBC, electrolytes, liver function tests; abdominal radiographic studies; blood cultures; stool leukocytes; stool cultures for enteric pathogens, ova, parasites; stool *Clostridium difficile* toxin titer

MANAGEMENT AND INTERVENTION

1. Mild to moderate diarrhea
   a. Maintain adequate fluid intake
   b. Provide antidiarrheal medication (*see* Figure 26–1)
2. Severe diarrhea
   a. Stop chemotherapy until resolution
   b. Admit to hospital if bloody stools, severe crampy abdominal pain, fever, dehydration
   c. Provide IV fluids, antibiotics, antidiarrheal medication

TOXICITY GRADING

1	2	3	4
Increase of 2–3 stools/d over pretreatment	Increase of 4–6 stools/d, or nighttime stools, or moderate cramping	Increase of 7–9 stools/d, or incontinence, or severe cramping	Increase of > 10 stools/d, or grossly bloody diarrhea, or need for parenteral support

CAUSATIVE AGENTS
Antimetabolites, particularly 5-FU, methotrexate, cytosine arabinoside

PATHOLOGIC PROCESS
Direct toxic effect on rapidly proliferating mucosal cells of the small and large intestine

DIFFERENTIAL DIAGNOSES
Direct toxic effect of chemotherapeutic agent; gastrointestinal infection—*C. difficile*, gram-negative enteritis, viral enteritis, parasitic infection; other drugs, especially antibiotics; malabsorption; large bowel obstruction; dumping syndrome

A classification of cancer-associated renal and metabolic abnormalities is shown in Table 27-1. Acute and chronic renal failure; proteinuria (the hallmark of glomerular involvement); hemorrhagic cystitis; fluid and electrolyte disorders, including hypercalcemia, hyponatremia, and syndrome of inappropriate antidiuresis (SIAD); and ectopic adrenocorticotropic hormone (ACTH) syndrome may all be associated with cancer or the treatment of malignant diseases (or both). This chapter highlights these renal and metabolic abnormalities, focusing on the clinical features, causes, and treatment of these disorders.

RENAL COMPLICATIONS

ACUTE RENAL FAILURE

Prerenal Azotemia

Cancer-associated acute renal failure affects the clinical management of patients and has an impact on patient morbidity and mortality. Acute renal failure can be classified into prerenal, postrenal, and intrinsic causes of renal dysfunction (Table 27-1). This classification serves as a framework for diagnostic and therapeutic management.

Table 27-1. Cancer-Associated Renal Abnormalities

Acute renal failure
Prerenal
Obstruction
  Urethral
  Bladder neck — prostatic or bladder cancer
  Bilateral ureteral — cervical or testicular cancer
Intrinsic
  Vascular
  Interstitial nephritis
    Allergic interstitial nephritis
    Tumor infiltration
    Radiation nephritis
  Glomerulonephritis
  Acute tubular necrosis
    Nephrotoxic
      Endogenous — uric acid, myoglobin, immunoglobulins, hypercalcemia
      Exogenous — contrast, antibiotics, analgesics, antineoplastic agents
    Ischemic (sepsis, prolonged prerenal)
  Associated with bone marrow transplantation

Chronic renal failure
Prolonged obstruction — prostate, cervical, uterine, testicular, primary renal cancers or retroperitoneal lymphoma; stones
Nephrotoxic — antineoplastic agents and radiation

Glomerulonephropathies (proteinuria)
With Hodgkin's disease (minimal change GN)
With solid tumors (membranous GN)
With antineoplastic agents

Hemorrhagic cystitis

Metabolic disorders
Hyponatremia and SIAD
Hypercalcemia
Ectopic ACTH syndrome

ACTH—adrenocorticotropic hormone; GN—glomerulonephritis; SIAD—syndrome of inappropriate antidiuresis.

Anorexia, vomiting, and diarrhea associated with either tumor involvement or chemotherapy may cause volume depletion resulting in prerenal azotemia. Clues to the development of acute renal failure because of volume depletion include a history suggesting volume loss, signs of volume depletion on physical examination, an elevated BUN-to-creatinine ratio (> 20:1), and a low urinary sodium value and fractional excretion of sodium (< 20 mEq/L and < 1%). Patients with cardiomyopathy causing decreased renal perfusion and patients with a reduced effective circulating volume (as in cirrhosis, nephrotic syndrome, or sepsis with vasodilation) also may develop prerenal acute renal failure characterized by an elevated BUN-to-creatinine ratio and low urinary sodium. Nonsteroidal antiinflammatory drugs may potentiate acute renal failure in patients with reduced effective circulating volume and should be avoided in such patients. The treatment of prerenal acute renal failure is volume repletion or correction of the reduced renal perfusion (*eg*, improving cardiac function).

Obstruction

Obstruction may occur at any site along the urinary tract and cause postrenal acute renal failure. Common causes of postrenal acute renal failure in patients with cancer are cervical and testicular (especially seminoma) carcinomas that cause ureteral obstruction, lymphoma with periaortic lymphadenopathy causing ureteral obstruction, and prostate and bladder carcinomas causing bladder outlet obstruction. Metastatic carcinoma also may infiltrate the retroperitoneal space and tissues and obstruct the ureters [1]. A history of urinary urgency, frequency, and reduced urine output with physical findings of a distended bladder and abdominal or pelvic mass suggests obstruction of the lower urinary tract, such as bladder outlet obstruction. The acute onset of flank pain may occur with rapid dilation of the renal pelvis and ureter proximal to an obstruction. Many cases of obstruction, however, are asymptomatic and diagnosed serendipitously by routine radiographic studies done for tumor monitoring (*eg*, bone scan, computed tomographic [CT] scan).

In acute renal failure caused by obstruction, the BUN-to-creatinine ratio is usually elevated. Obstruction is confirmed by finding hydronephrosis on ultrasound examination of the kidneys. On rare occasions, postrenal acute renal failure may result from ureteral encasement. In such cases, obstruction may occur without hydronephrosis. Clinically suspected obstruction requires further urologic investigation, usually by contrast retrograde radiologic studies. Relief of obstruction can be accomplished by placement of either ureteral stents or nephrostomy tubes. The degree of resolution of the acute renal failure depends in part on the duration of the obstruction. In some cases, such as advanced cervical carcinoma, uremia may develop. Aggressive intervention for the renal failure (relief of obstruction, dialysis) must be discussed candidly in view of the overall prognosis.

Once prerenal and postrenal causes for acute renal failure are excluded in the azotemic patient with cancer, intrinsic causes of acute renal failure must be considered (Table 27-1). Intrinsic acute renal failure is characterized by a preserved BUN-to-creatinine ratio (10–20:1) and can be due to thrombosis or infarction of the renal vessels (a rare cause for acute renal failure), interstitial inflammation (acute allergic interstitial nephritis or lymphomatous infiltration), glomerulonephritis (characterized by proteinuria), or acute tubular necrosis (ATN) caused by ischemia or nephrotoxins [1]. ATN due to either ischemic (prolonged prerenal failure or sepsis) or nephrotoxic (aminoglycoside or contrast agent) causes is the most common form of acute renal failure. Certain types of intrinsic acute renal failure are more common to patients with cancer and are discussed briefly.

TUMOR INFILTRATION AND RADIATION NEPHRITIS

Tumor and lymphomatous infiltration of the kidneys rarely cause renal failure but should be considered in cases of unexplained acute renal failure in predisposed patients [2]. Renal biopsy may be required to make the diagnosis. Treatment of the underlying malignancy may improve renal function [2]. Radiation can cause a spectrum of renal problems, including malignant hypertension and acute and chronic renal failure. Radiation-induced chronic renal failure occurs with exposure to more than 2500 rads and is characterized by hypertension, anemia, fatigue, and proteinuria more than 1 g per 24 hours [3]. Histologically, interstitial nephritis accompanied by widespread glomerular sclerosis, tubular atrophy, and arteriolar fibrinoid necrosis is seen [3]. The recognition of radiation nephritis and limiting renal exposure to radiation have reduced the incidence of this form of renal failure.

ACUTE TUBULAR NECROSIS

Acute tubular necrosis can be characterized etiologically as ischemic or nephrotoxic. The classic finding in either type of ATN is dirty brown casts on urinalysis. Because with ATN renal tubular function is impaired, little tubular reabsorption of sodium occurs. Thus, urinary sodium concentration and fractional excretion of sodium are high in ATN. The endogenous toxins associated with intrinsic acute renal failure include hypercalcemia, myoglobin (seen in cases of rhabdomyolysis), uric acid (as in the tumor lysis syndrome), and immunoglobulins, such as in multiple myeloma and amyloidosis, in which light chains, for unexplained reasons, are nephrotoxic. Acute renal failure associated with hypercalcemia is likely multifactorial in origin but includes a direct effect of hypercalcemia that reduces glomerular filtration and volume depletion as a result of the natriuretic effect of hypercalcemia [1]. Reduction of serum calcium and repair of volume deficits generally reverse the acute renal failure. The pathophysiologic contribution of myoglobin to the development of acute renal failure in rhabdomyolysis is poorly understood. Nontraumatic rhabdomyolysis may occur in the cancer patient in a variety of settings, including electrolyte disorders (hypokalemia and hypophosphatemia) and prolonged immobilization [1]. Appropriate treatment includes urinary alkalinization and maintenance of urinary output with mannitol and/or diuretics.

Exposure to exogenous renal toxins is perhaps the most common cause of acute renal failure in patients with cancer. The widespread use of intravenous contrast agents, aminoglycoside antibiotics, amphotericin, and potentially nephrotoxic antineoplastic agents may contribute to the development of ATN in patients with cancer. The elderly (serum creatinine underestimates renal impairment caused by nephron loss with age) and those with baseline renal functional impairment from any cause are at particular risk for ATN with contrast agent or aminoglycoside exposure. Appropriate dosing of medications, hydration, and perhaps administration of acetylcysteine before contrast administration may reduce the potential for nephrotoxic ATN.

The nephrotoxicity of antineoplastic agents is shown in Table 27-2. Acute renal failure is the most commonly seen nephrotoxic complication of antineoplastic agents but cases of chronic renal failure occurring distant to chemotherapy exposure have been seen in a dose-related fashion with the nitrosureas and cisplatin. Cisplatin and high-dose methotrexate are the agents that most often cause acute renal failure. Biologic response modifiers, particularly interleukin, also may cause acute renal failure through a variety of mechanisms, including prerenal factors and glomerular and interstitial involvement [1] (Table 27-2). Brief discussions of the specific antineoplastic agents causing nephrotoxicity follow.

ALKYLATING AGENTS

Cisplatin and Carboplatin

Cisplatin (*cis*-diaminedichloroplatinum II) is among the most widely used chemotherapeutic agents with efficacy against germ cell and solid tumors [1]. Nephrotoxicity is the limiting factor in the use of cisplatin and undoubtedly is related to the renal excretion of the drug [1,4]. Reduced glomerular filtration rate and polyuria and hypomagnesemia caused by renal magnesium wasting frequently are seen with cisplatin administration [1,4]. The risk of cisplatin-induced acute renal failure can be reduced by hypertonic saline hydration and forced diuresis with mannitol or furosemide, or both [1,4]. Careful attention to baseline renal function before treatment with cisplatin is required for appropriate dosing (Table 27-3). Because renal effects of cisplatin are cumulative, clinical practice has been to discontinue cisplatin once the serum creatinine is greater than 1.5 mg/dL. However, recent studies have show that amifostine (a phosphorylated aminothiol prodrug) can reduce the frequency of cumulative cisplatin damage to the kidney without decreasing its antitumor efficacy [5]. Carboplatin appears to be less nephrotoxic than cisplatin but also can cause acute renal failure and requires careful monitoring of renal function with appropriate predosage adjustment for renal insufficiency in addition to pretreatment hydration [6].

Cyclophosphamide

Cyclophosphamide and Ifosfamide has been used for many years to treat hematologic malignancies, lymphomas, and various solid tumors. The main nephrologic-related toxicities of cyclophosphamide are hemorrhagic cystitis and impaired water excretion after high-dose (50 mg/kg body weight) therapy [1]. A sustained diuresis after high-dose cyclophosphamide therapy is needed to avoid hemorrhagic cystitis. Because of the risk of hyponatremia secondary to cyclophosphamide-induced water retention, half-normal saline infusion before and throughout cyclophosphamide administration is recommended [1].

Ifosfamide (isomeric with cyclophosphamide and activated via the same metabolic pathway) is now widely used because early studies have shown superior results. However, ifosfamide can cause proximal tubular atrophy resulting in Fanconi syndrome. This has not been seen with cyclophosphamide. In one study, 5% developed Fanconi syndrome with 15% developing subclinical tubular atrophy. Risk factors include a high cumulative dose, unilateral nephrectomy, and therapy with platinum derivatives [7,8]. The pathophysiology of ifosfamide-induced Fanconi syndrome is not known and mesna does not prevent Fanconi syndromes [9].

Nitrosureas

Streptozotocin is unique among the nitrosureas for its effects on the proximal tubule and the development of Fanconi's syndrome [1,10]. Monitoring of proteinuria is required when streptozocin is given (usually in the treatment of islet cell carcinoma of the pancreas and carcinoid tumor) [10]. Discontinuation of the drug is recommended when proteinuria develops to avoid permanent impairment of renal function [1,10]. Hypophosphatemia may be an initial manifestation of renal tubular dysfunction caused by streptozocin [1,10], and hypericosuria without hyperuricemia has been postulated as a causative event in streptozotocin-induced renal failure [11].

Chronic renal failure is the primary manifestation of nephrotoxicity of the other nitrosureas (BCNU, CCNU, methyl-CCNU), which vary in their potential for renal dysfunction, with semustine (methyl-CCNU) most commonly causing renal failure (Table 27-2). Cumulative doses of nitrosureas totaling more than 1200 to 1400 mg/m^2 are associated with irreversible renal failure that can progress to end-stage renal disease and the need for dialysis [12,13]. Such cases of renal failure may present months to years after the completion of treatment with nitrosureas, particularly with methyl-CCNU, and often in the absence of underlying or transient acute renal failure [12,13].

ANTIMETABOLITES

High-Dose Methotrexate

Although conventional-dose methotrexate rarely causes nephrotoxicity, high-dose methotrexate (25–50 mg/kg to 1–7 g/m^2) has been associated with nonoliguric acute renal failure [1]. Because methotrexate primarily is excreted renally, any alteration in renal function affects plasma methotrexate levels and the rate of methotrexate elimination. With prolonged elevation of plasma methotrexate levels, bone marrow

and gastrointestinal toxicity may occur [14]. Maintaining a high urinary volume and pH by alkalinization of the urine reduces the nephrotoxicity of high-dose methotrexate [15] and is integral to therapy with this agent. Methotrexate is poorly dialyzed [16], making management of patients with elevated methotrexate levels and renal insufficiency difficult and emphasizing the need for careful dosing of methotrexate in patients with renal dysfunction (Table 27-3).

Other Antimetabolites

Table 27-2 shows the other antimetabolites capable of causing nephrotoxicity; renal dysfunction is much less common with these agents than with high-dose methotrexate. 5-Fluorouracil has been reported to cause acute renal failure as a result of hemolytic-uremic syndrome but only when given in combination with mitomycin [1]. Gemcitabine (nucleoside analogue structurally related to cytarabine) is a new cytotoxic agent effective against pancreatic cancer. It is also being used in metastatic non–small cell lung cancer, advanced ovarian cancer, and other malignancies. There have been case reports of acute renal failure from hemolytic-uremic syndrome associated with the use of gemcitabine [17]. Abnormalities of both proximal and distal tubular function may occur with 5-azacytidine. These are manifested by hypophosphatemia, low serum bicarbonate, polyuria or glucosuria, and renal salt wasting, which can result in volume deple-

Table 27-2. Possible Nephrotoxicity of Antineoplastic Agents

Drug	High	Int	Low	Renal Effects
Alkylating agents				
Carboplatin			X	ARF
Cisplatin	X			ARF: decrease risk with hydration and forced diuresis, mannitol; CRF dose related
Cyclophosphamide			X	Doses > 50 mg/kg: impaired water excretion; hemorrhagic cystitis
Ifosfamide	X			ARF, CRF, Fanconi syndrome
Nitrosoureas				
Streptozotocin	X			Fanconi's syndrome; may cause CRF
Carmustine (BCNU)			X	CRF: delayed effects, dose related
Lomustine (CCNU)			X	CRF: delayed effects, dose related
Semustine (Methyl-CCNU)		X		CRF: delayed effects with cumulative dose > 1200 mg/m^2
Antimetabolites				
High-dose methotrexate	X			ARF
Cytosine arabinoside			X	ARF
Gemcitabine			X	HUS
5-Fluorouracil*			X	ARF
5-Azacytidine			X	ARF: proximal and distal tubular dysfunction
6-Thioguanine			X	ARF
Vincristine, vinblastine				Impaired water excretion
Antitumor antibiotics				
Mitomycin			X	Hemolytic-uremic syndrome
Mithromycin	X			ARF: dose related; rare in doses used for hypercalcemia
Doxorubicin			X	ARF: case with proteinuria, glomerular proliferation
Biologic agents				
Interferon alfa			X	AFT: interstitial nephritis; proteinuria—minimal change; MPGN
Interferon gamma		X		ARF: ATN; proteinuria
Interleukin-2		X		RF: prerenal azotemia with low fractional excretion of Na
Corynebacterium parvum			X	ARF: proliferative GN

*Given with mitomycin C.
ARF—acute renal failure; CRF—chronic renal failure; Int—intermediate; RF—renal failure.
Adapted from Weber et al. [119].

tion with hypotension and mild azotemia [18]. Supportive therapy with replacement of the lost electrolytes and minerals is required. Resolution of the acquired defects of tubular function occurs with discontinuation of 5-azacytidine [18].

ANTITUMOR ANTIBIOTICS

Mitomycin

Two patterns of mitomycin C–associated renal failure occur: a relatively uncommon dose-related acute renal failure seen with administration of mitomycin C alone [19] and a hemolytic-uremic type of renal failure seen when a combination of mitomycin C and 5-fluorouracil is given [1,20]. The latter is characterized by a microangiopathic hemolytic anemia and thrombocytopenia with acute renal failure, which on renal biopsy shows microthrombi [1,20]. Renal failure may persist and result in end-stage renal disease; fatal cases are not unusual [20]. Plasma exchange may be useful in some cases [21]. The renal failure seen with high-dose mitomycin C alone is characteristically less fulminant and related to cumulative drug dosage [1,20]. Microangiopathic hemolytic anemia is less frequent with this type of mitomycin C–induced renal dysfunction, but renal biopsy shows similar changes [20]. Mortality with this type of renal failure is also high, usually occurring within 3 to 8 months [20].

Mithromycin

Nonrenal toxicity generally limits the use of high-dose (25–50 μg/kg daily for 5 days) mithramycin [1]. Nephrotoxicity, defined as a BUN more than 25 mg/dL or a reduction in creatinine clearance, was noted in 22 of 54 patients (40%) given high-dose mithramycin for a variety of tumors [22]. Qualitative proteinuria (1+ on urine dipstick) also was noted in 78% of the patients. Underlying renal insufficiency and higher cumulative doses of mithramycin increased the risk of nephrotoxicity [22]. Histopathologic examination of renal tissue was consistent with ATN. Currently, low-dose mithramycin (25 μg/kg) is more commonly used (to treat hypercalcemia) [1]. Renal failure is much less likely with this dosage regimen. There are case reports of renal failure

associated with single doses of mithramycin used to treat hypercalcemia [23]. Renal function should be monitored with mithramycin therapy, especially in patients with underlying renal dysfunction.

Despite the development of specific renal lesions (glomerular vacuolation) in animals given anthracycline antibiotics, such as doxorubicin and daunomycin [24], nephrotoxicity rarely occurs in humans. A single case report suggested that doxorubicin causes renal toxicity [25], but there are no confirming data. Cardiac toxicity is the dose-limiting factor for doxorubicin administration and may occur at lower cumulative doses than the nephrotoxicity, thereby limiting the development of renal toxicity [1].

BIOLOGIC AGENTS

Interferons

The literature on interferon alfa–induced nephrotoxicity consists primarily of case reports documenting proteinuria and renal failure [26–28] or immune complex membranoproliferative glomerulonephritis [29]. Proteinuria and renal failure with focal segmental glomerulosclerosis and ATN on renal biopsy have been reported in a child treated with interferon gamma [30]. In addition, one of the cases of interferon alfa nephrotoxicity described acute interstitial nephritis with minimal change nephropathy on biopsy [28]. Interferons are unique in that glomerular involvement is a common feature of their nephrotoxicity. Immune complex glomerulonephritis in an HIV–positive patient treated with interferon alfa was reported [31]. The authors suggested that a disruption in immunoregulation at the renal tissue level may underlie the observed pathologic responses seen with interferon therapy [31]. Additional study of the renal effects of interferons is needed.

Interleukin-2, with or without lymphokine-activated killer cells, can cause prerenal azotemia characterized by oliguria, hypotension, and a low fractional excretion of sodium [32]. Fluid retention with edema formation also occurs, suggesting a leaky capillary syndrome associated with renal hypoperfusion [1]. The rapid development and resolution of the renal failure in most patients suggests a hemodynamic cause [33]. A case study showing reduced renal prostaglandin synthesis in the setting of increased plasma renin activity supports

Table 27-3. Dosing of Antineoplastic Agents in Patients with Renal Failure

Drug	Excreted Unchanged, %	Half-Life (Normal/ESRD Hours)	Dose for Normal Renal Function	Dose Adjustment for Renal Failure as % Reduction GFR		
				> 50	10–50	< 10
Bleomycin	60	9/20	10–20 U/m²	100	75	50
Carboplatin	50–70	6/increased	360 mg/m²	100	75	50
Cisplatin	27–45	0.3–0.5/unknown	20–50 mg/m²/d	100	50	25
Cyclophosphamide	10–15	4–7.5/10	1.5 mg/kg/d	100	75	50
Hyroxyurea	Substantial	Unknown	20–30 mg/kg/d	100	100	75
Melphalan	12	1.1–1.4/4–6	6 mg/d	100	50	20
Methotrexate	80–90	8–12/increased	15 mg/d to 12 g/m²	100	75	50
Mitomycin C	Unknown	0.5–1/unknown	20 mg/m² q 6–8 wk	100	50	Avoid
Nitrosureas	Substantial	Short/unknown	Varies	100	100	75
Prototype — methyl-CCNU		Metabolites with variable T 1/2	Irreversible toxicity at dose more than 1500 mg/m²	100	75	25–50
Streptozotocin	None	0.25/unknown	500 mg/m²/d	100	75	50

ESRD — end-stage renal disease.
Adapted from Bennett et al. [120].

this theory [34]. Patients particularly at risk for interleukin-2 acute renal failure are those with underlying renal insufficiency; the degree of renal failure was greater and the duration of renal impairment was longer in such patients [32]. Recognition of the syndrome and appropriate fluid resuscitation are required. Nephrotoxicity is less likely with constant infusion of interleukin [35].

Treatment with *Corynebacterium parvum* immunotherapy caused an immune complex proliferative glomerulonephritis acute renal failure in a small number (three of 87) of patients [36]. The renal failure resolved in all patients with discontinuation of the immunotherapy. Although *C. parvum*–induced acute renal failure is uncommon, attention to the renal function of patients treated with this antineoplastic agent is needed.

RENAL FAILURE ASSOCIATED WITH BONE MARROW TRANSPLANTATION

Renal failure that occurs in the setting of bone marrow transplantation may be caused by entities unique to this patient population. The timing of the development of acute renal failure following bone marrow transplantation may be important in defining the causative events and subsequent treatment related to the renal failure. In addition to prerenal azotemia and ATN, bone marrow transplant recipients may develop acute renal failure as a result of tumor lysis and stored marrow infusion, a hepatorenal-like acute renal failure associated with hepatic venoocclusive disease, or hemolytic-uremia syndrome as a result of cytoreductive therapy and/or with use of cyclosporine or tacrilumus [37]. The hepatorenal-like form of acute renal failure typically occurs 10 to 21 days following transplant and often is associated with amphotericin therapy and sepsis. Recently, nephrotic syndrome has been described as a manifestation of chronic graft-versus-host disease in bone marrow transplant recipients [38]. This is the most common form of acute renal failure unique to the bone marrow transplant patient. Diagnosis of this syndrome can be difficult, and dialysis is often needed. Despite such measures, mortality remains high.

CHRONIC RENAL FAILURE

As noted previously, chronic renal failure in the cancer patient may result from nephrotoxic exposure, notably from radiation and certain antineoplastic agents, particularly the nitrosureas and cisplatin (Table 27-2). Chronic renal failure in the cancer patient, however, is much more likely to be caused by obstruction. As with acute renal failure secondary to obstruction, cervical, testicular, bladder, and prostate cancers most commonly cause chronic renal failure by obstruction. The extent and duration of the obstruction are the primary factors affecting the degree of renal functional recovery with relief of the obstruction. As with obstruction-induced acute renal failure, diagnosis usually is made by ultrasound examination showing hydronephrosis. Treatment is relief of the obstruction through urologic intervention.

GLOMERULONEPHROPATHIES

The nephrotic syndrome can occur as a paraneoplastic manifestation in patients with solid tumors and lymphomas. Proteinuria is the cardinal finding, and the nephrotic syndrome (> 3.5 g protein in 24-h urine collection, hypoalbuminemia, edema) confirms glomerular involvement. The type of glomerulopathy tends to be related to the cancer: membranous glomerulopathy often is seen in patients with solid tumors (*eg*, colon and lung cancer), and minimal-change

glomerulopathy occurs in patients with Hodgkin's lymphoma [39,40]. Nephrotic syndrome also has been reported in patients with non-Hodgkin's lymphomas but occurs less commonly [39,41] and often is associated with more extensive glomerular involvement and renal failure [42]. Leukemias are less frequently associated with nephrotic syndrome; chronic lymphocytic leukemia is the type of leukemia most often associated with the nephrotic syndrome [41]. The nephrotic syndrome may precede, occur concurrently, or follow the diagnosis of cancer or lymphoma and is unrelated to the stage of the disease [41]. There is some evidence for tumor-related antigens as pathogenetic triggers in the glomerulopathies of cancer, but the precise mechanisms for the development of these syndromes are not understood [39]. Frequently, remission of the tumor results in resolution of the proteinuria, and tumor recurrence is accompanied by relapse of the proteinuria [39,41].

As discussed previously, some antineoplastic agents have been associated with the development of proteinuria (Table 27-2). The interferons and *C. parvum* are the agents most often associated with the development of proteinuria. The single case report of glomerulonephritis in a patient given doxorubicin has not been confirmed by additional reports.

UROLOGIC COMPLICATIONS

HEMORRHAGIC CYSTITIS

Uncontrolled urinary tract hemorrhage in the cancer patient is less common today because of improvements in radiation therapy dosing and the use of reducing agents such as mesna cyclophosphamide or ifosfamide therapy [43]. With both alkylating agents and radiation therapy, urothelial damage is the initiating event resulting in hemorrhagic cystitis. Underlying bleeding diathesis or the concomitant use of anticoagulants may potentiate urothelial damage and exacerbate medication-induced or radiation-induced genitourinary bleeding. Other antineoplastic agents implicated in the development of hemorrhagic cystitis include L-asparaginase, dactinomycin, mitomycin C, mithramycin, and 6-mercaptopurine [43]. The management of hemorrhagic cystitis from cancer therapy includes bladder catheterization for drainage and continuous irrigation. Intravesical cauterization and surgical intervention also may be required in refractory cases [43].

METABOLIC COMPLICATIONS

SYNDROME OF INAPPROPRIATE ANTIDIURESIS

Although there are multiple causes for this syndrome, including abnormalities of the central nervous system, various respiratory diseases, and certain pharmacologic agents, the most common cause remains malignancies, particularly small cell carcinoma of the lung. In 1957, Schwartz *et al.* [44] described two patients with bronchogenic cancer who manifested hyponatremia and continued urinary loss of sodium and postulated that this syndrome may be caused by inappropriate secretion of an antidiuretic substance. In several instances, inappropriately high circulating levels of antidiuretic hormone (ADH) have been reported, hence the term *inappropriate secretion of antidiuretic hormone* (SIADH). Because in some cases ADH may not be the causative agent, the syndrome is best referred to as SIAD.

The diagnosis requires the presence of hyponatremia, hypoosmolality, inappropriately concentrated urine, and exclusion of other conditions that can cause hyponatremia, such as renal, adrenal, thyroid, cardiac, and hepatic abnormalities and volume depletion, edematous states, and diuretic use. Other features that are characteristic but not necessary for the diagnosis include a low blood concentration of urea and uric acid and continued renal excretion of sodium [45].

PHYSIOLOGY OF ANTIDIURETIC HORMONE SECRETION

Antidiuretic hormone, also called arginine vasopressin, is a peptide that is synthesized within the hypothalamus and stored in the posterior lobe of the pituitary gland. ADH release is regulated by hypothalamic osmoreceptors. An increase in plasma osmolality triggers release of ADH, which acts at the renal distal tubule and collecting duct to promote retention of free water and restore normal plasma osmolality. Conversely, a decrease in plasma osmolality suppresses ADH release. Increases in plasma osmolality of 2% to 3% above the normal (282 mOsm/kg) trigger ADH release. In humans this generally occurs at a plasma osmolality of 287 mOsm/kg, which is termed the osmotic threshold for ADH release [46].

Volume stimuli also regulate ADH release. A decrease in plasma volume as a result of hemorrhage, peripheral vasodilation, sustained quiet standing, and positive pressure ventilation all stimulate release of ADH by decreasing the left atrial inhibitory impulses directed at the hypothalamus. This compensatory mechanism restores plasma volume. In contrast, increases in plasma volume inhibit ADH release by increasing left atrial inhibitory input to ADH release. In the absence of ADH, diuresis occurs. Other conditions that inhibit ADH release include negative pressure ventilation, recumbency, lack of gravity, submersion in water, and exposure to cold. Volume stimulation overrides osmotic stimuli. Thus, the osmotic threshold for ADH release is increased by volume expansion and decreased by volume contraction.

In addition to volume and osmotic stimuli, several pharmacologic agents can stimulate ADH release, such as chlorpropamide [47], serotonin reuptake inhibitors [48], carbamazepine, nicotine, certain tricyclic antidepressants [49], and the chemotherapeutic agents cyclophosphamide [50,51], vinblastine [52], and vincristine [53]. Elderly patients treated with serotonin reuptake inhibitors appear to be especially prone to the development of hyponatremia [48]. ADH release also can be triggered by nausea, pain, and surgery [46].

Pathophysiology

The hallmark of SIAD is the inability to dilute the urine maximally in the presence of hyponatremia. Urinary osmolality in SIAD is typically higher than plasma osmolality. Because the inability to dilute the urine maximally in the face of hyponatremia also can occur in the absence of abnormalities in ADH secretion, such as in elderly patients, patients with renal disease, or patients using diuretics, these conditions must be excluded before making the diagnosis of SIAD. Assessment of volume status is critical to differentiate volume contraction from SIAD. Patients with SIAD are euvolemic. In volume-contracted patients, the decrease in effective blood volume provides a nonosmotic, volume-responsive stimulus for ADH release. As a result of ADH release, hyponatremia can occur, and the urine can become inappropriately concentrated.

Ingestion of water in patients with SIAD leads to a prompt natriuresis [54]. Although it was originally thought that the natriuresis was the result of aldosterone suppression by expansion of the extracellular volume [44], it was shown subsequently that circulating levels of aldos-

terone are normal and respond normally to stimuli [55,56]. Atrial natriuretic factor levels, which increase with modest volume expansion following acute water ingestion and correlate with the prompt increase in sodium excretion [57], may cause natriuresis in this syndrome. Patients with SIAD who have low sodium intake or who develop extracellular volume contraction are able to conserve sodium. In these instances, patients with SIAD may have low urinary concentrations of sodium. Once the volume contraction is corrected, urinary sodium excretion increases. By monitoring the response to isotonic saline infusion, patients with simple dehydration can be differentiated from patients with dehydration superimposed on SIAD. The former dilute their urine, whereas the latter do not dilute their urine once the volume deficit is corrected.

Patients with SIAD develop hyponatremia only if water intake is excessive. Although these patients rarely report excessive thirst, continued ingestion of water during hypoosmolality is considered to be inappropriate. Hypoosmolality should suppress thirst and thus prevent hyponatremia. The factors that lead to the continued ingestion of water in this syndrome have not yet been identified, but ADH itself is not dipsogenic.

In some cases of SIAD, especially in patients with cancer who develop this syndrome, frank hyponatremia may not develop. Rather, patients may manifest excess ADH secretion with impairment of urinary dilution but without hyponatremia. In these instances, water intake appears to be more appropriate for the degree of hyponatremia. Why this should occur more often in cancer-related than other causes of SIAD remains unknown.

SYNTHESIS AND SECRETION OF ANTIDIURETIC HORMONE

Peptide and messenger RNA for ADH have been identified in the tumors of several patients with clinical SIAD, and circulating plasma levels of ADH are frequently increased. ADH is synthesized and processed in these tumors in a manner similar to its synthesis in the hypothalamus [58,59]. Only a small percentage of patients with SIAD have undetectable levels of plasma ADH, and in these instances their tumors may make other antidiuretic substances that have not yet been identified. Although small cell (oat cell) carcinoma of the lung is most frequently associated with SIAD [59], carcinomas of the head and neck [60,61], bladder [62], cervix [63,64], colon [65,66], ovary [67,68], pancreas [69], and prostate [70,71], as well as neuroblastomas [72–74], Ewing's sarcoma [75], reticulum cell carcinoma [76], mesothelioma [77], and histocytosis [78] have been associated with this syndrome. The list is not inclusive, but it highlights the diversity of cancers reported with SIAD. In patients with malignancies and SIAD, the source of the ADH may not invariably be the tumor but may arise from the posterior pituitary gland via nonosmotic stimuli, such as nausea, pain, drugs, or chemotherapeutic agents.

Treatment

Because elevated levels of ADH lead to hyponatremia only if water intake exceeds its excretion, restriction of water intake is the cornerstone of therapy. To achieve a negative water balance, fluid intake should be restricted to approximately 800 mL/d. Correction of hyponatremia should be done slowly. Overzealous correction can lead to the rare but disabling condition known as central pontine myelinolysis [79,80]. Patients are at risk for this disorder if serum sodium is corrected more rapidly than 2 mEq/L/h, especially if the hyponatremia is chronic. More rapid correction can take place if the hyponatremia has been acute. The correction of hyponatremia with isotonic (0.9%) saline is usually ineffective because the sodium is excreted and the water is retained, which results in a paradoxic lowering of the serum sodium. Saline should be used only when given together with a loop diuretic, which impairs urine concentrating ability by facilitating free water excretion. The use of hypertonic (3%) saline should be reserved for emergencies in which neurologic symptoms such as seizures or coma occur or if the sodium level is below 110 mEq/L. The following are a list of guidelines for therapy. First, hyponatremia can be corrected at a rate of 0.5 mEq/L/h when not emergent. Second, in emergent situations the rate of correction should not exceed 2 mEq/L/h. Third, once the serum sodium is above 120 mEq/L the rate of correction can be slowed. During correction, the serum sodium must be monitored frequently.

Outpatient long-term treatment is directed at fluid restriction, but in instances of noncompliance or if impractical because of obligate fluid requirements, long-term daily furosemide with sodium chloride tablets to compensate for sodium loss can be used [81]. An alternate approach is to use an agent such as demeclocycline in doses of 600 to 1200 mg/d, which produces ADH-resistant nephrogenic diabetes insipidus, which is fully reversible on withdrawal of the medication [82]. Nonsteroidal anti-inflammatory agents also should be discontinued because they potentiate the effect of ADH by blocking prostaglandin synthesis.

Other therapies are directed at decreasing tumor synthesis and secretion of ADH by reducing tumor burden with surgery, radiotherapy, or chemotherapy. Because several of the chemotherapeutic agents may themselves promote ADH release, careful attention to fluid management is necessary. For example, cyclophosphamide can cause SIAD and is used with large volumes of fluid to prevent bladder toxicity. Thus, it is necessary to monitor serum sodium and fluid status carefully during such regimens. If large volumes of fluid must be given with chemotherapy, the coadministration of demeclocycline or furosemide may be useful to lessen or prevent hyponatremia. In addition, because the nausea that may accompany chemotherapy is a potent stimulus to ADH release, antiemetic agents may be administered to diminish this side effect.

HYPERCALCEMIA ASSOCIATED WITH MALIGNANCY

Clinical Features

Hypercalcemia is the most common life-threatening metabolic disorder associated with malignancy and typically results in neuromuscular, renal, and gastrointestinal symptoms as well as impaired cognitive function. Marked dehydration and severe mental status changes accompany greater degrees of hypercalcemia. Hypercalcemic crisis with dehydration, renal insufficiency, and obtundation may be the first clinical manifestation of malignancy. More often, hypercalcemia of malignancy occurs late in the course of the disease. The symptoms of hypercalcemia may mimic those of the underlying malignancy, such as anorexia, weight loss, muscle weakness, and altered mental status. The severity of the hypercalcemic symptoms often correlates with the degree of hypercalcemia.

Causes

Hypercalcemia of malignancy can be caused by local osteolytic hypercalcemia (LOH) or humoral hypercalcemia of malignancy (HHM). In certain patients, both of these mechanisms may be operative.

Humoral hypercalcemia of malignancy is associated with the production of a factor termed *parathyroid hormone (PTH)–related peptide* (PTHrP) by the tumor [83–86]. PTHrP is secreted into the circulation [83–88] and leads to osteoclastic bone resorption. The clinical HHM syndrome is characterized by hypercalcemia, hypercalciuria, hypophosphatemia, reduced levels of PTH, increased nephrogenous cyclic AMP, reduced plasma 1,25-vitamin D levels, and increased levels of PTHrP. Skeletal biopsy reveals a marked increase in osteoclastic bone resorption with a marked reduction in osteoblastic activity [89,90]. This dissociation of osteoclastic and osteoblastic activities contrasts with the bone morphology in primary hyperparathyroidism, in which osteoclastic and osteoblastic activities are increased in a coupled fashion. The tumors that usually are associated with HHM are squamous cell carcinomas of the lung, skin, ears, nose and throat, esophagus, and cervix [91]. HHM also is associated with renal, breast, bladder, ovarian, and endometrial carcinomas and HTLV-1 lymphomas. In contrast, prostate, colon, stomach, and pancreatic adenocarcinomas are rarely associated with HHM.

The absence of PTHrP in the sera of some patients with hypercalcemia of malignancy coupled with the observations that tumors are capable of making many factors that increase osteoclastic resorption of bone indicates that PTHrP is not the sole mediator of hypercalcemia of malignancy [92–94]. Several growth factors have been proposed as osteoclast-activating factors, including interleukins 1 and 2, tumor necrosis factor-α, transforming growth factors, and prostaglandins [95–98]. A number of these factors may lead to local bone resorption in LOH.

Treatment

Treatment of hypercalcemia is summarized in Table 27-4. Severe hypercalcemia requires emergent treatment [99,100]. Patients with hypercalcemic crisis are severely dehydrated and require intravascular volume repletion with forced saline diuresis. The addition of a loop diuretic should not be done until volume is first restored. Loop

Table 27-4. Treatment of Hypercalcemia

Treatment	Onset of Action	Duration of Action	Normalization, %	Advantages	Disadvanteges
Saline	Hours	During infusion	10	Rehydration	Cardiac compromise, intensive monitoring, hypokalemia, hypomagnesemia
Saline and loop diuretic	Hours	During treatment	10	Enhanced renal calcium excretion	Cardiac compromise, intensive monitoring, hypokalemia, hypomagnesemia
Calcitonin	Hours	2–3 d	10–20	Nontoxic, rapid onset of action in life-threatening hypercalcemia	Only lowers calcium by 2 mg/dL, tachyphylaxis
Gallium nitrate	48–72 h	10–14 d	70–80	Potent	Length of intravenous administration, renal impairment
Pamidronate	24–48 h	10–14 d	70–100	Potent, relatively nontoxic	Fever, hypophosphatemia, hypomagnesemia, hypocalcemia

diuretics given before volume restoration may worsen dehydration and increase serum calcium because of enhanced proximal sodium and calcium reabsorption. Serum calcium is rarely normalized by saline diuresis alone, however, and is a short-term, not long-term, treatment. Because the mechanism of hypercalcemia of malignancy is due to increased bone resorption, patients require an antiresorptive agent, such as a biphosphonate, gallium nitrate, mithramycin, or calcitonin. The most effective treatment for hypercalcemia of malignancy is to treat the underlying disease.

Biphosphonates are analogues of pyrophosphate that bind to bone hydroxyapatite. The compounds are taken up by osteoclasts and inhibit osteoclast action [101,102]. Pamidronate inhibits osteoclast-mediated bone resorption yet does not cause mineralization defects. Recommendations are for a single 45-to 60-mg IV dose over 24 hours [102,103]. Serum calcium levels gradually decline beginning 24 to 48 hours after the dose and remain normal for weeks. Serum calcium is monitored serially after treatment. The duration of effects appears to be shorter in patients with HHM than in patients with LOH [104,105]. Hypocalcemia and hypomagnesemia occur in 10% of patients and hypophosphatemia in 10% to 30% of patients. Transient fever is also a side effect.

Calcitonin therapy has its greatest utility within the first 24 to 36 hours of the treatment of severe hypercalcemia and should be used in conjunction with more potent, slower therapies while waiting for these effects. For example, the combined use of calcitonin with biphosphonates reduces serum calcium more quickly than if biphosphonates are used alone [99,100]. It is given as a dose of 4 U/kg body weight intramuscularly or subcutaneously every 12 hours. Tachyphylaxis often develops with calcitonin therapy. Calcitonin is considered only as an adjunctive therapy because calcium usually falls only by 2 mg/dL.

Gallium nitrate is another bone antiresorptive agent for the treatment of hypercalcemia. Normocalcemia ensues for 10 to 14 days after a 5-day infusion [99,100,106]. A disadvantage is the need for 5-day infusion and the concern for its adverse effects on renal function. It is less favored than biphosphonates.

Glucocorticoids have their greatest efficacy in patients with glucocorticoid-responsive diseases, such as myeloma or lymphoma, or in patients whose hypercalcemia is associated with increased 1,25-vitamin D absorption of calcium and resorption of bone. A dose of 200 mg of hydrocortisone or its equivalent is given IV for 3 to 5 days [99,100].

ADRENOCORTICOTROPIC HORMONE

Cushing's syndrome resulting from the ectopic production and secretion of ACTH by a tumor accounts for about 10% of all patients diagnosed with Cushing's syndrome [107]. As a result of the excess secretion of ACTH by the nonpituitary source, the adrenal gland becomes hyperplastic, and overproduction of cortisol ensues. Cortisol inhibits the biosynthesis and secretion of hypothalamic corticotropin-releasing factor (CRF) and pituitary ACTH in a classic fashion that exemplifies the negative feedback of hormones. The secretion of ACTH by the nonpituitary tumor, however, is usually not suppressed by the excess cortisol. This feature of nonsuppressibility of ACTH by the tumor is useful to differentiate ACTH secretion from a pituitary source, which is suppressible. ACTH in the normal pituitary as well as in nonpituitary tumors is derived from processing of the proopiomelanocortin (POMC) gene. Ectopic secretion of ACTH likely results from abnormal gene expression [108].

Clinical Features

The first step in the diagnosis is to establish that the patient has signs and symptoms compatible with Cushing's syndrome. The clinical presentation of patients with this disorder is varied and appears to reflect the tumor type and the rapidity and severity of the hypercortisolism. The acute syndrome consists of rapid onset of hypertension, hypokalemia, edema, and glucose intolerance, and is most often associated with small cell lung carcinoma, which accounts for about three fourths of all cases of ectopic ACTH secretion [109,110]. In contrast, the chronic syndrome is indistinguishable from Cushing's syndrome and is associated with indolent tumors, most frequently bronchial carcinoids but also pancreatic or thymic carcinoids, medullary carcinoma of the thyroid, pheochromocytoma, or other neuroendocrine tumors [111].

Biochemical and Radiologic Diagnosis

The diagnosis involves demonstrating hypercortisolism by elevated 24-hour urinary free cortisol excretion and failure of cortisol suppression following a standard low-dose dexamethasone suppression test (Fig. 27-1). To distinguish ectopic ACTH from other forms of Cushing's syndrome requires additional tests (Fig. 27-1). Distinguishing ACTH-dependent from non–ACTH dependent causes of Cushing's syndrome usually is done easily with determination of serum ACTH and cortisol levels. In ACTH-dependent causes, such as ectopic ACTH syndrome, serum levels of ACTH are measurable to elevated, whereas in the latter, ACTH levels are suppressed. The major differential diagnosis is distinguishing pituitary-dependent Cushing's syndrome from the ectopic ACTH syndrome. Patients with rapidly progressive ectopic ACTH syndrome usually can be diagnosed without difficulty. Patients who harbor more indolent nonpituitary tumors present a diagnostic challenge. Differentiation of these two entities requires the use of dynamic tests that are based on the assumption that pituitary-dependent disease retains some degree of responsiveness to cortisol feedback, whereas ACTH produced ectopically in nonpituitary tumors is not responsive to this feedback regulation.

The dynamic tests that are used include the cortisol response to high-dose dexamethasone suppression, the ACTH response to CRF during inferior petrosal sinus sampling, and the cortisol response to metyrapone. Typically, patients with pituitary-dependent Cushing's syndrome demonstrate suppression of ACTH and cortisol in response to high-dose dexamethasone suppression. In contrast, the expected response in patients with the ectopic ACTH syndrome is no suppression. Typically, malignant ectopic ACTH-secreting neoplasms, such as small cell lung carcinoma, almost always fail to suppress with high-dose dexamethasone. More indolent ectopic ACTH-secreting tumors, especially bronchial carcinoids, frequently demonstrate suppression [108,112].

Inferior petrosal sinus sampling has been proposed because of this latter problem. The test involves placing cannulae in the bilateral inferior petrosal sinuses that drain the pituitary gland. During the test, concurrent ACTH levels before and after CRH stimulation in both petrosal veins and at a distant peripheral site are obtained. The ratio of basal petrosal to peripheral ACTH of more than 2 is highly predictive (> 95%) of pituitary-dependent disease. Ratios of more than 3 obtained 5 minutes after CRH stimulation have an even greater sensitivity and specificity of nearly 100% [109].

Once a diagnosis of ectopic ACTH syndrome is considered, radiographic studies, including chest radiograph, CT scan, or magnetic resonance (MR) imaging of the chest, are indicated. Small cell carcinoma of the lung is usually apparent on plain film or CT scan. Bronchial carcinoids, because of their small size, may require MR imaging of the thorax, which is a more sensitive technique than CT scanning. Ectopic ACTH-secreting tumors may not become clinically apparent for many years after the diagnosis of Cushing's syndrome has been established.

Treatment

Management of this syndrome must be done in light of the severity of the illness and the long-term prognosis because of the underlying tumor. Management is directed at both the ACTH-secreting tumor and the hypercortisolism. Malignant neoplasms responsible for the ectopic ACTH syndrome, such as small cell carcinoma, are usually

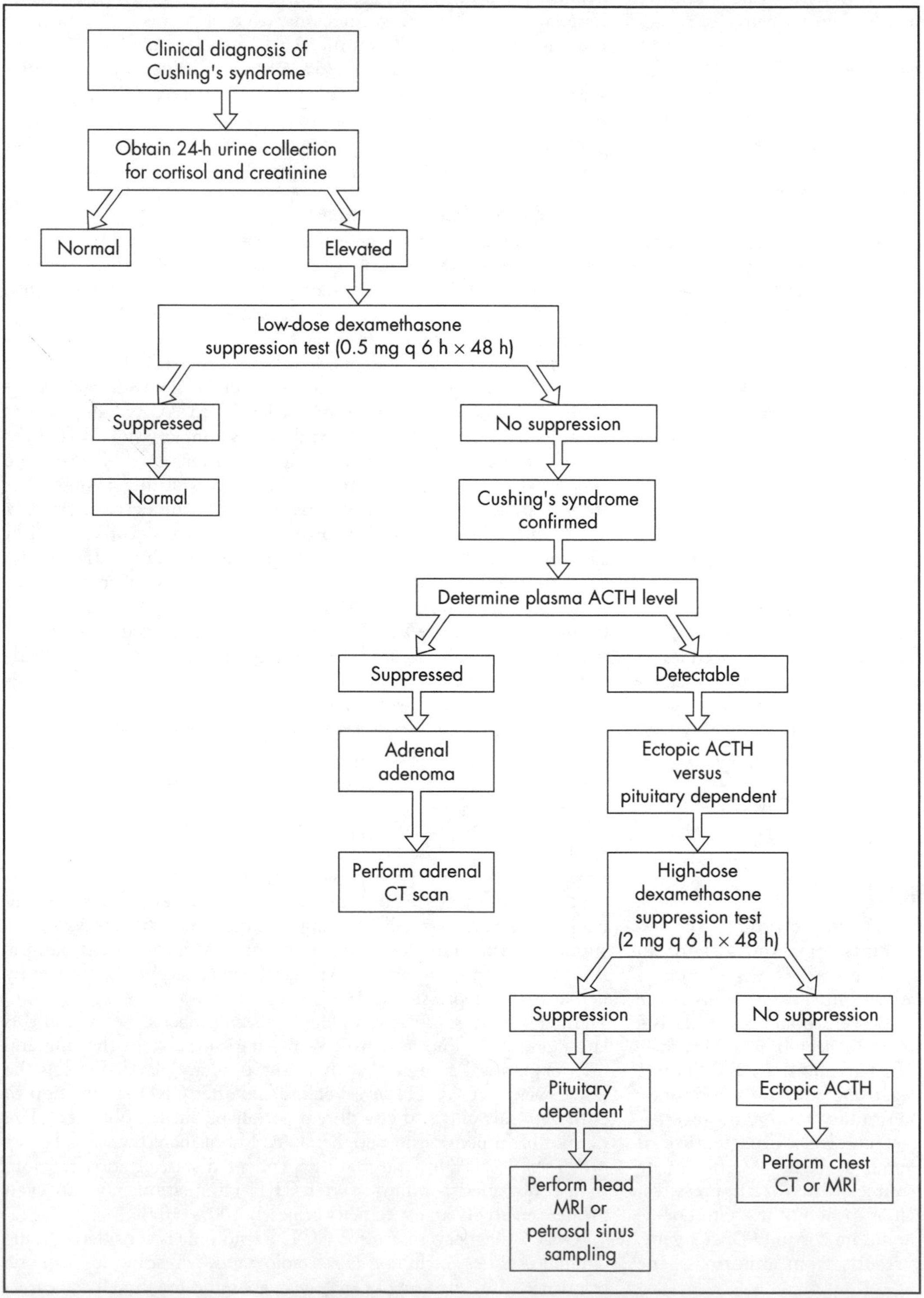

FIGURE 27-1.

Diagnosis of Cushing's syndrome and its causes. Occasional patient with indolent ectopic ACTH—producing tumor (*eg*, bronchial carcinoid) will not suppress.

Clinical diagnosis of Cushing's syndrome → Obtain 24-h urine collection for cortisol and creatinine → Normal / Elevated → Low-dose dexamethasone suppression test (0.5 mg q 6 h × 48 h) → Suppressed → Normal / No suppression → Cushing's syndrome confirmed → Determine plasma ACTH level → Suppressed → Adrenal adenoma → Perform adrenal CT scan / Detectable → Ectopic ACTH versus pituitary dependent → High-dose dexamethasone suppression test (2 mg q 6 h × 48 h) → Suppression → Pituitary dependent → Perform head MRI or petrosal sinus sampling / No suppression → Ectopic ACTH → Perform chest CT or MRI

unresectable and have extensive metastases at the time of diagnosis. Surgical and medical interventions have been used to control the hypercortisolism associated with inoperable ectopic ACTH production. Bilateral adrenalectomy is of questionable benefit in patients with malignant ectopic ACTH syndrome whose life expectancy is measured in months from the time of diagnosis. The prognosis of small cell carcinoma of the lung also appears to be worse when the tumor is associated with the ectopic ACTH syndrome, perhaps because of increased aggressiveness of these tumors as well as many of the complications secondary to hypercortisolism (eg, weakness, hypokalemia, secondary infection).

Medical therapy of hypercortisolism is directed at the adrenal gland and involves use of both inhibitors of steroid biosynthesis (ketoconazole, metyrapone, aminoglutethamide) and adrenolytic (mitotane) agents. Ketoconazole, an antifungal agent that inhibits P-450 enzymes that are involved in the synthesis of cortisol, aldos-

terone, and sex steroids, has been used with variable results [113]. In general, mild hypercortisolism is easier to control than severe disease. Metyrapone can also block steroidogenesis, but it is associated with gastrointestinal side effects and allergic reactions. Aminoglutethamide is also associated with skin rash, sedation, dizziness, ataxia, and gastrointestinal irritation. Adrenolytic agents, such as mitotane, have been reported to result in biochemical and clinical improvement in a few cases. This agent, however, has a slow onset of action and significant side effects. Another agent that has been tried in a small number of patients is octreotide, a long-acting somatostatin analogue. Few patients have been studied, and results are highly variable [114–117]. A glucocorticoid receptor antagonist, such as RU486, offers a method of alleviating excessive glucocorticoid action [118]. Little information is available regarding its effectiveness in this syndrome, and further studies are necessary to determine its efficacy.

REFERENCES

1. Rieselbach RE, Garnick MB: Renal diseases induced by antineoplastic agents. In *Diseases of the Kidney*, edn 3. Edited by Schrier RW, Gottschalk CW. Boston: Little Brown & Co, 1993:1165–1186.

2. Kanfer A, Vandewalle A, Morel-Maroger L, et al.: Acute renal insufficiency due to lymphomatous infiltration of the kidneys: report of six cases. *Cancer* 1976, 38:2588–2592.

3. Luxton RW: Radiation nephritis: a long-term study of 54 patients. *Lancet* 1961, 2:1221–1223.

4. Safirstein R, Winston J, Goldstein M, et al.: Cisplatin nephrotoxicity. *Am J Kidney Dis* 1986, 8:356–367.

5. Capizzi R: Amifostine reduces the incidence of cumulative nephrotoxicity from cisplatin: laboratory and clinical aspects. *Semin Oncol* 1999, 26:72–81.

6. Reed E, Jacob J: Carboplatin and renal dysfunction. *Ann Intern Med* 1989, 110:409.

7. Rossi R, Godde A, Klreinebrand A, et al.: Unilateral nephrectomy and cisplatin as risk factors of ifosfamide-induced nephrotoxicity: analysis of 120 patients. *J Clin Oncol* 1994, 12:159–165.

8. Rossi R, Kleta R, Ehrich JH: Renal involvement in children with malignancies. *Pediatric Nephrology* 1999, 13:153–162.

9. Sangster G, Kaye SB, Calman KC, et al.: Failure of 2-mercaptoethane (Mesna) to protect against ifosfamide nephrotoxicity. *Eur J Cancer* 1984, 20:435–436.

10. Weiss RB: Streptozotocin: a review of its pharmacology, efficacy, and toxicity. *Cancer Treat Rep* 1982, 66:427–438.

11. Hricik DE, Goldsmith GH: Uric acid nephrolithiasis and acute renal failure secondary to streptozotocin nephrotoxicity. *Am J Med* 1988, 84:153–156.

12. Schacht RG, Feiner HD, Gallo GR, et al.: Nephrotoxicity of nitrosureas. *Cancer* 1981, 48:1328–1334.

13. Micetich KC, Jensen-Akula M, Mandard JC, Risher RI: Nephrotoxicity of semustine (methyl-CCNU) in patients with malignant melanoma receiving adjuvant chemotherapy. *Am J Med* 1981, 71:967–972.

14. Pitman SW, Parker LM, Tattersall MHN, et al.: Clinical trial of high-dose methotrexate (NSC-740) with citrovorum factor (NSC-3590): toxicologic and therapeutic observations. *Cancer Chemother Rep* 1975, 6:43–49.

15. Pitman SW, Frei E III: Weekly methotrexate-calcium leucovorin rescue: effect of alkalinization on nephrotoxicity; pharmacokinetics in the CNS; and use in CNS non-Hodgkin's lymphoma. *Cancer Treat Rep* 1977, 61:695–701.

16. Thierry FX, Vernier I, Dueymes JM, et al.: Acute renal failure after high-dose methotrexate therapy: role of hemodialysis and plasma exchange in methotrexate removal. *Nephrology* 1985, 51:416–417.

17. Flombaum CD, Mouradian JA, Ephraim SC, et al.: Thrombotic microangiopathy as a complication of long-term therapy with gemcitabine. *Am J Kidney Dis* 1999, 33:555–562.

18. Peterson BA, Collins AJ, Vogelzang NJ, Bloomfield CD: 5-Azacytidine and renal tubular dysfunction. *Blood* 1981, 57:182–185.

19. Hamner RW, Verani R, Weinman EJ: Mitomycin-associated renal failure: case report and review. *Arch Intern Med* 1983, 143:803–807.

20. Hanna WT, Krauss S, Regester RF, Murphey WM: Renal disease after mitomycin C therapy. *Cancer* 1981, 48:2583–2588.

21. Price TM, Murgo AJ, Keveney JJ, et al.: Renal failure and hemolytic anemia associated with mitomycin C: a case report. *Cancer* 1985, 55:51–56.

22. Kennedy B: Metabolic and toxic effects of mithramycin during tumor therapy. *Am J Med* 1970, 49:494–503.

23. Benedetti RG, Heilman KJ, Gabow PA: Nephrotoxicity following single-dose mithramycin therapy. *Am J Nephrol* 1983, 3:277–278.

24. Fajardo LF, Eltringham JR, Stewart JR, Klauber MR: Adriamycin nephrotoxicity. *Lab Invest* 1980, 43:242–253.

25. Burke JF, Laucins JF, Brodovsky HS, Soriano RZ: Doxorubicin hydrochloride associated renal failure. *Arch Intern Med* 1977, 137:385–388.

26. Selby P, Kohn J, Raymond J, Judson I: Nephrotic syndrome during treatment with interferon. *Br Med J* 1985, 290:1180.

27. Lederer E, Truong L: Unusual glomerular lesion in a patient receiving long-term interferon alpha. *Am J Kidney Dis* 1992, 20:516–518.

28. Averbuch SD, Austin HA, Sherwin SA, et al.: Acute interstitial nephritis with the nephrotic syndrome following recombinant leukocyte A interferon therapy for mycosis fungoides. *N Engl J Med* 1984, 310:32–35.

29. Hermann J, Gabriel F: Membranoproliferative glomerulonephritis in a patient with hairy-cell leukemia treated with alpha II interferon. *N Engl J Med* 1987, 316:112–113.

30. Ault BH, Stapleton FB, Gaber L, et al.: Acute renal failure during therapy with recombinant human gamma interferon. *N Engl J Med* 1988, 319:1397–1400.

31. Kimmel PL, Abraham AA, Phillips TM: Membranoproliferative glomerulonephritis in a patient treated with interferon-alpha for human immunodeficiency virus infection. *Am J Kidney Dis* 1994, 24:858–863.

32. Bellegrun A, Webb DE, Austin HA, *et al.*: Effects of interleukin-2 on renal function in patients receiving immunotherapy for advanced cancer. *Ann Intern Med* 1987, 106:817–822.

33. Textor SC, Margolin K, Blayney D, *et al.*: Renal, volume, and hormonal changes during therapeutic administration of recombinant interleukin-2 in man. *Am J Med* 1987, 83:1055–1061.

34. Christiansen NP, Skubitz KM, Nath K, *et al.*: Nephrotoxicity of continuous intravenous infusion of recombinant interleukin-2. *Am J Med* 1988, 84:1072–1075.

35. West WH, Tauer KN, Yannelli JR, *et al.*: Constant infusion recombinant interleukin-2 in adoptive immunotherapy of advanced cancer. *N Engl J Med* 1987, 316:898–905.

36. Dosik GM, Gutterman JU, Hersh EM, *et al.*: Nephrotoxicity from cancer immunotherapy. *Ann Intern Med* 1978, 89:41–46.

37. Zager RA: Acute renal failure in the setting of bone marrow transplantation. *Kidney Int* 1994, 46:1443–1458.

38. Oliveira JS, Bahia D, Franco M, *et al.*: Nephrotic syndrome as a clinical manifestation of graft-versus-host disease (GVHD) in a marrow transplant recipient after cyclosporine withdrawal. *Bone Marrow Transpl* 1999, 23:99–101.

39. Martinez-Maldonado M, Benabe JE: Nonrenal neoplasms and the kidney. In *Diseases of the Kidney*, edn 5. Edited by Schrier RW, Gottschalk CW. Boston: Little Brown & Co, 1993:2265–2285.

40. Dabbs DJ, Morel-Maroger L, Mignon F, Striker G: Glomerular lesions in lymphomas and leukemias. *Am J Med* 1986, 80:63–70.

41. Zimmerman SW, Vishnu-Moorthy A, Burkholder PM, *et al.*: Glomerulopathies associated with neoplastic disease. In *Cancer and the Kidney*. Edited by Rieselbach RE, Garnick MB. Philadelphia: Lea & Febiger, 1982:306–378.

42. Rault R, Holley JL, Banner BF, El-Shawy M: Glomerulonephritis and non-Hodgkin's lymphoma: a report of two cases and review of the literature. *Am J Kidney Dis* 1992, 20:84–89.

43. Garnick MB: Renal and metabolic complications. In *Current Cancer Therapeutics* edn 3. Edited by Kirkwood JM, Lotze MT, Yasko JM. Philadelphia: Current Medicine; 1994:264–269.

44. Schwartz WB, Bennett W, Curelop S, *et al.*: A syndrome of renal sodium loss and hyponatremia probably resulting from inappropriate secretion of antidiuretic hormone. *Am J Med* 1957, 23:529–542.

45. Beck LH: Hypouricemia in the syndrome of inappropriate secretion of antidiuretic hormone. *N Engl J Med* 1979, 301:528–530.

46. Reeves BW, Andreoli TE: The posterior pituitary and water metabolism. In *Williams Textbook of Endocrinology*. Edited by Wilson JD, Foster DW. Philadelphia: WB Sanders; 1992:311–356.

47. Garcia M, Miller M, Moses AM: Chlorpropamide-induced water retention in patients with diabetes mellitus. *Ann Intern Med* 1971, 75:549–554.

48. Siegler EL, Tamres EL, Tamres D, *et al.*: Risk factors for development of hyponatremia in psychiatric patients. *Arch Intern Med* 1995, 155:953–957.

49. Moses AM: Drug-induced states of impaired water excretion. In *The Posterior Pituitary: Hormone Secretion in Health and Disease*. Edited by Baylis PH, Padfield RL. New York: Marcel-Dekker, 1985:227–260.

50. DeFronzo RA, Braine H, Colvin OM, *et al.*: Water intoxication in man after cyclophosphamide therapy: time course and relation to drug activation. *Ann Intern Med* 1973, 78:861–869.

51. Stahel RA, Oelz O: Syndrome of inappropriate ADH secretion secondary to vinblastine. *Cancer Chemother Pharmacol* 1982, 8:253–254.

52. Berghmans T: Hyponatremia related to medical anticancer treatment. *Support Care Cancer* 1996, 4:341–350.

53. Stuart MJ, Cuaso C, Miller M, *et al.*: Syndrome of recurrent increased secretion of antidiuretic hormone following multiple doses of vincristine. *Blood* 1975, 45:315–320.

54. Goldberg M: Hyponatremia and the inappropriate secretion of antidiuretic hormone. *Am J Med* 1963, 35:293–298.

55. Bartter FC, Schwartz WB: The syndrome of inappropriate secretion of antidiuretic hormone. *Am J Med* 1967, 42:790–806.

56. Fichman MP, Michaelakis AM, Horton R: Regulation of aldosterone in the syndrome of inappropriate antidiuretic hormone secretion (SIADH). *J Clin Endocrinol Metab* 1974, 39:136–144.

57. Cogan E, DeBieve MF, Pepersack T, *et al.*: Natriuresis and atrial natriuretic factor secretion during inappropriate antidiuresis. *Am J Med* 1988, 84:409–418.

58. North WG, Ware J, Chahinian AP, *et al.*: Clinical evaluation of the neurophysins as tumor markers in small cell lung cancer. *Recent Res Cancer Res* 1985, 99:187–193.

59. Sorensen JB, Anderson MK, Hansen HH: Syndrome of inappropriate secretion of antidiuretic hormone (SIADH) in malignant disease. *J Intern Med* 1995, 238:97–110.

60. Ferlito A, Rinaldo A, Devaney KO: Syndrome of inappropriate antidiuretic hormone secretion associated with the head neck cancers: review of the literature. *Ann Otol Rhinol Laryngol* 1997, 106:878–883.

61. Talmi YP, Wolf GT, Hoffman HT, Krause CJ: Elevated arginine vasopressin levels in squamous cell cancer of the head and neck. *Laryngoscope* 1996, 106:317–321.

62. Kaye SB, Ross EJ: Inappropriate antidiuretic hormone (ADH) secretion in association with carcinoma of the bladder. *Postgrad Med J* 1977, 53:274.

63. Kothe MJC, Prins J, Dewit R, *et al.*: Small-cell carcinoma of the cervix with inappropriate antidiuretic-hormone secretion: case report. *Br J Obstet Gynecol* 1990, 97:647.

64. Ishibashi-Ueda H, Imakita M, Yutani C, *et al.*: Small cell carcinoma of the uterine cervix with syndrome of inappropriate antidiuretic hormone secretion. *Mod Pathol* 1996, 9:397–400.

65. Cabrijan T, Skreb F, Suskovic T: Syndrome of inappropriate secretion of antidiuretic hormone (SIADH) produced by an adenocarcinoma of the colon: report of one case. *Rev Rheum Med Endocrinol* 1985, 23:213.

66. Elisaf MS, Konstantinides A, Siamopoulous KC: Chronic hyponatremia due to reset osmostat in a patient with colon cancer. *Am J Nephrol* 1996, 16:349–351.

67. Lam SK, Cheung LP: Inappropriate ADH secretion due to immature ovarian teratoma. *Aust N Z J Obstet Gynaecol* 1996, 36:104–105.

68. Taskin M, Barker B, Calanog A, Jormark S: Syndrome of inappropriate antidiuresis in ovarian serous carcinoma with neuroendocrine differentiation. *Gynecol Oncol* 1996, 62:400–404.

69. Nagashima Y, Iino K, Oki Y, *et al.*: A rare case of ectopic antidiuretic hormone-producing pancreatic adenocarcinoma: new diagnostic approach. *Intern Med* 1996, 35:280–284.

70. Ghandur-Mnaymneh L, Satterfield S, Block NL: Small cell carcinoma of the prostate gland with inappropriate antidiuretic hormone secretion: morphological, immunohistochemical and clinical expressions. *J Urol* 1986, 135:1263–1266.

71. Gasparini ME, Broderick GA, Narayan P: The syndrome of inappropriate antidiuretic hormone secretion in a patient with adenocarcinoma of the prostate. *J Urol* 1993, 150:978–980.

72. Ahwal M, Jha N, Nabholtz JM, *et al.*: Olfactory neuroblastoma: report of a case associated with inappropriate antidiuretic hormone secretion. *J Otolaryngol* 1994, 23:437–439.

73. Asada Y, Marutsuka K, Mitsukawa T, *et al.*: Ganglioneuroblastoma of the thymus: an adult case with the syndrome of inappropriate secretion of antidiuretic hormone. *Hum Pathol* 1996, 27:506–509.

74. Argani P, Erlandson RA, Rosai J: Thymic neuroblastoma in adults: report of three cases with special emphasis on its association with the syndrome of inappropriate secretion of antidiuretic hormone. *Am J Clin Pathol* 1997, 108:537–543.

75. Zimbler H, Robertson GL, Bartter FC, *et al.*: Ewing's sarcoma as a cause of the syndrome of inappropriate secretion of antidiuretic hormone. *J Clin Endocrinol Metab* 1975, 41:390–391.

76. Miller R, Ashkar FS, Rudzinski DJ: Inappropriate secretion of antidiuretic hormone in reticulum cell sarcoma. *South Med J* 1971, 64:763–764.

77. Siafakas NM, Tsirogiannis K, Filadeitaki B, *et al.*: Pleural mesothelioma and the syndrome of inappropriate secretion of antidiuretic hormone. *Thorax* 1984, 39:872–873.

78. Simpson CD, Aitken SE: Malignant histiocytosis associated with SIADH and retinal hemorrhages. *Can Med Assoc J* 1982, 127:302–303.

79. Sterns RH, Riggs JE, Schochet SS: Osmotic demyelination syndrome following correction on hyponatremia. *N Engl J Med* 1986, 314:1535–1542.

80. Ayus JC, Krothapalli RK, Arieff AI: Treatment of symptomatic hyponatremia and its relation to brain damage: a prospective study. *N Engl J Med* 1987, 317:1190–1195.

81. Decaux G, Waterlot Y, Genette F, *et al.*: Treatment of the syndrome of inappropriate secretion of antidiuretic hormone with furosemide. *N Engl J Med* 1981, 304:329–330.

82. Cherril DA, Stote RM, Birge JR, *et al.*: Demeclocycline treatment in the syndrome of inappropriate antidiuretic hormone secretion. *Ann Intern Med* 1975, 83:654–656.

83. Heath DA, Senior PV, Varley VM, *et al.*: Parathyroid hormone–related protein in tumors associated with hypercalcemia. *Lancet* 1990, 335:66–69.

84. Ratcliff WA, Hutchesson ACJ, Bundred NJ, *et al.*: Role of assays for parathyroid-hormone–related protein in investigation of hypercalcemia. *Lancet* 1992, 339:164–167.

85. Burtis WJ, Brady TG, Orloff JJ, *et al.*: Immunochemical characterization of circulating parathyroid hormone–related protein in patients with humoral hypercalcemia of malignancy. *N Engl J Med* 1990, 32:1106–1112.

86. Goltzman D, Henderson JE: Parathyroid hormone-related peptide and hypercalcemia of malignancy. *Cancer Treat Res* 1997, 89:193–215.

87. Rankin W, Grill V, Mardin JJ: Parathyroid hormone-related protein and hypercalcemia. *Cancer* 1997, 80(suppl):1564–1571.

88. Guise TA: Parathyroid hormone-related protein and bone metastases. *Cancer* 1997, 80(suppl):1572–1580.

89. Stewart AF, Vignery A, Silverglate A, *et al.*: Quantitative bone histomorphometry in humoral hypercalcemia of malignancy: uncoupling of bone cell activity. *J Clin Endocrinol Metab* 1982, 55:219–227.

90. Nakayama K, Fukumoto S, Takeda S, *et al.*: Differences in bone and vitamin D metabolism between primary hyperparathyroidism and malignancy-associated hypercalcemia. *J Clin Endocrinol Metab* 1996, 81:607–611.

91. Stewart AF, Horst R, Deftos LJ, *et al.*: Biochemical evaluation of patients with cancer associated hypercalcemia: evidence for humoral and non-humoral groups. *N Engl J Med* 1980, 303:1377–1383.

92. Mundy GR: Malignancy and the skeleton. *Horm Metab Res* 1997, 29:120–127.

93. Roodman GD: Mechanisms of bone lesions in multiple myeloma and lymphoma. *Cancer* 1997, 80:1557–1563.

94. Mundy GR: Mechanisms of bone metastasis. *Cancer* 1997, 80:1546–1556.

95. Bertolini DR, Nedwin GE, Bringman TS, *et al.*: Stimulation of bone resorption and inhibition of bone formation in vitro by human tumor necrosis factor. *Nature* 1986, 319:516–518.

96. Black KS, Mundy GR, Garrett IR: Interleukin-6 causes hypercalcemia in vivo and enhances the bone resorbing potency of interleukin-1 and tumor necrosis factor by two orders of magnitude in vitro. *J Bone Min Res* 1990, 5(suppl):S271.

97. Mundy GR: Hypercalcemic factors other than parathyroid hormone–related protein. *Endocrinol Metab Clin North Am* 1989, 18:795–806.

98. Sato K, Fujii Y, Kasono K, *et al.*: Parathyroid hormone–related protein and interleukin 1β synergistically stimulate bone resorption in vitro and increase serum calcium concentration in mice in vivo. *Endocrinology* 1989, 24:2172–2178.

99. Bilezikian JP: Management of acute hypercalcemia. *N Engl J Med* 1992, 326:1196–1203.

100. Chisholm MA, Mulloy AL, Taylor AT: Acute management of cancer-related hypercalcemia. *Ann Pharmacother* 1996, 30:507–513.

101. Canfield RE: Rationale for diphosphonate therapy in hypercalcemia of malignancy. *Am J Med* 1987, 82(suppl):1–5.

102. Merlini G, Turesson I: Utility of bisphosphonates in treating bone metastases. *Med Oncol* 1996, 13:215–221.

103. Vinholes J, Guo CY, Purohit OP, *et al.*: Evaluation of new bone resorption markers in a randomized comparison of pamidronate or clodronate for hypercalcemia of malignancy. *J Clin Oncol* 1997, 15:131–138.

104. Dodwell DJ, Abbas SK, Morton AR, *et al.*: Parathyroid hormone–related protein and response to pamidronate therapy for tumor-induced hypercalcemia. *Eur J Cancer* 1991, 27:1629–1633.

105. Gurney H, Kefford R, Stuart-Haarris R: Renal phosphate threshold and response to pamidronate in humoral hypercalcemia of malignancy. *Lancet* 1989, 2:241–244.

106. Warrell RP Jr.: Gallium nitrate for the treatment of bone metastases [review]. *Cancer* 1997, 80(suppl):1680–1685.

107. Findling JW, Tyrrell JB: Occult ectopic secretion of corticotropin. *Arch Intern Med* 1986, 146:929–933.

108. DeKeyzer Y, Bertagna X, Lenne F, *et al.*: Altered proopiomelanocortin gene expression in adrenocorticotropin-producing nonpituitary tumors: comparative studies with corticotropic adenomas and normal pituitaries. *J Clin Invest* 1985, 76:1892–1898.

109. Tsigos C, Chrousos GP: Differential diagnosis and management of Cushing's syndrome. *Annu Rev Med* 1996, 47:443–461.

110. Gizza G, Chrousos GP: Adrenocorticotropic hormone-dependent Cushing's syndrome. *Cancer Treat Res* 1997, 89:25–40.

111. Orth DN: Ectopic hormone production. In *Endocrinology and Metabolism*, edn 2. Edited by Felig P, Baxter JD, Broadus AE, Frohman LA. New York: McGraw-Hill, 1987:1692–1735.

112. Malchoff CD, Orth DN, Abboud C, *et al.*: Ectopic ACTH syndrome caused by a bronchial carcinoid tumor responsive to dexamethasone, metyrapone, and corticotropin-releasing tumor. *Am J Med* 1988, 84:760–764.

113. Farwell AP, Devlin JT, Stewart JA: Total suppression of cortisol excretion by ketoconazole in the therapy of the ectopic adrenocorticotropic hormone syndrome. *Am J Med* 1988, 84:1063–1066.

114. Woodhouse NJW, Dagog-Jack S, Ahmed M, *et al.*: Acute and long-term effects of octreotide in patients with ACTH-dependent Cushing's syndrome. *Am J Med* 1993, 95:305–308.

115. de Herder WW, Lamberts SW: Is there a role for somatostatin and its analogues in Cushing's syndrome? *Metabolism* 1996, 45:830.

116. Vignati F, Loli P: Additive effect of ketoconazole and octreotide in the treatment of severe adrenocorticotropin-dependent hypercortisolism. *J Clin Endocrinol Metab* 1996, 81:2885.

117. Christin-Maitre S, Bouchard P: Use of somatostatin analog for localization and treatment of ACTH secreting bronchial carcinoid tumor. *Chest* 1996, 109:845–846.

118. Sartor O, Cutler GB Jr: Mifepristone: treatment of Cushing's syndrome. *Clin Obstet Gynecol* 1996, 39:506–510.

119. Weber B, Gasnick MB, Rieselbach R: Nephropathies due to antineoplastic agents. In *Textbook of Nephrology*, edn 2. Edited by Massry SC, Glassock RJ. Baltimore: Williams & Wilkins; 1989.

120. Bennett WM, Arnoff GR, Golpher TA: *Drug Prescribing in Renal Failure: Dosing Guidelines for Adults*, edn 3. Philadelphia: American College of Physicians; 1994.

URINARY TRACT OBSTRUCTION

Retroperitoneal tumors causing ureteral obstruction can occur with any solid neoplasm. Urologic and gynecologic cancers, together with lymphomas, are the most common causes of obstruction. The effects of obstruction on kidney function result in an early inability to concentrate the urine maximally. Renal blood flow is also markedly diminished, particularly in the setting of unilateral obstruction. Regardless of the precipitating neoplasm, the presenting clinical manifestation is usually excruciating pain.

MANAGEMENT OR INTERVENTION

1. Establish histologic diagnosis of the underlying neoplasm
2. Introduce appropriate therapeutic modalities based on primary disease and obstruction:
   a. For prostate cancer causing bilateral obstruction, consider urethral catheterization, suprapubic cystostomy, immediate bilateral orchiectomy, or other endocrine therapeutic approaches
   b. For lymphomas causing retroperitoneal obstruction, radiation therapy or combination chemotherapy can be employed
   c. For isolated metastases, localized radiation therapy can be effective
   d. For retroperitoneal metastases or lymphoma with loss of renal function, if the neoplasm has not been controlled, immediate percutaneous nephrotomy with placement of antegrade or retrograde stents in the immediate future should be considered
   e. For sensitive neoplasms and testicular cancer, the presence of renal function abnormalities mandates consideration of temporary percutaneous nephrotomies
3. Inhibit xanthine oxidase with allopurinol to prevent a surge of uric acid, which could compromise renal function during systemic treatment
4. Minimize likelihood of infectious complications during manipulation of the obstructed urinary tract
5. Carefully manage postobstructive diuresis and natriuresis with intensive metabolic monitoring

CAUSATIVE FACTORS

Retroperitoneal tumors; urologic cancers, gynecologic cancers, and lymphomas causing lymphadenopathy in the paraaortic, paracaval, and periureteral locations; prostate and advanced cervical cancers commonly causing distal urinary tract obstruction; testicular cancers, especially seminoma, capable of obstructing both ureters simultaneously; metastatic neoplasms forming a plaque-like sheet of tumor

PATHOLOGIC PROCESS

Dilatation of proximal anatomic regions due to obstruction; kidney increases in weight and size and gradually atrophies; inability to concentrate urine maximally and marked dimunition of renal blood flow

DIFFERENTIAL DIAGNOSES

Retroperitoneal fibrosis, ureteral metastases, bladder neck obstruction, lymphadenopathy, kidney stones

PATIENT ASSESSMENT

Ultrasonography (method of choice); radionuclide studies; bone scans with technetium concentration to quantify renal blood flow; on occasion, retrograde and antegrade pyelography; cystoscopy and other interventional approaches for staging purposes; FE_{na} to determine duration of obstruction.

TOXICITY GRADING

	0	1	2	3	4
BUN or serum creatinine	$\leq 1.25 \times N$	$1.26-2.5 \times N$	$2.6-5 \times N$	$5.1-10 \times N$	$> 10 \times N$
Proteinuria	No change	1+ < 0.3 mg/dL < 3 g/L	2–3+ $0.3-1.0$ mg/dL $3-10$ g/L	4+ > 1.0 mg/dL > 10 g/L	Nephrotic syndrome
Hematuria	No change	Microscopic	Gross	Gross + clots	Obstructive uropathy

N — upper limit of normal value of population under study.

GENITOURINARY HEMORRHAGE

Hemorrhage into the genitourinary tract is a problem often seen with certain malignancies. It requires vigilant anticipation and specialized care. Specific antineoplastic agents, such as cyclophosphamide and ifosfamide, are associated with this complication. Management differs according to the site of the process, tumor involvement, and status of the patient.

MANAGEMENT OR INTERVENTION

1. Hemorrhagic cystitis
   Catheter drainage and continuous irrigation
   Intravesical cautery
   Intravesical therapy with formalin
2. Refractory bleeding
   Cystotomy with instillation of phenol and ligation of the bladder vessels
   In severe cases, urinary diversion and removal of the organ to stop life-threatening bleeding are necessary

TOXICITY GRADING

	0	1	2	3	4
Hematuria	No change	Microscopic	Gross	Gross + clots	Obstructive uropathy

CAUSATIVE AGENTS

Cyclophosphamide, ifosfamide, L-asparaginase, actinomycin D, mitomycin C, mithramycin, 6-mercaptopurine, anticoagulants

PATHOLOGIC PROCESS

Toxic metabolites of certain chemotherapeutic agents have direct effect on urethral surface; high concentrations of these metabolites can cause erosion of the bladder mucosal system, leading to microscopic and gross bladder hemorrhage

DIFFERENTIAL DIAGNOSES

Chemotherapeutic agents, tumor involvement, prostate disorders

PATIENT ASSESSMENT

Clinical examination, urinalysis, cystoscopy, urinary irrigation and drainage.

PULMONARY COMPLICATIONS OF CANCER THERAPY

Pulmonary complications arising from antineoplastic drugs range from asymptomatic, mild abnormalities (detected by chest radiograph or pulmonary function tests) to fatal pulmonary fibrosis. The incidence and severity of pulmonary toxicity depend on the characteristics of the responsible drug as well as host factors. It is useful to consider three major syndromes that may result from the pharmacologic treatment of cancer: 1) acute drug reactions (usually hypersensitivity), 2) noncardiogenic pulmonary edema, and 3) interstitial pneumonitis/pulmonary fibrosis. Table 28-1 provides a list of the drugs associated with pulmonary complications [1].

HYPERSENSITIVITY PNEUMONITIS/ACUTE DRUG REACTIONS: METHOTREXATE, PROCARBAZINE, AND VINCA ALKALOIDS

Acute hypersensitivity pneumonitis with dyspnea, cough, and a variety of symptoms (*eg*, fever, chills, malaise, arthralgias, rash, pleuritic chest pain, and headache) may be seen with the administration of methotrexate, procarbazine, and bleomycin. Peripheral blood eosinophilia and diffuse pulmonary infiltrates are characteristic. The incidence is highest with methotrexate, occurring in approximately 8% of patients. Withdrawal of the drug and the administration of steroids may produce rapid resolution of symptoms, and the overall prognosis is good, although approximately 10% of patients may develop pulmonary fibrosis.

Acute respiratory distress with the administration of vinca alkaloids is unusual, occurring in fewer than 1% of patients, but it may be fatal. Many of the reported reactions have occurred when the vinca alkaloid was administered concurrently with mitomycin. The rapid administration of steroids is likely beneficial.

NONCARDIOGENIC PULMONARY EDEMA: CYTARABINE AND GEMCITABINE

High-dose cytarabine, given as consolidation treatment for a variety of hematologic malignancies (usually 3.0 g/m^2 every 12 h for 8–12 doses), may result in noncardiogenic pulmonary edema. Patients present with dyspnea and physical and radiographic signs of pulmonary edema, but they lack other signs of heart failure. This complication appears related to the cumulative dose of cytarabine, occurring in 10% to 12% of patients receiving 12 to 18 g/m^2 compared with 21% to 32% of patients receiving 24 to 26 g/m^2.

Much more rarely, the syndrome occurs in association with teniposide, methotrexate (including intrathecal administration), and cyclophosphamide. The mechanism underlying the syndrome is unknown but has been postulated to be via central nervous system effects on pulmonary capillary permeability. Treatment is supportive; close attention to volume status and the judicious use of diuretics and supplemental oxygen are mainstays. There is a suggestion that high-dose intravenous methylprednisolone may be beneficial. In spite of the high reported incidence with cytarabine, the outcome is usually favorable, and most patients do not require ventilatory support.

Gemcitabine, a nucleoside analogue similar in structure to cytarabine, has also been associated with a syndrome of pulmonary infiltrates and noncardiogenic edema consistent with diffuse alveolar damage. A recent safety review of gemcitabine revealed an incidence of grade 3 or 4 pulmonary toxicity of only 1.4%; however, there have been reported fatalities due to gemcitabine pulmonary toxicity [2,3]. As with cytarabine-induced pulmonary toxicity, treatment is supportive.

INTERSTITIAL PNEUMONITIS/PULMONARY FIBROSIS: BLEOMYCIN, MITOMYCIN, NITROSOUREAS, ALKYLATING AGENTS, AND METHOTREXATE

Bleomycin

The pulmonary toxicity of bleomycin has been studied extensively. The fundamental insult appears to be oxidant damage to pulmonary endothelial cells and type I pneumocytes, resulting in an inflammatory exudate within alveoli and a subsequent fibrotic reaction that may permanently impair diffusion and reduce lung volumes. The activation of various cytokines, particularly tumor necrosis factor α and transforming growth factor β, may also be important. In reported series, the incidence of clinically significant lung injury ranges from 2% to 40%, depending on several factors that are listed in Table 28-2 [4,5].

Patients typically present with dyspnea and, occasionally, a nonproductive cough. Dry rales and a pleural friction rub may be present on examination, and low-grade fever may be present. Chest radiograph typically reveals diffuse interstitial infiltrates but may be

---

Table 28-1. Commonly Used Anti-Cancer Drugs Associated with Pulmonary Toxicity

Antibiotics
Bleomycin, mitomycin
Nitrosoureas
Carmustine (BCNU), lomustine (CCNU), semustine (methyl-CCNU)
Alkylating agents
Busulfan, cyclophosphamide, chlorambucil, melphalan
Antimetabolites
Methotrexate, cytarabine
Miscellaneous
Procarbazine, etoposide, vinblastine, vindesine

Table 28-2. Risk Factors for Pulmonary Toxicity from Bleomycin

Increased cumulative dose (> 400 U there is a 10% incidence of fibrosis)
Increased age (especially > 70 y)
Supplemental oxygen
Prior or concurrent radiotherapy to the chest
Renal dysfunction (concurrent cisplatin administration)
Concurrent administration of other drugs with pulmonary toxicity
Administration of hematopoietic growth factors or other cytokines (controversial, under investigation)
Bolus administration (some evidence that continuous infusion schedules result in less pulmonary toxicity, but data are limited and inconsistent)

---

normal and, rarely, may show pulmonary nodules that can cavitate and be mistaken for metastases.

On pulmonary function tests, the earliest change is a decrease in diffusing capacity (D_LCO) followed by a loss of lung volumes consistent with a restrictive pattern. Mild subclinical toxicity may not predict for the development of clinically significant fibrosis, and loss of lung function may occur suddenly long after treatment has been discontinued. Therefore, the usefulness of serial D_LCOs is limited. Although the routine use of D_LCO to detect subclinical toxicity is controversial, it is important to recognize early clinical signs and symptoms of bleomycin toxicity (eg, dyspnea, dry cough, fine rales, and the development of subtle reticulonodular infiltrates on chest radiograph) [6,7]. Bleomycin should be discontinued when any of these signs or symptoms is present until drug toxicity can be reasonably excluded as a cause of the finding.

Because the treatment of bleomycin-induced pulmonary toxicity is unsatisfactory and its morbidity and mortality are substantial, it is imperative to recognize the risk factors for its development and to weigh the risks and benefits of treatment for all patients. Toxicity is most common after cumulative doses of 400 to 450 U of bleomycin have been administered, but fatal toxicity has been reported with cumulative doses as low as 50 U. Subclinical renal impairment, as associated with the administration of cisplatin, may significantly heighten the risk of bleomycin-induced pulmonary toxicity.

The potential of granulocyte colony–stimulating factor (G-CSF) and granulocyte–macrophage colony–stimulating factor (GM-CSF) to increase the inflammatory or fibrotic response to bleomycin in the lung remains a significant question. Several small case series suggest that G-CSF or GM-CSF enhances bleomycin toxicity, particularly when given as part of the ABVD regimen (doxorubicin, bleomycin, vinblastine, and dacarbazine) for Hodgkin's disease [8]. A retrospective analysis of patients who received bleomycin for germ cell tumors, however, showed an equal incidence of pulmonary toxicity regardless of whether patients received G-CSF [9]. Nonetheless, caution should be exercised in the administration of cytokines to patients who have received bleomycin. Whether continuous infusion schedules reduce the pulmonary toxicity of bleomycin when compared with IV bolus schedules remains an unanswered question.

Withdrawal of bleomycin is the mainstay of management of bleomycin-induced pulmonary toxicity. Although steroids are commonly given and clearly can produce clinical responses, their overall efficacy in preventing progressive fibrosis has not been documented. Tapering of steroids may result in a recurrence of symptoms and should be done slowly. Mortality is reported to be as high as 30% among patients who develop bleomycin-induced pulmonary toxicity. Patients who survive may require long-term supplemental oxygen and may benefit from a formal program of pulmonary rehabilitation.

Mitomycin

In contrast to bleomycin, mitomycin-induced pulmonary toxicity is not dose dependent. The incidence of mitomycin-induced pulmonary toxicity is 3% to 12%, with mortality as high as 50% [10]. The clinical presentation is similar to that caused by bleomycin. Treatment includes the withdrawal of mitomycin and the administration of steroids.

Nitrosoureas

Carmustine (BCNU) is associated with dose-dependent pulmonary fibrosis that occurs in 20% to 30% of patients and may become clinically evident many years after treatment. Toxicity is rare in patients who receive less than 960 mg/m^2 but is seen in 30% to 50% of patients when the cumulative dose is greater than 1500 mg/m^2 [11]. Symptoms include dyspnea, dry cough, and bibasilar rales. Histologically, fibrosis predominates, and the inflammatory picture seen early in bleomycin toxicity is usually absent. Mortality is reported to be 24% to 90%. Steroids may be beneficial. Pulmonary toxicity resulting from other nitrosoureas, lomustine (CCNU) and semustine (methyl-CCNU), has rarely been reported.

Alkylating Agents

Pulmonary toxicity occurs with several alkylating agents but is most often associated with busulfan, occurring in approximately 4% of patients [12]. The onset of the typical symptoms of dyspnea, cough, and a low-grade fever may occur up to 10 years after the administration of busulfan. Although a clear dose-response curve has not been demonstrated, a threshold for toxicity may exist at a cumulative dose of approximately 500 mg. Steroids administered concurrently with busulfan do not appear to decrease the risk of fibrosis and are minimally effective in halting its progression. Mortality is approximately 50%.

Cyclophosphamide is reported to cause pulmonary toxicity similar to that of busulfan, but the incidence is less than 1%. The syndrome may be precipitated by the withdrawal of steroids that are commonly included in combination drug regimens for hematologic malignancies. Case reports of pulmonary toxicity resulting from melphalan or chlorambucil are rare.

HIGH-DOSE REGIMENS REQUIRING BONE MARROW OR PERIPHERAL-BLOOD STEM CELL SUPPORT

The use of high-dose chemotherapy regimens requiring bone marrow or peripheral-blood stem cell support has increased dramatically in the past decade. Although multiple organs are susceptible to nonhematologic toxicity from high-dose therapy, the lungs are often at greatest risk. The likelihood of developing pulmonary toxicity depends on several factors: 1) the conventional dose chemotherapy the patient has received, 2) the particular drugs used in the high-dose regimen, 3) whether the hematopoietic graft is allogeneic or autologous, and 4) the patient's exposure to radiation. The differential diagnosis of pulmonary abnormalities in the setting of high-dose therapy is complex and includes both infectious and noninfectious complications. The most serious complications are associated with allogeneic transplant in which high doses of alkylating agents and/or total-body irradiation are employed and prolonged immune suppression is required. The STAMP V regimen (cyclophosphamide, thiotepa, and carboplatinum), commonly used before autologous stem cell transplants in breast cancer, produces a decrease in DLCO of more than 20% in 32% of patients; 11% of patients have symptomatic pneumonitis that appears to respond to prednisone [13].

For a summary of syndromes occurring with chemotherapy, see Table 28-3.

PULMONARY COMPLICATIONS OF RADIOTHERAPY

Due to the focal nature of radiation therapy, pulmonary complications tend to be less severe than those resulting from chemotherapy [14]. Nonetheless, approximately 5% to 15% of patients who receive radiation to the chest develop pulmonary complications, and significant morbidity and rarely mortality are seen.

The changes that result from radiation have been studied extensively and are well characterized histopathologically, although the precise

Table 28-3. Summary of Pulmonary Syndromes Resulting from Chemotherapy

Syndrome (Drugs)	Clinical Presentation	Treatment Guidelines
Hypersensitivity pneumonitis/acute drug reactions (methotrexate, procarbazine, and vinca alkaloids)	Dyspnea, cough, and a variety of symptoms (including fever, chills, malaise, arthralgias, rash, pleuritic chest pain, and headache) in a patient who is receiving chemotherapy; peripheral blood eosinophilia may occur	Discontinue offending drug; the administration of steroid (usually prednisone 1–2 mg/kg/d) is beneficial; acute drug reactions involving vinca alkaloids may require intravenous steroids and aggressive bronchodilator therapy; prognosis is usually good, although occasional patients with hypersensitivity pneumonitis go on to develop pulmonary fibrosis
Noncardiogenic pulmonary edema (cytarabine; rarely gemcitabine, methotrexate, cyclophosphamide, and teniposide)	Dyspnea and respiratory failure in a patient who is receiving high-dose cytarabine; rales may be present on examination	Discontinue offending drug; close attention to volume status and the judicious of diuretics to maintain a "dry" weight are important; prognosis is good
Interstitial pneumonitis/pulmonary fibrosis (bleomycin, mitomycin, nitrosoureas, alkylating agents, and methotrexate)	Dyspnea and, occasionally, a nonproductive cough and low-grade fever; presentation may be weeks, months, or years after chemotherapy; dry rales and a pleural friction rub may be present on examination	Prednisone 1–2 mg/kg/d may relieve symptoms of pneumonitis but does not appear to prevent the development of fibrosis; tapering should be done slowly because symptoms may be exacerbated by steroid withdrawal; outcome is often poor, chronic low-flow oxygen, bronchodilators and formal pulmonary rehabilitation may be required; cor pulmonale is a common late complication

mechanisms of damage are not yet defined. Six to 12 weeks following exposure to ionizing radiation, an exudate is seen in pulmonary alveoli, followed quickly by an infiltration of inflammatory cells and sloughing of epithelial cells from alveolar walls. These changes may be asymptomatic and resolve completely or may be associated with the clinical picture of acute radiation pneumonitis. Subsequently, the exudate is organized, and to varying degrees, progressive fibrosis of alveolar septa occurs. The syndrome of acute pneumonitis is usually followed by some degree of pulmonary fibrosis, whereas pulmonary fibrosis may occur months following radiation without any antecedent clinical pneumonitis. Injury to pulmonary capillary endothelial cells and type II surfactant-producing pneumocytes, as well as the activation of various cytokines, appears to be important in inducing and sustaining the fibrotic reaction. Risk factors for the development of radiation toxicity are summarized in Table 28-4.

Because of the large number of variables, the occurrence of pulmonary toxicity can be difficult to predict. Although chronic obstructive pulmonary disease is not a risk per se, baseline pulmonary function obviously has important implications regarding the degree of radiation fibrosis that may be tolerated.

Acute Radiation Pneumonitis

Dyspnea that occurs 2 to 3 months following the completion of chest radiation is usually the chief complaint of patients with acute radiation pneumonitis. Rarely, symptoms occur as early as 1 month following radiation, and sometimes the development of symptoms may occur as late as 6 months after radiation. A cough with scant, occasionally pink-tinged sputum may be present, although frank hemoptysis is unusual. Fever may be present. Physical examination is usually unremarkable, although occasionally moist rales or a pleural friction rub is detectable over the irradiated area. The earliest radiographic change associated with acute pneumonitis is a hazy "ground glass" appearance to the irradiated area. As the pneumonitis progresses, patchy infiltrates with varying degrees of consolidation are seen.

Corticosteroids are the mainstay of treatment for acute radiation pneumonitis. No controlled clinical trials have been conducted to

Table 28-4. Factors Influencing the Development of Radiation Pneumonitis and Fibrosis

Factor	Influence
Total dose	In whole lung irradiation, there is a threshold and a steep dose-response curve once the threshold is met
Volume irradiated	The higher the volume irradiated, the greater the risk
Fractionation and rate	Increased rate of irradiation and decreased fractionation; increased risk
Chemotherapy	Concurrent or prior chemotherapy, especially with drugs with established pulmonary toxicity; increased risk
Supplemental oxygen	Increases pulmonary toxicity

document their efficacy, but animal data and nonrandomized series suggest a benefit. Although steroids clearly may produce symptomatic improvement, it is unclear whether their use during acute radiation pneumonitis reduces the severity of subsequent fibrosis. It is common practice to begin prednisone, 1 mg/kg/d, once the diagnosis of radiation pneumonitis is reasonably certain. Prednisone is administered at this dose for 2 to 3 weeks and then tapered very slowly over several additional weeks. Tapering too rapidly may cause relapse of symptoms.

Chronic Pulmonary Fibrosis

Radiologic evidence of fibrosis is seen in most patients who received chest radiation regardless of whether they experienced acute radiation pneumonitis. Radiation changes (linear streaking in mild cases; frank consolidation in more severe cases) are usually confined to the area irradiated but may be more extensive. It is sometimes difficult to determine whether the radiographic abnormality represents fibrotic changes or recurrent malignancy, and biopsy may be necessary to answer the question.

Corticosteroids appear to be of no benefit once fibrosis has developed, and treatment is supportive. In severe cases, the development of cor pulmonale and heart failure are consequences that may result in significant morbidity and mortality.

CARDIOVASCULAR COMPLICATIONS OF CANCER THERAPY

The use of chemotherapy in the cancer patient produces a wide range of direct and indirect cardiovascular effects. Significant concerns regarding the use of such agents in an older population—many of whom bear the overlapping risk factors for cancer and cardiovascular disease—should be under constant consideration at the time of therapy and, even more critically, at the time of toxic events. The role of underlying cardiovascular disease predisposing to more significant and even life-threatening toxicity should similarly be under constant consideration. Cardiovascular complications of chemotherapy fall into the following major categories: general cardiovascular concerns, anthracycline cardiomyopathy, other cardiomyopathies, anginal syndromes, arrhythmias, and pericardial disease.

GENERAL CARDIOVASCULAR CONCERNS

Some of the general cardiovascular factors to be considered when caring for the oncology patient include underlying ischemic heart disease, valvular heart disease, idiopathic hypertrophic subaortic stenosis (IHSS) or asymmetrical septal hypertrophy, diastolic dysfunction, existing arrhythmia, and use of diuretics. However, the use of chemotherapeutic agents that produce significant diarrhea and electrolyte loss (eg, fluoropyrimidines and irinotecan), probably cause the most frequent acute cardiovascular problems in everyday practice (ie, dehydration and hypotension). Electrolyte loss may produce additional complications, such as exacerbation of mental status change, ileus, and cardiac arrhythmias. Hypomagnesemia, resulting from cisplatin-induced tubular dysfunction, may predispose to ventricular arrhythmias. Furthermore, repletion of whole-body potassium stores may be difficult until normal total-body magnesium levels are restored, due to continuing renal potassium wasting.

Table 28-5 lists some underlying cardiovascular diseases that predispose to vascular instability and complications. Treatment of these problems should be directed to rapid resuscitation with physiologic electrolyte solutions and/or blood products. Volume depletion may also occur in elderly or cachectic patients with decreased intake of fluids, particularly in the setting of diuretics. The practice

of prescribing diuretics in an attempt to alleviate patient discomfort from mild peripheral edema should be discouraged, particularly in the elderly cancer patient. Dehydration from any cause may precipitate unstable angina and myocardial infarction. In the setting of IHSS or diastolic dysfunction, volume depletion and reduction of preload may precipitate overt congestive heart failure. Here, the physician must correctly administer fluids and blood products rather than diuretics.

Chemotherapy-induced anemia is also an important factor in exacerbating anginal syndromes or producing high-output cardiac failure. Acute anemia should be treated with transfusion of packed red blood cells, whereas chronic anemia may be treated with blood products or the use of recombinant human erythropoietin (Procrit [Ohio Biotechnology, New Brunswick, NJ] and Epogen [Amgen, Thousand Oaks, CA]) 5000 to 10,000 U SQ three times per week or 20,000 to 60,000 U/weekly. Many patients will have improved exercise tolerance and a greater sense of well-being with the use of growth factors preventing chronic anemia. These common problems must be considered in the differential diagnosis prior to diagnosing more direct cardiac complications of cancer therapy.

Biologic therapies may also have considerable cardiovascular consequences in cancer patients, particularly when given at higher doses (Table 28-6). Interleukin-2 is the cytokine most widely known for its cardiovascular effects when given on the common high-dose schedules (12 MU IV every 8 h). When given in this dose and schedule, a full 70% of patients will require ICU-level care with the use of

Table 28-5. Predisposing Cardiovascular Conditions in the Cancer Patient

Cardiac conditions
  Atherosclerotic heart disease
  Valvular heart disease
  Congestive heart failure
  Diastolic dysfunction
Vascular events
  Dehydration (diarrhea or diuretics)
  Anemia
Metabolic complications (predisposing to arrhythmia)
  Hyponatremia
  Hypernatremia
  Hypocalcemia
  Hypercalcemia
  Hypomagnesemia

Table 28-6. Cardiac Complications of Anticancer Drugs

Agent	Cardiac Effect
Chemotherapeutic	
Amsacrine	Arrhythmias
Anthracyclines	Arrhythmias; congestive cardiomyopathy; pericardial effusion
Anthrapyrazoles	Congestive cardiomyopathy
Bleomycin	Raynaud's phenomenon
Cyclophosphamide	Acute congestive heart failure; hemorrhagic myocarditis; pericardial effusions
5-Fluorouracil	Myocardial ischemia; arrhythmias
Mitoxantrone	Congestive cardiomyopathy
Taxol	Arrhythmias (bradycardia); electrocardiogram changes; ischemia; increased cardiomyopathy
Vinca alkaloids	Angina; Raynaud's phenomenon
Biologic response modifier	
Interferon α	Hypotension; tachycardia
Interferon β	Hypotension
Interferon γ	Hypotension
Interleukin-1 α	Hypotension
Interleukin-2	Congestive heart failure; hypotension; arrhythmias; ischemia
Interleukin-4	Congestive heart failure
Tumor necrosis factor	Hypotension; ischemia
GM-CSF	Hypotension; pericardial effusion
Trastuzumab	Congestive heart failure (in combination)
Radiation therapy	Congestive heart failure; coronary artery disease; pericarditis/effusion

GM-CSF—granulocyte–macrophage colony-stimulating factor.
Adapted from Speyer and Freedberg [15].

pressor agents for development of hypotension, shock, and pulmonary edema, presumably due to capillary leak syndrome. Additional effects, including angina and myocardial infarction, have been reported. Other biologics that may produce hypotension and cardiovascular collapse include the interferons and GM-CSF. Interleukin-4 has been associated with direct cardiac toxicity and pathologic myocardial changes in both humans and animals [16].

ANTHRACYCLINE CARDIOMYOPATHY

The most well-known and feared cardiac complication of chemotherapy is anthracycline-induced cumulative cardiomyopathy [17,18]. This complication has been the subject of considerable research and is reviewed in detail elsewhere [15,19]. Although anthracyclines such as doxorubicin generally act as DNA-damaging agents (as intercalating agents and through inhibition of topoisomerase II), they have a unique damaging effect on myocardium through a mechanism based on accelerated production of free radicals [20]. The four-ring chromophore moiety of the anthracycline is easily reduced to a semiquinone through a "red-ox" cycle that simultaneously induces the formation of oxygen and peroxide free radicals. Under normal conditions, free radical damage is limited by cellular defenses, including superoxide dismutase, catalase, and glutathione peroxidase. However, myocardium possesses fewer of these enzymes than other tissues. Myocardial enzymatic defenses become overwhelmed in the presence of ferric (Fe^{+3}) cations that form a stable, noncovalent complex with doxorubicin, thereby increasing the rate of free radical formation several hundred–fold. These free radicals then cause widespread membrane damage by lipid peroxidation. Subcellular targets include the nuclear and cellular membranes and, in the myocardium, the sarcoplasmic reticulum. This damage to the myocyte sarcolemma results in decreased bound calcium and decreased contractility via the actin–myosin complex.

Clinically, the result of this free radical damage to the myocardium is a global cardiomyopathy, resulting in biventricular congestive heart failure (CHF). This cumulative process has been reported to result in a 5% to 10% incidence of clinical CHF at a cumulative doxorubicin dose of 450 to 500 mg/m² in retrospective studies [17,21]. This figure, however, has been underestimated due to inconsistent cardiac monitoring and the retrospective nature of these studies. In the more recent prospective studies that have required consistent gated pool monitoring of cardiac function every one to two cycles, the true incidence of clinical CHF at a cumulative doxorubicin dose of 450 to 500 mg/m² is 20% to 25% [15,21–23]. Also, using the common definition of cardiac toxicity based on gated heart-pool scanning to quantitate the left ventricular ejection fraction (LVEF) (ie, 10% drop from baseline LVEF or fall in LVEF to < 50%), the incidence of cardiac toxicity is approximately 35% at a cumulative doxorubicin dose of 450 mg/m² in these same studies. The cumulative dose for development of cardiomyopathy varies according to anthracycline. These clinical changes are associated with pathognomonic electron micrographic findings described by Billingham *et al.* [25] and are quantitated on a scale from 0 to 3 (Table 28-7).

In practice, patients should have baseline LVEF determination at a cumulative doxorubicin dose of 300 and 450 mg/m² and every cycle thereafter until LVEF criteria for cardiac toxicity dictate discontinuing doxorubicin. Alternatively, many oncologists have not exceeded a lifetime cumulative doxorubicin dose limitation of 450 mg/m². It should be borne in mind that cardiac toxicity may progress for up to 2 months after the last dose of doxorubicin and some patients with falling LVEF may go on to develop clinical CHF. Some risk factors associated with development of CHF include prior myocardial infarction and age greater than 65 years.

In addition, the coadministration of other drugs may potentiate the cardiac toxicity of anthracyclines in unexpected ways. This was recognized when clinical investigators administered doxorubicin and paclitaxel in combination to patients with advanced breast cancer and encountered a higher incidence of CHF than anticipated [26,27]. Gianni *et al.* and other investigators subsequently found that paclitaxel interferes with the plasma elimination of doxorubicin and its metabolite doxorubicinol [28]. This effect is highly dependent on the time interval between the drugs and the sequence of their administration [29]. To avoid excess cardiac toxicity, doxorubicin should be administered before paclitaxel, and a waiting period of 15 minutes between the completion of doxorubicin and the initiation of paclitaxel observed. Docetaxel, another taxane, does not appear to interfere with doxorubicin pharmacokinetics and coadministration of the drugs does not increase cardiac toxicity [30]. Another example of an unexpected high rate of CHF was when an anthracycline (doxorubicin or epirubicin) was administered with trastuzumab (Herceptin; Genentech, South San Francisco, CA), a humanized monoclonal antibody targeting the HER2 receptor in advanced breast cancer. Although the combination of trastuzumab and anthracycline demonstrated a greater antitumor effect than anthacycline alone in a randomized trial, 28% of patients who received combination therapy developed cardiac toxicity (including 19% with NYHA class III or IV congestive heart failure), compared with only 7% of patients who received anthracycline alone [31]. Trastuzumab thus cannot be safely administered concurrently with doxorubicin or epirubicin. As discussed later, there is less cardiac toxicity when trastuzumab is administered as a single agent or in combination with paclitaxel.

Although these considerations have dictated the clinical boundaries of doxorubicin use in the past, anthracycline cardiomyopathy may now largely be prevented through the use of dexrazoxane (ICRF-187, Zinecard [Pharmacia and Upjohn, Kalamazoo, MI], Cardioxane [Eurocenter, Amsterdam, Holland]). Prospective randomized studies conducted at New York University [32], the National Cancer Institute (NCI) [24] (in children), and in industry-sponsored multicenter studies [31,33,34] have demonstrated the efficacy of this bisdioxopiperazine compound. Dexrazoxane is converted

Table 28-7. Histopathologic Scale of Doxorubicin Cardiomyopathy

Grade	Description
0	Within normal limits
1	Less than 5% of cells with early changes (myofibrillar loss and distended sarcoplasmic reticulum)
1.5	Small groups of cells (5%–15%) involved with definitive changes (marked myofibrillar loss and/or vacuolization)
2	Groups of cells (16%–25%) involved with definitive changes (marked myofibrillar loss and/or vacuolization)
2.5	Groups of cells (26%–35%) involved with definitive changes (marked myofibrillar loss and/or vacuolization)
3	Diffuse cell damage (> 35%) with marked change, including degeneration of organelles, mitochondria, and nucleus and loss of contractile elements

intracellularly to a bidentate chelator analogue of EDTA. This form of the drug is able to strip the Fe^{+3} cations from the Fe^{+3}:doxorubicin complex, thereby preventing cardiomyopathy. In these prospective randomized placebo and nonplacebo controlled clinical trials dexrazoxane has been shown to prevent anthracycline-induced cardiac toxicity based on clinical CHF, LVEF, and biopsy criteria. As approved in the United States, the drug is administered at a dose of 500 mg/m^2 (ratio of 10:1 to doxorubicin) over 15 minutes beginning 30 minutes prior to doxorubicin administration. Using this dose and schedule, no clinically significant myelosuppression was found for dexrazoxane together with the FAC regimen (ie, fluorouracil, doxorubicin, and cyclophosphamide).

Nearly all trials have shown that dexrazoxane does not change the response rate seen with doxorubicin. However, because of concern raised in one multicenter breast cancer trial [23,33], the drug has been approved for use in the United States beginning after a cumulative doxorubicin dose of 300 mg/m^2 has been reached in those patients continuing with the drug. In practice, it would be reasonable to begin use of dexrazoxane as soon as there is evidence of antitumor activity for doxorubicin, assuming it is the oncologist's goal to continue doxorubicin until evidence of tumor progression. For example, in the New York University study, which used dexrazoxane at the dose of 1000 mg/m^2 and started treatment from the first cycle, 15% of all women treated with dexrazoxane were able to tolerate cumulative doxorubicin doses in excess of 1000 mg/m^2 and several doses at more than 2000 mg/m^2, with the major cause of treatment termination being progression (rather than cardiac toxicity) [21].

Other strategies for abrogation of anthracycline cardiomyopathy include less cardiotoxic analogues, such as 4'-epi-doxorubicin (epirubicin). This agent is widely used in Europe as the anthracycline of choice due to its somewhat improved toxicity profile. Epirubicin is cardiotoxic through the same mechanisms as doxorubicin, although at a reduced level. Dexrazoxane also provides cardiac protection against epirubicin-induced cardiomyopathy when administered in a ratio of 10:1 [35]. Another approach has been the use of prolonged (durations of up to 96 h) infusion of doxorubicin. This method avoids the higher peak concentrations of doxorubicin produced by bolus administration, allowing tolerance of a somewhat greater cumulative dose [36]. Others have suggested that weekly administration may also lower the risk of cardiomyopathy [37]. Most recently, doxorubicin packaged in pegylated-liposomes (Doxil; Alza Pharmaceuticals, Mountain View, CA) has been approved for the treatment of Kaposi's sarcoma and ovarian cancer. This compound has significantly different pharmacokinetics compared with free drug, with effective circulation time of weeks. It also produces a very different toxicity spectrum compared with doxorubicin. To date, animal studies have not shown an association with cardiotoxicity. Human studies are limited, but patients with Kaposi's sarcoma often have exceeded normally cardiotoxic doses of free doxorubicin (500–1000 mg/m^2) without evidence of cardiac toxicity by LVEF. A study comparing endomyocardial biopsies in these patients with age-matched controls receiving equal doses of doxorubicin showed a median score of 0.50 for Doxil compared with 2.25 for the doxorubicin-treated group [38]. Additionally, in 29 women with breast cancer receiving a median of 550 mg/m^2, the median biopsy score was 0 (range 0.0–1.5).

OTHER CARDIOMYOPATHIES

Trastuzumab, which is a humanized monoclonal antibody that targets the HER2 receptor, is approved for use in patients with advanced breast cancer with HER2 overexpression. The development of the drug was complicated by the unexpected finding of cardiac toxicity, particularly when trastuzumab was administered with an anthracycline as already described. Although the precise mechanism for the toxicity has not been elucidated, clinically it appears no different from the global cardiomyopathy seen with classic anthracycline cardiomyopathy. In a randomized trial comparing paclitaxel alone with paclitaxel plus trastuzumab, patients in the combined therapy group had an 11% incidence of cardiac toxicity (4% NYHA class III or IV), compared with only 1% in the control arm that received paclitaxel alone [31]. All patients in the study had previously received anthracycline in the adjuvant setting, and the cardiotoxic potential of trastuzumab in anthracycline-naive patients has not been well defined.

Mitoxantrone, an anthracenedione compound, is structurally similar to the anthracyclines but lacks their characteristic daunosamine sugar moiety. The cardiac toxicity of mitoxantrone is not related to the free radical mechanism described for the anthracyclines. Clinically, however, this cardiomyopathy presents in a similar fashion to doxorubicin, although at a reduced incidence based on equitoxic cumulative dosing. At a cumulative dose of 160 mg/m^2, approximately 5% of patients may develop CHF; therefore, cumulative dosing should be limited, especially in patients with prior anthracycline exposure.

Other agents associated with cardiomyopathy include drugs causing direct myocardial injury. This has been documented most commonly with high-dose alkylating agents, particularly cyclophosphamide, in the setting of bone marrow transplantation or stem cell rescue. Effects associated with high-dose alkylating agents include acute hemorrhagic myocarditis, CHF, and death [39]. The majority of patients receiving doses of 120 to 240 mg/kg over 1 to 4 days have electrocardiogram changes consisting of a decrease in the QRS voltage associated with an asymptomatic decrease in systolic function [40]. This is usually reversible unless hemorrhagic myocarditis occurs. Postmortem and animal-model studies suggest that direct endothelial injury results in capillary microthrombosis and interstitial fibrin deposition.

Radiation therapy may also cause cardiomyopathy due to dose-related interstitial myocardial fibrosis. This long-term complication results from capillary and microcirculatory damage, exudation of fibrin, and eventual fibrosis [41]. Doses greater than 6000 cGy and treatment with a single anterior-posterior portal have been associated with increased risk of this complication, which may occur 5 to 20 years after radiation. This form of biventricular myocardial failure should be differentiated from radiation-induced chronic pericarditis by echocardiography.

ANGINAL SYNDROMES

5-Fluorouracil (5-FU) is the chemotherapy drug associated with the highest reported incidence of myocardial ischemia. The proposed mechanism is by direct induction of coronary artery spasm. Clinically, 5-FU produces angina with typical symptoms, electrocardiogram changes, and response to nitroglycerin, although some patients studied have had normal coronary angiograms, even with ergonovine [42]. Moreover, there have been reports of patients who, after experiencing an anginal syndrome during 5-FU, have successfully been reexposed at lower doses without significant subsequent toxicity [43].

In a review of 1000 patients receiving 5-FU, a 4.5% incidence of cardiac ischemia or arrhythmia was noted in patients with a history of coronary artery disease versus a 1.1% incidence of cardiac toxicity in those patients with no previous cardiac history. This association is more striking in those patients who receive a continuous infusion of 5-FU and in those patients who receive concomitant cisplatin [44]. Akhtar *et al.* [45] noted an 8% incidence of cardiac side effects in patients without cardiac history who were treated with 96-hour 5-FU infusion in combination with mitomycin-C or cisplatin. These side effects included angina (5 patients), palpitations (3 patients), diaphoresis (2 patients), and syncope (1 patient). There was no relationship between cardiotoxicity and age, sex, tumor, or drug combination.

ARRHYTHMIAS

Bone Marrow Transplantation

Cardiovascular toxicity has been reported to be related to the infusion of cryopreserved grafts for use in bone marrow transplantation. Keung *et al.* [46] noted an 82% incidence of transient cardiac arrhythmias, including sinus bradycardia and complete heart block, although all the patients remained asymptomatic. Another study, however, did not find a relationship between cryopreserved cell administration and cardiac arrhythmias in 44 consecutive patients [47].

The etiology of cardiac toxicity associated with graft infusion is probably multifactorial and may include underlying defects in cardiac conduction, electrolyte abnormalities, cell lysis products of the infusate, mechanical effects of a large volume load, and cardiotoxic effects of the cryopreservative dimethyl sulfoxide.

5-Fluorouracil

5-FU has been associated with arrhythmia as well as anginal syndromes. The incidence of cardiac side effects has been estimated at 5% to 8%, with arrhythmias accounting for approximately half of these episodes (*see* Anginal Syndromes section). Although most of the documented cases have included ventricular arrhythmias, a prospective evaluation of the specific nature and incidence of these arrhythmias with the use of Holter monitors remains to be performed.

Paclitaxel

Intravenous infusion of paclitaxel (Taxol; Bristol-Myers Squibb Company, Stanford, CT) was initially associated with a high inci-

dence of bradyarrhythmias [48]. As a result initial NCI-sponsored studies eliminated all patients with cardiac risk factors and required cardiac monitoring. With these precautions, a reassessment of the 3400 patients in the NCI database demonstrated only a 0.29% incidence of grade 4 or 5 cardiac toxicity, including heart block (4 patients), atrial arrhythmias (3 patients), ventricular tachycardia (9 patients), and myocardial infarction within 14 days of Taxol infusion (7 patients) [49]. Ten of these patients had prior cardiac risk factors. At present, routine cardiac monitoring for Taxol administration is not recommended, although it may be considered for patients with known cardiac conditions.

Cisplatin

Cisplatin induces renal tubular dysfunction, resulting in urinary magnesium and potassium loss. These electrolyte abnormalities may result in prolongation of the QT interval and subsequent ventricular arrhythmia. Oral supplementation with both magnesium (*eg*, Slow-Mag 64 mg twice daily) and potassium salts may be necessary chronically.

PERICARDIAL DISEASE

Pericardial disease with a malignant pericardial effusion causing tamponade and CHF should always be considered in the cancer patient. Routine chest radiograph may demonstrate a clearly enlarged and symmetric cardiac shadow. The presence of pericardial disease should be confirmed with echocardiography. This complication has been associated with malignant mediastinal adenopathy, resulting in lymphatic obstruction and pericardial tumor involvement, most commonly in patients with non–small cell lung cancer and breast cancer. Pericardial effusion has also been associated with the use of anthracyclines [50] and high-dose cyclophosphamide [40] generally in the setting of other manifestations of cardiac toxicity. Radiation-induced acute and chronic pericarditis has also been described. Acute pericarditis is dose related, with an estimated 10% to 15% incidence reported in patients with Hodgkin's disease who received greater than 40 Gy to the mediastinum [51]. A smaller proportion of these patients will go on to develop long-term, chronic constrictive pericarditis due to radiation-induced fibrosis. More modern radiation techniques should result in an incidence of less than 2.5% for these complications [52].

REFERENCES

1. Twohig K, Matthay R: Pulmonary effects of cytotoxic agents otherthan bleomycin. *Clin Chest Med* 1990, 11:31–54.

2. Aapro MS, Martin C, Hatty S: Gemcitabine: a safety review. *Anti-Cancer Drugs* 1998, 9:191–201.

3. Pavlakis N, Bell DR, Millward MJ, *et al.*: Fatal pulmonary toxicity resulting from treatment with gemcitabine [see comments]. *Cancer* 1997, 80:286–291.

4. Crooke S, Bradner W: Bleomycin: a review. *J Med* 1976, 7:333–428.

5. Jules-Elysee K, White D: Bleomycin-induced pulmonary toxicity. *Clin Chest Med* 1990, 11:1–20.

6. Comis R: Bleomycin pulmonary toxicity: current status and future directions. *Semin Oncol* 1992, 19(suppl 5):64–70.

7. Comis R: Detecting bleomycin pulmonary toxicity: a continued conundrum. *J Clin Oncol* 1990, 8:765–767.

8. Lei K, Leung W, Johnson P: Serious pulmonary complications in patients receiving recombinant granulocyte colony-stimulating factor during BACOP chemotherapy for aggressive non-Hodgkin's lymphoma. *Br J Cancer* 1994, 70:1009–1013.

9. Saxman S, Nichols C, Einhorn L: Pulmonary toxicity in patients with advanced-stage germ cell tumors receiving bleomycin with and without granulocyte colony stimulating factor. *Chest* 1997, 111:657–660.

10. Buzdar A, Legha S, Luna M, *et al.*: Pulmonary toxicity of mitomycin. *Cancer* 1980, 45:236–244.

11. Weinstein A, Deiner-West M, Nelson D, *et al.*: Pulmonary toxicity of carmustine in patients treated for malignant glioma. *Cancer Treat Rep* 1986, 70:943–946.

12. Gibson S, Comis R: The pulmonary toxicity of antineoplastic agents. *Semin Oncol* 1982, 9:34–51.

13. Abdel-Razeq H, Overmoyer B, Pohlman B, *et al.*: Pulmonary toxicity of STAMP V preparative regimen in high-dose chemotherapy (HDC) and autologous bone marrow transplantation (ABMT) for breast cancer [abstract]. *Proc Annu Meet Am Soc Clin Oncol* 1997, 16:100.

14. Rosiello R, Merrill W: Radiation-induced lung injury. *Clin Chest Med* 1990, 11:65–71.

15. Speyer J, Freedberg R: *Clinical Oncology.* New York: Churchill Livingstone, Inc.; 1995.

16. Trehu EG, Karp DD, Atkins MB: Possible myocardial toxicity associated with Interleukin-4 therapy. *J Immunother* 1993, 14:348–351.

17. Von Hoff D, Layard M, Basa P, *et al.*: Risk factors for doxorubicin-induced congestive heart failure. *Ann Intern Med* 1979, 91:710–717.

18. Von Hoff D, Rozencweig M, Layard M, *et al.*: Daunomycin-induced cardiotoxicity in children and adults: a review of 110 cases. *Am J Med* 1977, 62:200–208.

19. Hochster H, Wasserheit C, Speyer J: Cardiotoxicity and cardioprotection during chemotherapy. *Curr Opinion Oncol* 1995, 7:304–309.

20. Gianni L, Myers C: The role of free radical formation in the cardiotoxicity of anthracycline. In *Cancer Treatment and the Heart.* Edited by Muggia F, Green M, Speyer J. Baltimore: The Johns Hopkins University Press; 1992:9–46.

21. Bristow M, Mason J, Billingham M, *et al.*: Dose-effect and structure-function relationships in doxorubicin cardiomyopathy. *Am Heart J* 1981, 102:709–718.

22. Speyer J, Green M, Zeleniuch-Jacquotte A, *et al.*: ICRF-187 permits longer treatment with doxorubicin in women with breast cancer. *J Clin Oncol* 1992, 10:117–127.

23. Swain S, Whaley F, Gerber M, *et al.*: Cardioprotection with dexrazoxane for doxorubicin-containing therapy in advanced breast cancer. *J Clin Oncol* 1997, 15:1318–1332.

24. Wexler L, Andrich M, Venzon D, *et al.*: Randomized trial of the cardioprotective agent ICRF-187 in pediatric sarcoma patients treated with doxorubicin. *J Clin Oncol* 1996, 14:362–372.

25. Billingham M, Mason J, Bristow M, *et al.*: Anthracycline cardiomyopathy monitored by morphologic changes. *Cancer Treat Rep* 1978, 62:865–872.

26. Gianni L, Munzone E, Capri G, *et al.*: Paclitaxel by 3-hour infusion in combination with bolus doxorubicin in women with untreated metastatic breast cancer: high antitumor efficacy and cardiac effects in a dose-finding and sequence-finding study [abstract]. *J Clin Oncol* 1995, 13:2688–2699.

27. Dombernowsky P, Gehl J, Boesgaard M, *et al.*: Doxorubicin and paclitaxel: a highly active combination in the treatment of metastatic breast cancer. *Semin Oncol* 1996, 23 (suppl 11):23–27.

28. Gianni L, Bigano L, Locatelli A, *et al.*: Human pharmacokinetic characterization and in vitro study of the interaction between doxorubicin and paclitaxel in patients with breast cancer. *J Clin Oncol* 1997, 15:1906–1915.

29. Holmes FA, Madden T, Newman RA, *et al.*: Sequence-dependent alteration of doxorubicin pharmacokinetics by paclitaxel in a phase I study of paclitaxel and doxorubicin in patients with metastatic breast cancer [abstract]. *J Clin Oncol* 1996, 14:2713–2721.

30. Bellot R, Robert J, Dieras V, *et al.*: Taxotere does not change the pharmacokinetic profile of doxorubicin and doxorubicinol [abstract]. *Proc Am Soc Clin Oncol* 1998, 17:221.

31. Genentech: *Herceptin Investigator's Brochure.* South San Francisco: Genentech; 1999.

32. Speyer J, Green M, Kramer E, *et al.*: Protective effect of the bispiperazine ICRF-187 against doxorubicin-induced cardiac toxicity in women with advanced breast cancer. *N Engl J Med* 1988, 319:745–752.

33. Swain S, Whaley F, Gerber M, *et al.*: Delayed administration of dexrazoxane provides cardioprotection for patients with advanced breast cancer treated with doxorubicin-containing therapy. *J Clin Oncol* 1997, 15:1333–1340.

34. Lopez M, Vici P, Lauro LD, *et al.*: Randomized prospective clinical trial of high-dose epirubicin and dexrazoxane in patients with advanced breast cancer and soft tissue sarcomas. *J Clin Oncol* 1998, 16:1–7.

35. Sorensen B, Bastholt L, Mirza M, *et al.*: The cardioprotector ADR-529 and high-dose epirubicin given in combination with cyclophosphamide, 5-fluorouracil, and tamoxifen: a phase I study in metastatic breast cancer. *Cancer Chemother Pharmacol* 1994, 34:439–443.

36. Legha S, Benjamin R, Mackay B, *et al.*: Reduction of doxorubicin cardiotoxicity by prolonged continuous intravenous infusion. *Ann Intern Med* 1982, 96:133–139.

37. Torti F, Bristow M, Howes A, *et al.*: Reduced cardiotoxicity of doxorubicin delivered on a weekly schedule: assessment by endomyocardial biopsy. *Ann Intern Med* 1983, 99:745–749.

38. Berry G, Billingham M, Alderman E, *et al.*: Reduced cardiotoxicity of Doxil in AIDS Kaposi's sarcoma patients compared to a matched control group of cancer patients given doxorubicin [abstract]. *Proc Annu Meet Am Soc Clin Oncol* 1996, 15:A843.

39. Gottdeiner J, Appelbaum F, Ferrans V, *et al.*: Cardiotoxicity associated with high-dose cyclophosphamide therapy. *Arch Intern Med* 1981, 141:758–763.

40. Cazin B, Gorin N, Laporte J, *et al.*: Cardiac complications after bone marrow transplantation: a report on a series of 63 consecutive transplantations. *Cancer* 1986, 57:2061–2069.

41. Stewart JR FL: Radiation-induced heart disease: an update. *Cardiovasc Dis* 1984, 27:27–35.

42. Freeman N, Costanza M: 5-Fluorouracil associated cardiotoxicity. *Cancer* 1988, 61:36–45.

43. Weidmann B, Teipel A, Niederle N: The syndrome of 5-Fluorouracil cardiotoxicity: an elusive cardiopathy. *Cancer* 1994, 73:2001–2002.

44. Forni MD, Malet-Martino M, Jaillais P, *et al.*: Cardiotoxicity of high-dose continuous infusion fluorouracil: a prospective clinical study. *J Clin Oncol* 1992, 10:1795–801.

45. Akhtar S, Salim K, Bano Z: Symptomatic cardiotoxicity with high-dose 5-fluorouracil infusion: a prospective study. *Oncology* 1993, 50:441–444.

46. Keung YK, Lau S, Elkayam U, *et al.*: Cardiac arrythmia after infusion of cryopreserved stem cells. *Bone Marrow Transplantation* 1994, 14:363–367.

47. Lopez-Jimenez J, Munoz A, Hdez-Madrid A, *et al.*: Cardiovascular toxicities related to the infusion of cryopreserved grafts: results of a controlled study. *Bone Marrow Transplantation* 1994, 13:789–793.

48. Rowinsky E, McGuire W, Guarnieri T, *et al.*: Cardiac disturbances during the administration of Taxol. *J Clin Oncol* 1991, 9:1704–1712.

49. Arbuck S, Strauss H, Rowinksy E, *et al.*: A reassessment of cardiac toxicity associated with Taxol. *Monogr Natl Cancer Inst* 1993, 15:117–130.

50. Bristow M, Thompson P, Martin R, *et al.*: Early anthracycline cardiotoxicity. *Am J Med* 1978, 65:823–832.

51. Lawmore-Luria H, Kohn K, Pasternack R: Radiation heart disease. *J Cardiovasc Med* 1993, 8:113–125.

52. Tarbell N, Thompson L, Mauch P: Thoracic irradiation in Hodgkin's disease: disease control and long-term complications. *Int J Radiat Oncol Biol Phys* 1990, 18:275–282.

Neurologic symptoms and signs in cancer patients have several causes, such as metastatic involvement of the central nervous system (CNS) or peripheral nervous system, paraneoplastic disorders, or therapy-related neurotoxicity. Peripheral and central neurotoxicity is a common side effect of chemotherapeutic drugs. Vinca alkaloids, cisplatin, and the taxanes are among the most important agents inducing peripheral neurotoxicity, whereas, for instance, methotrexate and ifosfamide are primarily known for their central neurotoxic side effects. Neurotoxicity due to chemotherapy is frequently dose related. In most chemotherapeutic regimens, bone marrow toxicity is the major limiting factor. Strategies, such as bone marrow transplantation and the administration of growth factors, are being developed to overcome the toxic effects of chemotherapy on bone marrow. This will allow use of higher chemotherapy doses and, consequently, the risk of neurotoxicity will also increase. Peripheral and central neurotoxicities caused by several cytostatic compounds are reviewed in this chapter together with some data on neuroprotection. Comprehensive reviews of neurotoxic effects of chemotherapy have been written by several authors [1,2]. An overview of chemotherapeutic agents causing peripheral and/or central neurotoxicity is given in Table 29-1.

VINCA ALKALOIDS

The vinca alkaloids comprise two natural alkaloids, *vincristine* and *vinblastine*, and semisynthetic compounds, such as *vindesine* and *vinorelbine*. Vinca alkaloids arrest cell division by inhibiting microtubule formation in the mitotic spindle. They bind to tubulin and prevent its polymerization from soluble dimers into microtubules. The initial physiologic lesion in vinca alkaloid–induced neuropathy may be disruption of axoplasmic flow due to breakdown of micro/neurotubules, eventually leading to axonal degeneration. In early clinical studies, myelosuppression was mild, but dose-related neurotoxicity limited use of vincristine, which induces peripheral and autonomic neuropathy, cranial nerve palsy, and CNS toxicity. Other reported nonhematologic toxicities comprise alopecia, tightness of jaw or pharynx muscles, and abdominal pain.

Vinblastine produces a similar clinical spectrum of neurotoxicity, but, unlike vincristine, it also produces a severe degree of bone-marrow suppression that usually precedes neurotoxicity as the dose-limiting factor. **Vindesine** and **vinorelbine** normally produce only mild neurotoxicity, mainly consisting of a dose-dependent loss of deep tendon reflexes.

Neuropathic signs and symptoms are observed frequently with vincristine with early loss of ankle reflexes. Paresthesias can be the initial symptom and develop usually first in the fingers and later in the toes. Later, mild sensory loss for each type of superficial sensation may appear in fingers and toes, rarely spreading to the wrist or ankle. Vibration sensation is rarely severely impaired. Attendant weakness may be more disabling than sensory loss. It may require dose reduction or cessation of vincristine therapy. Motor impairment usually begins with clumsiness of the hands due to involvement of finger and wrist extensor muscles. The dorsiflexors of the toes and ankles are the most frequently involved muscles of the lower limb, leading to difficulties in walking [3].

In one study, motor weakness developed in 36%, and sensory complaints (numbness, burning, and tingling in hands and feet) in 46% of patients [4]. Paresthesias occurred in 57% of 392 patients treated with vincristine 12.5 to 75 µg/kg/wk and were evenly distributed over different dose levels but with shorter time to onset in the high-dose group. Weakness occurred in 23% of patients with decreased hand grip strength, hand clumsiness, wrist or foot drop, and slapping gait, particularly in the high-dose group.

Apart from symmetric and distal sensorimotor polyneuropathy, mononeuropathies can occur, such as unilateral femoral and peroneal neuropathy. Cranial nerve palsies have been recognized (vocal cord paresis, diplopia, ophthalmoplegia, ptosis, facial palsy, loss of corneal reflexes and paroxysmal jaw pain probably indicating trigeminal involvement, optic nerve dysfunction, or sensorineural hearing loss).

Autonomic neuropathy is not infrequent and gastrointestinal (GI) side effects are common. Troublesome constipation was reported in one third of patients with a higher frequency, greater severity, and earlier onset with high-dose vincristine. Reduction of GI tract motility can lead to paralytic ileus or megacolon. Other autonomic side effects include bladder atony with urinary retention, impotence, orthostatic hypotension, and disturbed heart rate variability.

Central nervous system (CNS) toxicity is rare, possibly due to poor penetration of vincristine. Mental depression, agitation, insomnia, confusion, hallucinations, transient cortical blindness, transient ataxia, syndrome of inappropriate antidiuretic hormone secretion (SIADH) with hyponatremia, seizures, and coma have all been reported in small numbers of patients.

An accidental massive overdose of intravenous vincristine causes more pronounced peripheral and CNS toxicity and resulted in death in four of 10 reported patients. Accidental intrathecal administration of vincristine almost invariably leads to a lethal ascending radiculomyeloencephalopathy, except for one patient who survived with residual lower extremity neuropathy, and another who survived in a vegetative state.

Unusually severe neurotoxicity has been described in three patients treated with vincristine and subsequently with isoniazid or L-asparaginase, and in patients with Charcot-Marie-Tooth syndrome [5].

With evidence of hepatic insufficiency, a severe neuropathy can occur after receiving relatively low doses of vincristine, probably due to impaired vincristine inactivation by the liver or delayed biliary excretion. Higher age may be a risk factor for the development of vincristine-induced neuropathy, although some authors dispute this. In children, neuropathy was less frequent than in adults.

The natural course of vincristine-induced neuropathy after discontinuation is usually favorable [6]. Improvement of paresthesias is the first sign of recovery. Cranial nerve palsies resolve within 4 months in most patients, although visual and hearing loss may persist. Electrophysiologic studies show distal axonal neuropathic changes with decreased distal motor and sensory nerve action potentials, whereas the response of proximal muscles is not clearly modified. Only slight reduction of motor and sensory nerve conduction velocities was found, even in patients with severe neuropathy [3].

Sural nerve biopsy in vincristine-treated patients shows primarily axonal or wallerian degeneration, accompanied by segmental demyelination and reduction of large- and small-diameter fiber density.

In general, neurotoxicity is less severe when smaller doses of vincristine or longer intervals between administrations are employed. Several attempts have been pursued to ameliorate or prevent vincristine-induced neurotoxicity. Gangliosides attenuate vincristine neurotoxicity in vitro, and substantially reduce vincristine-induced electrophysiologic alterations in rabbit sciatic nerve. Gangliosides 40 mg intramuscularly (IM) twice weekly prevented vincristine neurotoxicity in two of seven patients. Glutamic acid, 1.5 g orally (PO) daily, seemed to be able to reduce vincristine neurotoxicity. The adrenocorticotropic hormone (ACTH) (4-9) analogue Org 2766 modulated vincristine-induced neurotoxicity in an experimental snail model. In a randomized, double-blind, placebo-controlled pilot study, Org 2766 seemed to have a neuroprotective effect, but results were possibly influenced by a significant age difference between study groups [7].

Nerve growth factor prevented neurotoxic effects of vincristine on adult rat sympathetic ganglion explants. Neuroprotective effects of nerve growth factor in humans are not known at present.

PLATINUM ANALOGUES

Cisplatin and carboplatin are the most commonly used agents in this group. The mechanism of action is related to platinum binding to DNA and the formation of interstrand and intrastrand crosslinks. These platinum compounds are used against various tumor types. In combination therapy, they can be curative for testicular and ovarian cancer.

Cisplatin, in use since 1972, can be administered as intravenous bolus infusion in a dose range of 50 to 100 mg/m², but doses up to

Table 29-1. Peripheral and Central Neurotoxicity Caused By Chemotherapeutic Agents

Drug	Peripheral neurotoxicity	Central neurotoxicity	Comments
Vinca alkaloids			
Vincristine	Sensorimotor, autonomic neuropathy, mononeuropathy, cranial neuropathy	Agitation, somnolence, seizures, coma, SIADH	Usually favorable outcome, dose dependency; much less neurotoxicity compared to vincristine
Vinblastine			
Vindesine			
Vinorelbine			
Platinum analogues			
Cisplatin	Sensory neuropathy, autonomic neuropathy, cranial neuropathy, plexopathy, ototoxicity	Headache, cortical blindness, encephalopathy, seizures, focal deficit	Frequent off-therapy worsening, often residual symptoms/signs; dose dependency
Carboplatin	Peripheral neuropathy	Cortical blindness, focal deficit	Peripheral neuropathy is rare, with high dose
Taxanes			
Paclitaxel	Predominantly sensory neuropathy, sensorimotor neuropathy (high-dose), cranial neuropathy	Seizures, encephalopathy	Dose dependency, usually partial recovery, CNS toxicity only with high dose
Docetaxel	Predominantly sensory neuropathy, proximal extremity weakness		Sometimes off-therapy worsening; dose dependency
Methotrexate	Radiculopathy (rare)	Encephalopathy, seizures, aseptic meningitis, leukoencephalopathy	Depending on dose, route of administration, relation with RT
Adriamycin	Only preclinical evidence	Cerebrovascular events	Related to cardiotoxicity
Misonidazole	Sensory neuropathy	Encephalopathy	Usually recovery
Metronidazole	Sensory neuropathy	Confusion, somnolence, seizures, cerebellar dysfunction	Related to dose and long-term administration
Etoposide	Sensory neuropathy	—	—
Procarbazine	Sensory or sensorimotor neuropathy	Encephalopathy, drowsiness, stupor, coma	Usually reversible
Hexamethylmelamine	Sensory neuropathy	Ataxia, tremor, parkinsonism, mood changes	Usually mild
Ifosfamide	Painful neuropathy	Encephalopathy, cerebellar dysfunction, seizures, delirium, coma	Neuropathy only sporadic, with high dose
Cytosine-arabinoside	Sensory neuropathy, plexopathy	Cerebellar dysfunction, confusion, lethargy, somnolence	Meningitis, seizures, myelopathy after IT administration
Suramin	Sensorimotor neuropathy, Guillain-Barré–like syndrome	—	Dose dependency, incomplete recovery occasionally
5-Azacytidine	"Neuromuscular toxicity"	Encephalopathy, somnolence	
Mitotane	"Neuromuscular dysfunction"	Ataxia, neuropsychologic deficit	
Purine analogues	Motor and sensory neuropathy	Encephalopathy, dementia, coma, cortical blindness	Dose dependency
Fludarabine			
Cladribine			
Pentostatin			
Amsacrine	Sensory neuropathy	—	Sporadic
Immunomodulating agents	Motor and sensory neuropathy, auditory impairment, plexopathy, cranial nerve palsy	Encephalopathy, anxiety, tremor, akathisia, depression, confusion, seizures	
Interferon-α			
Interleukin-2			
Cyclosporin			
Tacrolimus			

CNS—central nervous system; IT—intrathecal; RT—radiotherapy; SIADH—syndrome of inappropriate antidiuretic hormone.

200 mg/m^2 per cycle may be given. Renal dysfunction, nausea and vomiting, auditory impairment, and myelosuppression are frequently observed. Peripheral neuropathy is considered an important side effect and may be dose limiting.

A survival analysis in ovarian cancer patients who were treated with cisplatin indicated that neuropathy may lead to persistent symptoms [8].

Sensory symptoms are common and most patients have no muscle weakness. The first symptoms usually consist of paresthesias in the feet and numbness of toes and fingers. These symptoms worsen with increasing cumulative doses and tend to spread proximally. Eventually paresthesias and dysesthesias may become extremely disabling. Impaired proprioception may lead to ataxia, clumsiness of fine movements, and gait disturbances. A positive Lhermitte sign has been experienced by many patients, presumably due to involvement of posterior tracts. Symptoms of autonomic neuropathy are infrequent and may consist of dizziness of postural change, palpitations, GI abnormalities, or impotence.

On neurologic examination, decreased vibratory sense and decreased ankle reflexes are the first signs. Reduction of patellar reflexes and reflexes in the arms and loss of vibratory sensation in the fingers follow when treatment continues. Joint position sense, light touch, and pin prick sensation are only slightly affected.

Cisplatin neuropathy is predominantly of a pure sensory axonal type, affecting large-diameter and, to a lesser extent, small-diameter sensory fibers. Motor signs (ie, muscular atrophy or impaired muscle strength) are usually not observed, although isolated cases with sensorimotor neuropathy have been reported.

Incidence of sensory neuropathy following cisplatin largely depends on the cumulative dose. Onset of symptoms occurs at cumulative doses of 300 to 400 mg/m^2, and after completion of treatment (usually at a total dose of 600 mg/m^2) up to 90% of patients may have clinical signs and symptoms. Cavaletti *et al.* [9] found that not only cumulative dose but also single-dose intensity is relevant.

A striking clinical characteristic of cisplatin-induced neuropathy is neurologic deterioration after cessation of therapy. This deterioration may continue for several months. Frequency of such off-therapy deterioration, which has only been studied in small numbers of patients, ranges from 31% to 100%. Neurotoxic side effects often show little tendency to improve over time.

Apart from sensory neuropathy, other manifestations of neurotoxicity have been reported (eg, optic disc swelling, loss of myelinated fibres, gliosis of dorsal columns).

Cranial nerve impairment was observed in patients who received intraarterial cisplatin, and intracarotid administration of cisplatin for CNS tumors may lead to serious optic toxicity. Lumbosacral plexopathies were observed after intraarterial cisplatin administration in the external or internal iliac arteries.

The CNS is occasionally involved. Headache, transient cortical blindness, encephalopathy, focal deficits, stroke, and generalized tonic-clonic epileptic seizures may occur. That cortical blindness may have a vascular cause is suggested by the sudden onset of symptoms. Cerebral herniation and coma have been reported in patients who are treated for intracranial tumors with intravenous cisplatin. Acute hypoosmolality with fluid shifts in combination with cerebral edema may contribute to this condition but direct neurotoxicity of cisplatin may also play a role.

Several studies report similar electrophysiologic abnormalities resulting from cisplatin therapy. Motor nerve conduction velocities and motor unit action potentials remain normal during therapy.

Distal sensory latencies become prolonged or disappear completely and sensory action potentials are reduced. Sensory nerve conduction velocity is only mildly impaired. These findings are consistent with an axonal rather than with a demyelinating neuropathy. Postmortem morphologic examination may reveal a mild degree of neuropathy in proximal nerves and a moderate to severe degree in distal nerves. Ultrastructurally, one may observe axonal degeneration and secondary myelin breakdown.

The exact mechanism of cisplatin neurotoxicity remains unclear. In a postmortem study of patients treated with cisplatin, the highest concentrations were found in the dorsal root ganglia [10], containing the cell bodies of the sensory nerves. Neural tissue concentrations correlated well with cumulative dose. Histopathologic signs of neurotoxicity occurred with higher accumulations of cisplatin. Moreover, platinum levels did not show a tendency to decrease with time. Evidence suggests platinum is tightly bound within nerve tissue, leading to dorsal root ganglia neurotoxicity [10,11].

Dose escalation may be possible by addition of cytoprotective agents that prevent cisplatin-related side effects without interfering with antitumor activity. Amifostine and glutathione are compounds that contain sulfhydryl. Amifostine is a prodrug that is turned into an active protecting agent by dephosphorylation. This compound acts as a scavenger of oxygen-free radicals, which may protect against cisplatin-induced neuropathy. One study reports significant reduction in the severity of cisplatin-induced neuropathy in patients pretreated with amifostine [12]. In a rat model, glutathione prevented cisplatin-related neuropathy, and a low degree of neurotoxicity was found in patients with ovarian cancer who were treated with 160 mg/m^2 cisplatin (4 days 40 mg/m^2) per cycle for five cycles in combination with glutathione (1500 mg/m^2). In two prospective randomized trials, glutathione treatment reduced cisplatin-induced peripheral neurotoxicity [13,14].

Org 2766 prevented or lessened cisplatin-induced neurotoxicity in experimental models. In humans, this compound was tested in a randomized, double-blind, placebo-controlled study. An increase in vibration perception threshold was not observed in the high-dose group of Org 2766 compared with findings in placebo-treated patients. Clinical signs and symptoms were less frequent in patients treated with Org 2766. The protective effects of Org 2766 were less prominent in patients treated with relatively lower doses [15]. This potential beneficial effect was not observed in a study with 131 ovarian cancer patients randomized to Org 2766 or placebo.

Carboplatin is a cisplatin analogue that provides more myelosuppressive effects but is significantly less neurotoxic than the parent compound. However, when cisplatin and carboplatin are combined, peripheral neuropathy is prohibitive, and severe neuropathy has been described in patients treated with high-dose carboplatin [16]. Furthermore, cortical blindness and thrombotic microangiopathy that lead to multiple cerebrovascular infarcts have been described.

TAXANES

Two taxanes are currently used as antineoplastic agents. Paclitaxel (Taxol; Bristol-Myers Squibb Oncology/Immunology Division; Princeton, NJ) was developed first for the treatment of cancer. Docetaxel (Taxotere; Rhône-Poulenc Rorer Pharmaceuticals, Inc.; Collegeville, PA) was introduced a few years later.

Paclitaxel is derived from the Western Yew, *Taxus brevifolia*. Paclitaxel acts as a potent inhibitor of eukaryotic cell replication, blocking cells in the late G2 mitotic phase of the cell cycle, through its action on microtubules. Microtubules are an essential component of the mitotic spindle and are required for maintenance of cell shape and various cellular activities such as cell motility and axoplasmic transport. Paclitaxel induces polymerization and stabilization of microtubules, which renders them less effective. At the molecular level, the mechanism by which paclitaxel interacts with microtubules and blocks cells in mitosis is still poorly understood. In 1989, Lipton et al. [17] were the first to report paclitaxel-induced neuropathy. Hypersensitivity reactions, neutropenia, myalgia/arthralgia, and mucositis are other frequently reported side effects. Paclitaxel is administered intravenously in courses of 1, 3, 6, 24 or 96 hours, usually once every 3 weeks. Neurologic symptoms are predominantly sensory, developing as early as 48 hours after treatment, usually beginning with paresthesias, numbness, and sometimes painful sensations in hands or feet. Difficulties with hand function (writing, doing up buttons), walking (unsteadiness), or problems with operating the foot pedals in an automobile may occur. The patient's motor symptoms are usually mild or absent. Myalgia and arthralgia occur temporarily after therapy, especially with higher dosage.

Large-diameter nerve fiber abnormalities are observed more frequently than small-diameter nerve fiber abnormalities. Motor signs are mild, although with higher doses per cycle (250 mg/m^2), some patients develop decreased hand grip strength and minor extensor hallucis weakness. With higher doses, the ankle reflex may disappear after only a single course, followed by patellar reflex depression. Vibration perception thresholds (VPT) increase primarily in feet, but with higher doses this effect may also be found in hands. Patients with diabetes seem to be at higher risk for development of paclitaxel-induced neuropathy.

Orthostatic hypotension and paralytic ileus have been described with doses over 170 to 250 mg/m^2. A mild myopathy has been recognized with high dose paclitaxel/cisplatin combination therapy [18]. Freilich et al. [19] suggested a neuropathic origin for paclitaxel-induced proximal weakness. Perioral numbness and optic nerve toxicity have been reported with dosages between 175 and 225 mg/m^2, and bilateral facial nerve palsy with high-dose paclitaxel [20].

The CNS is only rarely involved; in a few patients epileptic seizures occurred shortly after paclitaxel infusion, and in high-dose therapy, acute encephalopathy with obtundation, coma, confusion, and abnormal findings on magnetic resonance imaging may occur [21].

After discontinuation of therapy, neuropathic signs usually resolve, but this may take months: permanent residual neuropathy has been reported. In some patients, neuropathy may progress for 1 to 3 weeks after the end of treatment.

A clear correlation exists between neuropathic signs and symptoms and between cumulative dose and dose intensity per course. Neuropathy is the major dose-limiting toxicity with 250 to 300 mg/m^2 per course [22]. In a comparative study, the dose-limiting toxicity was myelosuppression in patients treated with paclitaxel at 250 mg/m^2, whereas neuropathy was the dose-limiting toxicity in patients treated with paclitaxel at 300 mg/m^2 if combined with granulocyte-colony stimulating factor for bone marrow support [23].

Most reports agree that higher dose per cycle, higher cumulative dose, and antecedent neuropathy are risk factors for development of paclitaxel-induced neuropathy. Infusion time may also influence findings.

Electrophysiologic studies show reduction of sensory nerve action potentials in a symmetric, distal, length-dependent fashion. Sural sensory nerve action potentials are nearly always reduced or absent in symptomatic patients. Abnormal peroneal motor action potentials, median and ulnar nerve conduction velocities, tibial motor nerve conduction velocity, and denervation on needle examination have all been described in a relatively few cases.

A sural nerve biopsy in a symptomatic patient revealed fiber loss, lack of axonal sprouting, and axonal atrophy associated with secondary demyelination and remyelination [24].

In conclusion, paclitaxel leads to a predominantly sensory, symmetrically distributed, distal axonal neuropathy, which clearly depends on dosage but may also depend on schedule.

Experimental models have shown that in dorsal root ganglion-spinal cord cultures, exposure to paclitaxel results in an unusual abundance of microtubules in neurons. Injection into rat sciatic nerve leads to slow accumulation of microtubules in Schwann cells and axons, altered Schwann cell behavior, axonal swelling, and combined retraction and disruption of myelin with significantly affected axoplasmic traffic. Paclitaxel's ability to induce clinical neuropathy seems in agreement with its effects on microtubules, but it is not clear whether the primary site of toxicity is the cell body (neuronopathy) or the axon (axonopathy). Some evidence suggests that with low or intermediate doses of paclitaxel, this neuropathy results in length-dependent axonal loss, similar to that seen in dying-back neuropathy (axonopathy), whereas with higher doses, the quick onset of symptoms in upper and lower extremities combined with increased vibration perception threshold suggest a neuronopathy. In experimental models paclitaxel accumulated preferentially in the dorsal root ganglia [25], and fast axonal transport was blocked [26].

In nonhuman animal studies, nerve growth factor attenuates or prevents neurotoxic effects of paclitaxel. Data on neuroprotection nerve growth factor with respect to paclitaxel-induced neuropathy are not yet available in humans. Administration of the cytoprotective agent amifostine with high-dose paclitaxel in patients with advanced cancer showed promising results, which were not, however, confirmed in a recent randomized study in patients with metastatic breast cancer [27].

Docetaxel (Taxotere) is a semisynthetic taxoid derived from a precursor extracted from the needles from the European Yew, *Taxus baccata*. Like paclitaxel, docetaxel is a potent inhibitor of cell replication. It promotes in vitro assembly of stable microtubules and induces microtubule bundle formation in cells. Response rates to 35% have been reported in non–small cell lung cancer and platinum-refractory advanced ovarian cancer. Hematologic toxicity is frequently encountered. Nonhematologic toxicities include alopecia, skin rash, fluid retention, diarrhea, hypersensitivity reactions, and peripheral neuropathy. The drug is administered intravenously over a 1- to 6-hour infusion time, usually 100 mg/m^2, once every 21 days.

Neuropathy resulting from docetaxel is mild to moderate in most cases with paresthesias, loss of deep tendon reflexes, and loss of vibration sensation usually occurring with higher cumulative dosage. Neuropathy occurred in about one third of chemotherapy-naive patients, but in two thirds of those patients who had previously been treated with cisplatin or vinblastine. Some patients experienced motor signs, possibly related to associated diseases such as connective tissue disease.

Of 40 patients treated with docetaxel (dose escalation 10 to 115 mg/m^2) once every 21 days in a 6-hour infusion, five patients (12%) developed peripheral neuropathy. Neuropathy developed in 16 of 146 patients (11%) treated with 100 mg/m^2 docetaxel in a 2-hour infusion every 21 days. Patients became symptomatic at a wide range of cumulative doses (50 to 720 mg/m^2) and dose levels (10 to 115 mg/m^2). More severe clinical and electrophysiologic abnormalities were noted at cumulative doses of 400 mg/m^2 or higher [28].

Symptoms are predominantly sensory with distal stocking-glove paresthesias, which begin in the feet and later progress to the fingers. The commonest abnormalities on electrophysiologic examination consist of low amplitude motor and sensory potentials, moderately slow motor conduction velocities (peroneal and tibial), and absent sural sensory nerve potentials. Fibrillary potentials may be registered on needle electromyography (EMG). A superficial peroneal nerve biopsy showed loss of large myelinated fibers and occasional fibers undergoing axonal degeneration. Follow-up data show improvement of sensory and motor symptoms as early as 6 to 8 weeks after therapy. One patient had progression of neuropathic symptoms and signs during more than 4 months after discontinuation of docetaxel. Hilkens *et al.* [29] reported a predominantly sensory neuropathy in half the patients treated with a 1-hour infusion of 100 mg/m² docetaxel once every 21 days. Paresthesias (51%), pain, numbness, unsteady gait, positive Lhermitte's sign (5%), objective sensory loss (30%), loss of ankle reflex (51%), and loss of both ankle and patellar reflexes (41%) were found. Symptoms, although mild in most patients, could be moderate or severe in patients treated with cumulative doses of more than 600 mg/m². Off-therapy deterioration was observed in 4 of nine patients. Predominantly proximal motor weakness has been described as well. Pyridoxine may ameliorate docetaxel-induced paresthesias and dysesthesias. Clinical, electrophysiologic, and pathologic data are consistent with an axonal sensorimotor neuropathy.

MISCELLANEOUS CYTOSTATIC DRUGS

Methotrexate is known for its central neurotoxic side effects, which can be categorized into immediate, acute to subacute, and chronic neurologic syndromes, in part depending on dosage level and on route of administration. After intrathecal administration, transient aseptic meningitis with headache, stiff neck, low grade fever, and CSF pleocytosis may occur. Rarely, paraplegia with spinal cord necrosis or anterior lumbosacral radiculopathy have been described [30]. After intravenous administration, acute or subacute encephalopathy (within days) can occur with somnolence, confusion, and focal deficits or seizures. The commonest long-term side effect of methotrexate is leukoencephalopathy, which is related to multiple intrathecal or high-dose intravenous administration of methotrexate, and especially to the combination of radiotherapy with subsequent methotrexate therapy. On computed tomography (CT) and MRI nonenhancing diffuse white matter abnormalities, atrophy, and small calcifications can be seen.

Adriamycin is a glycoside anthracycline drug that interferes with RNA-DNA synthesis by intercalating between base pairs of DNA, thus causing breaks in the helical strands. In a dose of 10 mg/kg, it can cause posterior limb ataxia in rats related to changes in dorsal root ganglion cells. Injection into rat sciatic nerve results in demyelination secondary to focal Schwann cell degeneration. Despite these laboratory findings on neurotoxicity, no clear evidence confirms peripheral neuropathy in patients treated with adriamycin. The drug may cause cardiotoxicity, which has been related to cerebrovascular events due to cardiac emboli.

Misonidazole, a 2-nitroimidazole, is used as a drug adjuvant to radiotherapy; it may cause painful paresthesias in feet or fingers, difficulties in walking, loss of deep sensation, or weakness. Conduction studies revealed evidence of axonal damage, especially in the lower limbs, and that affected sensory more than motor fibers with severe reduction of sensory action potentials. Sural nerve biop-

sies may reveal a decreased number of large-diameter myelinated fibers. After cessation of therapy, recovery or improvement has been observed. Encephalopathy has been described as well.

Metronidazole therapy is associated not only with CNS toxicity, but also with sensory neuropathy after long-term administration and high cumulative doses. Nerve biopsy shows axonal degeneration with secondary segmental demyelination [31]. Transient confusion, alterations of consciousness, seizures, headache, tinnitus, and cerebellar dysfunction may occur with reversible abnormalities found on MRI.

Podophyllin derivatives are also employed as anticancer agents.

Etoposide (VP-16) is a semisynthetic derivative of podophyllotoxin with established antineoplastic activity. This drug can cause sensory neuropathy in mice with dose-related changes in dorsal root ganglion cells, axonal degeneration of their distal and proximal processes in peripheral nerves, dorsal spinal roots, and dorsal spinal funiculi. Sensory neuropathy has been recognized in patients receiving intensive therapy with etoposide and melphalan. When etoposide is administered at higher doses, headache, seizures, and somnolence can occur.

Teniposide (VM-26) is not clearly associated with either peripheral or CNS neurotoxicity.

Procarbazine is used against hematologic malignancies and brain tumors. Peripheral neuropathy and CNS toxicity have been reported. Peripheral neuropathy with paresthesias of the extremities and depressed tendon reflexes occurred in 17% of patients. Ataxia, orthostatic hypotension, and weakness of intrinsic hand muscles are recognized findings. Peripheral neuropathy was rarely a significant problem during oral administration and was usually reversible. Encephalopathic symptoms range from mild drowsiness to confusion or stupor. In patients with recurrent glioma treated with prior radiotherapy, treatment with the combination of procarbazine, CCNU (lomustine), and vincristine may lead to partly reversible CNS side effects [32].

Hexamethylmelamine is used as a second-line agent in ovarian cancers. Mild to moderate peripheral sensory neuropathy has been reported in 36% of patients, but 96% of these patients had been treated previously with cisplatin-based chemotherapy [33]. Reversible CNS toxicity-related side effects include ataxia, tremor, parkinsonism, and mood changes.

Ifosfamide may cause acute, but usually reversible, encephalopathy with cerebellar dysfunction, extrapyramidal signs, hallucinations, seizures, delirium, and coma. These effects usually begin within hours of administration but may be delayed up to 6 days after treatment. Severe painful axonal peripheral neuropathy associated with high-dose ifosfamide has been described [34].

Cytosine arabinoside (cytarabine, Ara-C) may cause sporadic cases of painful sensory peripheral neuropathy, particularly in combination with daunorubicin and asparaginase. Brachial plexus neuropathy related to cytosine-arabinoside therapy has been reported. In an isolated case of severe neuropathy, axonal degeneration and scattered destruction of myelin sheaths were observed. After intrathecal administration of Ara-C, aseptic meningitis and myelopathy may occur, similar to findings seen with methotrexate, and, more rarely, seizures or (sub)acute encephalopathy. After intravenous administration, cerebellar dysfunction, confusion, lethargy, and somnolence have been described. Cerebellar atrophy and white matter abnormalities on CT or MRI can be seen. Neuropathology showed loss of Purkinje cells.

Suramin was originally developed as an antiparasitic. Later, it was found to have antineoplastic properties. It can prevent or inhibit binding of several growth factors to the associated receptors, and thus suramin antagonizes the ability of these factors to stimulate tumor growth. Various side effects have been described, such as acute reversible demyelinating polyneuropathy with a clinical picture resembling that found in Guillain-Barré syndrome. Patients may develop a transient flaccid paralysis with involvement of bulbar and respiratory muscles. Development of this neuropathy correlated with maximal levels of suramin in plasma [35]. Initially, progressive weakness mainly affected the proximal muscles of the legs, spreading distally and to arm muscles. Muscle weakness worsened over 4 to 9 weeks with occasional incomplete recovery.

Suramin may induce dorsal root ganglia damage that can be ameliorated by administration of high doses of nerve growth factor, which suggests a competition between both agents for the nerve growth factor receptor. Muscle weakness during suramin treatment may also be associated with hypophosphatemia and mitochondrial myopathy. CNS toxicity does not occur.

5-Azacytidine has been associated with reversible neuromuscular toxicity producing muscle tenderness, weakness, and lethargy. Confusion, irritability and somnolence have been observed too. It is not clear whether this neurotoxicity is due to a direct effect on neuromuscular function or due to a toxic encephalopathy.

Mitotane can cause neuromuscular dysfunction, cerebellar ataxia, and neuropsychological impairment.

Three purine analogues—**fludarabine, cladribine, pentostatin**—can produce severe, predominantly CNS toxicity with high-dose therapy (delayed progressive encephalopathy with cortical blindness, dementia, coma) and to generally transient and reversible CNS toxicity and peripheral neuropathy with standard therapy. Motor and sensory neuropathies have both been recognized [36].

Amsacrine leads sporadically to transient stocking-glove paresthesias in patients previously treated with cisplatin.

Interferon-α is used in the treatment of hairy cell leukemia; polyneuropathy and encephalopathy as side effects of this treatment have been reported. Neuralgic amyotrophy and bilateral oculomotor nerve paralysis may also develop. Auditory impairment (tinnitus, hearing loss, or both) was found in 45% of patients receiving long-term treatment with interferon. Audiometry-documented sensorineural hearing loss was found in approximately one third of patients. Anxiety, action tremor [37], akathisia, depression, confusion, somnolence, and lack of initiative have been described.

Interleukin-2 is used in the treatment of renal cell cancer and melanoma. Neurologic side effects involving the CNS include transient focal deficits, reversible encephalopathy, cerebral edema, and, rarely, painful brachial plexopathy.

The immunosuppressants **cyclosporine** and **tacrolimus (FK 506)** can cause motor and sensorimotor neuropathy in addition to CNS toxicity. Cyclosporine therapy may cause tremor, seizures, ataxia, paraparesis, quadriparesis, psychological disorders, and leukoencephalopathy. One case of recurrent acute inflammatory demyelinating polyradiculopathy, possibly related to cyclosporin therapy, has been reported.

REFERENCES

1. Posner JB: Side effects of chemotherapy. In *Neurologic Complications of cancer*. Edited by Posner JB. Philadelphia: FA Davis Company; 1995: 282–310.

2. Hammack JE, Cascino TL: Chemotherapy and other common drug-induced toxicities of the CNS in patients with cancer. In *Handbook of Clinical Neurology: Neuro-Oncology*, Part III, vol. 25 (69). Edited by Vecht ChJ. Amsterdam: Elsevier Science BV; 1997:481–514.

3. Casey EB, Jellife AM, Le Quesne PM, Millett YL: Vincristine neuropathy. Clinical and electrophysiological observations. *Brain* 1973, 96:69–86.

4. Sandler SG, Tobin W, Henderson ES: Vincristine-induced neuropathy. A clinical study of fifty leukemic patients. *Neurology* 1969, 19:367–374.

5. Hildebrandt G, Holler E, Woenkhaus M, *et al.*: Acute deterioration of Charcot-Marie-Tooth disease IA (CMT IA) following 2 mg of vincristine chemotherapy. *Ann Oncol* 2000, 11:743–747.

6. Postma TJ, Benard BA, Huijgens PC, *et al.*: Long term effects of vincristine on the peripheral nervous system. *J Neurooncol* 1993, 15:23–27.

7. van Kooten B, van Diemen HAM, Groenhout KM, *et al.*: A pilot study on the influence of a corticotropin (4-9) analogue on vinca alkaloid-induced neuropathy. *Arch Neurol* 1992, 49:1027–1031.

8. Willemse PHB, van Lith J, Mulder NH, *et al.*: Risks and benefits of cisplatin in ovarian cancer: a quality-adjusted survival analysis. *Eur J Cancer* 1990, 26:345–352.

9. Cavaletti G, Marzorati L, Bogliun G, *et al.*: Cisplatin-induced peripheral neurotoxicity is dependent on total-dose intensity and single-dose intensity. *Cancer* 1992, 69:203–207.

10. Gregg RW, Molepo JM, Monpetit VJA, *et al.*: Cisplatin neurotoxicity: the relationship between dosage, time, and platinum concentration in neurologic tissues, and morphologic evidence of toxicity. *J Clin Oncol* 1992, 10:795–803.

11. Meijer C, de Vries EGE, Marmiroli P, *et al.*: Cisplatin-induced DNA-platination in experimental dorsal root ganglia neuronopathy. *Neurotoxicology* 1999, 20:883–887.

12. Kemp G, Rose P, Lurain J, *et al.*: Amifostine pretreatment for protection against cyclophosphamide-induced and cisplatin-induced toxicities: results of a randomized control trial in patients with advanced ovarian cancer. *J Clin Oncol* 1996, 14:2101–2112.

13. Bogliun G, Marzorati L, Marzola M, *et al.*: Neurotoxicity of cisplatin +/- reduced glutathione in the first-line treatment of advanced ovarian cancer. *Int J Gynecol Cancer* 1996, 6:415–419.

14. Cascinu S, Cordella L, Del Ferro E, *et al.*: Neuroprotective effect of reduced glutathione on cisplatin-based chemotherapy in advanced gastric cancer: a randomized double-blind placebo-controlled trial. *J Clin Oncol* 1995, 13:26–32.

15. Gerritsen van der Hoop R, Vecht CJ, van der Burg MEL, *et al.*: Prevention of cisplatin neurotoxicity with an ACTH (4-9) analogue in patients with ovarian cancer. *N Engl J Med* 1990, 322:89–94.

16. Heinzlef O, Lotz J-P, Roullet E: Severe neuropathy after high dose carboplatin in three patients receiving multidrug chemotherapy. *J Neurol Neurosurg Psychiatry* 1998, 64:667–669.

17. Lipton RB, Apfel SC, Dutcher JP, *et al.*: Taxol produces a predominantly sensory neuropathy. *Neurology* 1989, 39:368–373.

18. Chaudhry V, Rowinsky EK, Sartorius SE, *et al.*: Peripheral neuropathy from taxol and cisplatin combination chemotherapy: clinical and electrophysiological studies. *Ann Neurol* 1994, 35:304–311.

19. Freilich RJ, Balmaceda C, Seidman AD, *et al.*: Motor neuropathy due to docetaxel and paclitaxel. *Neurology* 1996, 47:115–118.

20. Lee RT, Oster MW, Balmaceda C, *et al.*: Bilateral facial nerve palsy secondary to the administration of high-dose paclitaxel. *Ann Oncol* 1999, 10: 1245–1247.

21. Nieto Y, Cagnoni PJ, Bearman SI, *et al.*: Acute encephalopathy: a new toxicity associated with high-dose paclitaxel. *Clin Cancer Res* 1999, 5:501–506.

22. Postma TJ, Vermorken JB, Liefting AJM, *et al.*: Paclitaxel-induced neuropathy. *Ann Oncol* 1995, 6:489–494.

23. Schiller JH, Storer B, Tutsch K, *et al.*: Phase I trial of 3-hour infusion of paclitaxel with or without granulocyte colony-stimulating factor in patients with advanced cancer. *J Clin Oncol* 1994, 12:241–248.

24. Sahenk Z, Barohn R, New P, Mendell JR: Taxol neuropathy. Electrodiagnostic and sural nerve biopsy findings. *Arch Neurol* 1994, 51:726–729.

25. Cavaletti G, Cavalletti E, Oggioni N, *et al.*: Distribution of paclitaxel within the nervous system of the rat after repeated intravenous administration. *Neurotoxicology* 2000, 21:389–393.

26. Nakata T, Yorifuji H: Morphological evidence of the inhibitory effect of taxol on the fast axonal transport. *Neurosci Res* 1999, 35:113–122.

27. Gelmon K, Eisenhauer E, Bryce C, *et al.*: Randomized phase II study of high-dose paclitaxel with or without amifostine in patients with metastatic breast cancer. *J Clin Oncol* 1999, 17:3038–3047.

28. New PZ, Jackson CE, Rinaldi D, *et al.*: Peripheral neuropathy secondary to docetaxel (Taxotere). *Neurology* 1996, 46:108–111.

29. Hilkens PHE, Verweij J, Stoter G, *et al.*: Peripheral neurotoxicity induced by docetaxel. *Neurology* 1996, 46:104–108.

30. Koh S, Nelson MD, Jr, Kovanlikaya A, Chen LS: Anterior lumbosacral radiculopathy after intrathecal methotrexate treatment. *Pedriatr Neurol* 1999, 21:576–578.

31. Neundörfer B: Neurologische Begleiterkrankungen des M. Crohn. *Fortschr Neurol Psychiatr* 1992, 60:481–486.

32. Postma TJ, van Groeningen CJ, Witjes RJGM, *et al.*: Neurotoxicity of combination chemotherapy with procarbazine, CCNU and vincristine (PCV) for recurrent glioma. *J Neurooncol* 1998, 38:69–75.

33. Manetta A, MacNeill C, Lyter JA, *et al.*: Hexamethylmelamine as a single second-line agent in ovarian cancer. *Gynecol Oncol* 1990, 36:93–96.

34. Patel SR, Vadhan-Raj S, Papadopolous N, *et al.*: High-dose ifosfamide in bone and soft tissue sarcomas: results of phase II and pilot studies: dose-response and schedule dependence. *J Clin Oncol* 1997, 15:2378–2384.

35. Chaudry V, Eisenberger MA, Sinibaldi VJ, *et al.*: A prospective study of suramin-induced peripheral neuropathy. *Brain* 1996, 119:2039–2052.

36. Cheson BD, Vena DA, Foss FM, Sorensen JM: Neurotoxicity of purine analogs: a review. *J Clin Oncol* 1994, 12:2216–2228.

37. Caraceni A, Gangeri L, Martini C, *et al.*: Neurotoxicity of interferon-alpha in melanoma therapy: results from a randomized controlled trial. *Cancer* 1998, 83:482–489.

CHAPTER 30: EVALUATION OF QUALITY OF LIFE IN CANCER CLINICAL TRIALS

Bernard F. Cole, Richard D. Gelber, Shari Gelber

Quality of life is an important consideration when making treatment decisions [1–3]. The choice of one treatment option over another for an individual patient may hinge on how the treatments affect quality of life. Therefore, it is important that the practicing oncologist has a thorough understanding of the potential impacts that treatments can have on quality of life in general as well as an understanding of the individual patient's needs and preferences. To help address these issues, the evaluation of quality of life is taking on an increasingly larger role in cancer clinical research. In particular, patient-oriented quality-of-life assessments are frequently being included in clinical trials as study endpoints for treatment comparisons. The purpose of this chapter is to provide an overview of the most common methods used in cancer clinical trials for the evaluation of quality of life.

HISTORICAL BACKGROUND

Early measures of quality of life in cancer focused on quantifying a patient's physical functioning. The Karnofsky Performance Status (KPS) measure, introduced in 1948 [4,5], is generally considered to be the first measure of physical functioning and has been widely used in cancer clinical research. KPS is measured on an 11-point scale from 0% to 100% (in 10% increments) in which 0% denotes death, 100% denotes normal function, and other values denote the approximate percentage of normal physical performance. The KPS assessment is made by the clinician. In 1960, the Eastern Cooperative Oncology Group (ECOG) converted the KPS into a six-point scale, often called the Zubrod scale [6].

Subsequent efforts in quality-of-life evaluation incorporated patients' perspectives of their illnesses and therapeutic regimens. For example, in 1971, Izsak and Medalie [7] developed a multidimensional scale that measured physical, social, and psychological variables in cancer patients. The scale was tailored to specific cancers and designed to assist clinicians in determining rehabilitation needs and evaluating patient progress. In 1975, a trial for patients with acute myelogenous leukemia used a six-level assessment of quality of life, ranging from "hospital stay throughout illness" to "no symptoms, normal life" [8]. The assessments were based on patient reports of their symptoms and functioning.

The modern era of quality-of-life assessment in cancer clinical trials research is generally cited to have begun in 1976 when Priestman and Baum [9] studied breast cancer treatment. They used 10 questions to assess patients' general feeling of well being, mood, level of activity, pain, nausea, appetite, ability to perform housework, social activities, general level of anxiety, and overall treatment assessment. Their results indicated that this instrument could be used to assess the subjective benefit of treatment in individual women, to detect changes over time, and to compare different treatments within a clinical trial.

MEASURING QUALITY OF LIFE

Many instruments are available for descriptively measuring quality of life in clinical trials. In general, these can be divided into two main categories: general quality-of-life instruments and disease-specific quality-of-life instruments. Examples of general instruments include the SF-36 [10], the Sickness Impact Profile [11], the SCL-90-R [12], and the World Health Organization Quality-of-Life Assessment Instrument [13], which is currently being developed. Each of these instruments includes general questions relating to a patient's health and functioning, and they can be applied in a wide range of disease settings. Table 30-1 presents a list of instruments that are cancer-specific. These instruments include specific items that are relevant for cancer patients.

Regardless of the instrument used, the goal is to provide measures of quality of life in various domains and, usually, an overall measure of global quality of life. The three most frequently measured domains are physical, social, and mental health. Other domains include disease symptoms, pain, general health perceptions, vitality, and role functioning. The last column of Table 30-1 shows the domains assessed by the cancer-specific quality-of-life instruments. Each quality-of-life instrument usually includes several individual questions or items that pertain to a particular domain, and the domain score (also called scale score) is obtained by summarizing the responses from the associated items (ie, average of the item responses). Each instrument has its own rules regarding the computation of the domain scores, and these rules are established after careful testing. The second column of Table 30-1 shows the total number of items used in each cancer-specific instrument. Each item is generally measured on a Likert scale or a linear

Table 30-1. Cancer-Specific Quality-of-Life Measurement Instruments

Instrument	Items, n	Domains Assessed
Breast Cancer Chemotherapy Questionnaire (BCQ) [14]	30	Attractiveness, fatigue, physical symptoms, inconvenience, emotional, hope, social support
Cancer Rehabilitation Evaluation System (CARES) [15]	93–132	Physical, psychosocial, medical interaction, marital, sexual, symptom- and treatment-specific items
European Organization for Research and Treatment of Cancer scale (EORTC: QLQ-C30) [16]	42	Five functional scales (physical, role, cognitive, emotional, social), three symptom scales (fatigue, pain, nausea), disease-specific items, global quality of life
Functional Assessment of Cancer Therapy (FACT) [17]	36–40	Physical, social/family, relationship with doctor, emotional, functional, well-being, disease-specific items
Functional Living Index — Cancer (FLIC) [18]	22	Psychological, social, disease symptoms, global well-being, treatment and disease issues, physical functioning
International Breast Cancer Study Group Quality of Life Questionnaire (IBCSG-QL) [19]	10	Physical well-being, mood, fatigue, appetite, coping, social support, symptoms, overall health
Linear Analogue Self Assessment (LASA) (Priestman and Baum [9])	25	Physical, psychological, social
Quality of Life Index (QLI) [20]	5	Physical activity, daily living, health perceptions, psychological, social support, outlook on life

analogue self-assessment (LASA) scale. The Likert scale is a categorical scale consisting of a limited choice of clearly defined responses. The most frequently employed scales use either four or five categories. In contrast, the LASA scale is an unmarked line, usually 10 cm long, with text at either end describing the extremes of the scale. Patients are asked to place a mark on the line in a position that best reflects his or her response.

MEASURING PATIENTS' PREFERENCES AND UTILITIES

In addition to measuring descriptive quality of life, there are methods for measuring a patient's preference, or utility, for particular health states. These methods attempt to measure how a patient might value one health state compared with another based on the quality-of-life attributes of the health states. For example, two patients might report similar symptoms with similar frequency and duration, but they may differ on how important these symptoms are in their daily lives. Descriptive quality-of-life instruments will correctly provide similar scores for the two patients, whereas a measurement of preference or utility will differentiate them.

Utility is measured on an interval scale from zero to one, where zero denotes a health state that is as bad as death, and one denotes a health state as good as best possible health. Values between zero and one denote degrees between these extremes. A simple interpretation of a utility for a specific health state (*eg*, state A) is that the utility represents the amount of time in a state of perfect health for which a patient values equally as one unit of time in state A. For example, suppose that state A has a utility of 0.7; the patient then values one month in state A as being equivalent to 0.7 months of perfect health. This interpretation leads to the idea of quality-of-life–adjusted time, which can be obtained by multiplying a health state duration by its utility coefficient. For example, if a patient experiences 6 months of toxicity and has a utility weight of 0.8 for time with toxicity, then the quality-adjusted time spent with toxicity is 4.2 months. This adjustment allows treatments that have different impacts on quality of life to be compared in a meaningful way.

Classically, utility assessment is carried out using interview techniques. The "standard gamble" technique gives patients a choice between a chronic health state with certainty or an uncertain health state that is either perfect health (with probability p), or death (with probability 1-p). The probability p is varied until the patient is indifferent between the certain and the uncertain choice, and the final p is taken as the utility value. The "time trade-off" technique gives patients a choice between living for a certain amount of time in a state of less than perfect health or a shorter amount of time in a state of perfect health. The duration of the perfect health state is varied until the patient expresses indifference in the choice. The utility is then taken as the ratio of the final health state durations. For a detailed overview of utility assessment, *see* Bennett and Torrance [21].

These interview techniques are cumbersome to use in practice. Fortunately, there are procedures for obtaining utility data from quality-of-life instruments. Generally, these procedures were developed by administering both the instrument and the interview to a study sample and building a statistical model for predicting the utility value from the instrument responses. Instruments that can be used for this purpose include the EuroQol [22], Health Utilities Index (HUI) [23], and Spitzer's Quality of Life Index (QLI) [20,24].

STUDY DESIGN IN CLINICAL TRIALS

As a "gold standard" study design, the authors propose a cancer clinical trial including the following outcomes: 1) usual clinical endpoints such as progression-free survival and overall survival, 2) usual assessment of toxicity/adverse event frequency and grade, 3) measurements of the timing and duration of all toxicities and adverse events, 4) longitudinal assessment of quality of life using a general instrument and a specific instrument, 5) a procedure for estimating patient utility or preference, and 6) a procedure for estimating health care cost. By including all of these components in a clinical trial, it becomes possible to address the clinical benefits of a new therapy as well as its impact on quality of life and whether it is cost-effective.

Of course, due to constrained resources, few studies will include all of these components. In addition, clinical trials that began in the 1980s or early 1990s will generally not include components for measuring quality of life or utility because methods for assessment were not as well established as they are today. To fill this potential gap, researchers use other methods to address pressing clinical issues. The best approach is to launch a smaller study that collects quality-of-life and utility data from a group of patients. Such a study can be longitudinal or cross-sectional. The advantage of the cross-sectional design is that the study can be completed more quickly. The disadvantage is that longitudinal effects on quality of life cannot be estimated. Inferior ancillary study designs include those that use proxy data for subjective quality-of-life domains.

Another approach that is described in more detail later is to retrospectively evaluate the duration of major health states that are thought to affect quality of life (*eg*, toxicity, disease progression). By combining clinical-outcome data with patient-level, cycle-by-cycle toxicity data (both of which are typically collected in cancer clinical trials), it is often possible to obtain estimates of durations of the health states. Utility weights can then be assigned to the health states, and this health-state utility model can be used to compare treatments in terms of quality-adjusted time. The utility weights can be estimated from a secondary cross-sectional study or they may be left unspecified. In the latter case, the results of the analysis should be displayed for a wide variety of choices for the utility weight values, not for just one or two arbitrary selections.

For new clinical trials currently being designed, it is critical that quality-of-life components be prospectively incorporated. At a minimum, a general quality-of-life instrument should be administered longitudinally; however, a disease-specific instrument will likely have better sensitivity to changes in quality of life. The timing of assessments should be designed to measure quality of life for the various clinical health states that a patient might experience both during and after therapy (*eg*, treatment-related toxicity, disease progression). For randomized studies, a baseline assessment should take place prior to treatment randomization. In addition, patients should be able to self-report troublesome adverse events and symptoms and their durations using a diary. These data could be used to validate the physician-reported adverse-event data typically collected. The diary idea is particularly appealing from a quality-of-life perspective because it is likely that a patient will self-report a particular adverse event that is causing him or her some distress and, therefore, represents a decrement in quality of life. As a result, diary data are useful for estimating the duration of time spent with adverse events—an outcome necessary for a health-state utility model.

ANALYSIS OF QUALITY-OF-LIFE DATA

Once data have been collected in a clinical trial or perhaps in a secondary cross-sectional study, the next step is to analyze the data to make inferences about the quality-of-life treatment effect. A number of standard statistical procedures are available. The most common approach is a *t* test or an analysis of variance (with repeated measures if the data are longitudinal). These procedures compare the mean quality-of-life scores across the treatment groups. In the longitudinal setting, the analysis can evaluate trends over time and test for a treatment by time interaction. The interaction test evaluates whether quality-of-life score changes differ over time according to treatment group. Analysis of variance can adjust the treatment comparison for other factors that may differ across the treatment groups. This is particularly important if the factors influence (confound) the quality-of-life assessments. For example, prognosis, demographic outcomes, and health care institution are potential confounders. A helpful visual display of this information can be obtained by plotting the (adjusted) mean quality-of-life scores over time according to treatment group.

The main difficulty in analyzing quality-of-life scores is missing data. Assessments may be missing more often when a patient's quality of life is deteriorating. For example, a patient was not feeling well and, therefore, was unable to concentrate on the form. Missing data that are related to the actual (unobserved) quality-of-life score are called nonignorable missing data. This term reflects the notion that the missing data cannot be ignored in the analysis. Therefore, an appropriate analysis of quality-of-life data will give a thorough description of the pattern of missing data. In particular, the rates of missing data across treatment groups are important statistics. If the rates of missing data are similar across treatment groups, then it is likely that the estimation bias within each treatment group will be balanced by the estimation bias in the other treatment groups. In other words, the biases will likely cancel, and the difference in quality-of-life scores between two treatments will be an accurate estimate of the treatment effect. If the pattern of missing assessment differs across the treatment groups, then the situation becomes more complex. If the higher rate of missing data is observed in the treatment group that has the lower quality-of-life scores, then the difference in quality-of-life scores is likely to be an underestimate of the true treatment effect. If this estimate is large in magnitude and statistically significantly different from zero, then the analysis gives a meaningful result. New statistical procedures are currently being developed to better analyze quality-of-life data that are nonignorably missing [25], but these approaches are not yet widely applied. These methods require additional assumptions concerning the mechanism of missing data.

COMBINING QUALITY AND QUANTITY OF LIFE

An endpoint that is increasingly being used in cancer clinical research is quality-of-life–adjusted survival time. Generally, this endpoint represents a patient's survival time weighted by the quality of life experienced, in which the weightings are based on utility values. Because utility is measured on a scale from zero to one, the quality-adjusted survival time is measured in the same time units as overall survival. The main advantage of a quality-adjusted endpoint is that it allows treatments that differ in their quality-of-life effects and their effects on survival to be compared in a metric that accounts for both of these differences. This is a common issue in cancer clinical research in which a new therapy may improve overall or progression-free survival but is also associated with more toxicity.

One approach to evaluating quality-adjusted survival time is the Quality-adjusted Time Without Symptoms or Toxicity method (Q-

TWiST) [26]. Q-TWiST evaluates treatments by computing the time spent in a series of clinical health states that may differ in terms of quality of life. Each health state is then weighted by a utility value to adjust the health-state duration according to its value in terms of quality of life.

The three steps involved in a Q-TWiST analysis are briefly described below. To make the procedure more concrete, we also provide a specific example that compares high-dose interferon alfa-2b administered for 1 year versus clinical observation for the adjuvant therapy of malignant melanoma. These data are obtained from 280 patients who participated in the ECOG clinical trial EST1684 [27,28]. The original report of this study indicated that high-dose interferon improved overall survival and relapse-free survival, but the regimen was also associated with significant toxicity that may cause a decrement in quality of life [27]. A Q-TWiST analysis was used to evaluate the clinical benefits after adjusting for the toxicity associated with high-dose interferon [28].

Step 1: Define Clinical Health States

The first step in the analysis is to define quality-of-life–oriented health states that are relevant for the disease setting and the treatments being studied. Typically, the health states reflect changes in clinical status that may be associated with changes in quality of

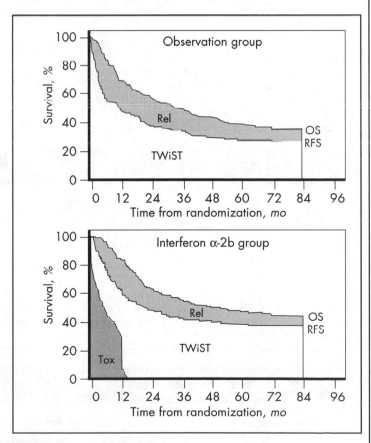

FIGURE 30-1.

Partitioned survival plots for the Eastern Cooperative Oncology Group trial. OS — overall survival; Rel — time following disease relapse; RFS — relapse-free survival; Tox — time with severe or life-threatening side effects of treatment toxicity; TWiST — time without severe or life-threatening treatment toxicity and without disease relapse.

life. For example, one health state may be associated with toxicity due to therapy, whereas another health state may be associated with disease progression. Usually, the health-state model includes a state of best possible health (given that the patient was diagnosed with cancer) represented by toxicity related to all time spent without treatment and without disease progression. Different health states may be defined for different treatment regimens when appropriate. For example, if two chemotherapy regimens are being compared and one of the regimens has a different toxicity profile than the other, then separate health states can be used to account for this in the model.

For example, in the ECOG trial comparing high-dose interferon versus observation for malignant melanoma, the following health states were defined: *Tox* represents all time with severe or life-threatening side effects of high-dose interferon, *TWiST* represents all time without severe or life-threatening treatment toxicity and without symptoms of disease relapse, and *Rel* represents all time following disease relapse. These health states reflect the major clinical changes in quality of life that are important for evaluating the impact of high-dose interferon.

Step 2: Partitioning Overall Survival

The second step in the analysis is to estimate the times at which patients make transitions from one health state to the next. This is accomplished by partitioning the overall survival time into the time spent in each of the health states. Kaplan-Meier survival curves are plotted for each health-state transition time and time to death on the same graph. A separate graph is used for each treatment group.

For example, using the health states Tox, TWiST, and Rel, one would plot the overall survival curve, a curve corresponding to the end of treatment toxicity (and the beginning of TWiST), and a curve corresponding to the disease relapse (indicating the end of TWiST

and the beginning of Rel). This technique allows one to visualize the health state durations as a portion of the overall survival time and compare them across the treatment groups. Most importantly, this procedure provides estimates of the mean duration of each health state. These estimates are derived from the areas between the curves. In the example, the mean duration of toxicity is given by the area under the toxicity curve, the mean duration of TWiST is the area between the relapse-free survival (RFS) curve and the toxicity curve, and the mean duration of Rel is the area between the overall survival (OS) curve and the relapse-free survival curve.

Figure 30-1 shows the partitioning of overall survival into the health states according to treatment group in the ECOG study. For each graph, the area beneath the overall survival curve is partitioned into the health states Tox, TWiST, and Rel as indicated. This partitioning was restricted to the median follow-up interval of 84 months. Table 30-2 shows the mean health state durations, the mean survival time, and the mean relapse-free survival time within the first 84 months from randomization in the study. The results indicate that patients in the interferon group experienced more time in TWiST and less time in Rel as compared with the observation group; however, the interferon group also experienced more time with severe or life-threatening toxicity.

Step 3: Comparing the Treatments

The third step is to compare the treatments using a weighted sum of the health-state durations. For example, in the Tox, TWiST, and Rel health-state model, the quality-adjusted survival endpoint (Q-TWiST) is defined by the equation Q-TWiST = $(u_{\text{Tox}} \times \text{Tox}) + \text{TWiST} + (u_{\text{Rel}} \times \text{Rel})$ in which *Tox*, *TWiST*, and *Rel* denote the mean time spent in each of the respective health states and u_{Tox} and u_{Rel} represent the utility weightings assigned to the states Tox and Rel, respectively.

Table 30-2. Mean Time for the Components of Q-TWiST Restricted to 84 Months of Median Follow-up in the ECOG Trial EST1684

Treatment Group	Treatment Group		Difference, mo	95% CI, mo	P value (2-sided)
	Observation, mo	Interferon alfa-2b, mo			
Tox	0.0	5.8	5.8	5.0–6.7	< 0.001
TWiST	30.0	33.1	3.1	-4.8–11.0	0.400
Rel	12.4	10.4	-2.0	-6.2–2.3	0.400
OS	42.4	49.3	7.0	-0.6–14.5	0.070
RFS	30.0	38.9	8.9	0.8–17.0	0.030

OS—overall survival; Rel—time following disease relapse; RFS—relapse-free survival; Tox—time with severe or life-threatening side effects of treatment toxicity; TWiST—time without severe or life-threatening treatment toxicity and without disease relapse.

Table 30-3. Mean Q-TWiST Within 84 Months of Median Follow-up in the ECOG Trial for Arbitrary Sets of Utility Weight Values

Utility Values		Treatment Group		Difference, mo	95% CI, mo	P value (2-sided)
u_{Tox}	u_{Rel}	Observation, mo	Interferon alfa-2b, mo			
0.5	0.5	36.2	41.2	5.0	-2.4–12.5	0.20
0.9	0.4	34.9	42.5	7.6	0.0?–15.1	0.05

u_{Rel}—utility weighting assigned to the time following disease relapse; u_{Tox}—utility weighting assigned to the time with severe or life-threatening side effects of treatment toxicity.

Q-TWiST is calculated separately for each treatment group, and the treatment effects are obtained by subtracting the Q-TWiST estimate for one treatment group from the Q-TWiST estimate for another treatment group. If data are available for the utility weightings, then these data can be incorporated into the analysis, and the estimated treatment effects can be tested for statistical significance. In the case in which utility data are not available, the treatment comparison can still be evaluated by computing the treatment effect for varying values of the utility weights. In the case in which two utility weights are unknown and two treatments are being compared (A vs B), the treatment comparison can be plotted across all possible values of the utility weights in a two-dimensional graph called a threshold plot. A solid line can be used to illustrate the set of utility weight pairs for which the two treatments have equal amounts of Q-TWiST on average. This "threshold line" will separate the utility space into two regions that correspond to "greater Q-TWiST on average for treatment A" and "greater Q-TWiST on average for treatment B." Dashed lines can be used to plot a confidence region for the threshold line. The confidence region will indicate pairs of utility-weight values for which treatment A gives significantly more Q-TWiST than treatment B and vice versa. In addition, contour lines can be used to illustrate the magnitude of the treatment effect. This allows an examination of how the treatment effect is influenced by the values of the utility weightings.

Table 30-3 shows the computation of Q-TWiST for two possible selections of the utility weights u_{Tox} and u_{Rel}. Figure 30-2 illustrates the threshold plot for the treatment comparison. Note that in this case, the interferon group experienced more quality-adjusted time than the control group, regardless of the utility values used. Therefore, the threshold line does not appear on the graph. However, the upper 95% confidence band for the threshold line does

appear in the graph, so that the utility space is divided into two regions corresponding to "interferon is significantly better ($P < 0.05$)" and "interferon is better but the comparison is not statistically significant ($P \geq 0.05$)." The contour lines indicate that the treatment effect ranges from approximately +1 month to +9 months.

The Q-TWiST analysis of the ECOG trial indicates that high-dose interferon can be beneficial for patients even after accounting for its side effects. However, the magnitude of the benefit for an individual patient depends on his or her utility weight values for the health states Tox and Rel. This is illustrated in Table 30-3 and the threshold plot in Figure 30-2. For example, the results indicate that for patients with a low utility weight for toxicity, there may be a quality-adjusted (Q-TWiST) benefit for high-dose interferon, but the comparison is not statistically significant. The optimal treatment for an individual patient is also influenced by the disease stage and nodal status (*see* Kirkwood *et al.* [27] for a full description).

DISCUSSION

In this chapter, we provided an overview of the basic components of quality-of-life research in cancer clinical trials, and there are a number of excellent references for further reading. In particular, the large volume edited by Spilker [29] is a thorough reference covering quality-of-life measurement, analysis, cross-cultural and cross-national issues, health policy issues, and pharmacoeconomics. This book is particularly well suited to the quality-of-life researcher who is involved with study design and analysis. Another, more compact reference is the chapter by Gelber and Gelber [30]. This chapter reviews methods used in clinical research and provides more detail regarding statistical analysis methods.

We also provided an example illustrating the use of quality-of-life-adjusted survival time (Q-TWiST) in cancer clinical research. The Q-TWiST analysis of the ECOG trial EST1684 improved the clinical usefulness of the information obtained from the clinical trial. Moreover, the evaluation illustrates the need to consider quality-adjusted survival comparisons in clinical research and develop better ways to evaluate patient preferences for incorporation in the decision-making process. Kilbridge *et al.* [31] recently demonstrated the use of computerized interview to elicit utility weights from a cross-sectional sample of patients with melanoma. They then combined these utility data with the Q-TwiST results from the ECOG trial to further interpretation of the clinical trial with respect to patient valuations of the quality of life associated with the health states "Tox" and "Rel."

The use of assessment tools and procedures similar to those described in this chapter is becoming increasingly important in cancer clinical research. At a minimum, future clinical trials should carefully collect data regarding toxicity grade and duration in addition to the usual clinical outcomes. The longitudinal use of a quality-of-life instrument is also strongly recommended, as is the tracking of individual health care costs over the course of a study. With these components in place, we can expect to have a meaningful evaluation of the treatments being compared in terms of clinical outcome, quality of life, and cost.

ACKNOWLEDGMENTS

Partial support for this work was provided by Grant #PBR-53 from the American Cancer Society.

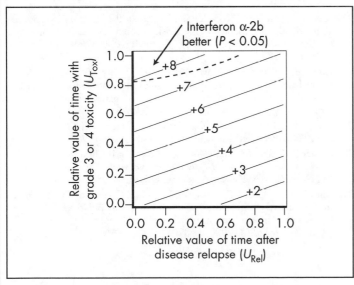

FIGURE 30-2.

Threshold utility analysis for the Eastern Cooperative Oncology Group trial. Utility pairs above the *heavy dashed line* correspond to a significant ($P < 0.05$) gain for interferon treatment in terms of Q-TWiST. The *dotted contour lines* indicate the magnitude of the gain in months. u_{Rel}—utility weighting assigned to the time following disease relapse; u_{Tox}—utility weighting assigned to the time with severe or life-threatening side effects of treatment toxicity.

REFERENCES

1. Schumacher M, Olschewski M, Schulgen G: Assessment of quality of life in clinical trials. *Stat Med* 1991, 10:1915–1930.

2. Cox DR, Fitzpatrick R, Fletcher AE, *et al.*: Quality of life assessment: can we keep it simple? *J R Stat Soc A* 1992; 155:353–393.

3. Gelber RD, Goldhirsch A, Hürny C, *et al.*: Quality of life in clinical trials of adjuvant therapies. *J Natl Cancer Inst Monogr* 1992, 11:127–135.

4. Karnofsky DA, Abelmann WH, Craver LF, Burchenal JH: The use of nitrogen mustards in the palliative treatment of carcinoma. *Cancer* 1948, 1:634.

5. Yates JW, Chalmer B, McKegney FP: Evaluation of patients with advanced cancer using the Karnofsky Performance Status. *Cancer* 1980, 45:2220–2224.

6. Zubrod CG, Schneiderman M, Frei E, *et al.*: Appraisal of methods for the study of chemotherapy in man. *J Chron Dis* 1960, 11:7.

7. Izsak FC, Medalie JH: Comprehensive follow-up of carcinoma patients. *J Chron Dis* 1971, 24:179–191.

8. Burge PS, Prankerd TA, Richards JD, *et al.*: Quality and quantity of survival in acute myeloid leukemia. *Lancet* 1975, 2:621–624.

9. Priestman TJ, Baum M: Evaluation of quality of life in patients receiving treatment for advanced breast cancer. *Lancet* 1976, 1:899–900.

10. Ware JE Jr: The SF-36 health survey. In *Quality of Life and Pharmacoeconomics in Clinical Trials*, edn 2. Edited by Spilker B. Philadelphia: Lippincott-Raven Publishers; 1996:337–345.

11. Damiano AM: The sickness impact profile. In *Quality of Life and Pharmacoeconomics in Clinical Trials*, edn 2. Edited by Spilker B. Philadelphia: Lippincott-Raven Publishers; 1996:347–354.

12. Derogatis LR, Derogatis MF: SCL-90-R and the BSI. In *Quality of Life and Pharmacoeconomics in Clinical Trials*, edn 2. Edited by Spilker B. Philadelphia: Lippincott-Raven Publishers; 1996:323–335.

13. Szabo S: The World Health Organization quality of life (WHOQOL) assessment instrument. In *Quality of Life and Pharmacoeconomics in Clinical Trials*, edn 2. Edited by Spilker B. Philadelphia: Lippincott-Raven Publishers; 1996:355–362.

14. Levine MN, Guyatt GH, Gent M: Quality of life in stage II breast cancer: an instrument for clinical trials. *J Clin Oncol* 1988, 6:1789–1810.

15. Ganz PA, Schag CAC, Lee JJ, *et al.*: The CARES: a generic measure of health-related quality of life for patients with cancer. *Qual Life Res* 1992, 1:19–29.

16. Aaronson NK, Bullinger M, Ahmedzai S: A modular approach to quality-of-life assessment in cancer clinical trials. *Recent Results Cancer Res* 1988, 111:231–249.

17. Cella DF, Bonomi AE: The functional assessment of cancer therapy (FACT) and functional assessment of HIV infection (FAHI) quality of life measurement system. In *Quality of Life and Pharmacoeconomics in Clinical Trials*, edn 2. Edited by Spilker B. Philadelphia: Lippincott-Raven Publishers; 1996:203–214.

18. Clinch JJ: The functional living index—cancer: ten years later. In *Quality of Life and Pharmacoeconomics in Clinical Trials*, edn 2. Edited by Spilker B. Philadelphia: Lippincott-Raven Publishers; 1996:215–225.

19. Hürny C, Bernhard J, Gelber RD, *et al.*: Quality of life measures for patients receiving adjuvant therapy for breast cancer. *Eur J Cancer* 1992, 28:118–124.

20. Spitzer WO, Dobson AJ, Hall J, *et al.*: Measuring the quality of life of cancer patients. *J Chron Dis* 1981, 34:585–597.

21. Bennett KJ, Torrance GW: Measuring health state preferences and utilities: rating scale, time trade-off and standard gamble techniques. In *Quality of Life and Pharmacoeconomics in Clinical Trials*, edn 2. Edited by Spilker B. Philadelphia: Lippincott-Raven Publishers; 1996:253–265.

22. Kind P: The EuroQoL instrument: an index of health-related quality of life. In *Quality of Life and Pharmacoeconomics in Clinical Trials*, edn 2. Edited by Spilker B. Philadelphia: Lippincott-Raven Publishers; 1996:191–201.

23. Feeny DH, Torrance GW, Furlong WJ: Health utilities index. In *Quality of Life and Pharmacoeconomics in Clinical Trials*, edn 2. Edited by Spilker B. Philadelphia: Lippincott-Raven Publishers; 1996:239–252.

24. Weeks J, O'Leary J, Fairclough D, *et al.* The 'Q-tility index': a new tool for assessing health-related quality of life and utilities in clinical trials and clinical practice. *Proc Am Soc Clin Oncol* 1994, 13:436.

25. Proceedings of the Workshop on Missing Data in Quality of Life Research in Cancer Clinical Trials: practical and methodological issues: July 1-3, 1996, Bad Horn, Switzerland. *Stat Med* 1998, 17:511–796.

26. Gelber RD, Cole BF, Gelber S, Goldhirsch A: The Q-TWiST method. In *Quality of Life and Pharmacoeconomics in Clinical Trials*, edn 2. Edited by Spilker B. Philadelphia: Lippincott-Raven Publishers; 1996:437–444.

27. Kirkwood JM, Hunt Strawderman M, Ernstoff MS, *et al.*: Interferon alpha-2b adjuvant therapy of high-risk resected cutaneous melanoma: the Eastern Cooperative Oncology Group Trial EST1684. *J Clin Oncol* 1996, 14:7–17.

28. Cole BF, Gelber RD, Kirkwood JM, *et al.* Quality-of-life-adjusted survival analysis of interferon alfa-2b adjuvant treatment of high-risk resected cutaneous melanoma: an Eastern Cooperative Oncology Group Study. *J Clin Oncol* 1996, 14:2666–2673.

29. Spilker B (ed): *Quality of Life and Pharmacoeconomics in Clinical Trials*, edn 2. Philadelphia: Lippincott-Raven Publishers; 1996.

30. Gelber R, Gelber S: Quality-of-life assessment in clinical trials. In *Recent Advances in Clincial Trial Design and Analysis*. Edited by Thall PF. Norwell, MA: Kluwer Academic Publishers; 1995.

31. Kilbridge KL, Cole BF, Kirkwood JM, *et al.*: Quality-of-life-adjusted survival analysis of high-dose adjuvant interferon alfa-2b (HDI) for high-risk melanoma patients (pts) based on E1690 and E1684 (abstract). *Proc ASCO* 2000, 19:570a.

CHAPTER 31: SYSTEMIC MANIFESTATIONS OF CANCER AND PARANEOPLASTIC SYNDROMES

Jayesh Desai, Michelle Gold, Sonia Fullerton, Jonathan Cebon

For the majority of patients with cancer, clinical features are directly attributable to the local effects of the primary tumor or metastases. In about 5% to 10% of cases, however, distant effects occur that are not due to the direct effects of tumor. These systemic effects or paraneoplastic syndromes are mediated by a variety of mechanisms: either "ectopic" or "inappropriate" hormone secretion, or the production of inflammatory mediators such as cytokines, interleukin, or growth factors. Immune effects mediated by the production of antibodies or T-cells that cross-react with normal host tissue are particularly seen with the neurologic syndromes.

Because paraneoplastic syndromes can be the presenting feature of cancer, their recognition can assist earlier diagnosis and treatment. They may cause significant symptoms that require treatment independent from the treatment of the underlying neoplasm. They may also act as a marker of disease activity, thus affecting prognosis, and they can provide unique insights into tumor biology and immunology.

Paraneoplastic syndromes generally fulfil the following criteria: 1) direct association between the syndrome and the presence of cancer; 2) presence of an identifiable mediator in the circulation or within tumor cells (effective treatment of the tumor should lead to a reduction in this mediator); and 3) clinical improvement of the paraneoplastic effects following treatment of the primary malignancy, although this is not often the case.

The systemic effects of cancer are often multifactorial and profound physiologic or systemic effects can occur, even in the absence of a well-defined syndrome. This chapter summarizes the clinical features, mechanisms, and management of the main systemic and paraneoplastic manifestations of cancer.

CONSTITUTIONAL SYMPTOMS

Cachexia and Anorexia Syndrome

Cachexia and anorexia represent the most common systemic syndrome seen in patients with malignancy. It has been estimated that approximately one quarter of patients suffer from either weight loss, anorexia, or both at the time of diagnosis and these are almost universal in the presence of widely metastatic disease.

The importance of these syndromes lie in their effect on survival and their influence on the quality of life of cancer patients and their families. Furthermore, prognosis and ability to tolerate treatment are both often influenced by nutritional status. Malnutrition is a significant cause of mortality, contributing to some 20% of deaths not due to direct tumor effects [1]. Loss of lean body mass (as distinct from adipose tissue), which is the predominant effect of starvation has been demonstrated to be an important predictor of early mortality.

Cachexia may be caused by multiple factors:

Nutrition may be reduced due to the direct effects of tumor (eg, head and neck or gastrointestinal tumors), or treatment (nausea, vomiting, anorexia, and altered taste sensation commonly accompany chemotherapy and radiotherapy).

Metabolic abnormalities often occur secondary to cancer. These can include glucose intolerance, increased hepatic gluconeogenesis and increased protein breakdown, and increased lipolysis. Whole body protein turnover is increased, resulting in muscle catabolism. Hyperlipidemia may result from elevated lipoprotein lipase levels.

Metabolic requirements in patients with cancer, in contrast to those seen in starving patients, are higher than in normal subjects.

Cytokines: under normal circumstances, the production of these glycoprotein regulators of cell and tissue function such as growth and differentiation, wound repair, immune responses, and angiogenesis, is regulated by a variety of tightly controlled mechanisms. Increasingly, they have been recognized as key mediators of many systemic manifestations of cancer. No single cytokine is consistently elevated in the blood of cancer patients; however, clinically detectable levels are not required for these molecules to have an effect because much of their activity occurs at a local tissue level. Common syndromes such as cachexia, anorexia and asthenia are likely to be caused, at least in part, by the actions of various cytokines.

The host's production of inflammatory cytokines in response to the tumor mediates a series of complex interrelated steps that can lead to a chronic state of wasting, malnutrition, and death. Tumor necrosis factor (TNF), a macrophage-derived cytokine, is the best understood of these, and has a clear role in cachexia associated with malignant and also nonmalignant disease. Other cytokines implicated include interleukins (IL)-6, -1 and interferon gamma. In various studies both have been shown to be associated with the signs of cancer cachexia and to be elevated in patients with cancer.

Tumor necrosis factor (TNF)-α, also known as cachectin, has a role in cancer cachexia and anorexia as well as the weight loss associated with chronic infection. Administration of TNF to experimental animals stimulates changes associated with cancer cachexia, which can be blocked by antisera [1]. Experimental infusion of TNF into the third ventricle of rats results in the suppression of glucose-sensitive neurons in the lateral hypothalamus and suppressed food intake [2]. TNF-neutralizing antibodies are able to reverse weight loss in mice with tumors, suggesting an important pathophysiologic role for TNF-α [3].

Interleukin-1 (IL-1) has similarly been associated with anorexia. Intracerebroventricular administration of IL-1 in rats suppressed food intake via an effect on neurons in the lateral hypothalamus [2]. Schwarz et al. [4] postulated that IL-1 impairs appetite by increasing hypothalamic corticotrophin-releasing hormone (CRH) production as well as suppressing neuropeptide Y, which has a stimulating effect on appetite. A rise in IL-1 levels detected in patients undergoing radiotherapy was associated with increased fatigue [5].

Interleukin-6 (IL-6) also appears to play a role in the production of anorexia-cachexia. Administration of IL-6 to humans can be associated with weight loss, nausea, and anorexia [6]. In a small study, the administration of anti–IL-6 monoclonal antibody to patients with HIV and lymphoma resulted in weight gain for eight of 11 patients [7]. Oral medroxyprogesterone reduced IL-6 levels in breast cancer patients, and those with more significant reductions in IL-6 levels were more likely to achieve weight gain and increased appetite [8]. A potential mechanism for this effect is once again via the hypothalamus. IL-6 has been shown to stimulate release of cortisol, ACTH, and ADH, suggesting activation of the hypothalamic-pituitary-adrenal axis [9].

Management

Because metabolism is altered, attempts to halt the weight loss by nutritional means are often unsuccessful. Treatment of the anorexia and cachexia syndrome is difficult. Classes of agents used include orexigenic (appetite stimulants), anticatabolic, and antimetabolic (primarily hormonal). Agents with proven efficacy include appetite stimulants such as corticosteroids, *eg*, dexamethasone 4 mg/d. They do not appear to improve survival. The mechanism is thought to be through their anti-inflammatory and euphorogenic effects. Megestrol acetate in doses of between 240 and 1600 mg/d is the other drug proven to be effective; it increases appetite and causes weight gain by downregulating the synthesis and release of cytokines [10].

Research is currently being undertaken into the effects of dronabinol, a cannabinoid, in cancer cachexia. Cyproheptadine appears not to be effective [11].

Asthenia

From the Greek words for "absence of strength," asthenia involves three distinct symptom complexes: 1) fatigue or lassitude (easy tiring and decreased ability to maintain performance); 2) generalized weakness defined as the anticipatory sensation of difficulty in initiating a certain activity; and 3) mental fatigue (including impaired concentration, memory loss, and emotional lability) [12].

Asthenia is a common feature of advanced malignancy. It may, however, occur with less advanced disease and has been reported in over 80% of patients receiving chemotherapy [13]. Other estimates have ranged from 40% to 75%, the variation likely to be due in part to the population studied and the definition of asthenia used.

In general, the specific mechanism of asthenia is not well understood. Cytokine production, such as TNF or IL-1, either by the tumor itself or as part of a host response to the tumor may play a role in the development of asthenia via alterations in intermediary metabolism.

It has been suggested that impaired muscle function may play a major role in producing asthenia [14], and abnormalities in both function and structure have been documented in cancer patients. Atrophy of type-2 muscle fibers, reductions in maximum strength, decreased reaction velocity, and increased fatigue have all been recorded. It is also common to see loss of muscle mass in cancer patients, particularly those with anorexia-cachexia. Bolus injections of TNF are associated with evidence of muscle catabolism in human subjects [15].

Several potentially reversible factors may contribute to asthenia in an individual patient:

1. Infection. Chronic infections may induce common cytokines. Such infections may complicate the disease or its treatment.
2. Psychologic distress. The incidence of depression in cancer patients has been found to be in the order of 25% [16]. Asthenia can be a feature of a major depressive episode or of an adjustment disorder.
3. Treatment side-effects. Antineoplastic treatment, particularly radiotherapy and chemotherapy, can cause asthenia although the means by which they do this is not well understood. Biologic therapies such as IL-2 and interferon-alfa predictably cause asthenia, especially at higher doses. Other medications such as opioids or benzodiazepines also commonly cause sedation and asthenia.

Table 31-1. Possible Causes of Fever in Patients With Cancer

Infection
Drug related
Transfusion
Tumor related (cytokines)
Necrotic tumor mass

4. Anemia. In many cases, the correction of anemia does not result in improvement in asthenia. The exception may be when the hemoglobin has fallen rapidly or is extremely low.
5. Endocrine/metabolic abnormalities. Diabetes, Addison's syndrome, hypercalcemia, hyponatremia, hypokalemia, and hypomagnesemia should be identified and treated appropriately.
6. Overexertion. This factor may be important in those patients undergoing treatment and attempting to continue social and work commitments.
7. Paraneoplastic neurologic syndromes. Although less common, syndromes such as myasthenia gravis, Guillain-Barré and Eaton-Lambert syndromes are important to identify as they may respond to specific intervention or treatment of the primary tumor.

Cachexia-related loss of muscle mass or muscle dysfunction, renal or hepatic failure are among contributing causes that are not easily reversed.

Management

Reversible causes should be identified and treated appropriately. Unfortunately, in many patients no specific cause for asthenia is identified. In others, there are multiple contributing factors, so treatment should be individualized.

Nonpharmacologic interventions are important in all patients and will often involve members of the multidisciplinary team. Occupational therapists provide advice about energy-conserving strategies and can provide assistive devices. Physiotherapy interventions may include an individualized program of exercise that aims to avoid deconditioning.

Education is a crucial factor in managing asthenia. Ensuring that the patient and the care-givers are aware of the causes of asthenia, the presence or absence of therapeutic interventions and what to expect in the future will assist in the establishment of realistic goals. Practical suggestions (eg, delegating household tasks or scheduling regular rest periods) can be particularly valuable.

Corticosteroids: Methylprednisolone (31 mg/d) has been demonstrated in a randomized trial to improve activity levels in cancer patients, albeit for a limited period [17]. Most responders noted a benefit within 72 hours; therefore it is reasonable to initiate a short trial of steroids and to cease treatment if no improvement is noted after 3 days. Because of the immunosuppressive and metabolic effects of corticosteroids, such treatment is best reserved for the latter stages of the patient's life. Dexamethasone is commonly used for this indication, with doses of 1 to 4 mg daily.

Amphetamines: No definitive trials have directly examined the effect of amphetamines on asthenia in cancer patients. Methylphenidate may have a role in the management of asthenia in patients on high doses of opioids.

Fever

Fever is common in patients with cancer and may be due to a variety of causes (Table 31-1). It is important to look for and exclude infection. The neutrophil count is important: in neutropenic patients, infection is responsible for more than two thirds of fevers, whereas only 20% of fevers in non-neutropenic patients are caused by infection. Malignancies classically associated with fever include renal cell carcinoma, hepatoma, metastases involving the liver, lymphoma, acute leukemia, myxoma, and osteogenic sarcoma. The mechanism of fever may relate to the action of cytokines TNF, IL-1, and IL-6 on the hypothalamus, stimulating release of prostaglandin E_2 [18].

Management firstly involves excluding infection. If the fever is deemed to be due to malignancy, nonsteroidal anti-inflammatory drugs (NSAIDS) (eg, indomethacin 25 mg three times daily or naproxen sodium 250 mg three times daily can be useful. NSAIDS reduce fevers via an effect on the anterior hypothalamus, thus reducing the "set point," which is elevated in inflammatory fevers. If this is unsuccessful or there is a contraindication to NSAIDS, steroids may be used. Paracetamol (acetaminophen) may also be tried. Effective treatment of the underlying malignancy is the most effective definitive management. Nonpharmacologic measures (fans, sponging) can be a useful adjunct.

METABOLIC AND ENDOCRINE PARANEOPLASTIC SYNDROMES

Hypercalcemia

Hypercalcemia is a potentially life threatening metabolic disorder commonly seen in cancer. It is seen in up to 30% of patients [19], most commonly in breast cancer, squamous cell carcinoma of the lung, and multiple myeloma. It is due to an increase in bone resorption and release of calcium from the mineralized bone matrix, either by osteolytic or humoral pathways.

The normal range for corrected calcium is 8.8 to 10.3 mg/dL (2.2 to 2.6 mmol/L). In hypoalbuminemic patients, the serum calcium must be corrected according to the following formula:

Corrected calcium = serum calcium (mg/dL) + 0.8 × (40 serum albumin [g/L]).

Three major mechanisms are involved:

1. Tumor secretion of parathyroid hormone-related peptide (PTHrP). The tumor secretion of PTHrP is the most common mechanism involved in the syndrome of hypercalcemia of malignancy. PTHrP shares 80% homology with the first 13 amino acids of parathyroid hormone (PTH), which in turn is responsible for binding to the same skeletal and renal receptors as PTH, and therefore has the same effect on calcium and phosphorous metabolism (see below).
2. Osteolytic metastases with local release of cytokines. Osteolytic metastases release several growth factors and cytokines, including tumor necrosis factor and interleukin-1, which stimulate differentiation of osteoclasts, thereby increasing bone resorption.
3. Tumor secretion of calcitriol. This mechanism is rare. It is seen in Hodgkin's and non-Hodgkin's lymphomas.

Normal Calcium Homeostasis

Parathyroid hormone controls calcium levels in the short term. Release of PTH is stimulated by hypocalcemia. It acts to increase calcium levels by several mechanisms, including 1) increasing the efficacy of renal tubular calcium resorption, 2) increasing calcium resorption from bone, 3) converting vitamin D to its active form (calcitriol), which increases intestinal absorption of both calcium and phosphorous, and 4) in hypercalcemia (whether caused by PTH or PTHrP), sodium and water resorption is decreased, leading to dehydration as dilute urine is excreted. Nephrocalcinosis, the precipitation of calcium in the tubules, can lead to irreversible renal compromise.

Signs and Symptoms

Malaise, fatigue, and altered conscious state are among the most common symptoms reported by patients. Other symptoms are anorexia, nausea, and vomiting accompanied by polyuria and bony pain. Neurologic signs reflect a decrease in neuronal excitability. Weakness, hyporeflexia, delirium and cognitive decline may be seen. Signs of dehydration include dry mucous membranes, altered skin turgor, postural hypotension and tachycardia and decreased jugular venous pressure. Cardiovascular events relate to irritability and increased contractility seen in the heart. Slowed conduction results in ECG changes such as increased PR interval and QRS prolongation, which can ultimately progress to bradycardia, bundle branch block, asystole and cardiac arrest. Depression of the autonomic nervous system leads to smooth muscle hypertonicity in the gastrointestinal tract, causing anorexia, nausea and vomiting, and abdominal pain.

Management

Patients at risk of hypercalcemia due to their underlying malignancy, immobility, dehydration, nausea or vomiting need to be educated about the symptoms and prevention of hypercalcemia. Advice should include encouraging fluid intake to 3 L/d if tolerated, increased mobility, and seeking early medical advice should symptoms appear. Thiazide diuretics should be ceased and calcium supplements and antacids avoided.

Treatment of hypercalcemia entails several approaches:

1. Increase urinary calcium excretion. Proximal tubule resorption of calcium is inhibited by volume expansion with intravenous saline. Monitoring of serum electrolytes and calcium should be carried out regularly. The volume infused and the speed at which it is administered will depend on volume depletion and comorbidities such as congestive cardiac failure. After euvolemia has been established, gentle use of a loop diuretic such as frusemide (eg, 20 mg orally twice daily) may be used if needed to prevent or treat fluid overload while hydration continues. Loop diuretics inhibit calcium resorption in the ascending limb of the loop of Henle. Thiazide diuretics are contraindicated as they enhance calcium resorption. In mild cases of hypercalcemia, hydration alone may suffice.
2. Decrease bone resorption. Bisphosphonates are the treatment of choice and act by binding to hydroxyapatite in calcified bone. They decrease the number of osteoclasts in sites undergoing resorption and may prevent osteoclast differentiation, therefore decreasing bone resorption. Pamidronate is more effective than etidronate [20], reducing calcium in 90% of patients [21], and has fewer side effects [22]. Bisphosphonates have also been proven to reduce skeletal complications of malignant disease when used prophylactically. Pamidronate (90 mg IV monthly) has been shown to decrease skeletal complications in patients with metastatic breast cancer or multiple myeloma with skeletal involvement. Corticosteroids (eg, dexamethasone 16 mg/d in divided doses) may be useful in sensitive tumors, particularly hematologic malignancies. Calcitonin (4 IU/kg subcutaneously twice daily) is safe but expensive and only effective in 60% to 70% of cases, with many patients swiftly developing tachyphylaxis, rendering it ineffective. Mithramycin (25 µg/kg IV) is rarely used due to its toxicity. It is, however, reliable and effective, and doses can be repeated. Gallium (200 mg/m^2 per 24 hours) is effective, but requires infusion over 5 days, and is nephrotoxic.

The mortality in malignancy-associated hypercalcemia is as high as 75% at 3 months despite treatment, reflecting the poor prognosis of the underlying malignancy [24]. Other poor prognostic factors identified include older age, lower serum albumin, and serum calcium level after treatment. Treatment of the hypercalcemia enhances survival if systemic treatment for the malignancy is available. In others, the aim of treatment should be symptom control [25].

Hyponatremia

Hyponatremia (serum sodium < 135 mmol/L) is a common electrolyte disturbance in patients with cancer and may have a variety of causes, including conditions unrelated to the tumor (Table 31-2). The syndrome of inappropriate antidiuretic hormone secretion (SIADH) is the most common cause of hyponatremia in cancer patients.

Defining the cause of hyponatremia can be challenging. The first step is to assess the volume of extracellular fluid (ECF) as increased, decreased, or normal on the basis of history, physical examination, and plasma creatinine and urea. (ECF comprises plasma volume [25%] and interstitial fluid [75%]). Serum osmolality (normal is 280 to 296 mosmol/L of water) and urinary sodium are also useful.

Reduced ECF causes decreased tissue turgor, dry mucous membranes with or without hypotension, tachycardia, and elevated serum urea. In this condition, hyponatremia is associated with dehydration. Low urinary sodium suggests extrarenal losses, whereas levels above 20 mmol/L occur with diuretics, hyperglycemia, and hypoaldosteronism.

Increased ECF causes peripheral edema, and ascites with or without raised jugular venous pressure. In this condition, hyponatremia occurs in association with edema and may be due to hepatic failure, congestive cardiac failure, or renal disease.

Hyponatremia with normal ECF. The main causes of hyponatremia with normal ECF include SIADH, renal disease, and endocrine causes (adrenal failure, hypothyroidism).

In SIADH, the serum osmolality is low, with inappropriately high urine sodium excretion (< 20 mmol/L) and osmolality.

Clinical Features and Diagnosis

Many patients are asymptomatic and hyponatremia is detected on routine blood tests. Symptoms usually appear at sodium levels of less than 125 mmol/L but the rate of decline is also important. Fatigue, anorexia, nausea and confusion occur initially and can progress to coma, seizures, and eventually death if untreated.

Management

The treatment initiated will depend on the rate of decline in sodium levels, the severity of hyponatremia, and the presence of symptoms. In most cases, fluid restriction (500 mL to 1000 mL/d, depending on severity) is a useful initial strategy. Treatment of the underlying cause is the most effective way of correcting hyponatremia and chemotherapy for small-cell lung cancer is generally effective treatment for SIADH. Drugs that may be responsible should be ceased.

In symptomatic patients or those with a rapid onset, hypertonic saline (3%) with or without IV furosemide should be used to increase the serum sodium by a rate not exceeding 12 mmoL/L/d or 1 mmoL/L/h. More rapid correction can result in central pontine myelinolysis [14].

When these measures are unsuccessful or undesirable, pharmacologic therapy may be instituted. Demeclocycline is a tetracycline analogue that acts by blocking the effect of ADH on the distal tubule, thereby causing nephrogenic diabetes insipidus. The usual regimen is 600 to 1200 mg/d in divided doses. Side effects include photosensitivity, gastrointestinal disturbance, and hypersensitivity reactions. Lithium has also been used and acts in a similar manner but has greater potential for toxicity.

Cushing's Syndrome

In its classic form, Cushing's syndrome is easily recognized. However, in the setting of neoplasia the clinical appearance may be confounded by other features of cancer such as weight loss. A high index of suspicion is required. The most common cancer associated with Cushing's syndrome is small-cell lung cancer (about 50% of cases) with carcinoid tumors, neural crest tumors, and bronchial carcinoid also contributing significant numbers. Tumors may be occult at presentation.

Clinical features include hypertension, hirsutism, and myopathy with muscle weakness and wasting. Hyperpigmentation is more common than in Cushing's disease (adrenal overproduction of cortisol). Truncal obesity may occur but is often hidden by weight loss. Severe hypokalemic alkalosis can occur.

The molecules involved in the syndrome in the setting of malignancy are precursors of adrenocorticotropin (ACTH), arising from the pro-opiomelanocortin (POMC) gene on the short arm of chromosome 23. These include pro-ACTH, endorphins, and melanocyte-stimulating hormone (MSH).

A step-wise approach to diagnosis is helpful:
1. Establish the presence of hypercortisolism. Screening tests for cortisol overproduction are 24-hour urinary free cortisol and a low-dose dexamethasone test (2 mg dexamethasone at 2300 h and measure cortisol at 0800 h; morning cortisol is suppressed in normal people.)
2. Distinguish between primary adrenal pathology and ACTH-dependent disease. Measure ACTH levels: in primary adrenal disease, ACTH will be suppressed compared with normal or elevated levels in pituitary disease or ectopic ACTH production.
3. Distinguish between pituitary disease and ectopic ACTH. Failure of cortisol suppression with the high-dose dexamethasone suppression test (8 mg at 2300 h and measure 0800 h cortisol) suggests ectopic ACTH production, as cortisol will be suppressed in pituitary disease. Because the sensitivity and specificity of this test are not perfect, other investigations may include corticotropin-releasing hormone (CRH) stimulation, metyrapone stimulation and inferior petrosal sinus sampling.
4. Localize site of ectopic ACTH production. Imaging of the chest with plain X-rays and CT scanning will detect the majority of lung carcinoma and bronchial carcinoid. Octreotide receptor scintigraphy has also been utilized for localizing ACTH-producing tumors [26].

Table 31-2. Causes of Hyponatremia

SIADH	CNS origin: infection, vasculitis, stroke, head injury, tumor, psychologic stress
	Pulmonary: infection, tumor, asthma, chronic obstructive pulmonary disease, pneumothorax
	Drugs: carbamazepine, chlorpropamide, tolbutamide, haloperidol, amitriptyline, vincristine, morphine
Organ failure	Adrenal insufficiency, hepatic dysfunction, cardiac failure, renal disease, hypothyroidism
Gastrointestinal losses	Gastrointestinal losses: vomiting, diarrhea, fistulas
Other drugs	Diuretics, cisplatin

Management

Where possible, treatment of the underlying tumor should be undertaken. Resection is preferred if feasible, otherwise standard treatment should be offered. In small-cell lung cancer chemotherapy or radiotherapy may be associated with a decline in ACTH levels although high levels may persist in long-term survivors.

Medical therapy revolves around the inhibition of adrenal steroid synthesis.

- Ketoconazole inhibits cytochrome P450 dependent steroid hydroxylases and can be used in doses of 400 to 1200 mg/d. Side effects include nausea, headache, rash, and hepatic dysfunction. There are several important drug interactions, and hepatic impairment is a contraindication to its use.
- Aminoglutethamide is an aromatase inhibitor, which at high doses (500 to 2000 mg/d) inhibits production of glucocorticoids, mineralocorticoids, and androgens. Side-effects are significant at this dose.
- Metyrapone (250 to 750 mg four times daily) acts by inhibiting the final step in cortisol synthesis. Toxicity is predominantly gastrointestinal and it may not be effective when levels of ACTH are very high.
- Combining low doses of metyrapone (250 mg four times daily) and aminoglutethamide (250 mg twice daily) may be an effective treatment that minimizes the toxicities of the two agents. Replacement therapy with fludrocortisone and prednisolone may be required.

Suppression of ACTH production may be achieved with the use of octreotide. Surgical adrenalectomy is also an effective palliative procedure.

PARANEOPLASTIC NEUROLOGIC SYNDROMES

Neurologic symptoms in patients with cancer are very common. Most of these can be directly attributable to the direct effects of the disease, eg, the compressive effects of tumor on neurologic structures, neurotoxicity of chemotherapy, or related to disorders of nutrition. True neurologic paraneoplastic syndromes are uncommon, occurring in around 3% of patients with cancer. They remain a challenge for the clinician, particularly if they occur before the appearance of the cancer, because they can affect almost any part of the nervous system.

Since the association between a small cancer and a remote and often profound neurologic effect was first made, our understanding of the processes involved has developed significantly. Several conditions exist in which there is a clear association with a specific tumor type, identification of target-specific autoantibodies, induction of clinical and pathologic features of the disease in passive transfer experiments, and improvement in the condition by treatment directed at reducing autoantibody levels. Lambert-Eaton myasthenic syndrome is a classic example of this: it is associated with antibodies, which interfere with presynaptic nerve endings. Infiltrates of lymphocytes in tumor and nervous system also suggests a role for cellular immune mechanisms in these conditions. Currently identified autoantibodies and their tumor associations and neurologic syndromes are listed in Table 31-3 below.

Paraneoplastic Encephalomyelitis

Paraneoplastic encephalomyelitis (PEM) is an inflammatory disorder that can affect the central nervous system at a number of different anatomic sites. The term *encephalomyelitis with carcinoma* was first coined by Henson in 1965 [27]; since then a number of other terms such as limbic encephalitis, subacute encephalomyelitis, or subacute cortical cerebellar degeneration have been used. It has since become apparent that all of these conditions describe a similar pathologic process, irrespective of site, that can affect a number of different cell types.

When the limbic system is involved, it is characterized by memory loss, confusion, hallucinations, and seizures. Paraneoplastic limbic encephalitis can occur as a distinct clinical entity or as part of the PEM syndrome. EEG and MRI changes are usually seen in the temporal lobes. Pathologic changes reflecting multifocal inflammatory changes with extensive loss of neurons and perivascular lymphocyte cuffing.

Brainstem involvement usually results in opsoclonus, vertigo, hearing loss, and central respiratory failure may ensue. The most commonly described variant of PEM, though, is with a disabling sensory neuropathy due to involvement of the dorsal root ganglia. Autonomic nervous system involvement is also seen, with postural hypotension, intestinal pseudo-obstruction and urinary retention.

A strong association between PEM and an autoimmune etiology has been well established. In patients with small-cell lung cancer (SCLC) who develop PEM, anti-Hu antibodies have been identified in the CSF in high titers (compared with serum levels), suggesting localized CNS production, in almost all patients. These antibodies, described as a polyclonal group of IgG type 1 anti-neuronal antibodies (ANNA-1) react against a number of RNA-binding proteins expressed by both neuronal cells and SCLC cells. In fact, patients expressing these antibodies appear to have a longer survival than those who are seronegative, suggesting the development of an antitumor immune response [28]. In this same study, which looked at anti-Hu antibodies in SCLC and neuroblastomas (both tumors of

Table 31-3. Antineuronal Antibodies in Paraneoplastic Neurologic Syndromes

Antibody	Target Cell	Main Tumor Association	Neurologic Syndrome
Anti-Hu	All CNS neurons	SCLC, breast	PEM, PCD, peripheral neuropathy
Anti-Yo	Purkinje cells	Ovarian, HD	PCD
Anti-Ri	All CNS neurons	SCLC, breast	Opsoclonus-myoclonus
Anti-retinal	Retinal photoreceptor cells	SCLS, melanoma	CAR
Anti-MAG	Myelin	Paraproteinemias (MGUS, MM, Waldenström's)	Peripheral neuropathy
Anti-VGCC	Presynaptic neuromuscular junction	SCLC	LEMS
Anti-Tr	Purkinje cell	HD	PCD

CAR—cancer-associated retinopathy; CNS—central nervous system; HD—Hodgkin's disease; LEMS—Lambert-Eaton myasthenic syndrome; MGUS—monoclonal gammopathy of undetermined significance; MM—multiple myeloma; PCD—paraneoplastic cerebellar degeneration; PEM—paraneoplastic encephalomyelitis; SCLC—small-cell lung cancer.

neuroectodermal origin, and which express high levels of the Hu antigen on their cell surfaces), in patients who expressed the antigen but had undetectable levels of the antibody, development of PEM was not seen. This would support the basis of the role of the immune response, rather than a primary antigenic effect, as the cause of the neurologic syndrome. Direct attempts have been made in mice, with passive transfer of anti-Hu IgG, to induce a neurologic syndrome. Although this has been unsuccessful, there is probably still enough evidence to support the antibody response to a tumor antigen and its paraneoplastic sequelae.

Neurologic symptoms often antedate tumor diagnosis, by an average of around 6 months, and although spontaneous remissions have been reported, most patients progress to widespread encephalomyelopathy. The median survival after onset of neurologic symptoms is about 1 year. A number of specific treatments including corticosteroids, intravenous immunoglobulin (IVIG) and plasmapharesis have been used, with little success [29]. Patients tend to die from respiratory and cardiac complications related to autonomic dysfunction rather than directly from their malignancy.

Paraneoplastic Cerebellar Degeneration

Paraneoplastic cerebellar degeneration (PCD) is the most common paraneoplastic neurologic disorder to affect the central nervous system, and is usually associated with small-cell lung cancer, breast cancer, ovarian cancer and Hodgkin's disease.

The onset of symptoms is usually abrupt, with severe truncal ataxia, dysarthria, dysphagia, and often nystagmus developing within days. Although the disorder is rare, developing in only 1% of patients with cancer, approximately 50% of patients who develop subacute pancerebellar degeneration will be found to have an underlying cancer.

Several autoantibodies have been identified in patients with PCD (Table 31-4). Patients found to be seropositive for anti-Yo antibodies (a cytoplasmic antibody directed against Purkinje cells) have been consistently found to be women with breast and gynecologic malignancies. In the largest series reported to date, 26 of 55 patients seropositive for anti-Yo Ab had ovarian cancer, 13 had breast cancer, and seven had other gynecologic malignancies [30]. Patients with high titers of anti-Hu antibodies tend to have PCD associated with PEM. Other autoantibodies associated with PCD alone include anti-Tr, usually associated with Hodgkin's disease.

PCD usually presents prior to the cancer itself, and almost always runs a course independent to that of the primary tumor. If a patient with known cancer presents with cerebellar dysfunction, a directly related cause is much more likely (eg, metastatic disease, chemother-apy toxicity) [31]. However, it has been recommended that women presenting with pancerebellar degeneration should be tested for anti-Yo antibodies, and if positive, be investigated for breast and gynecologic malignancies including exploratory surgery if required. Men with anti-Yo Ab and PCD are extremely rare.

Patients positive for anti-Yo antibody tend to have a much more abrupt and rapidly progressive onset than seropositive patients, although the differences are not as noticeable once the disease progresses. Treatment with corticosteroids, immunosuppressive drugs (eg, azathioprine), and plasma exchange have been largely unsuccessful to date.

Opsoclonus-Myoclonus

Opsoclonus, a form of ocular dyskinesia, consists of involuntary, high amplitude, chaotic saccadic eye movements that occur when there is loss of inhibitory neural control. Myoclonus of the extremities and trunk, ataxia and irritability often accompany this.

In children, opsoclonus is seen most commonly in nonmalignant diseases, eg, viral infections and trauma. Paraneoplastic opsoclonus is most commonly associated with neuroblastomas in children. In adults, it has been associated with a number of tumor types, in particular small-cell lung cancer, breast cancer, and ovarian cancer. Paraneoplastic opsoclonus typically has an acute onset. The condition usually predates the tumor by up to a year.

Diagnosis is largely clinical. A mild lymphocytic pleocytosis on CSF examination is common. Neuroimaging studies are usually normal. As with other paraneoplastic neurologic syndromes, an autoimmune pathogenesis is suspected, with Anti-Ri and Anti-Hu antibodies identified in a few cases in patients with cancer and opsoclonus. However, no consistent pattern or presence of antibody has, as yet, been identified.

Corticosteroids are often used to treat symptoms, with occasional initial responses. Symptoms may also improve with regression of the tumor in some cases, or spontaneously improve in others. Unfortunately, though, most affected individuals are usually left with residual neurologic deficits.

Cancer-Associated Retinopathy

Cancer-associated retinopathy (CAR) is rare, usually occurring in association with small-cell lung cancer, melanoma, and gynecologic tumors. It is characterized by subacute visual loss with night blindness, photosensitivity, and impaired color vision [31]. Visual symptoms usually predate the diagnosis of the tumor, with patients developing blurred vision, photopsias, scotomata (often with bizarre,

Table 31-4. Treatment Modalities in Paraneoplastic Neurologic Syndromes

Paraneoplastic Syndrome	Plasmapheresis	Corticosteroids	Immunosuppressive Drugs
Paraneoplastic encephalomyelitis	—	—	—
Paraneoplastic cerebellar degeneration	+	—	—
Opsoclonus-myoclonus	+	+++	+
Cancer-associated retinopathy	+	+	0
Sensory neuropathy	++	+	—
Autonomic neuropathy	0	+	0
Lambert-Eaton myasthenic syndrome	+++	++	++
Polymyositis/dermatomyositis	—	+++	++

— indicates treatment not shown to be effective; O indicates unknown efficacy; + indicates occasional reports of efficacy; ++ indicates treatment shown to be effective; +++ indicates standard of treatment.

episodic visual defects) followed by rapidly progressive painless loss of vision.

Fundoscopic examination may reveal arterial narrowing and abnormal mottling of the retinal pigment. The electroretinogram (ERG) is always abnormal, and is diagnostic. Different antiretinal antibodies have been identified; the best characterized of these is an antibody against recovering (a photoreceptor protein). Treatment with corticosteroids has lead to stabilization and improvement in some patients.

Peripheral Neuropathies

The development of peripheral neuropathy in cancer patients is commonly seen. In most of these patients, though, a direct cause is found such as compression or infiltration of the nervous system (eg, leptomeningeal disease), chemotherapy-induced (with cisplatin, vincristine and taxanes), or secondary to nutritional/metabolic causes (cancer cachexia, vitamin deficiency, uremia). Therefore, an underlying cause should be sought and excluded before a diagnosis of a paraneoplastic peripheral neuropathy is made.

Sensory Neuropathy

Subacute sensory neuropathy (SSN) is a rare paraneoplastic neurologic syndrome that is part of the PEM syndrome, with around 50% of patients having evidence of PEM elsewhere in the nervous system. Although it is much more commonly associated with Sjogren's syndrome, about 20% of affected patients have been found to have a cancer, in most cases small-cell lung cancer.

Clinically, patients usually present with rapidly developing sensory loss, affecting all four limbs, beginning distally and extending proximally. There may be associated areflexia, pain, and a debilitating sensory ataxia. There is a strong association between SSN and anti-Hu antibodies. Patients who develop a rapid onset of SSN should therefore be tested for anti-Hu antibodies, and a search for an underlying malignancy should be carried out if detected [33]. Diagnosis of SSN with nerve conduction studies shows markedly decreased or absent sensory potentials, while motor nerve conduction and F waves are usually completely normal.

Treatment is usually unsuccessful, although there have been reports of regression with antitumor treatment or with the use of intravenous immunoglobulin.

Motor Neuropathies and Motor Neuron Disease

Subacute motor neuropathy (SMN) is a very rare condition that is the motor counterpart to SSN. It is associated primarily with lymphomas, and also with small-cell lung cancer. Patients present with progressive motor weakness over weeks to months and have marked muscle atrophy with flaccid muscle weakness. Lower limbs are affected more than the upper limbs, and bulbar involvement is rare. Patients with SMN in association with small-cell lung cancer often have detectable anti-Hu antibodies.

Despite considerable debate, there appears to be an association between cancer and motor neuron disease (MND). In a recent report of 14 patients with both cancer and MND, the authors suggested that patients presenting with rapidly progressive MND and detectable Anti-Hu Ab had a paraneoplastic process as well as those found to have predominantly upper-motor neuron dysfunction (resembling amyotrophic lateral sclerosis), who were subsequently found to have breast cancer [34]. There have also been reports of an increased incidence of lymphomas in patients with MND, especially those presenting with ALS; therefore further investigation of these patients is warranted. The clinical presentation is usually identical to that of ALS, although the course tends to be a relapsing/remitting one subsequently.

Sensorimotor Neuropathies

The most common form of paraneoplastic neuropathy is a subacute or chronic sensorimotor neuropathy, representing 30% to 50% of peripheral neuropathies. Lung cancer (usually SCLC) is the most common underlying tumor; however, carcinomas of the breast, stomach, colon, and even lymphoproliferative disorders and myelomas have been implicated.

As opposed to Guillain-Barré syndrome, pathology specimens and nerve conduction studies usually reveal an axonal neuropathy rather than a demyelinating process. Clinically, mild motor weakness, hyporeflexia, and symmetrical distal sensory loss are seen, with the lower limbs more likely to be involved. As with the non-neoplastic presentation, CSF examination shows elevated protein with a normal cell count. A distinct autoantibody has not been identified, and the pathogenesis is not particularly well understood. This is in part due to the indistinct presentation compared with noncancer neuropathies such as that secondary to uremia, nutritional deficiencies, or diabetes. The clinical course tends to stabilize and remain chronic, although improvements have been reported with the use of immunosuppressive drugs.

Many patients also present with a neuropathy associated with monoclonal gammopathies including both the malignant (multiple myeloma, Waldenstrom's, B-cell lymphomas, and CLL) and nonmalignant (MGUS [monoclonal gammopathy of undetermined significance]) varieties. These patients typically have symmetrical sensory and motor loss affecting all limbs, often with tremor. Electrophysiologic studies show marked slowing of conduction velocity and conduction block with focal areas of axonal degeneration along with demyelination and remyelination on nerve biopsy. In patients with IgM monoclonal gammopathy, antibodies directed against myelin-associated glycoprotein (anti-MAG antibodies) lead to a slowly progressive sensory or sensorimotor neuropathy. Selective deposition of IgM gammaglobulin in areas of myelin where pathological changes occurred can be demonstrated on electron microscopy and further support for the immunologic basis has been gained by demonstrating a similar process occurring following passive transfer of human IgM anti-MAG antibodies to animals. In patients with an underlying malignant disease, the neuropathy occasionally improves with treatment of the underlying disease. Conversely, the neuropathy associated with MGUS usually responds well to plasmapharesis, IVIG, and immunosuppression.

Patients presenting with an acute neuropathy that is indistinguishable from Guillain-Barré have been shown to have an association with Hodgkin's disease. Response to treatment with plasmapharesis and IVIG is similar to the idiopathic variety.

Autonomic Neuropathy

Paraneoplastic autonomic neuropathy can occur as part of a more widespread paraneoplastic syndrome, such as anti-Hu antibody associated PEM or that associated with LEMS, or as an isolated disorder. It is most commonly associated with SCLC, but is also seen with lymphomas and pancreatic and stomach cancers. It can affect specific components, or all of the autonomic nervous system. Patients may develop dry mouth, postural hypotension, intestinal pseudo-obstruction, esophageal dysmotility, gastroparesis and urinary retention. The clinical course is variable, and specific treatments usually unsuccessful.

Lambert-Eaton Myasthenic Syndrome

Lambert-Eaton myasthenic syndrome (LEMS) is a myoneural disorder characterized by impaired release of acetylcholine from presynaptic nerve terminals resulting in muscle weakness. In two thirds of patients with LEMS, an underlying cancer is found [35]. Most of these have small cell lung cancer (SCLC); 1% to 3% of patients with SCLC develop LEMS [36].

The disorder is characterized by varying degrees of muscle weakness and fatigability. Unlike classic myasthenia gravis, the weakness does not usually involve the bulbar or ocular/orbital muscles to a significant extent. The first symptom is usually weakness and muscle aches of the thighs and pelvic girdle. Most patients also complain of autonomic symptoms including dry mouth, erectile dysfunction and constipation [35].

Electrophysiologic features of LEMS are pathognomic. With high rates of repetitive stimulation, marked increases in the amplitude of compound muscle action potentials occur, while they decrease at low frequencies of repetitive stimulation [37].

The pathogenesis of LEMS is well understood, and is caused by antibodies directed against the presynaptic nerve terminal, specifically against the voltage dependent calcium-channels, which thereby decreases the amount of acetylcholine released in response to an action potential.

Unlike most other paraneoplastic neurologic syndromes, LEMS responds well to treatment with plasmapharesis or intravenous immunoglobulin. Short-term use of steroids or immunosuppressives may also benefit. Others may benefit from treatment with drugs that increase acetylcholine release such as 3,4-diaminopyridine. Cholinesterase inhibitors, which are very effective in myasthenia gravis, are usually ineffective in LEMS, though. Treatment of the underlying malignancy itself may lead to neurologic response in some patients.

Polymyositis and Dermatomyositis

Polymyositis (PM) and dermatomyositis (DM) are inflammatory myopathies that have been associated with cancer since the early 1900s. Patients typically present subacutely with symmetrical proximal muscle weakness with or without pain and muscle tenderness. DM includes skin changes (with the classic heliotrope rash involving the eyelids, cheeks, elbows, knees, and knuckles) accompanying the myositis.

The diagnosis is based on clinical and laboratory abnormalities including elevated muscle enzymes (CK, LDH), a myopathic picture on electromyography, and inflammatory degeneration of muscle on biopsy.

Treatment, as with non–cancer-related patients, depends on the use of immunosuppressives including corticosteroids. The clinical course can be quite inconsistent and does not always parallel that of the cancer itself.

The association between PM/DM and cancer is still debated, although the strength of the association is certainly stronger with DM [38], with a risk of cancer association of approximately 10%. The most common cancers associated with DM/PM are lung cancer in men and ovarian and breast cancer in women. Certainly, patients

Table 31-5. Mucocutaneous Paraneoplastic Syndromes

Disease	Major Features	Associated Malignancies	Percent with Cancer	Comments
Disorders of Pigmentation				
Acanthosis nigricans	Dark, velvety plaques on neck, flexor areas	Adenocarcinoma, especially gastric cancer	Most	Appearance of skin condition may precede malignancy by many y
Sweet's syndrome	Fever, neutrophilia, erythematous raised plaques	AML, other hematologic malignancies	20	May precede or present concurrently with tumor; treat with corticosteroids
Paget's disease	Erythematous keratotic patch; classic Paget's cells on histopathology	Breast, anorectal	50	Malignancy usually arises in area underlying skin changes
Erythematous Conditions				
Exfoliative dermatitis	Progressive erythema followed by scaling	Cutaneous T cell, Hodgkin's lymphomas	20	
Flushing	Episodic reddening of the face, neck lasting for a few min at a time	Carcinoid, medullary thyroid carcinoma	Most	Caused by serotonin, other vasoactive peptides
Bullous Lesions				
Bullous pemphigoid	Large tense bullae	CLL, lymphomas	Unclear	Usually has poor prognosis
Pemphigus vulgaris	Intraepidermal bullae of skin, oral mucosa	Lymphoma, breast, Kaposi's	Unclear	
Dermatitis herpetiformis	Lifelong gluten-sensitive skin disorder with chronic, intensely itchy vesicles over elbows, knees, lumbosacral region	Non-Hodgkin's lymphoma, especially arising in jejunum	20–30	Unclear whether gluten-free diet reduces risk of malignancy
Conditions Characterized by Scaling and Hypertrichosis				
Acquired ichthyosis	Generalized dry cracking skin with scales on trunk and extremities	Hodgkin's disease; Kaposi's sarcoma	Unclear	Can occur in up to 30% of patients with AIDS
Other				
Clubbing and HPOA	Both digital clubbing and periostosis must be present for diagnosis of HPOA to be made	Lung	20	10%–20% of patients with clubbing also have HPOA; symptoms, signs may improve with treatment of tumor
Prorates	Commonest skin condition in patients with cancer	Lymphoma (typically), leukemias, myeloma	10	Usually associated with benign disease, but failure to elicit a cause necessitates a search for underlying malignancy

over the age of 40 presenting with DM should be investigated for malignancy. Although the degree of investigation remains controversial, it would be reasonable to pursue a primary cancer in this group. This should include chest radiography, mammography, pelvic assessment, and serum Ca-125 level in women.

Mucocutaneous Paraneoplastic Syndromes

Mucocutaneous paraneoplastic syndromes represent the most varied and diverse etiologic, pathologic, and morphologic manifestations of cancer. Detailed descriptions of each disorder are beyond the scope of this chapter; a selection of some of the more classic syndromes are therefore outlined in Table 31-5. The principles applying to other paraneoplastic syndromes also apply here, in that systemic manifestations may occur prior to, concurrently, or subsequent to the diagnosis of an underlying malignancy. It is therefore essential that, once a possible cutaneous paraneoplastic syndrome has been diagnosed, an appropriate search for an underlying malignancy takes place.

REFERENCES

1. Langstein HN, Norton JA: Mechanisms of cancer cachexia. *Hematol Oncol Clin North Am* 1991, 5:103–123.

2. Plata-Salaman CR, *et al.*: Tumor necrosis factor and interleukin-1β: suppression of food intake by direct action in the central nervous system. *Brain Res* 1988, 448:106–114.

3. Yoneda T, *et al.*: Evidence that tumor necrosis factor plays a pathogenic role in the paraneoplastic syndrome of cachexia, hypercalcaemia and leukocytosis in a human tumor in nude mice. *J Clin Invest* 1991, 87:977–985.

4. Schwarz MW, Dallman MF, Woods SC: Hypothalamic response to starvation: implications for the study of wasting disorders. *Am J Physiol* 1995, 269:R949–R957.

5. Greenberg DB, *et al.*: Treatment related fatigue and interleukin-1 levels in patients during external beam radiotherapy for prostate cancer. *J Pain Symptom Manag* 1993, 8:196–200.

6. Weber J, *et al.*: A phase 1 trial of intravenous interleukin-6 in patients with advanced cancer. *J Immunother* 1994, 15:292–302.

7. Emilie D: Administration of an anti-interleukin-6 monoclonal antibody to patients with acquired immunodeficiency syndrome and lymphoma: effect on lymphoma growth and on B clinical symptoms. *Blood* 1994, 84:2472–2479.

8. Yamashita J, *et al.*: Medroxyprogesterone acetate treatment reduces serum interleukin-6 levels in patients with metastatic breast cancer. *Cancer* 1996, 78:2346–2352.

9. Spath-Schwalbe E, *et al.*: Interleukin-6 stimulates the hypothalamus-pituitary-adrenocortical axis in man. *J Clin Endocrinol Metab* 1994, 79:1212–1214.

10. Mantovani G, *et al.*: Cytokine involvement in cancer anorexia/cachexia: role of megestrol acetate and medroxyprogesterone acetate on cytokine downregulation and improvement of clinical symptoms. *Crit Rev Oncol* 1998, 9:99–106.

11. Kardinal CG, *et al.*: A controlled trial of cyproheptadine in cancer patients with anorexia and/or cachexia. *Cancer* 1990, 65:2657–2662.

12. Watanabe S, Bruera E: Anorexia and cachexia, asthenia and lethargy. *Hematol Oncol Clin North Am* 1996, 10:189–206.

13. Irvine DM, Vincent L, Bubela N, *et al.*: A critical appraisal of the research literature investigating fatigue in the individual with cancer. *Cancer Nursing* 1991, 14:188–199.

14. Neuenschwander H, Bruera E: Asthenia. In *Oxford Textbook of Palliative Medicine*. Edited by Doyle D. New York: Oxford University Press Inc; 1998: 573–581.

15. Warren RS, Starnes HF, *et al*: The acute metabolic effects of tumour necrosis factor administration in humans. *Arch Surg* 1987, 122:1396–1400.

16. Pirl WF, Roth A: Diagnosis and treatment of depression in cancer patients. *Oncology (Huntingt)* 1999, 9:1293–1301.

17. Bruera E, Roca E, Cedaro L, *et al.*: Action of oral methylprednisolone in terminal cancer patients: a prospective randomized double-blind study. *Cancer Treatment Reports* 1985, 69:751–754.

18. Blatteis CM: Neuromodulative actions of cytokines. *Yale J Biol Med* 1990, 63:71–85.

19. Frolich A: Prevalence of hypercalcaemia in normal and hospital populations. *Danish Medical Bulletin* 1998, 45:436–439.

20. Eloma I: Diphosphonates for osteolytic metastases. *Lancet* 1985, 8430:1155–1156.

21. Body JJ: Current and future directions in medical therapy: hypercalcaemia. *Cancer* 2000, 88:3054–3058.

22. Zoger N: Comparative tolerability of drug therapies for hypercalcaemia of malignancy. *Drug Safety* 1999, 5:389–406.

23. Kanis JA: Bisphosphonates in multiple myeloma. *Cancer* 2000, 88 (S12):3022–3032.

24. Ralston SH, *et al.*: Cancer associated hypercalcaemia: morbidity and mortality. *Ann Intern Med* 1990, 7:499–504.

25. Ling PJ: Analysis of survival following treatment of tumour-induced hypercalcaemia with intravenous pamidronate (APD). *Br J Cancer* 1995, 1:206–209.

26. De Herder WW, Krennung EP, *et al.*: Somatostatin receptor scintigraphy: its value in tumour localization in patients with Cushing's syndrome caused by ectopic corticotropin or corticotropin-releasing hormone secretion. *Am J Med* 1994, 96:305.

27. Henson RA, Hoffman HL, Urich H: Encephalomyelitis with carcinoma. *Brain* 1965, 88:449–464.

28. Dalmau J, *et al.*: Major histocompatibility proteins, anti-Hu antibodies, and paraneoplastic encephalomyelitis in neuroblastoma and small cell lung cancer. *Cancer* 1995, 75:99–109.

29. Voltz RD, *et al.*: Paraneoplastic encephalomyelitis: an update of the effects of the anti-Hu immune response on the nervous system and tumour. *J Neurol Neurosurg Psychiatry* 1997, 63:133–136.

30. Posner JB: Paraneoplastic syndromes. *Neurol Clin* 1991, 9:919–36.

31. Anderson NE, *et al.*: Paraneoplastic cerebellar degeneration: clinical-immunological correlations. *Ann Neurol* 1988, 24:559–567.

32. Jacobson DM, *et al.*: A clinical triad to diagnose paraneoplastic retinopathy. *Ann Neurol* 1990, 28:162–167.

33. Dalmau JO, Posner JB: Paraneoplastic syndromes affecting the nervous system. *Semin Oncol* 1997, 24:318–328.

34. Forsyth PA, *et al.*: Motor neuron syndromes in cancer patients. *Ann Neurol* 1997, 41:722–730.

35. O'Neill JH, *et al.*: The Lambert-Eaton myasthenic syndrome: a review of 50 cases. *Brain* 1988, 111:577–596.

36. van Oosterhout AG, *et al.*: Neurologic disorders in 203 consecutive patients with small cell lung cancer: results of a longitudinal study. *Cancer* 1996, 77:1434–1441.

37. Sanders DB: Lambert-Eaton myasthenic syndrome: clinical diagnosis, immune-mediated mechanisms, and update on therapies. *Ann Neurol* 1995, 37(Sl):S63–S73.

38. Sigurgeirsson B, *et al.*: Risk of cancer in patients with dermatomyositis or polymyositis: a population-based study. *N Engl J Med* 1992, 326:363–367.

FLU-LIKE SYNDROME

Patients undergoing biologic therapy with aldesleukin, interferon α-2, sargramostim, oprelvekin, rituximab, and less frequently, BCG and levamisole develop a flu-like syndrome consisting of fever, chills, malaise, myalgias, arthralgias, headache, and occasionally nausea, vomiting, diarrhea, nasal congestion, dizziness, and light-headedness. For aldesleukin, interferon α-2, and sargramostim these side effects are dose related, occur 1–6 h after a dose, are more common with bolus administration, and resolve spontaneously within 24 h of administration of a single dose. With repeated daily doses (8 h for aldesleukin, daily for interferon α, oprelvekin, ritux-imab, sargramostim) there is a tendency to tachyphylaxis, with symptoms subsiding over time; however, with intermittent treatment, tachyphylaxis usually does not occur. With BCG, these side effects occur 6–12 h after intravesical administra-tion, and resolve within 1–2 d. The severity tends to parallel the intensity of the local reaction. With levamisole, side effects typically occur on the days of treat-ment. With epoetin α, the flu-like syndrome has occurred with IV but not SC administration. With any of these agents, fevers that occur after several days of therapy or that recur after resolution of early fevers are unusual and an infectious cause should be sought. Rarely are these constitutional symptoms dose limiting.

CAUSATIVE AGENTS

Interferon α, aldesleukin, sargramostim, oprelvekin, rituximab, BCG, levamisole, occasionally cytotoxic chemotherapy

PATHOLOGIC PROCESS

Release or generation of secondary cytokines (eg IL-1, TNF, IL-6) by lymphocytes or monocytes in response to aldesleukin and sargramostim; PGE$_2$ probably directly responsible for interferon-related constitutional symptoms; mechanism of levamisole and BCG toxicity is unclear, but may also be related to secondary cytokine release

DIFFERENTIAL DIAGNOSES

Coexisting viral, bacterial, or fungal infection, para-neoplastic syndromes

PATIENT ASSESSMENT

Rule out infections or neoplastic causes, especially if symptoms progress and are not closely related to administration of above agents

TOXICITY GRADING

	0	1	2	3	4
Fever in absence of infection	None	37.1°–38.0°C 98.7°–100.4°F	38.1°–40.0°C 100.5°–104.0°F	> 40.0°C > 104.0°F for < 24 h	> 40.0°C > 104.0°F for 24 h or accompanied by hypotension
Nausea	None	Able to eat reason-able intake	Intake significantly decreased but can eat	No significant intake	—
Vomiting	None	1 episode in 24 h	2–5 episodes in 24 h	6–10 episodes in 24 h	> 10 episodes in 24 h or requiring parenteral support
Diarrhea	None	Increase of 2–3 stools/d over pretreatment	Increase of 4–6 stools/d, nocturnal stools, moderate cramping	Increase of 7–9 stools/d, incontinence, or severe cramping	Increase of ≥ 10 stools/d, grossly bloody diarrhea, or need for parenteral support
Headache	None	Mild, no treatment required	Moderate non-narcotic treatment	Severe, narcotics required	—
Sinus congestion	None	Mild, no treatment required	Moderate	—	—
Chills, rigors	None	Mild, < 30 min, resolves sponta-neously	Moderate, < 30 min, requires inter-vention	—	—
Myalgia, arthralgia	None	Mild	Moderate	Severe	Intractable

MANAGEMENT

Agent	Dose	Maximum Dose	Action	Guidelines
Acetaminophen (Tylenol)	650 mg q 4 h PO or PR	4000 mg/d	Inhibits prostaglandin synthesis	Begin prior to the first dose of IL-2 or IFN and continue until completing treatment
Indomethacin (Indocin)	25 mg q 6 h PO or PR	200 mg/d	Inhibits prostaglandin synthesis	Begin prior to first dose of IL-2 and continue until com-pletion of treatment; PRN fever with acetaminophen
Diphenhydramine (Benadryl)	25–50 mg PO or IV q 8 h prn	400 mg/d	H$_1$ receptor antagonist	For fever, malaise, chills secondary to hypersensi-tivity reaction (especially with BCG)
Prochlorperazine (Compazine)	10 mg PO or IV, 25 mg PR q 6 h prn	40 mg/d	Dopamine receptor antagonist; affects the chemo-receptor trigger zone and vomiting center	For nausea and vomiting
Meperidine (Demerol)	25–50 mg IM or IV q 4 h prn	—	Central nervous system opioid agonist	For severe chills and rigors
Loperamide hydrochloride (Imodium)	4 mg followed by 2 mg after each unformed stool prn diarrhea	16 mg/d	Slows intestinal motility	For diarrhea
Diphenoxylate hydrochloride with atropine sulfate (Lomotil)	2 tablets q 6 h or 10 mL q 6 h prn (2.5–5.0 mg diphenoxylate Hcl and 0.025–0.05 mg atropine sulfate)	20 mg diphenoxylate HCl/d	Slows intestinal motility	For severe diarrhea

CHRONIC FATIGUE

The fatigue syndrome accompanying interferon α-2, aldesleukin, sargramostim, and oprelvekin therapy varies considerably from mild to severe and, in some cases, defines the maximum tolerated dose. Fatigue is dose-related and is often less when intermittent schedules and lower doses are used. Although individual variation in tolerance is wide, fatigue is often more profound in older patients or those with poor performance status.

MANAGEMENT OR INTERVENTION

1. Evening administration of interferon may reduce fatigue or improve tolerance
2. Moderate or severe fatigue with decreased performance status often improves with a 50% dose reduction of interferon α-2 or sargramostim; if no improvement, reduce drug doses an additional 10% of starting dose or discontinue therapy until fatigue resolves

TOXICITY GRADING SCALE

0	1	2	3	4
Asymptomatic	Symptomatic	Symptomatic, in bed < 50% of day	Symptomatic, in bed > 50% of day but not bedridden	Bedridden

CAUSATIVE AGENTS

Interleukin-2, interferon α-2, sargramostim, oprelvekin

PATHOLOGIC PROCESS

Unclear, but may be part of the broad constellation of CNS toxicity observed with these agents; may be related to IL-1 or other cytokine release

DIFFERENTIAL DIAGNOSES

Anemia; comorbid illness, especially chronic infections, thyroid dysfunction, hepatitis, renal dysfunction; tumor progression; other medications, particularly antiemetics, analgesics, sedatives, cytotoxic chemotherapy

PATIENT ASSESSMENT

Obtain hemoglobin, hematocrit, liver function tests, serum electrolytes (calcium), thyroid function tests, TSH, BUN, and creatinine; review other medications; assess for tumor progression

INFECTIOUS COMPLICATIONS

In patients receiving aldesleukin therapy bacteremia occurs in 10%–20%. The majority of these infections are related to the use of an indwelling intravenous catheter and occur toward the end of a course of aldesleukin treatment. If unrecognized or if institution of appropriate antibiotic therapy is delayed, these infections can be fatal. Antibiotic prophylaxis with several agents has greatly reduced both the incidence and severity of infections. Although uncommon, systemic BCG infections do occur and in rare cases have been fatal. Most septic and fatal cases are related to intravasation of intravesically instilled BCG, often from traumatic catheterization or instrumentation.

Interferon therapy has been associated with reactivation of herpes simplex infections in up to 10% of patients within the first several days of treatment. These infections generally clear within 10 d even while interferon therapy continues. Disseminated herpes has not been reported. Levamisole has only been associated with infections in patients who develop levamisole-induced agranulocytosis or neutropenia.

CAUSATIVE AGENTS

Aldesleukin, interferon α-2, BCG

PATHOLOGIC PROCESS

Aldesleukin infections: probably related to severely impaired neutrophil chemotaxis, resulting either directly or indirectly from aldesleukin administration; **Systemic BCG infections:** most likely related to intravascular disseminiation of BCG through an inflamed, friable, or bleeding urothelium; **Interferon α-2 therapy:** mechanism involved with reactivation of herpes simplex infections is unclear

DIFFERENTIAL DIAGNOSES

Flu-like syndrome associated with biologic agents, unrelated infectious process, drug reaction, paraneoplastic syndrome

PATIENT ASSESSMENT

Aldesleukin: obtain blood cultures from central venous catheter site and peripherally, examine central venous catheter site and skin for generalized reactions, check for lapse in antipyretic administration, assess fever pattern with prior doses; **Interferon α-2:** evaluate lesions, obtain herpes virus culture; **BCG:** rule out other infections causes, culture bacterial strains and biopsy of affected sites

MANAGEMENT OR INTERVENTION

Aldesleukin

1. Optimal intravenous catheter management; remove after ≤ 7 d
2. Surveillance cultures of intravenous catheter twice weekly
3. Prophylactic antibiotics (ciprofloxacin, 250 mg PO bid; cefazolin sodium, 250–500 mg IV q 8 h; or oxacillin, 500 mg IV q 6 h) for patients requiring central venous catheters
4. Prompt recognition of infections and initiation of appropriate antibiotics after obtaining cultures. Because of high risk for *S. aureus*, vancomycin hydrochloride, 1 g 12 h (dose adjusted for impaired renal failure) is empiric drug of choice; broader coverage may be indicated in some patients—particularly those with a history of urinary tract infections, biliary colic, abdominal discomfort, or neutropenia
5. Removal of intravenous catheter once infection is suspected or confirmed

Interferon α-2

Acyclovir, 200 mg PO 5 ×/d to manage pain associated with herpes labialis infection

BCG

1. Avoid use of BCG in immunosuppressed patients because of risk of systemic infection
2. Postpone BCG treatment until concurrent febrile illness, urinary tract infection, or gross hematuria resolves
3. Delay BCG dose for 7–14 d after traumatic catherization, biopsy, or transurethral resection
4. For fevers greater than 100°F or bladder-irritative symptoms lasting longer than 24 h and gross hematuria, administer isoniazid, 300 mg PO × 3 d; repeat isoniazid with subsequent administrations
5. Discontinue BCG if patient continues to have fevers while receiving isoniazid, recurrent elevations in liver function tests (related to isoniazid), or signs of prostatitis, orchitis, etc.
6. For systemic BCG infection, therapy should include: isoniazid 300 mg PO daily, rifampin 600 mg PO daily, and ethambutol 1200 mg PO daily for at least 6 mo. For patients with life-threatening BCG sepsis or "BCGosis," administer cycloserine 250–500 mg PO bid for first 3 d of treatment

TOXICITY GRADING

0	1	2	3	4
None	Minor, localized, antibiotics not required	Minor, antibiotics required	Severe, major organ infection	Disseminated, life-threatening

HEMODYNAMIC COMPLICATIONS

Hypotension is the most frequent dose-limiting side effect of high-dose aldesleukin therapy, particularly when administered by intermittent intravenous bolus. The sequence of hemodynamic effects is characterized by an initial vasodilatory phase occurring 2–4 h after a dose of aldesleukin, during which the systemic vascular resistance falls but vascular integrity is maintained. Subsequently, the capillary leak syndrome with third-space accumulation of fluid often develops. The decreased systemic vascular resistance persists until the completion of therapy.

Hemodynamic complications of GM-CSF are much less frequent and less carefully studied. A first-dose reaction, characterized by transient hypotension, hypoxemia, flushing, tachycardia, musculoskeletal pain, rigors, leg spasms, dyspnea, nausea, and vomiting has been observed with molgramostim (nonglycosylated, *E. coli*–derived GM-CSF) but rarely with sargramostim (glycosylated, yeast-derived GM-CSF). This reaction is limited to the first dose of each treatment cycle and is not dose limiting. The mechanism of the first reaction dose is unclear but appears unrelated to TNF. Hypotension also may occur late during a course of therapy and be related to vasodilation and the capillary leak syndrome, similar to what has been reported with aldesleukin.

Hypotension has occurred in up to 6% of patients with cancer treated with interferon α-2. It is generally mild and easily managed with intravenous fluids. Rarely are dose modifications required . Rituximab infusion is associated with mild to moderate hypotension in 10%–15% of patients. This usually occurs during administration of the antibody in conjunction with other acute systemic manifestations and usually can be effectively managed by slowing or interrupting the infusion and supportive measures, including administration of intravenous saline. The mechanism is most likely a hypersensitivity reaction, although secondary cytokine release cannot be excluded. Hypertension has been noted rarely in cancer patients treated with epoetin α. The hypertension has been associated with a significant increase in hematocrit often in a patient with preexisting hypertension. Epoetin α should not be administered to patients with uncontrolled hypertension.

CAUSATIVE AGENTS

Aldesleukin, sargramostim, interferon α-2, epoetim α, rituximab

PATHOLOGIC PROCESS

Decreased systemic vascular resistance and consequent hypotension are most likely related to a release of the secondary cytokine TNF; TNF is also responsible for the similar hemodynamic changes observed in early septic shock—may exert its effect on vascular smooth muscle through the synthesis of nitric oxide; mechanism of the first dose sargramostim reaction is unclear, but appears to be unrelated to TNF

DIFFERENTIAL DIAGNOSES

Bacterial sepsis; hypovolemia secondary to over-aggressive diuresis; vomiting, diarrhea, or bleeding; cardiac dysfunction; concomitant medications

PATIENT ASSESSMENT

Hemoglobin, hematocrit, ECG, BUN/creatinine; evaluate for infection, review daily weight

MANAGEMENT OR INTERVENTION

Aldesleukin

1. Administer normal saline for a weight gain of between 5%–10% of baseline weight over the 5-d course of aldesleukin therapy
2. In patients with preexisting essential hypertension, therapy with antihypertensive agents should be stopped
3. For hypotension, administer up to 3 normal saline fluid boluses (250 mL each); once weight reaches > 5% of baseline, initiate pressors rather than continue fluid boluses
4. If hypotension persists despite adequate fluid replacement, begin dopamine hydrochloride, 2–8 µg/kg/min; titrate dose to maintain a systolic BP 80–100 mm Hg; monitor for occurrence of atrial tachyarrhythmias—if they occur, and hypotension persists, change to phenylephrine hydrochloride
5. Phenylephrine hydrochloride, 0.1–2.0 µg/kg/min, may be used alone or with dopamine for persistent hypotension
6. Hold dose of aldesleukin if patient remains hypotensive despite pressors or if high doses of pressors are required to maintain blood pressure

Sargramostim

1. Symptomatic management of first-dose effect includes oxygen therapy, intravenous fluids for hypotension, NSAIDs for musculoskeletal pains, and morphine sulfate reserved for severe pain;
2. Prehydration may decrease incidence and severity of hypotension

TOXICITY GRADING

0	1	2	3	4
None or no change	Changes requiring no therapy (including transient orthostatic hypotension)	Requires fluid replacement only	Requires pressors, resolves within 48 h of stopping the agent	Requires pressors for > 48 h after stopping the agent

CAPILLARY LEAK SYNDROME

The capillary leak (vascular leak) syndrome is a common dose-limiting side effect of aldesleukin and occasionally sargramostim therapy. The administration of high-dose aldesleukin and, less frequently, sargramostim and oprelvekin, results in a generalized increase in vascular permeability and fluid extravasation into the tissues. The capillary leak syndrome is often first manifested as mild facial and ankle edema within 24 h of the initiation of treatment. It may subsequently progress to anasarca during the course of treatment. Weight gain equivalent to 5%–10% of baseline body weight due to fluid retention, ascites (especially in patients with extensive hepatic metastases), pulmonary edema, and pleural and pericardial effusions are commonly observed. The development of pulmonary edema is more frequent in patients with marginal pulmonary reserve (ie, in patients with a pretreatment FEV_1 of ≤ 2.0 L) and in those whose treatment is complicated by bacteremia. Edema of the CNS occurs as well and can be fatal in patients with brain metastases. The capillary leak syndrome occurs to some degree in all patients receiving standard high-dose aldesleukin therapy, but only rarely in patients receiving sargramostim in doses ≤ 250 µg/m^2/d or 6 µg/kg/d, and although more frequent, it is usually mild in patients receiving oprelvekin. The development of these potentially life-threatening side effects often contributes to decisions to withhold aldesleukin doses or otherwise limit the intensity or duration of a course of immunotherapy. Side effects resolve rapidly after the discontinuation of therapy, with most patients reverting to their baseline weight in 4 to 5 days after completion of a course of therapy.

CAUSATIVE AGENTS

Aldesleukin, sargramostim, oprelvekin

PATHOLOGIC PROCESS

Uncertain, but most likely a combination of several factors; direct endothelial injury mediated by aldesleukin activated leukocytes (NK and LAK cells, in particular), or their oxidative products; secondary cytokine release, TNF, and IL-1, which may induce various adhesion molecules necessary for attachment of activated leukocytes to endothelium) or systemic complement activation with resultant high plasma concentrations of anaphylatoxins such as C3a, which have potent effects on vascular permeability

DIFFERENTIAL DIAGNOSES

Bacterial sepsis; tumor progression with malignant effusions; IVC compression or thrombosis; hepatic dysfunction; congestive heart failure

PATIENT ASSESSMENT

Rule out infection; check radiograph, ECG, LFTs, albumin; evaluate for tumor progression with IVC compression; rule out IVC or other deep vein thrombosis

MANAGEMENT OR INTERVENTION

Aldesleukin

1. Select patients carefully. Patients should have no evidence of cardiac disease or brain metastases, adequate pulmonary reserve ($FEV_1 \geq 2.0$ L or $\geq 75\%$ of predicted for height and age), no significant pleural or pericardial effusions, and ECOG performance status of 0–1
2. Administer normal saline intravenously to limit weight gain to 5%–10% of baseline weight over 5-d course of aldesleukin
3. Give oxygen therapy for symptomatic pleural effusions or pulmonary edema
4. For severe cardiovascular or pulmonary compromise, hold aldesleukin until symptoms have resolved; for life-threatening complications, dexamethasone, 10 mg IV q 6 h may be given
5. Once treatment has been completed and blood pressure is normal off pressors, begin diuresis with furosemide, 20–40 mg PO or IV daily until edema has resolved and patient has returned to baseline weight

Sargramostim and oprelvekin

1. Select patients carefully. Patients should have no evidence of cardiac disease or brain metastases, adequate pulmonary function and no significant pleural or pericardial effusions
2. Give oxygen therapy for symptomatic pleural effusions or pulmonary edema
3. Reduce dose for moderate cardiovascular or pulmonary compromise
4. For severe cardiovascular or pulmonary compromise, hold sargramostim and oprelvekin therapy until symptoms have resolved; for life-threatening complications, dexamethasone, 10 mg IV q 6 h may be given

TOXICITY GRADING

	0	1	2	3	4
Weight gain	< 5%	5%–9.9%	10.0%–19.9%	20%–29.9%	≥ 30%
Pulmonary	None or no change	Asymptomatic, with abnormality in PFTs	Dyspnea on exertion	Dyspnea at rest	Severe symptoms not responsive to treatment, requiring intubation
Pericardial	None	Asymptomatic effusion, no intervention required	Pericarditis (rub, chest pain, ECG changes)	Symptomatic effusion; drainage required	Tamponade; drainage urgently required

ALLERGIC AND IMMUNE-MEDIATED COMPLICATIONS

Patients treated with aldesleukin, interferon α, rituximab, and less commonly, sargramostim, oprelvekin, filgrastim, levamisole, and BCG, may develop a variety of allergic and immune-mediated side effects. Although relatively common, local injection site reactions (cystitis with BCG, erythematous skin lesions at SC injection sites with the other agents) are generally self-limited. Acute serious hypersensitivity reactions, such as urticaria, angioedema, bronchoconstriction, and anaphylaxis have rarely been observed with these agents. Many of these agents have been associated with the development or exacerbation of preexisting autoimmune or chronic inflammatory diseases (eg, immune thrombocytopenia purpura, autoimmune hemolytic anemia, vitiligo, psoriasis, rheumatoid arthritis, vasculitis, thyroiditis, inflammatory bowel disease). In most cases, therapy must be discontinued.

Both neutralizing and nonneutralizing antibodies against aldesleukin, sargramostim, and interferon α-2 have been observed. The clinical significance of these antibodies remains unclear, but in several cases the development of neutralizing antibodies to interferon was associated with disease relapse. The development of autoantibodies to insulin, thyroid peroxidase, platelets, and other antigens has been described, and many of these autoantibodies may be associated with the development of autoimmune disease. For example, thyroiditis, which is seen in 10%–20% of patients undergoing high-dose aldesleukin therapy, is frequently associated with the development of antithyroid antibodies.

Unusual recall reactions to iodinated contrast medium and cytotoxic chemotherapy have occurred in patients receiving aldesleukin therapy. As many as 10% of patients undergoing routine IV contrast studies during follow-up for previous aldesleukin therapy and 50% of patients receiving combination cisplatin-based chemotherapy with aldesleukin therapy develop such reactions. These reactions usually occur at least 1 mo after initial exposure to aldesleukin and contrast medium or on second or subsequent chemotherapy cycles. Typical reactions begin 1–4 h after reexposure to the agent and consist of fever, chills, rash, diarrhea, nausea, vomiting, urticaria, dyspnea, weakness, and hypotension; resolution is within 24 hours. Reactions appear to be more common in patients who receive aldesleukin and radiographic contrast medium simultaneously.

CAUSATIVE AGENTS

Aldesleukin, interferon α-2, BCG, levamisole, sargramostim, filgrastim

PATHOLOGIC PROCESS

Poorly defined: release of secondary cytokines may induce expression of HLA-DR antigens on cells, eg, thyrocytes. These cells are then rendered competent to present cell-specific antigens, eg, thyroglobulin, to autoreactive T lymphocytes already present in the host. In some cases, administered cytokine may play a direct role in pathogenesis. Recall reaction may be related to enhancement by aldesleukin of an immune response to radiographic contrast material, followed by an anamnestic response on reexposure to the contrast material

DIFFERENTIAL DIAGNOSES

Allergic reactions or side effects of other medications, comorbid illnesses

PATIENT ASSESSMENT

Varies according to problem

MANAGEMENT OR INTERVENTION

1. Avoid biologic therapy or administer with great caution in patients with history of autoimmune or chronic inflammatory disease
2. Manage acute serious allergic reactions in a standard way with antihistamines, epinephrine, and, in some cases, corticosteroids
3. Discontinue therapy if severe reactions develop
4. Avoid or significantly decrease "recall reaction" to iodinated contrast medium by pretreatment with antipyretics and antihistamines
5. Because of the relatively high frequency of thyroiditis, monitor thyroid function for patients on aldesleukin or interferon α-2 therapy
6. BCG cystitis may be treated symptomatically with phenazopyridine hydrochloride, 200 mg PO tid, propantheline bromide, 15 mg PO before meals and 30 mg PO qhs, oxbutynin hydrochloride, 5 mg PO tid

TOXICITY GRADING

0	1	2	3	4
None	Transient rash, drug fever < 38°C, 100.4°F	Urticaria, drug fever > 38°C, 100.4°F, mild bronchospasm	Serum sickness, bronchospasm, requires parenteral meds	Anaphylaxis

Immune-mediated complications may be graded using standard toxicity grading criteria for the affected organ or organs.

Tissue wasting is a common and often devastating sequela of the cancer-bearing state. This loss in body mass can result in multiorgan derangements, including impaired immune function, impaired locomotive capacity, and ultimately impaired respiratory function. As little as 5% reduction in lean body mass has been associated with increased mortality in cancer patients. Numerous factors contribute to produce wasting and malnutrition in these patients (Table 32-1). Advances in understanding of these factors as well as improvements in nutrient delivery methods and availability of immunostimulatory nutrients and growth factors offer exciting potential modalities for specific treatment of cancer-related wasting.

CAUSES

The factors that produce malnutrition in the cancer patient are well-known. Gastrointestinal obstruction from tumor, perioperative gastrointestinal tract dysfunction, and the oral and esophageal mucositis that often complicates chemotherapy or radiation represent physical impediments to nutrient intake. In addition, anorexia or a decreased desire for food is a common finding in cancer-bearing states. The causes of the anorexia may be direct actions of tumor-related mediators on the hypothalamic satiety centers or result indirectly from depression, nausea, or vomiting. Gastrointestinal fistula formation as well as diarrhea and malabsorption can result not only from direct influences of certain tumors but can complicate surgical, chemotherapeutic, or radiation treatment plans. The effects of such malabsorption on nutritional status are obvious (Fig. 32-1).

Even without clear physical reasons, and often at low tumor burdens, the cancer-bearing state may be associated with a syndrome of anorexia, weight loss, anemia, and severe lean tissue wasting. Although the mechanisms underlying this syndrome of cancer cachexia remain elusive, the alterations in substrate handling that characterize this syndrome are well described [1] (Table 32-2) and are summarized briefly.

Glucose

Carbohydrate-related changes of the tumor-bearing state can be characterized by increases in glycolysis, anaerobic glycolysis by the tumor and certain host tissues, and insulin resistance. The increased glycolysis results in host glycogen depletion and is accompanied by an increase in liver gluconeogenesis. The resultant drain on body energy store is thought to be responsible, in part, for wasting of peripheral tissues.

Protein

The protein-specific changes associated with cancer cachexia are characterized by an increased peripheral skeletal muscle breakdown, decreased skeletal muscle protein synthesis, and an increased hepatic acute phase protein synthesis. The net result is an increased peripheral wasting. These protein metabolic changes often occur despite

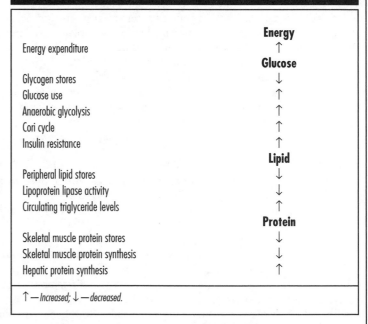

Table 32-2. Changes in Substrate Handling in the Cancer Patient

	Energy
Energy expenditure	↑
	Glucose
Glycogen stores	↓
Glucose use	↑
Anaerobic glycolysis	↑
Cori cycle	↑
Insulin resistance	↑
	Lipid
Peripheral lipid stores	↓
Lipoprotein lipase activity	↓
Circulating triglyceride levels	↑
	Protein
Skeletal muscle protein stores	↓
Skeletal muscle protein synthesis	↓
Hepatic protein synthesis	↑

↑ — Increased; ↓ — decreased.

Table 32-1. Causes of Malnutrition in Cancer Patients

Poor intake	Stress of surgery, chemotherapy, or radiation therapy
Anorexia	Perioperative intestinal dysfunction
Gastrointestinal dysfunction	Diarrhea
Blockage	Vomiting
Diarrhea	Anorexia
Malabsorption	Malabsorption
Altered substrate cycles	

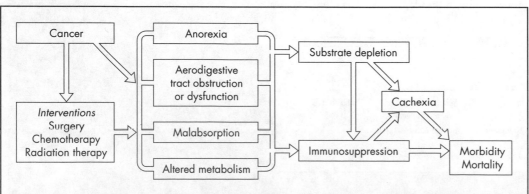

FIGURE 32-1.

Causes of malnutrition and cachexia in cancer patients.

decreased food intake, indicating an aberration in the normal mechanisms of protein preservation during starvation in these patients.

Fat

Central to the lipid-related changes in cancer is a decreased activity of lipoprotein lipase, which is a membrane-bound enzyme pivotal in triglyceride uptake by the peripheral adipocytes. The result is poor disposal of circulating triglycerides, peripheral lipid depletion, and hypertriglyceridemia. There also may be increased lipolysis, with the effect of loss of peripheral lipid stores, which is characteristic of the tumor-bearing state.

Vitamins

Patients with neoplastic disease are at a high risk for deficiency of vitamins. This deficiency results from a combination of poor intake, poor absorption, and increased requirements. Because of the limited stores of water-soluble vitamins within the body, deficiencies of these are more common and may occur even after relatively short-term dietary deprivation. Deficiency of fat-soluble vitamins usually results only after prolonged dietary deficiency or is related to compromised fat or bile absorption.

Vitamins may have a role in the prevention of cancers. Deficiencies of certain vitamins have been linked to an increased risk for malignancies. For example, deficiency of folate has been linked to increased risk of cancers of the esophagus, colon, bronchus, and cervix [2]. Therefore, experimental and clinical studies have sought to determine if vitamin supplementation may prevent development of cancer in high-risk groups. Administration of retinoids and β-carotene, which are synthetic analogues and precursors of vitamin A, have shown promise in the prevention of epithelial tumors [3,4]. In ulcerative colitis, an inflammatory condition that predisposes to colon cancer, folate supplementation has been shown to decrease the incidence of colonic neoplasia [5]. Although the definitive mechanisms by which each of these vitamins protects against tumor are incompletely defined, all of these vitamins have been shown to enhance anticancer immune function. Vitamins C and E and β-carotenes also have been shown to have antioxidant properties, whereas retinoids and folate have major roles in regulation of the cell cycles of normal and neoplastic cells. Further discussion of vitamins as a cancer prevention modality are beyond the scope of this chapter; interested readers are referred to reviews for a discussion of these issues [6,7]. This chapter concentrates on vitamin supplementation as it may relate to treatment of malnutrition.

ASSESSMENT

The simplest and most frequently used measures of nutritional status are the anthropometric measurements of weight, weight loss, arm circumference, and triceps skinfold thickness. Of these, weight loss has been found to be the most useful, with weight loss of more than 5% correlating with poor outcome. Arm circumference and triceps skinfold thickness are not good independent predictors of morbidity or mortality and therefore have limited use.

Circulating levels of serum proteins decrease with malnutrition and have been proposed as clinical markers of malnutrition. The most useful serum protein has been albumin, levels of which have been found to correlate inversely to complications. Because this protein has a circulating half-life on the order of 30 days, decreased circulating levels of this protein are a good index of persistent malnutrition but may not reflect acute changes. Measurements of prealbumin (half-life, 2 to 3 d) have been advocated as a better reflection of

acute changes in nutritional status. Costs of measuring proteins other than albumin, however, are still too high to consider using them as routine in assessment of the cancer patient.

Urinary creatinine excretion has been advocated as a parameter of nutritional status because creatinine excretion in normal subjects is related to lean tissue mass. Patients with a creatinine-to-height ratio of less than 60% ideal as determined by standard tables usually are considered severely malnourished. In cancer-bearing states, however, nitrogen excretion often does not correlate with lean tissue mass. Nitrogen excretion has been found to persist at high levels even as wasting progresses, indicating persistent catabolic influences and rendering the creatinine-to-height ratio of little use in assessing nutrition reserve in this population. Nitrogen excretion is indicative of the level of catabolism and may guide efforts in repletion.

Immune parameters also have been touted as a criterion for malnutrition. These include delayed hypersensitivity skin testing and determination of total lymphocytic counts. Three problems exist for using such parameters in cancer patients, however. Immunosuppression can be a primary consequence of malignancy. Second, host immune function may be altered by other disease-related conditions, such as infection, hemorrhage, or cirrhosis. Third, iatrogenic factors, such as chemotherapeutic agents or surgical procedures, also may alter host immune function.

More sophisticated assessments of nutritional status, such as isotopic measurements of body composition or protein metabolism, are much too costly and complicated to be used routinely in the assessment of the cancer patient and are relegated to the research arena. Of the above-mentioned parameters, the major correlates to outcome are weight loss [8] and albumin levels. In fact, there are studies showing that a clinical history and clinical assessment are as good as any laboratory or physical parameter in predicting outcome [9]. Nevertheless, certain clinical findings should alert the clinician to significant malnutrition and need for repletion, particularly if major surgical or chemotherapeutic intervention is planned (Table 32-3). These include weight loss of greater than 10%, weight loss of greater than 0.5 kg/week, evidence of muscular weakness, and serum albumin less than 3.2 g/dL [10]. A simple grading scale for the degree of malnutrition using these simple clinical and laboratory parameters is presented in Table 32-4.

Table 32-3. Assessment of Malnutrition in Cancer Patients

Absolute Indicators of Malnutrition	Relative Indicators of Malnutrition
Weight loss > 10%	Immune parameters
Weight loss of 0.5 kg/wk	Anergy in delayed hypersensitivity testing
Clinically evident muscular weakness	T cell numbers < 1500/mL
Serum albumin < 3.2 g/dL	Decreased complement levels
	Hypoproteinemia
	Thyroxine-binding prealbumin
	Transferrin
	Retinol binding protein
	Creatinine:height ratio < 60% ideal
	Negative nitrogen balance
	Clinical
	Stomatitis
	Gastrointestinal dysfunction

In the clinical consideration of cancer patients, all patients should be assessed for vitamin deficiency. The most common symptoms for deficiencies of the various vitamins are summarized in Table 32-5. The patient history should be evaluated for risk factors predisposing to vitamin insufficiency. Dietary history should look specifically for poor oral intake. Assessment should be made for signs and symptoms of intestinal or biliary obstruction, symptoms of pancreatic insufficiency or fat malabsorption, or past history of intestinal resection. Any of these conditions may result in deficiencies of fat-soluble vitamins [11] because bile and fats are important for absorption of these vitamins. Vitamin B$_{12}$ deficiency also may result from disease or resection of the terminal small bowel because this vitamin is absorbed in this region. Patients on long-term antibiotic therapy or mechanical bowel cleansing also may develop deficiencies of vitamins normally produced by the intestinal flora, such as biotin and vitamin K. Although laboratory tests for deficiencies of individual vitamins are available (*see* Table 32-5), their routine use in the screening of asymptomatic patients is discouraged.

TREATMENT

Strategies with the aim to treat malnutrition associated with cancer-bearing states must be directed at repleting lean tissue losses that have already occurred and preventing further loss of vital tissues. Such strategies have to overcome two basic obstacles. First are the physical factors that prevent intake or absorption of nutrients and second are the alterations in host metabolic substrate handling that predispose to tissue wasting. Clinical and experimental strategies that have been devised and practiced can be divided into four main categories: elimination of tumor, increasing nutrient intake, use of

Table 32-4. Toxicity Scale for Malnutrition

Grade	Degree of Malnutrition	Clinical Findings	Laboratory Findings
0	None	No weight loss	Normal albumin Normal transferrin level Reactive delayed hypersensitivity skin test
1	Mild	Weight loss < 5%	Albumin < 3.5 Decreased transferrin level
2	Moderate	5%–10% weight loss	< 5 mm reactivity on skin test Albumin < 3.2
3	Severe	Weight loss > 10% Muscular weakness	Nonreactive skin test Albumin < 2.7

Table 32-5. Symptoms of Vitamin Deficiencies and Assays for Confirmation of Deficiencies

Fat-Soluble Vitamins

Vitamin	Symptoms of Deficiency	Toxicity	Test for Deficiency
A	Night blindness, conjunctival xerotosis, hyperkeratosis, immune dysfunction, increased cerebrospinal fluid pressure, anemia, hepatosplenomegaly, anorexia	Dry mucous membranes, hepatic fibrosis, anemia, pseudotumor cerebri, headache, vomiting, diplopia	Optic dark adaptation, plasma retinol level, retinol-binding protein
D	Osteomalacia, bone fractures	Nephrocalcinosis, renal insufficiency, metastatic calcifications	Plasma calcidiol levels, plasma calcitriol levels
E	Hemolytic anemia, neuromuscular damage, brain stem demyelination	Nausea, headache, fatigue	Blood total tocopherols
K	Bleeding disorder	Hemolytic anemia, vomiting, anaphylaxis	Prothrombin time

Water-Soluble Vitamins

Vitamin	Symptoms of Deficiency	Toxicity	Test for Deficiency
C	Anorexia, irritability, weight loss, hemorrhage, anemia	Nausea, vomiting, diarrhea, hemolysis	Plasma vitamin C level
Thiamine	Peripheral neuropathy, congestive heart failure, cardiomegaly, edema, confusion, ataxia, nystagmus	Anaphylaxis	Urinary thiamine level
Riboflavin (B$_2$)	Stomatitis, glossitis, dermatitis	None	Erythrocyte riboflavin content
Niacin	Dermatitis, diarrhea, dementia, anorexia	Flushing	Urinary niacin
B$_6$	Anemia, stomatitis, irritability	Liver injury, ataxia, peripheral neuropathy	Tryptophan loading test
Folate	Macrocytic anemia, leukopenia	Renal damage	Serum or RBC folate levels
B$_{12}$	Megaloblastic anemia, peripheral neuropathy, confusion, memory loss, dementia	None	Serum holotranscobalamin II level, serum B$_{12}$ level

growth factors, and use of pharmacologic agents (Table 32-6). Elimination of tumor, whether by surgery, chemotherapy, or radiation is paramount and may reverse many of the derangements associated with cancer cachexia.

Increasing Nutrient Intake

Total Parenteral Nutrition in the Surgical Patient

Since the landmark report of Dudrick *et al.* in 1965 showing that high caloric IV feeding alone can provide long-term sustenance for patients, total parenteral nutrition (TPN) has become a widely used part of the clinical armamentarium. At least 19 studies examining this modality in cancer patients have been published and reviewed [12]. Although the majority are negative studies that do not show improvements in outcome parameters even with aggressive feeding, most studies are flawed by poor control groups, small sample sizes, and heterogenicity of patient population. These shortcomings are discussed at length in the meta analysis of this literature by Detsky *et al.* [12]. A number of these studies are sufficiently well executed to deserve further discussion (Table 32-7).

Muller *et al.* [13] examined patients with TPN undergoing gastric or esophageal surgery and found that parenteral feedings for 10 days (*n* = 66) significantly reduced the rate of mortality and major postop-

erative complications when compared with control patients undergoing customary oral feedings (*n* = 59). A subsequent study by the Veterans Affairs Study Group [14] examined patients (*n* = 395) undergoing abdominal or thoracic surgery. Although no overall differences existed between the groups in terms of morbidity or mortality in this study of 7 to 10 days of preoperative TPN, in subset analysis, for patients with severe malnutrition as defined by clinical parameters (weight loss > 20%, serum albumin < 2.9), there was an advantage in preoperative TPN. Fan *et al.* [15] published a trial in which patients undergoing hepatectomy for hepatocellular carcinoma were randomized to receive or not receive preoperative TPN; they found patients receiving TPN to have a significantly lower complication rate. This may yet be another trial demonstrating the use of nutritional support in a severely malnourished patient population because patients suffering from hepatocellular carcinoma generally have cirrhosis and poor baseline nutritional status.

More recently, Jin *et al.* [16] conducted studies on the effects of TPN in the severely malnourished cancer patient, the proliferation of tumor cells, and the sensitivity of tumor cells to chemotherapy. Malnourished patients with operable gastrointestinal cancer were randomly assigned to receive one of four interventions that were administered for 7 days preoperatively: 1) TPN, 2) TPN plus chemotherapy, 3) chemotherapy, and 4) no intervention. Their findings suggest that combining chemotherapy and nutritional support preoperatively improves short-term nutritional status without increasing the proliferation of tumor cells. Bozzetti *et al.* [17] reported on a randomized clinical trial of perioperative TPN in malnourished gastrointestinal cancer patients to study the role of TPN in reducing surgical risk; they found that 10 days of preoperative TPN that is continued postoperatively is able to reduce the complication rate by approximately one third, including mortality.

Lacking further evidence, a reasonable recommendation is that in preoperative patients with greater than 10% weight loss, preoperative aggressive nutritional supplementation is reasonable, whether by the enteral or parenteral route. If the decision is to use the parenteral route, at least a 7- to 10-day course of TPN is warranted. There is no

Table 32-6. Potential Treatments of Malnutrition in Cancer Patients

Eradication of tumor	Growth factors
Increasing nutrient intake	Anabolic steroids
Enteral supplementation	Insulin
IV supplementation	Growth hormone
Specific nutrient administration	Insulin-like growth factors
Nucleotides	Pharmacologic agents
Specific amino acids	Megestrol
Polyunsaturated free fatty acids	Metoclopramide
	Dronabinol

Table 32-7. Major Studies of Nutritional Support in Cancer Patients

Study	Nutritional Support	Patient Population, *n*	Findings
Parenteral Nutrition			
Mullin, *Ann Surg* 1980, 192:604	TPN 10 d preoperatively	GI surgery patients, 145	Improved survival; reduced complications
Muller, *Lancet* 1982, 1:68	TPN 10 d preoperatively	Esophageal/gastric surgery, 125	Improved survival; reduced complications
VA Coop Group, *N Engl J Med* 1991, 325:525	TPN 7–10 d preoperatively	GI/thoracic surgery, 117	Reduced complications in severely malnourished subset
Brennan, *Ann Surg* 1994, 220:436	TPN postoperatively	Upper GI malignancies, 117	No benefit
Fan, *N Engl J Med* 1994, 331:1547	TPN preoperatively	Liver surgery patients	Improved survival
Jin, *J Parenter Enteral Nutr* 1999, 23:237	TPN 7 d preoperatively	GI malignancies; surgery/chemotherapy, 92	Improved nutritional status
Bozzetti, *J Parenter Enteral Nutr* 2000, 24:7	TPN 10 d preoperatively; 9 d postoperatively	GI surgery patients, 90	Improved survival; Shorter hospital stay
Evans, *J Clin Oncol* 1987, 5:113	Oral diet counseling and supplementation	Chemotherapy patients for lung or colon cancer, 192	Improved survival; reduced complications
Daly, *Surgery* 1992, 221:327	EN postoperatively	Upper GI malignancies, 85	Decreased infections and ward complications
Heslin, *Ann Surg* 1997, 226:567	EN	GI malignancies, 195	No benefit
Braga, *Crit Care Med* 1998, 26:24	Compared TPN vs EN postoperatively	GI/pancreatic surgery, 166	EN: reduced infections, shorter hospital stay

EN—enteral nutrition; TPN—total parenteral nutrition.

evidence that any shorter course has clinical efficacy, and TPN is certainly not without complications (Table 32-8). A more recent randomized, controlled trial evaluated the effect of early postoperative TPN on outcome of patients undergoing surgery for upper gastrointestinal cancers and found no benefit to TPN. The patients randomizing to postoperative TPN actually had a higher infection rate compared with controls [18]. Routine postoperative parenteral nutritional feeding therefore is not justified. Only in patients with prolonged intestinal dysfunction or with severe malnutrition should TPN be used. Typical orders for initiating TPN are outlined in Table 32-9.

Total Parenteral Nutrition in the Chemotherapy Patient

Common adverse effects of chemotherapy include anorexia, emesis, diarrhea, and intestinal mucosal sloughing that leads to malabsorption. These effects and the fact that chemotherapy patients tend to have more advanced disease and larger tumor burdens make this group attractive to treat with parenteral nutrition. Despite our clinical prejudice that supplemental nutrient administration should improve clinical status of these patients and animal experimental data suggesting that TPN improves outcome from chemotherapy, no clinical data exist to support this. A multitude of studies have been performed and are summarized by McGeer *et al.* [19]. The conclusions of this position paper by the American College of Physicians were that TPN in the mildly malnourished medical oncology patient may be more harmful than helpful, likely owing to catheter sepsis in this immunosuppressed population. Further, in the severely malnourished person, more data need to be gathered before a conclusion of the risk-to-benefit ratio of TPN can be determined.

Total Parenteral Nutrition in Radiation Therapy Patients

There have been relatively few studies examining the efficacy of nutritional supplementation and the results of radiation therapy for cancer. They can be described as small, poorly controlled studies that are inconclusive and have been reviewed [20]. Based on current clini-

Table 32-8. Common Complications of Total Parenteral Nutrition

Complication	Frequency, %
Central line–related	
Pneumothorax	1–3
Thrombophlebitis*	1–2
Brachial plexus injury	0.5–1
Carotid or subclavian artery injuries	0.25–0.5
Overall	4–15
Infectious	
Line sepsis	2–10
Metabolic	
Electrolyte abnormalities	
Hyperglycemia (including hyperglycemic hyperosmotic coma)	
Hyperkalemia	
Hypomagnesemia	
Hypophosphatemia	
Acid-base disturbances	
Most commonly hyperchloremic metabolic acidosis	
Congestive heart failure	
Altered liver function	
Overall†	5–10

*Clinically apparent thrombophlebitis, angiographically evident thrombophlebitis may be 25% to 30% in select populations.
†Severe metabolic complications.

Table 32-9. Typical Orders for Total Parenteral Nutrition

Makeup of Typical Total Parenteral Nutrition Solution (per 1000 mL)

Nutrients	
Mixed amino acid	50 g
Dextrose	250 g
Electrolytes	
Calcium gluconate	4.6 mEq
Magnesium sulfate	8 mEq
Potassium chloride	22.4 mEq
Potassium phosphate	12 mM
Sodium acetate	18 mEq
Sodium chloride	33.5 mEq
Trace elements (per day)	
Zinc	5 mg
Copper	2 mg
Manganese	0.5 mg
Chromium	10 µg
Multivitamins (per day)	
Vitamin A	1mg
Ergocalciferol (vitamin D)	5 µg
Vitamin E	10 mg
Thiamine	3 mg
Riboflavin	3.6 mg
Niacinamide	40 mg
Dexpanthenol	15 mg
Pyridoxine HCl	4 mg
Biotin	60 µg
Cyanocobalamin	5 µg
Folic acid	400 mg
Ascorbic acid	100 mg
Fat emulsions	500 mL of 10% solution twice a week (4% of total nonprotein calories)

Medical Orders Relating to Start of Total Parenteral Nutrition

Start infusion at 40 mL/h
Maximum incremental increase should be 40 mL/h
Routine catheter care
Infuse total parenteral nutrition via pump
Vital signs q 6 h
Urine by dipstick q 6 h
Stat glucose for > 2+ and call house officer
Strict input and output
Weight 3 times/week
Routine blood tests
3 times/week: Electrolytes, liver function tests, glucose
Once weekly: Prothrombin time, CBC, platelet count, cholesterol, triglyceride, transferrin

cal data, no conclusion with regard to intravenous nutritional supplement in this population can be made.

Enteral Feedings

The majority of studies concerning aggressive nutritional supplementation and the cancer patient are performed using parenteral nutrition. Certainly, in patients with nonfunctional gastrointestinal tracts, the intravenous route represents the only option. When the enteral route is an option, however, there is clear experimental evidence that this route is preferable from an immunologic and metabolic standpoint. Animal and human data indicate that feeding by the intravenous route particularly suppresses host immunologic function. Several clinical trials have examined the use of enteral feedings in the treatment of cancer patients, although clinical indication of benefits has been less than clear. In a study of 192 patients with unresectable colorectal or lung cancer, patients were randomized to three groups: nutritional intake without restriction, dietary counseling, and dietary counseling and enteral defined formula supplementation if goals of 1.7 to 1.95 times resting energy expenditure were not reached [21]. No difference in clinical outcome could be discerned among the groups in this study. It must be noted, however, that aggressive tube feedings were not pursued in this study. In 1992, Daly *et al.* [22] published a trial in which patients who underwent operation for upper gastrointestinal malignancies were randomly assigned to receive either a supplemental diet or standard enteral diet after surgery. Their results suggest that postoperative enteral nutrition with supplemental arginine, RNA, and ω-3 fatty acids instead of a standard enteral diet significantly improved immunologic and metabolic parameters. Patients also had a decreased infection rate as well as decreased clinical outcome. Heslin *et al.* [23] examined the use of early postoperative enteral nutrition in 195 patients with upper gastrointestinal cancers. Patients of all nutritional backgrounds were included and no improvements can be seen for patients with enteral feeding. Studies examining aggressive enteral feeding protocols for preoperative, chemotherapy, or radiation therapy patients are still largely lacking, and this is an active area of research. There is certainly a large selection of enteral supplements available for the nutritional treatment of the cancer patient (*see* Table 32-9).

Specific Nutrients

In addition to strategies that improve total caloric and nitrogen intake, there are also strategies aimed at delivering specific nutrients at high concentrations to the patients. These clinical strategies are based on experimental studies that demonstrate some nutrients to have particularly potent trophic or stimulatory effects on components of the host defense mechanism. Most of these strategies must be considered experimental.

Nucleotides

Nucleotides are essential components of cellular RNA and DNA. Dietary deficiency of nucleic acids alters host cellular immunity, as measured by natural killer cell activity, T-cell response to mitogens, and macrophage cytokine release. Exogenous administration of polynucleotides enhances natural killer cell activity and release of cytokines. One randomized trial on the use of nucleic acids on cancer patients has been performed. In a placebo-controlled trial of patients undergoing resection of breast cancer, there was enhanced survival in polyadenylic acid–treated postmenopausal patients [24]. Further studies need to be performed to verify these results and examine whether similar effects on patients with other tumor types exist. Even before such studies are performed, however, tube feedings supplemented with nucleotides are already commercially available (Table 32-10).

Amino Acids

GLUTAMINE

The amino acid glutamine is a primary nitrogenous substrate used by the gastrointestinal tract. It appears to be a particularly potent trophic factor for intestinal mucosa. Specific use of this amino acid has two goals: improvement of gut barrier function and improvement of intestinal absorptive capacity. For this reason trials are underway to examine the efficacy of adding this amino acid to parenteral and enteral feedings. Preliminary studies from bone marrow transplant patients have not shown a major beneficial role for this amino acid in protecting against complications [25]. Trials in other cancer populations are underway.

ARGININE

Arginine is another amino acid with established immunostimulatory effects. Administration of high doses of this amino acid to cancer

Table 32-10. Common Oral Nutritional Supplements

Product	Calories/mL	Nonprotein calories:gN	Osmolality	Tube/Oral	Taste	Cost	Advantage
Isocal	1.06	167:1	300	Both	Fair	+	Isotonic, tolerated well orally, inexpensive
Isocal HCN	2.00	145:1	690	Both	Fair	++	Useful in fluid restriction
Ensure	1.06	153:1	470	Both	Good	+	Taste suitable for oral supplement, inexpensive, low residue/can be used for bowel preparation
Ensure Plus	1.50	146:1	690	Both	Fair	++	Useful in fluid restriction, low residue
Sustacal HC	1.50	134:1	650	Both	Good	++	Low sodium content
Isosource HN	1.20	116:1	330	Both	Fair	++	Low residue
Specialty Formulas							
Pulmocare	1.50	125:1	520	Tube	Poor	+++++	Low nonprotein caloric content may be beneficial for patients with pulmonary compromise
Impact	1.00	71:1	375	Tube	Poor	+++++	Contains arginine, fish oils, nucleotides: suggested to improve immune function
Elemental Formulas							
Vivonex TEN	1.00	149:1	630	Tube	Poor	+++++	Elemental/predigested, low fat, low residue
Criticare HN	1.06	148:1	650	Tube	Poor	++++	Elemental/predigested, low fat, low residue

patients enhances in vitro parameters of lymphocyte function, including natural killer cell activity, lymphocyte response to stimulation, and increased T helper cell numbers [26]. Whether this translates to improved outcome during cancer therapy is uncertain. Active trials examining the use of this amino acid in the treatment of cancer patients are in progress.

Polyunsaturated Free Fatty Acids

Composition of the dietary fat also seems to have a major effect on host immune function. In particular, the contents of unsaturated free fatty acids appear to be a major determinant of lymphocyte function and macrophage cytokine production. Experimental studies have documented that diets containing fish oils that are high in ω-3 fatty acids can enhance not only measured host immune function but can protect against infection and sepsis. The effects of fish oils or the manipulations of the dietary fats on tumor-bearing states remain unexplored. The findings from studies on sepsis and infection as well as the prevalence of infection in the cancer-bearing populations encourage these lines of investigation.

Vitamins

The causes of vitamin deficiency in cancer patients can be classified into three broad categories: altered intake, altered absorption and metabolism, and increased requirements. These causes contribute to the frequency of vitamin deficiency in this population.

There are many causes of poor vitamin intake. Mechanical obstruction of the oral-digestive tract by certain malignancies is an obvious cause. During treatment, patients may be kept without oral intake either for diagnostic testing or therapeutic interventional procedures. Anorexia, nausea, and vomiting related to either tumor or treatment are other causes. Vitamins, by definition, must be obtained from dietary or parenteral routes. Fat-soluble vitamins (*see* Table 32-5) usually are stored in high amounts within the body; unless patients have other causes for deficiencies or poor intake is prolonged (> 3 months), it is unusual for patients to manifest a clinically significant deficiency of these vitamins. Water-soluble vitamins are more prone to deficiencies from short-term deprivation because, with the exception of vitamin B_{12}, water-soluble vitamins are stored in limited amounts within the body. Assessment of deficiency or empiric supplementation should be considered for any patient with mechanical obstruction of the oral-digestive tract.

Altered dietary fat content can have profound effects on the absorption of fat-soluble vitamins. Other alterations in fat absorption, such as exocrine pancreatic insufficiency, also could result in deficiency of fat-soluble vitamins. Additionally, these fat-soluble vitamins depend on bile acids for absorption. Any interruption of the enterohepatic circulation of bile affects body stores of these vitamins. Therefore, any patient who has biliary obstruction, external biliary drainage or fistula, or resection of the terminal ileum should be assessed clinically for deficiencies of vitamins A, E, D, and K. Many vitamins are manufactured partly by the bacterial flora in the gastrointestinal tract, but this source of vitamins is particularly important for vitamin K. In any patient in whom a significant portion of the large intestine is removed or who undergoes mechanical or antibiotic clearance of intestinal bacterial flora, exogenous supplementation with vitamin K may be necessary.

Patients with cancer may have an increased requirement for certain vitamins. In studies measuring levels of vitamins, patients with cancer may have a deficiency despite intakes judged adequate by recommended daily allowances (RDA) for normal people. In one study of

vitamin C nearly half of the patients with cancer had a deficiency of intracellular vitamin C when their leukocytes were assayed [27]. Stressed patients have particularly high niacin requirements [28]. Folate deficiency is also more common in patients with malignancy. More systematic studies are necessary before determining if an RDA for cancer patients should be adopted. Therapeutic interventions for cancer also can increase vitamin requirements. It is well accepted that surgical stress increased requirements for certain vitamins important for protein synthesis and wound healing, including vitamin C. Certain chemotherapeutic agents have been definitively documented to increase the requirements for vitamins. The use of 5-fluorouracil, for example, has been shown to increase the need for niacin [29].

Patients with clinically evident deficiencies of specific vitamins should be repleted according to the guidelines in Table 32-11. The assays listed in Table 32-5 allow confirmation of deficiencies of individual vitamins. Empiric supplementation with the RDAs of each vitamin through the use of multisupplement tablets for patients with no symptoms of vitamin deficiency is recommended for cancer patients undergoing therapy because this is more cost-effective than using the various assays to document subclinical deficiency. All patients on TPN should receive vitamin supplementation. The doses to be added to the TPN are elaborated in Table 32-9. Fat-soluble vitamins bind to the plastics on intravenous administration equipment, and bioavailability of the administered vitamins may be significantly lower than that intended. Additionally, certain vitamins, such as vitamin A, are light sensitive and should be added to the TPN solution immediately before administration or kept in shielded bags. Even with these precautions, only 25% to 30% of the administered parenteral dose reaches the patient.

Growth Factors

Advances over the last century have uncovered the important roles that peptide growth factors and steroids play in growth and develop-

Table 32-11. Recommended Daily Allowances of Various Vitamins and Treatment Recommendations for Deficiences

Vitamin	Male RDA*	Female RDA	Treatment for Deficiency
Fat-Soluble Vitamins			
A	3300 U	2600 U	100,000 U/day x 3 d, then 50,000 U/day x 2 weeks
D	200 U	200 U	1000–10,000 U/d orally or 10,000 U IM
E	10 mg	8 mg	40–50 mg/d orally or IM
K	80 µg	65 µg	10–15 mg SQ or IV q day x 3 d
Water-Soluble Vitamins			
C	60 mg	60 mg	100–250 mg tid orally, IM, or IV
Thiamine	1.5 mg	1.1 mg	5–10 mg tid or 5–100 mg IM/IV
Riboflavin	1.7 mg	1.3 mg	5–30 mg/d orally or 50 mg IM
Niacin	19 mg	15 mg	10–50 mg tid orally or IM
B_6	2.0 mg	1.6 mg	10–20 mg q day x 3 weeks, then 3–5 mg q day orally, or 30–600 mg IV or IM
Folate	200 µg	180 µg	1–5 mg/d orally, IV
B_{12}	2.0 µg	2.0 µg	1 mg IM q day x 7 days, then weekly

Recommended daily allowance for age 25 to 50.

The information here is provided as guidance only. Prescribers should always consult the manufacturer's current prescribing information.

448

ment. It was not until recently, however, with widespread application of molecular biologic techniques, that large-scale production of many growth factors was possible. Peptide hormones, such as insulin, growth hormone, and insulin-like growth factor, are available in large quantities and, along with anabolic steroids, represent potential therapeutic modalities for cancer cachexia. Although many studies have been performed examining the potential roles of growth factors in the cancer patient, their role in the clinical treatment of this population is poorly defined.

Insulin

This pancreatic hormone has major anabolic and catabolic effects. It promotes amino acid and carbohydrate uptake by many tissues, increases use of glucose for glycogen synthesis and lipogenesis and protein synthesis, and decreases gluconeogenesis and lipolysis. In these ways, insulin is a major determinant of normal metabolism and growth. Clinicians have long attempted to harness the tissue-sparing effects of this polypeptide in the treatment of catabolic disease. The three major clinical studies in the injured population involved either burn or trauma patients. In these populations, infusions of high doses of insulin along with high glucose intravenous feedings produced laboratory measures of protein sparing, such as decreased urinary nitrogen excretion or decreased 3-methyl histidine excretion. These studies were difficult to interpret because the treatment populations had significantly higher caloric intakes than the control populations. In addition, two possible complications associated with high-dose insulin infusions have deterred clinical use. First, when high doses of insulin are employed, life-threatening hypoglycemia is a possible complication. In some studies, monitoring of serum glucose has been as frequent as every hour [30]. Second, high-dose insulin and glucose infusions may produce marked increases in lipogenesis. Such an increase in lipogenesis may manifest sufficient increases of carbon dioxide production to overcome pulmonary reserve and product respiratory compromise and failure. An increased lipogenesis also may lead to fatty liver formation and hepatic dysfunction. High-dose insulin alone is unlikely to be a clinically useful adjunct to nutritional supplementation.

Growth Hormone

Growth hormone is a 191–amino-acid polypeptide secreted by the anterior pituitary gland and is a prime stimulus for growth during puberty. In adults, this hormone also is released in an intermittent pulsatile pattern that may be important in normal homeostasis. The actions of this hormone are complex but can be summarized briefly as protein anabolic lipolytic and gluconeogenic. It appears that this hormone redirects the body to use lipids as fuel in preference to proteins and is thus an attractive agent in the treatment of the catabolic patient. Despite these clear theoretic advantages, proving clinical use of growth hormone in the injured patient has been difficult.

The majority of clinical nutritional studies performed before the availability of synthetic human growth hormone in the mid-1980s were performed in orthopedic or burn patients. Since then numerous preclinical studies and three clinical studies in cancer patients have been performed (Table 32-12). A most impressive clinical testimony to the potent influences of growth hormone on nitrogen accrual is the study of Jiang et al. [31] demonstrating that even in the setting of hypocaloric feedings, growth hormone can produce positive nitrogen balance in patients after surgery for intra-abdominal tumor. It must be pointed out that the study by Tayek and Brasel [32] demonstrated improved nitrogen balance as a response to growth hormone only in those patients who were relatively well nourished. Although these studies in cancer patients as well as a majority of studies in other clinical populations provided evidence for improved nitrogen retention with growth hormone administration, none has provided evidence that this is accompanied by improved clinical outcome. This situation likely is due to the small sample sizes in all studies performed to date and the short follow-up in these studies. A large randomized trial of this hormone in the cancer patient is imperative because the cost of this hormone is not inconsequential.

Combination therapy consisting of growth hormone and insulin has been studied as adjuncts to nutritional supplementation. Preliminary studies in cancer patients [33] have shown that daily injections of growth hormone for 3 days followed by a constant infusion of insulin acutely promotes skeletal muscle and whole body

Table 32-12. Major Studies of Growth Factor Support in Cancer Patients

Study	Agent	Patient Population, n	Findings
Growth Hormone			
Ward, *Ann Surg* 1986, 206:56	hGH	GI surgery patients, 16	Increased fat oxidation; decreased protein oxidation
Jiang, *Ann Surg* 1989, 210:513	hGH	GI surgery patients, 18	Increased protein synthesis
Douglas, *Br J Surg* 1990	hGH	TPN patients, 25	Reduced protein loss
Tayek, *J Clin Endocrinol Metab* 1995, 7:2082	hGH	TPN cancer patients, 10	Increased nitrogen balance in well-nourished patients
Growth Hormone and Insulin			
Wolf, *Ann Surg* 1992, 216:280	hGH + insulin	GI surgery patients, 28	Reduced protein loss
Berman, *Ann Surg* 1999, 229:1	hGH; hGH + insulin	GI malignancies (TPN), 30	Improved protein kinetics
Anabolic Steroids			
Abels, *J Clin Endocrinol Metab* 1944, 4:198	Testosterone	Gastric cancer, 5	Improved nitrogen balance
Johnston, *Br J Surg* 1963, 50:924	Methandienone	GI surgery, 25	Improved nitrogen balance
Young, *J Parenter Enteral Nutr* 1982, 7:221	Nandrolone decanoate	Preoperative patients, 24	Decreased plasma amino acids
Hansell, *J Parenter Enteral Nutr* 1989, 13:349	Stanozolol	Colorectal surgery, 60	Improved nitrogen balance
Darnton, *Dis Esoph* 1999, 12:283	Nandrolone decanoate postoperatively	Esophageal cancer, 40	Increased muscle mass

hGH — human growth hormone.

nitrogen retention at doses of insulin that are of a long magnitude less than the previously discussed clinical studies of insulin alone. More recently, Berman *et al.* [34] conducted an investigation on the impact of growth hormone, alone and in combination with insulin, on the nutritional status of patients with gastrointestinal cancer who have underwent surgery and are receiving TPN. Patients (n = 30) were prospectively randomly assigned into one of three nutritional support groups receiving either TPN, TPN plus GH, or PRN plus GH plus insulin. Their findings demonstrated a marked improvement in protein kinetics in the groups receiving GH or GH plus insulin over the group receiving TPN alone. The mechanisms of the hormone interaction and whether this or other combinations of growth factors will be clinically useful await future studies.

Insulin-Like Growth Factor 1

Insulin-like growth factor 1 (IGF-1), originally isolated and called somatomedin-C, is an intermediary hormone that mediates many of the actions of growth hormone. IGF-1 exerts many of the effects of insulin, including hypoglycemia and inhibition of lipolysis. In vitro, IGF-1 stimulates protein synthesis, and in vivo this hormone inhibits proteolysis. With synthesis of this molecule by recombinant techniques, potentially limitless quantities are now available, facilitating in vivo studies and making large-scale clinical trials possible. Studies of this hormone as nutritional adjunct in animals have been encouraging. Results of initial clinical studies should be available in the near future.

Anabolic Steroids

Androgenic steroids have long been known to have potent anabolic activities. Pharmacologic modifications of the natural androgens have been performed with the aim to reduce their androgenic actions, increase the ease of administration, and enhance their anabolic actions. Such efforts have resulted in production of a class of synthetic compounds referred to as anabolic steroids.

These compounds have been tested in the clinical setting for a long time. As early as 1944, Abels *et al.* found testosterone propionate to enhance nitrogen balance in three patients with gastric cancer. Since then, the clinical use of anabolic steroids has been examined in diverse clinical populations. The study of Hansell *et al.* [34] deserves particular mention because it is the only study of even moderate size. In this study, 60 colorectal surgery patients were randomized to receive or not receive stanozolol along with either hypocaloric or eucaloric supplementation. Improved nitrogen balance was noted only in the group with hypocaloric nutrition. In 1999, Darnton *et al.* [35] conducted a double-blind trial randomly assigning 40 patients to receiving low-dose (50 mg for 3 weeks) nandrolone decanoate or placebo over 3 months starting 1 month after surgery for esophageal cancer. At this dose, no clinical effect was noted. The studies on cancer patients are summarized in Table 32-10. Although a number of studies have shown an improvement in serum or urine parameters of nitrogen retention, no study to date has shown an improvement in any clinical outcome parameter. This may again be the result of inadequate sample sizes in the studies. Additionally the varied nutritional regimens and the steroid preparations used make this literature particularly difficult to decipher. One must conclude that the question of whether anabolic steroids have any role as an adjunct to clinical nutrition remains unanswered. Certainly, a large trial, possibly in a multicenter fashion, is necessary to evaluate use of these compounds by clinical outcome.

Another major obstacle to using anabolic steroids in the clinical setting is the significant side effects of these compounds. Virilization is a potential side effect, often manifest by hirsutism, acne, clitoral hypertrophy, voice coarsening, and male pattern baldness. Alternatively, peripheral conversion of testosterone and androstenedione to estradiol and estrone may result in "feminizing" effects, such as gynecomastia. Other potential detrimental effects include hypogonadism; lipoprotein abnormalities, including increased low-density lipoprotein; sleep apnea; and hepatic complications, including development of hepatocellular carcinoma.

Nutritional Support and Growth Factors

A major goal of aggressive nutritional support is growth of normal tissues. A commonly voiced concern in nutritional support of the cancer patient, however, is disproportional growth of the neoplastic tissues. Such concerns are fueled by animal studies documenting disproportionately enhanced tumor growth by nutritional support. No clinical study in patients corroborates these animal models. Using stable isotope methods, Mullen *et al.* [36] could not demonstrate an increased synthetic rate in tumor tissues compared to normal tissues.

A major theoretic obstacle to routine use of growth factors in the clinical setting is fear that growth factors may stimulate cancer growth. Animal and in vivo studies have linked growth hormone to development of certain lymphoid malignancies [37]. IGF-1 has been shown to be a stimulus for in vitro growth of breast tumors [38] and lung tumors [39]. Data also exist that show that growth hormone administration in rats actually decreased the number of tumor metastases in a transplantable adenocarcinoma model in rodents [40]. The relative influences of the mitogenic effects of growth factors compared with their beneficial influence on host cancer surveillance through improvements in immunocompetence remain to be determined. Further, if certain growth factors are capable of shifting tumors into the proliferative phase, such action may render tumors more sensitive to radiotherapy or chemotherapy. Therapeutic investigations using this treatment strategy are currently underway in myeloid leukemia, in which colony-stimulating factors are being administered as priming agents to stimulate acute myeloid leukemic blast cells to become more sensitive to cell cycle–specific chemotherapy. No human study has examined the effects of growth factors on cancer appearance or growth. These studies will not only be interesting but also will be necessary before accepting growth factor therapy as a routine clinical modality. Trials of growth factors as adjuncts to chemotherapy or radiotherapy will undoubtedly be an area of fruitful future investigation.

Pharmacologic Agents

In addition to the various growth factors and anabolic steroids many pharmacologic agents have been proposed as potential agents for enhancing weight gain during treatment for malignancy. Following are three that have undergone the most extensive trials.

Megestrol Acetate (Megace)

Megestrol acetate is a synthetic progestational agent used in the therapy of advanced breast cancer. In this population, the clinical observation was made that this agent improved appetite and weight gain. Although the relative importance of the central nervous system appetite-stimulating effects of this compound versus the metabolic effects of megestrol on peripheral tissue metabolism are still being debated, clinical trials of this compound as a nutritional adjunct in cancer patients have begun. In one study, 89 patients with various tumor types were studied in a randomized, placebo-controlled study [41]. The patients receiving megestrol had a significantly improved appetite and food intake. Although clinical use of this medication as a modality in the treatment of disease-related malnutrition is far from proven, megestrol holds promise in such a capacity and is under investigation for a variety of disease states [42]. In 1998, McMillan *et al.* [43] from the Royal Infirmary in Edinburgh conducted a study using ibuprofen in combination with megestrol acetate over a 6-week period to treat cachexia in advanced gastrointestinal cancer patients (*n* = 15). The hypothesis was that downregulating the acute-phase response using ibuprofen and perhaps stimulating the appetite using megestrol acetate may be effective in reversing or halting weight loss. The results of this study demonstrated that the combination of ibuprofen and megestrol acetate is effective in decreasing inflammatory response, increasing weight gain, and appetite stimulation. Also in 1998, Loprinzi *et al.* [44] from the Mayo Clinic conducted a three-armed phase III clinical trial comparing megestrol acetate, dexamethasone, and fluoxymesterone for the treatment of cancer anorexia/cachexia. A total of 475 patients were randomly assigned to receive one of the three treatment options with baseline assessment guidelines being similar for all. The results of this large series

demonstrate the superiority of megestrol acetate and dexamethasone over fluoxymesterone for increasing appetite, muscle mass, and nutritional baseline status. Megestrol acetate and dexamethasone elicited similar appetite-stimulating results with dexamethasone showing a higher toxicity component. Fluoxymesterone was shown to be an inferior choice due to its high toxicity level and minimal appetite-stimulating efficacy.

Cyproheptadine (Periactin)

Cyproheptadine (Periactin) is an antihistamine that has been tested in the cancer population because the compound enhances appetite in humans without cancer. Early trials had suggested that cyproheptadine may increase appetite in tumor-bearing humans, but more recent studies have failed to verify this. In a randomized, blinded, placebo trial involving 295 patients with advanced malignancy, there was no improvement in anorexia or weight gain [45]. There is no role for this medication in the clinical treatment of cancer cachexia.

Metoclopramide (Reglan)

Primary effects of tumor-bearing states as well as effects of treatment may produce alterations in intestinal motility. The most prominent treatment-related factors are postsurgical ileus and intestinal dysmotility associated with narcotic administration. Metoclopramide has been proposed as an agent to alleviate intestinal dysmotility in these and other cancer-related situations. Although metoclopramide improves gastric emptying following gastrointestinal surgery and in select cancer-bearing states, whether administration of this medication can have an impact on any clinically measurable nutritional parameter remains undetermined. Future prospective trials with defined nutritional end points are necessary to ascertain the use of this agent in clinical practice.

Dronabinol (Marinol)

Whether from disease or treatment, nausea and vomiting are a significant part of the clinical course of cancer patients. Nausea and vomit-

---

Table 32-13. Current Recommendations for Nutritional Support in Cancer Patients

Eliminate tumor

Maintain adequate oral intake as possible

Consider TPN or tube feedings for patients with > 10% weight loss

In patients with > 10% weight loss, consider 7–10 d of TPN before surgical therapy

Minimize narcotic use

Consider medications that attenuate nausea and gastrointestinal dysmotility as supplemental agents in nutritional therapy

---

TPN — total parenteral nutrition.

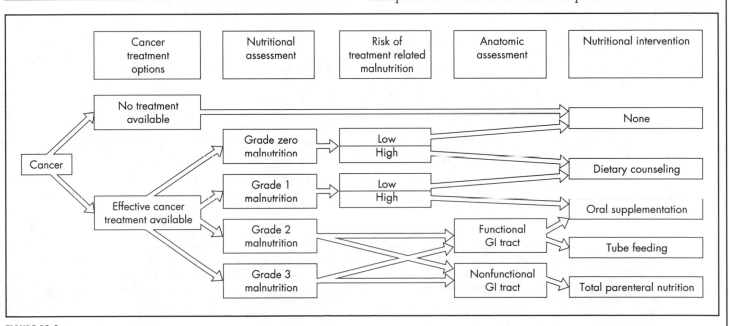

FIGURE 32-2.

The treatment of malnutrition in cancer patients.

ing can be a prime reason for reduced food intake. Strategies for improving nutritional status have been directed at mitigating nausea and vomiting. Dronabinol, the major active ingredient of the marijuana plant, is an effective agent in treating of otherwise refractory nausea and vomiting. This reduction in nausea is likely the mechanism of improved appetite that was noted in early studies using this medication. A small (n = 42) single-arm trial evaluating this medication with appetite and weight loss as clinical parameters has been performed. Administration of dronabinol improved appetite and reduced the rate of weight loss [46]. There is no doubt that marijuana and its derivatives stimulate appetite [47]. What is unknown is whether use of these will improve clinical outcome. Further controlled trials are needed to ascertain the efficacy of this medication in the nutritional treatment of cancer patients. Of interest, recent data suggest that cannabinoids may inhibit growth in transformed cells; this may have other benefits for cancer patients [48].

Other Agents

As the mechanisms of the anorexia and altered substrate cycles associated with cancer-bearing states are better understood, many other agents emerged as potential therapeutic modalities for cancer cachexia. For example, as the causative roles of cytokines such as tumor necrosis factor and interleukin-1 in mediating the anorexia and metabolic changes in cancer are elucidated, agents such as specific antibodies against these cytokines or pharmacologic agents such as pentoxyifylline that block the effects of these cytokines may emerge as useful modalities in clinical treatment of cachexia [49]. However, these must be regarded as experimental agents.

CONCLUSIONS

It is agreed that progressive nutritional depletion is often a major clinical feature of the cancer patient, at times dominating the clinical manifestations of the disease. Many strategies have been investigated in efforts to improve the nutritional status of the cancer patient. TPN can improve caloric intake and nitrogen balance of the patient, particularly those with dysfunctional gastrointestinal tracts. Pharmacologic agents may improve gastrointestinal dysmotility and attenuate nausea. Growth factors also may improve nitrogen and protein balance. Except in severely malnourished people none of these modalities alone have thus far been shown to improve clinical outcome.

A combination of the aforementioned strategies will likely prove most fruitful in the treatment of cancer patients; therefore, studies combining the various modalities are necessary. Areas of the greatest promise for future research include studies of the multitude of recombinant growth factors that are becoming available and studies of the gastrointestinal tract as the primary route of aggressive nutritional supplementation. In the meantime, a practical strategy can be recommended from available data (Table 32-13). Elimination of tumor is still of paramount importance, and effective responses to anticancer therapy are associated with more dramatic response to nutritional support. Patients with greater than 10% weight loss are likely to benefit from 7 to 10 days of aggressive intravenous nutritional support before major therapy (Fig. 32-2). Narcotic use should be minimized. Medications that attenuate nausea and gastrointestinal dysmotility should be considered as supplemental agents in the nutritional therapy of the cancer patient.

REFERENCES

1. van Eys J: Nutrition and cancer: physiologic interrelationships. *Ann Rev Nutr* 1985, 5:435–461.

2. Butterworth CE: Folate deficiency and cancer. In *Micronutrients in Health and Disease Prevention*. Edited by Bandich A, Butterworth CE. New York: Marcel Dekker, 1991:165–183.

3. Creagan ET, Moertel CG, O'Fallon JR, *et al.*: Failure of high dose vitamin C (ascorbic acid) therapy to benefit patients with advanced cancer. *N Engl J Med* 1979, 301:687–690.

4. Moertel CG, Fleming TR, Creagan ET, *et al.*: High dose vitamin C versus placebo in the treatment of patients with advanced cancer who have had no prior chemotherapy. *N Engl J Med* 1985, 312:137–141.

5. Lashner BA, Heidenreich PA, Su GL, *et al.*: Effect of folate supplementation on the incidence of dysplasia and cancer in chronic ulcerative colitis: a case control study. *Gastroenterology* 1989, 97:255–259.

6. Michels KB, Willet WC: Vitamins and cancer: a practical means of prevention. In *Important Advances in Oncology 1994*. Edited by DeVita VT, Hellman S, Rosenberg SA. Philadelphia: JB Lippincott, 1994:85–114.

7. Willet WC: Micronutrients and cancer risk. *Am J Clin Nutr* 1995, 59:1162S–1165S.

8. Dewys WD, Begg C, Lavin PT, *et al.*: Prognostic effect of weight loss prior to chemotherapy in cancer patients: Eastern Cooperative Study Group. *Am J Med* 1980, 69:491–497.

9. Baker JP, Detsky AS, Wesson DE, *et al.*: Nutritional assessment: a comparison of clinical judgment and objective measurements. *N Engl J Med* 1982, 306:969–972.

10. Hill GL: Malnutritional and surgical risk: guidelines for nutritional therapy. *Ann R Coll Surg Engl* 1987, 69:263–265.

11. Baker SJ, Kumar S, Swaminathan SP: Excretion of folic acid in bile. *Lancet* 1965, 1:685.

12. Detsky AS, Baker JP, O'Rourke K, Goel V: Perioperative parenteral nutrition: a meta-analysis. *Ann Intern Med* 1987, 107:195–203.

13. Muller JM, Brenner U, Dienst C, Pichlmaier H: Preoperative parenteral feeding in patients with gastrointestinal carcinoma. *Lancet* 1982, 1:68–71.

14. Perioperative total nutrition in surgical patients: the Veterans Affairs Total Parenteral Nutrition Cooperative Study Group. *N Engl J Med* 1991, 325:525–532.

15. Fan ST, Lo CM, *et al.*: Perioperative nutritional support in patients undergoing hepatectomy for hepatocellular carcinoma. *N Engl J Med* 1994, 331:1547–1552.

16. Jin D, Phillips M, Byles J: Effects of parenteral nutrition support and chemotherapy on phasic composition of tumor cells in gastrointestinal cancer. *J Parenter Enteral Nutr* 1999, 23:237–241.

17. Bozzetti F, Gavazzi C, Miceli R, *et al.*: Perioperative total parenteral nutrition in malnourished gastrointestinal cancer patients: a randomized, clinical trial. *J Parenter Enteral Nutr* 2000, 24:7–14.

18. Brennan MF, Pisters PWT, Posner M, *et al.*: A prospective randomized trial of total parenteral nutrition after major pancreatic resection for malignancy. *Ann Surg* 1994, 220:436–444.

19. Parenteral nutrition in patients receiving cancer chemotherapy: American College of Physicians. *Ann Intern Med* 1989, 110:734–736.

20. Heys SD, Park KG, Garlick PJ, Eremin O: Nutrition and malignant disease: implications for surgical practice. *Br J Surg* 1992, 79:614–623.

21. Chlebowski RT: Nutritional support of the medical oncology patient. *Hematol Oncol Clin North Am* 1991, 5:147–160.

22. Daly J, Lieberman M, Goldfine J, et al.: Enteral nutrition with supplemental arginine, RNA, and omega-3 fatty acids in patients after operation: immunologic, metabolic, and clinical outcome. *Surgery* 1992, 112:56–67.

23. Heslin M, Latkany L, Leung D, et al.: A prospective, randomized trial of early feeding after resection of upper gastrointestinal malignancy. *Ann Surg* 1997, 226:567–580.

24. Lacour J: Clinical trials using polyadenylic-polyuridylic acid as an adjuvant to surgery in treating different human tumors. *J Biol Resp Modif* 1985, 4:538–543.

25. Ziegler TR, Young LS, Benfell K, et al.: Clinical and metabolic efficacy of glutamine-supplemented parenteral nutrition after bone marrow transplantation: a randomized, double-blind, controlled study. *Ann Intern Med* 1992, 116:821–828.

26. Daly JM, Reynolds J, Thom A, et al.: Immune and metabolic effects of arginine in the surgical patient. *Ann Surg* 1988, 208:512–523.

27. Soukop M, Calman KC: Nutritional support in patients with malignant disease. *J Human Nutr* 1979, 33:179–188.

28. Inculet RI, Norton JA, Nichoald GE, et al.: Water-soluble vitamins in cancer patients on parenteral nutrition: a prospective study. *J Parenter Enteral Nutr* 1987, 11:243–249.

29. Aksoy M: Thiamin status of patients treated with drug combinations containing 5-fluorouracil. *Eur J Cancer* 1980, 16:1041–1055.

30. Hinton P, Allison SP, Littlejohn S, Lloyd J: Insulin and glucose to reduce catabolic response to injury in burned patients. *Lancet* 1971, 1:767–769.

31. Jiang ZM, He GZ, Zhang SY, et al.: Low-dose growth hormone and hypocaloric nutrition attenuate the protein-catabolic response after major operation. *Ann Surg* 1989, 210:513–524.

32. Tayek J, Brasel J: Failure of anabolism in malnourished cancer patients receiving growth hormone: a clinical research center study. *J Clin Endocrinol Metab* 1995, 80:2082–2087.

33. Wolf RF, Pearlstone DB, Newman E, et al.: Growth hormone and insulin reverse net whole body and skeletal protein catabolism in cancer patients. *Ann Surg* 1992, 216:280–290.

34. Berman R, Harrison L, Pearlstone D, et al.: Growth hormone, alone and in combination with insulin, increases whole body and skeletal muscle protein kinetics in cancer patients after surgery. *Ann Surg* 1999, 229:1–110.

35. Darnton SJ, Zgainski B, Grenier I, et al.: The use of anabolic steroid (nandrolone decanoate) to improve nutritional status after esophageal resection for carcinoma. *Dis Esoph* 1999, 12:283–288.

36. Mullen JL, Buzby GP, Gertner MH, et al.: Protein synthesis dynamics in human gastrointestinal malignancies. *Surgery* 1980, 87:331–338.

37. Rogers PC, Kemp D, Rogol A, et al.: Possible effects of growth hormone on development of acute lymphoblastic leukemia. *Lancet* 1977, 1:434–435.

38. Lippman ME, Dickson RB, Bates S, et al.: Autocrine and paracrine growth regulation of human breast cancer. *Breast Cancer Res Treat* 1986, 7:59–70.

39. Nakanishi Y, Mulshine JL, Kasprzyk PG, et al.: Insulin-like growth factor can mediate autocrine proliferation of human small cell lung cancer line in vitro. *J Clin Invest* 1988, 82:354–359.

40. Donoway RB, Torosian MH: Growth hormone inhibits tumor metastases. *Surg Forum* 1989, 40:413–415.

41. Tchekmedyian NS, Hickman M, Siau J, et al.: Megestrol acetate in cancer anorexia and weight loss. *Cancer* 1992, 69:1268–1274.

42. Tchekmedyian NS, Hickman M, Heber D: Treatment of anorexia and weight loss with megestrol acetate in patients with cancer or acquired immunodeficiency syndrome. *Semin Oncol* 1991, 18:35–42.

43. McMillan DC, Gorman PO, Fearon KCH, McArdle CS: A pilot study of megestrol acetate and ibuprofen in the treatment of cachexia in gastrointestinal cancer patients. *Br J Cancer* 1997, 76:788–790.

44. Loprinzi C, Kugler J, Sloan J, et al.: Randomized comparison of megestrol acetate versus dexamethasone versus fluoxymesterone for the treatment of cancer anorexia/cachexia. *J Clin Oncol* 1999, 17:3299–3306.

45. Kardinal CG, Loprinzi CL, Schaid DJ, et al.: A controlled trial of cyproheptadine in cancer patients with anorexia and/or cachexia. *Cancer* 1990, 65:2657–2662.

46. Plasse TF, Gorter RW, Krasnow SH, et al.: Recent clinical experience with dronabinol. *Pharmacol Biochem Behav* 1991, 40:695–700.

47. Voth E, Schwartz R: Medicinal applications of delta-9-tetrahydrocannabinol and marijuana. *Ann Intern Med* 1997, 126:791–798.

48. Roperh I, Sanchez C, Cortes M, et al.: Anti-tumoral action of cannabinoids: involvement of sustained ceramide accumulation and extracellular signal-related kinase activation. *Nature Med* 2000, 6:313–319.

49. Espat NJ, Moldawer LL, Copeland EM: Cytokine-mediated alterations in host metabolism prevent nutritional repletion in cachectic cancer patients. *J Surg Oncol* 1995, 58:77–82.

MALNUTRITION

Tissue wasting is a common and often devastating sequela of the cancer-bearing state. This loss in body mass can result in multi-organ derangements including impaired immune function, impaired locomotive capacity, and, ultimately, impaired respiratory function. As little as a 5% reduction in lean body mass has been associated with increased mortality in patients with cancer. Numerous factors contribute to produce wasting and malnutrition in patients with cancer. Recent advances in our understanding of these factors, as well as improvements in nutrient delivery methods and availability of immunostimulatory nutrients and growth factors offer exciting potential modalities for specific treatment of cancer-related wasting.

MANAGEMENT

1. Eradication of tumor
2. Increasing nutrient intake
   a. Enteral supplementation
   b. Intravenous supplementation
   c. Specific nutrient administration
      i. Nucleotides
      ii. Specific amino acids
      iii. Polyunsaturated free fatty acids
3. Growth factors
   a. Anabolic steroids
   b. Insulin
   c. Growth hormone
   d. Insulin-like growth factors
4. Pharmacologic agents
   a. Megestrol
   b. Cyproheptadine
   b. Metoclopramide
   c. Dronabinol

CAUSATIVE FACTORS

Poor intake: anorexia, gastrointestinal dysfunction (blockage, diarrhea, malabsorption); altered substrate cycles; stress of surgery, chemotherapy, or radiation therapy: peri-operative intestinal dysfunction, diarrhea, vomiting, anorexia, malabsorption

PATHOLOGIC PROCESS

Gastrointestinal obstruction from tumor, perioperative gastrointestinal tract dysfunction, oral or esophageal mucositis complicating chemotherapy or radiation therapy, anorexia, depression, nausea, vomiting, gastrointestinal fistula formation, diarrhea, malabsorption

PATIENT ASSESSMENT

Absolute indicators of malnutrition: weight loss >10%, weight loss of 0.5 kg/wk, clinically evident muscular weakness, serum albumin < 3.2 g/dL; **Relative indicators of malnutrition:** immune parameters—anergy in delayed hypersensitivity testing, T-cell numbers < 1500 /mL, decreased complement levels; hypoproteinemia—thyroxine-binding pre-albumin, transferrin, retinol-binding protein; creatinine-height ratio < 60% ideal; negative nitrogen balance; clinical—stomatitis, GI dysfunction

TOXICITY GRADING

	0	1	2	3
Degree of malnutrition	None	Mild	Moderate	Severe
Clinical findings	No weight loss	Weight loss < 5%	5–10% weight loss	> 10% weight loss, muscular weakness
Laboratory findings	Normal albumin, normal transferrin level, reactive delayed hypersensitivity skin test	Albumin < 3.5, decreased transferrin level, < 5 mm reactivity on skin test	Albumin < 3.2, nonreactive skin test	Albumin < 2.7

CHAPTER 33: CLINICAL TRIALS: MONITORING AND REPORTING OF TOXICITIES, AND EVALUATING TUMOR RESPONSE

Linda Barry Robertson

MONITORING AND REPORTING TOXICITIES

Data collection is an integral part of a clinical trial. The data collection process should be understood by those involved in collecting data. This understanding as well as recording of all study-related details will help to prevent the compromise of study validity.

A variety of methods are used to collect data for trials. Pharmaceutically supported and cooperative group trials generally have very specific data collection requirements with preprinted or on-line computerized forms. Individuals responsible for data collection have an opportunity to attend workshops that are offered periodically throughout the year or as new clinical trials are opened for accrual. These trials are also closely monitored by clinical site monitors, the sponsors, or the cooperative group so data queries and corrections or suggestions are made on a frequent basis. It is, however, the specific institution or facility's responsibility to maintain data prospectively. Because data collection was reviewed in the previous edition of this book [1], this section addresses the monitoring and reporting of expected and unexpected toxicities or adverse events of clinical trials.

An adverse event in the context of a clinical trial is any unwanted physical, psychologic, or behavioral change experienced by the individual enrolled in the trial. The adverse events are generally symptoms, physical findings, syndromes or diseases, abnormal laboratory values, or drug overdose. The evaluation of adverse events falls under three categories: medical, regulatory, and clinical evaluations. Patient care and safety is always the most important concern. Therefore, it is crucial that the study team be aware of the rules for reducing or withdrawing study treatment either temporarily or permanently if an adverse event occurs. It is also important that the trial guidelines for the use of concomitant medications be adhered to strictly if an adverse events occurs. Some adverse events will require special reports (discussed later in this chapter).

Baseline Evaluation

The patient should have an in-depth review of body systems as well as any current symptoms prior to beginning the actual study treatment. Each of the physical symptoms should be graded and documented on a form that permits grading because this information will be valuable while the patient is treated with the particular study drug(s). A form to document baseline findings is often provided by the sponsor or cooperative group; if not, then the institution should develop an internal form. Some trials provide an area on the Past Medical History Case Report Form to document baseline physical finding and symptoms. It is essential that the institutional database also have the mechanism to record the adverse event data at baseline and throughout the clinical trial.

Once the patient begins study treatment, any new finding should be recorded. These findings are often referred to as "side-effects" or "adverse events;" however, the direct cause-and-effect relationship to the finding and the study treatment might be unknown. It is anticipated that a clinical trial may cause a certain number of adverse events—some known, others unknown. It does not matter if these findings *may not* be study related; they should be recorded. Symptoms that existed at baseline and increase in intensity must also be recorded and graded appropriately, although this is often not an easy task. It is easier to document new findings because there is

generally not any uncertainty as to whether they existed prior to the initiation of the study treatment.

An example of an adverse event that is often not recorded as frequently as it should be are abnormal laboratory findings. This is a controversial issue for some sponsored trials because sponsors may have their own guidelines regarding when an abnormal laboratory value should be documented. In April 1998 the National Cancer Institute (NCI) defined an adverse event as any abnormal laboratory finding. This is the recommended guideline for institutionally sponsored and cooperative group trials unless otherwise indicated.

The coordinator or data manager should evaluate the patient during each visit to review the status of ongoing toxicities, including resolution and the possible development of any new toxicities. This is necessary because it is always better to collect these data when it is easily accessible then to attempt to retrieve it months or years later throughout the course of the trial. The patient or significant others play an integral role in the evaluation of toxicities because symptoms may occur between visits and resolve by the time of the actual visit. It is crucial that patients/significant others be educated regarding the importance of reporting information throughout the course of the study. It is recommended that they keep a journal or diary of such events and bring it with them at the time of their visit. Some studies actually provide study-specific diaries for the patient. If a diary or journal is not provided, the institution should have a generic diary that fits the needs of most studies available for the patient. Diaries should be reviewed with the patient by the coordinator or data manager at each visit so that the recorded information is clearly understood and can be accurately transcribed onto the case report forms (CRFs).

Grading Adverse Events

The national standard for grading adverse events is the NCI Common Toxicity Scale version 2.0. This scale is available on the Internet [2]. A variety of other toxicity scales have been used over the years for documenting toxicities; however, it is recommended that the NCI Common Toxicity Scale be used unless a trial otherwise indicates. The increasing acceptance of this scale as the standard has decreased the confusion for individuals involved in the conduct of clinical trials.

Adverse events should be graded objectively. If there is an adverse event documented that is not noted in the NCI Common Toxicity Scale, then it is recommended that this event be graded using mild (1), moderate (2), severe (3), life-threatening (4), and death (5). It is important that the documentation in the patient record/chart clearly define the adverse event so that the individual abstracting the data can easily grade it. The best scenario occurs when the physician, coordinator and patient review the adverse events and the documentation in the chart accurately reflects the actual severity of the event. It is important to avoid situations that can cause confusion. For example, the coordinator grades the toxicity objectively, but a note in the chart indicates that the event was graded either more or less severely then what was originally discussed. The patient chart serves as source documentation; thus it is important that information in both the CRFs and the patient's chart agree.

Grade 3 and 4 adverse events must be reported promptly to the investigator, because these events (depending on the phase of the trial) often require intervention. Grade 3 and 4 adverse events are classified as serious adverse events. Pharmaceutical and cooperative group trials provide detailed guidelines to be followed in the course of such events and the study team should strictly adhere to these guidelines. It is recommended that an individual be designated at the time of study implementation that will be responsible for reporting serious adverse events in the designated timely manner. Historically, this is generally the study coordinator or data manager. The entire study team as well as individuals involved in the care of the patient on study, the patient and significant others need to be well aware of the need to report such events immediately and to whom. If there is a breakdown in communication regarding the reporting of a serious adverse event, most often it is due to lack of understanding by one or all individuals involved in the study.

Serious Adverse Events

An adverse event is defined as serious (including abnormal laboratory values) throughout the course of a clinical trial if the study treatment is thought to have contributed to the following: a life-threatening event or death, permanent disability, inpatient hospitalization or prolonged hospitalization, a congenital anomaly, or an intervention was needed to prevent permanent impairment or damage.

Reporting Guidelines

Phase I Trials

The Food and Drug Administration (FDA) requires that *life-threatening reactions* that may be related to study drug(s), and all *fatal* reactions (during or within 30 days of study treatment) for phase I trials be reported immediately by telephone to the Investigational Drug Branch (IDB) of the NCI. Clinical trials that are sponsored generally mandate that the investigator or investigator's designee notify the sponsor. The sponsor will then assume responsibility for notifying the IDB. A written report must follow within 10 days of the initial telephone call. An *unexpected event* of any grade should be reported within 24 hours by telephone. If a clinical trial is nonsponsored or investigator initiated, then the investigator must adhere to the FDA guidelines.

Phase II and III Unknown Reactions

Grade 2 and 3 reactions that are classified as previously *unknown* for phase II and III studies are to be reported in writing within 10 working days to the IDB. Grade 4 and 5 unknown reactions must be reported to the IDB by phone within 24 hours and followed by a written report within 10 working days.

Phase II and III Known Reactions

Phase II and III studies are not required to have grade 2 and 3 *known* reactions reported but submitted as part of the study results. *Known* grade 4 and 5 reactions should be submitted in a written report within 10 working days to the IDB.

The cooperative group trials address the reporting of adverse events in detail in the clinical study. Generally these events are reported to the operations office. The Food and Drug Administration (FDA) guidelines (21 CRF 312.32 "IND Safety Reports") requires sponsors to submit an expedited report for both serious and unexpected toxicities associated with the study treatment. The timeliness of this reporting is very important because it may affect the care of future patients on study. Investigators who fail to report adverse events appropriately may have their studies terminated

by the FDA or lose investigator privileges. It is crucial that individuals involved in the care of the study patient, including the family, be made aware of the need for these events to be reported immediately to a designated member of the study team.

The forms required for submission for reportable adverse events may vary depending on the study. Copies of Med Watch forms can be obtained at the NCI website [2]. Information typically required for an adverse event is the date and time of onset, date and time of resolution if appropriate, the seriousness of the event, severity or grading of the event (grade 1 to 4), event outcome, relationship of the event to the study treatment, and any treatment the patient received as the result of the event. It is important that the information surrounding the event be reported but succinctly. Any supporting documentation (*eg*, diagnostic reports, laboratory values, notes from the patient record) should be copied and attached to the report when they are available. In the case that the event causes hospitalization, it is suggested that the patient's hospital record be copied every few days so that there are no prolonged delays in obtaining the information for the appropriate regulatory bodies. Once the appropriate adverse event form has been completed, the principal investigator is required to review the information and sign the report. A copy of the serious adverse event report should be placed in the patient's research chart, a copy sent to the local IRB and a copy maintained for filing the final report. It is always better to submit a report if the association of the event with the study treatment is unclear then to delay or not report the event. Studies that are sponsored by the pharmaceutical industry or cooperative groups often have resources available to answer questions when there is some uncertainty regarding reporting. Institutionally sponsored trials must adhere to the same FDA regulations for reporting serious and unexpected adverse events. The local Institutional Review Board (IRB) should be sent a copy of the adverse events report as well as periodic and final reports of all adverse events. The local IRB may require additional information and procedures if a serious adverse event should occur.

If the event is serious enough to warrant a 24-hour or 10-day report to the FDA, then it may be necessary for either the sponsor (in the case of sponsored studies) or investigator to revise the informed consent to accurately reflect all known risks. In some cases, the study may be terminated. This termination may be done by the sponsor, or the local IRB may recommend study suspension even in the case of sponsored trials if they view the risk as extreme.

The annual report that is submitted to the FDA on IND trials must be submitted within 60 days of the anniversary date of the IND. This report should include a narrative summary or tabulation of the most frequent and most serious adverse events, a summary of all IND safety reports submitted during the year, deaths and cause, and a list of patients who have withdrawn from the study due to adverse events.

Because many trials are conducted throughout a community network of research sites today, all sites participating in a clinical trial must adhere to the standard research practices. It should be the responsibility of the main institution to educate and to provide documented research guidelines to be adhered to by all that participate in clinical trials. These guidelines must also address the monitoring and reporting of adverse events.

Monitoring of adverse events can become an insurmountable task as the number of participants and clinical trials increase. It is important that a system be developed either on paper or be computerized to monitor the incidence of adverse events on participants and to track the follow-up activities. This information can be reviewed on a weekly or at least a monthly basis to determine what reporting and/or adverse event follow-up requirements are outstanding. It also provides information regarding ongoing missing data points. This system is vital for institutions with an active outreach program that participate in clinical trials.

A monthly report can provide whatever information is important to the specific institution. A suggestion is to develop the report so that individualized reports can be distributed to each clinical research coordinator/data manager and/or outreach site. This provides the individual with information that is specific for their studies. The report should provide information such as the study number, patient identification, and the specific type of data related to the adverse event that remains outstanding. Once the data have been collected, the report will be updated manually or entered into the computerized database by the main institution. This provides an excellent mechanism for keeping track of the adverse event data status for all clinical trials on a daily basis. It also facilitates data retrieval from outreach sites because it will provide information per investigator and participant at each specific facility. This information will provide a mechanism for determining the outreach sites where data need to be collected. When the institution sends a data manager to the outreach institution, data can be collected for all active studies by the same individual. This provides for an efficient system because data collection in outreach institutions is very labor intensive and a costly endeavor.

Adverse events should be reviewed on a routinely scheduled basis by the investigator, clinical research coordinator, and other research team members. This facilitates quality research as well as quality care of the participants. The review will provide the study team with possible positive or negative study trends, such as potential problems with unknown or serious adverse events. It should include adverse events from network sites participating in the clinical trial through the main institution. This also provides the opportunity to evaluate findings that should have been reported as adverse events. This review can be structured to meet an institution's data safety monitoring requirements.

EVALUATING TUMOR RESPONSE

Tumor response associated with clinical trials is generally assessed at prescribed intervals to assess response to study treatment. Restaging consists of repeating the same radiographic studies that were done at baseline and comparing the new results with the earlier results. Evaluating a patient's response can be complicated by other clinical factors; for example, a patient may experience resolution of clinical symptomology while the tumor has progressed. However, this section addresses the new evaluation criteria for solid tumors as it pertains to obtaining tumor measurements for clinical trials.

In 1979 the World Health Organization (WHO) published the criteria most commonly used by investigators nationally to assess tumor response. These criteria were not without problems, which led to modifications or clarifications to the WHO criteria over the years-the results being response criteria that were no longer universal. The WHO criteria were recently revised by representatives of several large research groups [3]. This new approach of evaluating tumor response simplifies the response evaluation process through the use of unidimensional tumor measurements and the sum of the longest diameters. Tumor responses previously were assessed using bidimensional tumor measurements and the sum of the products.

The new evaluation process is known as RECIST (response evaluation criteria in solid tumors). These guidelines were primarily developed for phase II trials whose prospective endpoint is tumor response.

Baseline Tumor Measurements

Measurable tumors at baseline are now defined as lesions that can be accurately measured in at least one dimension. The longest diameter should be recorded as > 20 mm with conventional techniques (ie, conventional CT, magnetic resonance imaging, chest radiography) or as > 10 mm with spinal CT scan. Nonmeasurable lesions are those lesions with the longest diameter (< 20 mm with conventional techniques or < 10 mm with spinal CT scan).

Measurable lesions are considered to be up to a maximum of five lesions per organ and no more then 10 total lesions. The measurable lesions, also known as target lesions, are to be measured and recorded at baseline. Measurable lesions should be evaluated by the same technique throughout the study and during follow-up.

It is recommend that all measurements be done with a ruler or calipers and recorded in metric notations. Baseline measurements should be done as close to the initiation of treatment as possible; generally this is specified with the study.

Response Criteria

The criteria for determining objective tumor response for target lesions has been adapted from the original WHO criteria: only the longest diameter for all target lesions is measured.

Complete response (CR) is indicated by the disappearance of all target lesions. Partial response (PR) is shown as a minimum of a 30% decrease in the sum of the longest diameter of target lesions; the baseline sum of target lesions is used as a reference. Progressive disease (PD) is indicated by a minimum of a 20% increase in the sum of the longest diameter of target lesions; the reference is the smallest sum longest diameter recorded since the initiation of treatment or the appearance of one or more new lesions. Stable disease (SD) is the smallest sum of the longest diameter is the reference; the criteria for PR or PD are not met. The best overall response is defined as that recorded from start of treatment until disease progression or recurrence. The reference used is the smallest measurement since the treatment started.

Tumor re-evaluation should be specified by the study. In phase II studies, follow-up is generally every 6 to 8 weeks. The duration of overall response is measured from the time that a CR or PR has been documented until the first date of recurrent or progressive disease.

Stable disease is measured from the start of treatment until progressive disease occurs.

CONCLUSIONS

The management and reporting of adverse events is essential for quality research and evaluation of tumor response. This can be best accomplished with the education of staff, a mechanism for determining specific data requirements per study, and an organized mechanism for monitoring data. Centralization of clinical trial coordination and data management, when possible, can facilitate these processes and ensure institutional consistency.

REFERENCES

1. Robertson LB: Clinical trial data collection. In *Current Cancer Therapeutics*, edn 3. Philadelphia: Current Medicine; 1998:437–438.

2. National Cancer Institute website: Investigator's Handbook: Appendix XII. Guidelines for reporting adverse drug reaction. Available at: http://www.ctep.info.nih.gov/handbook/HandBook Text/Appendix__XII.htm. Updated November 14, 2000.

3. James K, Eisenhower E, Christian M, *et al.*: Measuring response in solid tumors: unidimensional versus bidimensional measurement. *J Natl Cancer Inst* 1999, 91:523–528.

CHAPTER 34: SYNOPTIC PATHOLOGY REPORTS FOR STANDARDIZED REPORTING OF COMMONLY BIOPSIED OR SURGICALLY RESECTED NEOPLASMS

Michael J. Becich

The explosion of information and technology in medicine is changing the role of pathology and pathologists in patient care. Clinical pathology has kept pace with the rapidly changing medical environment, offering reliable, standardized, and timely results in simplified formats, using the available instrumentation and computer technology to maximum advantage, aided by an excellent Quality Assurance Program developed by the American Society of Clinical Pathologists (ASCP) and the College of American Pathologists (CAP). Anatomic pathology has become the focus of attention, as there is an urgent need to simplify and standardize all the pertinent information in a timely manner for the following reasons:

1. Many morphologic parameters such as type, grade, and extent of tumor, involvement of margins and lymphatic/vascular invasion have been investigated by cooperative clinical trials involving large number of patients, confirming them to be of clinical significance in predicting outcome.

2. A host of biologic tumor markers are available for fluid and tissue specimen testing. Attempts to characterize their predictive value should be correlated with morphologic parameters. In addition, markers of established clinical significance will need to become a part of routine histopathologic evaluation.

3. Diagnostic techniques, such as cytogenetics, flow cytometry, and polymerase chain reaction are being used more frequently as aids to tissue diagnosis. This information must be incorporated in the surgical pathology report.

4. Surgeons have a difficult time interpreting surgical pathology reports. In a recent study by Powsner *et al.* [1], the authors showed that surgeons misunderstood pathology reports 30% of the time. The authors attributed this to a communication gap and lack of familiarity with reporting formats. Standardized reports clearly could contribute to reducing the misunderstandings that clinicians have concerning pathology reports and, it is hoped, reduce medical errors.

5. It is important to understand that all information, even that which at present is seemingly of limited significance, may be important in the future and should be recorded. This would facilitate meaningful clinical research in future, dealing with large patient populations.

6. All data should be available in a format easily adaptable to various current computer information systems. This is a particularly important aspect, as we have supported the goal of having a national pathology cancer database that every potential researcher can tap into. In fact, the National Cancer Institute (NCI) has now funded our institution along with Harvard, the University of California at Los Angeles, and Indianapolis to develop a "Shared Pathology Informatics Network" (SPIN) [2] with this goal at the core of the program. If successful, SPIN will allow researchers interested in anatomic pathology specimens to use a browser to anonymously search for case material from the participating institutions. This is now a reasonable (and laudable) goal with the widespread use and availability of the Internet.

With these goals in mind, the pathologists from the University of Pittsburgh have developed synoptic templates to standardize the surgical pathology reporting. These reports present all the prognostically significant parameters in an easily interpretable manner, record information potentially useful for research, and introduce a format easily adaptable to various anatomic pathology computer information systems.

BACKGROUND

The idea of presenting surgical pathology reports in a synoptic form was initially described by Hutter and Rickert [3] in 1983. During the past decade, more interest been has shown by pathologists in this form of reporting, mainly because of the availability of computer information systems [4,5], recommendations [6], and implementation of a Q-Probe Quality Improvement Program [7,8] and development of protocols and checklists [9–17] by various individuals and committees under the aegis of the CAP; emphasis on improved quality control and quality assurance in patient care [18,19]; desire to present information in a consistent and unambiguous manner for proper staging, therapy selection and selection of patients for treatment protocols or other studies [20]; and the need to provide a cost-effective method of dispensing information to guide therapy and predict prognosis in an increasingly cost-conscious environment [21–25].

METHODS

Through review of literature for evaluation of morphologic features that have proven to be of predictive value for prognosis and effecting therapy, an initial draft template of the various organ systems listed was developed containing pertinent information [23]. Those gross parameters necessary for predicting outcome were included. This draft was circulated among the pathologists in the department, and a consensus draft was created based on their suggestions. This draft was then circulated to the surgeons, oncologists, and interns specializing in the particular system, and their input was solicited. These suggestions were discussed, and modifications were made to the draft. Next, specialists engaged in research in the particular organ/organ system were asked for their input as to the nature of special studies currently being performed in the department and the type of tissue required by them. These were incorporated in the special studies section of the template. Finally, the TNM staging [24] was added to the back side of the template. Any other staging system widely used in clinical practice, *eg*, Dukes' and Astler-Coller for colon cancers, was also added.

OBSERVATIONS

There has been a positive impact on the overall quality of surgical pathology reporting since the implementation of these synoptic templates. Fewer phone calls are made by clinicians questioning reports and requesting clarifications or additions. Introduction of the templates in the specimen-processing room has significantly decreased incorrectly or inadequately sectioned specimens and has also lessened the confusion arising in collection of tissue for special testing. A similar positive effect is seen at microscopic signout, where fewer parameters are missed during dictation, resulting in fewer returns of corrected reports to transcription. Fewer parameters being missed during dictation has resulted in a shorter turnaround time with complete and satisfactory reporting in a more efficient, productive, and cost-effective manner. The inclusion of a special testing section in the template has streamlined the availability of tissue for diagnostic and research purposes in a consistent manner, again resulting in more comprehensive reporting and satisfied researchers. The templates have proved to be invaluable in training residents, both in the gross room and at microscopic signout session.

A more comprehensive database has been developed since the introduction of these templates. Fewer cases have to be discarded from research work due to incomplete data. The final reporting is in free text, giving the signout pathologist freedom to vary reports as the needs of each case demand. The templates are being used by several regional and national community hospitals. This is a welcome step toward uniformity in reporting, opening the possibility of an effective regional and, ultimately, national pathology cancer database.

FUTURE POSSIBILITIES

Currently, there are many morphologic features that are proven prognostic and often independent predictors for different organs [5,21], making them cost-effective. This information is needed by the clinician to choose therapeutic protocols and to adhere to strict quality assurance regulations. Simultaneously, a host of new tests such as tumor markers, flow and image cytometry, immunohistochemistry, cytogenetics, and molecular biology have become available. These must be evaluated against proven morphologic features to be clinically significant [14]. This means that the pathologist has to include constantly increasing amounts of information in a clear, concise, and consistent manner in the surgical pathology report. The report should conform to quality assurance requirements and be generated with a quick turnaround time to reduce patient care costs and be an effective and comprehensive data source for clinical research. These objectives can be achieved successfully and easily without incurring any additional cost by adapting a synoptic template format.

Large-scale, multicentric cooperative clinical trials are needed to evaluate proposed new parameters for predicting clinical outcomes of disease. At present, different institutions are individually engaged in clinical research, often evaluating the same parameters, creating a measure of redundancy in research and an expenditure that can be better used. A standardized form of surgical pathology reporting available in a template format on a computer network through the Internet will minimize cost and duplication of effort. It will also lead to a better, time-saving, concerted effort in multicentric clinical trials. The template format as presented here can be easily adapted to any anatomic pathology computer information system, including voice-recognition systems.

Obviously, the templates will have to be modified and updated as newer information is forthcoming. A few centers are actively working in this area of anatomic pathology, including the CAP and ASCP. In addition, various academic institutions of excellence have their own inhouse developed synoptic templates. We suggest that a joint effort of different agencies and hospitals currently involved in developing the synoptic template format for standardized surgical pathology reporting form a consensus on a single format. This will reduce the time and effort spent, eliminate confusion and provide a single, standardized protocol for reporting. This will provide the community of pathologists with an invaluable service. If implemented, the format will prove to be an excellent quality assurance tool.

CONCLUSIONS

Surgical pathology reporting, using synoptic templates, is a comprehensive, efficient and cost-effective method resulting in improved patient care. They act as checklists for inclusion of important demographic, prognostic, therapeutic, and research parameters, decreasing professional and clerical errors and reducing turnaround time. They thereby result in improved customer (clinician) and supplier (pathologist) satisfaction. We have also found that synoptics are an effective method to guarantee quality assurance, as well as being an excellent tool in resident training. In addition, their use streamlines tissue processing for special studies. This adds to the comprehensiveness of the report and stimulates tissue acquisition for research and ancillary testing. Uniformity in reporting leads to a more detailed database with similar parameters included for a particular organ, making it easier to conduct large-scale clinical research in a timely manner. We have found that it is important to also allow for final reporting in a free text form, providing the pathologist the freedom to personalize the report. The templates can be easily adapted to a variety of anatomic pathology computer systems, including those utilizing voice recognition systems.

Much has to be accomplished in this field. Our effort was directed toward making templates for resections and biopsies of malignant neoplasms of the various organ systems. Now that this is complete we will focus our attention on automated methods for extracting this data for data warehouses and data mining purposes. Nevertheless, this is an initial small step toward the long journey that lies ahead.

REFERENCES

1. Powsner SM; Costa J; Homer RJ: Clinicians are from mars and pathologists are from venus: clinician interpretation of pathology reports. *Arch Pathol Lab Med* 2000, 124:1040–1046.

2. National Cancer Institute: Shared Pathology Informatics Network: Accessible at http://grants.nih.gov/grants/guide/rfa-files/RFA-CA-01-006.html. Accessed March 27, 2000.

3. Hutter RVP, Rickert RR: Organization and management of the surgical pathology laboratory. In *Principles and Practice of Surgical Pathology*, vol 1. Edited by Silverberg SG. New York: Wiley; 1983:17–18.

4. Markel SF, Hirsch SD: Synoptic surgical pathology reporting. *Hum Pathol* 1991, 22:807–810.

5. Rosai J and members of the Department of Pathology, Memorial Sloan Kettering Cancer Center: Standardized reporting of surgical pathology diagnoses for the major tumor types. *Am J Clin Pathol* 1993, 100:240–255.

6. Association of Directors of Anatomic and Surgical Pathology: Standardization of the surgical pathology report. *Am J Surg Pathol* 1992, 16:84–86.

7. Zarbo RJ: Interinstitutional assessment of colorectal carcinoma surgical pathology report adequacy: a College of American Pathologists Q-probes study of practice patterns from 532 laboratories and 15,940 reports. *Arch Pathol Lab Med* 1992, 116:1113–1119.

8. Zarbo RJ: The oncologic pathology report: quality by design. *Arch Pathol Lab Med* 2000, 124:1004–1010.

9. Henson DE, Hutter RVP, Sobin LH, Bowman HE: Protocol for the examination of specimens removed from patients with colorectal carcinoma: a basis for checklists. *Arch Pathol Lab Med* 1994, 118:122–125.

10. Fizgibbons PL, Connolly JL, Page DL : Updated protocol for the examination of specimens from patients with carcinomas of the breast: a basis for checklists. *Arch Pathol Lab Med* 2000, 124:1026–1033.

11. Compton CC : Updated protocol for the examination of specimens from patients with carcinomas of the colon and rectum, excluding carcinoid tumors, lymphomas, sarcomas, and tumors of the vermiform appendix: a basis for checklists. *Arch Pathol Lab Med* 2000, 124:1016–1025.

12. Fitzgibbons PL, Page DL, Weaver D, *et al.*: Prognostic factor in breast cancer: College of American Pathologists consensus statement 1999. *Arch Pathol Lab Med* 2000, 124:966–978.

13. Compton CC, Fielding LP, Burgart LJ, *et al.*: Prognostic factor in colorectal cancer: College of American Pathologists consensus statement 1999. *Arch Pathol Lab Med* 2000, 124:979–994.

14. Snigley JR, Amin MB, Bostwick DG, *et al.*: Update protocol for the examination of specimens from patients with carcinomas of the prostate gland: a basis for checklists. *Arch Pathol Lab Med* 2000, 124:1034–1039.

15. Bostwick DG, Grignon DJ, Hammond MEH, *et al.*: Prognostic factors in prostate cancer: College of American Pathologists consensus statement 1999. *Arch Pathol Lab Med* 2000, 124:995–1000.

16. Compton CC : Updated protocol for the examination of specimens from patients with carcinomas of the colon and rectum, excluding carcinoid tumors, lymphomas, sarcomas, and tumors of the vermiform appendix: a basis for checklists. *Arch Pathol Lab Med* 2000, 124:1016–1025.

17. Henson DE, Hutter RVP, Sobin LH, Bowman HE: Protocol for the examination of specimens removed from patients with colorectal carcinoma. *Arch Pathol Lab Med* 1994, 118:122–125.

18. Hutter RVP: Quality assurance in cancer care: pathology. *Cancer* 1989, 64:244–248.

19. Nash DB: Practice guidelines and outcomes: where are we headed? *Arch Pathol Lab Med* 1990, 114:1122–1125.

20. Ruby SG, Henson DE: Practice protocols for surgical pathology: a communication from the cancer committee of the College of American Pathologists. *Arch Pathol Lab Med* 1994, 118:120–121.

21. Kempson RL: The time is now: checklists for surgical pathology reports. [editorial]. *Arch Pathol Lab Med* 1992, 116:1107–1108.

22. Kempson RL: Checklists for surgical pathology reports: an important step forward [editorial]. *Am J Clin Pathol* 1993, 100:196–197.

23. Leslie KO, Rosai J: Standardization of the Surgical Pathology Report: Formats, Templates and Synoptic Forms. *Sem Diagnostic Pathol* 1994, 11:253–257.

24. Robboy SJ, Bentley RC, Krigman H, *et al.*: Synoptic reports in gynecologic pathology. *Int J Gynecol Pathol* 1994, 13:161–174.

25. Bale PM: A Comprehensive Microcomputer Network Program for Histopathology. *Pathology* 1991, 23:263–267.

26. Hammond MEH, Fitzbbons PL, Compton CC, *et al.*: College of American Pathologists conference XXXV: solid tumor prognostic factors: which, how and so what? Summary document and recommendations for implementation. *Arch Pathol Lab Med* 2000, 124: 958–965.

27. Taylor CR: The total test approach to standardization of immunohistochemistry. 2000, 124:945–951.

28. Rosai J: *Ackerman's Surgical Pathology*, edn 8. St. Louis: Mosby-Year Book, Inc.; 1996:1319–2732.

29. American Joint Committee on Cancer: *AJCC Cancer Staging Manual*, edn 5. Philadelphia: Lippincott-Raven;1997.

Primary Urinary Bladder/Urethra Tumors

A. Location of primary tumor: ____
1. Dome
2. Anterior wall
3. Posterior wall
4. Right wall
5. Left wall
6. Trigone
7. Ureter
8. Urethra
9. Multicentric
10. No residual tumor

B. Procedure: ____
1. Partial cystectomy
2. Total cystectomy
3. Cystoprostatectomy
4. Other

C. Size (if multicentric, size of the most deeply invasive or largest tumor): ____

D. Noninvasive neoplastic lesions: _____
1. Papilloma
2. Inverted papilloma
3. Papillary TCCa
4. Flat CIS
5. Other

E. Invasive neoplasia: ____
1. Transitional cell carcinoma
2. Squamous carcinoma
3. Adenocarcinoma
4. Sarcomatoid carcinoma
5. Small cell/neuroendocrine carcinoma
6. Mixed urothelial carcinoma
7. Lymphoma/leukemia
8. Sarcoma
9. Metastasis/direct extension from a contiguous primary
10. Other

F. Grade: ____ (Ash for TCCa grades 1–4) / n (WHO for TCCa grades 1–3): = n / n

G. Non-neoplastic and other conditions: ____
1. Von Brunn's nests, cystitis cystica/glandularis, intestinal metaplasia
2. Nephrogenic metaplasia/ adenoma
3. Granulomatous cystitis
4. Interstitial cystitis
5. Inflammatory pseudotumors
6. Carbuncle
7. Malakoplakia
8. Other

H. Margins of resection (positive/negative): ____

I. Angiolymphatic invasion (yes [1]; no [2]): ____

J. Perineural invasion (yes [1]; no [2]): ____

K. Mitotic activity: n per 10 HPF

L. Lymph node metastasis: n positive/total n lymph nodes = n / n

M. Prostate/seminal vesicles (if cystoprostatectomy)
1. Involved by bladder neoplasm (yes [1]; no [2]): ____
2. Concurrent primary invasive prostatic neoplasm (yes [1]; no [2]): ____
3. High grade PIN (yes [1]; no [2]): ____

N. TNM pathologic stage: T ____ N ____ M ____

O. TNM histopathologic grade: G____

HPF — high-powered fields.

SYNOPTIC PATHOLOGY REPORTS

Carcinoma In Situ of Breast

A. Laterality (right [1]; left [2]): ____

B. Procedure: ____
1. Excision biopsy/segmentectomy
2. Simple mastectomy
3. Modified radical mastectomy
4. Re-excision

C. Location: ____
1. Subareolar
2. UOQ
3. UIQ
4. LOQ
5. LIQ
6. Not specified

D. Size of the tumor (maximum dimension): ____ cm

E. Architectural type: ____
1. Cribriform
2. Solid
3. Papillary
4. Micropapillary
5. Apocrine
6. Comedo
7. Lobular
8. Other

F. Nuclear grade: ____
1. Low
2. Intermediate
3. High

G. Necrosis: ____
1. Zonal (comedo)
2. Nonzonal (punctate)
3. Absent

H. Polarization (yes [1]; no [2]; not assessable [3]): ____

I. Surgical margins involved (yes [1]; no [2]; not assessable [3]): ____

J. Non-neoplastic breast tissue: ____
1. ADH
2. ALH
3. Radical scar
4. FCD
5. Papilloma
6. Other

K. Microcalcifications: ____
1. Associated with CIS
2. Outside area of CIS

L. Cancerization of lobules (yes [1]; no [2]): ____

M. Pagetoid spread in ducts (yes [1]; no [2]): ____

N. Multicentricity (yes [1]; no [2]): ____

O. TNM pathologic stage: T____ N____ M____

P. TNM histopathologic grade: G____

ADH—atypical ductal hyperplasia; ALH—atypical lobular hyperplasia; CIS—carcinoma in situ; FCD—fibrocystic disease; HPF—high-powered fields; LIQ—lower inner quadrant; LOQ—lower outer quadrant; UIQ—upper inner quadrant; UOQ—upper outer quadrant.

Primary Invasive Carcinoma of Breast

A. Laterality (right [1]; left [2]): ____

B. Procedure: ____
1. Segmentectomy
2. Simple mastectomy
3. Modified radical mastectomy
4. Re-excision

C. Location: ____
1. Central subareolar
2. UOQ
3. UIQ
4. LOQ
5. LIQ
6. Not specified

D. Size of tumor (maximum dimension): ____ cm

E. Type (invasive component): ____
1. Not otherwise specified
2. Tubular
3. Mucinous
4. Medullary
5. Cribriform
6. Papillary
7. Lobular
8. Carcinoidlike
9. Metaplastic
10. Inflammatory
11. Other

F. If lobular carcinoma, specify type: ____
1. Classic
2. Solid
3. Alveolar
4. Signet ring
5. Trabecular
6. Tubulobular
7. Pleomorphic

G. Nottingham score: ____
1. Nuclear grade: ____
2. Tubule formation: ____
3. Mitoses per 10 HPF: ____
4. Total Nottingham score: ____

H. Vascular invasion (yes [1]; no [2]): ____

I. Calcification (no/yes [benign zones]/yes [malignant zones]): ____

J. Type of in situ component: ____
1. Cribriform
2. Solid
3. Papillary
4. Micropapillary
5. Apocrine
6. Comedo
7. Lobular

K. Surgical margins involved (no/yes [focal]/yes [diffuse]): ____

L. Paget's disease of nipple (yes [1]; no [2]): ____

M. Lymph nodes involved: *n* positive/total *n* examined = *n/n*

N. Skin involved (yes [1]; no [2]): ____

O. Non-neoplastic breast tissue: ____
1. ADH
2. ALH
3. Radical scar
4. Fibroadenoma
5. Papilloma
6. FCD
7. Other

P. Multicentricity of invasive foci (yes [1]; no [2]): ____

Q. TNM pathologic stage: T____ N____ M____

Primary Colon and Rectal Tumors

A. Location: ____
1. Ileocecal region
2. Ascending colon
3. Transverse colon
4. Descending colon
5. Sigmoid colon
6. Rectum

B. Procedure
1. Segmental colectomy
2. Total colectomy
3. Other

C. Size of tumor (maximum dimension): ____ cm

D. Type: ____
1. Adenocarcinoma, not otherwise specified
2. Adenocarcinoma arising in a background of an adenoma
3. Adenocarcinoma arising in a background of inflammatory bowel disease
4. Adenosquamous carcinoma
5. Carcinoid tumor (neuroendocrine tumor)
6. Mucinous adenocarcinoma
7. Signet ring cell–type adenocarcinoma
8. Neuroendocrine carcinoma
9. Squamous cell carcinoma
10. Undifferentiated carcinoma
11. Sarcoma
12. Smooth muscle tumor
13. Gastrointestinal stromal tumor
14. Lymphoma
15. Other

E. Grade: ____
1. Well differentiated
2. Moderately differentiated
3. Poorly differentiated

F. Extent of infiltration: ____
1. Limited to the mucosa
2. Into submucosa
3. Involving muscularis propria
4. Infiltrating through muscularis propria into serosal adipose tissue
5. Involving adjacent organs/pelvic wall

G. Angiolymphatic invasion (yes [1]; no [2]): ____

H. Surgical margins involved (yes [1]; no [2]): ____

I. Regional lymph node involvement (yes [1]; no [2]): ____

J. If regional lymph nodes involved, number positive examined: *n/n*

K. Extracapsular spread (yes [1]; no [2]): ____

L. Associated conditions: ____
1. Ulcerative colitis
2. Crohn's disease
3. History/presence of adenomatous polyps
4. Multiple polyposis syndromes
5. Diverticulosis

M. TNM pathologic stage: T____ N ____ M _____

N. TNM histopathologic grade: G____

O. Dukes' stage: ____
1. A (limited to mucosa and muscularis)
2. B (through muscularis into subserosa)
3. C (through subserosa and involving adjacent organ/pelvic wall/regional wall/regional or distant lymph nodes)

P. Astler-Coller stage: ____
1. A (mucosa but not into muscularis propria)
2. B1 (muscularis propria but not through, LN negative)
3. B2 (through muscularis propria into subserosal fibroadipose tissue, LN negative)
4. C1 (limited to muscularis propria but not through serosa, LN positive)
5. C2 (invades serosal adipose tissue, LN positive)

Esophageal Tumors

A. Size of tumor (maximum dimension): ____ cm

B. Location: ____
1. Upper third
2. Middle third
3. Lower third
4. Gastroesophageal junction

C. Procedure: ____
1. Partial resection
2. Esophagectomy and partial gastrectomy
3. Other

D. Type: ____
1. Invasive squamous cell carcinoma
2. Invasive adenocarcinoma
3. Invasive basaloid squamous cell carcinoma
4. In situ squamous cell carcinoma (without invasive component)
5. In situ adenocarcinoma (without invasive component)
6. Other

E. Grade: ____
1. Well
2. Moderate
3. Poor/undifferentiated

F. Maximal depth of invasion: ____
1. Into lamina propria
2. Into submucosa
3. Into muscularis propria
4. Into adventitia
5. Into adjacent tissues

G. Non-neoplastic mucosa: ____
1. Squamous dysplasia
2. Barrett's esophagus without dysplasia
3. Barrett's esophagus with dysplasia
4. Reflux change
5. Strictures

H. Vascular invasion (yes [1]; no [2]): ____

I. Perineural invasion (yes [1]; no [2]): ____

J. Surgical margins involved (yes [1]; no [2]): ____

K. If margins involved, specify: ____
1. Distal
2. Proximal
3. Deep (adventitial)

L. Lymph involvement (yes [1]; no [2]): ____

M. If yes, specify: n positive/total n examined = n/n

N. Extracapsular spread (yes [1]; no [2]): ____

O. TNM pathologic stage: T____ N ____ M ____

P. TNM histopathologic grade: G____

Primary Kidney/Renal Pelvis/Ureter Tumors

A. Side (right/left): ____

B. Location: ____
1. Kidney (parenchyma [cortex/medulla])
2. Kidney (pelvis)
3. Ureter
4. Kidney and ureter

C. Procedure: ____
1. Partial nephrectomy
2. Simple nephrectomy
3. Radical nephrectomy
4. Ureterectomy
5. Other

D. Size of neoplasm (maximum dimension in cm; if multicentric, size of largest mass): ____

E. Type of malignant neoplasm: ____
1. RCC, clear cell–type
   (includes non-papillary granular cell RCC)
2. RCC, chromophil cell type
   (papillary RCC, no clear cell component)
3. RCC, chromophobe cell type
4. RCC, oncocytic
5. RCC, sarcomatoid
6. Collecting duct carcinoma
7. Urothelial carcinoma, TCCa (noninvasive)
8. Urothelial carcinoma, TCCa (invasive ± in situ)
9. Urothelial carcinoma, squamous carcinoma
10. Urothelial carcinoma, adenocarcinoma
11. Urothelial carcinoma, small cell/neuroendocrine carcinoma
12. Urothelial carcinoma, mixed
13. Juxtaglomerular cell tumor
14. Wilms tumor
15. Rhabdoid tumor
16. Clear cell sarcoma
17. Congenital mesoblastic nephroma
18. Sarcoma (nonclear cell)
19. Lymphoma/leukemia
20. Other

F. Histologic grade: ____
1. Fuhrman grade (for RCC; grades 1–4): ____
2. Ash grade (grade 1–4): ____
3. WHO grade (grade 1–3) (for TCCa): ____
4. Other malignant neoplasms (grades 1–3): ____

G. Non-neoplastic and other conditions: ____
1. Glomerulopathy
2. Interstitial nephritis
3. Pyelonephritis
4. Nephrolithiasis
5. Papillary necrosis
6. Chronic parenchymal disease
7. Other

H. Margins of resection (positive/negative): ____

I. Mitotic activity: n per 10 HPF

J. Angiolymphatic invasion
1. Macroscopic (eg, renal vein thrombus): ____
2. Microscopic: ____

   1. Positive   2. Negative
   1. Positive   2. Negative

K. Lymph node metastasis: n Positive/total n: n / n

L. Adrenal gland:
1. Present (1), absent (2): ____
2. Involvement by renal neoplasm (yes [1]; no [2]; not applicable [3]): ____
3. Other adrenal pathology (yes [1]; no [2]; not applicable [3]): ____

M. TNM pathologic stage: T____ N____ M____

N. TNM histopathologic grade: G____

HPF—high-powered fields; RCC—renal cell carcinoma; TCC—transitional cell carcinoma; WHO—World Health Organization.

Larynx Resections

A. Type of laryngectomy: ____
1. Hemilaryngectomy   3. Total
2. Supraglottic   4. Extended

B. Predominant side of tumor (right [1]; left [2]; midline [3]): ____

C. Attached structures: ____
1. Neck dissection   3. Base of tongue   5. Thyroid
2. Pyriform sinus   4. Tracheotomy

D. Location of tumor: ____
1. Glottic   3. Base of tongue   5. Glottic-subglottic (> 1 cm)
2. Supraglottic   4. Transglottic

E. Greatest dimension of tumor in cm: ____

F. Histologic type of tumor: ____
1. Conventional squamous cell carcinoma   8. Mucoepidermoid or adenosquamous carcinoma
2. Papillary (exophytic) squamous cell carcinoma   9. Adenoid cystic carcinoma
3. Verrucous carcinoma   10. Lymphoepithelial carcinoma
4. Spindle cell carcinoma   11. Undifferentiated carcinoma
5. Basaloid squamous carcinoma   12. Sarcoma
6. Small cell carcinoma   13. Other (list)
7. Carcinoid or atypical carcinoid

G. Tumor differentiation: ____
1. Well   2. Moderate   3. Poor/undifferentiated

H. Structures involved: ____
1. True cord   9. Subglottis (> 1 cm subglottic extension)
2. Anterior commissure   10. Thyroid cartilage
3. False cord   11. Cricoid cartilage
4. Ventricle   12. Pre-epiglottic space
5. Epiglottis   13. Paraglottic space
6. A-E fold   14. Thyroid
7. Vallecula—base of tumor 15. Extralaryngeal soft tissue
8. Pyriform sinus   16. Tracheostomy site

I. Status of lymph nodes: n positive/total $n = n/n$

J. Intaperineural invasion (yes [1]; no [2]): ____

K. Vascular invasion (yes [1]; no [2]): ____

L. Surgical margins: ____
1. Free (≥ 2 mm)   3. Dysplasia (mild, moderate, severe)   5. In situ carcinoma
2. Positive (invasive tumor)   4. Close (within 2 mm)

M. TNM pathologic stage: T____ N____ M____

N. TNM histopathologic grade: G____

Primary Liver/Intrahepatic Tumors

A. Location: ____
1. Right lobe
2. Left lobe
3. Caudate lobe
4. Quadrate lobe
5. Multilobar
6. Not specified

B. Procedure: ____
1. Wedge/segmental
2. Lobectomy
3. Transplantation
4. Other

C. Size of tumor (maximum dimension): ____ cm

D. Multifocal (yes [1]; no [2]): ____

E. Type: ____
1. Hepatocellular carcinoma, NOS
2. Fibrolamellar carcinoma
3. Sclerosing hepatocellular
4. Squamous carcinoma
5. Carcinoid/neuroendocrine carcinoma
6. Mixed carcinoma
7. Hepatoblastoma
8. Bile duct adenocarcinoma
9. Adenosquamous carcinoma
10. Angiosarcoma
11. Cystadenocarcinoma
12. Clear cell carcinoma
13. Epithelioid hemangioendothelioma
14. Mesenchymoma
15. Sarcoma, NOS
16. Teratoma, NOS
17. Hemangioma
18. Other

F. Grade
FA. Predominant: ____
1. Well
2. Moderate
3. Poor/undifferentiated
FB. Worst: ____
1. Well
2. Moderate
3. Poor/undifferentiated

G. Encapsulation (yes [1]; no [2]): ____

H. Portal vein invasion (yes [1]; no [2]): ____

I. Angiolymphatic invasion (yes [1]; no [2]): ____

J. Mitotic activity (*n* per 10 HPF: ____

K. Elevated serum AFP (yes [1]; no [2]): ____

L. AFP expression by immunoperoxidase if performed (yes [1]; no [2]): ____

M. Perineural invasion (yes [1]; no [2]): ____

N. Surgical margins involved (yes [1]; no [2]): ____

O. Nodal involvement (yes [1]; no [2]): ____

P. Lymph nodes: *n* positive/ total *n* examined = *n/n*

Q. Underlying disease(s): ____
1. Cirrhosis, NOS
2. Viral-induced cirrhosis/liver disease
3. Liver cell dysplasia, large cell type
4. Liver cell dysplasia, small cell type
5. Adenomatous hyperplasia
6. Associated drug exposure, *eg*, steroids, Thorotrast

R. TNM pathologic stage: T ____ N ____ M ____

S. TNM histopathologic grade: G____

AFP—α-fetoprotein; HPF—high-powered fields; NOS—not otherwise specified.

Primary Lung Tumors

A. Location: ____
1. Right upper lung
2. Right middle lung
3. Right lower lung
4. Left lower lung
5. Left upper lung
6. Bronchus intermedius

B. Procedure: ____
1. Wedge/segmental
2. Lobectomy
3. Bilobectomy
4. Pneumonectomy

C. Size of tumor (maximum dimension): ____ cm

D. Satellite nodules (yes[1]; no [2]): ____

E. Type: ____
1. Invasive squamous carcinoma
2. Basaloid squamous carcinoma
3. Invasive adenocarcinoma
4. Bronchioalveolar carcinoma, nonmucinous type
5. Bronchioalveolar carcinoma, mucinous type
6. Large cell carcinoma
7. Clear cell carcinoma
8. Giant cell carcinoma
9. Sarcomatoid carcinoma
10. Blastoma
11. Fetal type adenocarcinoma
12. Oat cell carcinoma
13. Carcinoid
14. Atypical carcinoid
15. Sarcoma
16. Other

F. Grade: ____
1. Well
2. Moderate
3. Poor/undifferentiated

G. Bronchogenic (vs parenchymal) origin: (yes [1]; no [2]): ____

H. Visceral pleural invasion (yes [1]; no [2]): ____

I. Parietal pleural invasion (yes [1]; no [2]): ____

J. Chest wall invasion (yes [1]; no [2]): ____

K. Angiolymphatic invasion (yes [1]; no [2]): ____

L. Surgical margins involved (yes [1]; no [2]): ____

M. Inflammatory (desmoplastic) reaction: ____
1. Mild
2. Moderate
3. Severe

N. Hilar lymph node involvement (yes [1]; no [2]): ____

O. If hilar lymph nodes involved, n positive/n examined = n/n

P. Mediastinal nodes involved (yes [1]; no [2]): ____

Q. Mediastinal node group(s) involved: ____
1. Level 4R
2. Level 5R
3. Level 6R
4. Level 7R
5. Level 9R
6. Level 10R
7. Level 4L
8. Level 5L
9. Level 6L
10. Level 7L
11. Level 9L
12. Level 10L

R. Underlying disease(s): ____
1. Emphysema
2. Bronchiectasis
3. Tumorlets
4. Smoker's bronchitis
5. Asthma
6. Parenchymal scar

S. TNM pathologic stage: T____ N____ M____

T. TNM histopathologic grade: G____

Primary Cutaneous Melanoma

A. Age (*y*): ____

B. Sex (male [1]; female [2]): ____

C. Family history of melanoma/dysplastic nevus (yes [1]; no [2]): ____

D. Location: ____
1. Extremity
2. Head and neck
3. Trunk
4. Other

E. Type of excision: ____
1. Excision biopsy
2. Wide excision
3. Other

F. Gross description
1. Maximum size of tumor in cm: ____ 2. Gross ulceration (yes [1]; no [2]): ____ 3. Gross satellites: ____

G. Histologic type: ____
1. Nodular
2. Superficial spreading
3. Desmoplastic
4. Acral lentiginous
5. Lentigo malignant melanoma
6. Other

H. Histologic features: ____
1. Surface ulceration (yes [1]; no [2]): ____
2. Clarke level (1,2,3,4,5): ____
3. Breslow's maximum tumor thickness in mm: ____
4. Angiolymphatic/perineural invasion (yes [1]; no [2]): ____
5. Evidence of regression (yes [1]; no [2]): ____
6. Microscopic satellites (yes [1]; no [2]): ____
7. Preexisting nevus present (yes [1]; no [2]): ____
8. Intensity of tumor infiltrating lymphoid infiltrate (mild [1]; moderate [2]; severe [3]): ____
9. Mitotic rate: *n* per 10 HPF = *n*

I. LN dissection (yes [1]; no [2]): ____

J. Sentinel lymph node involvement (yes [1]; no [2]): ____

K. Lymph nodes: *n* positive/total *n* examined = *n*/*n*

L. Extracapsular spread (yes [1]; no [2]): ____

M. TNM pathologic stage: T____ N____ M____

N. TNM histopathologic grade: G____

HPF — high-powered fields.

SYNOPTIC PATHOLOGY REPORTS

Neck Dissection

A. Dissection site (right [1]; left [2]; bilateral [3]): ____

B. Type: ____
1. Selective
2. Modified rectal
3. Radical
4. Extended radical
5. Unknown

C. Sternocleidomastoid muscle (present [1]; absent [2]): ____

D. Sternocleidomastoid muscle involvement: ____
1. Free of tumor
2. Tumor present

E. Jugular vein: ____
1. Present
2. Absent

F. Jugular vein involvement: ____
1. Tumor involves wall but not lumen
2. Tumor involves lumen
3. Free of tumor

G. Right lymph nodes: n positive/total $n = n/n$
G1. Location of positive nodes: ____
1. Level I
2. Level II
3. Level III
4. Level IV
5. Level V
6. Level VI

H. Left lymph nodes: n positive/total $n = n/n$
H1. Location of positive nodes: ____
1. Level I
2. Level II
3. Level III
4. Level IV
5. Level V
6. Level VI

I. Largest lymph node (one dimension in cm): ____

J. Extranodal spread (yes [1]; no [2]): ____

K. Intraperineural invasion (yes [1]; no [2]): ____

L. Vascular invasion (other than jugular vein) (yes [1]; no [2]): ____

M. TNM pathologic stage: T____ N____ M____

N. TNM histopathologic grade: G____

Primary Orbital Tumors

A. Location: ____
1. Orbital bone
2. Orbital soft tissue
3. Optic nerve
4. Globe
5. Lacrimal gland

B. Procedure: ____
1. Wedge/segmental
2. Excision
3. Exenteration

C. Size of tumor (maximum dimension): ____ cm

D. Type: ____
1. Mucoepidermoid carcinoma
2. Adenoid cystic carcinoma
3. Adenocarcinoma
4. Carcinoma ex pleomorphic adenoma
5. Squamous cell carcinoma
6. Basal cell carcinoma
7. Rhabdomyosarcoma
8. Malignant melanoma
9. Lymphoma
10. Other

E. Grade: ____
1. Well
2. Moderate
3. Poor/undifferentiated

F. Limited to orbit (yes [1]; no [2]): ____

G. Angiolymphatic invasion (yes [1]; no [2]): ____

H. Perineural invasion (yes [1]; no [2]): ____

I. Surgical margins involved (yes [1]; no [2]): ____

J. Regional lymph node involvement (yes [1]; no [2]): ____

K. If regional lymph nodes are involved: n positive/n examined $= n/n$

L. If regional lymph nodes are involved: n with extracapsular spread $= n$

M. TNM pathologic stage: T ____ N ____ M ____

N. TNM histopathologic grade: G____

Primary Ovarian Tumors Including Borderline Tumors

A. Laterality: ____
1. Right
2. Left
3. Bilateral

B. Procedure: ____
1. Cystectomy
2. Salpingo-oophorectomy
3. Bilateral salpingo-oophorectomy
4. Total abdominal hysterectomy with salpingo-oophorectomy
5. Other

C. Size of primary tumor (maximum dimension): ____ cm

D. Histologic type: ____
1. Papillary serous tumor, borderline malignant
2. Papillary serous carcinoma
3. Mucinous tumor, border line
4. Mucinous carcinoma
5. Endometrioid tumor, border line
6. Endometrioid carcinoma
7. Clear cell tumor, border line
8. Clear cell carcinoma
9. Brenner tumor
10. Malignant Brenner tumor
11. Malignant mixed müllerian tumor
12. Undifferentiated carcinoma
13. Small cell carcinoma
14. Mature teratoma
15. Immature teratoma
16. Dysgerminoma
17. Embryonal carcinoma
18. Yolk sac tumor
19. Granulosa cell tumor, juvenile
20. Granulosa cell tumor, adult
21. Malignant lymphoma
22. Others

E. Histologic grade: ____
1. Well
2. Moderate
3. Poorly differentiated

F. Vascular invasion (yes [1]; no [2]): ____

G. Capsule (intact [1]; ruptured [2]): ____

H. Surface implants (yes [1]; no [2]): ____

I. Lymph nodes: n involved/n examined: n/n

J. Nodes involved: n/total n examined
1. External iliac: n/n
2. Obturator: n/n
3. Common iliac: n/n
4. Pelvic: n/n
5. Aortic: n/n
6. Inguinal: n/n

K. TNM pathologic stage: T ____ N ____ M ____

L. TNM histopathologic grade: G____

Primary Pancreas Tumors

A. Type of resection: ____
   1. Whipple
   2. Partial pancreatectomy
   3. Other

B. Tumor type: ____
   1. Acinar cell
   2. Adenocarcinoma
   3. Adenosquamous
   4. Carcinosarcoma
   5. Cystadenocarcinoma
   6. Duct cell carcinoma
   7. Giant cell carcinoma
   8. Islet cell (neuroendocrine) tumor
   9. Mucinous (colloid) carcinoma
   10. Pancreaticoblastoma
   11. Papillary carcinoma
   12. Sarcoma (type ____)
   13. Small cell (oat cell) carcinoma
   14. Undifferentiated carcinoma
   15. Mucinous tumor of uncertain potential
   16. Other

C. History of diabetes (yes [1]; no [2]): ____

D. If the patient has a history of MEN, which one?
   1. MEN 1
   2. MEN 2a
   3. MEN 2b

E. Tumor size (maximum dimension): ____ cm

F. Location: ____
   1. Head
   2. Body
   3. Tail
   4. Diffuse
   5. Indeterminate

G. Resection margins free of tumor (yes [1]; no [2]): ____

H. Histologic grade of differentiation: ____
   1. Well
   2. Moderate
   3. Poor
   4. Indeterminate

I. Tumor borders: ____
   1. Pushing
   2. Infiltrative

J. Vascular invasion (yes [1]; no [2]): ____

K. Lymphatic invasion (yes [1]; no [2]): ____

L. Perineural invasion (yes [1]; no [2]): ____

M. Tumor extends into adjacent organs (yes [1]; no [2]): ____

N. Mitoses per 10 HPF: ____

O. In situ carcinoma/dysplasia (yes [1]; no [2]): ____

P. Non-neoplastic pancreatic diseases: ____
   1. Chronic pancreatitis
   2. Pseudocyst
   3. Stones

Q. Lymph nodes: *n* positive/total *n* of nodes = *n/n*

R. Extracapsular invasion (yes [1]; no [2]): ____

S. TNM pathologic stage: T ____ N ____ M ____

T. TNM histopathologic grade: G____

HPF — high-powered fields.

Primary Prostate Tumors

A. Location: ____
   1. Right lobe   2. Left lobe   3. Both right and left lobes

B. Procedure: ____
   1. Radical prostatectomy   2. Cystoprostatectomy   3. Other

C. Size: greatest dimension in cm: ____

D. Percent of biopsy material involved by tumor: ____

E. Type: ____
   1. Adenocarcinoma   5. Small cell carcinoma
   2. Transitional cell carcinoma   6. Metastatic
   3. Large duct type carcinoma   7. Others
   4. Adenocarcinoma with neuroendocrine features

F. Gleason score ($n + n + n$): ____
   1. Primary grade (1–5): ____   2. Secondary grade (1–5): ____

G. Grade of tumor: ____
   1. Well differentiated (Gleason score: 2–4)   3. Poorly differentiated (Gleason score: 7–10)
   2. Moderately differentiated (Gleason score: 5–6)

H. Surgical margins involved (yes [1]; no [2]): ____

I. Perineural infiltration (yes [1]; no [2]): ____

J. Extracapsular penetration: ____
   1. No   2. Yes: focal   3. Yes: multifocal

K. Vascular invasion (yes [1]; no [2]) ____

L. Lymphatic invasion (yes [1]; no [2]) ____

M. Perineural invasion (yes [1]; no [2]) ____

N. Seminal vesicle status
   1. Involved by tumor   2. Free of tumor

O. Lymph node involvement (yes [1]; no [2]): ____

P. If regional lymph nodes involved, n positive/n examined = n/n

Q. Non-neoplastic conditions present: ____
   1. Benign prostatic hypertrophy   2. Basal cell hyperplasia   3. Atrophy

R. TNM pathologic stage: T ____ N ____ M ____

S. TNM histopathologic grade: G____

The information here is provided as guidance only. Prescribers should always consult the manufacturer's current prescribing information.

474

Primary Small Intestinal Tumors

A.* Small bowel segment in which tumor is identified: ____
1. Duodenum
2. Jejunum
3. Ileum

B. Tumor type: ____
Epithelial
1. Adenocarcinoma
2. Adenosquamous
3. Cystadenocarcinoma
4. Mucinous (colloid) carcinoma

Neuroendocrine
5. Adenocarcinoid
6. Atypical carcinoid
7. Carcinoid
8. Neuroendocrine carcinoma

Mesenchymal
10. Gastrointestinal stromal tumor
11. Leiomyoblastoma
12. Leiomyosarcoma
13. Malignant peripheral nerve sheath tumor
14. Sarcoma, unspecified

Other
15. Undifferentiated carcinoma
16. Small cell (oat cell) carcinoma

C. Tumor size (maximum dimension): ____ cm

D. Number of tumors: ____

E. Procedure: ____
1. Partial resection
2. Total resection
3. Other

F. Extent of invasion: ____
1. In situ
2. Intramucosal
3. Submucosal
4. Muscularis propria
5. Into subserosal fibroid adipose tissue

G. Resection margin: ____
1. Free of tumor
2. Involved by tumor

H. Histologic grade of differentiation: ____
1. Well 2.
Moderate
3. Poor

I. Tumor borders: ____
1. Pushing
2. Infiltrative

J. Vascular invasion (yes [1]; no [2]): ____

K. Lymphatic invasion (yes [1]; no [2]): ____

L. Perineural invasion (yes [1]; no [2]): ____

M. Mitoses per 10 HPF: ____

N. Lymph nodes: n positive/total n of nodes = n/n

O. TNM pathologic stage: T ____ N ____ M ____

P. TNM histopathologic grade: G____

*Appendix is evaluated using a separate form.
HPF — high power fields.

Primary Soft Tissue Tumors

A. Age: ____ years

B. Sex (male [1]; female [2]): ____

C. Family history of cancer (yes [1]; no [2]): ____

D. Location: ____
1. Extremity
2. Trunk
3. Body cavity
4. Head and neck

E. Tumor size (maximum dimension): ____ cm

F. Specimen size: ____ cm × ____ cm × ____ cm

G. Percent of gross tumor necrosis: ____

H. Proximity to major nerve, vessel, and bone: ____
1. Gross invasion
2. No invasion

I. Distance from closest margin: ____ cm

J. Lymph node involvement (yes [1]; no [2]; not applicable [3]): ____

K. Histologic type: ____
1. Alveolar soft-part sarcoma
2. Angiosarcoma
3. Epithelial sarcoma
4. Extraskeletal chondrosarcoma
5. Extraskeletal osteosarcoma
6. Fibrosarcoma
7. Leiomyosarcoma
8. Liposarcoma
9. Malignant fibrous histiocytoma
10. Malignant hemangiopericytoma
11. Malignant mesenchymoma
12. Malignant schwannoma
13. Rhabdomyosarcoma
14. Synovial sarcoma
15. Sarcoma, not otherwise specified
16. Other

L. Number of mitoses per 10 HPF: ____

M. Percent of microscopic necrosis: ____

N. Tumor satellites (yes [1]; no [2]): ____

O. Perineural invasion (yes [1]; no [2]): ____

P. Vascular invasion (yes [1]; no [2]): ____

Q. Microscopic margins involved (yes [1]; no [2]): ____

R. Histologic grade: ____
1. Well
2. Moderate
3. Poor

S. Lymph nodes involved (yes [1]; no [2]): ____

T. Number of positive nodes/total number of nodes: n/n

U. TNM pathologic stage: T ____ N ____ M ____

V. TNM histopathologic grade: G____

HPF — high-power fields.

Primary Stomach Tumors

A. Size of tumor (maximum dimension): ____ cm

B. Location: ____
1. Cardia/fundus
2. Corpus
3. Antrum/pylorus

C. Procedure: ____
1. Excision
2. Partial gastrectomy
3. Total gastrectomy

D. Type: ____
1. Invasive adenocarcinoma, not otherwise specified
2. Tubular (intestinal) type adenocarcinoma
3. Papillary type adenocarcinoma
4. Signet ring–type adenocarcinoma
5. Mucinous type adenocarcinoma (non–signet ring)
6. Adenocarcinoma with neuroendocrine features
7. Adenocarcinoma with squamous metaplasia
8. In situ adenocarcinoma (without invasive component)
9. Squamous cell carcinoma
10. Small cell carcinoma
11. Neuroendocrine carcinoma (carcinoid)
12. Malignant lymphoma
13. Gastrointestinal stromal tumor (malignant)
14. Gastrointestinal stromal tumor (uncertain potential)
15. Other

E. Grade: ____
1. Well
2. Moderate
3. Poor/undifferentiated

F. Maximal depth of invasion: ____
1. Into lamina propria
2. Into submucosa
3. Into muscularis propria
4. Into subserosal fibroadipose tissue
5. Into adjacent tissues

G. Non-neoplastic mucosa: ____
1. Chronic gastritis
2. Intestinal metaplasia
3. Dysplasia
4. Polyps separate from carcinoma
5. Atrophic gastritis
6. *Helicobacter* gastritis
7. Neuroendocrine cell hyperplasia

H. Vascular invasion (yes [1]; no [2]): ____

I. Perineural invasion (yes [1]; no [2]): ____

J. Surgical margins involved? (yes [1]; no [2]): ____

K. If margins positive, specify involved margin: ____
1. Distal
2. Proximal
3. Deep/adventitial

L. Lymph node involvement? (yes [1]; no [2]): ____

M. If node involvement, specify n positive/n examined: n/n

N. Extracapsular spread (yes [1]; no [2]): ____

O. TNM pathologic stage: T ____ N ____ M ____

P. TNM histopathologic grade: G____

The information here is provided as guidance only. Prescribers should always consult the manufacturer's current prescribing information

476

Primary Testicular Tumors

A. Location: _____
1. Undescended testes
2. Descended testes

B. Involved side: _____
1. Right
2. Left
3. Right and left

C. Procedure: _____
1. Biopsy
2. Orchiectomy
3. Radical orchiectomy

D. Size of tumor (maximum dimension): _____ cm

E. Tumor type: _____
1. Seminoma
2. Nonseminomatous germ cell tumor
3. Other

F. Histologic type: _____
1. Seminoma
2. Embyronal carcinoma
3. Yolk sac tumorv
4. Choriocarcinom
5. Lymphoma
6. Metastatic tumor
7. Sarcoma
8. Immature teratoma
9. Mature teratoma
10. Mixed germ cell neoplasma
11. Spermatocytic seminoma
12. Stromal tumor
13. Other

G. Tumor infiltration into tunica epididymis (yes [1]; no [2]): _____

H. Tumor infiltration into spermatic cord (yes [1]; no [2]): _____

I. Tumor infiltration into the scrotum (yes [1]; no [2]): _____

J. Vascular invasion (yes [1]; no [2]) _____

K. Lymphatic invasion (yes [1]; no [2]) _____

L. Perineural invasion (yes [1]; no [2]) _____

M. Lymph node involvement (yes [1]; no [2]): _____

N. Necrosis (yes [1]; no [2]): _____

O. History of undescended testis (yes [1]; no [2]): _____

P. If regional lymph nodes involved, number positive / number examined = n/n

Q. Size of largest lymph node involved: _____
1. < 2 cm
2. 2–5 cm
3. > 5 cm

R. TNM pathologic stage: T _____ N _____ M _____

S. TNM histopathologic grade: G_____

Thyroid Carcinoma

A. Specimen type: ____
   1. Right lobectomy
   2. Left Lobectomy
   3. Subtotal
   4. Total
   5. Isthmusectomy
   6. Other

B. Number of gross tumor nodules: ____

C. Size of tumor (maximum dimension of largest): ____ cm

D. Capsular penetration (yes [1]; no [2]): ____

E. Soft tissue extension (yes [1]; no [2]): ____

F. Tumor type: ____
   1. Papillary
   2. Follicular
   3. Medullary
   4. Anaplastic
   5. Metastatic
   6. Other

G. Nuclear grade: ____
   1. Well differentiated
   2. Moderately differentiated
   3. Poorly differentiated

H. Vascular invasion (yes [1]; no [2]): ____

I. Capsular invasion (yes [1]; no [2]): ____

J. Soft tissue invasion (yes [1]; no [2]): ____

K. Resection margins: ____
   1. Free
   2. Involved

L. Lymph nodes: n positive/total n of nodes = n/n

M. TNM pathologic stage: T ____ N ____ M ____

N. TNM histopathologic grade: G____

Primary Uterine Cervix Tumors: Hysterectomy and Conization Specimens

Invasive neoplasia (yes [1]; no [2]): ____

A. Type: ____
  1. Squamous cell carcinoma
  2. Adenocarcinoma
  3. Adenosquamous carcinoma
  4. Neuroendocrine small cell carcinoma
  5. Non-neuroendocrine small cell carcinoma
  6. Other (including metastasis)

B. Grade: ____
  1. Well differentiated
  2. Moderately differentiated
  3. Poorly differentiated

C. Size of neoplasm (maximum dimension): ____ cm

D. Location (epicenter): ____
  1. Ectocervix
  2. Endocervix
  3. Lower uterine segment

E. Depth of invasion: ____ cm

F. Structures involved:
  1. Parametrium (yes [1]; no [2]): ____
  2. Pelvic wall (yes [1]; no [2]): ____
  3. Upper third of vagina (yes [1]; no [2]): ____
  4. Lower third of vagina (yes [1]; no [2]): ____
  5. Causes of hydronephrosis of nonfunctioning kidney (yes [1]; no [2]): ____
  6. Mucosa of bladder or rectum (yes [1]; no [2]): ____

G. Intraepithelial neoplasia (yes [1]; no [2]): ____
G1. Type: ____
  1. Squamous intraepithelial lesion (SIL)
  2. Adenocarcinoma in situ
  3. Mixed squamous adenocarcinoma
G2. Grade: ____
  1. Low grade
  2. High grade
G3. Koilocytes (yes [1]; no [2]): ____
G4. Intraglandular involvement by SIL (yes [1]; no [2]): ____
G5. Horizontal spread: ____ mm

H. Non-neoplastic and other conditions: ____
  1. Endocervical polyp
  2. Microglandular hyperplasia
  3. Leiomyoma
  4. Endometriosis
  5. Other

I. Margins of resection (positive [1]; negative [2]): ____

J. Mitotic count: *n* per 10 HPF

K. Angiolymphatic lesion: (yes [1]; no [2]): ____

L. Lymph node metastases (yes [1]; no [2]): ____

M. Lymph node metastases: *n* positive/total *n* = *n*/*n*

N. Extranodal spread (yes [1]; no [2]): ____

O. Previous cervicovaginal cytology at UPMC (yes [1]; no [2]): ____

P. Distant metastasis (yes [1]; no [2]): ____

Q. TNM stage: T ____ N ____ M ____

R. TNM histopathologic grade: G____

S. FIGO pathologic stage: ____

HPF — high-powered fields.

Primary Uterine Endometrium Tumors: Hysterectomy Specimens

A. Invasive neoplasia (yes [1]; no [2]): ____
A1. Endometrial carcinoma (yes [1]; no [2]): ____
A2. Type: ____
   1. Endometrioid adenocarcinoma, not otherwise specified
   2. Endometrioid adenocarcinoma, secretory variant
   3. Endometrioid adenocarcinoma, ciliated variant
   4. Adenocarcinoma with squamous metaplasia (adenoacanthoma)
   5. Adenosquamous carcinoma
   6. Serous adenocarcinoma
   7. Clear cell adenocarcinoma
   8. Mucinous adenocarcinoma
   9. Squamous cell carcinoma
   10. Mixed carcinoma
   11. Undifferentiated carcinoma
   12. Other (including metastasis)

B. Nonepithelial tumors (yes [1]; no [2]): ____
B1. Type: ____
   1. Endometrial stromal nodule
   2. Low-grade stromal sarcoma
   3. High-grade stromal sarcoma
   4. Leiomyoma, not otherwise specified
   5. Leiomyoma variant (epithelioid, bizarre, lipoleiomyoma)
   6. Smooth muscle tumor of uncertain malignant potential
   7. Leiomyosarcoma, not otherwise specified
   8. Leiomyosarcoma variant (epitheloid myloid)
   9. Mixed endometrial stromal and smooth muscle tumors
   10. Neuroectodermal tumors
   11. Lymphoma
   12. Other nonepithelial tumors

C. Mixed epithelial-nonepithelial and other tumors (yes [1]; no [2]): ____
C1. Type: ____
   1. Adenofibroma
   2. Adenomyoma
   3. Adenosarcoma
   4. Carcinosarcoma (malignant mixed mesodermal tumor)
   5. Germ cell neoplasia
   6. Gestational trophoblastic disease
   7. Other tumors

D. Grade: ____
   1. Well differentiated   2. Moderately differentiated   3. Poorly differentiated

E. Size of neoplasm and percent of endometrium involved: n cm, n%

F. Depth of invasion and percent of myometrium involved: n cm, n%

G. Structures involved:
G1. Cervix (yes [1]; no [2]): ____
G2. Endocervical glands (yes [1]; no [2]): ____
G3. Cervical stroma (yes [1]; no [2]): ____
G4. Serosa and/or adnexa (yes [1]; no [2]): ____
G5. Ascites or peritoneal washing (yes [1]; no [2]): ____
G6. Vagina (yes [1]; no [2]): ____
G7. Bladder and/or bowel mucosa (yes [1]; no [2]): ____

H. Non-neoplastic or preneoplastic conditions: ____
   1. Endometrial polyp
   2. Simple endometrial hyperplasia without atypia
   3. Simple endometrial hyperplasia with atypia
   4. Complex endometrial hyperplasia without atypia
   5. Complex endometrial hyperplasia with atypia
   6. Adenomyosis
   7. Inflammatory pseudotumor
   8. Other

I. Margins of resection (positive [1]; negative [2]): ____

J. Mitotic count: n per 10 HPF

K. Angiolymphatic invasion (yes [1]; no [2]): ____

L. Regional lymph node metastasis: n of n pelvic and/or para-aortic lymph nodes contain metastasis

M. Distant lymph node metastasis: n of n distant lymph nodes contain metastasis (note: this is M1 disease)

N. Previous cervicovaginal, endometrial, or peritoneal cytology at UPMC: ____

O. Distant metastases (excludes metastasis to vagina, pelvic serosa, and adnexa; includes lymph nodes other than regional lymph nodes)

P. TNM stage: T ____ N ____ M ____

Q. TNM histopathologic grade: G____

R. FIGO pathologic stage: ____

HPF — high-powered fields.

Note: *Page numbers followed by* f *indicate figures; page numbers followed by* t *indicate tables.*